Therapeutic Exercise for Athletic Injuries

ATHLETIC TRAINING EDUCATION SERIES

PEGGY A. HOUGLUM, MS, PT, ATC
UNIVERSITY OF VIRGINIA, CHARLOTTESVILLE

DAVID H. PERRIN, PhD, ATC
SERIES EDITOR
UNIVERSITY OF VIRGINIA, CHARLOTTESVILLE

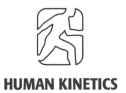

HUMAN KINETICS

Library of Congress Cataloging-in-Publication Data

Houglum, Peggy A., 1948-
   Therapeutic exercise for athletic injuries / Peggy A. Houglum.
     p. cm. -- (Athletic training education series)
   Includes bibliographical references and index.
   ISBN 0-88011-843-1
   1. Sports injuries--Exercise therapy. I. Title. II. Series.
RD97.H68 2000
615.8'2'088796--dc21

                                 00-036966

ISBN: 0-88011-843-1

Acquisitions Editor: Loarn D. Robertson, PhD
Series Developmental Editors: Kristine Enderle and Elaine Mustain
Developmental Editor: Joanna Hatzopoulos
Assistant Editors: Susan C. Hagan, Sandra Merz Bott, Stephan Seyfert, and Laurie Stokoe
Copyeditors: Joyce Sexton and Karen Bojda
Proofreader: Myla Smith
Indexer: Marie Rizzo
Permissions Managers: Sandra Merz Bott, Courtney Astle, and Heather Munson
Senior Graphic Designer: Stuart Cartwright
Senior Graphic Artist: Angela K. Snyder
Graphic Artists: Tara Welsch, Yvonne Griffith, Dawn Sills, Denise Lowry, Dody Bullerman, and Kathleen Boudreau-Fuoss
Photo Managers: Tom Roberts and Clark Brooks
Cover Designer: Stuart Cartwright
Photographer: All photos by Tom Roberts unless otherwise noted.
Models: Michael A. Curtis, Rosemary Dent, Tori Depp, Kate Fenner, Koren Forster, James Grimes, Taeyou Jung, Chelsea Kane, Jessica Kane, Kristie LaVanti, Ian McLeod, Susan Saliba, Fred Thomas, Tamara C. Valovich, and Lorraine Vizzuso
Art Manager: Craig Newsom
Illustrator: Argosy
Mac Artists: Angela K. Snyder and Dawn Sills
Printer: Sheridan Books, Inc.

Printed in the United States of America   10 9 8 7 6 5 4 3 2

Human Kinetics
Web site: www.humankinetics.com

United States: Human Kinetics
P.O. Box 5076
Champaign, IL 61825-5076
800-747-4457
e-mail: humank@hkusa.com

Canada: Human Kinetics
475 Devonshire Road, Unit 100
Windsor, ON N8Y 2L5
800-465-7301 (in Canada only)
e-mail: orders@hkcanada.com

Europe: Human Kinetics
Units C2/C3 Wira Business Park
West Park Ring Road
Leeds LS16 6EB, United Kingdom
+44 (0)113 278 1708
e-mail: hk@hkeurope.com

Australia: Human Kinetics
57A Price Avenue
Lower Mitcham, South Australia 5062
08 8277 1555
e-mail: liahka@senet.com.au

New Zealand: Human Kinetics
P.O. Box 105-231, Auckland Central
09-523-3462
e-mail: hkp@ihug.co.nz

To my mom (in memory) and dad,
who taught me the value of life,
the worthiness of self-respect,
the responsibility of doing what is right,
the merit of doing whatever you do to the best of your ability,
and the importance of appreciating all your blessings.
With special thanks
to Joel, Rita, Pam, Bob, Joan, Steve, Deanna, Dan, and Larry,
who have filled my life with perpetual laughter,
steadfast support, and unconditional love.

CONTENTS

INTRODUCTION TO THE ATHLETIC TRAINING EDUCATION SERIES

The five textbooks of the Athletic Training Education Series—*Introduction to Athletic Training, Assessment of Athletic Injuries, Therapeutic Exercise for Athletic Injuries, Therapeutic Modalities for Athletic Injuries,* and *Management Strategies in Athletic Training,* second edition—were written for student athletic trainers and as a reference for practicing certified athletic trainers. Many textbooks have been written that in one way or another address the competencies in athletic training. However, absent from these books has been a coordinated approach to the competencies that serves to optimally prepare student athletic trainers for the National Athletic Trainers' Association (NATA) certification examination. If you are a student athletic trainer, you must master the material included in each of the content areas delineated in the NATA publication *Competencies in Athletic Training.* The philosophy of the Athletic Training Education Series is to address these competencies in a comprehensive and sequential manner, while avoiding unnecessary duplication.

The series covers the educational content areas developed by the Education Council of the National Athletic Trainers' Association for accredited curriculum development. These content areas and the text (or in some cases, texts) of the series that primarily addresses each content area are as follows:

- Risk management and injury prevention (*Introduction* and *Management Strategies*)
- Pathology of injury and illnesses (*Introduction, Therapeutic Exercise, Therapeutic Modalities,* and *Assessment*)
- Assessment and evaluation (*Assessment* and *Therapeutic Exercise*)
- Acute care of injury and illness (*Introduction* and *Management Strategies*)
- Pharmacology (*Introduction* and *Therapeutic Modalities*)
- Therapeutic modalities (*Therapeutic Modalities*)
- Therapeutic exercise (*Therapeutic Exercise*)
- General medical conditions and disabilities (*Introduction* and *Assessment*)
- Nutritional aspects of injury and illness (*Introduction*)
- Psychosocial intervention and referral (*Introduction, Therapeutic Modalities,* and *Therapeutic Exercise*)
- Health care administration (*Management Strategies*)
- Professional development and responsibilities (*Introduction* and *Management Strategies*)

The authors for this series—Craig Denegar, Susan Hillman, Peggy Houglum, Richard Ray, Sandy Shultz, and I—are six certified athletic trainers with well over a century of collective experience as clinicians, educators, and leaders in the athletic training profession. The clinical experience of the authors spans virtually every setting in which athletic trainers practice, including the high school, sports medicine clinic, college, professional sport, hospital, and industrial settings. The professional positions of the authors include undergraduate and graduate curriculum director, head athletic trainer, professor, clinic director, and researcher. The authors have chaired or served on the NATA's most important committees, including the Professional Education Committee, the Education Task Force, Education Council, Research Committee of the Research and Education Foundation, Journal Committee, Appropriate Medical Coverage for Intercollegiate Athletics Task Force, Continuing Education Committee, and many others. The six authors of the series have created the most comprehensive and progressive collection of texts and related instructional materials presently available to athletic training students and educators. These materials, designed to accompany an accredited athletic training curriculum, will also serve to optimally prepare you for successful completion of the certification examination.

You will find several elements common to all the books in the series. These include

- chapter objectives and summaries tied to one another so that students can know and achieve their learning goals,
- chapter opening scenarios that illustrate the importance and relevance of the chapter content,
- cross-referencing among texts for a complete education on the subject, and
- thorough reference lists for further reading and research.

To enhance instruction, the series also includes Microsoft® PowerPoint® presentations and instructor guides that comprise features such as course syllabuses, lecture and chapter outlines, case studies, and test banks. Where most appropriate, laboratory manuals accompany texts. Other features vary from book to book, depending on the requirements of the subject matter, but all include various aids for assimilation and review of information, extensive illustrations, and material to help the student apply the facts in the text.

Beyond the introductory text by Hillman, the order in which the books should be used is determined by the philosophy of your curriculum director. In any case, each book can stand alone so that an entire curriculum doesn't need to be revamped to use one or more parts of the series.

When I entered the profession of athletic training nearly 25 years ago, one text—*Prevention and Care of Athletic Injuries* by Klafs and Arnheim—covered nearly all the subject matter necessary to pass the NATA Board of Certification examination and practice as an entry-level athletic trainer. Since that time we have witnessed an amazing expansion of the subject matter necessary to practice athletic training and an equally impressive growth of practice settings in which athletic trainers work. I trust you will find the Athletic Training Education Series an invaluable resource as you prepare for a successful career as a certified athletic trainer and a most useful reference in your professional practice.

David H. Perrin, PhD, ATC
Series Editor

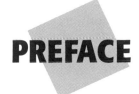

PREFACE

When Dave Perrin invited me to write this textbook, it wasn't the first time someone had broached the topic with me. It was, however, the first time I took the task to heart and decided to pursue the idea. Several years ago Pete Koehneke approached me with the idea. At that time there was no textbook on rehabilitation of athletic injuries. Since then, there have been textbooks written or edited on the subject.

Why, then, should I write one now? The answer is complex. Although several textbooks are now in print on the topic of athletic rehabilitation, none satisfies the needs of the sport rehabilitation specialist beyond the technical level. Over the past 10 years, a number of advances and revolutionary changes have occurred in how athletic injuries are rehabilitated. The advancement of surgical techniques has been accompanied by a concomitant advancement of rehabilitation techniques. The rehabilitation process is constantly evolving and becomes more sophisticated with changes in surgical techniques, equipment development, and newly acquired knowledge of human physiology.

In spite of the number of rehabilitation textbooks on the market today, instructors across the country have repeatedly told me that they do not use a textbook because those available are either incomplete or do not meet their needs. Others have told me that they use more than one because there is no single textbook that addresses all of their course's content. Additionally, the textbooks currently available are for technicians. They address how to perform rehabilitation techniques, but they do not tell what occurs physiologically, why applications are important, and how treatments are effective. Athletic trainers and others who rehabilitate sports-related injuries are medical professionals who are obligated to understand the therapeutic exercise and rehabilitation techniques used by the individuals they treat. This textbook differs significantly from other rehabilitation textbooks because it deals with information vital to these concepts. The reader is guided through a progression of information designed to reveal the whys, hows, whens, and whats of athletic rehabilitation and thus develop the essential building blocks to provide the rehabilitation specialist with the skills to safely and successfully rehabilitate injured individuals.

This text is divided into four parts. Each successive part builds on the information presented in previous parts. Part I deals with the basic concepts: what is important in a therapeutic exercise program, what factors affect it, the team members involved, and the components involved. It also addresses what happens physiologically to the injury site and emotionally to the individual following an injury, physics principles, assessment techniques, and record keeping. Part II presents specific techniques—including manual therapy, concepts involving range of motion, strength, proprioception, and functional activities—to serve as a foundation for parts III and IV. Reporting tools for findings and progressions are also discussed. These techniques are the cornerstone of the establishment, progression, and conclusion of a therapeutic exercise program for the injuries most commonly experienced by physically active people. Part III contains information on general therapeutic exercise application. These chapters cover topics such as posture evaluation, gait analysis, aquatic exercises, Swiss ball and foam roller exercises, and tendinitis treatment strategies. These techniques are all used throughout a treatment program and can be applied to many different body segments. This material is used as building blocks for the last section of the book, part IV, which deals with specific application to each body segment of the techniques discussed in parts I, II, and III. Specific rehabilitation techniques and progressions are presented for each area of the body, with special attention to common problems or unique programs that a body segment requires.

As medical professionals, we should be familiar with terms common to the medical community. As long as an injured athlete is under medical care, that individual is considered a patient first. Therefore, an injured athlete is referred to as a *patient*. The job title of the allied health professional who provides rehabilitative care is often *certified athletic trainer*, but since this textbook deals with athletic rehabilitation generally and therapeutic exercises specifically, the individual who offers this treatment is referred to as a *rehabilitation specialist*. Treatment is offered in a clinic. The clinic can be an athletic training room, an outpatient clinic, a conditioning facility, an industrial clinic; as long as the individual offering therapeutic exercise rehabilitation is a medical professional and the individual receiving that service is a patient, the facility is a clinic. The term used by the National Athletic Trainers' Association (NATA) to describe the individuals with whom certified athletic trainers are concerned is *physically active*. This is the term used in this textbook to refer to healthy individuals who engage in physical activity. NATA's definition of *physically active* refers to individuals "engaging in occupational, recreational or athletic activities that require physical skills and utilize strength, power, endurance, speed, flexibility, range of motion or agility" (National Athletic Trainers' Association Board of Directors, 1999).

This text is a compilation of nearly 30 years of experience in athletic training rooms and sports medicine clinics, and it provides what I believe is comprehensive information on therapeutic exercise for the physically active. It is meant to be an educational tool for the entry-level student as well as a reference text for the practicing rehabilitation clinician. It is meant to offer established and new information and to challenge both the neophyte and experienced rehabilitation clinician to provide a new level of insight and information about therapeutic exercise and our allied health profession.

This text does not provide a cookbook approach to therapeutic exercise. It does, however, provide the knowledge and tools you will need to develop the skills to determine what to use for each patient you encounter. It provides the instruments you will need for deciding the best course of action, the knowledge of why you are using it, what to expect when you use a technique, the dangers and advantages of applications, proper progressions, and how to apply the knowledge and techniques to specific injuries. Whereas each patient is different and responds differently to injury and treatment, it is neither fair to the patient nor realistic for you to believe that a cookbook approach would be helpful to the patient or to you as the person delivering care for that patient. The best course of action for you as a rehabilitation clinician is to provide the best therapeutic exercise program you can with your knowledge, skills, understanding, and appreciation of the whats, whys, and hows of therapeutic exercise. If you possess these attributes, you won't need or want a cookbook. This text provides you with the tools for developing your own therapeutic exercise programs for your patients. It is your responsibility to use those tools and your own imagination to provide a sound therapeutic exercise program that is fun for you and your patient.

National Athletic Trainers' Association Board of Directors. 1999. From the field. *NATA News* (March): 7.

ACKNOWLEDGMENTS

I would be remiss if I did not thank a few people who contributed in one way or another to this textbook. The staff at Physical Therapy of the North Shore, Northbrook, Illinois, and Dr. Glen Reinhart, orthopedic surgeon, all put up with me while I was writing this text. They were colleagues during the writing of this text. They provided me with encouragement, willingly rendered their impressions and information on various topics as I progressed in my writing, and consistently supported me throughout the entire process. Two individuals who were willing to find time in their busy schedules and apart from their own commitments, Julie Max, ATC, and Karen Toburen, EdD, ATC, provided me early suggestions for corrections and additions to this text in their very much appreciated reviews of the initial draft. The sports medicine staff at the University of Virginia extended themselves far beyond the call of duty while we took over their facility to shoot approximately 6000 photographs for this text. Ethan Saliba, Susan Saliba, Ian McCleod, Dr. Frank McCue III, and the entire sports medicine staff were not only patient and tolerant of the disruptions our presence and activities caused in their facility, but they went out of their way to accommodate and assist us in our efforts. Without their willing support and selfless sacrifice our task would have been exorbitantly difficult.

Long ago Pete Koehneke had confidence in my ability to produce a text like this. I am grateful to him for his persistent faith in me over the years. Dave Perrin has always demonstrated an assurance beyond my own in my ability to undertake such a project. I owe him a debt of gratitude for providing me with the final push to start and his patient nurturing that enabled me to create and complete the volume you have here.

Last but not least, I would like to thank the crew at Human Kinetics for their belief in this text, skillful support, professional persistence, and steadfast devotion to the project. This text has demanded the tireless efforts and long hours of many people at Human Kinetics. Their professional persistence and steadfast dedication have played an integral part in the completion of this project. Some of the people at Human Kinetics who have my gratitude are Tom Roberts, photographer, who has redefined the meaning of patience during endless hours of photo shoots for this text; Rainer Martens, publisher, who did not waver in his conviction of the importance of this series; Loarn Robertson, the acquisitions editor for the entire series, who had the daunting task of keeping all of the authors and editors on task and on time; Susan Hagan, Sandra Merz Bott, and a small army of other assistants who aided in the editorial process and permissions acquisitions; and most of all, Joanna Hatzopoulos, my developmental editor, who probably had the most difficult task of all, keeping me on task and on time.

CREDITS

Figure 1.1 Reprinted from J.M. Brinkly, P.W. Stratford, S.A. Lott, D.L. Riddle, and the North American Orthopedic Rehabilitation Research Network, 1999, "The lower extremity functional scale (LEFS): Scale development, measurement properties, and clinical application," *Physical Therapy* 79 (4): 383, with permission of the American Physical Therapy Association.

Figure 2.4 Adapted, by permission, from W.B. Leadbetter, 1994, Soft tissue athletic injury. In *Sports injuries: Mechanisms, prevention, treatment,* edited by F.H. Fu and D.A. Stone (Baltimore: Williams & Wilkins), 765. Copyright 1994 by Lippincott Williams & Wilkins.

Table 2.9 Adapted from J.E. Houglum, 1998, "Pharmacologic considerations in the treatment of injured athletes with nonsteroidal anti-inflammatory drugs," *Journal of Athletic Training* 33: 259–263.

Figures 3.10, 3.11, and 3.12 Adapted, by permission, from R. Groves and D.N. Camaione, 1983, *Concepts in kinesiology* (Philadelphia: Saunders).

Figure 5.1 Adapted, by permission, from S.L.-Y. Woo, J.V. Matthews, W.H. Akeson, D. Amiel, and F.R. Convery, 1975, "Connective tissue response to immobility," *Arthritis and Rheumatism* 18: 257–264.

Figures 5.2, 5.3, 5.4, 5.5, 5.6, 5.7, and 5.10 Figures from "Functional properties of collagenous tissue," by A. Viidik in *International Review of Connective Tissue Research* Volume 6, copyright © 1973 by Academic Press, reproduced by permission of the publisher.

Figure 5.8 Butler, D.L., Grood, E.S., Noyes, F.R., and R.F. Zernicke, 1978, "Biomechanics of ligaments and tendons," *Exercise and Sport Sciences Reviews* 6: 125–281.

Figure 5.9 Adapted, by permission, from N. Bogduk and L.T. Twomey, 1987, *Clinical anatomy of the lumbar spine* (New York: Churchill Livingstone).

Figure 5.11 Adapted from D.R. Brown, 1980, *Neurosciences for allied health therapies* (St. Louis: Mosby).

Figure 6.15 Adapted, by permission, from D.G. Simons, J.G. Travell, and L.S. Simons, 1999, *Travell & Simons' myofascial pain and dysfunction: The trigger point manual,* Vol. 1, 2nd ed. (Baltimore: Williams & Wilkins). Copyright 1999 by Lippincott Williams & Wilkins.

Figure 6.25 Adapted, by permission, from G. Maitland, 1991, *Peripheral manipulation,* 3rd ed. (Woburn, MA: Butterworth-Heinemann).

Figures 7.7 and 7.13 Adapted, by permission, from National Strength and Conditioning Association, 2000, *Essentials of strength training and conditioning,* 2nd ed., edited by T.R. Baechle and R.W. Earle (Champaign, IL: Human Kinetics), 6 and 17.

Figure 7.14 Reprinted, by permission, from J.H. Wilmore and D.L. Costill, 1999, *Physiology of sport and exercise,* 2nd ed. (Champaign, IL: Human Kinetics), 39.

Table 7.1 Adapted, by permission, from R.M. Enoka, 1995, "Morphological features and activation patterns of motor units," *Journal of Clinical Neurophysiology* 12(6):538–559.

Figures 7.23 and 9.1 Adapted, by permission, from P.-O. Åstrand and K. Rodahl, 1986, *Textbook of work physiology,* 3rd ed. (New York: McGraw-Hill). Copyright 1986 by P.-O. Åstrand.

Figure 11.20 Adapted, by permission, from J.K. Richardson and Z.A. Iglarsh, 1994, *Clinical orthopaedic physical therapy* (Philadelphia: Saunders).

Figure 11.22, b and c Reprinted, by permission, from J.K. Richardson and Z.A. Iglarsh, 1994, *Clinical orthopaedic physical therapy* (Philadelphia: Saunders).

Chapter 11 sidebar "An Example of the Feldenkrais Method" from *Mindful Spontaneity: Lessons in the Feldenkrais Method* by Ruthy Alon, copyright 1990. Reprinted with permission of North Atlantic Books.

Chapter 11 sidebar "An Alexander Technique Experiment" from *The Alexander Technique* by Wilfred Barlow. Copyright © 1973 by Wilfred Barlow. Reprinted by permission of Alfred A. Knopf, a Division of Random House, Inc.

Figure 12.9 Adapted, by permission, from M.P. Murray, A.B. Drought, and R.C. Kory, 1964, "Walking patterns of normal men," *Journal of Bone and Joint Surgery* 46-A:335–360, fig. 10.

Figure 12.16 Adapted, by permission, from Perry, J., *Gait analysis: Normal and pathological function*, 1992, with permission from SLACK Incorporated.

Figure 12.18 Adapted, by permission, from D.E. Klopsteg and P.D. Wilson, 1954, *Human limbs and their substitutes* (New York: McGraw-Hill). Courtesy of the National Academy of Sciences, Washington, DC.

Figures 12.19 and 12.22 Adapted, by permission, from S. Ounpuu, 1994, "The biomechanics of walking and running," *Clinics in Sports Medicine* 13: 843–862. Copyright 1994 by W.B. Saunders Company.

Figure 12.20 Adapted, by permission, from K.R. Williams, 1985, "The biomechanics of running," In *Exercise and sport sciences reviews,* vol. 13, edited by R.L. Terjung (Baltimore: Williams & Wilkins), 389–441. Copyright 1985 by Lippincott Williams & Wilkins.

Figures 12.21 and 12.23 Adapted, by permission, from R.A. Mann, and J. Hagy, 1980, "Biomechanics of walking, running, and sprinting," *American Journal of Sports Medicine* 8: 345–350. Copyright by American Orthopaedic Society for Sports Medicine.

Figures 13.1, 13.2, and 13.3 From A. Bates and N. Hanson, 1996, *Aquatic exercise therapy.* (Philadelphia: Saunders). Copyright 1996 by W.B. Saunders Company.

Figure 13.4 Reprinted, by permission, from R.A. Harrison, M. Hillman, and S. Bulstrode, 1992, "Loading of the lower limb when walking partially immersed: Implications for clinical practice," *Physiotherapy* 78 (3): 164–167. Copyright by Chartered Society of Physiotherapy.

Figure 15.2 Adapted, by permission, from P.A. Houglum, 1986, "A clinical view of causes and cures for Achilles tendinitis in runners," *Topics in Acute Care Trauma Rehabilitation* 1 (2): 65. © 1986 by Aspen Publishers, Inc.

Table 15.1 Adapted, by permission, from S. Curwin and W.D. Stanish, 1984, *Tendinitis: Its etiology and treatment* (Lexington, MA: Heath). Courtesy of Dr. William D. Stanish, Halifax, Nova Scotia.

Figures 16.1a and 16.6a Adapted, by permission, from D.G. Simons, J.G. Travell, and L.S. Simons, 1999, *Travell & Simons' myofascial pain and dysfunction: The trigger point manual,* Vol. 1, 2nd ed. (Baltimore: Williams & Wilkins). Copyright 1999 by Lippincott Williams & Wilkins.

PART ONE

Basic Concepts

I keep six honest serving-men
(They taught me all I knew)
Their names are What and Why and When
And How and Where and Who.

Rudyard Kipling, *The Elephant Child*

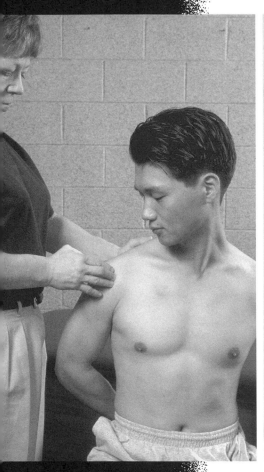
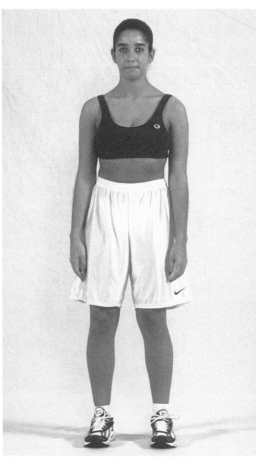
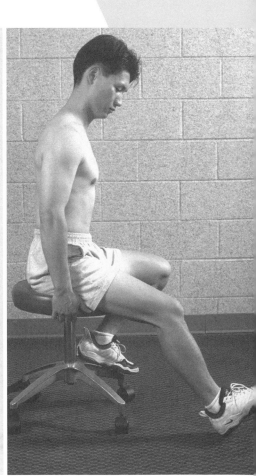

What, why, when, how, where, and who are questions that are continually asked in sports medicine. Knowing the answers to them is not always easy or even possible. Understanding them can be even more difficult. Attempting to know and understand the answers, however, is the goal of sports medicine providers. It is the difference between technicians and professionals.

It is one thing to merely do something, and another to understand why something is done. To be a true allied health professional, you must not only know how to perform the techniques and skills that are a part of that profession, but even more important, you must have the knowledge to appreciate why a technique or skill is used and understand the impact of their application. The challenge does not lie in applying a weight to an ankle but in knowing why it is done, when it should be done, and what impact this action has on the body. In a speech delivered in 1985, Diane Ravitch said, "The person who knows 'how' will always have a job. The person who knows 'why' will always be his boss." The allied health professional knows why; the technician knows how. A technician can apply the technique, but a professional knows, appreciates, and understands the technique.

To develop as a professional and gain this knowledge, appreciation, and understanding of therapeutic exercise, you must first establish a foundation. Once this foundation is established, the larger concepts of therapeutic exercise can be addressed.

The fundamentals on which therapeutic exercise is formulated include factors such as interpersonal relationships; ethical, moral, and legal considerations; principles, goals, and objectives of rehabilitation; psychological factors affecting the program; and the basic components of a program. These factors are building blocks for therapeutic exercise and are covered in **chapter 1.** Unfortunately, they are often neglected in the examination of therapeutic exercise programs but play important roles in the overall rehabilitation process.

In **chapter 2** you are introduced to what happens within the body when an injury occurs. Understanding this process is vital to appreciating the impact of therapeutic exercise on healing. You must be continually aware of the timing of the healing process during your administration of the rehabilitation program if the program is to be successful.

There are many different ways that therapeutic exercises can be applied to the body. Simply changing a patient's position from side-lying to supine can significantly change the stress of an exercise and therefore the effect of that exercise. In **chapter 3** you are introduced to forces that are applied to the body and how they can be changed. Understanding basic physics principles that directly apply to a therapeutic exercise program is fundamental to establishing a sound, beneficial program for the physically active.

How do you know whether what you are doing is working? How do you judge whether your efforts are producing the desired effect? One of the most important ways to answer these questions is to assess the results of your treatments. Even before you can determine what treatment techniques you should use, you must evaluate the patient. In **chapter 4** the aspects and techniques of evaluation and assessment that will guide your decisions for a treatment program are presented. Recording these findings is a part of the evaluation and assessment process and is also addressed.

Once these foundations have been established, we can move on to other factors that are critical to a total rehabilitation program. Specifically, we explore in detail techniques and applications for therapeutic exercise. First, however, as you read through part I, think of physically active people and situations you have either observed or in whose rehabilitation process you have been involved. You will begin to realize that these foundational concepts do indeed play a vital role on a daily basis for any rehabilitation specialist who works with physically active people. An understanding and appreciation of these basic concepts is imperative if you are to create and administer a successful rehabilitation program.

CHAPTER ONE

Concepts of Rehabilitation

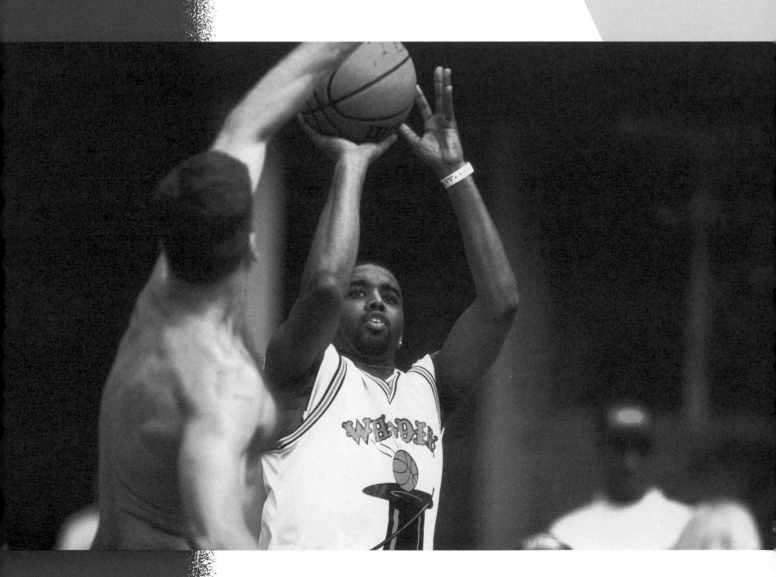

OBJECTIVES

After completing this chapter, you should be able to do the following:

1. Identify rehabilitation team members and their roles.

2. Discuss the qualities of professionalism in athletic training.

3. Discuss the principles, goals, and objectives of rehabilitation.

4. Describe the relationship among goals, progression, and assessment.

5. Outline the importance of outcomes-based rehabilitation.

6. Outline the basic components of a therapeutic exercise program and their interrelationship.

7. Identify the stages of grief and the certified athletic trainer's role in assisting the patient through the stages.

Joel Ritterson had been in his first athletic training position for three weeks. He felt good about his position as assistant certified athletic trainer at the Division I university and was excited about being the athletic department's first rehabilitation coordinator. Until now, the certified athletic trainers had delivered rehabilitation to patients in a haphazard, inconsistent manner, but it was Joel's task to organize and ensure consistent, efficient, and cooperative rehabilitation programs for all the patients.

Coincidentally, the athletic department also hired a new orthopedic surgeon, Dr. Owens, as the team physician. Dr. Owens came to the university with extensive experience at another school where there was good communication and cooperation between the doctor's office and the athletic training staff. Joel looked forward to establishing a good relationship with Dr. Owens.

Joel's first real challenge came early in the football season when the first-string tight end, Richard Jackson, underwent a surgical reconstruction of his anterior cruciate ligament (ACL). Richard was a promising patient whose future depended on good rehabilitation of the knee. Joel felt a lot of pressure and mistrust from the coaching staff, Richard's parents, and Richard himself. Joel wasn't sure whether these anxious feelings were because of the injury, the history of the department's care of these types of injuries, or his own limited experience. Joel felt the best way to gain their trust was to handle Richard's case well. Joel knew he must do a good job not only of rehabilitating Richard's knee, but also of communicating with all the people involved.

Learning without thought is useless; thought without learning is dangerous.

Confucius, *Analects*

The preceding quote by Confucius reminds us of the important relationship between education and critical judgment. A professional should think and analyze throughout the rehabilitation process. Thinking is based on knowledge and sound reasoning. It is my goal that the information you gain from this book prepares you better for the professional path you will follow as a sport rehabilitation specialist.

If you are ready to heed the wisdom of Confucius, read on. This chapter will provide you with an understanding of the basics of rehabilitation: professional interaction with others, the goals and objectives of rehabilitation, and the components of a good rehabilitation program.

This chapter includes varied topics, but they all form the foundation for the therapeutic exercise program that a certified athletic trainer provides a patient. To provide a program that works and is successful, you must understand who affects the process and what determines the patient's successful rehabilitation outcome.

THE ROLES OF REHABILITATION TEAM MEMBERS

The primary rehabilitation team members are the patient, sport rehabilitation specialist, athletic training student, physician, patient's family, coach, and additional medical and allied health personnel. Secondary members include others who play a less significant or less direct part in the patient's rehabilitation. The sport rehabilitation specialist plays a central role as coordinator of the rehabilitation team.

Rehabilitation of patients is not accomplished solely by the sport rehabilitation specialist. It takes a team of several different people working together. Some individuals have more involvement than others, and sometimes more people are involved in the process. The composition of the rehabilitation team depends on the situation and on the extent of the patient's injury.

For example, if the patient is a member of a high school interscholastic team, parents are often involved with even minor injuries. At the college level when the patient is away from home, parents are likely to play a more peripheral role during minor injuries. In severe injuries, specialists not normally consulted enter into the picture.

The injured athlete is part of the rehabilitation team. Without the patient, there would be no need for the team. Once the athlete becomes injured that athlete becomes a patient who is cared for by the rehabilitation team. Physicians and allied health personnel, including certified athletic trainers, use common medical terminology to communicate. An individual who receives medical care is referred to as a patient. The terms *patient* and *injured athlete* are used in this text when referring to the person receiving treatment and care from a certified athletic trainer, physician, or other rehabilitation team member. The sport rehabilitation specialist, athletic training student, physician, parents, coach, and additional medical and allied health personnel are the rest of the members of the primary team. In addition, there can be other team members who play an indirect, or secondary, role. These people do not usually affect the rehabilitation process directly but may have some impact on its ultimate result. These members include athletic administrators, sport team members, equipment managers, orthotists, pharmacists, nutritionists, teachers, and attorneys.

Primary and Secondary Rehabilitation Team Members

Primary Team Members
- Sport rehabilitation specialist
- Athletic training student
- Physician
- Parents
- Coach
- Patient
- Orthopedist
- Podiatrist
- Ophthalmologist
- Psychologist or counselor
- Physical therapist
- School nurse

Secondary Team Members
- Emergency medical technicians
- Orthotist
- Sport team members
- Pharmacist
- Equipment manager
- Kinesiologist
- Exercise physiologist
- Teachers
- Nutritionist
- Athletic administrator
- Attorney

SPORT REHABILITATION SPECIALIST

A sport rehabilitation specialist is a certified athletic trainer who rehabilitates sports injuries. In the course of a day's work, the certified athletic trainer may wear several hats. When dealing with patients who require rehabilitation before returning to full sports participation, the certified athletic trainer wears the hat of a sport rehabilitation specialist. This role is different from the role played during the immediate care and treatment of injuries on the field. As we will discuss, the sport rehabilitation specialist role requires many professional and interpersonal skills.

At the center of the rehabilitation team, regardless of who or how many people make up the team, is the sport rehabilitation specialist. As the individual who has daily contact with the patient and often is the only one who has contact with all the other involved parties, the sport rehabilitation specialist is the coordinator and leader of the rehabilitation team.

Interpersonal Skills

As a vital rehabilitation team member, the sport rehabilitation specialist must possess good interpersonal skills. Besides being dedicated to the rehabilitation process, the sport rehabilitation specialist must be competent and energetic, for the rehabilitation process can be very challenging and lengthy. The sport rehabilitation specialist's interest in the program and empathy for what the patient is enduring has a profound impact on the patient. The sport rehabilitation specialist must act professionally toward all rehabilitation team members. Your consideration, respect for others, confidence, honesty, and sincerity inspire the patient to comply with the rehabilitation program you provide and reassure parents, physicians, and other team members that you possess the knowledge, ability, and skill required to be the coordinator for their rehabilitation team.

Additional information on management and interaction with others can be found in *Management Strategies in Athletic Training*, second edition (Ray 2000).

The sport rehabilitation specialist also needs good active listening skills. Being an active listener means being involved in the conversation, participating appropriately, and understanding what the other person is saying. These qualities can be reflected by simply paraphrasing to the other person what he or she has just said. This technique imparts to the other person that you are listening and also helps you to understand clearly what is being said.

Record Keeping

One role of the sport rehabilitation specialist is to keep accurate records regarding the injury, evaluation, rehabilitation treatment, and response to treatment. Summaries, written or verbal, are communicated to the physician. Record keeping is a part of the process until the patient returns to competition. Record keeping is discussed in more detail in chapter 4.

Educating Others

Educating the patient, family members, and coach is an important task of the sport rehabilitation specialist as the rehabilitation team coordinator. Understanding the injury, its healing process, and the expected rehabilitation response is important to these individuals. Education prepares the patient for the rehabilitation process and prevents surprises. If the patient knows what to expect, he or she has less fear and is more compliant with the rehabilitation program. Family members' fears are calmed with education. If family members are informed, they are also more willing and able to assist the sport rehabilitation specialist in helping the patient achieve a successful rehabilitation outcome. Finally, educating the coach provides the coach with a better understanding of what the patient is going through and an appreciation of the time it may take to complete the rehabilitation process.

ATHLETIC TRAINING STUDENTS

Sport rehabilitation specialist students are in the unique position of acting as the rehabilitation specialist for a patient but not having the independence of a certified athletic trainer. They operate under the guidance of their approved clinical instructor (ACI), a certified athletic trainer. They must be aware of their own limitations and not hesitate to consult the certified athletic trainer whenever they feel they need advice or assistance.

PHYSICIAN

As the medical chief of the team, the physician diagnoses the patient's injury, determines the course of treatment, oversees the rehabilitation program, and determines when the patient is ready to resume sports participation. The physician and sport rehabilitation specialist must cooperate and have respect for and confidence in one another. Each should understand the other's role and appreciate the importance of good communication to a successful rehabilitation outcome.

Planning ahead, communicating, and working together to establish protocols and systems of rehabilitation treatment help to minimize conflicts later. It is important for physicians and sport rehabilitation specialists to know and understand each other's rehabilitation philosophies and preferred methods of treatment ahead of time. It is not unusual for sport rehabilitation specialists and physicians to differ in their perspectives, but it is important for them to reach an understanding and develop a common ground so that they can respect their differences and work with each other in achieving what they both ultimately want: the successful rehabilitation of a patient's injuries.

It is the responsibility of the physician to educate the sport rehabilitation staff, patient, and family members as the need arises. Communication is the key for everyone to have a good understanding of the injury and its expected course of recovery.

FAMILY

Family members are important rehabilitation team members at all levels of competition. When a patient lives at home, they play a vital role because they can assist the patient in complying with the home rehabilitation program. At the collegiate level the patient may not live at home, so family members have a less significant role in assisting with compliance, but they are frequently involved with more serious injuries. More often than not, the sport rehabilitation specialist maintains the most frequent contact with the family.

COACH

As a daily coworker of the certified athletic trainer, the coach relies on the certified athletic trainer for information on the current status of the injured athlete. The coach plays an important role on the rehabilitation team regarding the injured athlete's restrictions on participation in practice and competition, through communication with the certified athletic trainer. If participation is restricted, the coach can help the injured athlete continue to feel he or she is part of the team by including the injured athlete in practices, team meetings, and strategy sessions and having the injured athlete assist with sideline activities.

ATHLETE

The athlete should inform the certified athletic trainer of any injury he or she sustains and seek treatment as soon as possible following injury. Delay in treatment can often mean needless prolongation of an injury and can retard or prevent the individual's return to full athletic function.

When an injury occurs, it is important that the patient maintain good nutrition to enhance the healing process. Patients must take responsibility for their rehabilitation program's success by adhering to the recommendations of the physician and certified athletic trainer. Performing the home treatment regimen provided by the certified athletic trainer is crucial to the overall success of the rehabilitation program.

OTHER TEAM MEMBERS

Occasionally, other medical and paramedical professionals are included on the rehabilitation team. They are often called on as consultants by the primary or team physician when their special expertise is indicated to enhance the rehabilitation process. Examples of some ancillary team members include podiatrists, orthopedists, ophthalmologists, psychologists, physical therapists, and emergency medical technicians. Rehabilitation techniques that have been used to treat the patient, the plan for care, and the response to treatment may be among the information that is conveyed by the certified athletic trainer to the consulting medical professional.

Other peripheral team members include attorneys, school administrators, sports teammates, and other nonmedical team members. Which of these team members is involved varies according to the specific situation and circumstances. Attorneys may be involved in cases of negligence; school administrators may be active in a variety of situations, such as when rules and regulations require reassessment or when there is a conflict among involved parties; sports teammates can play an important support role for the injured athlete. The level of involvement of these team members ranges from no involvement to extensive involvement. When these team members do play a role, the certified athletic trainer should be aware of this and interact with them appropriately.

INTERACTING WITH TEAM MEMBERS

Courteous, professional, accurate, and appropriate communication among all rehabilitation team members is essential for a successful rehabilitation program.

Now that you have an awareness of the roles of each of the rehabilitation team members, the importance of good interaction among these members becomes apparent. Also apparent is why the certified athletic trainer is the coordinator for this team. The certified athletic trainer is easily accessed by the other team members, has daily contact with the patient, has a good understanding of the injury and the healing process, guides the patient along in the rehabilitation program, sees the response to treatment, and knows the expected progression of rehabilitation.

The certified athletic trainer is the center of the communication process. The certified athletic trainer communicates with the patient, the parents, the coach, the physician, the ancillary medical personnel, and the specialists. Each of these rehabilitation team members may speak with another, but the certified athletic trainer has contact with all of them.

With this position comes responsibility. The certified athletic trainer must be sure any information conveyed is accurate and not a guess. Saying "I don't know" generates more respect than guessing the correct response. "I don't know" accompanied by "but I'll find out and get back to you" is even more appreciated.

COMMUNICATING WITH THE PATIENT

Being responsible in communication also means knowing when to say something, when to withhold information, and how to communicate effectively and appropriately. When an athlete has just been injured and feels his or her athletic career is over, it is not the time to explain in detail the process that will occur during rehabilitation. Using big words and medical terminology is not practical when speaking with most patients or their family, especially if they are upset. In a good situation a person normally does not absorb more than seven new items of information. In a stressful situation the ability to understand or retain unfamiliar information is even less. Using good judgment about what to say and when to say it is a skill that is developed with practice by having sensitivity and observing others who are good at it. Be patient with yourself as you develop this skill. Contemplate what you will say before you say it, and put yourself in the place of the injured athlete or family member with whom you are talking. Ask yourself how you would like to be addressed at that time, what information you would want or be able to comprehend without any medical knowledge, and then proceed to listen and observe that person's responses as carefully as you listen to your own words to him or her.

You should communicate with the patient with sincere compassion, understanding of the individual situation, and confidence in your own knowledge of injuries and rehabilitation. It is important to instill in the patient confidence in your ability to treat the injury. This is done by providing the patient with the information he or she seeks about the extent of the injury, the time it will take to heal, and the treatment plan. As mentioned, not all of this information should be provided at once or at the time of injury. Your best judgment about when to provide this information is important in establishing confidence and trust.

COMMUNICATING WITH THE PHYSICIAN

You should not hesitate to contact the physician regarding the patient's injury or response to treatment. Communication between the certified athletic trainer and the physician is important to the outcome of rehabilitation. Both must be aware of the seriousness and extent of the injury, the patient's response to the injury and treatment, and his or her compliance with the rehabilitation program. Both must also agree with the treatment course and appreciate and respect each other's contributions to the rehabilitation process. This is accomplished by communicating and establishing a rapport with each other. Certified athletic trainers communicate with physicians by telephone, through e-mail, in person, and through written reports. Telephone and face-to-face, informal conversations are ways to understand general philosophies and develop rapport. Written and verbal patient reports are also vital to an ongoing professional relationship between the physician and the certified athletic trainer.

COMMUNICATING WITH FAMILY MEMBERS

Depending on the situation, communication with the patient's family varies considerably. At the high school level, parents commonly are intimately involved with an injured athlete's recovery process from the start. Communicating with family members at the time of injury is important because it is an opportunity for the certified athletic trainer to establish a rapport with the family if one has not been established already. It also will reassure parents and calm their fears about serious or lasting results of their son's or daughter's injury. When a patient lives at home, you can inform his or her parents of home activities that can expedite the rehabilitation program.

When the patient does not live at home, family members do not play as important a role in the rehabilitation program. Occasionally, however, when the patient's injury is more serious and the rehabilitation process is longer and more complicated, family involvement may be more direct. For example, if the patient is to have surgery, he or she may choose to go home for the surgery or following surgery. In other situations, patients may return home at the end of the school year when their rehabilitation program is not yet concluded. In these situations the family may be requested to assist with the rehabilitation program or consult with a local facility to continue the rehabilitation process you have started.

COMMUNICATING WITH THE COACH

When a coach has confidence and trust in the certified athletic trainer, cooperation in restricting the patient's workouts is more likely. Impressing upon the coach the extent of the patient's injury, the limitations placed on the injured part, and the importance of the coach's involvement in the rehabilitation process helps to ensure the success of the rehabilitation program.

COMMUNICATING WITH SECONDARY TEAM MEMBERS

When a patient is referred to other medical specialists, input from the certified athletic trainer is appreciated. It provides the specialist with information regarding the patient's injury because often the certified athletic trainer has witnessed the injury. It also provides the specialist with insight regarding the rehabilitation program thus far and the patient's response to it. The certified athletic trainer can also assist in and compliment the specialist's course of treatment.

Like all primary rehabilitation team members, secondary team members' communication with other team members should be honest, constructive, and professional. The ultimate goal of all team members should be to assist in whatever way appropriate for their position within the team in providing the patient with satisfactory and successful rehabilitation. Acting responsibly by performing their roles unselfishly, appropriately, and cooperatively ensures that this goal is achieved.

QUALITIES OF PROFESSIONALISM

Certified athletic trainers demonstrate their professionalism by maintaining a professional appearance and demeanor, continuing their education within the profession, contributing to the profession by being active in NATA, and adhering to legal and ethical standards.

Being a professional means looking and acting like one. A true professional gives something back to the profession by being an active member of the professional association, the National Athletic Trainers' Association (NATA), and making a positive contribution.

Being a professional also means adhering to the legal standards determined by the state's regulating body and complying with the ethical standards established by NATA. Awareness of these professional standards is the responsibility of every individual who considers himself or herself a member of the athletic training profession.

Using your knowledge to provide the patient with the best care possible is an undisputed precept of the profession. This means taking the responsibility to learn current information and practices in the profession and delivering only the care you feel confident in providing.

The years you spend in college to attain a degree and become a certified athletic trainer provide you with a base upon which you will build within the profession. There are more specialized techniques, more complicated information, and more sophisticated treatment application methods that will become available to you as you continue beyond your entry-level education in the allied health profession of athletic training. Attending postgraduate seminars, participating in professional meetings, and reading professional publications to learn current information regarding rehabilitation and other topics within the profession are means by which professionals keep up to date.

It is your responsibility to yourself and to the patients you treat to be aware of the new and ever-evolving methods of treatment and rehabilitation. Medical science is continually advancing, and research is continually being conducted around the world to lead us to better understanding of treatment methods. As a professional, you have an ethical and moral responsibility to provide the best care you can to a patient. Participating in different types of continuing education to optimize your allied health knowledge, techniques, and skills is an important aspect of fulfilling that responsibility.

Treating the patient with concern, respect, and a consistently professional attitude is vital. This attitude establishes the patient's confidence in your ability to give quality care and guide the patient to a successful rehabilitation outcome.

LOOKING LIKE A PROFESSIONAL

Dressing appropriately and being neatly groomed when working as a certified athletic trainer reflect not only your attitude toward yourself, but also your pride in being an allied health professional. If you dress professionally and are neat, clean, and well groomed, you present an appearance that encourages confidence and respect from others. If you are to be taken seriously, you should look like a professional.

ACTING LIKE A PROFESSIONAL

Showing respect and consideration for others, whether you work with them as colleagues or as patients, is part of acting like a professional. Acting professionally also involves being sensitive to the privacy of the patients you treat. Privacy is important when taking a patient's medical history or exposing a body part in the clinic. Acting professionally means being morally and legally responsible and conducting yourself in a manner that reflects well on the medical profession of which you are a member.

Qualities of Professionalism

- Looking professional
- Acting professionally
- Being professional

BEING A PROFESSIONAL

Being a professional goes beyond looking and acting like one. A true professional also attends professional meetings and becomes active in professional associations. The needs of professionals are met through the profession's association. The association's needs are met through the active participation of its members. It should be the professional responsibility of each certified athletic trainer to contribute at the local, state, regional, district, or national level to make the association effective and provide vitality to the profession. A professional cannot stand alone, and a profession needs the energy and dedication of its members to play a viable and convincing role in the medical arena today.

The certified athletic trainers' professional association is NATA. If you are not yet a member, I encourage you to ask the director of your athletic training curriculum program for information regarding student membership in NATA or to contact the NATA office directly to obtain a student membership application.

NATA National Contact Information

Phone: 800-TRY-NATA
Fax: 214-637-2206
Membership e-mail: **NataMIS@aol.com**
Web site: **http://www.nata.org**

ETHICAL AND LEGAL STANDARDS

As allied health professionals, certified athletic trainers have a responsibility to themselves, to their profession, to their employers, and to the patients they rehabilitate to act in a consistently professional manner, including following ethical and legal guidelines.

In today's medical environment the legal aspects of athletic training have become more important than in years past. Ethics, however, has always been an important part of this profession. NATA scripted its *Code of Ethics* in its very early days. The founders of NATA realized the importance of providing guidelines for standards of behavior and ensuring high-quality, principled care for patients by certified athletic trainers. The *NATA Code of Ethics* has since been revised to keep in stride with current issues, but the primary precepts have remained the same. I suggest that you obtain a copy of this document and familiarize yourself with it.

Ethics Guideline Resource

Code of Ethics
National Athletic Trainers' Association
1952 Stemmons Freeway
Dallas, TX 75247

Some of the topics presented here lie in the legal arena, some in the ethical arena, and some in both. These subjects are important enough in the rehabilitation of patients that you should spend a little time understanding them.

State Regulations

Each state has different legal guidelines. The majority of states now have some type of regulation in the form of licensure, certification, registration, or exemption that determines the legal parameters within which a certified athletic trainer must operate. It is your responsibility to know and operate within the regulations of the state in which you practice.

Consent

Certified athletic trainers use their professional skills, knowledge, and best judgment to decide the course of rehabilitation for a patient. Sometimes the patient may not wish to follow the course of treatment that the certified athletic trainer has proposed. The patient may refuse to perform a specific activity. Although you may attempt to convince the patient that the activity is appropriate for a variety of reasons, you must remember that if the patient refuses to perform the activity you request, you cannot force the patient to do it. For example, if a gymnast who suffered an ankle sprain refused to do the non-weight-bearing pool therapy that you recommend, you would probably attempt to make her understand why you want her to go into the water. Regardless of her reasons, if she continues to refuse, you cannot force her into the pool. It is up to you to find an alternative program for her. Likewise, if you wanted a basketball player with a subluxating shoulder to start doing medicine-ball work, but he refused because he lacked confidence that his shoulder could tolerate the exercise, the same policy would apply. You would attempt to explain why this is an important step and reassure him that you would not have him do it until you thought he was ready. If he continued to refuse, you would have to use a different type of exercise that would be less threatening to him yet still accomplish the same goal. You can attempt to reintroduce the activity later in the program, once the patient's confidence has improved and he is less likely to object.

In other words, the patient always has the last say on what is or is not done with his or her body. The patient gives consent for treatment by performing what is requested during the rehabilitation program, but the patient always has the right to say no. The patient's consent is assumed to be given in the treatment process until it is taken away. As a certified athletic trainer, you must always respect the patient's right to consent to or refuse treatment. If your best judgment tells you that a specific course of treatment is indicated but the patient refuses to comply, you should use your communication skills to explain why you are suggesting it. Generally, your knowledge, skill, and past experiences with the patient give the patient the confidence and trust in you so that he or she will not refuse to comply with your rehabilitation procedures. Occasionally, however, perhaps because the patient lacks confidence in himself or herself, has too much pain, or does not feel comfortable with the activity, he or she refuses to perform it. In those cases, you must respect the patient's refusal and remember that, even though you may disagree, it is the patient who has the final control. Your best defense against this situation is to possess the knowledge to create an appropriate rehabilitation program, self-confidence in your knowledge and mastery as an allied health professional, and an ability to create the same confidence in your patients.

Touch

Athletic training is a touching profession. We palpate injuries on a daily basis, feel for spasm and temperature, and touch painful and swollen areas routinely. For this reason, touch becomes something we often do not think about, but we must be continually sensitive to the patient's perception of our touch.

Touching a patient should always be purposeful, with a specific reason and goal in mind. For example, if you touch the thigh of a patient who has received a contusion to the quadriceps, the pressure applied and area palpated should be appropriate.

Touching is an integral and necessary part of a certified athletic trainer's duties, but you must be acutely aware that a patient may not be accustomed to the intimacy of touch in this context. Presenting yourself in a professional manner, being deliberate in how you touch, demonstrating respect for the patient, and having sensitivity for the patient's situation help to reassure the patient and permit you to perform your tasks appropriately.

If you are unsure of how a patient will respond to your touch, it is best to have another professional present. In today's litigious environment, touch—even when it is purely professional and necessary—can be questioned. Most injured athletes are treated in an athletic training facility where other people are around. However, in an isolated situation or when you feel that questions may potentially arise later, you should take precautions, such as having another professional or someone else present, keeping the treatment room door open, or providing the treatment in a common room where others are present. It is often wise to listen to your instincts; if you have an uneasy feeling about a situation, be cautious.

COMPONENTS OF A REHABILITATION PROGRAM

A rehabilitation program should be designed with seven essential principles, two main objectives, and individual long- and short-term goals in mind. The overall program and individual exercises should progress safely and effectively. Rehabilitation specialists should know how to assess the patient's status and evaluate the program's outcomes.

This section deals with the general principles, objectives, and goals of an athletic rehabilitation program. An overview of the components of a rehabilitation program is presented. We also take a brief look at assessing the patient's status, evaluating program progression, and measuring the outcomes of the program.

REHABILITATION PRINCIPLES, OBJECTIVES, AND GOALS

The principles of rehabilitation are used to achieve the goals and objectives of a therapeutic exercise program. The ultimate design of the therapeutic exercise program is based on these principles, goals, and objectives of rehabilitation. The principles and objectives are constants in a therapeutic exercise program. The goals are established for each individual patient in each situation.

Principles

There are seven principles of rehabilitation. Principles are the foundation on which rehabilitation is based. This mnemonic may assist you in remembering the principles of rehabilitation: ATC IS IT.

A: Avoid Aggravation

It is important not to aggravate the injury during the rehabilitation process. Therapeutic exercise, if administered incorrectly or without good judgment, has the potential to make the injury worse. A prime rule was put forth by Hippocrates when he said, "As to diseases, make a habit of two things: to help, or at least to do no harm." This precaution serves certified athletic trainers well.

Rehabilitating the injured athlete in a continually progressive manner without aggravating the injury is a primary concern throughout the therapeutic exercise program. Knowledge of how the body responds to injury, aptitude in determining which exercises to use, good judgment in deciding when the program should progress, and skill in observing the patient's response are needed to recognize when and how far to advance the therapeutic exercise program without aggravating the injury.

Principles of Rehabilitation

Avoid aggravation
Timing
Compliance

Individualization
Specific sequencing

Intensity
Total patient

T: Timing

The therapeutic exercise portion of the rehabilitation program should begin as soon as possible without aggravating the injury. The sooner the patient can begin the exercise portion of the rehabilitation program, the sooner he or she can return to full activity. Following injury, rest is sometimes necessary. Studies have demonstrated, however, that too much rest is actually detrimental to recovery. Appell (1990) reported the significance of inactivity when he estimated that during the first week of immobilization, 3% to 4% of an individual's strength is lost each day. This strength is not recovered in the equivalent amount of time, but takes much longer (Staron et al. 1991). In chapter 2 we investigate the deleterious effects of prolonged rest and immobilization.

Some studies indicate that the rate of recovery is much slower than the rate at which strength is lost. This finding emphasizes the importance of beginning a therapeutic exercise program as soon as is safely possible. The longer the initiation of therapeutic exercises is delayed, the longer the recovery process will take. In more concrete terms, if a patient is out for two days with an injury, it may take a week for full recovery to occur. If a patient is put on rest for four days, it may take perhaps as long as three weeks to return to competition.

C: Compliance

Without a compliant patient, the rehabilitation program will not be successful. To ensure compliance, it is important to inform the patient of the content of the program and the expected course of rehabilitation. The patient will be more compliant when he or she is better aware of the program to be followed, the work he or she will have to do, and what the whole rehabilitation process entails.

Often an injured athlete feels powerless after suffering an injury. That feeling of powerlessness can prevent a successful return to sport participation. Knowledge empowers the patient. Empowerment engenders compliance. Compliance leads to success.

Compliance means that the program is carried out consistently, which allows progressive recovery and improvement. Compliance means that the patient performs whatever exercises or tasks the certified athletic trainer has instructed the patient to perform outside of the athletic training facility. Compliance also means that the patient attends rehabilitation treatment sessions consistently and during those sessions performs whatever activities are included in the treatment to the best of his or her ability.

I: Individualization

Each person responds differently to an injury and to the subsequent rehabilitation program. Expecting a patient to progress in a program the same as the last patient you had with a similar injury will prove to be frustrating for both you and the patient. It is no more realistic to compare one patient to another than it is for a parent to compare one child to its sibling. It is first necessary to recognize that every person is different. It is also important to realize that even though an injury may seem the same in type and severity as another, undetectable differences can change an individual's response to the injury. Individual physiological and chemical differences profoundly affect a patient's specific responses to an injury. Several other non-physical variables can influence the recovery of the patient, including the outside support the patient has from friends, teammates, and family; the patient's psychological makeup and response to the injury; the degree and types of outside pressures the patient may feel to return to competition; and the goals and rewards the patient may want to achieve.

It is your responsibility to understand that these differences exist, be aware of the patient's responses to the injury and rehabilitation program, and design the therapeutic exercise program accordingly to guide the patient through the rehabilitation program as effectively, safely, and efficiently as you can.

S: Specific Sequencing

A specific sequence of events should be followed in a therapeutic exercise program. This specific sequence is determined by the body's physiological healing response.

This topic is covered later in this chapter in the section "Basic Components of Therapeutic Exercise."

I: Intensity

The intensity level of the therapeutic exercise program must challenge the patient and the injured area, but at the same time the intensity must not aggravate the injury. Knowing when to increase intensity without overtaxing the injury requires observational skill and knowledge of the healing process. The healing process is covered in chapter 2.

For you to use the correct exercise intensity in the therapeutic exercise program, knowledge of the progression of exercises and the amount of stress that each exercise imposes is also important. Along with this knowledge, you should have an imagination. This is important because if an exercise is too severe or too easy for the patient to perform, modifying it can permit the right intensity for the patient to progress appropriately. Sometimes all it takes is a slight modification, and other times the modification is more complex. For example, if a patient finds it easy to balance on one leg, having the patient perform the same activity on an unstable surface such as a mini-trampoline makes it more difficult. If doing this exercise on the floor is too easy but doing it on the trampoline is too difficult, you can have the patient perform the exercise on the floor but with eyes closed. Using your imagination and resourcefulness can also be vital if you have a limited equipment budget.

If you combine your knowledge and imagination, you can design a therapeutic exercise program that is challenging and provides the correct intensity level for achieving the goals that have been established. Being imaginative also makes the therapeutic exercise program more interesting for both you and the patient. Making the program interesting enhances the patient's desire to comply and therefore increases the likelihood of a successful outcome.

T: Total Patient

You must consider the total patient in the rehabilitation process. It is important for the injured athlete to stay finely tuned in the unaffected areas of his or her body. This means keeping the cardiovascular system at a preinjury level and maintaining range of motion, strength, coordination, and muscle endurance of the uninjured limbs and joints. When a patient is injured, the whole body must be the focus of the rehabilitation program, not just the injured area. Remembering that the total patient must be ready for competition and providing the patient with a program to keep the uninvolved areas in peak condition, not just rehabilitating the injured area, better prepares the patient physically and psychologically to return to competition when the injured area is completely rehabilitated.

Rehabilitation Objectives

1. Prevent deconditioning.
2. Rehabilitate the injured part.

Objectives

There are two basic objectives for any therapeutic exercise program. The first is related directly to the principle just discussed of treating the total patient. This objective is to prevent deconditioning of uninjured areas. The second objective is to rehabilitate the injured part in a safe, efficient, and effective manner.

Prevent Deconditioning

Preventing deconditioning includes providing exercises for the cardiovascular system, the uninvolved areas of the injured extremity or segment, and the uninvolved extremities. For example, if the patient has a knee injury preventing weight bearing on that leg, the patient can maintain cardiovascular conditioning by performing pool exercises or working out on an upper-body ergometer. The patient can also maintain good strength and range of motion of the upper body and uninvolved lower extremity by using weights and other exercises for these segments. Exercises for the involved extremity's hip and ankle can also be used to prevent deconditioning of those areas without applying undue stress to the injured knee.

Similarly, another patient who has suffered a left shoulder injury can exercise the left elbow, wrist, and hand. Even after surgery and immobilization a patient may be able to perform some type of wrist and hand exercise to help maintain that part's strength and range of motion.

Because of the nature of the injury or the medical restrictions involved, it may sometimes take some imagination on your part to develop exercises that challenge the uninjured parts while not harming the injured area, but it is important for you to design programs with the objective of maintaining current conditioning levels as much as possible.

Rehabilitate the Injured Part

Good knowledge of the injury, healing process, and methods of rehabilitation is paramount to achieving the objective of rehabilitating the injured part. You must use good judgment along with this knowledge to enable the patient to progress safely and effectively through the therapeutic exercise program.

Therapeutic exercise can be used effectively to enhance and promote recovery, but it can also be harmful and ineffective if used incorrectly. It is your responsibility to know the appropriate use of this highly effective yet potentially dangerous therapy.

Goals

Goals are results one strives to achieve. In therapeutic exercise the ultimate goal is the return of the patient to athletic competition. That return, however, should be safe yet quick, effective yet efficient, and pursued in an aggressive yet guarded manner. This means that you must work diligently with all the tools available to you to enhance the healing of the injury, restore the deficient parameters that have been lost because of the injury, and restore the patient's self-confidence to permit him or her to return to sport participation with at least the same level of competence as before the injury. This is done in the minimum amount of time that allows the healing process to occur and also provides enough time to rehabilitate the injured area without undue time lost away from the sport.

There is often a fine line between going too slowly and advancing too quickly. Once again, it is vital for you to use all your skill in application and your knowledge of medicine and how the individual's body responds to the therapeutic exercise program for the patient to progress at an appropriate rate. The program should stress the patient just enough to provide gains, not losses, as it progresses regularly. This image might help you to grasp this concept: Each day it is your responsibility to push the patient up a hill to its peak (applying enough stress to gain as much as possible in an exercise session) without pushing so far that the patient goes over the other side (applying so much stress that it causes deleterious effects).

Objective and Measurable Goals

Goals should be objective and measurable whenever possible. Goals are occasionally subjective; for example, pain is subjective. However, some objectivity is possible in measuring this subjective parameter by asking the patient to rate his or her pain on a 10-point scale. Other parameters such as girth, range of motion, and strength can be measured as objective and more concrete goals.

It is necessary to record these measurements at various stages in the therapeutic exercise program, most obviously at the beginning and conclusion of the program. Throughout the program, the patient is reassessed routinely as well. Any changes should be recorded. This is important in assisting you and the patient to identify improvements. This record can also help you more easily notice when changes do not occur as frequently as expected and decide what specific modifications to make to the program.

Short- and Long-Term Goals

When an athlete's injury is severe enough to restrict sport participation for at least a month, both long-term and short-term goals should be set. A long-term goal is the final, desired outcome of a therapeutic exercise program. Returning the patient to athletic competition is a long-term goal. Specifically, this involves returning the patient to normal levels of all parameters that allow full return to sport participation, including flexibility, strength, endurance, coordination, and skill execution. Definitive levels of these parameters are different for each patient and depend on the patient's sport, specific position, age, skill level, and level of participation. These parameters are discussed in more detail later in this chapter in the section "Basic Components of Therapeutic Exercise."

Short-term goals provide both you and the patient with objective aims to guide you toward the long-term goals. Short-term goals are established weekly or biweekly and depend on the patient's response to the injury and ability to progress, the stage of the rehabilitation process, and the severity of the injury. A short-term goal may be to reduce edema by 1 cm and increase range of motion by 15° in one week. Other short-term goals may be to increase strength by half a grade (the scoring system for muscle strength is discussed in chapter 7), reduce pain to 3 on a scale of 10, and achieve 90% of normal range of motion in two weeks.

Short-term goals are important because they give the patient something concrete to work toward and the psychological boost to achieve them. Looking at long-term goals can be overwhelming, but focusing on short-term goals gives the patient direction and establishes a logical progression for the rehabilitation process.

Short-term goals should be reasonable and attainable yet challenging for the patient. They should be realistic to allow the patient to achieve them within the time established without irritating the injury or frustrating the patient. Establishing realistic goals takes skill, knowledge, and judgment on your part. You must also be aware of additional factors that may affect the patient's ability to achieve these goals, such as the patient's personality and how he or she responds to injury, challenges, and discipline; outside pressures such as from scholarships, family, coach, and friends; the patient's other activities, including recreational activities, work, and school; the severity, type, and healing process of the injury; and the level of dysfunction involved.

Example Goals

These are examples of long- and short-term goals that could be set for a patient with a shoulder injury.

Long-term goal:
The patient will have full strength in all rotator cuff muscles at the conclusion of the rehabilitation program.
Short-term goal: Two weeks from today's treatment session, the patient will have 4/5 strength in the subscapularis, 3+/5 strength in the teres minor and infraspinatus, and 3/5 strength in the supraspinatus (using the scoring system discussed in chapter 7 in which 5 = full strength and 0 = complete loss of contractility).

An alternative short-term goal:
Two weeks from today's treatment session, the patient will increase strength in each rotator cuff muscle by 1/2 grade from today's evaluation scores.

All injuries involve precautions and contraindications. Complications can occur regardless of the quality of care provided. You must establish goals and place demands on the patient with these factors in mind.

ASSESSMENT

Certified athletic trainers continually assess injuries, from the time the injury occurs to the time the patient is ready to return to sport participation. Therapeutic exercise programs are one area in which certified athletic trainers make frequent assessments.

The only way to establish goals is to make an assessment of the patient's current condition. How much swelling is present? How much range of motion is lost? What is the status of the injured area's strength? These and other questions are assessed on the first day of rehabilitation. They are also reassessed regularly throughout the rehabilitation treatment.

To create short- and long-term goals, you must first establish the present status of the deficient parameters. Then you decide what realistic short-term goals the patient can achieve in a specific amount of time. Once those goals are achieved, you once again make an assessment to decide new and appropriate short-term goals.

You must continually assess the patient's condition to provide the patient with an accurate therapeutic exercise program with appropriate goals. This is only one area in which assessment skills are needed. Assessment and other contexts where it is necessary are covered in more depth in chapter 4.

PROGRESSION

A good therapeutic exercise program progresses in a challenging yet safe manner. Accurate assessment of the patient's response to the exercises and treatment is necessary for this to occur. The progression should be in accordance with the severity of the injury, the type of injury, and the patient's response to the injury and treatment. A good progression challenges the patient without causing deleterious effects such as increased pain or swelling or decreased ability to perform.

Exercise Progression

One level of progression is the progression of each exercise. For example, a strength progression may advance from **isometrics** to **isotonics** to **isokinetics** to **plyometrics**. The patient begins with a level that is challenging but not irritating to the injury, which is determined by the severity of the injury and the certified athletic trainer's assessment of the patient's current ability. A patient with a mild ankle sprain who is ambulating without crutches may be able to forgo isometrics and begin isotonics and weight-bearing resistive exercises. However, a patient with profound swelling who is on crutches may be able to tolerate only non-weight-bearing range-of-motion and isometric exercises.

Program Progression

Another level of progression involves the program itself: A program should be designed to emphasize different types of exercises as it progresses. This is discussed in the section "Basic Components of Therapeutic Exercise" later in this chapter. Keep in mind that you cannot expect a patient to perform advanced skill drills in his or her sport before flexibility and strength have been achieved and that full strength cannot be achieved until flexibility is restored.

OUTCOMES-BASED REHABILITATION

Today's buzz word in medicine is *outcomes*. Outcomes are important to the understanding of and justification for the programs used to treat patients. The outcome of a treatment program is often assessed using a tool that has been devised for measuring the patient's response and satisfaction following a treatment that is given for a specific injury or condition. The outcome tool is most often a questionnaire that is given before the start of the program, sometime during its course, and at its conclusion. Questions often relate to the patient's condition before and after treatment and to the patient's perception of different aspects of the treatment, including quality of care, professional attitudes, effectiveness of the program in achieving goals, and other items. Input from the professional providing the treatment program is also obtained. Figure 1.1 shows the Lower Extremity Functional Scale (LEFS), an example of a specific outcomes questionnaire. The results are then compiled and statistically analyzed to provide a variety of information to today's medical providers, patients, and payers.

Outcomes tools are divided into two categories—a general health status measurement tool and a region-specific measurement tool. A generic status measurement tool is used to assess a patient's physical, social, and emotional health and is used in a variety of illnesses and treatment environments. The gold standard for the generic health status tool is the SF-36, originally advanced by John E. Ware, Jr. (Ware and Sherbourne 1992; Ware et al. 1995). Although it has been demonstrated to be a reliable and valid tool, it is time consuming to administer and was not designed as a tool with which to make treatment decisions for individual patients (Binkley et al. 1999). A variety of condition-specific outcomes tools have been developed in an attempt to more accurately assess items that are related to the specific injury or illness and will reveal changes with treatment applications. For example, a commonly used condition-specific outcomes tool that assesses changes in back pain is the Roland-Morris Questionnaire (Stratford et al. 1998).

Some of the problems that are recognized in selecting an assessment tool that restricts the reliability of one tool to assess treatment effects for different conditions include the difficulty in using a tool's scale for different injuries, the shortcomings a tool has in its application to specific individuals, and the clinician's lack of confidence in the meaningfulness of the scores (Binkley et al. 1999). For example, a condition-specific tool that is designed to measure patellofemoral injury treatment outcomes may not be considered a reliable tool to measure outcomes of treatment for a shoulder dislocation, or a tool designed to measure treatment outcomes on a high school athlete may not be applicable to measuring treatment outcomes on a middle-aged athlete.

Outcomes are important in many fields of medicine. They are used in physicians' offices, outpatient clinics, and hospitals. They are used to modify treatment, justify treatment, evaluate the effectiveness of protocols, judge the appropriateness of treatment responses, and assist in authorization of payment. An outcome assessment tool can be provided by an outside agency, which analyzes the results from many different treatment providers around the country, or it can be devised and analyzed by a single facility.

A couple of the more commonly used outcome research tools used today in rehabilitation are the Functional Independence Measure (FIM) (Keith et al. 1987), a tool used primarily for inpatient rehabilitation facilities, and Focus on Therapeutic Outcomes (FOTO), a tool for outpatient rehabilitation facilities. The following resources are also used in assessment of outcomes.

Outcomes Resources

Guide for the Uniform Data Set for Medical Rehabilitation (Adult FIM), version 4.0. 1993. Buffalo, NY: University of New York at Buffalo/UB Foundation Activities.

Lewis, C., and T. McNerney. 1994. *The functional tool box.* Washington, DC: Learn.

McDowell, I., and C. Newell. 1996. *Measuring health.* 2nd ed. New York: Oxford University Press.

Medical Outcomes Trust approved instruments. 1996. *Medical Outcomes Trust Bulletin* 4(1).

Scientific advisory committee instrument review criteria. 1995. *Medical Outcomes Trust Bulletin* 3(Sept.).

Lower Extremity Functional Scale

We are interested in knowing whether you are having any difficulty at all with the activities listed below *because of your lower limb* problem for which you are currently seeking attention. Please provide an answer for **each** activity.

Today, *do you* or *would you* have any difficulty at all with:

(Circle one number on each line)

Activities	Extreme Difficulty or Unable to Perform Activity	Quite a Bit of Difficulty	Moderate Difficulty	A little Bit of Difficulty	No Difficulty
a. Any of your usual work, housework, or school activities	0	1	2	3	4
b. Your usual hobbies, recreational or sporting activities	0	1	2	3	4
c. Getting into or out of the bath	0	1	2	3	4
d. Walking between rooms	0	1	2	3	4
e. Putting on your shoes or socks	0	1	2	3	4
f. Squatting	0	1	2	3	4
g. Lifting an object, like a bag of groceries, from the floor	0	1	2	3	4
h. Performing light activities around your home	0	1	2	3	4
i. Performing heavy activities around your home	0	1	2	3	4
j. Getting into or out of a car	0	1	2	3	4
k. Walking 2 blocks	0	1	2	3	4
l. Walking a mile	0	1	2	3	4
m. Going up or down 10 stairs (about 1 flight of stairs)	0	1	2	3	4
n. Standing for 1 hour	0	1	2	3	4
o. Sitting for 1 hour	0	1	2	3	4
p. Running on even ground	0	1	2	3	4
q. Running on uneven ground	0	1	2	3	4
r. Making sharp turns while running fast	0	1	2	3	4
s. Hopping	0	1	2	3	4
t. Rolling over in bed	0	1	2	3	4

Column Totals:

Error (single measure) ± 5 scale points; MDC: 9 scale points; MCID: 9 scale points

Score_____/80

■ **Figure 1.1** Outcome assessment tools.

Reprinted from J.M. Binkley, P.W. Stratford, S.A. Lott, D.L. Riddle, and the American Orthopedic Rehabilitation Research Network, 1999, "The Lower Extremity Functional Scale (LEFS): Scale development, measurement properties, and clinical application," *Physical Therapy* 79(4): 383, with permission of the American Physical Therapy Association.

Different users of the assessment tool evaluate outcomes differently, depending on their perspective. For example, an insurance company may use outcome research results to decide what is usual and customary for expected duration and treatment cost of an injury. A patient may use them to see whether the treatment program met his or her needs. Health care providers may look at the results of the outcome study to assess whether the programs being used to treat specific injuries and individual patients in their facility are effective and cost efficient and achieve the goals of the professional administering the treatment. There are occasions, however, when outcome assessments are used incorrectly to generalize results to a larger population or different situation. Inappropriate inferences should be avoided, for they are misleading, unfair, and erroneous.

Because it is imperative for a certified athletic trainer to be as effective and efficient as possible in treating patients and returning them to sport participation, certified athletic trainers are inherently concerned with outcomes. Outcome assessments may not be as critical, however, for certified athletic trainers who practice in an athletic training clinic or industrial setting as for those who practice in other settings, such as orthopedic clinics or hospitals. As systems of allied health care and payment continue to change, however, all certified athletic trainers will eventually be compelled to deal with outcome assessments more formally than is currently typical.

BASIC COMPONENTS OF THERAPEUTIC EXERCISE

Therepeutic exercise must address the following physiological parameters in proper order: first, flexibility and range of motion, then muscular strength and endurance, and finally, proprioception and coordination.

In the total rehabilitation program, therapeutic exercise plays one of the more important roles in returning the patient to sport participation. If the therapeutic exercise program is to be effective, however, specific parameters must be addressed sequentially. Each of these parameters must be restored to at least preinjury levels if the patient is to return safely to participation and competition. Therapeutic exercise, correctly applied, restores deficient parameters to permit the patient to return to sport participation and also reduces the risk of reinjury.

The correct application of therapeutic exercise in a rehabilitation program emphasizes a sequence of physiological parameters, which must be restored to at least preinjury levels of function. These parameters in their proper sequence are

1. flexibility and range of motion,
2. strength and muscle endurance, and
3. proprioception and coordination.

Each of these parameters is based on the previous ones, much like a pyramid of building blocks. This concept will become clearer as we discuss each parameter.

FLEXIBILITY AND RANGE OF MOTION

There is a technical difference between flexibility and range of motion, but in functional terms the difference is minimal. The term **flexibility** is often used when referring to the mobility of muscles and the length to which they can extend. If a muscle is immobilized for a period of time, it tends to lose its flexibility, or degree of mobility. If stretching exercises are incorporated as part of a routine conditioning program, the muscle tends to maintain its flexibility or length. Inflexible often means that the muscles, not the joints, have limited mobility.

Range of motion, however, refers to the amount of movement possible at a joint. For example, the normal range of motion for shoulder **abduction** is 170°. Range of motion is affected by the flexibility of the muscles and muscle groups surrounding the joint. If a muscle lacks flexibility, the joint may not have full range of motion. Range of motion is also affected by other factors, including mobility of the joint capsule and ligaments, fascial restraints, and scar tissue in the area.

Range of motion is also affected by strength. For example, if a patient does not have the strength to lift the arm fully against gravity, the shoulder range of motion may not reach 170°. This is one reason why active and passive range-of-motion measurements are often different from each another, the passive range of motion being greater than the active. Active and passive ranges of motion are discussed in chapter 5.

Because of their close functional relationship, the terms *range of motion* and *flexibility* are often used interchangeably. We will treat these terms as synonyms here, but keep in mind that technical differences exist between them.

A properly designed therapeutic exercise program for rehabilitation places a priority on regaining lost range of motion and flexibility first. Achieving flexibility early in the therapeutic exercise program is necessary because of two important factors. First, the other parameters are based on the flexibility of the affected area. To make this point clear, consider how handicapped a hurdler would be if the hamstrings were inflexible. The patient's strength and timing would be of little importance if the flexibility necessary to extend the leg over the hurdle were lacking. A baseball pitcher with less than full shoulder range of motion is at a distinct disadvantage. Lacking full shoulder motion, the pitcher is at risk for reinjury, regardless of strength, endurance, or timing.

The second reason to emphasize regaining range of motion first in the therapeutic exercise program is the impact of the healing process (discussed in chapter 2). As tissue heals following injury, scar tissue is laid down. As the scar tissue matures, it contracts. This is important in eventually minimizing the size of the scar, but it also can be detrimental because as the tissue contracts, it pulls on the tissue around it, resulting in loss of motion.

During healing there is a window of opportunity during which the injured area's range of motion can be influenced and changed. Once that time frame has passed, the likelihood of successfully achieving full range of motion is diminished considerably. If efforts are not made during the remodeling phase, when the newly forming scar tissue is most easily influenced, attempts to improve range of motion will be very difficult and frustrating at best and futile at worst. Although restoration of other parameters is also sought during the first stage of rehabilitation, flexibility must be the primary emphasis.

STRENGTH AND MUSCULAR ENDURANCE

As the patient progresses, achieving normal strength and muscular endurance becomes the priority. With any injury some strength is lost. The amount of strength and muscular endurance lost depends on the area injured, the extent of the injury, and the amount of time the patient has been disabled by the injury.

Muscular strength refers to the maximum force that a muscle or a muscle group can exert. It is most often measured by determining the amount of weight that the muscle or group can lift in one repetition. **Muscular endurance** is the muscle's ability to sustain a submaximal force in either a static activity or a repetitive activity over a period of time. An example of muscular endurance in a static activity is the length of time a gymnast can maintain an iron-cross position on the rings (see figure 1.2). A runner in a marathon and a starting pitcher are examples of patients performing repetitive activities that require muscular endurance.

Of all the parameters achieved during therapeutic exercise, strength is probably the most obvious and the most frequently sought following an injury. It is obvious because it is easily understood that a weightlifter cannot return to competition following a sprain until full knee strength is achieved. It is just as obvious that a wrestler must have normal shoulder strength to return to competition after suffering a dislocation.

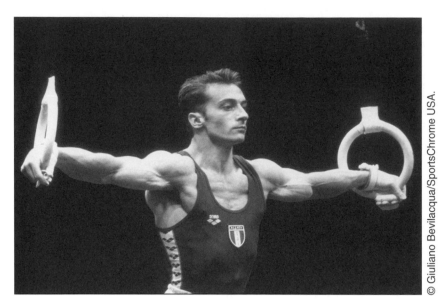

■ Figure 1.2 Gymnast in iron-cross position.

© Giuliano Bevilacqua/SportsChrome USA.

The need for muscular endurance and the relationship between muscular strength and endurance are sometimes not considered, however. If a baseball pitcher has good rotator cuff strength but no endurance beyond 10 repetitions, how is he going to manage pitching more than a couple of innings in a game? If a basketball center can leg press 225 kg (496 lb) but can last only five repetitions, will she be able to recover rebounds for an entire game?

Muscular strength and endurance are two dimensions within a continuum of muscle resistance. They also affect each other. When strength improves, there are also gains in endurance, and vice versa. This is an important factor to remember in establishing a therapeutic exercise program for patients. For example, if a patient is attempting to recover from patellofemoral pain syndrome, the patient may not be able to tolerate heavy weights to achieve the strength you would like to see. Exercises for endurance may be more tolerable and will still produce gains in strength until the patient becomes strong enough to tolerate higher resistance.

PROPRIOCEPTION AND COORDINATION

Proprioception and coordination are often neglected in the total rehabilitation program. It is too often assumed that because range of motion and strength have returned, the patient is ready to resume full sport participation. This is not the case at all. Impaired balance, proprioception, or coordination—either from injury to the structures controlling these parameters or from lack of practice in a specific sport skill—increases risk of injury.

A variety of factors affect a patient's proprioception and coordination. A number of factors in turn are affected by proprioception and coordination, including muscular power, skill execution, and sport performance. (The factors that affect and are affected by proprioception and coordination are discussed later in chapter 8.) To develop appropriate proprioception and coordination skills for sport participation, enough flexibility and strength must first be achieved. Coordination and skill execution are based on the patient's having enough flexibility to perform the skill through an appropriate range of motion and enough strength, endurance, and power to perform it repeatedly and correctly. This is the reason that proprioception and coordination are the last parameters to focus on: they need the foundations of good flexibility, strength, and endurance to be optimal.

Although not all allied health professionals emphasize this parameter, a total rehabilitation program must include the recovery of proprioception and coordination. Consider a tennis player who has suffered a back injury that has kept him out of competition for two months. The timing of his serve, his response to his opponent's serve, and the coordination of his feet in sudden lateral movements on the court may all be impaired. Exercises for proprioception are introduced early in the therapeutic exercise program, but proprioception and coordination are not emphasized until strength and range of motion are achieved. Development of execution skills is the last step before a patient's return to full sport participation. Accurate execution of sport-specific skills requires attainment of all parameters.

The final stage of emphasis on coordination and proprioception evolves into the execution of sport-specific drills that mimic the patient's actual sport activities. Functional activities, the final step before returning to competition, involves execution of these sport-specific activities. In this stage the patient regains the confidence necessary to perform at his or her prior level in the sport. When the patient can perform well and with confidence, the certified athletic trainer can be assured that the goal of fully rehabilitating the patient has been achieved.

RETURN-TO-COMPETITION CRITERIA

The physician determines when a patient is ready to return to competition based on the information provided by the rehabilitation specialist about the patient's status.

By the time the patient is ready to return to full sport participation, you have fully assessed the injured area, the patient's ability to withstand the demands of the sport, and the patient's readiness to return to competition. Full readiness to resume sport participation means that the injured area has no pain, swelling, or atrophy and has full range of motion, flexibility, strength, and endurance and that the patient can perform the sport skills and coordination tasks at an appropriate functional level.

You and the patient must remember that the physician has the final word on when the patient is able to return to competition. It is through your communication with the physician regarding the patient's response to treatment, the patient's ability to perform activities required in the sport, and the injured area's status that the physician can make that determination.

PSYCHOLOGICAL CONSIDERATIONS

A patient may go through four stages of grieving: denial, anger, depression, and acceptance. To ensure compliance with the therapeutic exercise program, the rehabilitation specialist must recognize the importance of the patient's psychological state, communicate effectively, educate, provide support, set goals cooperatively, establish rapport, and make the program interesting.

Many psychological factors have a direct and sometimes profound influence on the overall results of the rehabilitation program. The certified athletic trainer must be aware of these factors not only to be able to promote optimal results of the therapeutic exercise program, but also to encourage and provide needed support to the patient.

STAGES OF GRIEF

Kubler-Ross (1969) outlined stages of grief that people go through when confronted by the knowledge of their own death or that of a loved one. Although it has never been measured or conclusively proven, others (Peterson 1986; Rotella 1985) have suggested that patients who have experienced a disabling injury that keeps them out of competition also go through this process. Since anecdotal reports indicate injured athletes go through this process, it will be explained here. Kubler-Ross's stages of grief are denial, anger, depression, and acceptance.

1. **Denial.** At first, the patient doesn't believe that the injury is severe and feels that he or she will return to competition in a day or two.

2. **Anger.** As the reality of the severity and consequences of the injury sets in and the patient is forced to see the difficulty he or she is having in recovery, the patient expresses anger as a release of the genuine feelings of frustration and helplessness. This anger is often directed at whomever is present. It is helpful to remember that during this phase the patient is angry because of the injury and the situation he or she is in, not because of any action or words of those who are around. Attempts to calm, rationalize with, or help the patient see what is really happening are often futile at this point. The patient wants only to express this anger and does not want to be told why he or she should not be angry or that things will get better.

During this stage, you should attempt to prevent the injury from becoming aggravated by any harmful activities the patient may attempt. You should also be a sounding board for the patient, letting the patient express the feelings of frustration and anger at the loss of the ability to perform and the loss of power over the situation.

3. **Depression.** As the patient begins to realize the reality of the situation, depression is the next stage. The patient's self-worth declines during this time. The patient feels he or she has no physical or emotional control. Not participating with the team can cause feelings of isolation, further adding to self-doubt and low self-esteem. Hope is questionable at best because the patient sees no good results forthcoming.

It is during this phase that rehabilitation becomes the most difficult for both you and the patient. It becomes difficult for the patient to comply with the rehabilitation program. The patient may not attend scheduled treatment sessions or may not fully participate in them.

4. **Acceptance.** In this final phase the patient begins the battle of fighting the physical limitations and psychological downswing experienced during the previous stages.

PROGRESSION THROUGH THE STAGES

Throughout the grieving process there are no abrupt changes; rather, the patient goes through gradual transitions, and fluctuation between stages can occur. For example, a patient who has entered the depression phase may swing back into the anger phase in the beginning but later return to the depression phase. As the patient progresses through depression, he or she displays less and less anger. As the patient enters the acceptance phase, he or she may regress to depression before finally accepting the situation.

You must be aware that these swings occur and are natural. Seeing these stages on a continuum from the extreme ends of denial and acceptance, each phase overlapping with the adjacent one, may help you in dealing with the patient as he or she goes through these stages.

When a patient is unable to advance through the grieving process smoothly or you are concerned about the patient's emotional condition, it is your responsibility to support the patient and encourage him or her to seek additional psychological support from a counselor, psychologist, psychiatrist, or other psychological professional. You should never hesitate to refer a patient to an appropriate specialist.

THE CERTIFIED ATHLETIC TRAINER'S ROLE IN PSYCHOLOGICAL RECOVERY

Supporting the patient in psychological recovery is vital to achieving goals of therapeutic exercise and rehabilitation programs. The certified athletic trainer is crucial to this process because of the role he or she plays in the patient's response to injury and commitment to the rehabilitation program. A survey of certified athletic trainers (Fisher, Mullins, and Frey 1993) revealed the most important variables influenced by certified athletic trainers in patients' compliance with rehabilitation programs. At the top of the list is education and communication. If you educate the patient about the type and extent of the injury, inform him or her about the rehabilitation process, and communicate with him or her in a respectful, open, and honest manner, the patient will exhibit better compliance.

Communication

Using good communication skills throughout the rehabilitation process is important. Being a good and an active listener is a communication skill that every certified athletic trainer should possess. Repeating the patient's uncertainties, worries, and goals is an active listening skill that demonstrates to the patient your interest and concern. Making good eye contact is a simple yet important part of communication. Being aware of the environment and realizing whether it is conducive to good listening and communication are also necessary. Simply being at the same eye level, instead of standing and looking down at the patient, encourages communication.

As discussed earlier in the section "Communicating With the Patient," appropriate communication incorporates good judgment and interpersonal skills. Being timely with explanations and knowing how much to explain is often vital to the patient acceptance. The information you provide the patient educates him or her, enhances compliance with your treatment program, and gives him or her hope for a foreseeable end to the injury and return to competition.

Communication includes providing the patient with written and oral instruction and demonstration of any home exercises or activities. Having written descriptions of exercises along with illustrations or photos ensures optimal patient compliance with a home program.

Offering encouragement for the patient's physical efforts throughout the therapeutic exercise program positively impacts the patient's psychological response. Encouragement also improves compliance. When someone of authority and expertise whom the patient respects offers support and encouragement, the patient's performance and compliance are enhanced.

Goal Setting With the Patient

Goal setting is important in facilitating patient compliance. The patient's assistance in setting goals offers two benefits: the patient has some control over the situation, and working together to establish goals ensures mutual understanding of and agreement on those goals. It is natural for a patient to feel a loss of power or control when injured. Thus, regaining control is important. If a patient feels in control, he or she will be more compliant.

You and the patient should have the same goals. If one has a goal that conflicts with the other's, failure is certain. You and the patient should understand each other's goals, agree with them, and work together to achieve them. For example, if an injured alpine skier has no desire to return to skiing but instead wants to become a recreational cyclist, while your goal is to have the patient return to the slopes, you will be frustrated when the patient does not work as hard as you would like, and the patient will be frustrated that you are making her work harder than necessary to achieve her goal.

Monitoring the patient's progress, using goals, recording objective changes, and setting new and more challenging goals are all methods of providing the patient with additional incentives for adhering to the therapeutic exercise program. The patient may be able to feel some benefits from the program, but providing him or her with more objective, concrete measurements enhances his or her willingness and motivation to continue the rehabilitation program.

Supporting the Patient

Depending on the environment, the members of the patient's support system may vary. The certified athletic trainer is key to this support system, however, and acts as the coordinator of the patient's support system to assist him or her in a successful outcome. Support team members can assist the patient with home exercises, provide encouragement, and share with the certified athletic trainer observations or concerns noted outside the treatment environment.

Establishing Rapport With the Patient

Treating a patient on a frequent, if not daily, basis, the certified athletic trainer usually develops a rapport with the patient. This rapport results from the interaction between these two people, mutual respect, and desire to achieve the same goals. Establishing rapport can be a challenge when patients are hard to manage or have difficult personalities. In these cases it is the certified athletic trainer's responsibility to put aside his or her own prejudices and feelings and act in a professional manner. Usually, however, the challenge of the situation and the common bond between the patient and certified athletic trainer facilitate an easily established rapport. The patient is more compliant and willing to perform any activity requested when this rapport exists.

Making the Program Interesting

Personalizing the program, making its goals challenging yet achievable, and using your imagination to make it interesting are important to overall success and the patient's compliance. The therapeutic exercise program can be a treatment of drudgery or stimulation for both the patient and you. It is up to you to see to it that it is the latter if your common goals are to be achieved.

SUMMARY

1. *Identify rehabilitation team members and their roles.*

   A rehabilitation team consists of individuals who are closely related to the rehabilitation program or who have peripheral roles. Some of these individuals are the patient, certified athletic trainer, physician, family members, athletic training students, coach, team members, and specialists.

2. *Discuss the qualities of professionalism in athletic training.*

   The certified athletic trainer is an allied health caregiver who is responsible for looking, acting, and being professional. Being a professional means acting as a responsible certified athletic trainer and contributing within the professional organization. Being a professional carries with it the responsibility of continuing to learn new techniques and applications that are pertinent to the profession. It also means always treating others in a respectful and courteous manner.

3. *Discuss the principles, goals, and objectives of rehabilitation.*

   The mnemonic ATC IS IT can help you remember the principles of rehabilitation. The objectives of any therapeutic exercise program are to prevent deconditioning of the unaffected areas, including the cardiovascular system, and to rehabilitate the injured area safely, efficiently, and successfully.

   The goals established for each patient are based on achieving these objectives and are divided into short-term and long-term goals. The long-term goal is to restore the patient to at least former levels of function to permit the patient to return to sport participation. Short-term goals are used when the patient has a more severe injury and cannot participate in sports for a while.

   To achieve these goals and objectives, you must be sensitive to the patient and what the patient is going through psychologically.

4. *Describe the relationship between goals, progression, and assessment.*

   Short-term goals are based on measures as objective as possible, recorded to see the patient's progress, and changed when the patient achieves them until the final long-term goals are achieved. You must continually assess the patient's and the injured area's response to treatment. Using objective measures in this assessment and recording the results help the patient and you to realize the changes that are the product of the rehabilitation program and to know how the program should progress.

5. *Outline the importance of outcomes-based rehabilitation.*

   Outcome assessment investigates whether a program that you design for a patient produces the expected response and whether the program meets expectations and goals.

6. *Outline the basic components of a therapeutic exercise program and their interrelationships.*

   A rehabilitation program must progress in a sequential manner, since each parameter builds upon the components of the prior parameter so that a patient can ultimately return to sport participation. The sequential parameters include flexibility and range of motion, strength and muscle endurance, proprioception and coordination, leading to full functional activity.

7. *Identify the stages of grief and the certified athletic trainer's role in assisting the patient through the stages.*

   Although it has not been clearly demonstrated that an injured athlete follows the four stages of grief, they follow this sequence: denial, anger, depression, and acceptance. To ensure the patient's compliance with the therapeutic exercise program, the rehabilitation specialist must recognize the importance of the patient's psychological state, communicate effectively, educate, provide support, set goals cooperatively, establish rapport, and make the program interesting.

CRITICAL THINKING QUESTIONS

1. How would you handle a situation in which a certified athletic trainer with whom you work did not properly complete the requirements established by the NATA Board of Certification (NATABOC) to sit for the certification examination but was able to get his or her supervising certified athletic trainer to sign off on the required documents anyway? Would you report him or her to the NATABOC, discuss it with him or her or your supervisor, or ignore it?

2. If you were treating a patient whose injury was severe enough to doubt whether he or she would return to full sport participation at the preinjury level, how would you deal with the questions the patient would have regarding long-term goals? Would you tell the patient in the beginning that returning to his or her prior level of participation was questionable? Would you let the patient discover the reality him- or herself? Would you ease the patient into that reality?

3. If you were the certified athletic trainer for a college and a 17-year-old freshman was injured severely enough to require emergency room care, when would you inform the parents? Would you have obtained prior permission from the parents for such care?

REFERENCES

Appell, H.-J. 1990. Muscular atrophy following immobilization: A review. *Sports Medicine* 10:42–58.

Binkley, J.M., Stratford, P.W., Lott, S.A., Riddle, D.L., and North American Orthopaedic Rehabilitation Research Network. 1999. The Lower Extremity Functional Scale (LEFS): Scale development, measurement properties, and clinical application. *Physical Therapy.* 79:371–383.

Fisher, A.C., Mullins, S.A., and P.A. Frye. 1993. Athletic trainers' attitudes and judgments of injured athletes' rehabilitation adherence. *Journal of Athletic Training* 28:43–47.

Keith, R.H., Granter, C.V., Hamilton, B.B., and F.S. Sherwin. 1987. The functional independence measure: A new tool for rehabilitation. In *Advances in clinical rehabilitation,* ed. M.G. Eisenberg and R.C. Grzesink. New York: Springer.

Kubler-Ross, E. 1969. *On death and dying.* New York: Macmillan.

Peterson, P. 1986. The grief response and injury. *Athletic Training* 21:312–314.

Ray, R. 2000. *Management strategies in athletic training.* 2d ed. Champaign, IL: Human Kinetics.

Rotella, R.J. 1985. The psychological care of the patient. In *Sports psychology: Psychological consideration in maximizing sport performance.* Ann Arbor, MI: McNaughton and Gun.

Staron, R.S., Leonardi, M.J., Karapondo, D.L., Malicky, E.S., Falkel, J.E., Hagerman, F.C., and R.S. Kikada. 1991. Strength and skeletal muscle adaptations in heavy-resistance-trained women after detraining and retraining. *Journal of Applied Physiology* 70:631–640.

Stratford, P.W., Binkley, J.M., Riddle, D.L., and G.H. Guyatt. 1998. Sensitivity to change on the Roland-Morris Pain Questionnaire: Part 1. *Physical Therapy.* 78:1186–1196.

Ware, J.E., Jr., Kosinski, M., Bayliss, M.S., McHorney, C.A., Rogers, W.H., and A. Raczek. 1995. Comparisons of methods for the scoring and statistical analysis of the SF-36 health profile and summary measures: Summary of results from the Medical Outcomes Study. *Medical Care.* 33:AS264–279.

Ware, J.E., Jr. and C.D. Sherbourne. 1992. The MOS 36-Item Short Form Health Survey (SF-36), I: Conceptual framework and item selection. *Medical Care.* 30:473–483.

CHAPTER TWO

Concepts of Healing

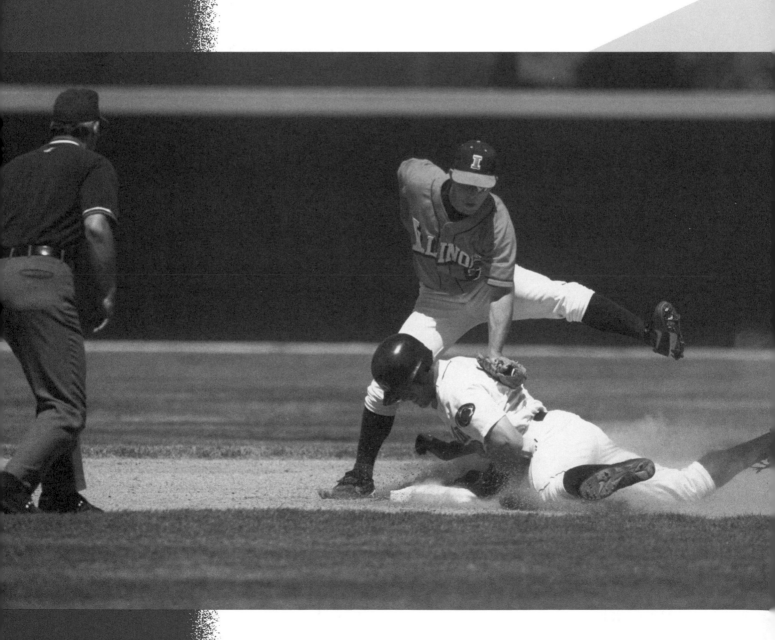

OBJECTIVES

After completing this chapter, you should be able to do the following:

1. Explain the differences between primary and secondary healing.

2. Identify the healing phases.

3. Describe the primary processes of each healing phase.

4. Discuss the causes for the signs of inflammation.

5. Explain the role of growth factors in healing.

6. Discuss the differences between acute and chronic inflammation.

7. Discuss healing characteristics of specific tissues.

8. Identify the relevance of tensile strength.

9. Discuss factors that can modify the healing process.

10. Explain the role NSAIDs play in inflammation.

11. Discuss the timing of treatment with the various stages of healing.

12. Identify the guidelines for treatment progression in acute and chronic injuries.

Deanna Daniels has been assigned to work with gymnast Roberta Kingsley, who underwent an Achilles tendon repair seven days ago and is now in the athletic training room for her first day of rehabilitation. Deanna's knowledge of healing allows her to judge where in the healing process such an injury should be and what rehabilitation techniques can be safely applied to the Achilles tendon at this time. She understands the tendon's tensile strength and the precautions that apply for repairs such as Roberta's. She also understands the status of the healing connective tissue and the processes that are now under way.

However, Deanna suspects that Roberta has poor eating habits. Before applying rehabilitation techniques, Deanna decides to discuss the importance of proper nutrition and the role proteins, vitamins, and minerals play in tissue healing.

The brain is like a muscle. When we think well, we feel good. Understanding is a kind of ecstasy.

Carl Sagan, *Broca's Brain*

Understanding the healing process goes beyond the words of Carl Sagan; it is vital if the sport rehabilitation specialist is to develop a safe and effective therapeutic exercise program for a patient. Performing an exercise before the injured area is ready can impede healing and cause additional injury. As a professional who rehabilitates sport injuries, you have a duty to understand healing and realize the impact of the therapeutic exercise and rehabilitation techniques you apply. There are many aspects to healing that are still unknown, even to experts. What is presented here is the most current information we have on the body's response to injury and the procedure it follows in an effort to return to normal.

It is common knowledge that an injury produces a scar when healing. Although there are occasions when the body actually replaces damaged tissue with normal tissue, more frequently in sport injuries, scar tissue is healing's end result. This chapter deals primarily with the healing process involved in scar-tissue formation following sport injuries. Keep in mind that there have been entire books written on healing, so this chapter is merely an overview and by no means a detailed description of the healing process.

In spite of all that has been written on healing, there is still a lot of information that eludes us. The information presented in this chapter has resulted from the research of a great many people. I have attempted to simplify this complex topic and to present what sports medicine specialists should know to safely apply therapeutic exercise and rehabilitation techniques to injured athletes.

This chapter introduces many terms that may be new and unfamiliar to you. To assist you in becoming familiar with these terms, table 2.1 defines the terms that appear in boldface in this chapter and indicates their most common function or their significance in the healing process.

PRIMARY AND SECONDARY HEALING

Healing by primary intention occurs through a bridge of tissue when the wound separation is small. Healing by secondary intention occurs by filling in the wound with new tissue from the sides and bottom when the separation is large.

When an injury occurs, the healing process that follows depends on the extent of the injury and the approximation of the wound site's stump ends. If the separation of tissue is small, a bridge of cells binds the ends together. This is called healing by **primary intention**. This type of healing commonly occurs in minor wounds. It is also seen in surgical incisions where the stump ends are sutured together.

In more severe wounds where the stump ends are farther apart and cannot be bridged, the wound heals by producing tissue from the bottom and sides of the wound to fill in the space created by the wound. This is called healing by **secondary intention**. This may occur in second-degree sprains where ligament tissue is torn

Table 2.1   Terminology of Wound Healing

Term	Definition	Significance/Function
acetylcholine	A neurotransmitter at the neuro-muscular junction of striated muscles.	Causes vasodilation.
adrenaline	See *epinephrine.*	
angiogenesis	Formation of blood vessels.	Provides for subsequent scar tissue formation and normal healing events that follow.
arachidonic acid	An unsaturated essential fatty acid.	A precursor in the production of leukotrienes, prostaglandins, and thrombaxanes.
basophil	See *granular leukocyte.*	
bradykinin	A local tissue hormone that is activated by the interaction of proteases with the Hageman factor.	A very potent local vasodilator. It increases vascular permeability and stimulates local pain receptors.
callus	Fibrous matrix formed at a bone fracture site.	Immobilizes the bone fragments and serves as the foundation for eventual bone replacement.
chemotactic factor	A chemical gradient. Also referred to as a chemotactin or chemo-attractant.	See *chemotactin.*
chemotactin	An agent that facilitates chemotaxis.	Must be present and function properly to promote the healing process.
chemotaxis	Movement or orientation of cells in response to a chemical stimulus after an injury, which occurs complex and not totally understood processes.	Cells either become oriented along a chemical concentration gradient or move in the direction of that gradient. For example, chemicals attract platelets, red blood cells, and PMNs into an injured area.
collagen	Major type of protein in the body. There are five types: I is most abundant, high in tensile strength, and found in dermis, fascia, and bone. II is found in cartilage. III is found in embryonic connective tissue. IV and V are found in basement membranes.	Forms inelastic bundles to provide structure, integrity, and tensile strength to tissues.
collagenase	An enzyme produced by newly formed epithelial cells and fibroblasts.	Involved in degradation of collagen during tissue repair. Important in controlling collagen content in a wound.
complement system	Various proteins found in serum.	Act as chemotactic factors for neutrophils and phagocytes.
drug interaction	When one drug enhances or reduces the effectiveness of other drugs also being taken.	It is important to know what drugs an individual takes so that they are not rendered harmful or ineffective by each other.
duration of drug action	Amount of time the blood level of the drug is above the level needed to obtain a minimum therapeutic effect.	Determined by the drug's half-life.

(continued)

Table 2.1 *(continued)*

Term	Definition	Significance/Function
elastin	An essential protein of connective-tissue elastic structures. Arranged in a wavy orientation.	Its wavy arrangement allows tissue to change shape with stress and resume normal conditions after stress removal. It plays an as yet unknown role in the remodeling phase.
endothelial cells	Large flat cells that line blood and lymphatic vessels.	Are restored during angiogenesis.
endothelial leukocytes	Large white blood cells that circulate in the bloodstream and tissues.	Act as phagocytes to remove debris from an injured area.
eosinophil	See *granular leukocyte*.	
epinephrine	A hormone. Also called adrenaline.	A potent stimulator of the sympathetic nervous system and a powerful vasopressor. Increases blood pressure, stimulates the heart muscle, accelerates the heart rate, increases cardiac output, and increases such metabolic activities as glycogenolysis and glucose release.
erythrocyte	An element of blood. Also known as red blood cell or corpuscle.	Used for oxygen transport.
extracellular matrix	The basic material from which tissue develops. Produced by fibroblasts in wounds. Composed of fibers and ground substance.	Serves as a foundation on which new tissue is cast.
exudate	Material that escapes from blood vessels following an injury. Contains high concentrations of protein, cells, and other materials from injured cells.	As PMNs die and decompose, exudate may resemble pus although no infection is present.
factor XII	See *Hageman factor*.	
fibrin	Insoluble fibrous protein formed by fibrinogen.	Important in clotting.
fibrinogen	A globulin present in plasma.	Converts to fibrin to form a plug at the injury site.
fibrinolysin	An enzyme in plasma released in later healing.	Converts fibrin into a soluble substance to unplug lymphatics.
fibroblast	A connective tissue cell that differentiates into chondroblasts, osteoblasts, and collagenoblasts.	Form the fibrous tissues to support and bind a variety of tissues.
fibrocyte	An inactive fibroblast. See *fibroblast*.	
fibronectin	An adhesive glycoprotein found in most body tissues and serum. Fibronectin is plentiful in early granulation tissue formation but gradually disappears during the remodeling phase.	Cross-links to collagen in connective tissue, thereby playing a role in the adhesion of fibroblasts to fibrin. Also involved in the collection of platelets in an injured area and the enhancement of myofibroblast activity.

Term	Definition	Significance/Function
glycoprotein	Protein–carbohydrate compounds. Elements of ground substance. Includes fibronectin.	Probably cross-links with collagen so tissue is able to withstand pressure.
glycosaminoglycan (GAG)	Compounds occurring mostly in proteoglycans. Nonfibrous elements of ground substance in the extracellular matrix. Examples: hyaluronic acid, proteoglycans.	Different GAGs have different functions: stimulating fibroblast proliferation, promoting collagen synthesis and maturation, contributing to tissue resilience, and regulating cell function.
granuloma	Hard mass of fibrous tissue.	Occurs in chronic inflammatory conditions when the body produces collagen around a foreign substance to protect itself from that substance.
granular leukocytes	White blood cells, which are divided into three groups of polymorpho-nuclear leukocytes: neutrophils, eosinophils, and basophils.	Among their functions, they are chemotactic and phagocytic and release histamine and serotonin to produce vasoactive reactions following injury.
granulation tissue	Newly formed vascular tissue that is produced during wound healing. Consists of fibroblasts, macrophages, and neovascular cells within a connective tissue matrix of collagen, hyaluronic acid, and fibronectin. It has the appearance of small, red, velvety, nodular masses seen in new tissue.	Eventually forms the scar of the wound.
ground substance	Gel-like material in which connective tissue cells and fibers are imbedded. Part of the connective tissue or extracellular matrix.	Reduces friction between the connective tissue fibers when forces are applied to the structure. Adds to the area's density.
growth factor	Components released by platelets and macrophages. Also referred to as growth hormone factor.	Performs numerous complex roles, the stimulation of reepithelialization, and is chemotactic for macrophages, monocytes, and neutrophils. Its role is not thoroughly understood, but it is believed to play an important role throughout tissue repair.
Hageman factor	An enzyme present in the blood.	Initiates the blood coagulation process following trauma by converting prothrombin to thrombin.
half-life	Amount of time it takes for the level of a drug in the blood-stream to diminish by one half.	Determines the frequency with which a medication is taken.
histamine	A local tissue hormone released by mast cells and granulocytes.	Increases vascular permeability to proteins and fibronectin.
hyaluronic acid	A major component of early granu-lation tissue. Greatest amounts are seen in a wound during the first 4-5 days. See also *glycosaminoglycan*.	Promotes cell movement and migration during repair. Stimulates fibroblast proliferation. Pro-duces edema by absorbing large amounts of water to increase fibroblast migration.

(continued)

Table 2.1 *(continued)*

Term	Definition	Significance/Function
kallikrein	A proteolytic enzyme found in blood plasma, lymph, and other exocrine secretions. Activated by the Hageman factor.	Forms kinins and activates plasminogen, a precursor of plasmin. Increases vascular permeability and vasodilation.
kinin	A generic term for polypeptides that are related to bradykinin. A potent local tissue hormone found in injured tissue, released from plasma proteins. Examples: bradykinin, kallidin.	Mediates the classic signs of inflammation. Acts like histamine and serotonin on the microvascular system in the early inflammation phase to cause increased microvascular permeability.
leukocytes	White blood cells or corpuscles. Different types include poly-morphonuclear leukocytes and mononuclear cells.	Have phagocytic properties to remove debris from an injury site.
leukotriene	Compound formed from arachidonic acid.	Regulates inflammatory reactions. Some stimulate the movements of leukocytes into the area.
lipid	A heterogeneous group of fats and fatlike substances, including fatty acids and steroids.	Serves as a source of fuel and is important to the structure and makeup of cells.
lymphocytes	Nonphagocytic leukocytes found in blood and lymph.	Serve in the body's immune system by producing antibodies.
macrophages	Mononuclear phagocytes that arise from stem cells in bone marrow.	Considered one of the regulators of the repair process. Serve to phagocytize injury areas of debris, kill microorganisms, and secrete substances into an injury site, including items such as enzymes, fibro-nectin, and coagulation factors. Play a role in keeping the inflammatory process localized; enhance collagen deposition and fibroblast proliferation.
mast cells	Connective tissue cells. Also referred to as mastocytes and labrocytes.	Store and produce various mediators of inflammation. Through their release of histamine, enzymes, and other mediators, mast cells increase local blood flow, attract immune cells, stimulate cell production of fibroblasts and endothelial cells, and promote and control remodeling of extracellular matrix.
matrix	Substance of a tissue. Can refer to intracellular or extracellular structure.	Forms the basis from which a structure develops.
monocyte	Mononuclear phagocytic leukocyte. Formed in the bone marrow and transported to tissues to become macrophages.	Removes debris from an injury site.

Term	Definition	Significance/Function
mononuclear phagocyte	Cells with only one nucleus, capable of ingesting particulate matter, i.e., monocytes.	Ingest microorganisms and remove debris from an injury site.
myoblast	A cell formed from myogenic cells in muscle.	Forms myotubes, which eventually evolve into muscle fiber.
myofibroblasts	Fibroblasts that have a combination of the ultrastructural features of a fibroblast and the qualities of a smooth muscle cell.	Responsible for wound contraction.
myogenic cells	Cells arising from muscle that later become myoblasts.	See *myoblast*.
neurotransmitters	Hormones such as norepinephrine, epinephrine, and acetylcholine, which are found in capillary, arteriole, and artery walls.	Released at the injury site to enhance platelet and leukocyte adherence to the vessel surface.
neutrophil	See *polymorphonuclear leukocyte*.	
norepinephrine	A hormone.	Acts as a powerful vasoconstrictor at the immediate onset of injury. It may last from a few seconds to a few minutes.
osteoblasts	Osteogenic cells from periosteum.	Lay down the callus of fractured bone. Convert later to chondrocytes.
osteoclasts	Large multinuclear cells.	Resorb dead, necrotic bone tissue.
osteocytes	Cells characteristic of adult bone.	Maintain new bone mineralization.
platelet-derived growth factor (PDGF)	Substance found in platelets.	Essential for the growth of connective tissue cells. Stimulates the migration of polymorphonuclear leukocytes.
PGE_1	See *prostaglandin*.	Increases vascular permeability by causing vasodilation.
PGE_2	See *prostaglandin*.	Is chemotactic to attract leukocytes to the area.
phagocyte	See *mononuclear phagocyte* and *polymorphonuclear leukocyte*.	
phospholipids	Lipids that contain phosphoric acid. Found in all cells and in layers of plasma membranes.	Stimulate the clotting mechanism.
plasmin	An enzyme that occurs in plasma as plasminogen. It is activated by kallikrein and other activators.	Converts fibrin to soluble substances.
plasminogen activator	See *fibrinolysin*.	
platelets	Irregular cell fragments found in blood.	The first cells seen at an injury site and considered one of the regulatory cells of healing. Releases growth factors. Forms a plug at the injury to stop bleeding.

(continued)

37

Table 2.1 *(continued)*

Term	Definition	Significance/Function
primary intension	Healing that occurs with minor wounds or surgical wounds.	Re-epithelialization closes the wound within 48 hr. Scarring is minimal when healing by primary intention occurs.
polymorphonuclear leukocyte (PMN)	A type of white blood cell. One of the granular leukocytes. Also referred to as neutrophil.	Chemotactic and phagocytic in the healing process.
prostaglandin (PG)	Hormones formed primarily from arachidonic acid as a result of cell membrane damage. Its release requires the Complement System and follows kinin formation. Specific PG compounds are designated by adding a letter, A through I, and a subscript number, 1 through 3, to designate the number of hydrocarbon bonds. Examples: PGE_1 and PGE_2.	Mediates cell migration during inflammation and modulates serotonin and histamine. Some PGs increase pain sensitivity, induce fever, and suppress lymphocyte transformation, thereby inhibiting the inflammatory reaction. Mediates myofibroblasts, initiates early phases of injury repair, and plays a role in later stages of inflammation.
protease	An enzyme.	Acts as a catalyst to split interior peptide bonds in protein. Activates kallikrein to release bradykinin, ultimately causing increased vascular permeability and an increase in concentration of proteins and cells in the wound spaces.
proteoglycan	Substances found in tissues, including synovial fluid and connective tissue matrix. Proteoglycan solutions are very viscous lubricants and are sulfated GAGs. See also *glycosaminoglycan*.	Provides a resilient matrix to inhibit cell migration. Regulates cell function and proliferation, and regulates collagen fibrillogenesis.
reticulin	Collagen-like fiber. Some consider it type III collagen fiber.	Forms the early framework for collagen deposition in a wound.
satellite cells	Cells present in muscle.	Regenerate new muscle tissue.
secondary intention	Healing that occurs in large wounds associated with soft-tissue loss. The wound heals with granulation tissue from the bottom and sides of the wound. Epithelial tissue does not form until granulation tissue has filled the wound.	Larger scar formation occurs with healing by secondary intention. Wound contraction is evident with this healing.
serotonin	A hormone released by mast cells and platelets.	Produces vasoconstriction in small vessels after norepinephrine activity is complete; occurs only when blood-vessel endothelial walls are damaged. In later phases, initiates reactions leading to collagen cross-linking. Also involved in granuloma formation.
steady state of a drug	Occurs when the average level of drug remains constant in the blood, and the amount of drug leaving the body is equal to the amount being absorbed.	On average, occurs after 5 doses; equals the drug's half-life.

Term	Definition	Significance/Function
tenocyte	Tendon cell.	Converts to fibroblasts during healing of tendons.
tensile strength	Maximal amount of stress or force that a structure is able to withstand before tissue failure occurs.	Varies as tissue healing occurs; must be taken into account when determining appropriate stress application in rehabilitation.
thrombin	An enzyme.	Converts fibrinogen to fibrin to form a fibrin plug early in the inflammation phase. In later inflammation, it stimulates fibronectin production and fibroblast proliferation.
thromboxane	A compound that is produced by platelets and is unstable. Its half-life is 30 s. Related to prostaglandins.	Acts as a vasoconstrictor and is a potent inducer of platelet aggregation.

and not surgically repaired. Healing by secondary intention usually takes longer and results in a larger scar.

HEALING PHASES

The three phases of healing are inflammation, proliferation, and remodeling. During inflammation, the injury is contained and stabilized and debris is removed. During proliferation, fibroblasts, myofibroblasts, and collagen peak to begin granulation tissue formation and angiogensis. During remodeling, wound contraction is well under way, and type III collagen is converted to type I collagen to stabilize and restore the injury site.

Whether the body heals by secondary or primary intention, the process through which it proceeds is consistent and predictable in most situations. We do not entirely understand the process, but we can determine the outcomes of each phase.

Healing is a changing continuum of events. To understand and clarify this process, researchers and clinicians divide the events into three different phases. Keep in mind, however, that as far as the body is concerned, the process is continuous, without clear-cut delineations. The body merely continues the process until the end is reached. The three phases designated by researchers and clinicians are

1. inflammation,
2. proliferation, or fibroplastic phase, and
3. remodeling, or maturation phase.

INFLAMMATION PHASE

When an injury occurs, the body attempts to stabilize the injured site by rushing chemicals and cells into the area. This is an extremely complex process that occurs within three to five days. A simplified version of the processes that occur is summarized in figure 2.1. The body is extremely busy during this phase in its attempt to protect the site and begin the return to status quo as well as possible.

Inflammation often has negative connotations. In reality, it is an important and necessary step in the healing process. Without inflammation, the body would be unable to complete the healing process. If inflammation did not occur, proliferation, maturation, and final resolution would not take place. The wound would remain unhealed. Inflammation becomes deleterious when it is prolonged, extending beyond the normal healing time. This condition is called *chronic inflammation* and is discussed later in this chapter.

The goal of sports medicine specialists is to allow inflammation to occur but to minimize it. This is done at the time of injury by applying initial first aid: ice, compression, elevation, and rest.

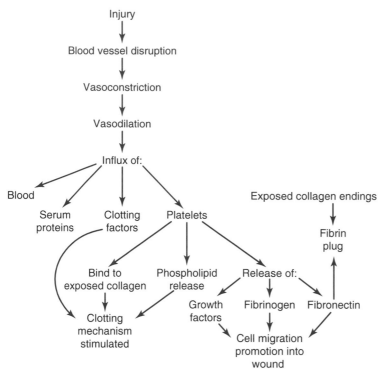

Figure 2.1 Immediate injury response.

As the injury's status changes in the first few days, the sports medicine specialist minimizes inflammation and encourages healing to continue along its normal path by using various treatment modalities that are discussed in the Athletic Training Education Series text *Therapeutic Modalities for Athletic Injuries* (Denegar 2000).

To make appropriate decisions about when to employ modalities and therapeutic exercise techniques, the rehabilitation specialist must first understand the events that occur in the healing process. Let us examine the series of events involved in the first phase of healing, the inflammation phase.

Vasoconstriction and Vasodilation

When an injury occurs, blood and lymph vessel walls suffer damage. The immediate local vasoconstriction that occurs in the small vessels is followed by vasodilation. You may have observed this if you have cut your skin. At first there is no bleeding, but within a few seconds the wound starts to bleed.

Cellular Reactions

It is at this moment that the inflammation phase begins. The vasodilation causes the release of blood and blood products into the injured site, including blood **platelets** and serum proteins as noted in figure 2.2a. As these products accumulate in the injury, chemicals are released, and other cells are attracted into the area. Platelets release **phospholipids**, which stimulate the clotting mechanism to stop the bleeding. Platelets also bind to the **collagen** fiber stumps that were exposed by the injury. Platelets release other important substances, such as **fibronectin**, **growth factors**, and **fibrinogen** (Koopman 1995). Each of these substances is important in the healing process.

Fibronectin binds together **fibrin** and collagen. Fibronectin and fibrin bind together in a cross-link arrangement with the exposed collagen ends to form a latticelike complex, which acts as a plug to stop the bleeding. This plug is temporary and fairly fragile, but in these early hours it provides the wound's only **tensile strength** (Martinez-Hernandez and Amenta 1990). As healing progresses, this plug is replaced by type III collagen.

In addition to blood vessels, the more fragile lymph vessels are also damaged at the time of injury. Leakage from these vessels is halted by the formation of a fibrin plug. Once fluid accumulates in the extracellular spaces, as it does during an injury, the only way it is removed is through the lymph system. Unfortunately, because the lymph vessels are plugged by the fibrin plug to stop leakage, their ability to remove the extra fluid from the area is compromised. Once the area becomes stable, **fibrinolysin** is released. Fibrinolysin is an enzyme that converts fibrin from an insoluble to a soluble protein to promote absorption of the fibrin plug and allow the lymph vessels to perform their normal function, draining the area of edema (excess fluid).

Within the first few hours of injury, the body attempts to remove debris from the site. This process is started by **neutrophils**, or **polymorphonuclear leukocytes (PMNs)**, within 5 to 6 h of injury. The inflammation phase is named after these cells. Neutrophils are the most plentiful white blood cells in the body and migrate into the

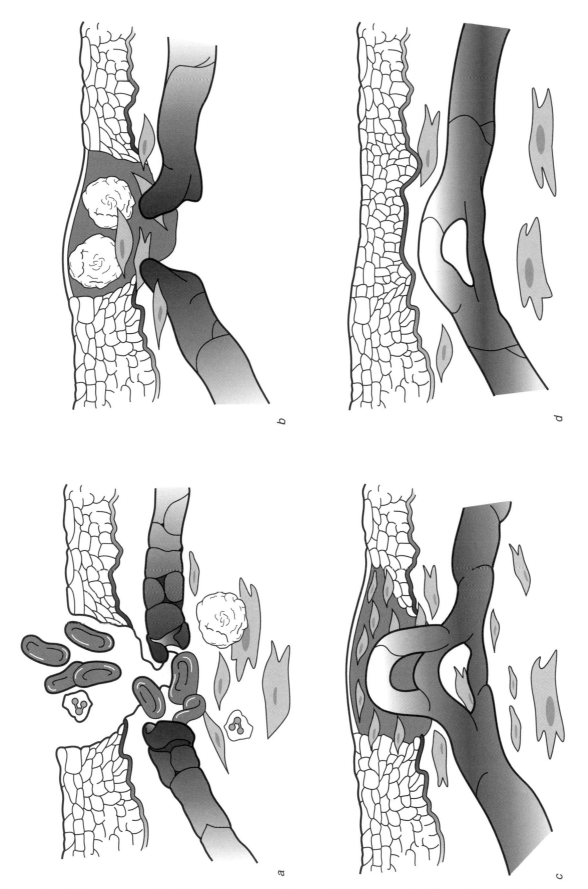

■ Figure 2.2 Epidermal wound healing. (*a*) Release of blood and blood products at time of injury. (*b*) Macrophages and fibroblasts in the area with capillary buds apparent. (*c*) Angiogenesis has caused anastamosis with new capillary growth. Fibroblasts are present in large numbers. (*d*) Reepitheliazation has occurred. Regression of earlier established capillaries is noted.

wound in great numbers, but their presence is short-lived. Other white blood cells in the granular leukocyte family include eosinophils and basophils.

The cells that replace the neutrophils are the **mononuclear phagocytes: monocytes** and **macrophages**. These become the predominant cells at the injury site within 24 to 48 h.

Both the PMNs and the macrophages act as **phagocytes** to remove debris and dead tissue from the area. As the inflammatory process proceeds, an inflammatory **exudate** is formed from the fluid escaping from the local vessels, dead tissue from the injury, and dying PMNs. Inflammatory exudate is commonly whitish and differs from the exudate seen in an infection, which contains bacteria. Although normally produced exudate is often referred to as pus, Peacock (1984, p. 2) feels that this is a misnomer and prefers to refer to this uninfected substance as *cell aggregation centers*, not pus.

Debridement (removal of debris) is necessary for healing to continue. Before the subsequent phases can occur, the injury site must be cleared of excess fluid and other waste materials that have accumulated. For this reason alone, macrophages are vital to the healing process, but they perform other important functions as well. Once in the injury site, they recruit and activate other macrophages to assist in debridement. Macrophages also release growth factors and may trigger the termination of tissue growth when the healing process is complete (DiPietro 1995).

Chemical Reactions

There is an intimate interaction between cells and chemicals throughout healing. Some cells stimulate the production of chemicals, and certain chemicals at the injury site stimulate the arrival or production of specific cells in the area. This process of attraction or stimulation is called **chemotaxis**.

A good example of chemotaxis is the series of events that causes vascular permeability. Vascular permeability is a crucial event that initiates the inflammation phase. It allows cells and chemicals that normally remain in the bloodstream to enter the injury site and perform their functions to ultimately heal the injured tissue and return the area to as close to normal as possible. Vascular permeability is initially caused by **histamine** in the area. Histamine is released by cells that enter the area, such as platelets, PMNs and **mast cells**. Histamine is **chemotactic** for **leukocytes**, or white blood cells, causing them to enter the area. Histamine is a short-lived, local hormone whose function of vascular permeability is continued by **serotonin** and **kinins** that also enter the area. Serotonin is released by mast cells and platelets, and kinins are released by plasma.

The presence of kinins in the injury site is short term, but they are followed by **prostaglandin (PG)** formation. Once kinins are released and a **Complement System** is formed from serum proteins, PGs are discharged by cells that have been damaged. There are two PGs that are most evident and perform important functions: PGE_1 and PGE_2. The function of PGE_1 is continuing the vascular permeability in the local area. PGE_2 is responsible for attracting leukocytes to the site. As healing progresses, they both appear to stimulate repair of the damaged area and permit advancement to the proliferative phase. They also seem to have a role in continuing inflammation at the same time (Salter et al. 1980). It is these compounds that are influenced by anti-inflammatory drugs, discussed later in this chapter.

During all of this activity, additional chemical reactions are also occurring. **Hageman factor**, sometimes referred to as **factor XII**, is produced in the area. It acts to stimulate production of the enzyme **kallikrein**, which increases vascular permeability and vasodilation (Peacock 1984, p. 4).

Signs of Inflammation

Many complex events go on during the inflammation phase. The injured area undergoes intense activity during this time. We see evidence of the degree of activity as common signs of inflammation, including localized redness, edema, pain, increased temperature, and loss of normal function. Redness, increased local temperature, and edema are caused by the leakage of fluid, cells, and chemicals into the area because of the local vasodilation and increased vascular permeability. The increase in local cellular and chemical activity increases local temperature. Histamine and other released hormones and vasodilation cause redness. Edema is the result of increased substances in the area and blockage of lymph vessels whose normal responsibility of drainage is restricted by the newly formed fibrin plug. The chemical substances that are released at the site, such as histamine, prostaglandins, and **bradykinin** (Christie 1991; Kibler 1990), make the local nerve endings hypersensitive and irritable, causing pain. Pressure from edema on nerve endings also causes pain. Pain causes a withdrawal reflex, which reduces the function of surrounding structures, limiting the athlete's normal functional ability. Direct damage to tissues also prevents them from functioning normally (Kibler 1990).

PROLIFERATION PHASE

There is an overlap of phases as the injury site heals. Figure 2.3 demonstrates that there is no clear-cut delineation between one phase and another. Rather, as the body steadily accomplishes the tasks in one phase, the next phase evolves.

Although many cells and chemicals are involved during the inflammation phase, the macrophages are most responsible for removing debris from the area. Once this task is accomplished, the next step in the healing process is the development and growth of new blood vessels and **granulation tissue**. This transition from debridement to **angiogenesis** and formation of granulation tissue marks the beginning of the proliferation phase. Angiogenesis occurs at a rapid rate during this phase. This is important, for scar tissue formation requires vascular production and supply if subsequent events of healing are to follow.

The cells largely responsible for production of this new growth are **fibroblasts**. Fibroblasts are seen in greatly increased numbers three to five days following injury. Their increased numbers along with a decrease to minimal or nonexistent levels of PMNs are the hallmark of the wound site's transition from inflammation to proliferation. Other activities that indicate that the injury has started the transition into the proliferation phase include a significant increase in extracellular collagen production, increased **proteoglycans**, and epithelial cell mitosis (cell division). The duration of the proliferation phase depends on factors such as the size and site of the injury and the tissue type involved. Generally, the phase is thought to last two to four weeks (Peacock 1984, p. 13).

As is true during the inflammation phase, during the proliferation phase there is an interactive response among cells and chemicals in the area. Growth factors, for example, enter into the area through the chemotaxis produced by platelets and macrophages. In turn, these growth factors are responsible for the local migration and proliferation of fibroblasts, **myofibroblasts**, and **endothelial cells**.

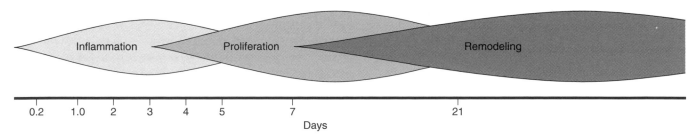

▌Figure 2.3 Tissue healing phases. Note the overlap of these phases.

The migration of fibroblasts is important during proliferation because these cells are primarily responsible for the development of new capillaries and the **extracellular matrix**. Fibroblasts produce substances that will eventually make up the matrix. These substances, which include collagen, proteoglycans, and elastin, are required for ultimate scar tissue formation and maturation (Kirsner and Eaglstein 1993).

Granulation tissue is the combination of the matrix and newly formed capillary buds. Granulation tissue is typically a bright, beefy red color. This is because the new capillary buds make up a significant part of the granulation tissue. Endothelial cells, the most important cell in the formation of these capillaries, contain a **plasminogen activator**. The plasminogen activator breaks down and removes the fibrin network that was formed during the inflammation phase so that lymphatic flow for removing local excess fluid can be restored.

The matrix has two components: fibrous and nonfibrous elements. The nonfibrous element is called **ground substance**. This is a gel-like substance composed of **glycosaminoglycan (GAG)**, proteoglycans, and **glycoproteins**. The ground substance fills in the spaces between the fibrous elements of the matrix and reduces friction between the fibers when stress is applied to the tissue.

Fibrous elements of the matrix include collagen, **reticulin**, and **elastin**. Collagen and reticulin are inelastic while elastin has elastic qualities. The combination of these types of fibers provides tensile strength and some resilience to stresses applied to the tissue.

During the proliferation phase, in the first five to seven days following injury, the fibroblasts produce both of these elements of the extracellular matrix. They form ground substance and rapidly lay down collagen. The activity during this phase is the result of new capillary growth by the fibroblasts. Capillary growth is followed by epithelial advancement across the granulating wound. As the epithelium progresses across the wound, epithelial cells and fibroblasts stimulated by the epithelial cells both release **collagenase**. Collagenase is an enzyme that prevents overproduction of collagen in the wound. This is an important process in normal tissue healing. An example of uncontrolled collagen production is keloid formations (excessive scar-tissue formations), a condition sometimes seen in dermal injuries.

Collagen produced in these early days of healing is type III collagen. It is seen as early as 48 to 72 h after the injury occurs (Kirsner and Eaglstein 1993). The fiber structure of type III collagen is weak and thin. Although it is relatively weak, it is the substance that provides the wound's primary tensile strength in the early stages of healing. Type III collagen is laid down in a haphazard manner, without organized arrangement, further reducing its strength. It is later replaced by type I collagen, a stronger and more durable collagen.

Tensile strength is directly related to the amount, type, and arrangement of collagen. By day 7 there is a significant amount of collagen in the area. By day 12 the immature type III collagen begins to be replaced by the stronger type I collagen. Both these occurrences add significant strength to the injury site.

While these processes are going on, a GAG known as **hyaluronic acid**, a part of the extracellular matrix, draws water into the area. This provides additional room for the proliferating fibroblasts in the wound site.

External signs of this phase demonstrate this ongoing activity. The combination of increased capillaries and additional water volume accounts for the redness and swelling in the area. Pressure-sensitive nerve endings cause the site to be sensitive to pressure just as the tension-sensitive nerve endings make the area painful when it is stretched.

REMODELING PHASE

Some of the activities that begin during the proliferation phase continue during the remodeling phase. One example of this is wound contraction. Myofibroblasts are responsible for this activity. They have been observed in wounds by the fifth day and have been seen later than two months after the injury (Betz et al. 1992). Some of the fibroblasts convert to myofibroblasts to contract the wound's size. The entire mechanism is very complex and yet to be fully understood.

Wound contraction makes the scar smaller. This is advantageous, but it can be detrimental in situations in which joints are affected. If an injury occurs at or near a joint, scar tissue contraction and adhesions can cause a loss of motion at that joint. Indirect effects of wound contraction may occur if the wound is large and affects adjacent areas. The importance of preventing the adverse effects of scar-tissue contraction is discussed later in this chapter in the section "The Role of Therapeutic Exercise in Healing."

Another activity that begins during the proliferation phase and continues into the remodeling phase is collagen transition. As type I collagen is synthesized, type III collagen is destroyed. When the construction rate equals the destruction rate, the healing process evolves to the final and longest phase, remodeling. This phase is generally thought to be about 12 months long, but may range from 6 months to 18 months (Connolly 1988).

A number of activities diminish as the area becomes more stable and more permanent in its cellular and structural arrangement. The large number of capillaries that were produced during the proliferation phase to promote tissue growth are no longer needed and begin to recede. They will eventually disappear entirely (Peacock 1984, p. 13). Glycoproteins, GAGs, and the cells responsible for them—fibroblasts—in the extracellular matrix decrease significantly. Myofibroblasts also diminish.

With these cellular changes, visible changes can also be observed. These include the loss of the scar's red color with progressive change to white and eventually more normal skin tones. With the loss of extracellular matrix substances, the swelling is diminished. Wound sensitivity is also lessened.

As collagen is converted to predominantly type I, it becomes more insoluble and less resistant to destruction. As fluid is reduced in the area, the collagen fibers can produce more cross-links with each other, further strengthening the scar's structure. This collagen cross-linking becomes the primary source of the scar's tensile strength.

The maturation of the wound's collagen structure and arrangement is the primary activity during the remodeling phase, hence its name. Collagen strength is enhanced by the arrangement of collagen fibers. When collagen fibers are aligned in an organized, parallel fashion, collagen can form the greatest number of cross-links and thereby possess optimal strength. The greatest degree of function

Phases of Healing

Here is a summary of the three phases of healing, when they occur, their characteristics, and the goals during each phase.

Phase	Duration	Characteristics	Goal
Inflammation	Up to about 5 days	At onset of injury area is warm, red, swollen, and tender.	Stabilize and contain area of injury.
Proliferation	Up to about 21 days	Scar tissue is red and larger than normal because of edema.	Dispose of dead tissue, mobilize fibroblasts, and restore circulation.
Remodeling	Up to 1 year or more	Water content of the scar is reduced; vascularity and redness are reduced; scar-tissue density increases.	Stabilize and reestablish the area.

and mobility is also provided when collagen has this organized arrangement (Peacock 1984, p. 188). Properly applied external forces enhance this arrangement.

Table 2.2 summarizes in chronological order the phases of healing and identifies the primary activities and their time line.

GROWTH FACTORS

Growth factors assist healing by causing cell proliferation and attracting fibroblasts, macrophages, and other cells needed for healing.

Growth factors are proteins that serve many functions. They interact with each other and other substances to promote the healing process. Their role is complex and not yet fully understood. One reason their function is difficult to understand is that their action in vitro is different than in vivo, so what is observed in the laboratory is not necessarily what occurs in the body. Another clouding factor is that what they are seen doing in laboratory animals is not necessarily what occurs in humans.

Specific growth factors perform specific tasks that affect specific cells to speed and enhance the healing process. Growth factors are named for the target cell they affect, their source, or their behavior. For example, the growth factor affecting the epidermis is called epidermal growth factor (EGF), the growth factor derived from platelets is

Table 2.2   Chronology of Wound Healing

Phase	Day	Activity	Purpose/Result
Inflammation	1	Neutrophil migration	Fight contamination. Release growth factors and biologically reactive substances.
Inflammation	1	Fibrin bridge creation	Area is red, warm, swollen, tender to touch.
Inflammation	1–2	→Monocyte migration	Phagocytose bacteria.
Inflammation	2	Angiogenesis	Ingrowing fibroblasts.
Inflammation	2–3	Fibroblasts produce type III collagen.	
Proliferation	3–4	→Rapid increase in fibroblasts Increased epithelial cell mitosis Increased synthesis of extracellular collagen Increased proteoglycans	
Proliferation	5	→Myofibroblast production	Wound contraction.
Proliferation	5–7	→Collagen synthesis very active	
Remodeling	5–9	Reduction in fibroblasts Reduction in macrophages Reduction in wound vascularity →Reduction in fibronectin in proportion to the amount of type I collagen formed	Less redness.
Remodeling	10	Wound contraction	
Remodeling	12	→Type III collagen converting to type I	
Remodeling	6–18 wk	→Reduction in capillaries	Reduced fluid content, increased scar density.
Remodeling	6–18 mo	Completion of all healing	

→ = key activities of each phase.

called **platelet-derived growth factor (PDGF)**, and transforming growth factors (TGFs) transform substances. Many of these growth factors work together to cause desired results in healing. Some of them are chemotactic, and others stimulate cell production.

Growth factors play a role in several key activities of healing. They control the migration and proliferation of cells vital to wound healing, including fibroblasts, macrophages, epithelial cells, and endothelial cells. Some growth factors are important in the early hours of inflammation, acting as stimulators of vasoconstriction and vasodilation. Growth factors also affect the formation of the fibrin plug. Others play roles in controlling macrophages and prevent phagocytization of healthy cells. In the proliferation phase, some growth factors assist and coordinate the capillary endothelial production. A number of growth factors are responsible for angiogenesis, granulation tissue, and collagen production. Growth factors in the remodeling phase stimulate the degradation of type III collagen and the synthesis of type I collagen.

A few growth factors stand out as primary players in healing and are worth identifying. One group is the EGFs. They stimulate production of a number of cells, including epithelial cells, endothelial cells, and fibroblasts. EGFs also draw epithelial cells into the damaged area and stimulate fibroblasts to produce GAG.

Another important group of growth factors is the fibroblast growth factors (FGF). They are believed to be primarily responsible for formation of the new vascular and granulation tissue following injury. They promote angiogenesis by stimulating fibroblasts and capillary endothelial cell proliferation. They also stimulate production of chondrocytes (cartilage cells), keratinocytes (keratin-producing epidermal cells), and myoblasts.

The PDGF group is a family of growth factors that facilitate production of collagenase by stimulating fibroblast activity. The PDGFs are particularly active during the remodeling phase, when they prepare the extracellular matrix. They are produced by a variety of cells, including macrophages, fibroblasts, epithelial cells, and vascular endothelial cells.

The primary TGF in wound healing is TGF-beta. This growth factor has a number of responsibilities. It is involved in stimulating extracellular matrix production and coordinating the process of neovascularization. TGF-beta also coordinates other growth factors to regulate the healing process.

Keep in mind that many other growth factors play roles in wound healing. As mentioned, their function is not entirely understood, but their presence is vital if healing is to occur. Table 2.3 summarizes the most common growth factors in the healing process.

Table 2.3 Common Growth Factors in Healing			
Growth Factor	**Source**	**Target**	**Cell proliferation and chemotactic activity**
EGF	Epithelial cells Macrophages Platelets	Fibroblasts Epithelial cells	Re-epithelialization Angiogenesis Collagenase activity
FGF	Macrophages Endothelial cells	Fibroblasts Endothelial cells	Angiogenesis Granulation tissue
PDGF	Platelets Macrophages Endothelial cells Epithelial cells	Fibroblasts	Fibroblast production Deposition of extracellular matrix
TGF	Macrophages Platelets Epithelium	Endothelial cells Fibroblasts Epithelial cells	Deposition of extracellular matrix Inhibition of epidermal proliferation

Chronic Inflammation

Normal healing of tissue occurs in the sequence just described. Occasionally, the injury does not progress along this normal time line. It gets stuck in the inflammation phase and is unable to proceed in healing. This condition is referred to as *chronic inflammation*. Recall that in acute inflammation, the large number of granular leukocytes that initially invades the area is replaced with mononuclear phagocytes. The cells are transformed into larger macrophages and giant cells to debride the area. As the area is cleared of waste and foreign matter, these cells diminish in number, but in chronic inflammations they persist at the site.

The continued presence of macrophages and giant cells is a key characteristic of chronic inflammation. The granular leukocytes have not been successful in fully debriding these areas, so the mononuclear phagocytes persist to rid the area of unwelcome substances. Their proliferation continues as long as these irritating substances prevail at the injury site.

In open wounds the persistence of foreign substances, such as bacteria, causes continued inflammation. If an insoluble, nonphagotizable foreign substance, such as a sand grain or unabsorbed extracellular blood, is the cause of chronic inflammation, the area's response is the formation of a **granuloma**. The macrophages become chemotactic for fibroblasts to invade the area. The foreign substance becomes surrounded by the collagen that these fibroblasts produce to isolate the substance and form a granuloma.

It has been shown that chronic wounds have deficient growth factor levels (Hom 1995). The introduction of growth factors such as PDGF, TGF-beta, and others has improved healing. According to Hom, studies have also revealed that **protease** occurs at higher levels in chronic wounds. Protease degrades growth factors to prevent their presence in the wound. The studies that have investigated chronic wounds and growth factors have looked at several different effects, causes, and preventions and have all come up with one conclusion: Growth factors are necessary for proper healing, and when they are not present, healing is impaired or prevented.

Although not technically a chronic wound condition, overuse injuries are frequently so classified. Overuse and overloading activities lead to cumulative trauma that exceeds the area's stress resistance. This is actually a continual reinjury, not a chronic wound. Overuse and overloading conditions are discussed in chapter 15.

HEALING OF SPECIFIC TISSUES

Although all tissues follow the same general steps in healing, the course of healing in different tissues—such as ligaments, tendons, muscles, cartilage, and bone—varies and involves events specific to the tissue.

Specific types and compositions of tissue show some variations in the healing sequence, although each tissue proceeds from inflammation to proliferation to remodeling generally following the time line. Given structural, cellular, and chemical differences, however, it is not reasonable to expect muscle tissue, for example, to proceed along the exact recovery time line that bone or ligament follows. Let's take a look at some of the differences in tissues that we commonly see traumatized in athletic injuries.

LIGAMENTS

When a ligament is torn, frayed stump ends are present where the ligament has been separated. The ligament undergoes the expected inflammation process, including local edema formation. The injured ligament stumps become surrounded with fluid, causing the ends to become friable, or easily crumbled. Vascular permeability increases and permits the normal inflammatory products, including PMNs and **lymphocytes**, to invade the area. **Erythrocytes** and other cells accumulate to fill the gap between the stump ends. Within the first day, macrophages and monocytes enter the area to begin debridement. Table 2.4 summarizes the time line of ligamentous tissue healing.

Within 48 to 72 h after the injury, the proliferation phase begins with extracellular matrix development and proceeds through production of collagen and ground substance by the fibroblasts. This phase continues for up to six weeks (Andriacchi et al. 1988). Other routine processes occur during this phase, including

Table 2.4	Ligament Healing Time Line
Time	**Activity**
First few hours	The injury site fills with erythrocytes, leukocytes, and lymphocytes. The ligament stumps become progressively more friable with the accumulation of serous fluid in the area.
24 h	Monocytes and macrophages infiltrate the area. Fibroblasts begin to appear and eventually become significant in number.
48–72 h	Fibroblasts produce extracellular matrix.
1–2 wk	Fibrocytes and macrophages are numerous. Random collagen fibers and abundant ground substance are seen. Fragile vascular granulation tissue is seen at the injury site. The extracellular matrix continues to be synthesized by fibroblasts. Macrophages, mast cells, and fibroblasts continue to predominate. Vascular buds appear in the wound to communicate with existing capillaries. Elastin is seen in the area.
2–3 days to 6 wk	Proliferation phase occurs, during which cellular and matrix structures replace the blood clot formed during inflammation.
6 wk–12 mo	Macrophages and fibroblasts diminish.
Up to 12 mo	Collagen concentration stabilizes with type I collagen replacing type III and collagen cross-links increasing in number. Ligament becomes more normal.
40–50 wk	Near-normal tensile strength restored.

capillary-bud formation that eventually join with existing vessels. Phagocytosis also continues during this time. The quantity of collagen being synthesized is greater than the amount being degraded, so that there is an increase in net collagen during this time.

Several weeks later the remodeling phase is heralded by the conversion of type III collagen to type I collagen and an increase in the number of collagen cross-links. There is also a reduction of edema, fibroblasts, and macrophages, and the area takes on a more normal appearance. This final stage may take one year or more to complete.

TENDONS

As with ligaments, the tendon inflammatory phase is approximately three days long (Gelberman, Banes, and Goldberg 1988). Tendons have support from local structures that aid in the initial healing process. These structures include the periosteum of underlying bone, the synovial sheath, the epitenon, and the endotenon. They provide the vascular supply and fibroblasts that are needed for healing. The epitenon and endotenon provide macrophage-like cells and fibroblasts to begin debridement. Table 2.5 summarizes the tendon healing time line.

Within the first week, collagen synthesis begins and continues at a rapid rate for the first four weeks (Gelberman, Banes, and Goldberg 1988). During the second week, the collagen starts to become more organized, so that by the end of the second week the cells are beginning to align themselves in the direction of stress. Collagen synthesis continues until day 35 (Peacock 1984, p. 319). Granulation tissue produced by fibroblasts migrating from surrounding connective tissue and from the tendon sheath is also seen in rapidly forming quantities. By day 28 collagen and active fibroblasts producing the collagen are clearly aligned along the tendon's long axis. This assists the remaining collagen to form in a proper orientation.

Table 2.5   Tendon Healing Time Line

Time	Activity
First 3 days	Cells that originate from extrinsic peritendinous tissue and from intrinsic tissue from the epitenon and endotenon are active.
5 days	Wound gap is filled by phagocytes.
1 wk	Collagen synthesis is initiated, with new collagen fibers placed in a random and disorganized way.
10 days	Collagen synthesis is maximal.
3 wk	The endotenon provides significant fibroblast proliferation in the injury site. Significant revascularization occurs. Synovial sheath is reconstituted. The synovial sheath is rebuilt, and a smooth gliding surface develops. Fibroblasts also start to become oriented in line with the tendon's axis.
4 wk	Fibroblasts predominate in the healing area. Collagen content increases. Collagen is fully oriented with the tendon's long axis.
35 days	Collagen synthesis is completed.
42 days	Fibroblasts that have proliferated from the endotenon are the primary cells, simultaneously synthesizing collagen while contributing to collagen resorption.
2 mo	Collagen is mature and realigned along the tendon's axis.
112 days	Fibroblasts have reverted to tenocytes, type III collagen has been replaced by type I, and maturation is complete.
40–50 wk	Strength is 85%–95% normal.

During the first three weeks, the area undergoes a significant revascularization. Because of this restoration of blood supply, it is possible to begin mobilization of a surgically repaired tendon by day 21. Immobilization prior to this time is important to allow reconstruction and restoration of local circulation because circulation is so vital to the tendon's successful recovery and function. Thus, immobilization is necessary not for the tendon to reconnect, but for the blood supply to be restored.

Also by three weeks the synovial sheath has been reconstituted. This is important so the tendon has a smooth gliding surface within which to move. When type III collagen has been replaced with type I collagen and the fibroblasts revert to their original status as **tenocytes**, the remodeling phase is finished. This occurs by day 112 (Gelberman, Banes, and Goldberg 1988).

When a tendon is surgically repaired, the tendon and the surrounding soft tissue, including blood vessels, fascia, and skin, all become one wound. The area is filled with a sticky gel. This gel is viscous and has the potential to become a thick, dense scar. If formed, the scar will limit the gliding of the tendon and thereby impede function of the muscle, ultimately limiting the success of rehabilitation (Peacock 1965). For normal function to return, the scar tissue must not bind together the normally separate structures at the site but instead allow the tendon to glide within its sheath, the skin to move freely from subcutaneous structures, and the blood vessels and nerves to have normal mobility so that all structures can function normally. One major factor that determines the success of this separation of elements is how long immobilization is maintained and when motion is initiated. The effects of immobilization are discussed in further detail in chapter 5.

MUSCLES

Although muscle tissue may heal like the other tissues we have discussed, following the same three phases to ultimately produce scar tissue, muscle also has unique structures within it that permit it also to regenerate. These structures are called **satellite cells**. These cells fuse with adjacent myofibers to repair and regenerate muscle tissue. It is believed that some destruction of muscle tissue occurs daily in routine activities. This destruction also occurs when an individual exercises without injury. The satellite cells play a role in the restoration and replacement of muscle cells routinely damaged during activity (Caplan et al. 1988). If an injury is sufficiently small, revascularized, and reinnervated and involves a muscle type that can regenerate, satellite cells replace injured muscle tissue with new muscle tissue. Table 2.6 summarizes the muscle's healing time line.

In the early hours of healing, injured muscle tissue appears to follow the same route of other tissue: Phagocytes, primarily macrophages, invade the site within 6 h following an injury. Macrophages are the predominant cell in the area for the next 10 days as they work to debride the area. In the proliferation phase, muscle tissue regeneration is begun as **myogenic cells** are activated. These evolve into **myoblasts**, which fuse together to form myotubes. Myotubes are seen in the injury site by day 13. Through a complex progression of events, these myotubes become muscle fibers and are apparent in the area by day 18. The final muscle regeneration is completed with the development of the neural aspect of the neuromuscular structure. When the process is complete, satellite cell levels return to normal and resume their daily function of less-intensive, ongoing muscle tissue replacement.

Larger muscle injuries are unable to repair by regeneration and must resort to scar tissue as the means of healing. When the mass of damaged muscle is larger than 3 g (0.1 oz), the muscle heals via the scarring process and goes through the normal sequence of healing.

CARTILAGE

There are different types of cartilage. Hyaline cartilage dissipates loads in joints. Commonly referred to as articular cartilage, it lines the surfaces of the diarthrodial joints. Fibrocartilage transfers loads between the tendons and ligaments and the bone.

Table 2.6	Muscle Healing Time Line
Time	**Activity**
6 h	Fragmentation of injured muscle fibers begins. Macrophages appear.
1–4 days	Fibroblasts appear. Ability to produce muscle tension is progressively reduced.
1 wk	Scar tissue is seen in large muscle injuries. Muscle is able to produce near-normal tension.
7–11 days	Tensile strength reaches near normal.
10 days	Large number of phagocytes, primarily macrophages, are seen at the injury site.
13 days	Regenerating myotubes are seen.
18 days	Cross-striated muscle fibers appear.
6 wk–6 mo	Contraction ability is 90% normal.

Examples of fibrocartilage are found in the intervertebral disks and the temporo-mandibular joint. Elastic cartilage provides a flexible support to external structures and is similar to hyaline cartilage.

As a rule, cartilage is composed primarily of type II collagen. When tissue healing occurs, type I collagen is the primary resulting collagen, so the ultimate structure changes if scar tissue is produced. Cartilage does have some regenerative capability. The difficulty in cartilage healing is that cartilage is regenerated at a slower rate than scar tissue is deposited. Fibrocartilage seems to have a better capacity to regenerate than articular cartilage (Silver and Glasgold 1995).

Whether cartilage regeneration or scar tissue occurs depends on three variables: the depth of the defect, the maturity of the cartilage, and the location of the defect (Silver and Glasgold 1995). Small, full-thickness defects are repaired by regeneration of fibrocartilage, but partial-thickness defects are repaired with scar tissue. For this reason, a surgeon may opt to place burr holes in an arthritic joint to stimulate the production of fibrocartilaginous tissue to repair the defect.

The healing course of articular cartilage once again follows a sequence of events initiated with macrophages and fibrin-plug formation. Fibroblasts appear in the area to perform their rebuilding tasks. As the site advances into the remodeling phase, collagen becomes the prevalent structure. See Table 2.7 for a general outline of the sequence of events in cartilage healing.

For regeneration of cartilage to occur, the following conditions must be present (Buckwalter et al. 1988):

• Cells that will proliferate and differentiate into chondrocytes must be located in or migrate to the wound site.

• A mechanical stimulus that enhances articular cartilage formation must be present.

• Protection from excessive loads must be sufficient to allow cartilage repair without causing damage.

• A normal joint conformation must be maintained or restored.

A procedure to replace articular cartilage with homogeneous cartilage was reported by Brittberg et al. (1994) from the University of Gloteborg, Sweden. Some hyaline cartilage is first removed from the patient's unaffected joint area, then grown in a lab to increase the quantity before finally being reimplanted in the cartilage defect site. This is known as the Swedish procedure. The procedure is currently being used in isolated situations and has not yet obtained approval by the Food and Drug Administration (FDA) for standard use in the United States.

Table 2.7	Articular Cartilage Healing Time Line
Time	**Activity**
48 h	Fibrin clot is formed to fill the defect.
5 days	Fibroblasts are in the area and combine with collagen fibers to replace the clot.
2 wk	Fibroblasts differentiate, and islands of chondrocytes appear.
1 mo	Fibroblasts have been completely differentiated.
2 mo	Satisfactory repair has occurred, with the defect resembling cartilage in appearance. The majority of collagen present, however, is type I.
6 mo	A combination of type I and type II calcified cartilage has a normal appearance.

Even more recent attempts have been made at the Stone Foundation for Sports Medicine and Arthritis Research in San Francisco using homogeneous grafts to transplant articular cartilage into arthritic joints without culturing the hyaline cartilage in a laboratory. This procedure is still at the experimental stage, but results have been promising.

BONE

As with other tissues, bone tissue has an inflammation phase that lasts three to four days (Heppenstall 1980), during which time fibroblasts and macrophages invade the area. The necrotic ends of the fractured bone and metabolic wastes are debrided by osteoclasts to clear the way and set the stage for the next phase.

During this next phase the bone demonstrates its ability to regenerate. **Osteoblasts**, bone-generating cells, invade the area via the periosteum. As these cells go to work, a **callus** is formed at the site of each bone fragment end. This soft callus, whose formation takes three to four weeks, is a fibrous **matrix** of collagen that eventually becomes bone. The callus has an internal component and an external component. The external callus immobilizes the fragment ends, eventually bridges the two fragments, and allows stress to be applied to the bone without harming the fracture site before it is completely healed. By the third week, the bony ends have become united. It takes approximately 40 days from the time of injury for the fracture site to become mechanically stable. Table 2.8 demonstrates the healing time line of bone.

As the osteoblasts move along the stump ends and farther away from the blood supply, they convert to chondrocytes, which produce a layer of cartilage. The chondrocytes are in turn covered by osteogenic cells, which are also covered by a fibrous layer. This process occurs simultaneously on the external and internal layers in the bone's marrow cavity. The soft callus matures into a hard callus as the fibrous matrix converts into spongy bone. In a not fully understood process, the spongy bone converts to normal compact bone over time. In the long bones of adults, this routinely takes three to four months (Heppenstall 1980, pp. 42–44).

Table 2.8 Bone Healing Time Line

Time	Activity
Immediately	PMNs, plasma, and lympocytes occur.
First few hours	Fibroblasts invade the area.
3–4 days	Hematoma forms. Fractured edges become necrotic. Mast cells occur at the site. Macrophages remove debris. Osteoclasts mobilize in the area.
Up to 4 wk	Osteoclasts proliferate to form soft callus. Cartilage cells are seen.
3–4 wk	Hard callus develops. Osteoclasts continue to remove dead bone. Endosteal blood supply continues to develop.
4–6 wk	External blood supply dominates.
6–10 wk	Medullary circulation is re-established.
3–4 mo	Fracture is healed, but remodeling continues.
12 wk	Near-normal strength is attained.

During the remodeling phase, the callus size is reduced, the medullary canal is reestablished, the conversion to bone tissue is finalized, and normal oxygen and electrical levels are restored (Lane and Werntz 1987, p. 55).

TENSILE STRENGTH DURING HEALING

Tensile strength takes a year or more to reach near-normal levels after an injury and seldom returns to its preinjury level, but the strength of surrounding tissues may permit a return to sport participation sooner than that.

Tensile strength is the maximal amount of stress or force that a structure is able to withstand before tissue failure occurs. In other words, it is the amount of outside force that can be applied to a muscle, tendon, ligament, or bone before it tears or breaks. Healthy tissue is able to withstand high amounts of tensile force. Once injured, however, tissue's tensile strength seldom returns to 100% of its prior level.

This is about the only fact on which researchers of tensile strength agree. Disagreements arise because research techniques, the animals and specific structures investigated, the degrees of the injury, and the results of in vitro versus in vivo studies all vary. It is difficult to extrapolate findings of research with animals to humans, and it is even more difficult to obtain humans who are willing to be injured to study the in vivo effects of injury on tensile strength. Studies investigating tensile strength are limited because the tensile strength of a structure can be affected by surrounding tissues that contribute strength through their own framework, function, configuration, or attachment in the area.

The contributing strength of surrounding tissues may explain why athletes often return to full competition without becoming reinjured six months after reconstructive surgery, even though the tissue does not regain its full tensile strength for one year or more after injury. There are many unanswered questions about the tensile strength of healing and healed tissue; nevertheless, rehabilitation specialists must be aware of current knowledge, incomplete though it may be.

During the inflammation phase, normal tensile strength declines rapidly to 50% (Gelberman et al. 1988; Gelberman et al. 1982). Depending on the tissue type involved, this decline occurs in 24 h to 48 h. In the very early stage of healing, the injured site's strength derives from the fibrin clot, which is insufficient to withstand much stress. Tensile strength is at its lowest during this time. Around day 5, tensile strength begins to increase. Without significant collagen, the injured tissue relies on other structures in the area, including the granulation tissue and ground substance, for this increase in strength.

As collagen becomes more plentiful and cross-links develop, the area's tensile strength becomes greater. Collagen conversion from type III to type I along with the increased number of cross-links are the core reasons for tensile strength development.

Studies of tensile strength in muscle have demonstrated that it varies in time, depending on the animal investigated. Rat studies show that by six weeks after injury, 90% of normal tensile strength is achieved, and in the cat it takes six months (Caplan et al. 1988). Bone strength is returned to 83% of normal 12 weeks after injury (Grundnes and Reikeras 1992). Ligaments and tendons vary in the time it takes to achieve near-normal strength, depending on the specific structure. These tissues approach near-normal levels anywhere from 17 to 50 weeks after injury (Nordin and Frankel 1980).

Researchers agree that once an injury occurs, the structure involved never regains full tensile strength. Tensile strength initially increases rapidly after an injury, then slows and even regresses as type III collagen degrades and is replaced with type I collagen. Depending on the structure, it may take a year or more for an injured part to regain maximal tensile strength.

FACTORS THAT AFFECT HEALING

Factors that affect healing include the treatment modality, drugs, surgical repair, patient's age, systemic diseases suffered by the patient, injury size, infection, nutrition, spasm, and swelling.

A number of outside influences can profoundly or subtly affect the healing process. Some of these factors can be applied by sport rehabilitation specialists to assist or stimulate the healing process. Others can be controlled by the patient, parents, or physician. Still others, such as age and systemic diseases, cannot be controlled.

Figure 2.4 outlines the injury and healing process and the difference an effective rehabilitation program can have on tissue healing and its outcome. It is important for a sports medicine specialist to know appropriate techniques that positively influence the healing process.

TREATMENT MODALITIES

Some of the treatment modalities most frequently used to enhance healing are electrical stimulation, ice, superficial heat, and deep heat.

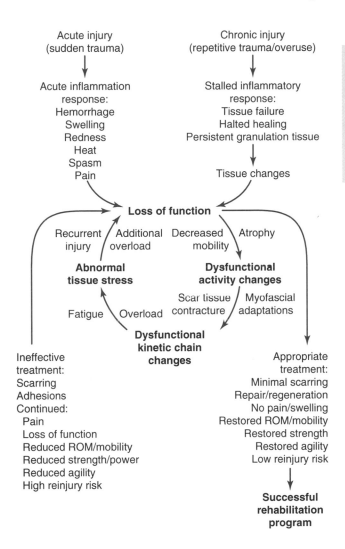

■ Figure 2.4   Effects of treatment on healing.

Adapted, by permission, from W.B. Leadbetter, 1994, Soft tissue athletic injury. In *Sports injuries: Mechanisms, prevention, treatment*, edited by F.H. Fu and D.A. Stone (Baltimore: Williams & Wilkins), 765. Copyright 1994 by Lippincott Williams & Wilkins.

There is an excellent profile of modalities and their effects on tissue healing in Craig Denegar's (2000) Athletic Training Education Series text, *Therapeutic Modalities for Athletic Injuries.* Refer to his text for specific information on how modalities can affect the signs of inflammation.

Ice is used during rehabilitation to reduce inflammation caused by therapeutic exercise. Occasionally after therapeutic exercise such as vigorous stretching or strengthening, signs of new inflammation, such as increased edema, occur. Although ice will not affect existing edema, it can reduce new edema resulting from overstretching or overstrengthening exercises. Remember that tissue irritation should be avoided; however, there may be occasions when it is unavoidable. At such times, ice should be used preemptively to quell new pain and edema.

Electrical stimulation during the first week after injury has been shown to enhance protein synthesis to help promote healing. It also increases the tensile strength of tendons (Enwemeka 1989). Because tendon and ligament structures are similar, it may also have the same effects when applied to ligaments.

Electrical stimulation can also be applied to muscles to relax muscle spasm. When facilitating muscle contraction, electrical stimulation may also assist in relieving local edema by pumping fluid into the lymph system, which reduces pain. With less pain, the athlete may exercise more willingly.

Muscle atrophy following injury or prolonged inactivity can be retarded by electrical stimulation. After prolonged inactivity, electrical stimulation is often used to facilitate muscle contraction and encourage reactivation and recruitment of dormant fibers. During short-term denervation, it may be used to facilitate muscle contraction until nerve function is restored.

After the inflammatory phase, heat can be advantageous when applied prior to exercise. It can increase circulation to better exchange nutrients and waste products and encourage healing, relax muscles to allow better exercise execution with less pain, and reduce tissue viscosity to make an area more pliable for stretching.

Ultrasound has the benefit of producing thermal as well as mechanical effects. A contraindication to continuous ultrasound is in the acute inflammatory phase, when heat is deleterious. At that time, pulsed ultrasound is indicated. It is believed that ultrasound promotes collagen, neovascular, and myofibroblast production. As a source of deep heat, it may be a useful prestretch application for tendon and capsular adhesions that lie deeper than superficial heat can reach effectively.

It is important for the sport rehabilitation specialist to know the desired results and choose a modality that best facilitates those results. As the patient progresses in the rehabilitation program, fewer modalities are required because the injury is more closely approaching normal function and metabolism. For example, as the patient enters the final stages of therapeutic exercise, ice is not needed following the therapeutic exercise program. If the patient continues to have swelling or pain that requires ice application following a therapeutic exercise routine, the cause for these symptoms should be examined because these symptoms should not occur late in rehabilitation.

DRUGS

The injured athlete often consults with a sport rehabilitation specialist for information about the drugs that have been prescribed after an injury. Therefore, the sport rehabilitation specialist should have a basic understanding of medications, be aware of his or her own limited knowledge, and readily refer the athlete to either the physician or the pharmacist for information beyond the scope of his or her knowledge.

Sport rehabilitation specialists should remember certain general rules of thumb about medication. All drugs, even vitamins, have the potential to produce undesirable side effects. Any drug should be used with caution and taken according to recommendations of the physician, pharmacist, or manufacturer of over-the-counter (OTC) medications. If undesirable side effects occur, the physician should be contacted for instructions to either discontinue the medication or alter its administration. All drugs have a **duration of action**, the length of time that the amount of drug in the blood is above the level needed to obtain a minimal therapeutic effect. This length of time is determined by the half-life of the drug. The **half-life** is the amount of time it takes for the level of the drug in the bloodstream to diminish by half. The frequency with which the drug is administered is based on the half-life. The shorter the half-life, the more frequently the drug must be administered to obtain a minimal therapeutic effect. The example given in Houglum (1998) demonstrates this concept: Naproxen, with a half-life of about 14 h, is administered twice a day, whereas ibuprofen, with a half-life of around 2 h, is administered three to four times a day.

A goal of drug administration is to achieve a steady state. A **steady state** occurs when the average level of drug remains constant in the blood, that is, when the amount absorbed into the blood equals the amount removed through metabolism or excretion. After the first few administrations of the drug, the amount of drug in the bloodstream increases until this steady state is achieved. As a rule of thumb, a steady state is achieved after the number of doses of the drug administered equals at least five half-lives. For example, if a drug has a half-life of 12 h and is given twice a day, a steady state is achieved by the middle of the third day (5×12 h). If a drug has a half-life of 2 h and is administered every 6 h, a steady state occurs following the third dose (5×2 h), because the first dose is at time 0, the second is at 6 h, the third at 12 h, and so on. (Houglum 1998). A patient's compliance in taking medication is important for achieving a steady state and the desired results. If a patient fails to take prescribed medication, the intended results may not be achieved. By the same token, taking more than the prescribed dosage may not produce better results faster. In fact, it can be deleterious. "More is better" does not apply to drugs. Taking higher or more frequent doses of a drug causes higher concentrations and may cause toxic side effects. Taking two different anti-inflammatory drugs, whether they are prescription or OTC medications, should also be avoided because it is equivalent to increasing dosage and can be dangerous. These important precautions should be pointed out to the patient when medications are given.

Most drugs taken by mouth are absorbed in the small intestine. If medication is taken with liquid, a full glass of liquid is advisable, not just a swallow. The liquid helps dissolve the medication and also increases the speed with which the drug moves from the stomach to the small intestine. If a drug is to be taken with food, it is absorbed at a slower rate, but the food may reduce otherwise irritating effects on the stomach.

Other factors that alter drug absorption include exercise immediately following ingestion, since blood normally allotted to the gastrointestinal tract is shunted to working muscles. With delayed release of medication from the stomach, irritation of the stomach lining may increase (Houglum 1998). For this reason, it may not be a good idea to take an anti-inflammatory medication immediately before exercise, especially when the stomach is empty.

NSAIDs

The most commonly prescribed drugs in medicine today are anti-inflammatories (Leadbetter 1990). The most frequently used of these are the nonsteroidal anti-inflammatory drugs (NSAIDs). Although research does not demonstrate a significant advantage of NSAIDs for athletic injuries, there is enough evidence to warrant their use. The NSAIDs are used to reduce pain and promote healing by minimizing inflammation in both acute and chronic athletic injuries. The NSAIDs reduce inflammation by inhibiting the enzymes cyclooxygenase-1 (COX-1) and cyclooxygenase-2 (COX-2). The primary reason for NSAID use in sport injury therapy is to reduce pain by inhibiting prostaglandin (PG) production. PGs stimulate local nociceptors (pain-causing nerve endings) and enhance edema formation by increasing vascular permeability. By limiting PG production, NSAIDs can encourage healing progression from the inflammation phase to the proliferation phase. By reducing edema and pain, range-of-motion and other therapeutic exercises can begin sooner to promote recovery.

Several prescription and OTC NSAIDs are now available on the market. Refer to table 2.9 for a list of commonly used NSAIDs. Individuals respond differently to each of these drugs. As a general rule, the amount of NSAID in the OTC dosage is half the equivalent prescription medication. One person may find better results from aspirin, whereas another may find aspirin ineffective but have great relief from ibuprofen. Another person may find that naproxen upsets the stomach but have no problem with tolmetin. Physicians commonly try a different NSAID if a patient does not respond appropriately to the first. Because each person responds differently, trial and error is often used to discover the medication that is most effective in achieving desired therapy goals.

Steroid medication is also used to control inflammation, but its use is currently limited because of its severe side effects. It is usually prescribed in large doses for a

Table 2.9 NSAIDs			
Generic name	**Trade name**	**Doses/day**	**Maximum daily adult dose (mg)[1]**
Nonselective COX Inhibitors:			
Aspirin[2]	many	4	6000
Fenoprofen	Nalfon	3–4	3200
Flurbiprofen	Ansaid	2–3	300
Ibuprofen[2]	Advil	3–4	3200
Indomethacin	Indocin	2–3	200
Ketoprofen[2]	Actron	3–4	300
Naproxen Na[2]	Aleve	2	1375
Piroxicam	Feldene	1	20
Sulindac	Clinoril	2	400
Tolmetin Na	Tolectin	3–4	2000
COX-2 Inhibitors: Celecoxib	Celebrex	1–2	NA[3]
Meloxican	Mobic	1	7.5
Rofeoxib	Vioxx	1	NA[4]

[1]Typical daily dose may be considerably less.

[2]Available without prescription.

[3]Max. daily adult dose not available yet. Typical dosage for osteoarthritis is 200 mg/day.

[4]Max. daily adult dose not available yet. Recommended dosage for osteoarthritis is 12.5–25 mg/day.

Adapted from J. Houglum 1998.

short amount of time. Administration is closely monitored by the prescribing physician because of the possible side effects.

Because NSAIDs inhibit the production of PGs through alteration of **arachidonic acid** metabolism, other physiological functions are also affected. Besides affecting the inflammation phase of local injuries, PGs play an important role in protecting the stomach lining. Therefore, one of the most common side effects of NSAIDs is stomach upset. For this reason, people with a history of ulcers or allergy to aspirin should not use NSAIDs. Stomach upset, nausea, and vomiting are possible side effects and may be reason for the patient to discontinue NSAID use. Generally, the tendency for stomach upset and ulcers increases the longer a person uses NSAIDs.

NSAIDs may also be harmful to kidney and cardiac functions. Arachidonic acid plays an important role in renal physiology, so people with renal disease may not be able to use NSAIDs. Because of the heart's relationship to renal function, people with congestive heart failure should avoid NSAIDs.

Like most drugs, NSAIDs should be avoided by women who are pregnant or nursing infants since NSAIDs may be harmful to the fetus or infant.

A new family of NSAIDs was recently approved by the FDA. These drugs primarily inhibit COX-2 enzymes, by their influence on arachidonic acid metabolism. The more traditional NSAIDs are nonselective and affect both COX-1 and COX-2 enzymes to varying degrees. Function of the COX-2 enzymes occurs primarily in the inflammation process, so the newer NSAIDs COX-2 inhibitors reduce inflammation with less impact on gastric or kidney cells.

As a rule, disregarding side effects, a drug should be continued as long as desired results are obtained. Researchers disagree about the length of time an NSAID should be administered. Generally, NSAIDs should be administered during the first two phases of healing. There is some indication that continued use of these drugs into the third phase may slow healing (Almekinders and Gilbert 1986). It seems obvious that the most effective time for using anti-inflammatory medication is during the inflammation phase, when production of PGs is the greatest. The use of NSAIDs during the first week after injury, therefore, may be most crucial. If an individual continues to respond to the medication beyond that time, however, it may be useful to continue it into the proliferation phase. This decision, of course, is made by the physician.

Drug Interactions

Any drug can interact with other drugs also being taken to either enhance or reduce their effectiveness. This is known as **drug interaction**. For example, NSAIDs increase blood-clotting time by affecting the role of arachidonic acid in platelet aggregation and therefore magnify the results of drugs used in anticoagulant therapy. NSAIDs may also decrease the effectiveness of other drugs such as diuretics (medication to increase urine excretion, usually to relieve systemic swelling), beta blockers (medication to slow heart rate), angiotensin-converting enzyme inhibitors (medication to lower blood pressure), and oral hypoglycemic agents (medication taken orally to control non-insulin-dependent diabetes). Antacids delay the rate at which an NSAID is absorbed.

Other Drugs

Some medications may delay the healing process. Antibiotics, antineoplastic drugs, heparin, nicotine, and corticosteroids can all delay healing.

OTHER MODIFYING FACTORS

A number of other factors affect healing. Some of the factors over which the sport rehabilitation specialist has no control include the surgical repair, the patient's age, systemic diseases from which the patient suffers, and wound size. Other factors, including infection, spasm, and swelling, can be reduced by appropriate and timely treatment. Nutrition can be influenced through instruction and advice to the injured athlete.

Surgical Repair

The physician's surgical and sterile techniques have a direct effect on the healing of injuries that are repaired surgically. Infection complicates and delays the healing process. The quality of the surgeon's repair technique and follow-up care directly influences when rehabilitation can be started. If a surgeon's technique results in increased rather than decreased postoperative edema, tissue repair is delayed. If a surgeon immobilizes an injury for three months rather than three weeks, rehabilitation will be slower.

Age

Age can be a factor that alters healing. A good blood supply is crucial for any injury to heal properly. A poor blood supply delays or prevents an injury from healing properly. Blood supply is often impaired with age. Diseases associated with age also can affect healing.

Disease

Certain systemic diseases can impede healing. If an athlete has diabetes, HIV, arthritis, endocrine disease, connective tissue disease, carcinoma, or other systemic diseases, extra care should be taken with healing wounds. Additionally, conditions not often seen in athletes that can delay healing include renal, hepatic, cardiovascular, and autoimmune diseases. If an athlete has any of these conditions, the certified athletic trainer is wise to be especially cautious.

Wound Size

Generally, the greater the injury, the more time necessary for healing to occur. If an athlete suffers a first-degree ankle sprain, he or she may be able to participate in practice the next day. However, if an athlete has a second-degree ankle sprain, he or she may be unable to return to practice for one week.

The larger the destruction of tissue and separation of tissue ends, the longer it will take for the body to debride the area and connect the stump ends. Similarly, the greater the injury, the greater the scar tissue. Scar tissue can impede rehabilitation, depending on where the scar tissue is and how long the injured site is immobilized before exercises begin.

Infection

Infection is a possibility any time an open wound occurs, whether is it an abrasion, a surgical wound, or a needle stick from an injection or aspiration. Precautions should always be taken to prevent infection, regardless of the source of the wound. Infection always delays healing. When an infection occurs, the ultimate healed structure will have more scar tissue than it would otherwise have had.

Nutrition

Nutrition plays an important part in healing. The certified athletic trainer should encourage the patient to have good nutrition through well-balanced meals to enhance healing. Diets lacking in protein, vitamins (especially A and C), or minerals (especially the trace minerals zinc and copper) make healing more difficult.

Muscle Spasm

Spasm is a reflex that occurs with injury as the body attempts to minimize the injury by immobilizing the area. Pain and muscle inhibition combine to diminish function. Spasms result in ischemia by restricting blood flow. Applying immediate first aid to the area is important in reducing spasm and ultimately improving the rate of tissue healing and the function of the injured part.

Swelling

The more severe the injury, the greater the swelling, although the amount of swelling for similar injuries varies from one person to another. Swelling, or edema, is caused by fluid in the interstitial spaces and can include blood, watery fluid from damaged cells, and plasma fluids. The body interprets extracellular blood as a foreign substance and works to rid the area of it. Edema also puts pressure on sensitive nerve endings, causes reflex muscular inhibition, and negatively affects nutrient exchange at the site of injury. These factors ultimately increase pain, reduce function, and slow healing. The greater the amount of accumulated extravascular blood and fluid, the greater the symptoms of inflammation and the longer it will take the body to progress from inflammation to proliferation. It therefore is crucial for the certified athletic trainer to apply immediate treatment to minimize the edema and promote healing. Minimizing edema also reduces inflammation, pain, and loss of function.

THE ROLE OF THERAPEUTIC EXERCISE IN HEALING

Application of therapeutic exercise components must be carefully coordinated with the phases of healing. Respecting tissue healing must always be a tantamount consideration when planning a successful rehabilitation program.

Now that you understand the healing process, it is time to see how this knowledge can help in designing therapeutic exercise programs for injured athletes. Your knowledge of the events and timing of the healing cycle should help you know what to do and when to do it to promote the athlete's safe and timely return to competition.

The sport rehabilitation specialist can influence healing positively or negatively, depending on the treatment and when it is applied. Knowledge plays a vital part in the delivery of treatment. Knowing how to apply a treatment is the easy part. Knowing when to apply it and the consequences or benefits of applying it are more difficult and just as important.

Although immediate treatment after an injury is considered first aid, it is really the first step in rehabilitation. Sue Hillman's (2000) Athletic Training Education Series book, *Introduction to Athletic Training,* provides an excellent description of first-aid procedures. Therefore, they are not addressed here; refer to her text for a review.

Rehabilitation involves two aspects of treatment following on-field evaluation and immediate care. Passive therapeutic modalities are often first applied. They are used to promote healing, reduce spasm and pain, and allow the next phase of rehabilitation—therapeutic exercise—to begin. Therapeutic exercise is necessary to allow the patient to resume full sport participation. Various aspects of therapeutic exercise are discussed in detail throughout this text. This section covers only general principles. It is important to realize that rehabilitation actually involves the use of both modalities and therapeutic exercise. Each serves a very different purpose but they are used to achieve a common goal, the full recovery of the injured athlete.

TIMING OF TREATMENT

Once the injury has been stabilized, efforts to control the edema and pain are important in the early rehabilitation phase. Even at this time, efforts can be made through therapeutic exercise to encourage the healing process. Care must be taken, however, not to disturb the newly formed, tenuous fibrin plug, which provides the injured site's primary stability and strength. Recall that in the first three days after injury, there is a lot of physiological activity at the injury site. Among other activities, macrophages are attempting to clear the site of debris so that the fibroblasts can start their task of rebuilding. Undue stress to the injury at this time reinjures the site, disconnects the fibrin clot, and causes additional edema.

In severe injuries, the sport rehabilitation specialist must be cautious about the amount of stress applied to the area, especially in the early healing phases. During these phases even patients with surgically repaired injuries can begin therapeutic exercise early. Even though the injury is unable to tolerate high stresses, the patient can work toward one of the goals of rehabilitation (discussed in chapter 1): maintaining the conditioning status of uninjured parts and the cardiovascular system. For example, if a patient has had surgery on the right knee, he or she can maintain cardiovascular conditioning by performing activities such as one-legged cycling or upper-body ergometric activities. Upper-body weight lifting and left-lower-extremity resistance exercises can also be a part of the program at this time. Some evidence indicates that exercising the contralateral limb provides some gains in strength in the involved extremity (Steadman, Forster, and Silferskiold 1989).

By the end of the first week, the injured site is already entering the remodeling phase. Type I collagen is being produced, and the area becomes stronger and able to withstand more stress than in the first few days. The site of injury is still very weak compared to normal tissue, but it is able to tolerate some controlled stress. At this time, depending on the injury and the tissue involved, flexibility exercises and some strengthening activities are used, although there are some exceptions to this general rule.

Tendon repair is one exception. Some physicians permit range-of-motion exercises but no strengthening exercises until the third week. Others prefer to wait six weeks or longer to begin strengthening. Some physicians allow strengthening exercises after one week because collagen fibers are being synthesized rapidly and reach their maximum levels by day 10. They feel that the collagen is strong enough at this time to start mild resistive exercises, often in the form of isometrics. Other physicians prefer to wait three weeks because it is then that the synovial sheath has been rebuilt to provide a smooth gliding surface for the tendon. Physicians who wait six weeks presumably do so because by then the new collagen is fairly mature and risk of rupture is significantly less. The risk of waiting too long to initiate activity following surgery is that the tendons will become bound by the collective scar tissue formed following surgical disruption of skin, fascia, surrounding soft tissue, and the tendon. It is important to know the physician's preferred protocol regarding initiation of therapeutic exercise.

As mentioned in chapter 1, flexibility must be achieved before the other physical parameters. After reading this chapter, you should appreciate the reasons for this sequence. By the end of the first week of healing, collagen is transforming from weak type III to stronger, permanent type I. The cross-links are increasing, and the bonds between the collagen are becoming stronger. As a general rule, the most effective gains in range of motion are made during the first three weeks after injury. Changes in motion can be made relatively easily during the first two months following surgery or severe injury. After that time the collagen becomes fairly mature and more resistant to change. This is the reason that an ankle that has been immobilized for three months following a non-surgically repaired tibial fracture is much more difficult to restore to its former range of motion than one that has been immobilized for three weeks.

Different techniques for achieving flexibility are used at different times in the rehabilitation process. Specific flexibility techniques depend on how mature the scar tissue is. These techniques are described and differentiated in chapter 5.

Once a therapeutic exercise program has begun and flexibility activities have been initiated, strength activities should begin when it is safe to do so. Depending on the severity of the injury and the status of the patient, early strength exercises may include only isometrics. Progression of strengthening exercises is discussed in more detail in chapter 7. The sport rehabilitation specialist must be cognizant of the stresses applied by strengthening activities. Care must always be taken to stress the tissues enough to provide the desired results without overstressing them and causing damage. The most dangerous time for strength activities is during the inflammation phase, when there is little tensile strength in the injured area except the fibrin clot holding the injury site together. Care must also be taken during the remodeling phase, when collagen is converted from type III to type I, especially following surgical repair, when tendons and ligaments are particularly vulnerable.

The therapeutic exercise program should progress as described in chapter 1. Once flexibility is achieved, emphasis is placed on progressive strength and muscular endurance activities. These exercises become more intense as the injured area increases in tensile strength through healing and the muscles, tendons, ligaments, and bones themselves gain strength from the exercises.

As the injured area's supporting structures, especially the muscles that provide dynamic control, increase their strength, exercises progress to improve the next parameter, proprioception. These activities emphasize balance, agility, speed, and coordination. The exercises become more advanced until the patient can transit into functional activities that replicate the motions and stresses of normal sport performance.

The timing of the injured part's healing should always be considered in determining when the patient should progress in the program. Stresses applied to the injured part must be assessed and correlated with tissue's healing time line.

ACUTE AND CHRONIC INJURIES

Rehabilitation programs for chronic injuries involve different strategies from those for acute injuries because the timing of events and healing progression for chronic and acute injuries differ. These differences are discussed in more detail in chapter 15. A rehabilitation program must always be designed with the healing of injured tissue in mind.

Often, a chronic injury is caused by continual irritation to an area. The aggravating factor must first be changed before a successful treatment program can be instituted. Once the cause has been determined, healing can begin, although it is often slower than the healing of acute injuries. Even though the rehabilitation process is different, the same observations should be made in both chronic and acute injuries.

For any injury, two considerations determine the appropriate course of therapeutic exercise. The first is the usual healing sequence and timing. Knowing when the tissue is most vulnerable and how long it takes for various tissues to go through their normal healing process determines what stresses can be applied safely.

The second consideration is the individual's unique response to injury and treatment. To evaluate each person's response, examine the area for negative and positive responses to treatment. Increased edema, increased pain, and diminished function are signs that the exercise was too severe for the injury to tolerate. Asking the patient for his or her response to exercise is helpful. "Did your knee have more swelling last night?" "Was there more pain in your shoulder after you left the athletic training facility yesterday?" "Was it easier or more difficult to walk on one crutch after the last treatment?" If you determine that an exercise produced undesirable effects, the appropriate action is to exclude that exercise until the injured area further improves. If no deleterious effects occur, the current course of treatment is appropriate.

SUMMARY

1. *Explain the differences between primary and secondary healing.*

   Primary healing produces a minimal scar and occurs when the damaged edges of a wound are close to each other, whereas secondary healing produces a greater scar because the wound must heal by filling in tissue from the bottom and sides of the wound.

2. *Identify the healing phases.*

   The body follows a very complex and not entirely understood process of healing, going through the three phases of healing: inflammation, proliferation, and remodeling.

3. *Describe the primary processes of each healing phase.*

   During inflammation, neutrophil migration begins the process, fibrin-plug production prevents fluid and blood from escaping, monocyte migration rids the area of debris, angiogenesis restores blood flow, and type III collagen is produced. Proliferation occurs when fibroblasts, myofibroblasts, and collagen synthesis are at their peak. During remodeling, healing slows, wound contraction is well under way, and type III collagen is converted to type I collagen.

4. *Discuss the causes for the signs of inflammation.*

   Redness, localized warmth, swelling, pain, and dysfunction are all signs of inflammation. Redness occurs because of increased circulation and released chemicals, localized warmth and swelling are caused by interstitial fluid leakage and increased metabolic activity in the area, pain is caused by pressure on nerve endings from edema and damage to nerves in the area. Dysfunction occurs because of the physical restrictions of swelling, damage to structures, and the muscular inhibition from the pain.

5. *Explain the role of growth factors in healing.*

   Growth factors are not well understood, but present knowledge indicates that they play an important role in tissue healing. They assist in causing cell proliferation and chemotactic activity that are vital to healing.

6. *Discuss the differences between acute and chronic inflammation.*

   Acute inflammation occurs through a systematic progression of chemical and cellular activity. Chronic inflammation occurs when the site is unable to proceed from the inflammatory phase to the proliferation phase because granulocytes are unable to fully debride the area so that mononuclear cells persist.

7. *Discuss specific tissue healing characteristics.*

   Ligaments, tendons, muscle, bone, and cartilage all follow the general healing process, but their healing also has aspects unique to their own cellular makeup. For example, muscle has myogenic cells that are able to regenerate muscle tissue, bone has osteoblasts, and tendons have tenocytes.

8. *Identify the relevance of tensile strength.*

   Tensile strength enables a structure to withstand stresses. Once an area is damaged, the tensile strength is not restored to 100% normal. In spite of this, an athlete is able to safely return to sport participation if the injury has properly healed and a proper rehabilitation program has been followed.

9. *Discuss factors that can modify the healing process.*

   Healing of any tissue is influenced by a number of factors. Factors that can be influenced include the use of medications (especially anti-inflammatories), the use of various treatment modalities, the application of first aid, edema and pain, infection, and nutrition. Other factors over which the certified athletic trainer has no control include the physician's surgical technique and the patient's age and general health.

10. *Explain the role NSAIDs play in inflammation.*

    NSAIDs reduce the effects of inflammation by altering chemical production or the impact of specific chemicals on the healing process. If administered correctly, they can positively reduce the inflammation phase to promote healing.

11. *Discuss the timing of treatment with the various stages of healing.*

Therapeutic exercise must be administered appropriately without causing harm to the healing tissues if the rehabilitation program is to be successful. It is important to use exercises carefully and watch for adverse effects from the exercises.

12. *Identify the guidelines for treatment progression in acute and chronic injuries.*

The application of therapeutic exercise is different for acute and chronic injuries, because the healing of each is different, but the signs to watch for and avoid are the same.

CRITICAL THINKING QUESTIONS

1. If you were Deanna in the opening scenario, how would you approach Roberta to discuss whether or not she has anorexia? How could anorexia affect Roberta's healing process? What could you do to counteract her anorexia? What precautions should you take to "do no harm"?

2. If an athlete presented to you with Achilles tendinitis that began two weeks ago, at what stage would you estimate the tendinitis to be? What would be your criteria for determining whether it is acute or chronic?

3. A patient who undergoes an outpatient surgical repair of the elbow comes to you three days after the surgery to begin rehabilitation. Where in the healing process do you estimate this patient to be, and what healing activities are occurring? What would you do for treatment in the first three days of your treatment program? What would you do for treatment in the first three weeks of your treatment program? What factors would you consider to determine when to change the treatment program?

4. A patient with a second-degree ankle sprain that occurred four days ago comes to you for rehabilitation. If the athlete was 50 years old; had diabetes, severe swelling, and cramps in the calf muscles; was on Coumadin and an oral hypoglycemic medication; and had been taking oral anti-inflammatories for the past three days, what would your treatment program include? How would your treatment be different if the patient was 22 years old; had severe swelling and cramps in the calf muscles; and had been taking oral anti-inflammatories for the past three days?

REFERENCES

Almekinders, L.C., and J.A. Gilbert. 1986. Healing of experimental muscle strains and the effects of non-steroidal antiinflammatory medication. *American Journal of Sports Medicine* 14:303–308.

Andriacchi, T.P., Sabiston, K., DeHaven, K., Dahners, L., Woo, S., Frank, C., Oakes, B., Brand, R., and J. Lewis. 1988. Ligament: Injury and repair. In *Injury and repair of the musculoskeletal soft tissues,* ed. S.L.-Y. Woo and J.A. Buckwalter. Park Ridge, IL: American Academy of Orthopaedic Surgeons.

Betz, P., Norlich, A., Wilske, J., Tubel, J., Penning, R., and W. Eisenmenger. 1992. Time-dependent appearance of myofibroblasts in granulation tissue of human skin wounds. *International Journal of Legal Medicine* 150:99–103.

Brittberg, M., Lindahl, A., Nilsson, A., Ohlsson, C., Isaksson, O. , and L. Peterson. 1994. Treatment of deep cartilage defects in the knee with autologous chondrocyte transplantation. *New England Journal of Medicine* 331:889–895.

Buckwalter, J.A., Rosenberg, L., Coutts, R., Hunziker, E., Reddi, A.H., and V. Mow. 1988. Articular cartilage: Injury and repair. In *Injury and repair of the musculoskeletal soft tissues,* ed. S.L.-Y. Woo and J.A. Buckwalter. Park Ridge, IL: American Academy of Orthopaedic Surgeons.

Caplan, A.B., Carlson, J., Faulkner, J., Fischman, D., and W. Garrett, Jr. 1988. Skeletal muscle. In *Injury and repair of the musculoskeletal soft tissues,* ed. S.L.-Y. Woo and J.A. Buckwalter. Park Ridge, IL: American Academy of Orthopaedic Surgeons.

Christie, A.L. 1991. The tissue injury cycle and new advances toward its management in open wounds. *Athletic Training* 26:274–277.

Connolly, J.F. 1988. *Fracture complications, recognition, prevention, and management.* Chicago: Year Book Medical.

Denegar, C. 2000. *Therapeutic modalities for athletic injuries.* Champaign, IL: Human Kinetics.

DiPietro, L.A. 1995. Wound healing: The role of the macrophage and other immune cells. *Shock* 4:233–240.

Enwemeka, C.S. 1989. Inflammation, cellularity, and fibrillogenesis in regenerating tendon: Implications for tendon rehabilitation. *Physical Therapy* 69:816–825.

Gelberman, R., An, K.-A., Banes, A. , and V. Goldberg. 1988. Tendon. In *Injury and repair of the musculoskeletal soft tissues,* ed. S.L.-Y. Woo and J.A. Buckwalter. Park Ridge, IL: American Academy of Orthopaedic Surgeons.

Gelberman, R.H., Woo, S.L.-Y., Lothringer, K. Akeson, W.H., and D. Amiel. 1982. Effects of early intermittent passive mobilization on healing canine flexor tendons. *Journal of Hand Surgery* 7:170–175.

Grundnes, O., and O. Reikeras. 1992. Blood flow and mechanical properties of healing bone. *Acta Orthopaedica Scandinavica* 63:487–491.

Heppenstall, R.B. 1980. Fracture healing. In *Fracture treatment and healing,* ed. R.B. Heppenstall. Philadelphia: Saunders.

Hillman, S. 2000. *Introduction to athletic training.* Champaign, IL: Human Kinetics.

Hom, D.B. 1995. Growth factors in wound healing. *Otolaryngologic Clinics of North America* 28:933–953.

Houglum, J.E. 1998. Pharmacologic considerations in the treatment of injured athletes with nonsteroidal anti-inflammatory drugs. *Journal of Athletic Training* 33:259–263.

Houglum, P.A. 1992. Soft tissue healing and its impact on rehabilitation. *Journal of Sport Rehabilitation* 1:19–39.

Kibler, W.B. 1990. Concepts in exercise rehabilitation of athletic injury. In *Sports-induced inflammation*, ed. W.B. Leadbetter, J.A. Buckwalter, and S.L. Gordon. Park Ridge, IL: American Academy of Orthopaedic Surgeons.

Kirsner, R.S., and W.H. Eaglstein. 1993. The wound healing process. *Dermatological Clinics* 11:629–638.

Koopman, C.F. 1995. Cutaneous wound healing: An overview. *Otolaryngologic Clinics of North America* 28:835–845.

Lane, J.M., and J.R. Werntz. 1987. Biology of fracture healing. In *Fracture healing,* ed. J.M. Lane. New York: Churchill Livingstone.

Leadbetter, W.B. 1994. Soft tissue athletic injury. In *Sports injuries: Mechanisms, prevention, treatment,* ed. F.H. Fu and D.A. Stone. Baltimore: Williams & Wilkins.

Martinez-Hernandez, A., and P.S. Amenta. 1990. Basic concepts in wound healing. In *Sports-induced inflammation,* ed. W.B. Leadbetter, J.A. Buckwalter, and S.L. Gordon. Park Ridge, IL: American Academy of Orthopaedic Surgeons.

Nordin, M., and V.H. Frankel. 1980. Biomechanics of collagenous tissues. In *Basic biomechanics of the skeletal system,* ed. V.H. Frankel and N. Nordin. Philadelphia: Lea & Febiger.

Peacock, E.E. 1965. Physiology of tendon repair. *American Journal of Surgery* 109:283.

Peacock, E.E. 1984. *Wound repair.* 3rd ed. Philadelphia: Saunders.

Salter, R.B., Simmons, D.F., Malcom, B.W., Rumble, E.J., Macmichael, D., and N.D. Clements. 1980. The biological effect of continuous passive motion on the healing of full-thickness defects in articular cartilage. *Journal of Bone and Joint Surgery* 62A:1232–1251.

Silver, F.H. and A.I. Glasgold. 1995. Cartilage wound healing. *Otolaryngologic Clinics of North America* 28:847–864.

Steadman, J.R., Forster, R.S., and J.P. Silferskiold. 1989. Rehabilitation of the knee. *Clinics in Sports Medicine* 8:605–627.

CHAPTER THREE

Concepts in Physics

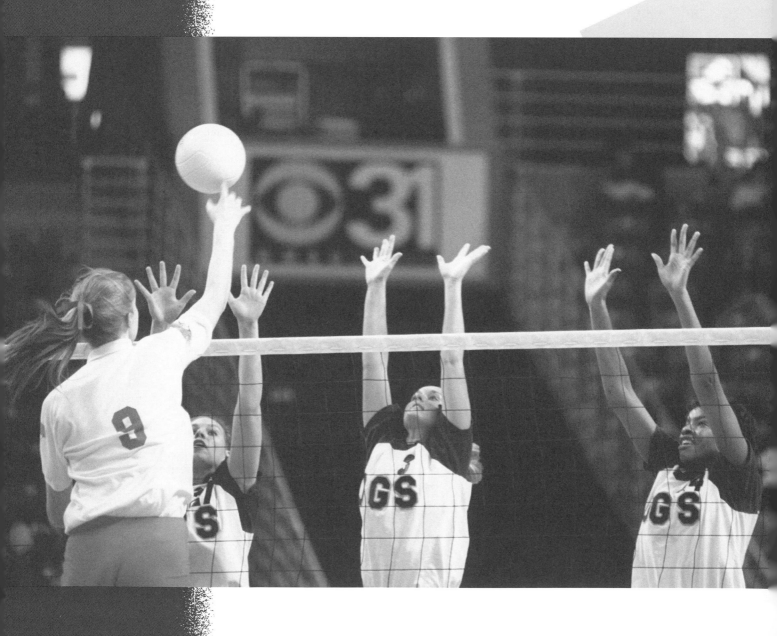

OBJECTIVES

After completing this chapter, you should be able to do the following:

1. Define force and give an example of an internal and an exernal force.

2. Explain the relevance to therapeutic exercise of Newton's first, second, and third laws of motion.

3. Explain how center of gravity changes with movement.

4. Discuss how a change in base of support can change a person's stability.

5. Explain the relationship between line of gravity and base of support.

6. Explain two ways of increasing stability.

7. Identify the difference between stabilization and fixation.

8. Explain how torque can be altered in the body.

9. Identify how varying position changes a muscle's mechanical advantage.

10. Discuss the difference between mechanical and physiological advantage of a muscle.

11. Explain the importance of positioning in exercising two-joint muscles.

12. Distinguish between velocity and acceleration.

13. Discuss the relevance of elasticity, stress-strain, creep, and friction to therapeutic exercise.

Michael Mattson is working to rehabilitate Robin, a swimmer with a shoulder injury. The facility where Michael works has an adjustable pulley system, and he wants to use it for the series of scapular strengthening exercises he has planned for today's program with Robin. He wants to exercise the lower trapezius, middle trapezius, rhomboids, and serratus anterior on the pulleys. He realizes that the muscle's physiological length, lever-arm length, and angle of pull all influence the amount of work that is done by the muscle and understands that stabilization must be a consideration, but he is at a loss as to where the pulleys should be placed to obtain the best results. Robin is scheduled to begin the program in 30 min, so Michael must be efficient in figuring out the pulley placement for the exercises he has in mind for today's program.

Education is our passport to the future, for tomorrow belongs to the people who prepare for it today.

Malcolm X

Knowing why we do what we do in therapeutic exercise is vital. Only with an understanding of theory and precepts can we adjust exercises to each injured athlete's needs and develop soundly structured, knowledge-based therapeutic exercise programs. It is easy to know the hows, but knowing the whys is the difference between a technician and a professional. A professional knows what is important and why. The concepts presented in this chapter provide the whys of therapeutic exercise so that the hows become logical and simple.

The physics concepts in this chapter are not new; they have successfully endured the test of centuries. Many of the ideas that Sir Isaac Newton and other engineers and philosophers introduced during the 1600s have profound impact on the delivery of therapeutic exercise in sports medicine today. These concepts are another vital part of the foundation of knowledge that you will need to guide a patient through a therapeutic exercise program. Without this knowledge it is difficult to apply forces correctly for stretching and strengthening, use your own body efficiently and effectively, or develop a successful therapeutic exercise program.

As you read through this chapter, you should develop an appreciation of basic physics principles that will affect the application of your clinical skills daily. These principles are not complicated, but they are vital for sport rehabilitation specialists. First, concepts are presented; then examples of direct applications to daily tasks in therapeutic exercise are provided.

FORCE

A force causes movement and has direction and magnitude. Gravity is a pervasive external force that affects every movement.

A **force** is something that causes movement and has direction and magnitude. A mass is moved in a specific direction when a specific amount of force is applied. In the human body, the force can be either internal or external and is generally considered to produce either a push or a pull. Internal forces, of course, are generated by the muscles. External forces can be applied by a wide variety of sources, the most basic being gravity.

Gravity is probably the most basic external force; we all deal with gravity continuously. Whether you realize it or not, it affects your every move. If there were no gravity, sports as we know them would be drastically different. Although Sir Isaac Newton didn't formulate his law of gravity until the late 1600s, gravity has been around since before the beginning of earth.

Sir Isaac Newton's law of gravity states that every object attracts every other object with a force proportional to the product of their masses and inversely proportional to the square of the distance between them. Because the earth is so massive compared with the objects on its surface, gravity is commonly thought of as the force of attraction that the earth exerts on an object. Gravity is counterbalanced by the supporting surface on which a person is standing, sitting, or lying. In other words, without surfaces such as a floor, bed, or chair to balance our weight on, we would simply fall. This concept leads us to Newton's third law of motion, which will be discussed later.

NEWTON'S LAWS OF MOTION

Newton's first and second laws of motion describe inertia, momentum, and acceleration. These laws explain that the faster an object already moves, the less force is needed to move it in the same direction. His third law, action-reaction, states that for every action there is an equal and opposite reaction.

The mathematician Sir Isaac Newton (1642–1727) formulated laws of motion and gravity that are used to explain movement. The three laws of motion discussed here are inertia, acceleration and momentum, and action-reaction.

INERTIA

Newton's first law of motion deals with **inertia:** A body remains at a state of rest or remains in uniform motion until an outside force acts on it. This is one reason why it is difficult for a weak muscle to initiate the lifting of a limb, but once movement begins, it becomes easier for the muscle to continue the movement. The muscle must have enough strength not only to lift the weight of the limb but also to overcome inertia. For example, if you give assistance in the beginning of a weightlifting exercise, such as a straight-leg raise, the patient may be able to continue the exercise on his or her own once the motion has begun, provided that there is enough strength to lift the limb.

ACCELERATION AND MOMENTUM

Newton's second law of motion deals with **acceleration** and **momentum**. It states that the acceleration of an object is directly proportional to the force causing motion and inversely proportional to the mass of the object being moved. Momentum is the

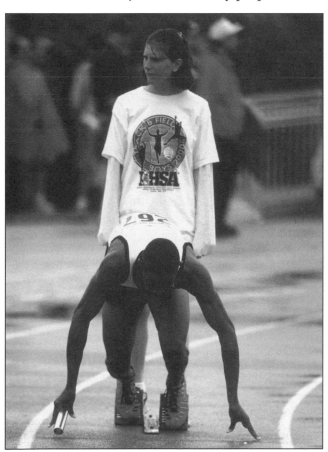
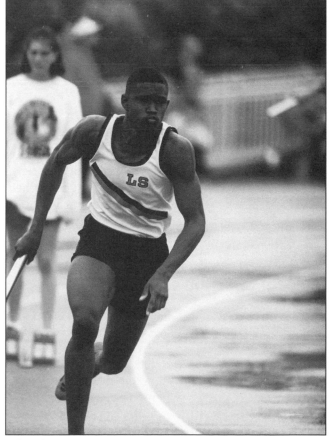

When starting and stopping motion, a runner must first overcome inertia.

amount of motion that a moving object has. The formulas used to calculate acceleration and momentum make it easy to understand:

$$\text{Momentum} = \text{mass} \times \text{velocity}$$

$$\text{Mass} = \text{weight}/\text{acceleration due to gravity}$$

$$\text{Linear velocity} = \text{distance}/\text{time}$$

This concept is important in therapeutic exercise because a slow, controlled motion of an extremity requires more strength than a quickly executed movement. If strength gain is the goal, it is better to have the patient move the extremity through the motion in a slow, controlled manner.

ACTION-REACTION

The force of gravity is commonly referred to as *weight*. If this force is counter-balanced, a body does not fall to the earth. This demonstrates **Newton's third law of motion**: An object reacts to a force with a force of equal magnitude in the opposite direction. Simply stated, for every action there is an opposite and equal reaction. Here are a couple of everyday applications of this law: If you hold a book in your hand, your muscle force counteracts the force of gravity and prevents the book from going to the ground. Another example is a patient's lying on a treatment table: The force of gravity on the patient is counterbalanced by the upward force of the treatment table.

Newton's Three Laws of Motion

Here is a summary of Newton's first three laws:

1. **Newton's first law of motion: inertia.** A body remains at a state of rest or remains in uniform motion until a force acts on it.
2. **Newton's second law of motion: acceleration and momentum.** The acceleration of an object is directly proportional to the force causing motion and inversely proportional to the mass of the object being moved.
3. **Newton's third law of motion: action-reaction.** For every action there is an equal and opposite reaction.

Let's consider the next step, what happens when a force that is stronger than gravity causes a body to move in the direction of that force. For example, a basketball being shot is propelled by a force strong enough to move the basketball up and toward the basket. The force must not only be applied with enough intensity to get the ball to the basket, but the force must be applied in the correct direction or angle to reach the target accurately. As another example, a volleyball player jumping to block at the net must produce enough force to overcome the force of gravity; the more force applied, the higher the volleyball player jumps. To perform a straight-leg raise, a patient must exert enough muscle force in the hip to counteract gravity's pull on the lower extremity.

CENTER OF GRAVITY

Center of gravity refers to the point in the body or object around which its weight is balanced. Knowing the center of gravity of a body or object can lead to understanding how to increase its stability.

Every object has a **center of gravity**. It is the point in the body or object around which its weight is balanced. If we look at a symmetrical, rigid pole, the center of gravity is easy to find; it is the point toward the middle at which the pole balances when suspended. Each body part, as well as the human body itself, has its own center of gravity, as noted in table 3.1. Knowing where the center of gravity is, is important for knowing where to apply force and how much force to apply to move or maintain a position.

In the human body, the center of gravity is harder to find because of the body's irregular shape. In the anatomic position, the center of gravity of the body is generally considered to be at about the level of the S2 vertebra. It is slightly higher in men

Table 3.1 Parts of the Human Body and Their Centers of Gravity

Body part(s)	Segmental weights and percentage of total body weight for 68-kg (150-lb) man			Location of center of gravity
	kg	lb	%	
Upper Limb (just above elbow joint)				
Head	4.7	10.3	6.9	In sphenoid sinus, 4 mm beyond anterior inferior margin of sella (on lateral surface, over temporal fossa, or on near nasion-inion line)
Head and neck	5.4	11.8	7.9	On inferior surface of basioccipital bone or within bone 23 ± 5 mm from crest of dorsum sellae (on lateral surface, 10 mm anterior to supratragic notch above head of mandible)
Head, neck, and trunk	40.1	88.5	59.0	Anterior to 11th thoracic vertebra
Lower limb (just above knee joint)				
Arm	1.9	4.1	2.7	In medial head of triceps, adjacent to radial groove; 5 mm proximal to distal end of deltoid insertion
Forearm	1.1	2.4	1.6	11 mm proximal to most distal part of pronator teres insertion; 9 mm anterior to interosseus membrane
Hand	0.4	0.9	0.6	Hand: (in rest position) On axis of metacarpal III, usually 2 mm deep to volar skin surface; 2 mm proximal to proximal transverse palmar skin crease, in angle between proximal transverse and radial longitudinal creases
Entire body (anterior to second sacral vertebra)				
Thigh	6.6	14.5	9.7	In adductor brevis muscle; 13 mm medial to linea aspera, deep to adductor canal, 29 mm below apex of femoral triangle and 18 mm proximal to most distal fibers of adductor brevis
Leg	3.1	6.8	4.5	35 mm below popliteus, at posterior part of posterior tibialis; 16 mm above proximal end of Achilles tendon, 8 mm posterior to interosseus membrane
Foot	1	2.1	1.4	In plantar ligaments, or just superficial in adjacent deep foot muscles; below proximal halves of second and third cuneiform bones; on a line between ankle joint center and ball of foot in plane of metatarsal II
Lower limb	10.6	23.4	15.6	
Leg and foot	4.1	9.0	6.0	

than in women and varies with individual variations in shape. It also is different in children, because their body-weight distribution is different from that of adults.

As the body or part of the body moves, the center of gravity changes, as seen in figure 3.1. When a sprinter is on the starter blocks, the center of gravity is much lower than when running. When a rhythmic gymnast reaches out to catch a baton, her center of gravity changes as the arm extends forward and the baton's weight is added to her body weight.

The center of gravity also changes when weight is added to the body. For example, if a track and field athlete picks up a 15.9-kg (35 lb) hammer in his left hand, his center of gravity shifts to that side. If a 91-kg (200 lb) weightlifter jerks a 68-kg (150 lb) barbell overhead, his center of gravity becomes significantly higher than vertebra S2; this is why some weightlifters have a difficult time stabilizing themselves in this maneuver.

The lower the center of gravity, the more stable the object. We see this commonly in athletics. For example, a football lineman protects himself from being pushed by an opponent by lowering his center of gravity.

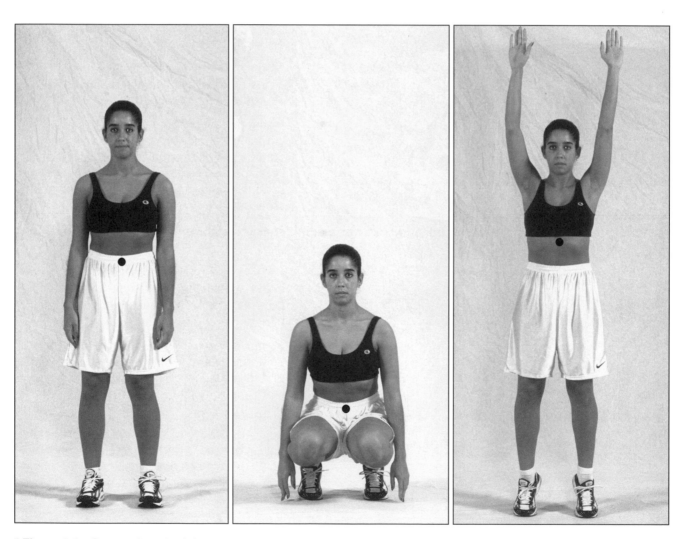

∎ **Figure 3.1**   Center of gravity (●) changes with changes in body position.

STABILITY AND FIXATION

Stability is a state in which a person or object is not easily thrown off balance. Fixation is a state of stabilization in which motion is restricted or prevented.

A number of factors determine a person's or object's **stability**. They all relate, however, to the relationship between the line of gravity and the base of support.

The **line of gravity** is an imaginary line that runs through the center of gravity toward the center of the earth. This line is used as a point of reference when discussing posture and is investigated in chapter 11. The line of gravity is also used to determine stability of an object. An object is most stable when the line of gravity falls within the object's base of support, as demonstrated in figure 3.2.

The **base of support**, simply referred to as the base, is the two-dimensional area between and including an object's points of contact with the supporting surface. As the example in figure 3.3 demonstrates, when you stand with your feet 15 cm (6 in.) apart, your base of support is the area of the surface that your feet contact and the area between your feet. If you spread your feet 46 cm (18 in.) apart, your base becomes larger.

STABILITY

An object is most stable when the line of gravity falls within the base of support. A person is stable when standing upright with the line of gravity within the base of support, but if the line of gravity falls outside of that base, it is difficult to maintain

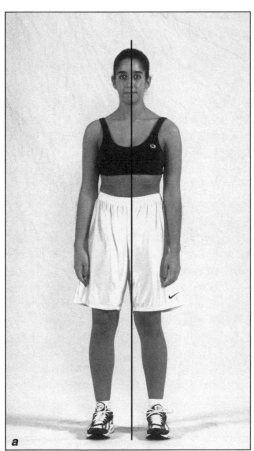
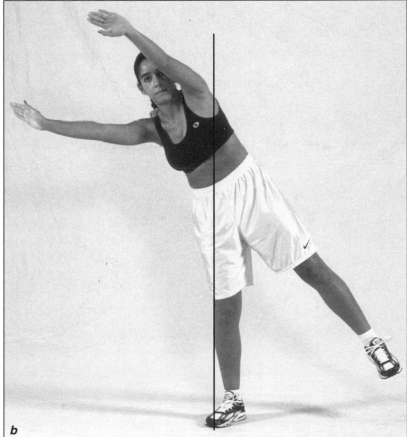

■ **Figure 3.2** Line of gravity must fall within the base of support for the object to be stable. The larger the base of support is, the more stable the object is. According to the description above, is this patient more stable in *(a)* or *(b)*?

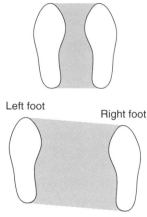

Figure 3.3 Base of support.

Left foot

Right foot

Normal stance

Larger base of support

Lateral force application →

Stance to increase stability from lateral force

↓ Force application

Stance to increase stability from anterior force

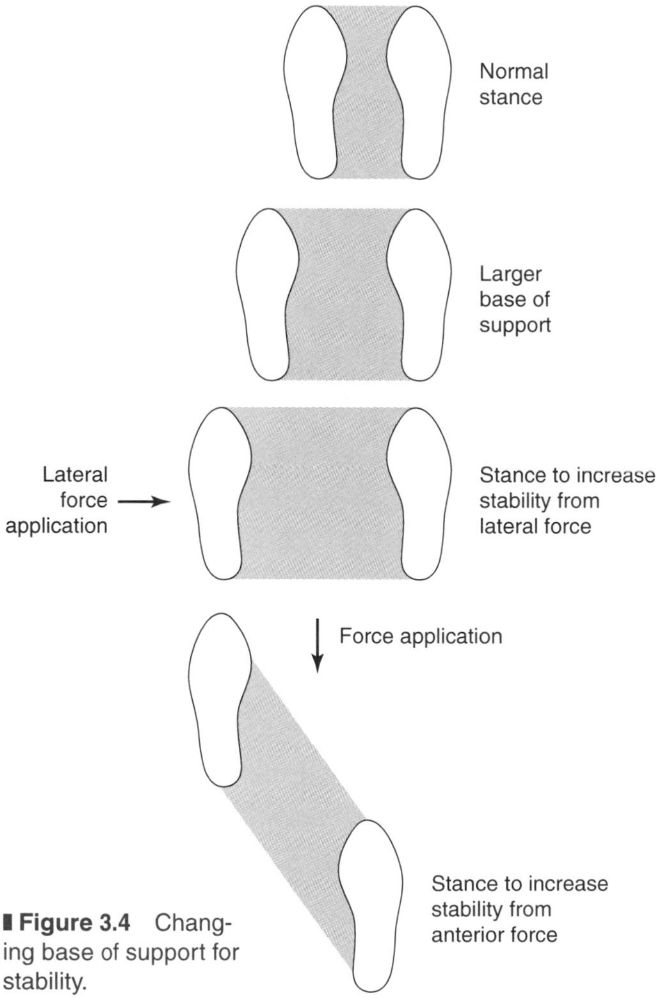

Figure 3.4 Changing base of support for stability.

balance. For the hammer thrower of the earlier example to maintain his balance while holding the hammer with his left hand, his center of gravity must remain inside his base of support. So what does he do to keep himself upright? He leans to the right to shift the center of gravity over his feet. The size and shape of the base of support also determines stability. The larger the base of support, the more stable the object. If you stand with your feet together, it is relatively easy for someone to push you over. If you spread your feet to give yourself a larger base of support, it is easier for you to maintain your stability and harder for someone to push you over.

The shape of the base can give additional support against external forces. A football lineman has more success in resisting an opponent's force if his feet are spread apart and in line with the direction of the oncoming player. In this position he is more likely to keep his center of gravity within his base of support and maintain stability. Most of us make these unconscious adjustments when we ride the bus or train while standing; we position our feet depending on our relation to the forward motion of the vehicle, either standing with feet side by side if we are standing sideways or positioning them in a tandem stance (one farther forward than the other) if we are facing forward, as shown in figure 3.4. In therapeutic exercise the shape and position of your base of support determines the ease with which you can provide manual resistance to a patient. For example, it is easier for you to provide manual resistance to a biceps curl while facing a seated patient if you position your feet in a forward-backward stance rather than a side-by-side stance.

FIXATION

Fixation is a state of stabilization in which motion is restricted or prevented. This condition is a degree of stability optimal for efficient muscle function and is also desirable in certain therapeutic exercise situations. Fixation can be produced by either active muscle contraction or application of an external force. In performing an arm curl, fixation of the upper arm allows movement of the lower arm to produce the desired goal of elbow flexion. When referring to the act of fixating a body segment to produce a desired motion, stabilization is the term often used, since the desired effect—stabilization—is the result of fixation of a body part.

Fixation is often needed in a therapeutic exercise to produce a desired result. If fixation of a body segment and stabilization of the body are not applied during exercise, substitution of unwanted muscles or muscle groups can result in exercising a muscle other than the one intended, and desired results are diminished. For example, when you give manual resistance to hip abductors for a side-lying patient, it is important that the hip is stabilized in a position to prevent the patient from using hip flexors during the exercise. On an isokinetic machine the thigh strap is the external fixator used to stabilize the leg and prevent the patient from using hip flexors to lift the leg when the knee is moved into extension.

A muscle can produce motion from either its proximal or distal attachment. One end of the muscle must be fixated to achieve a desired motion. For example, the upper trapezius can move its proximal end to produce cervical extension and rotation or its distal end to cause scapular and clavicular elevation. To provide the greatest cervical motion, the scapula must be stabilized, and to provide the best scapular elevation, the neck must be stabilized. This stabilization is usually performed by other muscles.

Using a muscle as a stabilizer to fixate a body segment can be one way of strengthening it, especially in the early stages of a therapeutic exercise program. For example, if injured abdominal muscles are too weak or painful to perform an abdominal curl, they may tolerate a straight-leg raise; the abdominals work to fixate the trunk during this activity but do not work as hard as they would in a trunk curl.

BODY LEVERS

A lever is a simple machine consisting of a rigid bar that rotates about a fulcrum. Levers are classified as first class, second class, or third class, depending on the relative positions of the fulcrum and the points where resistance and force are applied. Levers in the body can affect the force, speed, or distance of a movement.

A **lever** is a simple machine that contains a rigid bar and a fulcrum, or point of movement. The body moves through the function of its levers. It is important to know the types of levers since levers are used continually in therapeutic exercise to produce resistance or to enhance movement. You need to know about levers in the body and also how to apply external levers to provide the desired therapeutic results.

There are three classes of levers. Each lever, regardless of its classification, has three primary components (shown in figure 3.5): the force arm (and force point), the resistance arm (and resistance point), and the fulcrum. The fulcrum is the point at which the bar rotates. In the body, the fulcrum is the joint and the bar is the bone. The resistance point in the body's lever system is the center of gravity of the body part being moved. If an external object such as a weight is attached to the part, the center of gravity for that part, and thus the resistance point, changes. For example, the center of gravity for an average forearm and hand is approximately $3/_7$ the distance from the elbow to the fingertips. If the athlete grasps a weight in the hand, the center of gravity resistance point moves more distally. The resistance arm is the distance from the fulcrum to the resistance point. The force point is the point at which the force moving the lever is applied, and the force arm is the shortest distance from that point to the fulcrum. The generic term for resistance arm and force arm is lever arm. Two lever arms and a fulcrum comprise a lever system. The relationship among the positions of these components determines the class of lever that is being used.

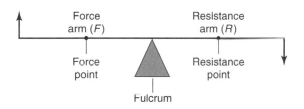

■ Figure 3.5 Basic lever system.

FIRST-CLASS LEVER

A **first-class lever** is one in which the fulcrum is located between the resistance and the force. A simple example is the seesaw. In the body an example of a first-class lever is the triceps, shown in figure 3.6: Its point of force is at its insertion on the olecranon, proximal to the joint, and the resistance force is at the center of gravity of the forearm, down the forearm $3/_7$ of the distance between the elbow and the fingertips.

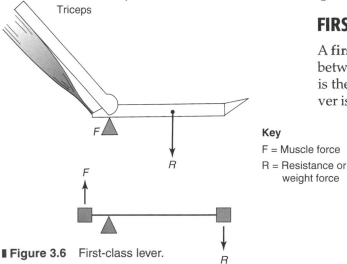

Key
F = Muscle force
R = Resistance or weight force

■ Figure 3.6 First-class lever.

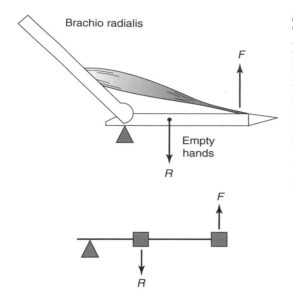

■ **Figure 3.7**   Second-class lever.

SECOND-CLASS LEVER

In a **second-class lever** the resistance point is between the fulcrum and the force. This class of lever always has a longer force arm than resistance arm. It is efficient in production of force, because the amount of force needed to move a resistance with this type of lever is always less than the resisting force. A typical example is the wheelbarrow. In the human body the brachioradialis, seen in figure 3.7, is an example of a second-class lever because it inserts on the forearm distal to the forearm's center of gravity.

THIRD-CLASS LEVER

A **third-class lever** has the force between the fulcrum and the resistance. This is an inefficient lever since the force arm is always shorter than the resistance arm, so more force is always required to move the resistance. Many of the levers in the body fall into this class. The elbow can once again be used as an example of this class of lever: As seen in figure 3.8, the biceps tendon inserts on the forearm between the elbow joint and the center of gravity of the forearm.

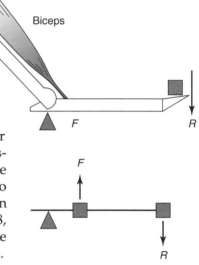

■ **Figure 3.8**   Third-class lever.

EFFECTS OF LEVERS

All these classes of levers determine the body's mechanical response. They can increase or decrease the forces produced, the speed of movement of a body part, and the range of motion of the joint. If one or more of these factors increases, the remaining factors decrease. Conversely, if one or more decreases, the others increase. Figure 3.9 shows two people of equal weight at opposite ends of a seesaw. If person A is 6 ft from the fulcrum and person B is 8 ft from the fulcrum, person B can exert more torque (discussed later in this chapter) than person A, and person A moves more slowly and over a shorter distance than person B.

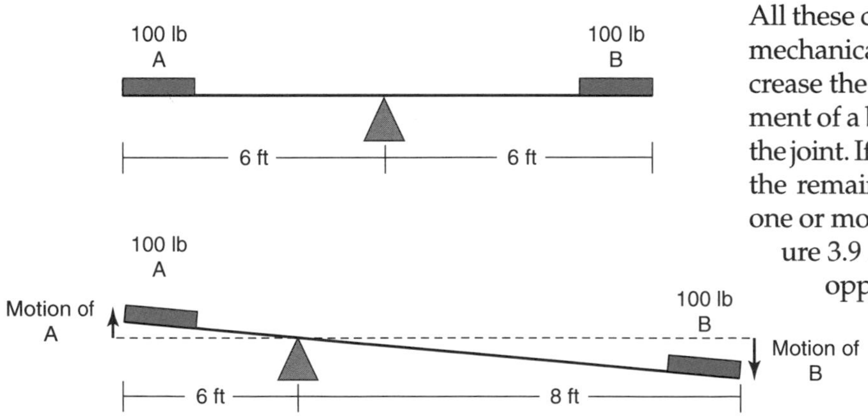

■ **Figure 3.9**   Second-class lever.

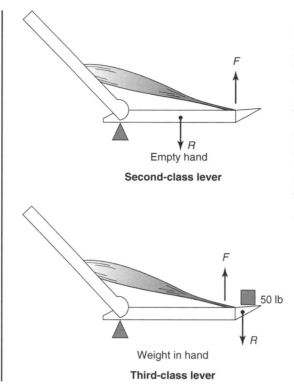

Second-class lever

Third-class lever

■ Figure 3.10 Changing from a second-class to a third-class lever.

Adapted from Groves and Camaione 1983.

Levers are classified according to the relative location of the fulcrum, force point, and resistance point. Sometimes when an outside resistance—such as a weight in a hand—is added, the class of lever changes. Recall that the brachioradialis is normally a second-class lever. If a weight is placed in the hand, however, as seen in figure 3.10, the center of gravity (resistance point) moves more distally and can change the brachioradialis from a second-class to a third-class lever.

LEVERS AND FORCE

The ability of a force to cause a rotational movement, or torque, is affected by the angle at which the force acts on a body part.

Linear motion is movement in a straight line, whereas **angular motion** is rotational movement through an arc. All joints in the body produce angular motion, but movement of the entire body through space is often linear. In other words, the rotational movement of the hips, knees, and ankles causes the body to move forward linearly, a motion known as walking.

TORQUE

The ability of a force to cause a rotational movement is referred to as **torque**. Torque is the product of the force and length of the force arm. Torque is commonly expressed in units such as newton-meters ($N \cdot m$), foot-pounds (ft-lb), or inch-pounds (in.-lb).

An increase in the length of the lever arm increases the torque produced by a force. For example, if you apply manual resistance at the thigh to a straight-leg raise, your torque is less (or you have to produce more force for the same torque) than if you positioned your hand at the ankle. With your hand at the ankle, your effort is less for the same torque because your lever arm is longer. If a patient has a difficult time performing a straight-leg raise against gravity, bending the knee to shorten the leg's resistance arm length may permit the patient to lift the leg without assistance.

Torque can also be altered by changing the force. Placing a 4.5 kg (10 lb) weight on an ankle produces twice as much torque as a 2.25 kg (5 lb) weight on a knee-extension exercise.

As a joint goes through its range of motion, a muscle's torque changes. This is related in part to the change in the muscle's line of pull and the angle of pull.

LINE OF PULL

The **line of pull** of the muscle is the long axis of the muscle. The **angle of pull** is between the long axis of the bone (lever arm) and the line of pull of the muscle. The

Key

A = Direction of biceps force
B = Angle of pull

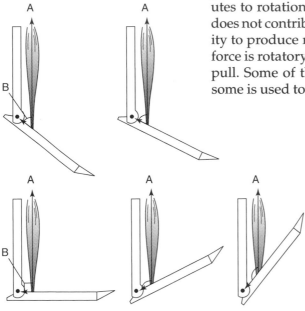

angle of pull changes as the joint goes through its range of motion. As demonstrated in figure 3.11, the maximal amount of torque is produced when the angle of pull of the muscle is 90°. As the muscle's angle of pull increases or decreases from 90°, the part of the force that contributes to rotational motion (rotatory force) decreases, and the part that does not contribute to rotation (nonrotatory force) increases, so the ability to produce rotational motion—or torque—diminishes. How much force is rotatory and how much is nonrotatory depends on the angle of pull. Some of the nonrotatory force is used to stabilize the joint, and some is used to produce a dislocating force, depending on the angle of pull. The farther the angle of pull is from 90°, the more force is used to stabilize or destabilize the joint. For example, the biceps, seen in figure 3.12, has a nonrotatory force component that is pushing the ulna into the elbow and provides stability to the joint. It also has a rotatory component causing the forearm to move through its arc of motion. In therapeutic exercise the mechanics of each joint and the angle of pull of the muscles surrounding the joint should be appreciated. A recently dislocated shoulder, for example, should not be placed in positions that encourage surrounding muscle to destabilize it. For this reason, early rehabilitation of this condition warrants avoiding overhead or full-external-rotation positions.

■ **Figure 3.11** The angle of pull changes as range of motion changes. The most rotatory force occurs when the muscle's angle of pull is 90°.

Adapted from Groves and Camaione 1983.

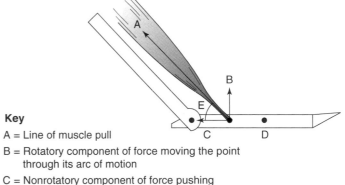

Key

A = Line of muscle pull

B = Rotatory component of force moving the point through its arc of motion

C = Nonrotatory component of force pushing the ulna into the elbow

D = Resistance point (center of mass of forearm)

E = Angle of pull

■ **Figure 3.12** Rotatory and nonrotatory components of force.

Adapted from Groves and Camaione 1983.

ANGLE OF PULL

Angle of pull of a muscle is an important concept in therapeutic exercise. If you want to produce the maximal torque from a muscle, the joint must be positioned so that the muscle being worked has a 90° angle of pull on the extremity.

This concept also works for external forces applied to the body. With pulleys, the maximal resistance occurs when the angle of pull of the pulley's rope is 90° to the extremity being resisted, as shown in figure 3.13. With free weights, the maximal resistance occurs when the pull of the weight is perpendicular

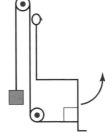
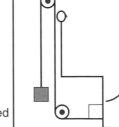

■ **Figure 3.13** With this pulley arrangement, the greatest resistance is produced at 90° knee flexion.

Key

B = Weight in hand
A = Resistance lever
     arm length

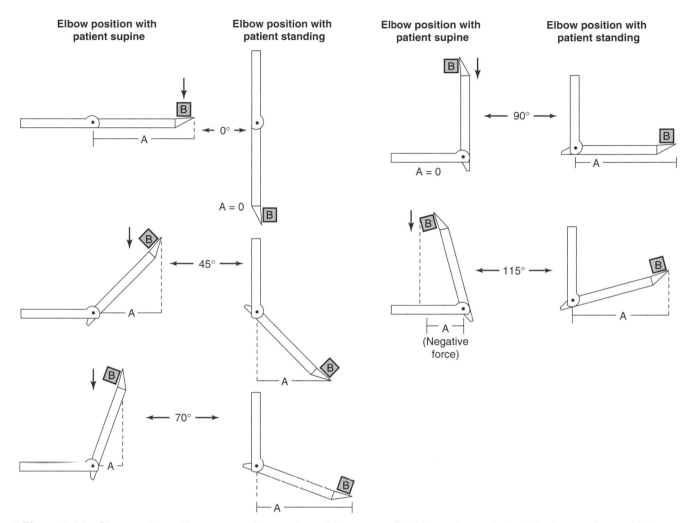

Elbow position with patient supine

Elbow position with patient standing

Elbow position with patient supine

Elbow position with patient standing

0°

A = 0

45°

70°

90°

A = 0

115°

A (Negative force)

■ **Figure 3.14**   Changes in position causes changes in resistance arm. Resistance is greatest at 0° when supine and 90° when standing.

to the ground regardless of the extremity's position. For example, when a patient performs elbow flexion with a weight, the greatest resistance is at the start of the motion if the patient is supine, when the patient's elbow goes from full extension to flexion , as seen in figure 3.14. If the patient is standing or sitting, however, the maximal resistance from the weight is when the elbow is at 90°.

PHYSIOLOGICAL MUSCLE ADVANTAGES

A muscle's ability to shorten is its physiological advantage. A two-joint muscle will have a better physiological advantage when it is placed on stretch at one joint while it is moving the other.

What we have been discussing thus far is the mechanical advantage of muscles, which relates to the angle of pull of the muscles and the amount of resistance a muscle must overcome to produce motion. **Physiological advantage** is a muscle's ability to shorten. This is an important functional concept in therapeutic exercise. A muscle has the most physiological advantage when it is at its resting length. The resting length of a muscle is the length to which a muscle can be lengthened in a relaxed condition without producing tension or any additional stretch. For example,

Key

A = Combination of stretch of connective tissue and muscle elasticity
B = Active tension of muscle fiber as it is stretched
C = Passive stretch of connective tissue

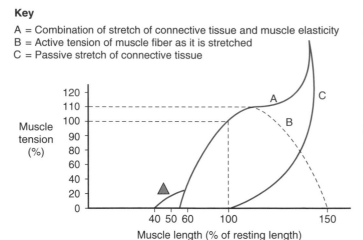

Figure 3.15 Physiological advantage of muscles.

the greatest physiological advantage of the brachialis is with the elbow in full extension, and the greatest physiological advantage for the soleus is with the ankle in dorsiflexion.

As a muscle shortens, its physiological advantage becomes progressively less until it is unable to produce a force, as illustrated in figure 3.15. A muscle shortens to no less than about 50% of its resting length. At that point, all the muscle's energy is used to shorten it, so no external force can be exerted.

MULTIJOINT MUSCLES

If a two-joint or multijoint muscle is to be worked, its position at the inactive joint is important for it to work optimally at the injured joint. For example, when you want to maximize efforts of the hamstrings during an exercise, the best position for the patient is sitting. If the patient is prone, the hamstrings are already shortened at the hip and will be unable to fully contract at the knee. When you want to produce as much force from a two-joint muscle as possible, the muscle should be placed on stretch at one joint as it moves the other joint. This permits all its available physiological length to be used at the desired site. When working with the finger flexors and other multijoint muscles, care must be taken to stabilize the multiple joints they cross when attempting to isolate their activity.

SUMMATION OF FORCES

Summation of forces is especially important during the functional rehabilitation phase of a therapeutic exercise program. The **summation of forces** is a sequence of movements timed so that each movement contributes to the next movement to produce a desired outcome. For the summation of forces to be successful, the forces from each part must be correctly timed, and each successive joint from which the activity occurs must be stabilized. This is more easily understood with an example: A baseball pitcher goes through a series of sequential movements starting with the hips, progressing to the trunk, then the shoulder, the elbow, and finally the wrist and hand. Acceleration of the ball is produced by a series of rotations and extensions in each of the joints. If a ball is tossed with movement only from the wrist, it does not go as far as when it is thrown correctly using a summation of forces from all body segments. Even using only the upper extremity and not the hips and trunk produces a far less effective throw than a full summation of forces. The forces applied by the muscles in each of the joints must be precisely timed to build on the previous forces. If correct timing does not occur, the pitcher ends up using forces primarily from the arm, not the hip and trunk, and risks injury to the shoulder or elbow.

For summation of forces to occur, each joint must be stabilized by the previous joint. If this does not occur, the transfer of forces generated fails. Once a joint's desired motion is produced and the muscle's forces have been transmitted, the joint must be stabilized by a static contraction of the muscles for summation to occur. If the pitcher does not have good hip strength for stabilizing the hip and back during pitching, the pitch will be weak and demand higher forces from the upper extremity to compensate for the hip's weakness. This example not only demonstrates summation of forces but also points out the importance of two concepts in therapeutic exercise: (1) maintaining normal parameters in uninjured parts and (2) achieving normal parameters of factors, including strength, before functional activities can be resumed.

OTHER CONCEPTS IN PHYSICS

Other concepts that relate to movement and the way the body responds to force include strength, work, power, energy, velocity, acceleration, elasticity, stress, strain, creep, structural fatigue, and friction.

Many physics terms have been used in this chapter. To improve your understanding and because these terms are used in later chapters, terms that are commonly used in therapeutic exercise and rehabilitation programs are defined here.

STRENGTH

Strength is a muscle's relative ability to resist or produce a force. The greater the strength, the greater the ability to produce a force. The muscle's angle of pull, the angle of the resisting force, the muscle's length, and the speed of contraction and movement are factors that determine a muscle's strength.

The measure of a muscle's strength varies, depending on these factors and also on the method of measurement used. Using free weights to determine strength assesses the strength of the muscle at its weakest point in the range of motion. For example, if a patient is able to perform a forearm curl with 14 kg (30 lb), this is the weight that the forearm flexors are able to lift at their weakest point. Although the weight of the dumbbell does not change as the forearm goes through its range of motion, the muscles' strength changes with the changing angles of pull and lever-arm lengths of the muscles and dumbbell and the changing physiological length of the muscles.

Using an isometric contraction evaluates the muscle's strength only at the specific joint position tested. The quantity of strength produced in an isometric contraction changes as the joint is positioned differently in its range of motion because of the changes in the muscle's lever-arm length, angle of pull, and physiological length. A more complete discussion of strength can be found in chapter 7.

WORK

Work is the product of the amount of force (F) and the distance (d) through which the force is applied:

$$W = Fd$$

Work is measured in foot-pounds (ft-lb) in the English system and joules (1 J = 1 N · m) in the metric system. If you lift a 20 lb (89 N) weight from the floor to a shelf 6 ft (1.8 m) above the floor, you would do 120 ft-lb (about 160 J) of work (6 ft × 20 lb, or 89 N × 1.8 m). When a weightlifter lifts a 250 lb (1112.5 N) barbell overhead to a height of 6.5 ft (2 m), he produces 1625 ft-lb (2225 J) of work.

POWER

Power is the work per unit of time, or how fast the work is produced:

$$P = Fd/t$$

Work is done regardless of how much time it takes to perform the work. Power is a measure of the work done in a specific amount of time. In the English system it is measured in foot-pounds per second or in horsepower (1 horsepower = 550 ft-lb/s). In the metric system it is measured in joules per second or newton-meters per second. Power is sometimes inaccurately interchanged with force.

In sports the most frequently used tests for power include the standing vertical jump and the softball throw. These activities require a sudden contraction of muscles to move the body or object in a short amount of time, thus generating a large force and great power.

Power requires strength to produce the force necessary to perform an activity and neuromuscular control to contract the muscles rapidly. The proprioception and functional aspects of therapeutic exercise programs for patients involved in sports that should include power activities. Power training is sport specific and requires you to understand the requirements of the athlete's sport.

ENERGY

Energy is the capacity to do work. There are different types of energy. The law of conservation of energy states that energy can neither be created nor destroyed. Energy can, however, be converted from one form to another. For example, when a volleyball player serves the ball, some of the mechanical energy is converted to sound energy, but no energy is lost.

In sports and sport rehabilitation the two energy classifications that we are interested in are potential energy and kinetic energy. Potential energy and kinetic energy are often converted from one to the other. **Potential energy** is the capacity to do work that is stored in a body. **Kinetic energy** is the energy a body has because of its motion. When a moving body stops, the kinetic energy is all converted to potential energy. It is important in sports to absorb this energy in a way that prevents injury. For example, when a gymnast dismounts from the high bar, he bends his knees to absorb the kinetic energy. When a patient performs plyometrics in the final stages of the therapeutic exercise program, the patient should move to safely absorb the kinetic energy produced by the movements in the exercise.

VELOCITY

Velocity is the rate of change of position. It is expressed in miles per hour (mph), feet per second (ft/s), or meters per second (m/s). *Velocity* is often interchanged with *speed*, which is not entirely accurate, but in most instances the difference is inconsequential. We use velocity to assess how well a sprinter runs the 100 m or how well a basketball player can get to the other end of the court on a fast break. Part of the functional assessment before allowing an injured athlete to return to activity may include an evaluation of the athlete's velocity in functional sport activities.

ACCELERATION

Acceleration is the rate at which velocity changes. It is expressed in feet per second per second (ft/s^2) or meters per second per second (m/s^2). A sprinter coming out of the blocks at the start of a race accelerates, increasing velocity as she continues. In the final stages of a therapeutic exercise program, it is important for you to work on acceleration activities with injured athletes in sports in which acceleration is a factor. The therapeutic exercise program for an injured sprinter needs to include explosive strength development in the starting positions of hip flexion and knee flexion if the sprinter is to have the acceleration necessary to get out of the starting blocks as well as possible.

Negative acceleration is called **deceleration**, the process of an object's slowing down rather than speeding up. After a baseball is pitched, the pitcher's arm goes from sudden acceleration to deceleration until the arm stops moving. It is the follow-through on an activity that provides as smooth a transition as possible from acceleration to deceleration. Poor follow-through increases the risk of injury because of the more rapid change from acceleration to deceleration. This is an important concept to recall in the final stages of the therapeutic exercise program, when sport-specific activities are part of the program.

Gravity provides a constant acceleration of 9.8 m/s² (32 ft/s²). In other words, every second that an object falls it moves 9.8 m/s (32 ft/s) faster than it did in the previous second. If you drop a golf ball from a sufficient height, after the first second it falls at a velocity of 9.8 m/s (32 ft/s). After the next second it falls at a velocity of 19.6 m/s (64 ft/s), and after the third second it has a velocity of 29.4 m/s (96 ft/s). As Galileo discovered during the late 1500s when he dropped objects from the Tower of Pisa, this occurs regardless of the object's weight if the effect of air resistance is disregarded. If you drop a Ping-Pong ball from the same height as the golf ball, its acceleration will be the same as the golf ball. If you let them drop at the same time, they will hit the floor at the same time.

Conversely, a diver who jumps off a 3-m board will not hit the water at as great a speed as one who jumps off a 10-m board. Their acceleration is the same, but the diver from the 3-m board has a shorter distance to go before hitting the water; therefore, the time during which he accelerates is shorter, so his velocity by the time he hits the water is less than that of the 10-m diver.

ELASTICITY

Elasticity is the ability of an object to resume its former shape after a deforming or distorting force is applied. A muscle has elasticity because it can be stretched but returns to its normal length when the deforming force is discontinued. Rubber tubing or bands used in therapeutic exercise have a lot of elasticity. Steel has elasticity but less than asphalt. Ligaments have more elasticity than bone but less than muscles.

STRESS AND STRAIN

Stress is a force that changes the form or shape of a body. **Strain** is the amount of change in the size or shape of the object caused by the stress. **Hooke's law**, developed during the 1600s by the physicist and mathematician Robert Hooke, deals with the relationship of stress and strain to elasticity: The strain is proportional to the stress producing it (so long as the strain is not too great—once the elastic limit is exceeded, permanent deformation occurs).

This concept is demonstrated in figure 3.16. The *OA* curve segment represents the elastic range. If a load is released in this range of the stress-strain curve, the object returns to its normal length. *A* is called the elastic limit, beyond which Hooke's law is no longer valid. Beyond the elastic range is the plastic range *AM*. When a load stresses an object into this range, a permanent change in the object's size or shape occurs. Any load that goes beyond the plastic range ultimately causes a failure of the object, *F*.

The size of these ranges varies from material to material and from structure to structure. In sports medicine it is important to realize the differences in the stress-strain curves of structures such as bone, muscle, tendons, cartilage, and ligaments. This knowledge is important in prevention and treatment of injuries. Some ligaments contain more elastic fibers than others, so they can withstand more stress, whereas others have fewer elastic fibers and provide more stability to a joint. Recently formed scar tissue has more elasticity than more mature scar tissue.

Key

A = Elastic limit
Y = Yield point
0A = Elastic range
M = Maximum strength
AM = Plastic range
F = Failure point

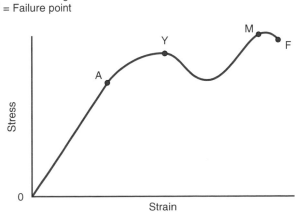

■ **Figure 3.16** Stress-strain curve.

Knowing the maturity of scar tissue determines the amount of stress and the length of time the stress should be applied to effect a change in the scar tissue's size.

CREEP

Creep occurs when a low-level stress, usually in the elastic range of the tissue, is applied over a long enough period of time to cause a deformation of the tissue. Increasing the temperature of the tissue increases the rate of creep. For this reason, applying heat to an area before stretching may make the stretch more effective. This concept also indicates that longer stretches produce better results. It also demonstrates why poor posture over time causes changes in the muscles, joints, and connective tissue; sitting with your head forward for a prolonged period of time as you read this book will cause the ligaments and muscles of your posterior neck and upper back to lengthen, making it ultimately more difficult to resume a proper posture. Over time and with repetition of this position, permanent changes in tissue length result.

STRUCTURAL FATIGUE

All tissues and objects are subject to structural fatigue. **Structural fatigue** is the point at which a tissue or object can no longer withstand a stress, and breaks. This can occur in a sudden movement, as when a ligament is suddenly stressed and torn, or it can occur over time with an accumulation of stress. The point at which tissue failure results from long-term stress is sometimes referred to as the **endurance limit** or **fatigue failure**. Breakdown of bone from cumulative trauma is called a stress fracture. Injuries caused by repeated stress, such as carpal tunnel syndrome, are called repetitive stress syndromes or overuse syndromes. Treatment of cumulative-trauma injuries is different from that of acute-trauma injuries and is discussed more thoroughly in chapter 15.

FRICTION

Friction is the relative resistance between two surfaces. It can be advantageous or deleterious, depending on the circumstances. A patient who is very weak and unable to abduct the thigh while lying supine because of friction of the leg against the treatment table may be able to perform the motion if the surface is made smoother by applying a friction-reducing agent such as talcum powder.

Standing with a wide base of support, with the feet wider than the hips, stabilizes the body but requires friction. If a person takes that same stance on ice, he or she will fall because ice provides less friction than many other surfaces.

Sometimes we want to increase friction to obtain more traction and apply more force. Cleats on football shoes or tread on basketball shoes are good examples of this. When decreasing friction is desirable, such as on the uneven parallel bars in gymnastics, substances such as chalk are used to reduce friction and the chance of blisters.

In therapeutic exercise, friction may not be desirable in pulley exercises because it wears out the system more quickly and makes exercises more difficult. On the other hand, it may be advantageous to have more friction to increase resistance in other exercises. For example, an exercise to work the hamstrings is a rolling stool sitting on it and propelling it with one foot while seated on it, as in figure 3.17a. If a patient can propel the stool without much difficulty, you can attach a weight that is dragged behind the stool; the increased friction as well as the added weight provide more resistance to the movement (figure 3.17b).

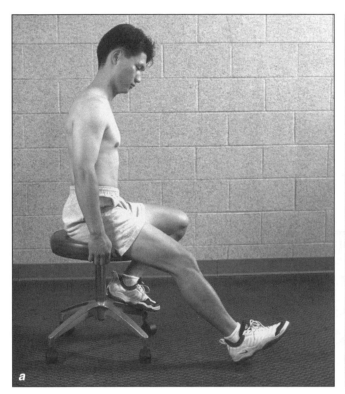 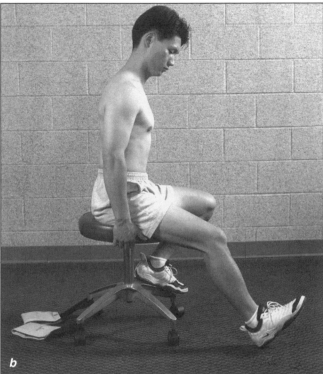

■ Figure 3.17 Use of friction in therapeutic exercise.

SUMMARY

1. *Define force and give an example of an internal and an external force.*

   Force is energy that causes movement and has direction and magnitude. Internal forces are generated by muscles. An example of an external force is gravity.

2. *Explain the relevance to therapeutic exercise of Newton's first, second, and third laws of motion.*

   Newton's first law of motion deals with inertia, the second law of motion deals with acceleration and momentum, and the third law of motion concerns action and reaction. All these laws govern how the body moves and reacts to forces that are applied to it.

3. *Explain how center of gravity changes with movement.*

   The body's center of gravity becomes higher if the arms are raised overhead and lower if the body crouches. If a weight is carried at the side, the center of gravity shifts to the side with the weight; to maintain balance and keep the center of gravity over the feet, the body must lean away from the weight.

4. *Discuss how a change in base of support can change a person's stability.*

   The narrower the base of support, the less stable is the object, and the wider the base of support, the more stable it is.

5. *Explain the relationship between line of gravity and base of support.*

   An object is stable when the line of gravity is within its base of support.

6. *Explain two ways of increasing stability.*

   A person can increase stability by placing the feet in the direction of the force being applied or lowering the center of gravity while keeping it within the base of support.

7. *Identify the difference between stability and fixation.*

   Stability is a state in which a person or object is not easily thrown off balance. Fixation is a state of stability where motion is being restricted or prevented. When referring to the act of fixating a body segment to produce a desired motion, stabilization is the term often used, since the desired effect, stabilization, is the result of fixation.

8. *Explain how torque can be altered in the body.*

   Torque produced by the body can be altered most easily by changing the force-arm length, the force applied, or the angle of pull.

9. *Identify how varying position changes a muscle's mechanical advantage.*

   As a joint moves through its range of motion, the angle of pull of a muscle changes, altering the length of the muscle's lever arm, which changes its mechanical advantage.

10. *Discuss the difference between mechanical and physiological advantage of a muscle.*

    A muscle's mechanical advantage has to do with its line and angle of pull and the forces it must produce or overcome, while the physiological advantage is the muscle's ability to shorten.

11. *Explain the importance of positioning in exercising two-joint muscles.*

    The ability of a muscle that crosses two joints to produce force is affected by its relative length at both joints. A muscle is able to shorten to no less than 50% of its resting length, so its position at one joint affects its ability to produce force at the other joint.

12. *Distinguish between velocity and acceleration.*

    Velocity is the rate of change of position, whereas acceleration is the rate at which velocity changes.

13. *Discuss the relevance of elasticity, stress and strain, creep, and friction to therapeutic exercise.*

    Elasticity, stress and strain, and creep are all qualities that affect a tissue's ability to change its length or shape. These factors influence the type of stretch that is applied to a structure and the effectiveness of that stretch. Friction can be advantageous or detrimental, depending on the exercise and its goal.

CRITICAL THINKING QUESTIONS

1. Explain how Newton's first three laws of motion and gravity affect therapeutic exercise programs. In other words, how do inertia, acceleration, action-reaction, and gravity determine how you have a patient perform an exercise?

2. Using the concepts about base of support discussed in this chapter, describe how you can improve your base of support while giving manual resistance to hip flexion and extension on a patient who is supine. Use a partner and try the changes in your base of support to demonstrate how those changes give you an advantage or disadvantage in the manual-resistance exercise.

3. Explain how the different classes of levers apply to therapeutic exercise. Give an example of each class of lever with a different therapeutic exercise, and explain how the class of lever can change with a change in the exercise position or resistance application.

4. Describe how an elbow-flexion exercise changes when the technique or equipment used is manual resistance, rubber banding, pulley, dumbbell, weight machine, and hydraulic machine. Does the type of resistance change? What about the kind of muscle activity? What advantage of each exercise makes it different from the others?

5. In what position would you put a patient to provide maximal muscle shortening during an exercise for the hamstring? In what position should the patient be to maximize hamstring activity at the knee? at the hip?

6. Throw a ball as far as you can while standing on one foot and then with both feet on the ground. In which position are you able to throw the ball farther? What mechanical concepts come into play here?

SUGGESTED READING

Brunnstrom, S., Lehmkuhl, L.D., and L.K. Smith. 1983. *Clinical kinesiology.* Philadelphia: Davis.

Cornwall, M.W. 1984. Biomechanics of noncontractile tissue. *Physical Therapy* 64:1869–1873.

Dumbelton, J.H., and J. Black. 1975. *An introduction to orthopedic materials.* Springfield, IL: Charles C Thomas.

Frankel, V.H., and M. Nordin. 1980. *Basic biomechanics of the skeletal system.* Philadelphia: Lea & Febiger.

Frost, H.M. 1973. *Orthopedic biomechanics.* Springfield, IL: Charles C Thomas.

Gardiner, M.D. 1981. *The principles of exercise therapy.* London: Bell.

Groves, R., and D.N. Camaione. 1983. *Concepts in kinesiology.* Philadelphia: Saunders.

Luttgens, K., and N. Hamilton. 1998. *Kinesiology: Scientific basis of human motion.* 9th ed. Boston: McGraw-Hill.

Rasch, P.J., ed. 1989. *Kinesiology and applied anatomy.* Philadelphia: Lea & Febiger.

Strauss, R.H., ed. 1979. *Sports medicine and physiology.* Philadelphia: Saunders.

Wilmore, J.H., and D.L. Costill. 1994. *Physiology of sport and exercise.* Champaign, IL: Human Kinetics.

CHAPTER FOUR

Evaluation and Assessment

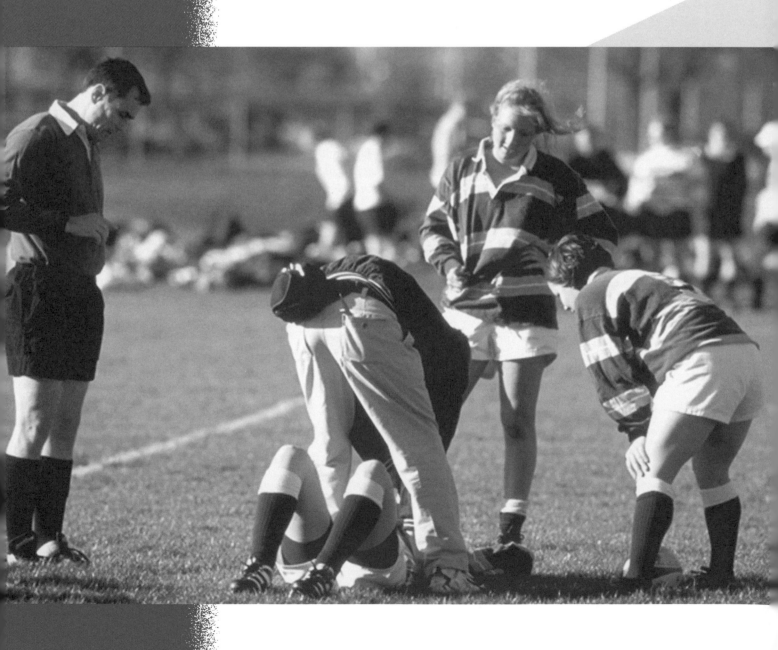

OBJECTIVES

After completing this chapter, you should be able to do the following:

1. Identify the primary factors of subjective evaluation.

2. Outline an objective evaluation procedure that includes all primary factors.

3. Explain the different types of end-feel and distinguish between normal and pathological end-feels.

4. Explain how a treatment plan is designed and upon what factors it is based.

5. Define the SOAP note and explain its significance to rehabilitation.

6. Identify two other records used in rehabilitation and demonstrate their importance.

Joan Stevenson instructs incoming athletic training students on the evaluation procedure for rehabilitation. She has found in the past that the students' primary point of confusion is identifying the difference between evaluation of an acute injury for first aid and evaluation of an injury for rehabilitation. Instruction with the new class begins today. Her first goal is to identify the differences between an acute-injury evaluation and a rehabilitation evaluation. She will then itemize the procedures for a rehabilitation evaluation, explain how to identify the patient's problems, how to base goals on those problems, and how to develop a plan of treatment based on the problems and goals.

Although many of the students have been exposed to record keeping for initial injuries in the athletic training clinic, few of them know the record-keeping procedures for rehabilitation. Some of them have seen SOAP notes during their observations in their freshman year, but not many of them understand what they are and how they function. In addition to SOAP notes, Joan will introduce students to the other records used in rehabilitation. Many new students are overwhelmed with their first sight of what seems like a mountain of paperwork, but Joan knows from experience that the paperwork becomes routine and is not the insurmountable task students initially think it to be.

A doctor who cannot take a good history and a patient who cannot give one are in danger of giving and receiving bad treatment.

Paul Dudley White, U.S. physician, 1886–1973

Assessment and evaluation of an injury serve as the foundation for a treatment program. For the sport rehabilitation specialist to design the most appropriate therapeutic exercise program, the patient must first be evaluated. Without an evaluation to know where deficiencies lie, the extent of the injury, and other factors that may affect a therapeutic exercise program, the sport rehabilitation specialist has no basis on which to decide what should or should not be incorporated in the rehabilitation program. The term *evaluation* is commonly replaced with *examination*. Although either term would suffice, this text uses **evaluation** to indicate the means by which a sport rehabilitation specialist seeks information on the severity, irritability, nature, and stage of a patient's injury. The evaluation is composed of subjective and objective elements. The **subjective evaluation** is the history of the injury and the patient's experience of pain and other symptoms. It is obtained from the patient and serves to guide the objective portion of the assessment. The **objective evaluation** discovers the observable signs and effects of the injury and involves observing, testing, and palpating the injury. The results of the subjective and objective evaluations allow the sport rehabilitation specialist to assess the patient's injury and determine the most appropriate treatment for achieving whatever goals are established for the patient. An **assessment** is a conclusion based on the gathering of information. At the time of an initial evaluation, assessment is used to design a therapeutic exercise program. Once the program has been instituted, the results of the treatment are evaluated to assess the treatment's effectiveness. Finally, before the patient returns to full sport participation, the patient is evaluated and his or her readiness and ability to perform and withstand the stresses of the sport are assessed. In short, an evaluation, or examination, must precede an assessment, and both are required not only at the commencement and conclusion of a rehabilitation program, but frequently throughout the program as well.

This chapter is divided into three parts. The first part deals with subjective and objective aspects of evaluation, the second part discusses assessments that are based on the evaluations, and the third part introduces records of these evaluations and assessments that should be kept throughout the rehabilitation process. This chapter concludes the presentation of the basic concepts needed to understand the whys of therapeutic exercise.

EVALUATION: MAKING A PROFILE

Information from the patient regarding the history of the injury and subjective symptoms is gathered during the subjective evaluation. The objective evaluation involves inspecting, palpating, and testing to determine the extent and severity of the injury.

The first part of performing an initial evaluation to determine the extent and involvement of the injury, the patient's deficiencies, and a course of treatment is to create a profile of the injury. This is accomplished by performing a subjective and an objective evaluation.

It is important to take an accurate and complete history before the objective evaluation. As Dr. White indicated in the opening quotation of this chapter, a complete and accurate exchange of information between the injured individual and the examiner is crucial to a successful treatment program. A history is only as good as the questions asked. If you expect a thorough history from the patient, you must ask questions that will reveal all that is necessary to obtain a complete picture.

Once the subjective evaluation is made, an objective evaluation follows. This includes observations of abnormalities, palpation, and measurements of deficiencies in range of motion, strength, proprioception, and other parameters, which provide you with a clear picture of problems. A treatment program cannot be planned and delivered until you identify and assess the problems and deficiencies that the injury has caused. Problems are identified by thorough and accurate subjective and objective evaluations.

SUBJECTIVE EVALUATION

The subjective evaluation is essentially the history of the injury and patient's report of pain and other symptoms. The subjective evaluation can assist in determining the extent of the injury, how aggressively the objective evaluation can be performed, and what to include in the objective evaluation. The specific questions to ask during the history vary, depending on a variety of factors such as the area injured and the severity and nature of the injury.

To obtain a thorough and accurate history, it is best to ask questions that do not lead the patient to an anticipated answer. For example, rather than ask, "Is it painful to walk?" a better question is, "What activities cause you more pain?"

The questions should be simple and straightforward. They should be presented in a logical and systematic sequence. It is best for each sport rehabilitation specialist to develop his or her own method or system of sequential questions that is consistent and easy to remember. This is not to say that the questions should be rigid and unchanging, because each patient's history is different, so the line of questioning will be different in each situation. The idea is to make history-taking procedures a habit that results in a consistent overall profile. When you first start out, you may need to write questions down to establish a routine for yourself, but listening to patients' responses and taking a logical and thorough history will become more automatic with experience.

History of the Injury

Allow the patient to explain in his or her own words how the injury occurred. The goal is to get an idea of the mechanism of injury, tissues involved, and extent of involvement. The patient should tell when the injury occurred, whether it occurred suddenly or gradually, immediate signs and signs that occurred later (e.g., immediate swelling or swelling only 24 h later), and what treatment has been provided. The patient should also say whether he or she was able to continue sport participation, if the injured part remained functional (e.g., was the patient able to walk?), and what, if anything, has changed between the time of the injury and the time of your examination. Information of this type can help you determine the severity of the injury and the tissue type involved. Knowing whether ice or heat has been applied may change your impression of the injury. The involved area may be very swollen because no treatment was given, heat was applied, or the patient swells easily. If the patient has taken medication, it may mask pain or change the results of the tests you perform.

Medical History

Getting a medical history of previous injury to the area is also crucial. If a prior injury has occurred, it is important to know previous treatments. Did the patient seek medical care? Did the patient receive treatment, and if so, what treatment was given, how long was it provided, and what was the outcome? How many subsequent injury episodes has the patient experienced? Is the pain the same this time as it was in the past?

Recurring episodes may affect your assessment of the current problem and the treatment program you establish. For example, recurring ankle sprains may result in additional scar tissue in or around the joint, restricted soft-tissue mobility, reduced strength and proprioceptive abilities, or increased laxity and instability of the joint. Repeated muscle strains may cause tendinitis. Recurring knee meniscus lesions may lead to chronic synovitis. Over the long term, repetitive injuries to a joint may result in arthritis.

In the case of prior injuries, a report of the previous treatments provided is necessary to get a picture of prior injury management. Good management may have minimized previous injuries and left the patient with a good impression of rehabilitation, but poor management may prejudice the patient into having little confidence in rehabilitation outcomes and may also complicate the current picture. For example, if a patient presents with a knee injury and a history of prior similar injuries that were not treated, the current injury may have been caused by a weakness of the muscles and other knee structures that may prolong the current treatment, because you must deal with effects of both the current injury and the prior injury.

Special Questions

Special questions, such as whether the patient is taking any medications and the general health of the patient, can reveal factors that influence your understanding of the injury and your treatment plan. Does the patient have any systemic diseases that may affect treatment, such as diabetes, asthma, HIV? Has there been any unexpected weight loss lately? This may be a sign of unsuspected cancer and should be referred to the physician. Is the patient taking steroids? This can interfere with the healing process. With back injuries, questions regarding difficulty with bowel or bladder control are important, because a positive answer may indicate an injury to the cauda equina, which needs immediate medical attention. Knowing what tests have been performed, such as X rays or MRI, can help you focus your evaluation on related tests.

Additional Information

Additional information is also useful in completing an accurate profile of the injury and the patient's expectations of the treatment program. The patient's normal level of activity and the activities to which the patient wishes to return after rehabilitation give you an idea of the patient's expectations and the physical requirements for meeting those expectations. For example, if a runner presents with a knee injury that has been getting worse over time, what does he want to be able to resume doing once the treatment is over? How far, fast, and frequently was he running before the injury? What terrains was he running on? What kind of shoes does he use? Has he had any changes in his workouts, terrain, or other activities? Questions like these help you create an accurate profile of the patient and determine the cause of injury.

Other general questions include the patient's sport and position in that sport. These questions give you an idea of the amounts and kinds of stresses that may have caused the injury and also the level of stress that the patient's body must withstand on returning to the sport.

When working with high school or college athletes, the sport rehabilitation specialist often knows the age of the patient. In a clinic, however, the ages of patients can vary greatly. The patient's age is important in identifying certain injuries and also in deciding what treatment to apply. For example, osteoarthritis is a common problem among individuals over the age of 40. Ultrasound is not a treatment choice for a 13-year-old patient with a knee injury because of the open epiphyseal plates in the knee at that age.

Does the patient hear **crepitus** (clicking or snapping) from the injured part? These are what I call the Rice Krispies sounds: the snap, crackle, and pop of injury. Crepitus in a joint can sound either light or coarse, depending on whether the roughening of cartilage surfaces is slight or significant. A fine crepitus sometimes can be palpated in a joint with synovial thickening, as in synovitis. Crepitus can also be felt or heard in tendinitis because of the increased thickening and friction between the tendon and its sheath. A creaking sound is heard in joints that are in the later stages of joint-surface degeneration. A clicking or popping sound can be heard with meniscal displacement in either the temporomandibular joint or the knee joint; if the clicking is painful, the meniscus may be torn. Nonpainful clicks heard in joints, especially hypermobile joints, may be a normal vacuum click and of no consequence. Nonpainful but sometimes loud snapping sounds are frequently the inconsequential result of a ligament or a tendon slipping over a bony prominence as a joint moves. A clunking sound is produced by a joint that is unstable and subluxes as it moves through a particular part of its motion. Repeated subluxation making this sound can eventually cause degeneration of the joint.

Pain Profile

A profile of the patient's pain assists in determining the nature and severity of the injury and what to include in your objective examination and initial treatment plan. Several questions should be asked to obtain this profile:

• *Where is the pain?* Can it be located with one finger, or is it over a larger area? Does it stay localized, or does it go to other areas? Is the pain deep or superficial? Is it in a joint or in the surrounding area? A small, pinpoint area of pain is probably a localized, minor injury or a chronic injury. A larger, more diffuse or deep area of pain probably indicates a larger or more serious injury or an acute injury.

Pain that radiates into other areas may be referred pain caused by pressure on a nerve or myofascial referral from stimulation of trigger points. This pain and its cause need to be identified and further assessed during your objective evaluation.

• *Did the pain come on suddenly or gradually?* This question helps determine the cause of injury. A sudden pain is most often seen in sport injuries and occurs with a sudden overstress of tissue, as occurs with a muscle strain or a ligamentous sprain. Gradual onset of pain occurs more often with tendinitis and other inflammations. With gradual pain, patients commonly do not seek medical assistance until the pain interferes with sport performance or less stressful daily activities.

If the pain occurred gradually, how long has the patient had the pain? This determines whether the problem is acute or chronic. Acute pain is treated differently from chronic pain.

• *Is the pain constant or intermittent?* Most pain is intermittent or varies in intensity with either activity or time of day. The cause of pain that is constant and unchanging must be suspected as something other than musculoskeletal injury. Pain that is initially constant becomes intermittent with treatment that successfully reduces pain.

• *How intense is the pain?* Have the patient rate the pain on a scale of 0 to 10, where 0 is no pain and 10 is "take me to the hospital, I'm dying" pain. Pain is very subjective and varies greatly from one person to another. Trying to quantify pain by assigning a number to it does not make it an objective measure but does allow relative comparisons. The patient's pain rating gives you an idea of the patient's pain tolerance and can be used later to assess changes in the patient's pain. If a patient rates pain initially as 8 and three days later as 4, your treatment program is achieving the desired goal of reducing the patient's pain. This numerical system gives both you and the patient a method of gauging changes. It would be improper and useless to compare one patient's pain to another's, but there is some value in reassessing the patient's pain ratings as the treatment program progresses.

• *How does the patient describe the pain? What kind of pain is it?* There are a variety of descriptors that can be used to identify pain, such as sharp, dull, aching, burning, tingling. Musculoskeletal pain is usually deep, dull, or an ache. The pain of more acute or severe muscle injuries can be described as sharp, stabbing, or throbbing.

• *What are aggravating and easing factors? What does the patient do that causes or intensifies the pain? What relieves or reduces it?* In general, musculoskeletal pain occurs with movement and is relieved with rest. Pain from inflammation may not be relieved with rest. Prolonged positioning, such as poor sitting posture, can irritate soft tissues by applying prolonged or abnormal low-level stress to them.

• *Does the pain vary with time of day? How does the area feel in the morning? as the day progresses? by evening?* Stiffness in the morning can be related to inflammation. If the pain increases as the day progresses, it may be that the injured area lacks sufficient strength and endurance to carry on activities and becomes fatigued. Spasm and pain may intensify as the day progresses, especially in acute injuries.

• *Does the pain awaken the patient at night?* Musculoskeletal pain can worsen at night enough to disturb the patient's sleep. Inflammation and bone pain can also cause sleep disturbances. Inflammation pain that causes sleep disturbances indicates a bigger problem than pain that does not disturb sleep. If pain disturbs sleep, ask the patient how many times this occurs in a night and how long it takes to return to sleep. The answers to these questions give you an idea of the irritability of the injury. The more frequent the disturbances and the longer it takes the patient to return to sleep, the more irritated the injury is.

The intensity of the pain, the kinds of activities that aggravate it, how long a patient can perform an activity before the pain increases, and how long it takes to reduce the pain once it has increased also indicate the **irritability** of the injury. The more irritable an injury is, the higher the pain, the more easily it is increased with even low-level activity, and the longer it takes to ease. Corrigan and Maitland (1989) define an injury as being irritable when only a moderate amount of activity increases the pain and pain lasts for an hour. When an injury is not irritable, the patient feels only a momentary pain after stress.

OBJECTIVE EVALUATION

Once you have completed your subjective evaluation by taking the history of the injury, determining the patient's activity level and performance expectations, and profiling the pain and injury, it is time to perform your objective examination. Your goal is to determine exactly the structure or structures involved and the extent of the injury's effects so that you can determine your course of treatment.

Before you begin your physical examination, you already have a lot of information about the injury. This information guides your objective examination. From your subjective evaluation you have an idea of the nature of the problem, the severity and irritability of the injury, how aggressive or cautious you should be in performing your examination, which special tests to use, and which contraindications to consider. Although you may expect certain findings from your objective evaluation, it is important to keep an open mind and look at all possibilities for the injury and the tissues involved. Do not assume that you know what the problem is until you have a total picture based on the accumulated information from both the subjective and objective evaluations. Narrowing your scope of vision may lead you to an inaccurate conclusion and to create an inappropriate rehabilitation program.

If an injury is irritable, your examination should be brief, relatively gentle, and less stressful to the injury. On the other hand, if an injury is not irritable, your examination can be more aggressive. A second-degree sprain that occurred two days ago, that now exhibits a lot of swelling, causes persistent pain that increases with any active or passive range of movement, and causes pain with weight bearing is considered irritable and requires a gentle, brief examination to determine initial treatment. At a later stage when the injury is less irritable, a more aggressive and complete evaluation can be performed. Right now, however, your evaluation goal is to determine what treatment will best relieve current symptoms so that the patient can begin exercises as soon as safely possible.

If a patient is able to walk without pain and has minimal edema, your objective evaluation can be more aggressive to determine the extent of the injury, the tissues involved, and the treatment approach that will most effectively return this patient to sport participation.

A **comparable sign** is an active or passive movement that reproduces the patient's pain symptom, (Maitland 1991). Although it is not always easy to achieve a comparable sign in an objective evaluation, the sport rehabilitation specialist usually attempts to produce one.

Observation and Visual Inspection

Your visual inspection starts the moment you see the patient enter your facility. How is the patient walking? What is the posture and gait? General observations give you information about the severity of the injury and the items to inspect in your evaluation. For example, if the patient complains of medial knee pain and has excessively pronated feet, part of the problem may come from the feet and not the knee. If a patient has hip pain and genu valgus, weakness or structural anomalies at the knee may be contributing to the hip pain.

Other general observations include noting whether the patient requires any assistive devices, such as a brace or crutches. Is the patient reluctant to move the injured part? Noting any abnormal movements, posture, or behavior helps you complete your picture of the injury. For example, if a patient enters your facility walking with crutches, you already know that gait training will be a part of your treatment program. If you see a patient limping into the room, you should assess the entire lower extremity for weakness, because limping can cause weakness of improperly used muscles very quickly.

Your visual inspection of the injured area includes noting any abnormalities in the extremity that need more discriminate examination. Is there edema present, and if so, how much? Is there any discoloration, rash, wound, deformity, or atrophy present? If there is discoloration, does it appear distal to the injury, indicating that the patient probably did not elevate and correctly treat the injury when it occurred, or is the discoloration around the injury or proximal to it? Is there a scar, and if so, is it healed, does it look infected or excessive, and how recent does it appear to be?

Range of Motion

Range of motion of any joint can be normal, excessive (hypermobile), or less than normal (hypomobile). Normal ranges of motion for specific joints and how to measure them are discussed in chapter 5. Evaluation of the quality and quantity of available joint mobility investigates the capsule and ligamentous stability of the joint.

Active Range of Motion

Active range of motion (AROM) is the amount of movement produced by an individual without assistance (figure 4.1). Active range of motion depends on the amount of pain caused by active movement of the part, the willingness of the patient to move it, the strength of the muscles moving the joint, and the available range of motion of the joint. Pain may not be the only reason a patient is reluctant to move a part through its range of motion. The patient may be apprehensive of reinjury or other problems with movement. When evaluating active range of motion, the sport rehabilitation specialist must consider the patient's position and be aware of gravity's effect on movement. For example, in a test of shoulder-flexion range of motion, a sitting patient has to overcome the greatest resistance to gravity

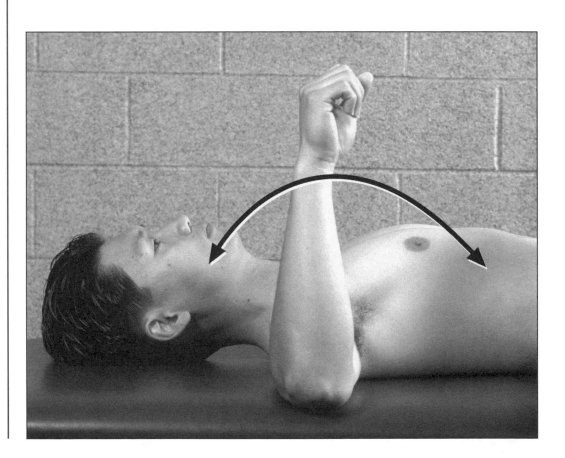

▌ Figure 4.1 Active range of motion.

at midrange, but in a supine position gravity's effect is greatest in the initial stages of movement. If a patient is unable to raise her arm overhead when sitting, the rehabilitation specialist should have the patient lie supine to see whether additional active motion is possible when gravity has less impact on shoulder-flexor strength in that position.

Range of motion may be restricted by a number of causes. Swelling, tightening of the joint capsule and ligaments, loss of flexibility in muscles, and a mechanical blockage, such as a loose body or osteophyte, can by themselves or in combination prevent a patient from achieving full range of motion. As your evaluation proceeds, the cause should be revealed.

It is also important to observe the quality of movement. Is the movement full and fluid, or is it irregular, hesitant, or jerking? Does it occur through substitution of improperly used muscles? If active motion causes pain, where in the motion does it occur? Does the pain occur midrange through an arc of motion? This often indicates a structure's being irritated, as can occur in the shoulder's supraspinatus tendon or when a disk protrusion of the back causes nerve root compression.

Information regarding the patient's ability to move helps you to determine what to include in your rehabilitation program, such as pain-relief measures, joint motion and strength exercises, and coordination and functional activities.

Passive Range of Motion

Passive range of motion is the amount of movement produced without any active participation by the patient (figure 4.2). Passive joint motion can be divided into two categories: physiological and accessory. **Physiological joint motion** is movement that can also be performed actively by the individual. Physiological motion is also called cardinal motion. **Accessory joint motion** is motion that cannot be performed actively but is necessary for full active motion to occur.

Passive physiological range of motion is the motion a joint attains when you move it while the patient remains relaxed. It is usually greater than the active range of motion in both injured and uninjured joints. As you move the joint through its motion, the patient should tell you when and where pain occurs in the motion. You should observe the patient's facial expressions, which also may indicate pain. The joint should be moved as far into the pain and through the range of motion as the patient can tolerate.

Once again, note the quantity and quality of the motion, whether passive motion causes pain, and if so, where in the motion the pain occurs. Pain that occurs with passive movement may be the

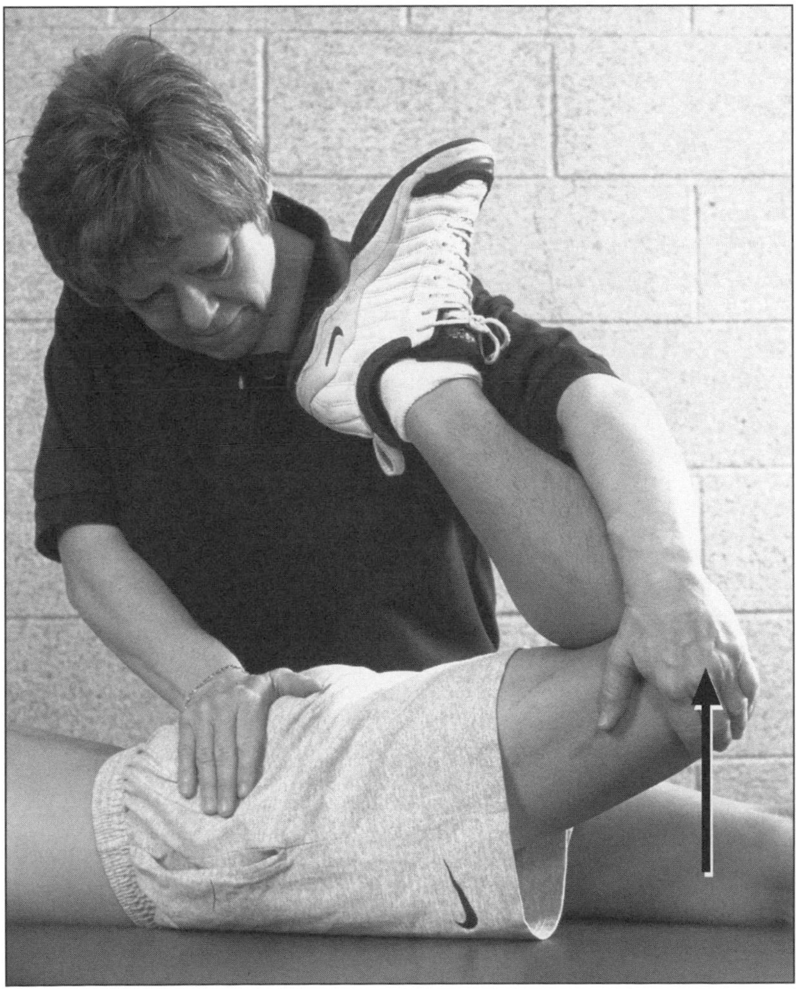

Figure 4.2 Passive range of motion.

result of stretching either inert structures, such as ligaments and capsules, or active structures, such as muscles. As you move the part through its motion, it is also important to note the end-feel of the movement.

If a joint's movement is normal and painless, **overpressure** is applied to truly assess full, painless motion. The pressure should be moderate and achieve slightly more motion as the joint is brought to its end range, but the motion should remain painless. To truly consider a joint as normal, firm overpressure must produce a painless and full range of motion (Maitland 1991).

End-Feel of Movement

The **end-feel** of a joint's movement is the nature of resistance that is felt at the end of a range of movement. The end-feel can be normal or pathological, depending on the particular joint and the extent of its range of motion compared to what's expected. Kessler and Hertling (1983) list normal and pathological end-feels for a variety of tissues. End-feels that can be either normal or pathological include capsular, bony, soft-tissue approximation, and muscular. Some end-feels are pathological because they occur only when there is tissue injury. These include muscle spasm end-feel, boggy end-feel, springy end-feel, and empty end-feel.

A capsular end-feel is a firm, leathery sensation when bringing a joint to the end of its motion. It is firm but not hard. If you move a normal, uninjured shoulder into full external rotation you will feel a firm, leathery end-feel. A capsular end-feel can also be felt in a pathological joint, such as a knee that does not have edema or inflammation but has limited mobility.

The most common example of a normal bony end-feel is that of the elbow in full extension with the olecranon process moving against the fossa. It is a sudden-stop end-feel. In pathological states the sensation is the same, but it occurs because of an abnormal condition, such as a bony growth or fracture malunion, and the total motion is less than normal.

Soft-tissue approximation end-feels occur when two muscle bellies meet to prevent further movement. Normal examples are the upper arm and forearm meeting in elbow flexion. The sensation is soft at the end of the movement.

A muscular end-feel is softer, less abrupt, and more rubbery than a capsular end-feel. It has a spring to it, much like what is felt when performing a straight-leg raise that is restricted by the hamstring muscles. The muscular end-feel is different from a muscle spasm end-feel in that the muscle spasm end-feel is more abrupt and usually causes pain. A rebound of the muscle as it reflexes into a contraction in response to the stretch is felt only in pathological conditions.

A boggy, soft, mushy end-feel is usually observed with joint effusion, when fluid within the joint prevents full motion. While the sensation of movement is boggy, the fluid's pressure blocks normal motion. It is common for this sensation to follow capsular joint movements, but this sensation occurs before the capsular end-feel is achieved.

A springy end-feel occurs from the mechanical block of a loose body and indicates an internal derangement. It is most commonly seen in the knee, where loose bodies of cartilage or meniscal flaps can stop normal joint movement.

An empty end-feel is not common. There is no resistance to joint movement because the ligamentous and capsular restrictions are gone, and there is too much pain with muscular restriction for the patient to voluntarily stop the movement. In the absence of any ligamentous injury, acute bursitis or a neoplasm should be suspected with an empty end-feel.

Accessory Joint Mobility

The other portion of passive motion, accessory joint motion, must also be evaluated to determine overall joint mobility. Accessory joint motion is motion that cannot be produced actively by the patient but is necessary for full, normal motion of a joint. Ac-

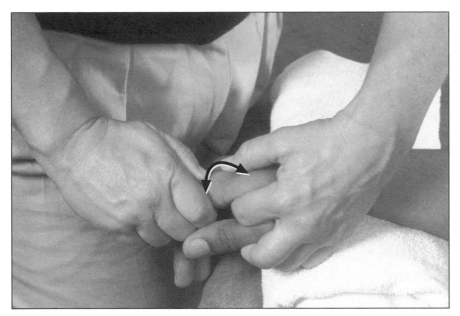

Figure 4.3 Accessory joint mobility.

cessory joint motion is evaluated by joint mobilization techniques. A good example of accessory joint motion is longitudinal rotation of the finger on the metacarpophalangeal joint (figure 4.3). It is not a motion that the patient can produce by any muscle activity, but you can rotate the phalanx easily by grasping the finger and rotating the proximal phalanx on its metacarpal. This accessory rotation must be present for full, active finger flexion-extension to occur. Specific joint mobilization techniques for treatment are the same as those used in evaluation and are discussed in chapter 6.

A joint can be normal in its mobility, hypermobile (excessive mobility), or hypomobile (restricted mobility). Joints that are hypomobile may be so because of muscle spasm protecting the area or because of restriction of ligamentous and capsular structures. Adhesions within the capsule can occur following injury, surgery, and immobilization. If you determine that a joint lacks full capsular mobility, part of your treatment plan should include joint mobilization techniques.

In evaluation of physiological and accessory joint mobility, you are looking for signs of stiffness in the joint, amplitude of available mobility, quality of motion, end-feel, and motion that is pain free. The best evaluation of the quality and quantity of stiffness and amplitude of motion is made by comparing the joint with its counterpart. Hypermobility of a joint can be considered normal for the individual if it is bilateral. Accessory joint motions should be pain free throughout a normal range of movement.

Muscle Performance

Evaluating muscles surrounding the injured area involves investigation of their strength and endurance in addition to their motion. There are a number of procedures that can evaluate muscular strength and endurance. The most common technique is isometric strength testing (figure 4.4). Other techniques can be used and are discussed in chapter 7.

Isometric testing for a quick assessment of muscular strength is usually performed in a midrange joint position to measure gross muscle-group strength. If there is any discrepancy, more detailed individual muscle testing is warranted.

Special Tests

Special tests are used in the evaluation to determine the aggressiveness of the treatment program and at what point the patient should begin the program. For example, if a patient has an ankle sprain with a positive anterior drawer test, you should avoid aggressive dynamic proprioception activities in weight bearing until the patient's ankle has increased strength sufficiently to keep the ankle stabilized during those activities. If, on the other hand, a patient has a mild sprain and a negative anterior drawer sign, you can initiate those activities sooner in the program.

Special tests are outlined in detail in Shultz, Houglum, and Perrin's (2000) book in the Athletic Training Education Series, *Assessment of Athletic Injuries.*

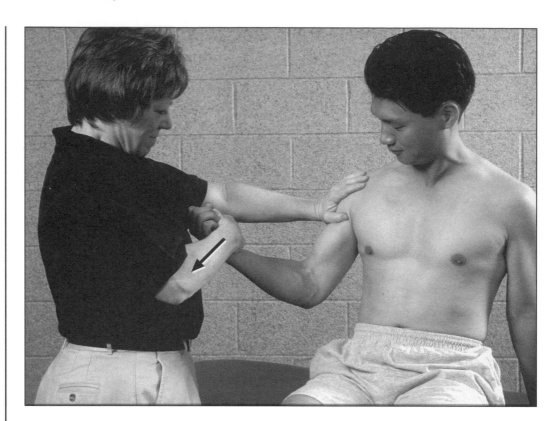

Figure 4.4 Muscular strength testing.

Neurological Tests

If your evaluation demonstrates neurological changes, neurological testing is warranted. These special tests include evaluation of sensory, motor, and reflex parameters (figure 4.5). Many professionals, including Corrigan and Maitland (1989), advocate using neurological testing for any signs or symptoms distal to the acromion in the upper extremity and distal to the gluteal fold in the lower extremity. This rule of thumb is especially warranted if you did not witness the injury incident and the patient is unsure of the nature of the injury. If neurological deficiencies are noted, impingement on the nerve root is possible and should be addressed in the treatment program.

Palpation

Palpation of the site is performed after the other tests are completed because palpation can irritate the tissues and cause inaccurate results in other tests. This sequence in a rehabilitation evaluation is different from that in an evaluation at the time of injury. One of the primary reasons for this is that it is not always clear during a rehabilitation evaluation what structures are involved until the evaluation is nearly complete, but if you have seen the injury occur, there is usually less question of what structures are involved. If palpation is performed early in a rehabilitation evaluation, before a good profile of the injury is obtained, the sport rehabilitation specialist may end up palpating a structure that is not actually injured, reducing the patient's confidence and wasting time.

Several structures are evaluated through palpation. Skin and subcutaneous tissue are examined by light touch for temperature, tone, and edema. Light movement of the skin and subcutaneous tissue against underlying structures shows any excessive rigidity or adhesions of tissue, as commonly seen following prolonged immobilization or excessive edema with immobilization. If movement between the subcutaneous tissue and underlying structures is impaired, a loss of motion results.

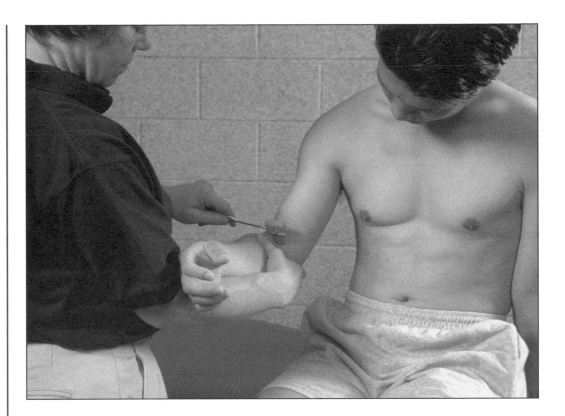

Figure 4.5 Special tests for neurological evaluation.

Deficiencies in this area warrant soft-tissue mobilization techniques as part of the treatment plan.

Palpation of fascia, muscles, ligaments, and tendons for tenderness, trigger points, and texture is important in evaluating causes of pain, motion restriction, and irritability (figure 4.6). Evaluation of these structures starts with light palpation of superficial structures; if the area's irritability permits, palpation pressure then increases to get to deeper structures. Palpation of deeper structures requires a sensitive touch, not heavy pressure. For example, in palpating the midback area, light palpation is first performed to evaluate skin and subcutaneous mobility. Then slightly deeper palpation allows examination of the rhomboids and trapezius. Even deeper palpation is required to examine the paraspinal muscles. The deepest palpation in this region allows examination of the costovertebral joints. If palpation is too vigorous, accurate evaluation of tender structures is not possible. Palpate only as deeply as necessary to obtain the information you seek.

Areas of tenderness are detected by palpation. Areas of spasm, areas of crepitus, nodules, and scar tissue can also be palpated. Palpation reveals specific sites of tenderness and the tissue type involved. Palpation is also used to evaluate consistency, mobility, and abnormalities of underlying tissue. Gaps, rigidity, loss of normal mobility, woodiness, nodules, and other textures and tissue quality are recorded and used later to form the assessment.

Functional Testing

Functional tests are not always performed at the time of the initial rehabilitation evaluation. When they are performed can vary. Sometimes they may be used after palpation and after other factors have been assessed, and sometimes they may be incorporated before palpation to assist you in further identifying deficiencies. The irritability and severity of the injury dictate if and when these tests are appropriate.

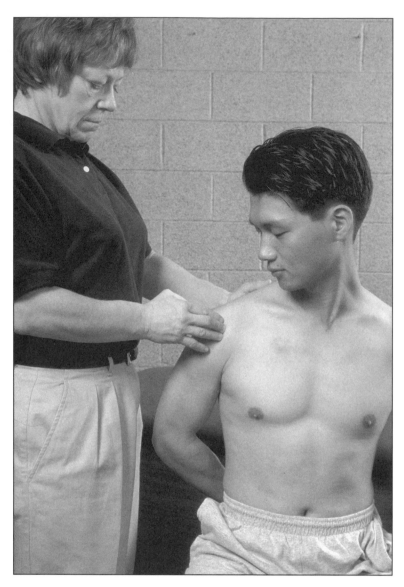

These tests determine whether specific activities produce pain, the injured part's ability to perform an activity, and the quality of movement during the activity. Agility, coordination, and proprioception play key roles in a patient's ability to perform functional tasks. Simple functional tests include having the patient perform a squat while you look for smoothness of movement, full motion, and an ability to keep the feet flat on the floor.

Standing on one foot (figure 4.7), standing on toes, walking on toes, walking on heels, jumping, running, and cutting are other functional tests used to determine functional ability and quality. More advanced functional testing can include sport-specific activities.

Evaluation Results

Once you have accumulated all the information from the subjective and objective portions of your evaluation, you can make a well-informed assessment and determine the problems that should be addressed in the treatment plan. The treatment program is designed to resolve these problems and achieve the goals that you and the patient set.

❚ **Figure 4.6**   Palpation.

ASSESSMENT: PLANNING FOR ACTION

Assessment involves identifying problems based on information from the evaluation, setting goals to address those problems, and planning the treatment program for achieving those goals.

Once the subjective and objective evaluations are complete, you assess the patient's status as it relates to the goals. This process includes creating a list of problems and a list of goals. The goals address the problems, and the problems are based on the findings of the evaluation.

PROBLEMS TO OVERCOME

After the evaluation, the sport rehabilitation specialist can identify the problems that the injured athlete must overcome in order to return to full competition. Several simultaneous problems may need to be addressed, including subjective findings of pain and swelling or objective findings of reduced joint mobility or strength. Inability to compete can be an additional problem.

GOALS FOR TREATMENT

Once the problems are identified, the treatment program and its goals can be outlined. The general goals most often are to remove or reduce the problems and return

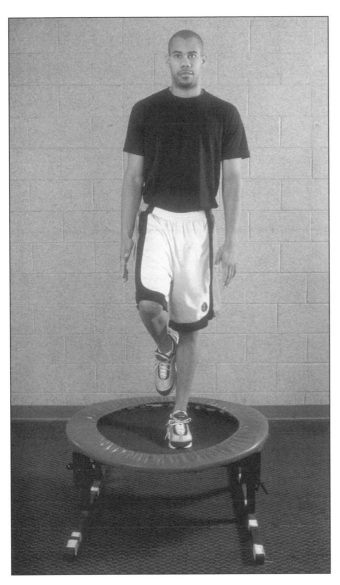

■ **Figure 4.7** Functional testing.

the patient to full competition. Specific goals may include relief of pain and swelling and restoring normal levels of joint mobility and strength. For every problem listed, there should be a goal to address and resolve it. A goal should not be listed if a problem has not been identified. For example, a goal to relieve spasm should not be listed if spasm is not present. There is a direct relationship between the problems identified by an evaluation and the goals that are sought through the treatment program.

Both short-term and long-term goals should be set, as discussed in chapter 1. The time it will take to achieve short-term and long-term goals should be estimated. A common duration for a short-term goal is two weeks. You should estimate how far the patient will progress in the next two weeks of your therapeutic exercise program and base your short-term goals on those estimates. The long-term goals are the final goals that the patient will achieve.

Some long-term goals are achieved sooner than others during the course of the treatment program. For example, full flexibility is achieved before full agility and coordination. A short-term goal for week 6 of a rehabilitation program following ACL reconstruction surgery might be 100% range of motion of the knee, 50% of normal quadriceps strength, and 30% of normal agility. Once full range of motion is achieved, the maintenance of full motion becomes a goal.

Plan for Treatment

After the goals have been outlined, a plan of action for achieving those goals can be designed. The **plan of treatment program** includes the frequency and duration of the treatment and the components included. Various factors are involved in the treatment program, depending on the problems and goals that have been identified. For example, if goals include relieving swelling and pain and increasing range of motion and strength, modalities to reduce swelling and pain are used. Active range of motion may also be used to relieve these problems. Joint mobilization, range-of-motion exercises, massage, and home exercises may all be used to increase range of motion, depending on the problems that caused loss of motion. Resistive exercises to increase strength may start with isometrics or more aggressive exercises, depending on the patient's ability at the time. Just as goals are designed to fit the problems, the plan is designed to achieve those goals.

A good therapeutic exercise program changes as the patient's problems decline and his or her status improves. As short-term goals are achieved, new short-term goals are set. To meet those goals, new treatment techniques must be planned. For example, if the patient achieves a short-term goal of balancing in a stork stand for 30 s, a new goal should be established to further challenge the patient to achieve normal balance and progress to agility tasks.

The final short-term goals are actually the long-term goals. The patient progresses in the treatment plan until only the long-term goals are left. Once these are achieved through the treatment plan, the final treatment goal of returning the rehabilitated athlete to competition becomes a reality.

CONTINUAL ASSESSMENT

Once the treatment plan is under way, the sport rehabilitation specialist continues to evaluate and assess the patient. Evaluation and assessment take place before treatment, after treatment, and periodically throughout treatment to determine whether a specific technique is achieving its goals. For example, an evaluation before applying modalities assesses the extent of muscle spasm present. An evaluation at the conclusion of the modality treatment assesses the success and efficacy of the modality. Similarly, an evaluation before applying a joint mobilization technique determines the quantity and area of joint restriction. An evaluation during the treatment determines whether joint mobility is improving as the mobilization technique is applied. An assessment following the joint mobilization technique determines its effectiveness: Did your treatment achieve the improvements in pain reduction, range of motion, and joint mobility that you expected? How much motion has been gained?

The only way to assess whether the treatment is producing the desired effects is to continually evaluate and reevaluate. Evaluation and assessment are also performed after exercise. Sometimes the exercise effects are determined immediately: Was the patient able to perform the exercise correctly? Could the patient have tolerated a higher resistance or more repetitions? Did the patient favor the injured extremity during the exercise? At other times the effectiveness and appropriateness of exercise are determined at the next treatment session: Did the patient suffer any unwanted side effects, such as more pain or edema after the exercise? Was there any muscle soreness without pain and edema? Your pretreatment evaluation findings determine your treatment for the day and also indicate whether you are providing the patient with an appropriate exercise program and what changes should be made in the exercises to achieve your goals.

The patient's response to the treatment must be assessed so that the program can be changed appropriately when necessary. Without ongoing evaluation and assessment, the sport rehabilitation specialist is unable to determine when to advance a patient, what techniques to use, how much force to apply in treatment techniques, and whether a treatment is beneficial or harmful to the patient. The process is also necessary for designing and following an appropriate treatment plan. An evaluation and an assessment based on it are made before, during, and after each treatment and from one treatment session to the next.

FUNCTIONAL ASSESSMENT

As the therapeutic exercise program advances, more and more functional activities are incorporated. Functional activities are covered in detail in chapter 10. As the patient nears the end of the therapeutic exercise program and is preparing to return to sport participation, it is important for the sport rehabilitation specialist to assess the patient's abilities and readiness to return to participation. This is accomplished through functional testing. Specific functional activities vary from sport to sport and from one position to another within a sport. For example, a soccer offensive wing and a soccer goalie perform different activities. A gymnast has different functional requirements and should be assessed differently from a basketball player. It is your responsibility to appreciate these differences, know functional assessment tools that appropriately test the necessary skills of different sports and positions, and accurately assess the patient's readiness to return to his or her sport.

KEEPING REHABILITATION RECORDS

Record keeping is essential for judging the treatment's effectiveness, for communicating with other care givers, as a reference in the event of reinjury, and as a legal document.

Record keeping sometimes can seem overwhelming to medical professionals, but it is a crucial part of the treatment process. It reports the patient's initial levels of ability and performance, the effects of treatments, and the final outcomes of a rehabilitation program. It is important to keep accurate records because they can be referred to later to determine progress, they can be used by other sport rehabilitation specialists to provide consistent treatment, and they are legal documents. Because medical records are legal documents, all records that are not typed must be recorded clearly and legibly in pen, not pencil. Recorded items should not be erased, blacked out, or covered with correction fluid; an error should be noted with one line drawn through it and your initials next to it, indicating that you have altered the record. You always sign or initial and date the record after completing notes.

RECORDING THE EVALUATION

Many different formats can be used to record the evaluation. Most directors of athletic training clinics and other health care facilities develop their own forms for use in the facility. Preprinted forms are easy to use and provide consistency and thoroughness in evaluations. Forms can offer a detailed list or a general outline, but they should include all the necessary information discussed in this chapter. A human figure on the form is also convenient so that the specific area of injury can be easily marked. Figures 4.8 and 4.9 are examples of detailed and general evaluation forms.

The record should include information from the patient's subjective assessment, including the injury site and onset; history and previous treatment of prior injuries; pain profile; additional medical problems; special questions; patient's activities, such as job or school demands; and the patient's sport and position. Any tests that have been ordered and their results should be included as well.

The objective portion of the form should include observations and inspections; evaluation findings on range of motion, strength, joint mobility, soft-tissue mobility, and neurological signs; palpation findings; and special test results.

A list of problems and a list of goals are a routine part of the evaluation form. The final portion of the evaluation form is the presentation of the treatment plan. A copy of the evaluation is frequently forwarded to the physician as a professional courtesy. It also completes the physician's records and helps the sport rehabilitation specialist and the physician to communicate and coordinate their treatment plans and goals.

RECORDING THE TREATMENT

Recording your treatment sessions is as important as recording your evaluation (figure 4.10). A common method of record keeping is the SOAP (subjective, objective, assessment, and plan) note, which is thoroughly described in Kettenbach (1990). SOAP notes are the most commonly used system of problem-oriented record keeping in the medical profession. SOAP notes are clear, concise, and easily understood, and they provide a plan of action for medical care and treatment.

Additional information on SOAP notes appears in *Management Strategies in Athletic Training,* second edition (Ray 2000).

S: Subjective

Subjective notes are what the patient says. Direct quotations should be used. A common mistake is to put the evaluator's impressions or assessments in this category. For example, a statement such as "The patient seems depressed" is incorrect. A more correct statement would be, "The patient states that he is having trouble sleeping, has lost his appetite, and doesn't feel like working on his rehabilitation program."

REHABILITATION EVALUATION

Name _____ Date _____

Diagnosis _____ DOI _____

Age _____ Occupation/Sport _____ M.D. _____

Activity level _____

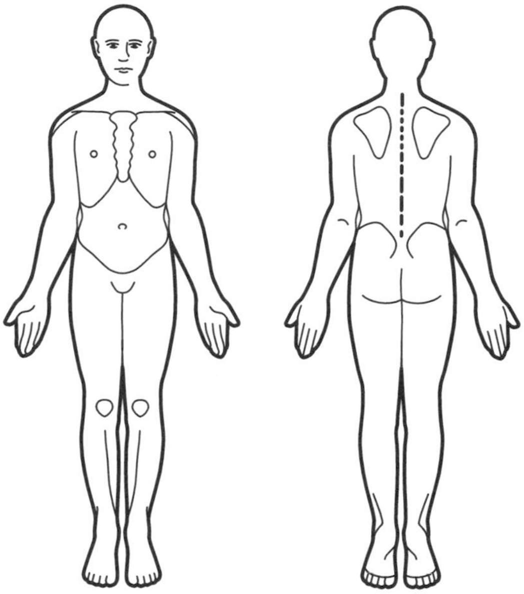

Current history:

Previous history:

Pain:

    Area:

    Description:

    Intensity: (0 = no pain; 10 = "take me to the hospital, I'm dying.")

    Aggravating factors:

    Easing factors:

    24-hour profile: A.M.:

        As day progresses:

            Evening:

                Night:

Special questions:

    GH: WL: X rays: CE:

                        Steroids: Meds:

Athlete's goals:

■ **Figure 4.8** Detailed evaluation form.

(continued)

OBJECTIVE EVALUATION

Observation/Inspection:

Range of motion/Flexibility:

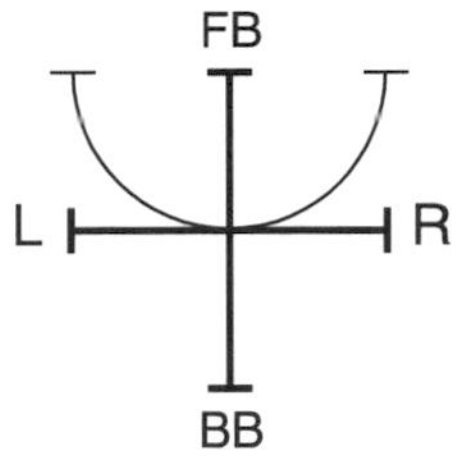

```
        FB
     ⌐  |  ¬
  L ├────┼────┤ R
        |
        BB
```

Strength/Endurance: Special tests:

Tension signs: Neurological signs:

Accessory movements:

Palpation:

Problems:

Goals:

Recommendations/Plan:

Initial treatment:

_____
Sport Rehabilitation Specialist

■ **Figure 4.8** *(continued)*

EVALUATION

Name:

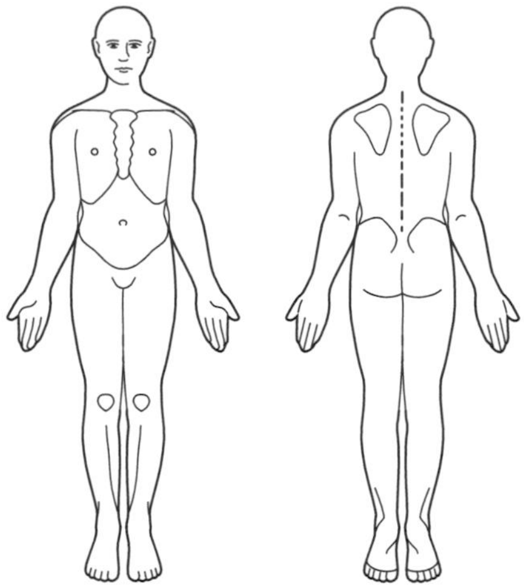

Subjective/History:

Objective/Findings:

Assessment/Problems:

Plan/Goals:

Date _____

_____
Sport Rehabilitation Specialist

▌**Figure 4.9** General evaluation form.

TREATMENT NOTES

Patient _____ Diagnosis _____

Date: _____

S: _____

O: _____

_____

_____

A: _____

_____

P: _____

_____

_____
Sport Rehabilitation Specialist

Date: _____

S: _____

O: _____

_____

_____

A: _____

_____

P: _____

_____

_____
Sport Rehabilitation Specialist

Date: _____

S: _____

O: _____

_____

_____

A: _____

_____

P: _____

_____

_____
Sport Rehabilitation Specialist

❚ **Figure 4.10**　Rehabilitation treatment form.

O: Objective

Objective notes record what is done in the treatment session. They also include any objective measurements or evaluations you perform, for example, "ROM L knee = 115°. Leg press, L with 90 lb, 3 × 15. Heel raises on L only, 3 × 20, no wt. Ice L knee × 15 min." Many organizations use an exercise record sheet as part of their objective reporting (figure 4.11). This is particularly useful in sport rehabilitation, where many exercises may be used from one treatment session to the next. It saves time by reducing paperwork and needless repetition, yet still provides an accurate record of treatment.

A: Assessment

The assessment is your interpretation of the problems being addressed and how the patient and the injury responded to the treatment. Here is an example: "Patient continues to walk with an antalgic gait secondary to pain in the medial knee joint. His range of motion and strength are improving but remain deficient. He seems to be depressed about the injury but is willing to perform all activities in the treatment session."

P: Plan

This is the treatment plan. What will you do with the patient at the next treatment session? Continuing with the patient in the previous examples, the plan may be written like this: "Add beginning agility activities of stork standing and balance board next treatment. If pain persists, use electrical stimulation to reduce pain. Continue in strengthening program progression as tolerated, add weight to heel raise, and increase repetitions on leg press."

ADDITIONAL RECORDS

Additional records help to form a complete synopsis of treatment and progression for a patient. They provide a well-rounded perspective of progress, a summary of overall results, and a reference in the event of future injury.

Progress Note

When the patient is seen for follow-up visits by the physician, a brief progress report in a SOAP format is often sent with the patient (figure 4.12), and a copy is kept in your records as well. The progress note provides the physician with a written record of the rehabilitation program and the patient's progress. It also allows communication between the sport rehabilitation specialist and the physician and helps to ensure that both are on common ground in the care of the patient.

Additionally, the progress note provides you with a regular summary of the changes in the patient's condition. Objective and subjective changes that occur over time are sometimes difficult to assess when working with a patient regularly but are easily seen with a glance at your progress notes. You can judge more easily whether the patient is progressing appropriately.

Discharge Summary

When the patient has achieved the long-term goals that were established at the outset of the rehabilitation program, a brief discharge summary is completed, one copy is sent to the physician, and another is kept in your files (figure 4.13). A discharge summary is important because it indicates the completion of the patient's rehabilitation program. It states the patient's condition at the time of discharge and summarizes the program and its duration. If the patient suffers another injury to the same area, the discharge summary also provides a quick reference to the patient's response to treatments, willingness to work in a therapeutic exercise program, and any deficiencies that may have resulted from the previous injury.

Diploma

An optional bit of paperwork that usually is a pleasure instead of a drudgery is a rehabilitation diploma (figure 4.14). A special diploma printed on special paper for a

EXERCISES												

Name _____   DX _____

M.D. _____   Precautions _____

DATE

EXERCISE												

▌**Figure 4.11** Exercise record sheet.

REHABILITATION PROGRESS REPORT

NAME _____ DATE _____

DIAGNOSIS _____

NUMBER OF TREATMENTS _____

===

SUBJECTIVE:

OBJECTIVE:

ASSESSMENT:

RECOMMENDATIONS/PLAN:

_____
Sport Rehabilitation Specialist

∎ **Figure 4.12** Rehabilitation progress report.

REHABILITATION DISCHARGE SUMMARY

NAME _____ DATE _____

DIAGNOSIS _____

NUMBER OF TREATMENTS _____

INITIAL TREATMENT DATE _____ FINAL TREATMENT DATE _____

==

DISCHARGE STATUS:

PAIN/SWELLING: _____

ROM: _____

_____

STRENGTH: _____

_____

FUNCTION: _____

_____

RECOMMENDED HOME PROGRAM: _____

_____

GOALS ACHIEVED: _____ YES _____ NO

REASONS FOR DISCHARGE: _____

_____

_____
Sport Rehabilitation Specialist

■ **Figure 4.13** Rehabilitation discharge summary.

patient who successfully completes a rehabilitation program is often well earned and coveted. It provides a bit of motivation for patients. Patients with whom I have worked have cherished and even framed their rehabilitation diplomas. Successful completion of a rehabilitation program involves dedication, hard work, and diligence, so a diploma is a well-deserved reward.

SUMMARY

1. *Identify the primary factors of subjective evaluation.*

   The subjective portion of the evaluation should include a history of the injury, pain profile, medical history, special questions, and additional questions about factors that may affect the injury.

2. *Outline an objective evaluation procedure that includes all primary factors.*

   The objective portion of the evaluation includes observation and visual inspection, evaluating active and passive physiological and accessory range of motion, strength tests, special tests, palpation, and functional tests if appropriate.

3. *Explain the different types of end-feel and distinguish between normal and pathological end-feels.*

   Typical normal end-feels include capsular, bony, soft tissue, and muscular, although these can also be abnormal, depending on the tissue involved. Other abnormal end-feels are springy, boggy, and empty.

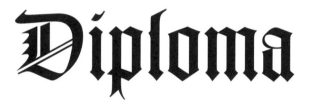

Diploma

this is to certify that

_____

Has satisfactorily completed and endured the rigors of rehabilitation and the trauma of treatment prescribed for graduation from this facility, and is awarded this diploma for rehabilitation of _____

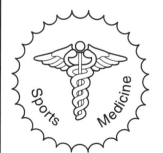

_____
SPORT REHABILITATION SPECIALIST

_____
DATE

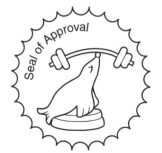

State University of Science and Technology

▌Figure 4.14 Rehabilitation diploma.

4, *Explain how a treatment plan is designed and upon what factors it is based.*

A treatment plan is developed after an assessment is made of the results of the evaluation. A list of problems based on the findings dictates a list of treatments to relieve those problems.

5. *Define the SOAP note and explain its significance to rehabilitation.*

A SOAP note is a common method of record keeping. It includes subjective reports from the patient, objective treatment provided, assessment of the results of and tolerance to the treatment, and plan of treatment for the next session. It provides a record of progress and allows consistency of treatment.

6. *Identify two other records used in rehabilitation and demonstrate their importance.*

A progress note to the physician, written when the patient returns to the physician for follow-up visits, and a discharge summary when the patient returns to sport participation are common rehabilitation records.

CRITICAL THINKING QUESTIONS

1. Describe the difference between an evaluation that occurs at the time of an injury and one that occurs before a rehabilitation program is started. Why are these differences important? What information may be different from one evaluation to the other?

2. Since pain is often the dominant complaint, an accurate pain profile provides you with a better idea of its source and how to proceed in your treatment program. Can you identify the most common types of pain and what they classically indicate? How does duration or intensity of pain influence the treatment you provide?

3. Your objective evaluation is based on the results of the subjective evaluation. How would your objective evaluation of a patient who reports severe pain most of the time compare with an evaluation of a patient who has minimal pain most of the time with occasional severe pain? If the patient's pain prevents you from performing all the tests you would like, what does your objective evauation include, and what do you do for treatment?

4. Is it possible to have a goal without a problem? Is it possible to have a problem without a goal? How are these two aspects of the assessment related? If the goals change, does that mean the problem has changed?

5. You have been newly hired at a university that has not kept medical records beyond the initial injury incident report and daily athletic training clinic visitation record. How would you change the system to make it more compliant with record-keeping standards for medical facilities? What forms would you develop to make the process as simple as possible? What minimum record-keeping requirements would you put into place? What are the justifications for these changes?

REFERENCES

Corrigan, B., and G.D. Maitland. 1989. *Practical orthopedic medicine.* London: Butterworth.

Kessler, R.M., and D. Hertling. 1983. *Management of common musculoskeletal disorders.* Philadelphia: Harper & Row.

Kettenbach, G. 1990. *Writing S.O.A.P. notes.* Philadelphia: Davis.

Maitland, G.D. 1991. *Peripheral manipulation.* London: Butterworth-Heinemann.

Ray, R. 2000. *Management strategies in athletic training.* 2d ed. Champaign, IL: Human Kinetics.

Shultz, S.A., Houglum, P.A., and D.H. Perrin. 2000. *Assessment of athletic injuries.* Champaign, IL: Human Kinetics.

PART TWO

Therapeutic Exercise Parameters and Techniques

It is not enough to have a good mind.
The main thing is to use it well.

René Descartes, *Discourse on Method*

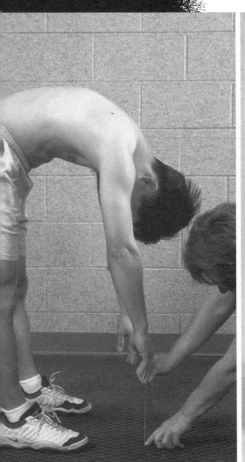
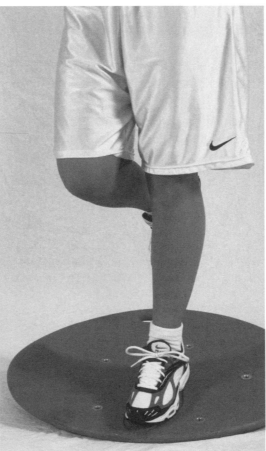
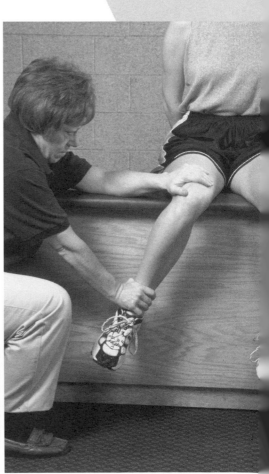

The next six chapters delve into specific techniques for restoring range of motion and flexibility, muscular strength and endurance, coordination and agility, soft-tissue and joint mobility, and functional activities.

Recall from part I that the parameters of normal function are emphasized in a logical sequence, each one building on the previous ones, throughout the therapeutic exercise program. This part follows that sequence in the presentation of topics. In **chapter 5**, range of motion and flexibility are discussed. What normal joint motion is and how to achieve it are presented. **Chapter 6** extends the material of chapter 5 in that it deals with soft-tissue and joint pathology that may interfere with normal motion. The various techniques commonly used to resolve problems in these areas are discussed.

Progressing along the rehabilitation sequence, strength and muscular endurance are discussed in **chapter 7**. The various types of strengthening techniques, equipment used, program progressions, and precautions are also introduced.

Proprioception—including balance, agility, and coordination—is discussed in **chapter 8**. Progression from a static to a dynamic program is also included.

Chapter 9 presents information on plyometrics—activities that require flexibility, strength, endurance, and proprioception. Plyometrics are often incorporated into a rehabilitation program before functional exercises.

Chapter 10 presents functional exercises and their concepts. Functional exercises are the final progression of a total therapeutic exercise program.

The words of Descartes apply directly to your education in sport rehabilitation. As you read through the chapters of this part, the relevance of the information presented in part I will become clear. By the time you complete part II, you will have the knowledge needed for parts III and IV, where general and specific programs for injuries are presented. Parts I and II are your gateway to understanding and appreciating the practical applications of the programs and concepts in parts III and IV. By the time you have completed this book, you will be able to use your mind to apply what you have learned in developing your own rehabilitation programs.

CHAPTER FIVE

Range of Motion and Flexibility

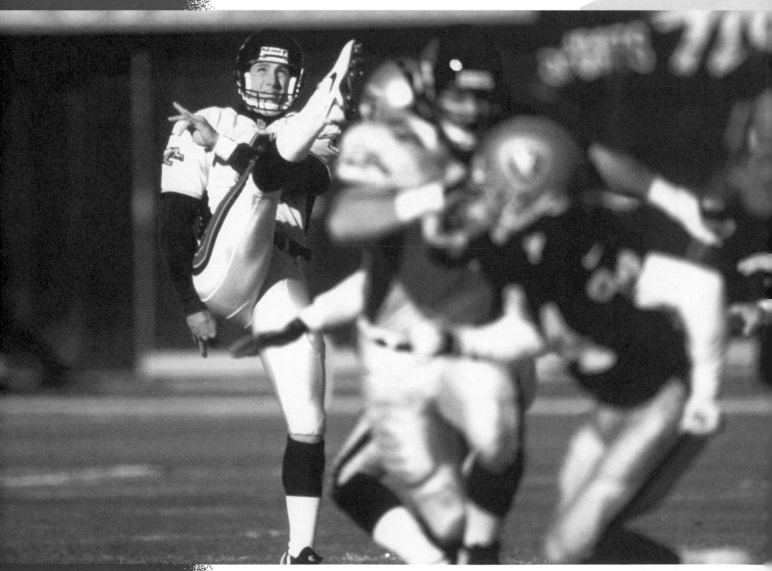

OBJECTIVES

After completing this chapter, you should be able to do the following:

1. Define the differences between range of motion and flexibility.

2. Explain the differences in structure of loose connective tissue and dense connective tissue.

3. List the deleterious effects of prolonged immobilization.

4. Discuss the mechanical properties of plasticity, elasticity, and viscosity of connective tissue.

5. Explain the physiological properties of creep and stress-strain and how they affect stretching techniques.

6. Discuss the neuromuscular influences of the muscle spindle and GTO on stretching muscle.

7. Explain the procedure for measuring range of motion with a goniometer.

8. Discuss the active and passive methods for stretching.

9. Identify two mechanical assistive devices used to increase range of motion.

10. List contraindications, indications, and precautions of stretching.

11. Discuss the progression of a stretching exercise program.

As a senior athletic training student, Larry Carlson is on his first sports medicine clinical rotation. His first patient today is a new shoulder patient. Larry knows from his past experience that he will measure the shoulder, elbow, and wrist ranges of motion in all their planes of movement. He also knows that the patient had a rotator cuff repair, but he does not know when the surgery was performed, what specific repair was used, or the physician's postoperative restrictions on shoulder motion. He anticipates, though, that there may be some limitations and precautions that must be respected. Although there should be no limitations on elbow and wrist motions, if the shoulder has been immobilized in a sling, there may be some loss of motion in the elbow that must be evaluated and addressed.

A mind that is stretched to a new idea never returns to its original dimension.

Oliver Wendell Holmes

By now you realize that a rapid restoration of range of motion and flexibility is important in a therapeutic exercise program. The aim of this chapter is to stretch your mind to new dimensions, as Oliver Wendell Holmes suggests, by showing you concepts and techniques designed to stretch tissue to new lengths. This chapter introduces the deleterious effects of prolonged immobilization, defines the differences between range of motion and flexibility, discusses the various methods and progressions for achieving full motion, identifies normal levels of motion throughout the body, and investigates the equipment that is used to evaluate motion.

At the conclusion of this chapter, the consequences of establishing or not establishing normal motion and of delaying the process should become clear. You will also know the techniques and skills needed for successfully restoring range of motion, and you will acquire an awareness of the precautions that should be taken and the progression that should be used.

DEFINING FLEXIBILITY AND RANGE OF MOTION

Flexibility is a musculotendinous unit's ability to elongate, whereas range of motion is a joint's mobility, which is affected by many tissues in and around the joint.

Range of motion and flexibility are closely related. Although the terms are often used interchangeably, their definitions are different.

Flexibility refers to the musculotendinous unit's ability to elongate with application of a stretching force. The amount of flexibility of an area is generally thought of as its stiffness, suppleness, or pliability. Prolonged loss of flexibility can cause reduced range of motion.

Range of motion is the amount of mobility of a joint and is determined by the soft-tissue and bony structures in the area. The status of soft tissues—including muscles, tendons, ligaments, capsule, skin, subcutaneous tissues, nerves, and blood vessels—all affect the range of motion of a joint. If a patient has impaired flexibility, range of motion is also limited.

Clinically, range-of-motion measurements are used to quantify both range of motion and flexibility. Although there is a technical distinction between the two, clinical interpretations make the differences less clear. For this reason, range of motion and flexibility are used interchangeably in this text.

CONNECTIVE-TISSUE COMPOSITION

Connective tissue supports the body and provides it with its framework. It is composed of many different kinds of cells and fibrous and ground substances that form in various combinations, depending on the specific connective tissue type. These connective tissues vary in the types, orientation, and linking of their fibers, which affect their flexibility and ability to withstand stress.

Mobility of the musculoskeletal system is determined by the composition of connective tissue and the orientation of the various soft-tissue structures. Connective tissue of soft-tissue structures is composed of collagen, elastin, reticulin, and ground substance. The quantities of these substances vary according to the specific structure and determine the characteristics of the structure. For example, there is more collagen in ligament and more elastin in skin.

Collagen provides tissue with strength and stiffness. Recall from chapter 2 that the collagen fibers bind themselves together, and the more binding between the fibers, the greater the tensile strength and stability of the structure. Collagen fibers are five times as strong as elastin fibers.

Elastin fibers provide the structure with extensibility. They are able to withstand elongation stress and to return to normal length. Tissues that have more elastin have more flexibility.

Reticulin fibers are essentially type III collagen fibers. They are weaker than type I and are considered temporary. They are particularly important during repair following injury.

Ground substance is a structureless organic gel that serves to reduce friction between the fibers, maintains spacing between the fibers to prevent excessive cross-linking, and transports nutrients to the fibers.

Connective-tissue composition varies according to structural differences and the amount of motion required. The fiber arrangement of **areolar (loose) connective tissue** is unorganized and loose with relatively long distances between the cross-links. Loose connective tissue's open network is composed primarily of thin collagen and elastic fibers that are interlaced in several different directions. This arrangement provides the structure with tensile strength as well as pliability. Skin is an example of areolar connective tissue.

Tendons are an example of a structure containing more highly organized connective tissue with parallel collagen fibers and more cross-links. This arrangement allows **dense connective tissues** to resist high-tensile loads and still provide some flexibility. Ligaments are similar to tendons in their structure except that their fiber arrangement is not as regular. Their collagen fibers are primarily parallel, but there are also spiral and oblique arrangements.

Between the structural extremes in the arrangement, orientation, and quantity of fibers and cross-links in skin and tendons are structures such as ligaments, capsules, and fascia. Even within these categories fiber arrangements vary. For example, ligaments that are able to resist higher forces have more organized fiber arrangements with greater quantities of cross-links.

Areolar connective tissue is present between the tissues in areas where motion occurs, such as joint capsular fascia, intermuscular layers, and subcutaneous tissue. Areolar connective tissue permits movement in all directions.

EFFECTS OF IMMOBILIZATION ON CONNECTIVE TISSUE

Immobilization causes changes that result in loss of motion in all tissues. Increased collagen cross-links, loss of ground substance, and fibrosis all impair the flexibility of connective tissue.

Connective tissue is continually replaced and reorganized as a part of normal body function. As a part of the reorganization process, connective tissue normally tends to shorten (Kottke, Pauley, and Ptak 1966). To combat this tendency, normal motion is maintained through daily activity. If motion is restricted, either voluntarily or passively, rapid changes in the structure and function of connective tissue can be seen. Immobilization following injury is sometimes necessary to protect the area and permit the healing process to occur unimpeded. Immobilization, however, can also be detrimental. Depending on how long an area is immobilized, the changes in connective tissue can be permanent or reversible. Although it does not take long for changes to occur, the longer the period of immobilization, the more difficult the restoration to normal becomes.

To understand the problems that must be addressed to restore normal range of motion and other lost parameters of an affected area, you must first be aware of the changes that occur with immobilization. Immobilization affects all tissue, from bone to soft tissue, including tendon, ligament, capsule, muscle, skin, and subcutaneous structures.

GENERAL CHANGES IN SOFT TISSUE

Soft-tissue changes are seen following even one week of immobilization and are increased by edema, trauma, and impaired circulation (Kottke, Stillwell, and Lehmann 1982). Immobilization causes a loss of ground substance, which in turn results in less separation and more cross-link formations between collagen fibers. The fiber meshwork contracts so that the tissue becomes dense, hard, and less supple. If a normal joint is immobilized for four weeks, the dense connective tissue that forms prevents normal motion.

In the presence of injury, the newly formed fibrin and collagen fibers are laid down in a haphazard way when the area is immobilized. The increase in newly formed cross-links impairs motion. Although cross-links are necessary for collagen strength, excessive cross-link formation can restrict normal movement of collagen tissue (figure 5.1).

Free gliding collagen fibers

Reduced gliding with increased cross-linking

Relaxed

Stretch applied

Loss of mobility with increased cross-links

▮ Figure 5.1 Collagen cross-links reduce mobility.

Adapted from Woo et al. 1975.

After two weeks of immobilization, an injured joint has reduced motion because of these connective tissue changes. Remember also that as scar tissue forms, the natural process of wound contraction augments the injured area's motion loss.

When edema is combined with immobiliza-tion, fibrosis increases, probably as a result of more tissue fluid protein and metabolites in the area along with deficient local metabolism. The end result is less tissue mobility. Fibrosis further increases when circulation is impaired, either because of age or local conditions. Edema acts like a glue to bind down tissue structures, especially if its presence is prolonged.

Even when an area is immobilized, connective tissue continues its process of remodeling and reorganizing. Without movement, as collagen is laid down, it forms a dense, hard meshwork of sheets or bands with a loss of normal suppleness. Collagen fibers then form between the connective tissue's reticular fibers and also from one structure to another, "gluing down" the area. The result is restricted motion where normal areolar connective tissue would have permitted one tissue type to freely flow over another. Muscle tissue becomes restricted by fascia, tendons lose their ability to move against subcutaneous tissue, and ligaments adhere to capsules.

Immobilization produces structural weakness as well as a loss of tissue mobility. Weakness occurs because of a decrease in collagen mass. This is believed to occur because of the reduction in applied load or stress when a part is immobilized. Klein et al. (1989) demonstrated that if motion is allowed in a non-weight-bearing extremity, the integrity of the ligaments is not lost. Immobilized, non-weight-bearing limbs also lose bone density. When possible, activity therefore should be instituted for non-weight-bearing extremities until weight bearing and a full therapeutic exercise program are allowed.

EFFECTS ON MUSCLE TISSUE

Changes in muscle tissue following immobilization include reductions in muscle fiber size, number of myofibrils in the muscle, and oxidative capacity. As these changes occur, there is an increase in the fibrous and fatty tissue in the muscle and a reduction in the intramuscular capillary density. These changes, which cause the muscle to become smaller and weaker, can be seen after two weeks of immobilization. The longer a muscle is immobilized, the greater the number of muscle fibers that degenerate and the greater the quantity of fibrous and fatty tissue. As the muscle becomes weaker, loses its motion, and is kept immobilized, the normal neural feedback system of movement is lost. The combination of these factors along with changes in the ligaments impairs proprioception (Montgomery and Steadman 1985).

Histological changes in immobilized muscle include decreased levels of adenosine triphosphate (ATP), adenosine diphosphate (ADP), creatine phosphate (CP), creatine, and glycogen. When the immobilized muscle works, more than the normal level of lactic acid is produced. These changes, along with a reduction in mitochondrial production and size, cause a reduction in the oxidative capacity of the muscle, which causes the muscle to fatigue more quickly and easily. Several clinical observations can be made of immobilized muscle. The most obvious change is that the muscle is smaller in size. It is also unable to produce as strong a contraction and cannot sustain activity for as long a time as before immobilization. Additionally, the muscle is slower to respond to a stimulus when it contracts.

Many of these changes occur within the first few days of immobilization. A decrease in muscle size (atrophy) and mitochondrial production are seen with-in the first five to seven days of immobilization. The rate of atrophy, however, varies from one muscle to another. For example, when the thigh is immobilized, the quadriceps becomes weaker and smaller at a faster rate than the hamstrings.

EFFECTS ON ARTICULAR CARTILAGE

Articular cartilage suffers changes from immobilization, as well as other soft-tissue structures. These changes depend on the position of immobilization, the duration of immobilization, and whether the joint bears weight or not during the immobilization. Generally, the mechanical properties decay: The cartilage becomes thinner, the proteoglycan concentration decreases, and the matrix organiza-tion is reduced (Buckwalter 1996). In joints where articular surfaces are not in contact with each other, the articular cartilage of those surfaces changes. In addition, necrosis of articular cartilage has been seen when constant pressure between the joint surfaces is maintained during immobilization. Immobilization also increases the amount of fibrofatty tissue that ultimately becomes scar tissue within the joint.

Buckwalter (1996) also indicated that with continued immobilization, joints suffer irreparable damage. These changes include contracture of the joint because dense, fibrous tissue forms around the joint and in muscles that cross the joint; reduction of the articular cartilage lining of the joint surfaces; and replacement of the normal joint cavity by fibrofatty tissue. How long before the process becomes irreversible has not yet been definitively established in humans. In rats it occurs after 60 days of immobilization (Evans et al. 1960). In rabbits irreversible changes were seen after immobilization for six weeks (Finsterbush and Friedman 1975). Studies performed on animals also demonstrate that the longer an extremity is immobilized, the longer it takes to establish preimmobilization parameters. It is presumed that, at least in this regard, human tissue is no different.

EFFECTS ON PERIARTICULAR CONNECTIVE TISSUE

Periarticular connective tissue is soft tissue surrounding the joint, such as ligaments, the joint capsule, fascia, tendons, and synovial membranes. As with muscle and articular cartilage, all these structures are adversely affected by immobilization. The connective tissue becomes thick and fibrotic. Normally, the ground substance, a viscous gel that contains GAGs and water, serves to separate the collagen fibers, lubricate the area, and keep the fibers gliding freely. During immobilization the GAG and water content of the ground substance is reduced, causing a diminution of extracellular matrix. The combination of changes in ground substance, increased collagen cross-links, and continued normal collagen processing diminishes tissue mobility. The clinical impact of these changes is a loss of motion of the affected joint.

With all these dramatic changes from immobilization, it makes sense to minimize the duration of immobilization. Immobilization is important and necessary after some injuries and surgeries, and some require longer immobilization than others. It is in the best interest of the patient, however, to base the time of immobilization on the time course of injury and healing that was discussed in chapter 2.

Recall that collagen formation is well under way after seven days. The injury has gone from inflammation to proliferation and is entering the start of the remodeling phase. By day 21 the remodeling phase is in full swing, and the permanent structure is emerging. Although there are exceptions, gentle range-of-motion activities can be started by day 7 and certainly should be instituted by the third week following injury or surgery. From a biological standpoint, the initiation of range-of-motion activities depends on the severity of the injury, the tissue and body part involved, and the surgical repair technique used. From a practical standpoint, it is also determined by the patient's ability and status, the philosophy of the physician, the physician's confidence in his or her own surgical repair, and the abilities of the sport rehabilitation specialist.

EFFECTS OF REMOBILIZATION ON CONNECTIVE TISSUE

Remobilization enhances recovery. It prevents abnormal collagen cross-link formation and increases fluid content in the extracellular matrix of connective tissue.

Recent awareness of the deleterious effects of immobilization has changed how acute and surgically repaired injuries are treated. It is now more rare to cast a knee after surgery than it was in the early 1980s. It is also uncommon to see injuries other than bone fractures immobilized for more than a few weeks.

Just as there are many disadvantages to prolonged immobilization, there are many advantages to early remobilization.

EFFECTS ON MUSCLE FIBERS

Muscle fibers generally recover from immobilization. Initially, the recovery is rapid, but as it continues, the rate of change slows until full recovery is achieved. Injured muscle responds best to a short period of immobilization followed by active motion. Movement causes a more rapid absorption of hematoma, an increase in tensile strength, and improved myofiber regeneration and arrangement for an effective overall recovery. Adhesions of muscle to fascia with immobilization can reduce the muscle's flexibility and affect joint range of motion. Techniques for treating these restrictions are discussed in chapter 6.

EFFECTS ON ARTICULAR CARTILAGE

Less articular cartilage degeneration occurs if both joint motion and weight bearing are allowed, even on a limited basis. Controlled weight bearing or loading of articular cartilage may even encourage repair of damaged cartilage. Overall, research findings consistently indicate that a joint, after injury, responds best to a rehabilitation program that provides controlled loading and movement, which stimulate proteoglycan and chondrocyte production.

EFFECTS ON PERIARTICULAR CONNECTIVE TISSUE

Remobilization of periarticular connective tissue prevents abnormal cross-link formation and helps to maintain the fluid content of the extracellular matrix so that proper fiber distance can be maintained (Donatelli and Owens-Burkhart 1981). Fatty tissue buildup around the joint limits mobility and must be broken by techniques such as stretching and joint mobilization. Stretching techniques are discussed later in this chapter, and joint mobilization is introduced in chapter 6.

MECHANICAL PROPERTIES AND TISSUE BEHAVIOR IN RANGE OF MOTION

A tissue's mechanical properties, such as plasticity, elasticity, and viscoelasticity, affect its response to force and thus to stretching.

Even when an extremity is not immobilized, injury or surgery causes scar-tissue formation, which can lead to adhesions of connective tissue and increased fibrosis. In most cases, whether in healthy or injured athletes, restricted range of motion is the result of limited connective-tissue extensibility. Connective tissue includes joint capsules, ligaments, tendons, and fascia. Although muscles are not composed primarily of connective-tissue like these other structures, they are surrounded by an extensive fascial network that affects their flexibility and response to stretch. The flexibility of all tissues that sport rehabilitation specialists deal with in the treatment of injuries is therefore affected by connective tissue.

To determine the most effective ways to increase the range of motion of injured parts, it is important to review the physiology of connective tissue. Stretching exercises affect the noncontractile element of all connective tissue. Because collagen gives a structure its tensile strength, resilience, and form, it is also the primary component that restricts range of motion and therefore should be the primary target of stretching exercises.

Remember that body parts are three-dimensional and respond to forces in three dimensions. When stress is applied, a structure's response depends on the direction, duration, and magnitude of the force and the specific fibers involved.

MECHANICAL PROPERTIES OF CONNECTIVE TISSUE

To effectively apply stretching forces to collagen, you must first understand its mechanical properties. Collagen is elastic, viscoelastic, and plastic. Connective tissue possesses all these qualities simultaneously (figure 5.2). When connective tissue is stretched, all three qualities may be affected. If we separate the properties and look at them individually, it might be easier to understand how collagen functions and what we can do to influence it. Plasticity allows the connective tissue's length to change, while elasticity allows some restoration of normal length. The effectiveness of the stretch depends on the amount of collagen and elastin in the gross structure. The effectiveness of the stretch also depends on the amount of force applied, the duration of the stretch, and the temperature of the tissue. The physical properties of collagen also influence the effectiveness of a stretch.

▌Figure 5.2 Connective tissue stretch model. Connective tissue possesses qualities of plasticity, viscoelasticity, and elasticity.

Reprinted from Viidik 1973.

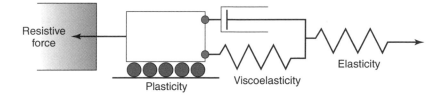

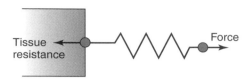

■ Figure 5.3   Elasticity.

Reprinted from Viidik 1973.

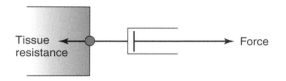

■ Figure 5.4   Viscosity.

Reprinted from Viidik 1973.

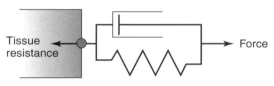

■ Figure 5.5   Viscoelasticity.

Reprinted from Viidik 1973.

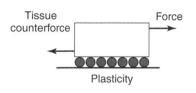

■ Figure 5.6   Coulomb friction model.

Reprinted from Viidik 1973.

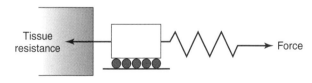

■ Figure 5.7   St. Venant body.

Reprinted from Viidik 1973.

Elasticity

Elasticity is the ability to return to normal length after an elongation force or load has been applied. This restoration of length occurs because of its stored potential energy. Elastic material is commonly symbolized by a spring in engineering models (figure 5.3). Elasticity is observed when you give a rubber band a brief pull; when you release the force, the rubber band returns to its normal length.

Viscoelasticity

Viscoelasticity is demonstrated by substances that have both elastic and viscous properties. **Viscosity** is the resistance to an outside force that causes a fluidlike, permanent deformation. No potential energy is stored in a viscous object, so there is no energy to permit its return to normal length; the energy is released as heat before it can be stored. Viscosity is represented by a hydraulic cylinder, as in figure 5.4. Elasticity provides some recovery to a former condition. **Viscoelasticity**, then, is the ability of a structure to resist change of shape when an outside force is applied but an inability to completely return to its former state after changing shape. Viscoelasticity is commonly represented as a combination of a spring and a hydraulic cylinder (figure 5.5).

Plasticity

Plasticity is the ability of a substance to undergo a permanent change in size or shape after a deforming force is applied. An example of plasticity is pulling a ball of putty; the putty changes in length and does not return to its former condition when you release your force. Plasticity is commonly represented by the Coulomb model of dry friction, as seen in figure 5.6. In the Coulomb model, if the force applied to a structure is greater than the friction, movement occurs; if the applied force is less than the friction force, no movement will take place. So it is with plasticity of collagen: Change in length occurs when the applied force is greater than the force holding collagen fibers attached to one another. The St. Venant body (figure 5.7), however, is a more practical representation of biological tissue, which has both plastic and elastic components. In this model, when a load is applied to the structure, it responds elastically until the friction force is exceeded. At that point a plastic deformation occurs. When the load is released, there is some change in the structure's length because of the plastic deformation, but there is some return toward normal length as well because of the elastic component of the tissue.

PHYSICAL PROPERTIES OF CONNECTIVE TISSUE

The physical behaviors of connective tissue include force relaxation and creep. They are both time-dependent responses that rely on the duration of the outside force and the rate at which it is applied. **Force deformation** is the amount of force that is applied to maintain a change of length or other deformation of tissue. It results in a relaxation of the tissue. If the force is applied too quickly and viscoelastic and plastic changes occur that are faster or greater than the tissue can tolerate, an injury can result (figure 5.2).

Creep

Creep is the elongation of tissue when a load, usually a low-level load in the plastic range, is applied over an extended period of time. The result is a permanent change in the tissue's length. Creep is time dependent, so a load that is applied for a longer time is more effective in causing a change in tissue length than a load that is applied and released quickly. Increasing the tissue's temperature increases the rate of creep. In functional terms, applying heat to a muscle before stretching it permits a better stretch.

If a load is applied in the elastic range, the structure gradually returns to normal length once the load is released. This does not cause a permanent change in tissue length.

A structure's length can also be affected by structural fatigue. Fatigue of a structure occurs when it is loaded repetitively below the failure point until the cumulative stress results in failure. The greater the load, the fewer the repetitions necessary for failure to occur. The point at which structural fatigue causes tissue failure is referred to as **fatigue failure** or **endurance limit**. When structural fatigue occurs in bones it is called a stress fracture; when it occurs in tendons, as an overuse injury, it is called tendinitis.

Stress-Strain

As was discussed in chapter 3, the load required to change the length of connective tissue is directly related to the tissue's strength, and the tissue's strength is directly related to its ability to resist a load. This relationship is defined by **Hooke's law**, which states that the strain (deformation) of an object is directly related to the object's ability to resist the stress (load), and is illustrated by the stress-strain curve. **Stress** is a force that changes the form or shape of a body. Connective tissue is subject to three types of stress: tension stress (stretching force), compression stress (from muscle contractions and weight bearing on joints), and shear force (force applied parallel to the cross section of the tissue).

Strain is the amount of deformation that occurs when a stress is applied. Each tissue has a stress-strain curve that represents its own specific ability to resist deforming forces. Although different tissues' stress-strain curves may differ in timing and magnitude, they share the same general characteristics. The specific reactions of a tissue to a load that are illustrated by this curve can be seen in figure 5.8.

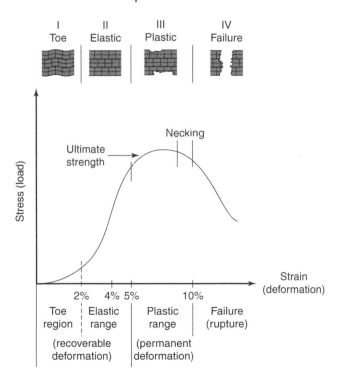

I Figure 5.8   Stress-strain curve.

Reprinted, by permission, from W.B. Butler, E.S. Grood, F.R. Noyes, and R.F. Zernicke, 1978, "Biomechanics of ligaments and tendons," *Exercise and Sport Sciences Reviews* 6:125-281.

The initial portion of the stress-strain curve is referred to as the toe region. In connective tissue the collagen fibers have a wavy crimp arrangement at rest. The toe region accounts for 1.5% to 4% of the total collagen fiber lengthening that is possible (Butler et al. 1978). As a force is applied, the fibers are stretched into the elastic range. As the slack in the collagen is taken up, it loses its wavy appearance. At a macroscopic level, no resistance is felt until the tissue is brought to the end of the elastic limit. In the elastic range a collagen fiber elongates to 2% to 5% of its total possible elongation (Butler et al. 1978). The tissue's full normal range of motion is in the elastic range. If the force is released in this range, the tissue will return to its prestretch length.

At the yield strength point, the stress loads the tissue beyond its elastic range and into its plastic range. Tissue loaded into this range undergoes permanent elongation. This is the result of the failure of a few of the collagen fibers to withstand the stress and a disruption of the cross-links. Collagen fiber can fail through a number of mechanisms, including a failure of the force-relaxation response when a load is applied too quickly for the collagen's viscoelastic and plastic adaptations to occur. Fibers also tear if the creep response causes too much deformation too quickly. This deformation can occur either in one episode or from accumulated stress from a number of lesser loads. This failure of isolated collagen fibers occurs unpredictably and results in an increase in range of motion.

Two factors within the plastic range should be respected. **Ultimate strength** is the greatest load that a tissue can tolerate. After this point the fiber length changes without application of any additional load. The point of ultimate strength is not always achieved. There may be a necking region prior to failure of the tissue, where the tissue's strength noticeably decreases so that less stress is needed to cause a change in the tissue's length. When this occurs, failure of the tissue is often imminent if the stress application continues.

Fatigue failure is the point at which the tissue is unable to tolerate continued stress and then ruptures. In collagen this occurs when the fiber is stretched to 6% to 10% beyond its resting length (Butler et al. 1978).

The general shape of the stress-strain curve is seen in figure 5.8, but the specific shape of the curve varies from one structure to another. Some additional factors influence the failure point of the whole structure rather than just the connective tissue. Tissue width is one of these factors. A structure's larger cross-sectional size indicates more fibers, so more stress is required to produce failure of the structure. The tissue's slack length is another factor. Longer tissues can withstand greater forces because they have more slack. For example, if two pieces of rope have the same number of fibers but one is twice as long as the other, the longer rope can tolerate greater deformation before breaking. The microstructure of the tissue and the orientation of the structure to the forces applied also influence the ability of the ligament or tendon to withstand deforming loads.

Given these physical and mechanical properties of connective tissue, some methods of stretching can be more effective than others for increasing range of motion. Using the principle of creep, a low load applied over a period of time can effectively remodel collagen bonds to increase range of motion. Stretches that take advantage of creep are more effective in remodeling collagen and maintaining range of motion increases than other stretching methods. This type of stretching is commonly referred to as prolonged stretching and is discussed later in this chapter.

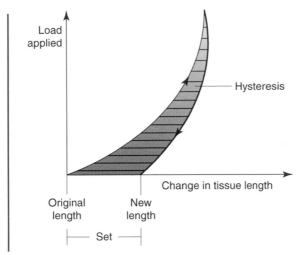

Figure 5.9
Hysteresis.

Adapted from Bogduk and Twomey 1987.

Hysteresis

Repetitive stretching with sub-maximal loads can also be effective in increasing range of motion. Energy in the form of heat is released when stress is applied to tissue. As the tissue is heated with repetitive stretches, the tissue is more easily stretched. When tissue is unable to keep pace with the forces, with each successive load application, it elongates more. This response is called **hysteresis**. When a load is released, the tissue returns to its normal length at a different rate from that of stretching it. When a new length is achieved with this process, the change in length is referred to as the *set*, as seen in figure 5.9.

As the tissue changes length and is heated with the stretch, higher-level loads are tolerated in later repetitions. In other words, the tissue's failure load increases, so that a greater force can be applied to produce a greater tissue deformation, as seen in figure 5.10. An example of this is when a **proprioceptive neuromuscular facilitation (PNF)** stretch is applied, released, then reapplied to a patient's hamstrings; in the second stretch, the patient's hamstring is stretched farther and the patient can tolerate a slightly greater stretch force.

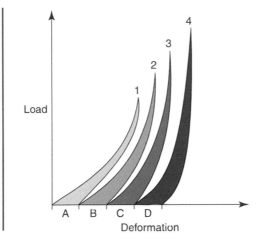

Figure 5.10 Deformation with hysteresis in repetitive stretching.
Reprinted from Viidik 1973.

NEUROMUSCULAR INFLUENCES ON RANGE OF MOTION

Muscle spindles and Golgi tendon organs are sensitive to tension in the muscle and its tendons, respectively, and protect these structures from abrupt changes in tension.

In addition to the physical and mechanical properties of connective tissue, neurological factors influence the effectiveness of stretching techniques in increasing range of motion of a structure. Neurological components that affect a muscle's ability to respond to a stretching force include the muscle spindle and the Golgi tendon organ (GTO). The muscle spindle is much more complex than the GTO.

MUSCLE SPINDLE

There is a variation in the ratio of muscle spindles to muscle fibers in each muscle. Generally, the more precise the movement required of a muscle, the lower the ratio of muscle fibers to muscle spindles. A typical muscle fiber is often referred to as an **extrafusal fiber**. Muscle spindles vary in length and diameter, but all lie between and parallel to the extrafusal muscle fibers. The muscle fibers contained by the muscle spindle are called **intrafusal fibers.**

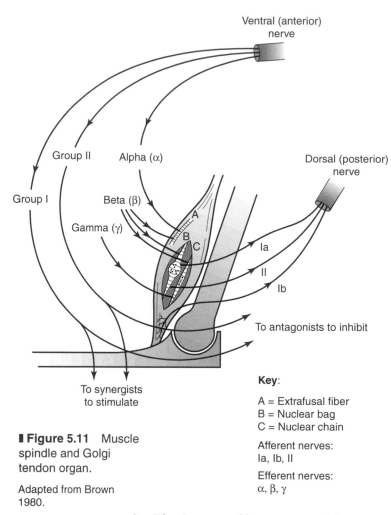

Ventral (anterior) nerve

Group II   Alpha (α)

Group I   Beta (β)

Gamma (γ)

Dorsal (posterior) nerve

A

B

C

Ia

II

Ib

To antagonists to inhibit

To synergists to stimulate

Key:

A = Extrafusal fiber
B = Nuclear bag
C = Nuclear chain

Afferent nerves:
Ia, Ib, II

Efferent nerves:
α, β, γ

▌**Figure 5.11** Muscle spindle and Golgi tendon organ.

Adapted from Brown 1980.

Entering the intrafusal muscle fiber are three nerve fibers: alpha, beta, and gamma nerves, as noted in figure 5.11. Exiting the intrafusal fibers are the Ia, Ib, and II afferent, or sensory, fibers. The muscle spindle is composed of these nerve fibers, the intrafusal muscle fibers, and the sac that surrounds these structures. There are two types of intrafusal fibers, and each has a different function within muscle spindles. One type, the **nuclear bag fiber,** has an enlarged center region with two or three nuclei stacked beside each other. The shorter, thinner fibers are called **nuclear chain fibers,** and their nuclei are arranged in single file in the center region. Although both are sensitive to stretch, the nuclear bag fiber has more elasticity and is therefore sensitive to the velocity of the stretch.

An afferent Ia nerve fiber wraps around the center region of the intrafusal fibers. This nerve ending is sometimes called a *primary ending* or an *annulospiral ending*. The secondary or II afferent nerve endings are at the ends of the intrafusal muscle fibers, primarily on nuclear chain, and are sometimes called *flower-spray endings* because of their appearance. Because of the structure of Ia nerve fibers, they respond much more quickly to stimulation than the II nerves. The Ia nerve fibers are sensitive to a quick stretch, and both Ia and II nerve fibers respond to a static stretch (Eldred 1967).

Because the intrafusal fiber is attached to the connective tissue surrounding extrafusal muscle fibers, the intrafusal muscle fiber is sensitive to changes in the muscle's length. Both the afferent nerve fibers in the muscle spindle transmit signals to the spinal cord regarding changes in the muscle's length and the velocity and duration of a stretch. An efferent response is sent to both the intrafusal and extrafusal muscle fibers to permit the muscle to react to the stimulation. Gamma efferent fibers transmit to the intrafusal muscle fibers, and alpha efferent fibers transmit to the extrafusal muscle fibers to cause a muscle contraction. Once the muscle contracts and shortens, stress and stimulation of the muscle spindles cease.

In addition to stimulating the muscle in which they lie, group I nerve fibers of a muscle send a branch to synergistic muscles and antagonistic muscles. The result is simultaneous stimulation of synergistic muscles and inhibition of antagonistic muscles. Group II nerve fibers also transmit to the synergistic and antagonistic muscles, but they use another neuron link to complete the transmission. The impact of stimulating synergistic muscles will become more apparent in chapter 7 during the discussion of proprioceptive neuromuscular facilitation (PNF).

GOLGI TENDON ORGANS

Like the muscle spindle, the **Golgi tendon organ (GTO)** also functions as a protective mechanism. GTOs are not as sensitive to stretch as muscle spindles are, but they are very sensitive to contraction and tension that occur in a muscle.

GTOs, located at the distal and proximal muscle-tendon junctions, are long, delicate, tubular capsules that contain a cluster of Ib nerve fibers. These nerve fibers originate on the tendon's fascicles. The protection performed by the GTO is known as **autogenic inhibition**. When the GTO is stimulated, its activity causes simultaneous inhibition of the alpha motor neuron of its own muscle and internuncial activation (between afferent and efferent neurons) of the antagonistic muscle.

The result of the combined reactions of the muscle spindle and the GTO is seen in functional activities. If a muscle is stretched quickly, the muscle spindle produces a **monosynaptic response**, which is a rapid reflex motor response resulting from a direct neural connection between a sensory (afferent) and motor (efferent) nerve without an intermediary neuron. A monosynaptic response is the most rapid response because an intermediary nerve is not involved. If a stretching force is applied too quickly, the muscle being stretched reflexively responds secondarily to stimulation of the muscle spindle. This is a potential problem with ballistic stretching that is discussed later in this chapter. On the other hand, if a stretch is applied slowly, the GTO inhibits muscular contraction. This may actually provide better relaxation of the muscle to improve the effectiveness of the stretch.

DETERMINING NORMAL RANGE OF MOTION

Normal range of motion is different for each joint, each patient, and each sport and position.

Before you can determine whether a joint has deficient range of motion, you must first know the normal range of motion. Only then can you decide whether stretching exercises should be included in the therapeutic exercise program. Table 5.1 demonstrates that there is some dispute among authors as to what is considered normal, though all are within close range of one another. Differences are probably due to the populations each author measured to achieve the data. Age and sex of the subjects and the positions in which measurements are taken all affect measurement results. Regardless of whose data are used, they can provide sport rehabilitation specialists with a guideline for expectations of normal range of motion.

Each patient's normal range of motion is actually determined by comparison with the contralateral part. It is also based on the demands of the individual's sport and position. For example, normal range of motion for shoulder external rotation is different for a baseball pitcher and for a football lineman.

It is important for you to become familiar with normal ranges of motion. Without this knowledge, it is impossible to determine when a problem exists. If problem areas are not identified, proper therapeutic exercise programs cannot be designed, and the rehabilitation program cannot be successful.

MEASURING RANGE OF MOTION

Range of motion is typically measured with a goniometer. Good technique is essential for measuring accurately and consistently.

Now that you have been introduced to the physiological constructs that determine range of motion and to the normal values of range of motion, you are ready to learn how to measure range of motion.

Table 5.1 Examples of Normal Ranges of Motion in Upper and Lower Extremities According to Various Authors

Joint Motion	Hoppenfeld (1976)	Daniels & Worthingham (1972)	A.A.O.S. (1965)	Kendall & McCreary (1983)	Kapandji (1980)	Esch & Lepley (1974)	Gerhardt & Russe (1975)
Shoulder							
Flexion	180	—	180	180	180	170	170
Extension	45	50	60	45	50	60	50
Abduction	180	—	180	180	180	170	170
External rotation	45	90	90	90	80	90	90
Internal rotation	55	90	70	70	95	80	80
Horizontal abduction	—	—	—	—	—	—	30
Horizontal adduction	—	—	135	—	—	—	135
Elbow							
Flexion	135+	145–160	150	145	145–160	150	150
Forearm							
Supination	90	90	80	90	80	90	90
Pronation	90	90	80	90	85	90	80
Wrist							
Extension	70	70	70	70	85	70	50
Flexion	80	90	80	80	85	90	60
Radial Deviation	20	—	20	20	15	20	20
Ulnar Deviation	30	—	30	35	45	30	30
Thumb, carpometacarpal							
Abduction	70	50	70	80	50	—	—
Flexion	—	—	15	45	—	—	—
Extension	—	—	20	0	—	—	—
Opposition	Tip of thumb to tip of 5th finger						
Thumb, metacarpophalangeal							
Flexion	50	70	50	60	80	—	—
Thumb, interphalangeal							
Flexion	90	90	80	80	80	—	—
Digits 2–5, metacarpophalangeal							
Flexion	90	90	90	90	—	—	—
Extension	45	30	45	—	—	—	—
Digits 2–5, proximal interphalangeal							
Flexion	100	120	—	—	—	—	—
Digits 2–5, distal interphalangeal							
Flexion	90	80	—	—	—	—	—
Subtalar joint							
Inversion	—	—	35	35	52	30	40
Eversion	—	—	20	20	30	15	20
Ankle							
Dorsiflexion	20	—	20	20	20–30	10	20
Plantar flexion	50	45	50	45	50	65	45
Knee							
Flexion	135	140–160	135	140	135	135	130
Hip							
Flexion	120	115–125	120	125	120	130	125
Extension	30	15	30	10	30	45	15
Abduction	45–50	45	45	45	45	45	45
Adduction	20–30	—	30	10	30	15	15
Internal rotation	35	45	45	45	45	33	45
External rotation	45	45	45	45	60	36	45

EQUIPMENT

Range of motion is usually measured with an instrument known as a **goniometer**. It is essentially a protractor with a stationary arm and a movable arm, as shown in figure 5.12. It can measure up to either 180° or 360°. Many varieties of goniometers have been designed to measure different joints. Other devices have been designed either to measure specific body segments or to make measurement easier. For example, the Leighton flexometer has a weighted, 360° dial with an enclosed needle; it

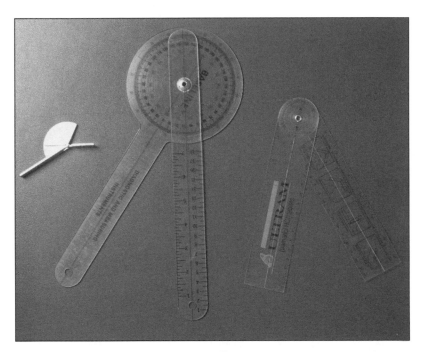

Figure 5.12 Goniometers come in different sizes to measure various body segments. They are most often 360° or 180°.

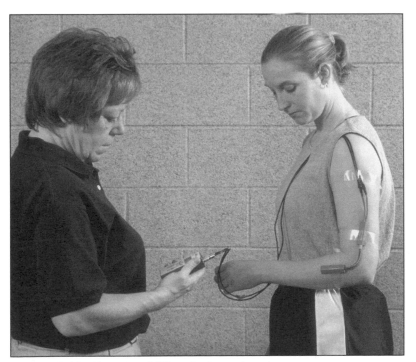

Figure 5.13 Penny and Giles electrogoniometer.

is attached with a strap to the body part that is being measured. An elgon, or electrogoniometer, was developed by Karpovich et al. (1959) and uses a potentiometer rather than a protractor. It is used to measure primarily dynamic motion, as it is less accurate with static motion. The number of joints that it can be used to measure is also limited. Another electrogoniometer, the Penny and Giles, is shown in figure 5.13.

Trunk motion is difficult to measure with a standard goniometer. Using the Moll and Wright (1971) method (figure 5.14), marks are made at the top and bottom of the lumbar spine. A metal tape measure is used to measure the difference in distance between the two marks in flexion, extension, and normal standing. This measure is relative to the individual being tested and cannot be used to determine an individual's deviation from normal, because standards have not been established and would probably be difficult to determine.

One of the most common methods for measuring trunk flexion is the fingertip-to-floor method, demonstrated in figure 5.15. The person stands with trunk flexed, and the distance between the fingertips and the floor is measured. Side bending (figure 5.16) also produces a relative measurement, recorded as the distance from the fingertips to either the fibular head or the floor. Although this method may not be as accurate as others and does not isolate the structure being assessed (i.e., the lumbar spine), it can be reproduced in the same individual so that changes can be evaluated.

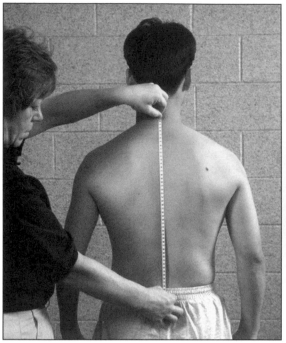
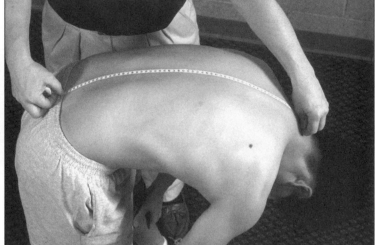

▌Figure 5.14 Moll and Wright spinal ROM method.

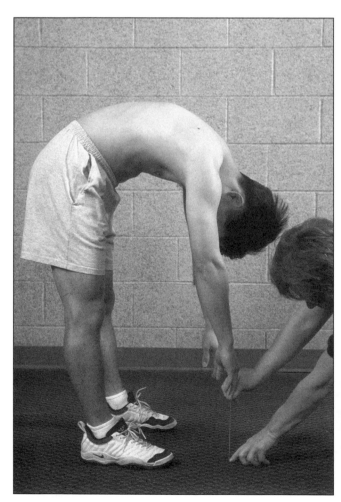
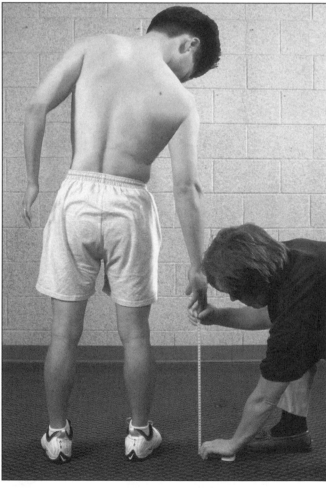

▌Figure 5.15 Measuring trunk flexion.

▌Figure 5.16 Measuring lateral trunk flexion.

APPLICATION

To measure accurately with a goniometer, the most common tool for evaluating range of motion, placement of the protractor and arms is important. The arms of the goniometer are placed along the length of the two limbs forming the joint. If placed correctly, the pivot point of the protractor should be lined up over the presumed axis of motion of the joint. For correct alignment, the limbs being measured should be exposed. With some exceptions, the goniometer is placed along the central lateral aspect of the limb. Figure 5.17 demonstrates measuring techniques for some joints.

Range of motion is measured in either a 180° or 360° system using either a 180° or 360° goniometer. In the 360° system, 0° is overhead and 180° is at the feet. In the 180° system, 0° is at the start of the range in the anatomical position

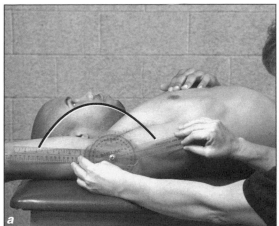
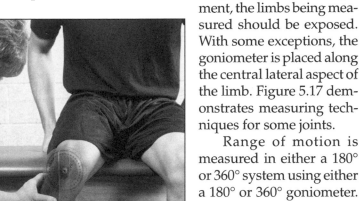
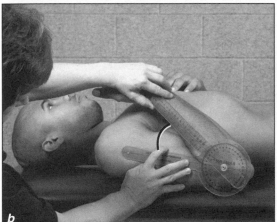
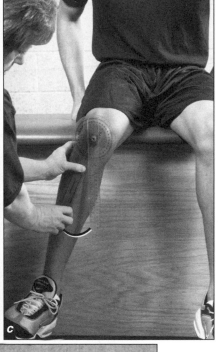
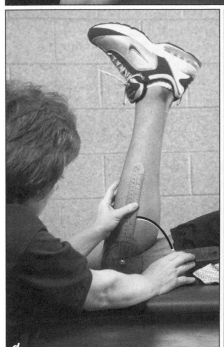
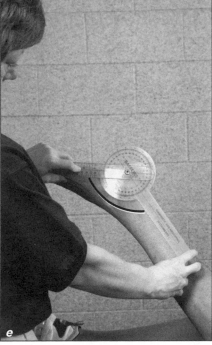
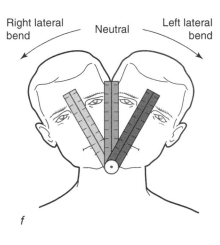

Right lateral bend   Neutral   Left lateral bend

■ Figure 5.17 Goniometer placement for measuring *(a)* shoulder flexion, *(b)* elbow flexion, *(c)* hip internal rotation, *(d)* knee flexion, *(e)* ankle plantar flexion, and *(f)* cervical lateral flexion. The center of the goniometer is placed over the joint's center (axis of motion). Alignment of the goniometer's stationary and movable arms and fulcrum must be accurate for reliable measurements.

and 180° is at the end. There is some variation in both systems for measurements of inversion, eversion, supination, pronation, and lateral flexion. Either system is valid and can be used to measure range of motion. The most common system used for sport injuries is the 180° system.

ACCURACY

A sport rehabilitation specialist's ability to accurately measure range of motion depends on his or her training, experience, and attention to detail. Even an experienced sport rehabilitation specialist with good equipment can expect accuracy only within 3° to 5° of true values. It is therefore vital to be as consistent as possible. Careful attention to the placement of the goniometer arms and making sure that the axis of the goniometer coincides with the joint's axis of rotation are very important in ensuring accurate measurements. Check the goniometer placement, adjust the patient's position if necessary to achieve correct body segment alignment, and then check again before recording your final measurement to help ensure accuracy. Consistent measurements depend on your attention to these details. If your technique is good, your measurements should be reliable. If your technique varies, your results will be inconsistent and therefore of no use to you, the patient, or anyone else. If your technique is accurate, other sport rehabilitation specialists (assuming their technique is also good) should obtain measurements that are the same or within 5° of yours.

Interpretation of range-of-motion measurements can be clouded by a variety of conditions. The position in which the patient is placed, whether active or passive motion is measured, pain occurring with motion, spasm, voluntary resistance to movement, wounds, and the patient's willingness to move the part can all affect measurements. You should note such conditions in your record.

TERMINOLOGY IN GONIOMETRY

Standard terminology and frames of reference to describe bodily movements and range of motion make your records usable by others.

To ensure accurate interpretation of your results by those to whom your report is sent or by those who refer to your notes, you and your readers should use common terminology. Table 5.2 gives common terms used in goniometry.

The bodily motion can be divided into three planes: sagittal, frontal or coronal, and horizontal or transverse. Their frame of reference is the anatomical position, which is the body standing erect with the hips and knees in extension, the feet facing forward, the elbows and wrists in extension, the hands at the sides, and the palms facing forward.

Motions of flexion and extension occur in the sagittal plane. Motions in the frontal plane include abduction and adduction at the shoulders and hips. Transverse plane movement includes hip and shoulder rotation, pronation, and supination in the anatomical position. Although discussions of range of motion refer to these planes, functional activities usually involve oblique planes of motion that include all three conventional planes.

STRETCHING TECHNIQUES

Stretching can be active, passive, or a combination of the two. Knowing the indications, contraindications, and proper precautions for stretching is necessary to safely and effectively use any stretching technique.

When an athlete has an injury that results in deficient range of motion, several techniques can be applied to restore range of motion, depending on your preference and skill, the type of tissue restriction involved, the extent of the injury, and the duration of the loss of motion. Continuous passive motion machines and other mechanical devices are discussed later in this chapter. Joint mobilization and various techniques of soft-tissue mobilization are investigated in chapter 6.

Probably one of the most common methods of increasing range of motion is using stretching exercises. Many researchers have investigated various methods and techniques in search of the best and most effective way to gain range of motion.

Table 5.2 Goniometric Terms

Term	Definition
saggital plane	The anterior-posterior vertical plane through which the longitudinal axis passes and that divides the body into right and left halves.
frontal (coronal) plane	Any vertical plane that divides the body into front and back parts.
transverse (horizontal) plane	A plane that divides a section of the body into upper and lower parts. It is parallel to the horizon.
flexion	Bending a joint so that the two body segments approach each other and decrease the joint angle.
extension	Straightening a joint so that the two body segments move apart and increase the joint angle.
abduction	Lateral movement of a limb or segment away from the midline of the body or part.
adduction	Lateral movement of a limb or segment toward the midline of the body or part.
internal rotation	Rotation of a joint around its axis in a transverse plane toward the midline of the body. Also called *medial rotation*.
external rotation	Rotation of a joint around its axis in a transverse plane away from the midline of the body. Also called *lateral rotation*.
supination	Movement of the palm forward or upward into the anatomical position. Also, the multiplanar rotation of the subtalar and transverse talar joints that includes plantar flexion, adduction, and inversion.
pronation	Movement of the palm backward or downward so that the palm faces in a posterior direction, opposite the anatomical position. Also, a multiplanar rotation of the subtalar and transverse talar joints that is the combination of dorsiflexion, abduction, and eversion.
inversion	Inward turning motion of the foot that causes the bottom of the foot to face medially.
eversion	Outward turning motion of the foot that causes the bottom of the foot to face laterally.
dorsiflexion	A flexion of the ankle that causes the dorsum (top) of the foot to move toward the lower leg so that the angle of the ankle decreases.
plantar flexion	An extension of the ankle that causes the dorsum (top) of the foot to move away from the lower leg so that the angle of the ankle increases.
radial deviation	A movement of the wrist toward the thumb side of the forearm. Also called *radial flexion*.
ulnar deviation	A movement of the wrist toward the little-finger side of the forearm. Also called *ulnar flexion*.
opposition	A diagonal movement of the thumb across the palm of the hand to permit it to make contact with one of the other four fingers.

(continued)

Table 5.2 *(continued)*	
Term	**Definition**
depression	A downward movement of the scapula
elevation	An upward movement of the scapula.
protraction	A forward movement of the scapula. Also called *scapular abduction.*
retraction	A backward movement of the scapula. Also called *scapular adduction.*
upward rotation	A movement of the scapula that causes the glenoid to face forward and upward. The inferior angle of the scapula moves laterally away from the spine, and the scapula slides forward.
downward rotation	A movement of the scapula that causes the glenoid to face downward and backward. The inferior angle of the scapula moves medially, and the scapula slides backward.
horizontal flexion	A motion of the upper extremity in a transverse plane toward the midline of the body. Also called *horizontal adduction.*
horizontal extension	A motion of the upper extremity in a transverse plane away from the midline of the body. Also called *horizontal abduction.*

Unfortunately, the answer remains elusive. One of the problems is that many of the research studies investigating stretching methods have been performed with normal, uninjured subjects or with animals. Some of the investigations are not sound, objective, or reproducible. Studies, as yet, have failed to provide answers regarding the best method of stretching for patients. Needless to say, we must rely on our knowledge of injury, healing, and the physiology of connective tissue more than on specific investigations to determine the best way to stretch an injured area.

Regardless of the type of stretch used, the application of heat before the stretch produces a better stretch. Heat can be applied either passively or actively. An example of a passive heat application is the application of a hot pack before stretching. A better method is active heat application, in which the patient performs a warm-up activity, such as exercising on a stationary bike, stair climber, or upper-body ergometer, before stretching. A hot pack provides superficial heat, but an active exercise increases the deeper tissues' temperature more effectively and more safely than a passive modality (Saal 1987).

ACTIVE STRETCHING

Stretching exercises can be divided into active stretching, passive stretching, and a combination of the two. Active stretching includes flexibility exercises that are performed by the patient without outside assistance from either a partner or a machine (figure 5.18). Depending on the duration and repetitions of the active stretch, it affects the elastic range of connective tissue and may have some effect on the plastic range. This type of stretch is commonly used and most effective when there is no injury or the injury is recent and minor with minimal scar tissue. Based on the results of four studies (Garrett 1990; Bandy et al. 1997; McNair and Stanley 1996; Taylor et al. 1990) and my clinical observations, I feel the best application of active stretching is a 15 to 30 s hold for four to five repetitions of an exercise. For patients who have significant loss of motion, repeated stretch sessions throughout the day may be beneficial; although there have not been any studies demonstrating that repeated sessions are beneficial, reason indicates the possibility that they may be,

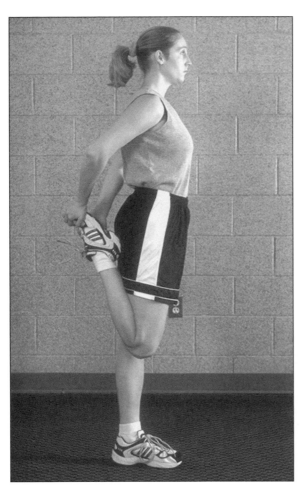

Figure 5.18   Active stretch.

especially during scar-tissue formation and contraction. If the individual is participating in sport activities, the stretches should also be performed after the activity.

Because of the phenomenon of antagonist inhibition, if the individual contracts the opposing muscle, relaxation of the muscle being stretched increases. This results in a more effective stretch. For example, a better stretch occurs when the patient actively contracts the quadriceps as the hamstrings are being stretched. It is believed that a strong relationship between muscles and their antagonists affects muscles' flexibility. Some researchers believe that an agonist muscle is shortened when its antagonist is weaker, preventing a balance between the two and resulting in a loss of range of motion. If the antagonist is facilitated, the agonist becomes inhibited, which allows a restoration of normal flexibility. You can perform this quick experiment on yourself to see the impact of antagonist inhibition on increasing muscle flexibility. Do not perform this activity if you have a lumbar disk injury. In a standing position, first evaluate your hamstring flexibility by attempting to touch your toes, keeping your knees straight. Return to an upright position. Now bend over at the waist to touch your toes but with your knees bent to prevent a stretch of the hamstrings. Keeping your hands on your toes, straighten your knees by tightening the quadriceps. Repeat this three or four times. Now return to a full standing position, and reevaluate your hamstring flexibility by attempting to touch your toes, keeping your knees straight. You should be able to reach farther than on your initial evaluation. This improvement occurs because the contraction of the quadriceps causes a reciprocal inhibition of the hamstrings, so the hamstrings are able to relax and allow elongation to occur.

The effects of reciprocal inhibition demonstrate the need to accompany any stretching technique with strengthening exercises to maintain newly acquired muscle length. Strengthening exercises also assist in restoring balance between agonists and their antagonistic muscle groups. This topic is discussed in later chapters.

PASSIVE STRETCHING

Passive stretching includes a variety of methods, including short-term and long-term stretches. Passive stretching involves the use of equipment or another person, and the patient does not assist in the stretch activity (figure 5.19). A typical example of a short-term passive stretch is when the sport rehabilitation specialist moves the

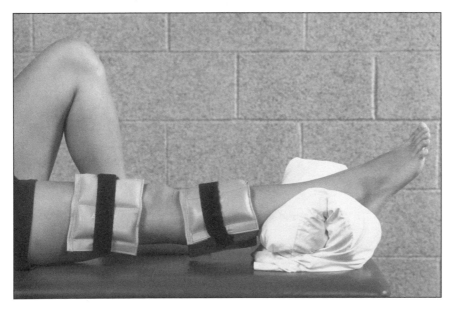

Figure 5.19   The patient does not assist in passive stretch. The stretch here is provided by gravity and further assisted with weights on the leg.

patient's injured part through its range of motion and applies a stretch at the end of the motion. Madding et al. (1987) reported that the most effective length of time to hold a short-term, passive stretch is 15 s. Although a short-term, passive stretch affects primarily the elastic range of connective tissue, it may be more effective in producing changes in the plastic range than an active stretch, because a passive stretch may be applied longer or with a slightly greater force than the patient can apply unassisted.

When applying a stretch, the part should be moved to the end of its free motion. The proximal segment of the joint being stretched should be stabilized to prevent its movement while a firm pressure is applied to the distal segment. A steady pressure is applied until the slack of soft tissue is taken up and the joint is tight. The joint is then moved slightly beyond this point. The patient should feel a stretch or tension, but not pain. If a two-joint muscle is being stretched, first one joint is positioned in the muscle's lengthened position, then the second joint, until maximum muscle length is achieved. The stretch is repeated four to six times.

The most effective stretches involve the steady application of force over a period of time. This prolonged stretch causes a better plastic deformation of connective tissue, primarily because of the length of time it is applied. Although research has yet to define how long a prolonged stretch should be applied, Kottke, Pauley, and Ptak (1966) suggested 20 min in clinical application. Although prolonged stretching is the most effective of all stretching techniques, it seems to be the least investigated (Light et al. 1984). A prolonged stretch is applied with a reduced load. Two articles by Warren, Lehmann, and Koblanski (1971, 1976) reported that the amount of time required for a prolonged stretch to change connective tissue length is inversely proportional to the amount of force used. A prolonged stretch is effective in increasing motion because of its impact on the stress-strain curves of tissue and the creep phenomenon, discussed earlier in this chapter.

When using prolonged stretches, the part being stretched should be stabilized to permit the load to stretch the correct tissue. This stabilization can be provided either by the weight of the body or part or by a mechanical device such as a weight or strap. The stretch is applied slowly and steadily to the point of joint tightness. The segment is then secured in this position and held for the desired amount of time. If a two-joint muscle is stretched, the secondary joint should be placed in a position that elongates the muscle. For example, if the knee is stretched in extension, the patient should sit so as to elongate the hamstrings at the proximal end where it crosses the hip joint. The patient commonly does not feel much, if anything, when the stretch is first applied. Within 5 to 10 min, however, the patient should feel the stretch's effect. The minimal prolonged stretch duration is usually about 15 to 20 min; if the patient cannot tolerate the stress, the force should be reduced to allow the patient to stretch for the desired time.

The part placed in a prolonged stretch can feel very stiff once the stretch load is removed. The patient should be cautioned about this. Gentle, active range-of-motion activities help to relieve the stiffness. The stretch should be released slowly. As the stretch is released, the patient's contracting the stretched muscle also helps to reduce the discomfort and stiffness.

PROPRIOCEPTIVE NEUROMUSCULAR FACILITATION

The combination of active and passive stretching is often referred to as neuromuscular facilitation or proprioceptive neuromuscular facilitation (PNF). Although PNF is used as a strengthening technique, it also is useful for gaining range of motion. A more extensive discussion of PNF principles is presented in chapter 7. Of the various PNF techniques used to increase motion, the most frequently used are the hold-relax, contract-relax, and slow reversal-hold-relax techniques (figure 5.20).

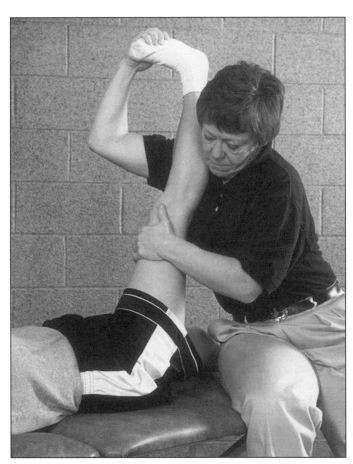

Figure 5.20   PNF stretch.

The hold-relax technique is a maximal isometric contraction of the antagonist followed by a relaxation of the muscle. The agonist is then used actively without resistance to increase motion. This technique is used to relax muscle spasm. For example, if a biceps is in spasm and limits elbow extension, the biceps is tightened progressively until a maximum effort against resistance is produced. The patient is then instructed to relax the muscle and actively extend the elbow without resistance. The patient then contracts the muscle isometrically for 5 to 10 s. This process is repeated four to five times or until the desired results are achieved. The isometric contraction of the muscle activates the GTO, which results in autogenic inhibition and thus better relaxation of the muscle. As the patient contracts the agonist, in this case the triceps to extend the elbow, additional relaxation of the antagonist (biceps) may occur.

The contract-relax technique is used with patients who have limited range of motion. With the patient's restricted joint placed at the point of limitation, the sport rehabilitation specialist provides maximal resistance against rotation and does not permit any other motion of the antagonist to occur. When the patient relaxes the muscle tension, the sport rehabilitation specialist moves the part passively through as much range as possible. The process is repeated several times. The patient then actively moves the agonist through its new range of motion.

The slow reversal-hold-relax technique uses concentric activity of the agonist followed by an isometric contraction of the antagonist in the shortened position against resistance provided by the sport rehabilitation specialist. This is followed by relaxation of the antagonist, then concentric activity of the agonist. The sport rehabilitation specialist provides maximal isometric resistance against the rotational component of the movement pattern and does not permit other motions to occur. All the PNF stretches are useful when the primary resisting factor is a shortening of the antagonist caused by muscle spasm or loss of motion.

Various investigations have compared the different types of short-term passive, active, and combination stretching procedures. Many investigators conclude that PNF stretches are more effective than other active or short-term passive stretches. Others conclude that there is no difference in the results of the various short-term stretching techniques. The body parts stretched, duration of stretches, frequency, and duration of studies vary widely among the investigations. With so many variables, it is not surprising that little or no consensus has been reached on specific methods, duration, and frequency of these stretching techniques.

BALLISTIC STRETCHING

Ballistic stretching is the use of quick, bouncing movement through alternating contraction and relaxation of a muscle to stretch its antagonist. This type of stretch is not used much in sport rehabilitation because of the damage it can cause to already injured tissue. The physiological characteristics of connective tissue and muscle discussed previously in this chapter provide an understanding of the dangers of ballistic stretching in therapeutic exercise:

• Ballistic stretching stimulates both the muscle spindles and GTOs. These structures normally oppose stretch reactions to protect the muscle from injury, but with uncoordinated firing, their protective mechanisms are ineffective.

• Control of the stretch is limited by the velocity of the force applied in the stretch. Plastic deformation is related to the magnitude and duration of the force. A greater force over a shorter period of time is likely to cause failure of the structure, risking injury to the connective tissue. Injury will result in more scar-tissue formation that ultimately decreases flexibility.

Ballistic stretching is used most often by normal, healthy people in sport activities and serves well to increase dynamic flexibility. In unhealthy tissue, however, the risk of causing further injury is too great for ballistic stretching to be considered a viable technique.

ASSISTIVE DEVICES

In addition to equipment such as weights, pulleys, and straps for providing prolonged stretch to areas of limited motion, many devices are commonly used to assist in regaining range of motion.

Continuous Passive Motion Machines

A continuous passive motion (CPM) machine is sometimes used following surgery to restore range of motion. Although now used less frequently, a CPM can help counteract the deleterious effects of immobilization and reduce pain and edema after surgery. Because range of motion is more quickly restored with the use of a CPM, the patient is able to begin active exercises sooner to ultimately shorten the recovery and rehabilitation time following surgery. CPMs are designed for a variety of joints, including the knee, ankle, elbow, wrist, and shoulder. An example of a CPM is seen in figure 5.21.

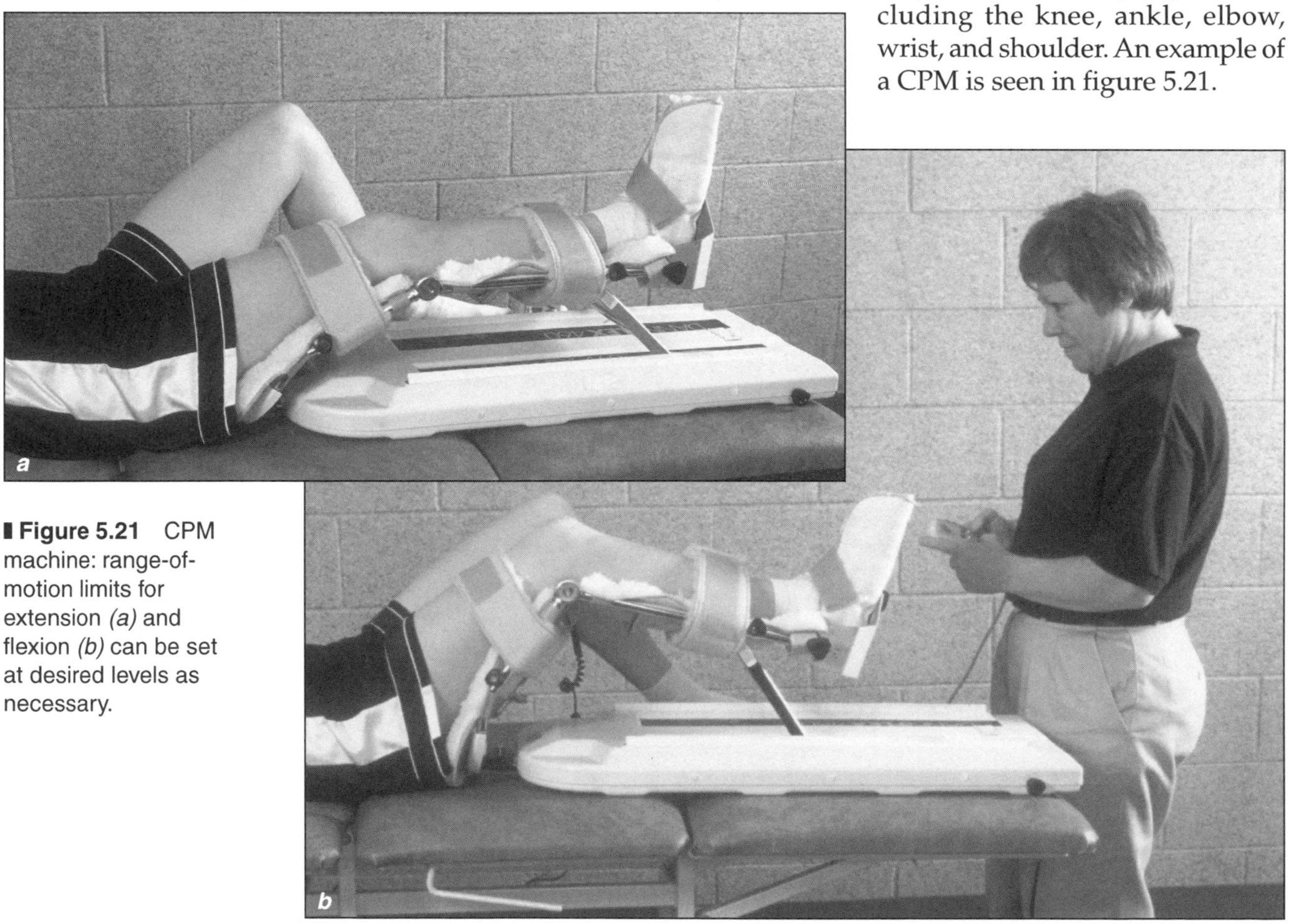

■ Figure 5.21 CPM machine: range-of-motion limits for extension (a) and flexion (b) can be set at desired levels as necessary.

Splints

Splints also assist in prolonged stretching of restricted joints. After injury the collagen and connective tissue that produce scarring become progressively more difficult to stretch as the cross-links become more numerous and the collagen more mature with time. Prolonged stretching for more than 20 min is often needed with very mature or restricted scar tissue. In such instances, various splints that apply a low-level, continual stretch force are often most beneficial. They commonly use a three-point lever-and-spring system to provide a low-level, continual load (figure 5.22). These devices are used to stretch connective tissue surrounding joints and not to change muscle length. The magnitude of the load and the angle at which it is applied can be adjusted to meet the individual patient's needs. A splint can be worn for several hours at a time to cause effective plastic deformation of connective tissue.

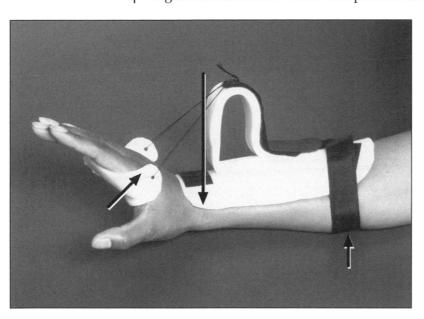

▌Figure 5.22 Splint to increase range of motion. Notice the 3-point system used to provide the stretch force.

INDICATIONS, CONTRAINDICATIONS, AND PRECAUTIONS

Before applying a stretch to increase range of motion, you must first know when stretching is indicated, when you should not use stretching, and precautions for its use.

Indications

The evaluation performed in sport rehabilitation determines deficiencies in range of motion, the structures causing the loss of motion, and the status of the tissue. Is the loss a result of recent scar-tissue formation, adherent and mature scar tissue, spasm, edema, postural deformities, or weakness of opposing muscles? If ligaments, capsules, muscles, fascia, skin, or other soft tissue is shortened because of scar tissue or adhesions, stretching exercises are indicated. Stretching is also indicated in the presence of contractures and structural deformities from injury or posture changes over time. If weak muscles are overpowered by opposing tight structures, flexibility of the restricted structures must accompany strengthening of the weak muscles for the treatment program to be effective. If muscle spasm or edema contributes to reduced motion, the rehabilitation program must include modalities and activities to address these problems.

Contraindications

Although stretching is usually safe, it is contraindicated when certain conditions are present. These include recent fractures when immobilization is necessary for healing and movement is detrimental to it, a bony block that restricts motion, infection in a joint, acute inflammation in a joint, extreme and sharp pain with motion, and when tightness of soft tissue actually contributes to an area's stability.

Precautions

Precautions should be taken to ensure the most effective application of the stretch and to prevent harm from the stretch. Before applying any treatment, you should always explain to the patient what you will do and the outcome and sensations to expect. A patient who is apprehensive and unable to relax will not receive an effective stretch treatment.

The force applied in a stretch should cause sensations of tension, perhaps unpleasant, in the part being stretched but not residual pain following release of the stretch. This is true for active and passive stretching. It is important that the patient understand that during active stretches the sensation of a stretch is necessary, but it should be without pain. Residual pain beyond a transitory tenderness, especially accompanied with new edema, is an indication that the stretch has been too aggressive. The stretch should be less forceful to cause proper plastic changes without unwanted damage.

Vigorous stretching of areas that have been immobilized for a period of time should be used with extreme caution or even avoided in the early stretching stages. Recall that immobilization reduces the tensile strength of many connective-tissue structures, including tendons and ligaments, so caution should be used when stretching these structures.

Stabilization of the area is necessary for properly applying the stretch force and thus for stretching the correct structures. During both active and passive stretches, the part should be positioned so that the force affects only the targeted structures. For example, if a patient is stretching the left hamstrings in a standing position with the left foot on a chair or bench, the foot should be facing the ceiling, not rotated so that the adductors rather than the hamstrings are stretched. When stretching a muscle that traverses two or more joints, the other joints must be positioned so that the muscle is elongated throughout its entire length. For example, to stretch the quadriceps, place the hip in extension with the knee in flexion to fully elongate the rectus femoris portion of the quadriceps.

In active and passive stretches, the muscle being stretched should be relaxed for optimal results. If a muscle tenses, it will resist the stretch and make it ineffective. For this reason, careful positioning and analysis of positions is important. For example, standing bent over from the waist to touch the floor with the fingertips is an ineffective position for stretching the hamstrings, since the hamstrings must work isometrically to hold the position and cannot relax. By the same token, if a passive stretch is too forceful and causes a reflex or voluntary muscle contraction, the stretch will be both ineffective and painful to the patient.

Once full range of motion is achieved following an injury, maintenance flexibility exercises need to be continued. With the continued contraction of connective tissue as scar tissue matures, loss of motion also tends to continue. This is why a patient can achieve full range of motion in one session of therapeutic exercise and can return the next day with less than full range of motion. Until the healing process is complete, special attention must be paid to maintaining full range of motion after achieving it.

The release of the stretch force is as important as its application. Both should be done slowly. A quick application or release of a stretch, especially release of a prolonged stretch, can be very uncomfortable. Begin applying the stretch slowly, and do not apply more force until you know the patient can tolerate it.

Some pain and stiffness are normal after release of a stretch, especially a prolonged stretch. As mentioned earlier, these symptoms can be relieved by contracting the agonist as the stretch is released and following the stretch with gentle, active range-of-motion exercises.

If stretch application is painful, gentle traction of the joint may relieve the pain. If this is not successful in relieving the pain, reduce the stretch load. A stretch should not be painful.

A stretch force affects all soft tissue in the area where the force is applied. Knowing exactly which tissues are affected has thus far eluded researchers. The structures affected may include the joint capsule, ligaments, surrounding tendons, muscles, fascia, nerves, skin, and subcutaneous tissue.

EXERCISE PROGRESSION

The choice of stretching technique depends on the tissues involved, the stage of healing, the patient's motivation, the time and facilities available, and other factors of the injury.

Common questions regarding therapeutic flexibility exercises are when to use them and which stretching exercises to use. The information presented in this chapter and in chapter 2 provides the answers. If motion is permitted immediately following injury, active range of motion may be all that is necessary to regain motion. Active motion is the first choice because it does not require outside assistance, so the patient can perform it frequently and independently throughout the day when it is convenient. Frequent flexibility exercise sessions throughout the day can be an effective way to increase flexibility.

Following major surgery, the physician may order the use of a CPM machine for involved areas that require close monitoring. A CPM machine does not harm the surgical site, yet provides immediate postoperative motion.

Other techniques may be needed after immobilization. To some extent, the method of stretching depends on the length of immobilization, the tissues affected by the immobilization, the patient's motivation, and the sport rehabilitation specialist's facilities and availability. Recall that collagen appears in a wound within three to five days following an injury. By the seventh day, collagen abounds, and the forming scar tissue begins to contract. This contraction continues into the final phase of healing and requires stretching exercises to maintain range of motion even after full motion has been achieved.

If scar tissue is relatively new and still pliable, active and short-term passive stretches are effective for increasing motion. PNF stretching techniques can also be utilized with success. If scar tissue is more mature and well into the remodeling phase, however, prolonged-stretching techniques should be the main part of the stretching program. Short-term and active stretches accompanying the prolonged stretches help to reinforce the effects.

In particularly difficult situations where scar tissue is more than three to four months old and range of motion is still deficient, prolonged-stretch machines can be used to achieve maximal range of motion. The degree of plastic deformation of connective tissue required at this point to effect a change in range of motion requires a very prolonged stretch.

SPECIAL CONSIDERATIONS

The anatomy of the specific structure to be stretched determines the most appropriate stretch application.

As with application of any therapeutic exercise technique, application of stretching techniques requires common sense and consideration of the specific structure to be stretched.

TRUNK

The most important consideration in stretching the trunk is to avoid any stretch that causes pain or a change in sensation down either leg.

UPPER EXTREMITY

When stretching the shoulder, the scapula must be stabilized. If it is not, the stretching force is distributed into the scapular muscles, and gains in motion may not be actual gains in the intended area.

When stretching the elbow, remember that several muscles acting at the elbow also cross the shoulder, so the shoulder should be positioned and stabilized before stretching. Because the elbow flexors and extensors work in both supination and pronation, stretches for those muscles should be performed in both positions. One possible side effect of vigorous elbow stretching is myositis ossificans, especially in youth. For this reason, elbow stretches should be performed with caution. Active stretches and reciprocal inhibition techniques may help to prevent this problem.

When stretching the wrist, the distal force should be applied over the metacarpals, not the fingers. The patient's fingers should remain relaxed during the stretch, since the extrinsic finger flexors and extensors cross the wrist and can affect the stretch if they are not relaxed.

LOWER EXTREMITY

The ankle and foot contain many joints and soft-tissue structures. When stretching these areas, the location where the joint's tendons cross and the appropriate force application must be considered to produce the desired results.

The position of the hip affects stretching the knee. Since both the knee flexors and extensors cross the hip joint, the effectiveness of the stretch is determined by the hip position.

When stretching the hip, the pelvis must be stabilized. If the pelvis is not stabilized, as with the scapula, movement occurs in this area, and an increase in hip range of motion is sacrificed to the pelvis.

Caution must be used when stretching hip rotators with the knee in flexion and the force applied at the lower leg. This position offers the sport rehabilitation specialist a tremendous lever-arm advantage and reduces the force required to cause hip joint subluxation, especially in patients who have undergone prolonged immobilization, recent fracture, or recent dislocation.

SUMMARY

1. *Define the differences between range of motion and flexibility.* Range of motion is the amount of mobility of a joint, and flexibility is the musculotendinous unit's ability to elongate with application of a stretching force. Both are closely related and are often used interchangeably.

2. *Explain the differences in structure of loose connective tissue and dense connective tissue.* The primary tissue that determines range of motion is connective tissue. The fiber arrangement of loose connective tissue, such as skin, is unorganized and loose with relatively long distances between the cross-links. Dense connective tissue, such as tendons and ligaments, is highly organized with parallel collagen fibers and more cross-links.

3. *List the deleterious effects of prolonged immobilization.* Each tissue type is affected by immobilization differently, but some general changes are seen in all tissues. These include a loss of ground substance, which in turn results in less separation and more cross-links between collagen fibers. The fiber meshwork contracts so that the tissue becomes dense, hard, and less supple. The more severe effects occur with more prolonged immobilization. If a normal joint is immobilized for four weeks, the dense connective tissue that forms prevents normal motion.

4. *Discuss the mechanical properties of plasticity, elasticity, and viscosity of connective tissue.* Connective tissue's plastic quality allows its length to change, while its elasticity allows some return toward normal length. Viscoelasticity is a combination of elastic and viscous properties that allows either a change in length or a return to former length after stretching, depending on the speed, duration, and magnitude of the stretch force applied.

5. *Explain the physiological properties of creep and stress-strain and how they affect stretching techniques.* Creep permits a gradual change in tissue length with the prolonged application of a stretch force, and the stress-strain curve describes a tissue's ability to withstand stresses and the strains they produce. If a stretch force is applied beyond a tissue's stress-strain limits, deformation occurs.

6. *Discuss the neuromuscular influences of the muscle spindle and GTO on stretching muscle.* The muscle spindle and GTO are neuromuscular protective mechanisms that attempt to reduce the stress-strain forces on the musculotendinous unit.

7. *Explain the procedure for measuring range of motion with a goniometer.* To measure a joint's range of motion, the goniometer's stationary arm is placed along one segment, and the movable arm is aligned along the segment on the other side of the joint. The protractor portion of the goniometer is placed over the joint's axis of rotation.

8. *Discuss the active and passive methods for stretching.* Active stretching uses the antagonistic muscles to provide the stretch force to the agonist. In passive stretching, outside assistive devices or another person provide the force to gain additional range of motion.

9. *Identify two mechanical assistive devices used to increase range of motion.* CPMs and splints are commonly used as external devices to gain additional motion. CPMs are sometimes used after surgery to counteract the deleterious effects of immobilization. Splints can be used to apply prolonged stretch to joints restricted by mature or very restricted scar tissue.

10. *List contraindications, indications, and precautions of stretching.* Indications for stretching include a shortening of ligaments, capsules, muscles, fascia, skin, and other soft tissue by scar tissue or adhesions. Some precautions include explaining to the patient the technique and expected sensations before application, applying and releasing the force slowly and steadily, and avoiding pain. Contraindications include recent fractures, inflammations, infections, and extreme pain.

11. *Discuss the progression of a stretching exercise program.* The type of flexibility exercise applied depends on a number of considerations, including the age of the scar tissue, the stage of healing, available equipment, the patient's motivation and pain tolerance, and the tissue involved. If the scar is recent and in the remodeling phase of repair, active exercises may be sufficient. If the scar tissue is more mature, a more prolonged stretch that affects the plastic range of the tissue is probably indicated.

CRITICAL THINKING QUESTIONS

1. How would you stretch the quadriceps muscle if you did not want to fully lengthen the rectus femoris? In what bodily position is the rectus femoris included in the quadriceps stretch? Try these two positions with a partner. Does the knee motion change in the different positions? If so, what does that tell you?

2. Over the course of a week, stretch a partner's hamstrings using a different technique each day: a passive technique with a 15 to 30 s hold, a contract-relax-stretch PNF maneuver, a ballistic stretch, and a prolonged stretch for 15 to 20 min. Measure the hamstring length immediately after the stretch is released. Which technique gives you the greatest change in hamstring length? Measure the hamstrings 24 h after each stretch and notice the change. Why does this occur? Do any of the physical properties of creep, stress-strain, or hysteresis influence the changes?

3. If you are measuring a patient's shoulder range of motion, in what position should he or she be for the most accurate measurements? Why? What position would be least accurate when measuring a weak shoulder? Why?

4. Explain why active range of motion is not usually as great as passive range of motion. Can you think of exceptions to this generalization and explain why they occur?

5. If a patient had a condition in which the GTOs did not respond to stimuli, what would be the result? Could this be harmful during normal activity?

6. If you did not have a goniometer small enough to measure finger joint range of motion, what could you use to record flexibility in each finger joint? How can you measure trunk motion without a goniometer?

7. What is the most effective stretch for a patient who has a tight Achilles tendon? Why would you select that stretch?

REFERENCES

American Academy of Orthopaedic Surgeons. 1965. *Joint motion: Method of measuring and recording.* New York: Churchill Livingstone.

Bandy, W.D., Irion, J.M., and M. Briggler. 1997. The effect of time and frequency on flexibility of the hamstring muscles. *Physical Therapy.* 77:1090–1096.

Buckwalter, J.A. 1996. Effects of early motion on healing of musculoskeletal tissues. *Hand Clinics* 12:13–24.

Butler, D.L., Grood, E.S., Noyes, F.R., and R.F. Zernicke. 1978. Biomechanics of ligaments and tendons. *Exercise and Sport Sciences Reviews* 6:125–281.

Daniels, L., and C. Worthingham. 1972. *Muscle testing.* Philadelphia: Saunders.

Donatelli, R., and A. Owens-Burkhart. 1981. Effects of immobilization on the extensibility of periarticular connective tissue. *Journal of Orthopaedic and Sports Physical Therapy* 9:67–72.

Eldred, E. 1967. Peripheral receptors: Their excitation and relation to reflex patterns. *American Journal of Physical Medicine* 46:69–87.

Esch, D., and M. Lepley. 1974. *Evaluation of joint motion: Methods of measurement and recording.* Minneapolis: University of Minnesota Press.

Evans, E.B., Eggers, G.W.N., Butler, J.K., and J. Blumel. 1960. Experimental immobilization and remobilization of rat knee joints. *Journal of Bone and Joint Surgery* 42A:737–758.

Finsterbush, A., and B. Friedman. 1975. Reversibility of joint changes produced by immobilization in rabbits. *Clinical Orthopaedics and Related Research* 111:290–298.

Garrett, W.E., Jr. 1990. Muscle strain injuries: Clinical and basic aspects. *Medicine and Science in Sports and Exercise* 22:436–443.

Gerhardt, J.J., and O.A. Russe. 1975. *International SFTR method of measuring and recording joint motion.* Bern: Huber.

Hoppenfeld, S. 1976. *Physical examination of the spine and extremities.* New York: Appleton-Century-Crofts.

Kapandji, I.A. 1980. *The physiology of the joints.* Vols. 1 and 2. New York: Churchill Livingstone.

Karpovich, P.V., Herden, E.L., Jr., Asa, M.M., and G.P. Karpovich. 1959. Electrogoniometer: A new device for study of joints in action. *Federation Proceedings* 18:79.

Kendall, F.P., McCreary, E.K., and P.G. Provance. 1993. *Muscles: Testing and function.* 4th ed. Baltimore: Williams & Wilkins.

Klein, L., Heiple, K.G., Torzilli, P.A., Goldberg, V.M., and A.H. Burstein. 1989. Prevention of ligament and meniscus atrophy by active joint motion in a non-weight-bearing model. *Journal of Orthopaedic Research* 7:80–85.

Kottke, F.J., Pauley, D.L., and R.A. Ptak. 1966. The rationale for prolonged stretching for correction of shortening of connective tissue. *Archives of Physical Medicine and Rehabilitation* 47:345–352.

Kottke, F.J., Stillwell, G.K., and J.F. Lehmann. 1982. *Krusen's handbook of physical medicine and rehabilitation.* Philadelphia: Saunders.

Light, K.E., Nuzik, S., Personius, W., and A. Barstrom. 1984. Low-load prolonged stretch vs. high-load brief stretch in treating knee contractures. *Physical Therapy* 64:330–333.

Madding, S.W., Wong, J.G., Hallum, A., and J.M. Medeiros. 1987. The effect of duration of passive stretch on hip abduction range of motion. *Journal of Orthopaedic and Sports Physical Therapy* 8: 409–416.

McNair, P.J., and S.N. Stanley. 1996. Effect of passive stretching and jogging on the series elastic muscle stiffness and range of motion of the ankle joint. *British Journal of Sports Medicine* 30:313–317.

Moll, J., and V. Wright. 1971. Normal range of spinal mobility: A clinical study. *Annals of the Rheumatic Diseases* 30:381–386.

Montgomery, J.B., and J.R. Steadman. 1985. Rehabilitation of the injured knee. *Clinics in Sports Medicine* 4:333–343.

Saal, J.S. 1987. Flexibility training. In *Rehabilitation of sport injuries,* ed. J.A. Saal. Philadelphia: Hanley & Belfus.

Shellock, F.G., and W.E. Prentice. 1985. Warming-up and stretching for improved physical performance and prevention of sports-related injuries. *Sports Medicine* 2:267–278.

Taylor, D.C., Dalton, J.D., Jr., Seaber, A.V., and W.E. Garrett, Jr. 1990. Viscoelastic properties of muscle-tendon units: The biomechanical effects of stretching. *American Journal of Sports Medicine* 18:300–309.

Warren, C.G., Lehmann, J.K., and J.N. Koblanski. 1971. Elongation of rat tail tendon: Effect of load and temperature. *Archives of Physical Medicine and Rehabilitation* 52:465–474.

Warren, C.G., Lehmann, J.K., and J.N. Koblanski. 1976. Heat and stretch procedures: An evaluation using rat tail tendon. *Archives of Physical Medicine and Rehabilitation* 57:122–126.

CHAPTER SIX

Manual Therapy Techniques

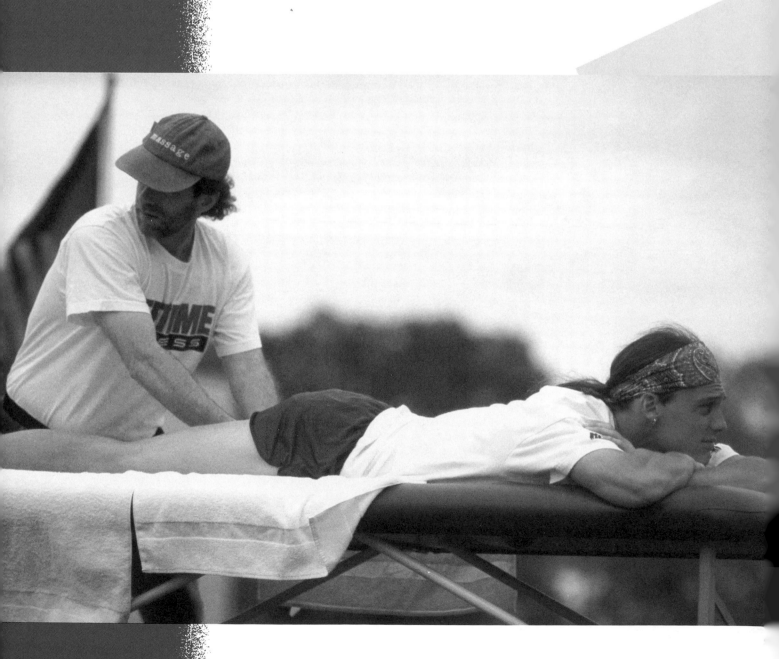

OBJECTIVES

After completing this chapter, you should be able to do the following:

1. Discuss the three techniques of massage and their indications, precautions, and contraindications.

2. Explain the progression of myofascial restriction after an injury.

3. Discuss the techniques for myofascial release.

4. Explain the theory of the mechanism of myofascial trigger points.

5. Discuss the ice-stretch trigger point release theory.

6. Explain the concave-convex and convex-concave rules.

7. Define joint mobilization grades of movement.

8. Discuss the direction of glide and traction in relation to the treatment plane.

9. Explain the double-crush syndrome.

10. Discuss the dangers of neural mobilization.

11. Describe one neural self-mobilization technique for the upper extremity and one for the lower extremity.

Dan Edwards, certified athletic trainer for a Division III college, had never seen scar tissue adhesions like the ones he encountered in his most recent rehabilitation case. Over six months ago, one of the softball players, Sara, had suffered a severe cleat laceration along her entire forearm when an opposing player sliding into second base ran the bottom of her shoe into Sara's forearm. The forearm required over 30 stitches. Although Sara hadn't suffered any immediate loss of motion from the scar, she was now losing some elbow and wrist motion because the scar tissue was pulling on both joints. When Dan palpated the forearm, he could feel a lot of hard, unyielding scar tissue adhesions below the skin. He knew he had to soften the scar tissue and mobilize the tissue below the skin if Sara was to have normal elbow and wrist motion. He also knew he would have to show Sara some soft-tissue techniques that she could perform on her own throughout the day to reinforce his efforts in the athletic training room.

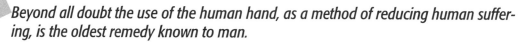

Beyond all doubt the use of the human hand, as a method of reducing human suffering, is the oldest remedy known to man.

James Mennel, *Manual Therapy*

Manual therapy is the use of hands-on techniques to evaluate, treat, and improve the status of neuromusculoskeletal conditions. A variety of structures, including joints and soft tissue, are affected by procedures that come under the category of manual therapy. The various procedures in this category are defined according to the tissues and structures they influence. This chapter discusses some of the more commonly used manual therapy procedures and techniques. Manual therapy techniques are considered by many medical professionals to be subjective because little quantitative research has been performed to investigate the efficacy of such treatment techniques. It is difficult to create an objective research design of these treatments because the specific application, direction, duration, and amplitude of a force can vary from one health care provider to another. With these variations come a variety of outcomes, so a truly objective assessment of treatment effectiveness is difficult, if not impossible. Most of the benefits recorded are considered anecdotal because of their subjective, rather than objective, basis. Manual therapy techniques, however, deserve attention and application because of these overwhelming clinical reports of successful outcomes. Certain common principles apply to all manual therapy techniques if they are to be used successfully.

It is important for you to keep in mind these common principles for applying all manual therapy techniques:

- The patient should be in a comfortable position.
- You should be in a comfortable position.
- You should always use good body mechanics.
- Feedback from the patient throughout the treatment is necessary for proper application of the technique and appropriate pressure.
- Your fingernails should be clean and trimmed. As a general rule, the nail should not extend beyond the fingertip pad.

- You should explain to the patient before applying the technique what will be done and what sensations to expect. The patient should be warned whether any discomfort may be felt and should tell you whether less pressure or discomfort is desired during the treatment.

- The patient's condition must be assessed before, during, and at the conclusion of the treatment.

- The appropriate manual therapy technique must be correctly applied for a successful result.

- Precautions and contraindications must always be respected.

- If you are unsure, do not perform the technique.

CRITICAL ANALYSIS

Evaluation and assessment are important for selecting appropriate manual therapy techniques.

The foundation of any manual therapy technique is your ability to critically think and to analyze the patient's condition to determine the best and most appropriate course of action. This practice involves understanding the injury and healing process, identifying the structures and problems involved, analyzing the situation and all its parameters to decide on a plan of action, and critically appraising the results of the treatment plan to determine its effectiveness or the need to change it. Critical analysis and assessment with continual reassessment is key to effective manual therapy application and outcomes.

There is no cookbook method for applying manual therapy. You must be able to use your skills of observation, palpation, analysis, and technique application. As with other aspects of sport rehabilitation, analysis and deductive reasoning are skills vital to a successful outcome of manual techniques. The sport rehabilitation specialist is a detective in search of answers to problems. Detective skills in the assessment of clinical findings and deduction of logical expectations must be continually used throughout the manual therapy process.

Depending on the specific injury and resulting impairments, you may choose to use more than one manual therapy technique. Evaluation and deductive reasoning allow you to select treatment techniques that can best reduce the impairment and improve the functional ability of the injured athlete.

Whatever techniques you choose, your selection should be based on individual findings, not on rote or cookbook decisions. Always approach an injury with an open mind and maintain flexibility in your treatment options. Each patient must be individually and objectively assessed to determine the best course of treatment. Two patients may have shoulder pain and loss of motion, but the causes and courses of treatment may be very different for each of them. A successful treatment program depends on your evaluation skills as much as on your treatment skills.

MASSAGE

Effleurage, petrissage, and friction massage are techniques that can relax muscles, improve blood and lymph flow to reduce edema, reduce pain, and improve soft-tissue movement.

Many types of massage are used in a number of applications to achieve a variety of goals. A sports massage is frequently used either before or after competition in what is known in nonmedical circles as a rubdown. Even though massage is used in nonmedical situations, it still produces a physiological effect. The use of massage for nonpathological conditions, however, is not discussed in this text. The range of techniques most commonly used in the injury treatment is briefly described in this section.

DEFINITION OF MASSAGE

Massage is the systematic and scientific manipulation of soft tissue for remedial or restorative purposes. Massage affects various systems of the body through its influence on reflex and mechanical processes to produce desired results.

EFFECTS OF MASSAGE

Massage produces reflex physiological and mechanical effects in the area treated. Repetitive pressure stimulation without irritation to the skin causes transmission from peripheral receptors to the spinal cord and brain, which results in relaxation of muscles and dilation of blood vessels. Mechanical effects improve blood and lymph flow, promote mobilization of fluid, and stretch and break down adhesions to ultimately assist in reducing edema and improving tissue mobility. The overall end result is relaxation of muscles, dilation of local capillaries, an increase in lymph flow to reduce edema, a reduction of pain, and an improvement soft-tissue movement. The specific effects vary, depending on the type of massage given.

TYPES OF MASSAGE

Although there are many different massage techniques, three primary techniques are used in treating injuries to achieve the effects mentioned earlier. The French terms for many of these techniques were first introduced by Peter Ling of Sweden, who traveled widely in Europe (Beard and Wood 1969).

Effleurage

Effleurage, or stroking, is a massage that is performed by running the hand lightly over the skin's surface. The direction of the stroke moves distally to proximally (figure 6.1). Effleurage is used to assist in venous and lymphatic flow to decrease edema and aid in muscle relaxation. If the technique is used primarily to treat edema, it

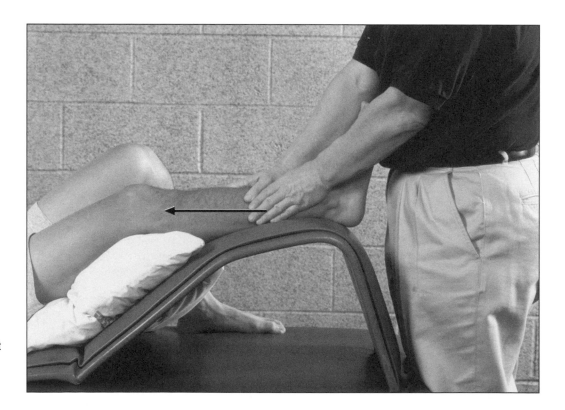

■ **Figure 6.1** Effleurage: stroking motion begins distally and moves proximally toward the heart. Elevating the segment during treatment further assists in edema reductions.

should be performed with the part in a position so that gravity can assist the flow. The pressure should be applied firmly and deeply but not heavily. The direction should be toward the heart.

Petrissage

Compression and kneading fall under the category of petrissage. In this technique the soft tissue is grasped and manipulated intermittently so that there is movement between the skin's underlying structure and the muscle itself (figure 6.2). Although the stroking movement is constant, the pressure is intermittent. The tissue is grasped and released with varying degrees of pressure so that the action's mechanical effects reduce edema.

This technique is often preceded and followed by a stroking technique for relaxation. Petrissage is used to promote circulation, relax muscle, mechanically assist fluid exchange, and improve mobility of muscle tissue.

Friction

Friction is a deep-pressure movement of superficial soft tissue against underlying structures (figure 6.3). Sometimes the underlying structure is bone or another hard surface, and sometimes it is soft tissue, such as muscle or fascia. The intent is to loosen scar tissue and adhesions of deeper parts, such as tendons, ligaments, and joint capsules, to improve movement and gliding of these structures. Friction also helps to stimulate circulation of the local area. It usually is applied through firm pressure by either the thumb or finger pads in a crisscross or circular motion.

INDICATIONS

The indications for massage are related to its effects. Relief of pain, muscle relaxation, reduction of swelling, and mobilization of adherent scar tissue are all appropriate indications for the use of massage. The specific technique selection is based

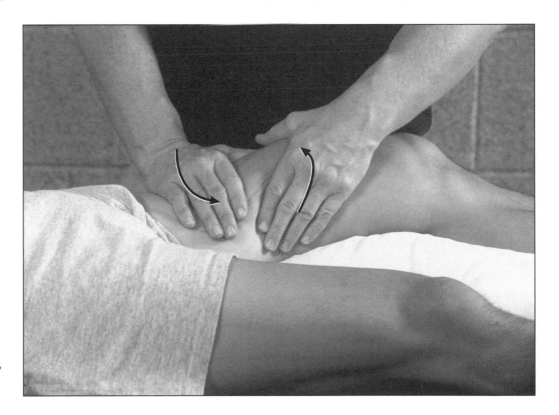

■ **Figure 6.2** Petrissage: skin and underlying tissue are kneaded and lifted to improve tissue mobility, relax muscle, and promote circulation.

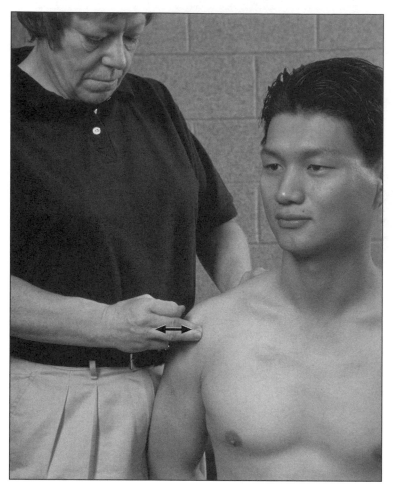

■ Figure 6.3 Friction massage across the biceps tendon will loosen adhesions and stimulate circulation.

on the evaluation findings. Recent edema secondary to trauma is an indication for effleurage and petrissage massage techniques. Friction massage is indicated when scar-tissue restriction of superficial tissue can be palpated and in inflammatory conditions where adhesions play a role in continued symptoms, such as tendinitis and bursitis.

CONTRAINDICATIONS

Massage is contraindicated when the technique may aggravate the condition or cause additional harm to the patient. Contra-indications include the presence of infection, malignancies, skin diseases, blood clots, and any irritations or lesions that may spread with direct contact.

PRECAUTIONS

When you apply massage to the patient, both the patient's skin and your hands should be clean. Your hands should be warm and your nails should be trimmed so as not to cause a laceration or abrasion. Rings, watches, and wrist jewelry should be removed for the same reason. A lubricant is used to reduce friction when using effleurage. Less lubricant is used with petrissage, and still less is used with friction massage. Too much lubricant with friction massage does not allow the presence of enough friction to be effective, and too much lubricant with petrissage makes it difficult to lift or grasp the tissue.

APPLICATION

Before beginning the massage, position the patient comfortably with the part to be massaged properly exposed. If the massage is to reduce edema, elevate the part to enhance lymphatic flow. Explain the procedure to the patient and instruct the patient to inform you if he or she feels pain with the massage.

When using effleurage or petrissage, the pressure of the massage strokes should be toward the heart, and the hands should not lose contact with the skin. On the return stroke, continue lightly touching the part. Keep your hand in good contact with the part and your fingers together, not spread apart. The rhythm of the stroke should be even and slow to promote relaxation. Maintain a comfortable position during the treatment and use proper body mechanics.

When using friction massage, it is important to warn the patient that some discomfort may be felt but that it will not be lasting. The thumb or finger pads are used on a small, localized surface in a cross pattern. A firm, consistent pressure and rhythm are also important. A small area at a time is massaged until the discomfort of the massage subsides and you can palpate an increase in tissue mobility. The massage is applied in a "cross" pattern perpendicular to the tissue's fiber arrangement.

MYOFASCIAL RELEASE

Myofascial release involves manual contact to evaluate and treat soft-tissue restriction and pain, relieve symptoms, and improve motion and function. It is commonly used to treat the restricted fascia associated with skin, subcutaneous tissue, and other superficial structures.

Myofascial release is a close relative to massage. They both involve manual contact with the patient, and they both use the sense of touch to evaluate the problem and the effectiveness of the treatment. They also both include the use of pressure and tissue stretch to produce results.

There are many different techniques of myofascial release, but they all are essentially variations of the same principle: The use of manual contact for evaluation and treatment of soft-tissue restriction and pain with the eventual goal of the relief of those symptoms to improve motion and function. There are different names for these techniques: myofascial release, myofascial stretching, strain-counterstrain, Rolfing, soft-tissue mobilization. Because of the individual variations in application, forces, duration, and precise technique, reliable research results on the efficacy of myofascial release remain elusive. Clinical observations and anecdotal reports of those who have recorded treatment results is currently the best barometer by which to judge the results of this type of treatment. Ultimately, treatment effectiveness must be assessed by the results of your own applications on the patients you treat. In this section, some of the more commonly used myofascial techniques are introduced briefly.

Before describing the various myofascial release techniques, their theoretical basis is discussed. The different myofascial release systems cannot be appreciated without understanding their basis.

FASCIA

Fascia is a continuous structure that surrounds and integrates tissues and structures throughout the body. Fascia varies in density and thickness and is interconnected with the structures it surrounds. It can affect the relationship among the structures it ensheaths (their physical orientation to each other, their chemical relationship, or their physiological relationship, e.g., what tissues are served by which blood vessels or nerves). Fascia is vital for tissue form, lubrication, nutrition, stability, integrity, function, and support.

Throughout the body, fascia is divided into three layers. The superficial layer is attached to the undersurface of the skin. Within this superficial layer lie capillaries, lymph vessels, nerves, and fat. Because this layer is a loosely knit structure made of fibroelastic and areolar connective tissue, it permits the skin to move in many directions over the underlying structures. It is also a place where edema accumulates following injury.

Deep fascia is dense connective tissue that surrounds and separates deeper structures, such as muscle, tendon, joints, ligaments, and bone. Because of its stiffer, firmer structure, deep fascia is less able to accommodate edema, which can cause problems, such as compartment syndromes in the lower leg.

The final layer is subserous fascia, which surrounds internal organs. Its loose areolar connective tissue contains channels where fluid assists in providing the organs with lubrication. Myofascial release techniques are not used to treat fascia surrounding visceral organs.

Fascia contains collagen, elastin, cellular components, and ground substance. The elastin within fascia allows the structure to return to its original shape when applied stresses are released. Fascia also responds with plastic deformation when prolonged forces are applied. Creep and hysteresis, discussed in chapters 3 and 5, are properties of fascia and are used in myofascial release techniques.

Although fascia has high tensile strength and is able to tolerate multidirectional compressive, stretch, and sheer forces, an injury can profoundly affect fascia. The fascia's normal biomechanics can be altered to cause either a temporary or permanent deformation, depending on the load, duration, and type of stress applied to the fascia. Injury to fascia causes a change in the biochemical structure of the ground substance, and the scar tissue that forms after injury can interfere with normal fascia functions. The fascia's reduced ability to provide skin, subcutaneous, muscle, and other tissue with normal motion, support, lubrication, and other functions can cause extended disability and prolonged symptoms following injury and repair if not treated properly.

Myofascia maintains an intimate relationship with the muscle it covers and surrounds. The two provide the combined contractile and noncontractile properties of muscle. Myofascia assists in increasing muscle strength during eccentric contractions. It helps provide structure and form to the muscle, lubrication between muscle fibers and muscles, and nutrition for the muscles. It also bears the blood and lymph vessels and nerves for the muscles. In short, myofascia provides vital support to permit normal muscle function.

NONACUTE BIOMECHANICAL FORCES

When injury or unbalanced biomechanical forces are applied to myofascia, its ability to support normal muscle function is impaired. This can lead to loss of motion, pain, and less than optimal performance by the athlete. Dysfunction causes additional changes in the myofascia.

In pathology that occurs over time—for example, the swimmer who has developed poor posture—muscle imbalances are often the cause. As noted in figure 6.4, the process may start with a minor trauma or injury. It causes a change in the muscle, perhaps as a part of its withdrawal reflex to the injury. This muscle change eventually causes an imbalance of muscle strength between an agonist group and its antagonist group. Muscle imbalances lead to changes in neuromuscular response and coordination, which lead to further imbalances, until the structure reaches a point where the imbalance and resulting increased tissue stress cause symptoms that impair performance and require treatment.

The athlete can inadvertently start this cycle through the activities he or she performs in sport participation. If the swimmer with poor posture concentrates on pectoralis strengthening without also working on antagonist strength, or uses only strokes that emphasize anterior and not posterior muscles, eventually a muscle imbalance will occur. Awareness of muscle imbalance is important in treating patients with loss of motion. Muscle imbalances are discussed more thoroughly in chapter 7.

I Figure 6.4 Pathology of myofascial restriction: myofascial restriction can occur within a short time from acute injury and scar-tissue formation or gradually from minor but progressive alterations from repeated low-level trauma.

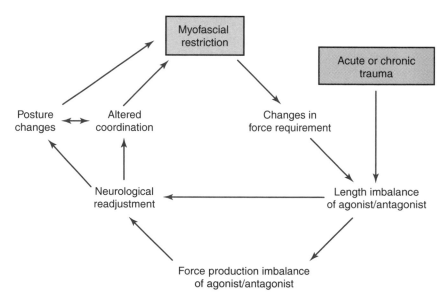

It is also important to realize that exercise is a vital collaborative adjunct of myofascial release treatments in a successful rehabilitation program. Myofascial techniques release restricted areas, but exercises for flexibility and strength reset neurological programming. Together they cause permanent positive changes in the affected tissues.

ACUTE BIOMECHANICAL FORCES

Previous chapters have already addressed the biomechanical causes of fascial restriction following acute injury. Scar tissue is less extensible and creates a localized connective-tissue meshwork that extends tentacles outward, much like a shattered plate glass window, to adjacent locations and can limit normal tissue mobility. Recall from the discussion of immobilization in chapter 5 that the scar-tissue matrix can restrict neurovascular and lymph vessels and reduce local metabolism. With reduced metabolism a fluid imbalance further adds to the area's reduced mobility and continued inflammation. Less motion causes a loss of GAGs and promotes increased cross-link formations. Interfiber mobility becomes restricted through this process.

In addition to the scarring that occurs with acute injury, spasm also can influence the myofascial system by producing prolonged tightness in one area that causes another area to compensate with prolonged looseness, initiating a cycle of imbalance and myofascial pathology. It is important to evaluate for fascial restrictions in both acute and nonacute injuries.

CONCEPTS

A few concepts are important for applying myofascial techniques appropriately.

Terminology

The term *myofascial release* is common and is frequently used in the techniques described here, but it is actually a misnomer. Myofascial release implies the treatment to myofascia. Although myofascia can certainly be the target of treatment, it is not always the targeted tissue nor the only tissue treated. For example, to relieve fascia contractures and restriction of skin and subcutaneous tissue mobility following edema and immobilization, myofascial release techniques actually commonly treat the fascia associated with skin, subcutaneous tissue, and other superficial structures that are limited in their mobility, not the muscle's fascia.

Even when the target tissue is myofascia, other structures may also be affected by treatment because of secondary restriction in the area. With subcutaneous restriction following edema and immobilization, for example, myofascial structures may be restricted and require myofascial release treatment, but the restricted subcutaneous and skin structures are also treated when the myofascia is treated.

Palpation

Palpation is fundamental in myofascial release. Not only is it required for an evaluation of the area, but continual palpation is performed during the treatment. The soft tissue's extensibility, movement, end-feel, and response to treatment are continually palpated during and after the treatment. Adjustments are made as the area is palpated and evaluated during the treatment.

Normal tissue has no tenderness when palpated. Normal tissue also has a springy end-feel that can be palpated when pressure to the tissue is released. This springy end-feel is present in normal tissue regardless of the tissue's excursion. Tissue mobility varies according to the body part and tissue type, but the springiness of the end-feel is consistent. In myofascial techniques, palpation also includes feeling the release in the tissues during the treatment. This release is the treatment goal and is necessary for restoring tissue mobility and balance. The release that is palpated has been described as the tissue giving way, letting go, relaxing, or melting like a hot knife going through ice.

Superficial to Deep Structures

When evaluating and treating with myofascial release techniques, you should move from superficial structures to deeper structures to avoid a mistake in identifying the structure or tissues that are restricted. Techniques should be applied with the least amount of force that is appropriate for achieving the established goals. More force is often indicated when scar-tissue adhesions and reduced mobility are present, but the additional force is applied only after assessing the area and determining the patient's tolerance.

Autonomic Effects

Neuroreflex changes can sometimes result from the use of myofascial techniques. Myofascial restriction can cause autonomic changes, so it is not surprising that when restriction is released, the autonomic system can be affected. If pain and myofascial restriction cause changes in skin color, moisture, temperature, and sensation, then their release will also cause changes in those signs and symptoms.

Afferent sensations are transmitted to the dorsal horn of the spinal cord. The dorsal horn is a processing center that receives and redirects information. It can send an impulse directly out the spinal cord as a reflex efferent response, or it can send the information to the subcortical or cortical level of the brain, where it is interpreted and a response formulated and returned down the spinal cord to the appropriate locale.

The patient may experience an autonomic response when the myofascial treatment is particularly effective. The patient's sympathetic system is stimulated, and the patient demonstrates symptoms such as increased pulse rate, sweating, and blood pressure changes. Less intense responses include sensations of burning, tingling, stinging, or heat in the area being treated (Sutton and Bartel 1994). Although these sympathetic responses are unusual, you should be aware that they may occur and be prepared to respond appropriately.

TREATMENT TECHNIQUES

Because there are many different ways to apply myofascial techniques, only general application techniques regarding time, frequency, pressure, and palpation are introduced here. This is by no means an exhaustive list of myofascial techniques. It is, however, a list of the more commonly used techniques.

General Guidelines

In the beginning, it may be necessary to restrict the treatment time to 3 to 5 min and increase it as the patient's tolerance and the response of the area indicate. Daily treatment can be beneficial. If bruising occurs, the technique is too aggressive. Because bruising causes additional scarring and adhesions, it should be avoided. Bruising is not a desirable reaction, but a short-term reddening of the skin in the area should be expected.

There are many different ways to apply myofascial release techniques (Manheim 1994). Palpation and relaxation by the sport rehabilitation specialist are basic to applying myofascial techniques. Relaxation allows you to have more sensitivity in your hands and fingertips for palpating the area being treated. An exercise to illustrate this idea is to take a dime in your fingertips, close your eyes, tense your arm from the shoulder to the fingers, and try to feel the nose on the portrait. Then relax your entire arm and try to feel the nose. It should be easier to locate the nose when your arm and hand are relaxed. To ensure both the patient's and your relaxation, you should both be in comfortable positions.

In one of the most frequently used techniques, both hands move longitudinally in opposite directions while stretching the tissue (figure 6.5). In another variation, only one hand applies the treatment while the other hand stabilizes or supports the tissue. The treatment hand applies pressure through the finger pads, thumb, knuckles, or heel of the hand (figure 6.6). The pressure can also be applied by the forearm or elbow, depending on the size and location of the area being treated. The stabilizing hand anchors the tissue so that the pressure can be applied in the direction of the restriction. The tissue's slack is taken up, and a steady pressure into the restriction is continued until the area releases or for about 90 s.

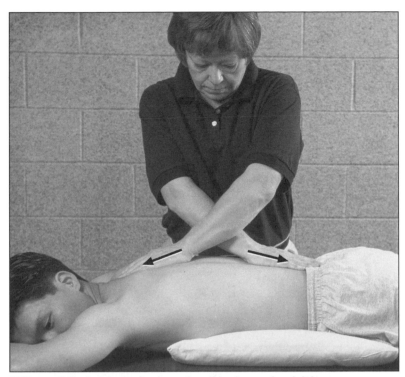

■ **Figure 6.5** In longitudinal myofascial release, fascial tissue between the hands is stretched.

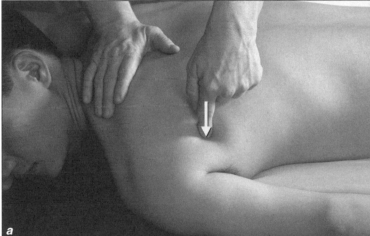

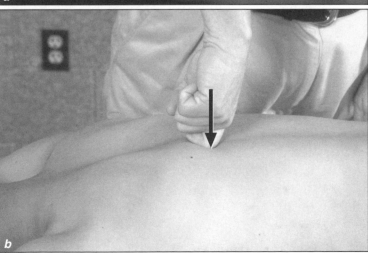

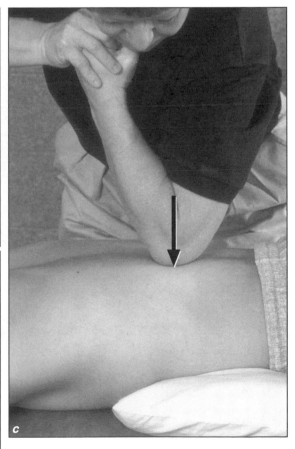

■ **Figure 6.6** Alternative myofascial release applications using finger pad (a), knuckle (b), or elbow (c).

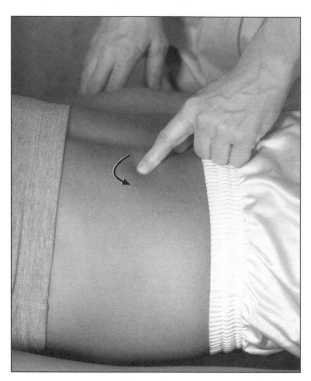

Figure 6.7 J-stroke.

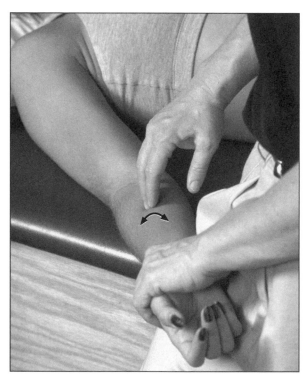

Figure 6.8 Oscillation.

The amount of pressure applied is determined by the tissue involved and the sensitivity of the area, but it is generally a low-load, sustained pressure.

J-Stroke

A J-stroke is a common technique that is used on limited areas of tightness and on longitudinal scars. The technique is used in these situations because of its multidirectional stretch. As shown in figure 6.7, the treatment hand draws short Js across the restricted area.

Oscillation

When muscle spasm is present, an oscillating pressure technique can be used. This technique involves a rhythmic, back-and-forth application of a low-load pressure while maintaining constant contact. It is designed to relax the muscle by reducing the spasm and relieving the patient's guarding of the area. It can be applied with finger pads for small areas, as shown in figure 6.8, or with the palms for larger areas.

Wringing

In areas of generalized or multidirectional restriction, a technique referred to as *wringing* can be effective. In this technique both hands are used for treatment. The hands are placed on the area in similar positions. They are then rotated on the extremity in opposite directions to twist or wring the tissue, as in figure 6.9. This same technique can be used on smaller areas using the two thumbs in the same manner.

Stripping

The stripping technique is used as a deep-tissue release. It is similar to the general technique described earlier, but it is applied to deeper tissue. Although the knuckles and elbow are frequently used in this technique (figure 6.10), in some instances the finger pads can also be effective. The pressure is slow, consistent, and deep. It is uncomfortable for the patient, but if it can be tolerated, it is effective in breaking up deep adhesions.

Arm Pull and Leg Pull

The arm pull and leg pull are gross techniques applied to generalized tightness in the upper and lower extremities, respectively. These techniques involve the application of longitudinal traction to the arm or leg from the hand or foot with the patient lying supine (figure 6.11). As the traction is applied, the extremity is slowly moved into abduction and rotation. When tissue resistance is felt, the motion is stopped, and the position is maintained

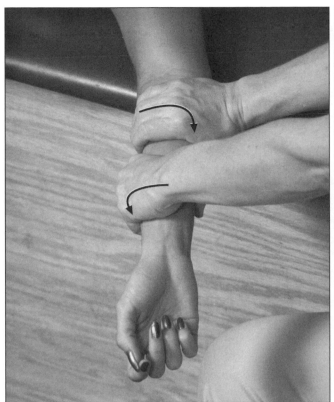

Figure 6.9 Wringing: a generalized, multidirectional release technique.

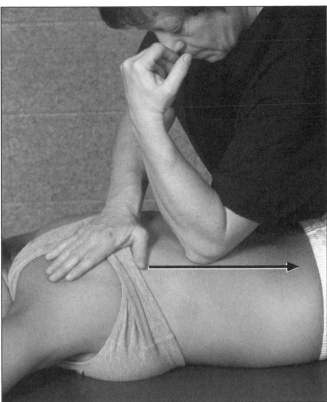

Figure 6.10 Stripping: a deep tissue release using one hand to stabilize and the elbow to treat.

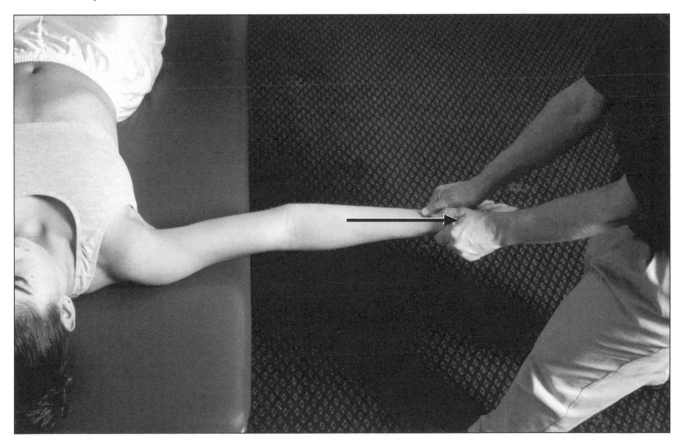

Figure 6.11 Arm pull: a generalized technique in which traction is applied to the arm while moving it into abduction and rotation to the point of resistance. Movement through an arc of motion continues following the resistance after the extremity releases.

until you feel the extremity release. Once the area releases, the extremity is moved through its arc of motion into the new area of restriction, and the sequence is repeated until an end position is reached.

PRECAUTIONS

As with any treatment, you should take precautions with this application. Myofascial release should be used cautiously on new scars. The new tissue is fragile because of its reduced tensile strength. It also may have increased sensitivity and limited tolerance to pressure.

Care should also be used with patients with reflex sympathetic dystrophy (RSD). RSD is exacerbated with pain, so treatments should be designed to avoid pain.

Bruising should be avoided. This is especially true when the purpose of the treatment is to improve scar-tissue mobility, because bruising produces more scar tissue.

The patient should be warned that sensations of pain, tingling, burning, and warmth are normal for this technique. The patient should also be instructed to inform you if any additional sensations are felt.

CONTRAINDICATIONS

Contraindications for the use of myofascial techniques include malignancy, hypermobile joints, recent fractures, hemorrhages, sutures, osteoporosis, local infections, and acute inflammations (Sutton and Bartel 1994). As always, contraindications should be respected, and treatment in the presence of these conditions should be avoided.

MYOFASCIAL TRIGGER POINTS

A myofascial trigger point is an area of tenderness in a muscle or its fascia that can cause referred pain and is palpated as a taut band with a nodule. Ice stroking, ischemic compression, stripping, and PNF are techniques often used to treat trigger points.

Probably the most recognized names in the study of myofascial trigger points are Janet Travell and David Simons. They devoted their professional lives to understanding and treating trigger points and are world-recognized leaders on the topic. Most of the information presented here is the result of their findings. For additional information on trigger points, see Travell (1976), Simons (1981), and Travell and Simons (1983, 1992).

Myriad terms are often used interchangeably with myofascial trigger point. Some of the more commonly used terms include myalgia, fibrositis, muscular rheumatism, fibroplastic syndrome, myositis, and myofascitis.

DEFINITION OF TRIGGER POINT

Travell and Simons (1983) define a **trigger point** as a "focus of hyperirritability in a tissue that, when compressed, is locally tender and, if sufficiently hypersensitive, gives rise to referred pain and tenderness, and sometimes to referred autonomic phenomena and distortion of proprioception." Trigger points can be located in myofascial, cutaneous, fascial, ligamentous, and periosteal tissue. The discussion here is limited to myofascial trigger points.

A myofascial trigger point involves a taut band of muscle tissue and its surrounding fascia, hence the name. A central focal point of local tenderness can be palpated as a nodule within the taut band. Compression of this point often refers pain to other areas or causes an autonomic response.

Travell and Simons (1983, 1992) identify two types of trigger points: active and latent. An **active trigger point** is one that is always tender and can produce referred pain whether the muscle is active or inactive. The muscle can also display weakness and reduced motion. When an active trigger point is palpated with a rolling pressure crosswise against the muscle fibers, the muscle fibers are stimulated to produce a localized twitch response. This palpation technique is called a snapping palpation and is performed using firm constant pressure and moving the fingertips across the muscle fibers as if plucking a guitar string. The local twitch response is an involuntary contraction of the muscle fibers in response to the snapping palpation (Travell and Simons 1983). Sometimes this response is incorrectly called a **jump sign**. A jump sign is also a reflex response but is a reaction of wincing or withdrawal.

A **latent trigger point** is painful only when it is palpated. Normal muscles do not have areas of tenderness, sites that elicit a local twitch response, or palpably taut bands.

TRIGGER POINT CHARACTERISTICS

Trigger point tenderness is often described as a dull ache and can be merely uncomfortable or very intense. Pressure on the trigger point can elicit a referred pain that is specific for each muscle. The more irritable the trigger point, the more severe and extensive is the referral pattern. For detailed trigger point referral patterns, refer to the two texts that Simons and Travell have written on this topic (1983, 1992). The earlier publication deals with referral patterns of the upper extremities, and the more recent text is concerned with lower-extremity referral patterns.

The referral patterns do not follow neurological referral patterns; this is an important distinction. The sensation of trigger point referral pain is also different from neurologically referred pain. Trigger point pain is often described as a deep ache. Occasionally, a trigger point pain is described as a sharp or stabbing pain, and rarely it is described as burning. Referred sensation from peripheral nerve entrapment or nerve root irritation, however, is evidenced by prickling, tingling, or numbness.

Myofascial trigger point pain becomes amplified by muscle activity (especially strenuous activity), passive stretch of the muscle, direct pressure of the trigger point, prolonged stationary periods followed by moving (such as getting up in the morning or standing after prolonged sitting), repeated or sustained muscle activity, and cold. On the other hand, myofascial trigger points are relieved with short periods of rest; heat accompanied by slow and sustained stretches; short-term, low-level activity; and specific treatment techniques that are discussed later in this chapter.

TRIGGER POINT CAUSES

Trigger points can be activated by various factors, including injury, overload, fatigue, and chilling. Acute conditions that can activate trigger points include fractures, sprains, dislocations, muscle impact injuries, and the stress of excessive or unusual exercise that the body is unable to tolerate. Overload of the muscles from a prolonged stationary posture, prolonged muscle immobilization in a shortened position, and nerve compressions are the most common causes of gradual trigger point onset. The exact mechanism of production of trigger points, however, is only theoretical at this time. Travell and Simons (1983) have proposed a theory that involves the contractile activity of a muscle: During contraction of a normal muscle fiber, calcium that is stored in the fiber's sarcoplasmic reticulum is rapidly released when the contraction begins and then reabsorbed in the presence of ATP when the contraction terminates. This process is triggered by a brief nerve impulse called an action potential. The contraction is the result of the shortening of the sarcomere when its cross-bridges pull the actin and myosin filaments over each other (figure 6.12). If an injured muscle fiber's sarcoplasmic reticulum is damaged, its calcium stimulates the sarcomere to produce a sustained contraction as long as ATP is present to provide the energy for the activity. This runaway metabolic activity no longer needs an action potential to continue the sustained contraction; it can continue on its own as long as the calcium and ATP are present together. Once the calcium becomes depleted, the trigger

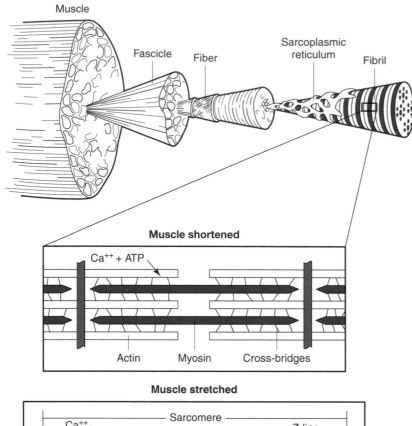

Muscle shortened

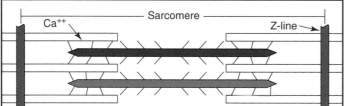

Muscle stretched

Figure 6.12 Normal skeletal muscle structure and a sarcomere in shortened and lengthened conditions.

point may continue to exist, but the mechanism for its persistent presence remains theoretical as yet. It is proposed that with a near exhaustion of local ATP levels, localized muscle contractions that do not require action potentials may take over. Without any ATP, the sarcomere's filaments cannot release from each other and remain rigid in their contracted position.

Vasoconstriction of the area occurs probably either because of a localized reflex response or stimulation of the central nervous system and autonomic system through the trigger point. This simultaneously reduces local circulation and increases metabolic needs. The release of nerve-sensitizing and ischemia-causing substances such as histamine, serotonin, kinins, and prostaglandins (mentioned in chapter 2) may be the cause of continued, localized, runaway metabolic activity. Travell and Simons (1983, 1992) propose that these substances, which are released following an injury, increase the metabolic demands and sensitize afferent nerve endings to make them hyperirritable to mediate referred pain, autonomic response, motor neuron response, and cause trigger points.

TRIGGER POINT EXAMINATION

As part of the total treatment plan, the causes of the patient's pain must be accurately assessed to rule out trigger points as a possible factor. Observation and evaluation of the patient's posture, range of motion, weakness patterns, pain areas, and history are all required to determine the patient's injury and rehabilitation needs. It is sometimes easier to identify patterns if the areas of pain are indicated on a figure drawing like the one in figure 6.13.

A compression test over the muscle can detect taut bands, nodules, and local and referred pain. A local twitch response confirms the presence of a trigger point. A taut band is palpated by stretching the muscle until the taut fibers are pulled to the point of discomfort without pain while the overall muscle remains slack. The taut band feels like a cord within the muscle. Begin at the distal attachment and palpate with either the pad of the thumb or two or three fingers along the taut band toward the fibers' proximal attachment to locate the trigger point within the band. It is an area of increased tenderness and feels like a hard ball within the taut band.

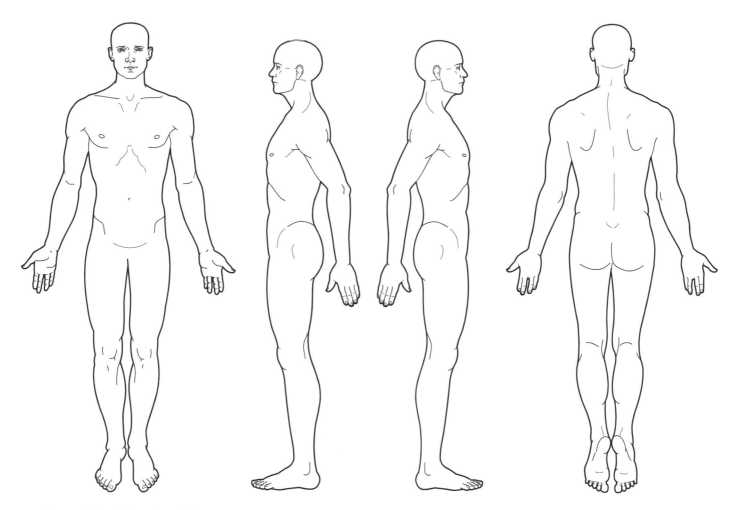

Figure 6.13 Pain-referral figure.

A local twitch response can be elicited along the taut band by performing a snapping palpation of the band. A snapping palpation is done by placing the muscle in a relaxed, neutral position and strumming the fibers with pressure perpendicular to the fiber alignment, much like strumming a guitar. In a positive response the taut band twitches. The more closely the pressure is applied to the trigger point of the taut band, the more vigorous is the response. This technique works most effectively on superficial muscles.

TRIGGER POINT TREATMENT

Travell and Simons (1983, 1992) and Cyriax (1977) advocate the use of trigger point injection as an effective method of treatment, but this treatment is not appropriate nor legal for sport rehabilitation specialists. When an active trigger point does not respond to the treatment techniques presented here, it may be useful to refer the patient to a physician who may use the injection technique.

Three primary methods of myofascial trigger point treatments are discussed briefly here. For additional information, refer to the Travell and Simons texts (1983, 1992).

Ice-Stretch

Fluori-Methane was formerly used as a common treatment for myofascial trigger points. Now that we are more aware of the harm that chlorofluorocarbons cause to the atmosphere, Fluori-Methane is no longer used in many facilities and has been replaced by the use of ice stroking. An "icicle" is made by placing a tongue depressor in a cup of water and freezing the water. Before applying the icicle to the skin, the cup is torn back and covered with thin plastic wrap to avoid getting any cold water on the patient's skin; keeping the skin dry throughout the treatment maintains the contrast between the warm skin and the cold ice.

Before application the patient should be instructed to relax. Applying enough pressure on the trigger point area to produce the referred pain may help the patient understand why your treatment is not applied directly to the area of pain. The patient is placed in a comfortable position with the skin exposed and the body part supported to permit full relaxation. Before treatment the part is moved through its range of motion so that you and the patient can judge changes made by the treatment. With the muscle anchored at one end, the ice is applied in a sweeping motion in parallel strokes in only one direction over the length of the muscle and then over the referred pain pattern. As the ice is applied in a rhythmic, unhurried fashion, a slow, continual, passive stretch is applied progressively to the muscle. Any one area of the skin should receive only two to three strokes of ice before rewarming to achieve optimal results of the ice and stretch technique (figure 6.14). The rate at which the ice is moved over the skin is approximately 4 in./s (10 cm/s). The stretch force should be light enough that it does not elicit a stretch reflex from the muscle. As a muscle releases, you must be able to detect the relaxation and place the muscle in a new stretch position that takes up the slack and provides the same level of tension on the muscle. The application and release of the stretch force should be done smoothly and gradually, not quickly. A hot pack can be immediately applied to further relax the muscle. The patient can also assist the stretch by contracting the antagonist, but you must monitor the contraction so as to prevent a co-contraction of the agonist and antagonist. The ice-and-stretch technique can be repeated for several cycles after the skin has been rewarmed, depending on the results of treatment, the patient's response, and desired goals.

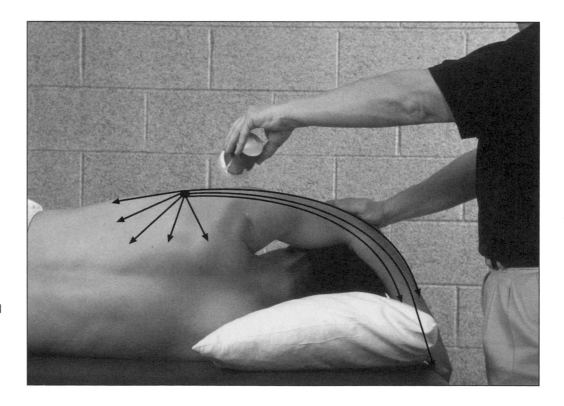

▌Figure 6.14 In the ice-and-stretch technique, ice strokes are applied in sweeps that include the muscle, its trigger points, and its referred pain areas. The ice is applied in a rhythmic fashion while a gentle stretch is applied to the muscle.

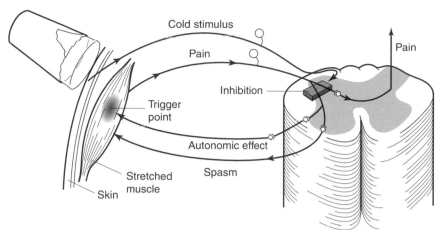

■ **Figure 6.15** Effect of trigger point release on neural pathways: The sudden cold and touch afferent stimulation facilitates a presynaptic inhibition to "close the gate" to pain transmission.

Adapted, by permission, from D.G. Simons, J.G. Travell, and L.S. Simons, 1999, *Travell & Simons' myofascial pain and dysfunction: The trigger point manual*, Vol. 1, 2nd ed. (Baltimore: Williams & Wilkins).

Theory of Effectiveness

It is believed that this technique is effective because of two mechanisms, although they have not been confirmed through research. The gate theory of pain presented by Melzak (1973) postulates that sudden cold and touch sensations inhibit the pain cycle by blocking transmission of pain signals. Active trigger points activate the pain-spasm response. Ice stroking inhibits the pain-spasm cycle and allows the muscle to respond to the stretch (figure 6.15).

The second factor is mechanical: If a muscle is stretched, its sarcomere elongates and releases the actin and myosin elements enough to end the sustained muscle-fiber contraction.

Ischemic Compression

Another myofascial trigger point release is ischemic compression. In this technique, pressure is applied slowly and progressively over the trigger point as the tension in the trigger point and its taut band subsides. Pressure is maintained until the tenderness is gone or the tension is released. This is followed by stretching the muscle. Before application, the patient should be informed that some discomfort may occur.

Stripping

A third technique is stripping massage, a deep-stroking massage applied with minimal lubrication on the fingertips. A firm pressure is used along the length of the taut band. The pressure increases progressively with each successive pass along the muscle. A milking movement from the distal to proximal end of the muscle goes over the trigger point at the rate of about 1 in. (2.5 cm) every 3 s. As the effects of the technique become apparent, the taut band relaxes, the trigger point nodule softens, and the area ceases to be tender and no longer refers pain.

The ischemia produced by the pressure of both the ischemic compression and stripping massage techniques is believed to cause a reflexive hyperemia that returns the site to a normal condition (Travell and Simons 1983).

Proprioceptive Neuromuscular Facilitation and Other Techniques

The PNF techniques of contract-relax and reciprocal inhibition, which were introduced in chapter 5 and are discussed further in chapter 7, are also effective in relaxing myofascial trigger points. In addition, various other techniques are used in the treatment of myofascial trigger points. Modalities such as hot packs, ultrasound, and electrical stimulation are also frequently used as adjuncts to enhance the effectiveness of treatments.

PRECAUTIONS

Before application, an accurate history should be taken and the patient's condition assessed to determine whether trigger point therapy will be effective. Trigger point therapy is not as effective on scar tissue adhesions as on myofascial restrictions.

The patient should relax for optimal treatment results. The stretch applied should be passive without any contraction of the agonist. If the patient is able to isolate the antagonist and if you can monitor the patient's response, contraction of the antagonist may improve treatment results, as long as the stretched muscle remains relaxed. Cold is not as effective if it is applied too quickly or repetitively over the same area. The stretch should be applied slowly and should not cause painful spasm or prevent the patient from relaxing, but it should be sufficient to produce the desired results.

The cause of the myofascial trigger point must be corrected for the treatment to be successful, particularly if the cause is poor posture or chronic stress of the muscle. The cause can be corrected with flexibility and strengthening exercises and patient education and instruction.

Prolonged direct pressure over nerves and blood vessels should be avoided. The pressure should be discontinued if the patient complains of tingling or numbness.

MUSCLE ENERGY

Muscle energy techniques are used to treat joint malalignments. These techniques involve the precise and controlled voluntary contraction of a muscle against a counterforce provided by the sport rehabilitation specialist, followed by a passive stretch.

Like most manual therapy techniques, muscle energy techniques have their origin in osteopathic medicine. Fred Mitchell, DO, originally developed muscle energy techniques, which others have since modified.

DEFINITION OF MUSCLE ENERGY

According to Greenman (1996), muscle energy is a manual technique that involves the voluntary contraction of a muscle in a precisely controlled direction, at varying levels of intensity, against a distinct counterforce applied by the sport rehabilitation specialist. Essentially, muscle energy is the use of muscle contraction to correct a joint's malalignment.

MUSCLE ENERGY THEORY

Muscle energy theory is based on the premise that joint malalignments occur when the body becomes unbalanced. Malalignment may be the result of a muscle spasm, a weakened muscle overpowered by a stronger muscle, or restricted mobility. The muscle contraction used to correct a malalignment may be **isometric, concentric,** or **eccentric.** The patient controls the magnitude of contraction, and the sport rehabilitation positions the patient and provides the resistance to change the treated joint's alignment.

In malalignments, movement is restricted by what Mitchell identifies as a barrier. A **barrier** is not the end of the existing range of motion, but a resistance that is felt when a part is moved through its passive range of motion. For example, you can passively move the leg of a patient with a tight hamstring in a straight-leg raise. Although the hip may be able to go through its full motion, you will feel a resistance because of tightness in the hamstring at some point before the end of its motion. Where in the motion this resistance is felt depends on how tight the hamstring is.

Isometric muscle contraction is most commonly used when treating the spine with muscle energy techniques, whereas isotonic contraction is more frequently used when treating the extremities. Briefly reviewing muscle physiology principles can help you understand how muscle energy techniques work. When the patient contracts a muscle against an external resistance, the contracting muscle causes the neurological response of reciprocal innervation. In other words, the contracting muscle causes relaxation of the antagonist and contraction of synergists through responses of Golgi tendon organs and muscle spindles via spinal cord and cortical reflexes. After the isometric contraction, the antagonist relaxes enough to permit a stretch. Its relaxation also impedes its inhibition of the contracting muscle to permit a more normal force-counterforce balance between the agonist and antagonist. Repeated contractions combined with passive stretches then provide additional motion gains and improved muscle balance.

It is believed that these muscle contractions and changes in muscle length affect the surrounding fascia and connective tissue. Since the technique is an active one, requiring the active participation of the patient, muscle physiology is affected and can result in postexercise soreness secondary to metabolic waste buildup and a change in the fascial length. You should warn the patient that muscle soreness may occur and avoid overpowering the patient or overdoing the activity. Because the forces used are relatively low and the techniques involve an active motion and a passive stretch, the only contraindications to muscle energy techniques are recent or non-union fractures.

COMPONENTS OF MUSCLE ENERGY TECHNIQUE

The components necessary for muscle energy techniques are an accurate assessment of the cause and best treatment of the malalignment, a specific joint position, a precise active muscle contraction performed by the patient, an appropriate counterforce produced by the sport rehabilitation specialist, and an applied stretch force that results in increased motion without pain.

Before you can determine the appropriate muscle energy technique to apply, you must determine through an evaluation the presence of a malalignment and the cause of the malalignment.

Once you determine that muscle energy would assist in correcting the deficiency, you must determine the most effective position for the muscle energy technique. The patient's injured part is then positioned at the end of the barrier, and the patient is instructed on the type of muscle contraction desired. While the patient actively contracts the muscle, you apply the appropriate resistive force with the correct direction, duration, and magnitude.

If the contraction is isometric, you should provide enough force to prevent movement but not overpower the patient's contraction. The isometric contraction is not strong but should be sustained and light. It should be sustained for 5 to 10 s, and the length of the muscle should not change.

If an isotonic contraction is used, enough counterforce should be provided to allow motion at an even, controlled speed. The muscle contraction should be forceful and through the muscle's full range of motion.

For either an isometric or isotonic contraction, it is important for you to permit full relaxation of the muscle after the contraction before stretching the joint to a new barrier position. This allows the muscle to enter its refractory period (time of relaxation) following its contraction and achieve optimal stretch results. The technique is repeated three to five times for the best results. The greatest changes are seen after three repetitions; clinical observations indicate that more than five repetitions produce little additional benefit.

APPLICATION

A couple of examples can demonstrate the application of muscle energy techniques. In the first example, an isotonic contraction is illustrated. Let us look at a basketball player who has undergone rehabilitation after an ACL reconstruction. After many varied attempts to attain full motion, she still lacks full extension. You must investigate possible alternative methods for relieving the problem:

1. *Assessment of the problem.* You have determined that the lack of extension is the result of restricted external rotation of the tibia on the femur.

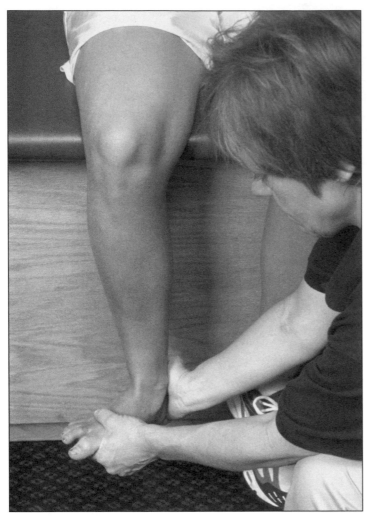

Figure 6.16 Muscle energy release to gain knee extension: With the lower leg in external rotation and the foot in dorsiflexion, the patient rotates the lower leg internally while you provide a smooth resistance throughout the full movement. Once the patient relaxes the muscles, the lower leg is externally rotated to its new barrier.

2. *Specific joint position.* The patient sits with the lower legs hanging over the table. You position the ankle in dorsiflexion and the lower leg in external rotation to their barrier (figure 6.16).

3. *Precise active contraction by the patient.* The patient contracts the thigh muscles to move the lower leg into internal rotation through the full range of motion.

4. *Appropriate counterforce.* While the patient contracts the muscles and moves the joint, you offer resistance that permits a smooth, controlled movement into internal rotation for 5 s. Guide the lower leg through the correct plane of motion while offering resistance.

5. *Stretch force.* Instruct the patient to relax while holding the lower leg at its end position, wait to feel the muscles fully relax, then apply a stretch into external rotation to a new joint position where the new barrier is felt. This technique is repeated three to five times. Reassess for range of motion changes.

In the next example, isometric contractions are used in a muscle energy technique applied to a soccer player who collided with another player and suffered a direct blow to the right anterior ilium. The contusion is resolved, but he continues to complain of groin pain that goes down his leg. The physician has ruled out a disk injury and reports to you that the problem may be coming from his pelvis. You are given the challenge of evaluation and treatment of the patient's injury:

1. *Assessment of the problem.* Your evaluation reveals that there is an inflare of the right ilium. Other tests for lumbar dysfunction have ruled out injury to the low back. You determine that muscle energy techniques would be an appropriate treatment.

2. *Specific joint position.* With the patient lying supine, his right leg is placed in a figure-4 position with the right knee flexed, the hip abducted and flexed, and rotated so the outside of the ankle is placed on the distal left thigh to the barrier point. Stabilize the patient's pelvis by placing your left hand on the left anterior superior iliac spine and the right hand on the patient's medial right knee. Then apply enough pressure on the knee to move the right hip to its end position of external rotation.

3. *Precise active contraction by the patient.* Ask the patient to attempt to move the leg into internal rotation pulling the knee toward the left shoulder as you provide resistance to prevent the motion from occurring. The isometric contraction is held for 5 to 10 s.

4. *Appropriate counterforce.* The amount of resistance applied by the patient is not great: less than a pound of resistance. Since the contraction is isometric, you must instruct the patient to match your force and not to overpower the resistance you provide (figure 6.17).

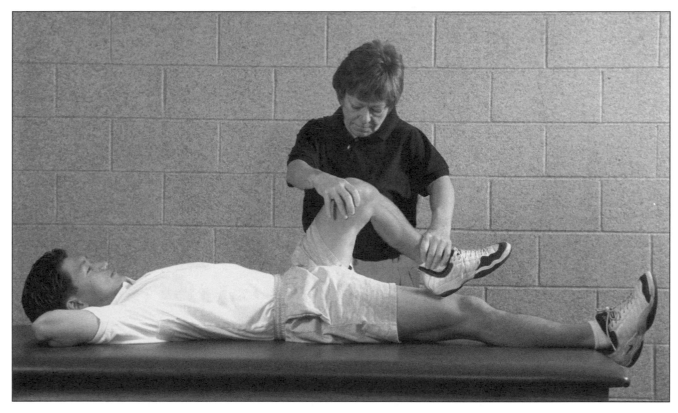

■ Figure 6.17 Muscle energy release to correct ilium inflare.

5. *Stretch force.* As in the previous example, instruct the patient to relax while you support the extremity at its end position, wait to feel the muscles fully relax, then apply a stretch into external rotation and abduction by pushing the right knee toward the table to the new barrier. The process is repeated three to five times. After the final repetition, passively return the leg into hip and knee extension. Reassess for alignment and pain.

The majority of muscle energy techniques must be accompanied by exercise to effectively treat the problem. You must understand the mechanics of the change that occurs with muscle energy treatment in order to correctly use accompanying active stretches. As an example, you could instruct the soccer player with the iliac inflare to perform a stretch similar to the position used in the treatment. It is also necessary for the patient to progress to strengthening exercises that support the stretching exercises, such as hip external rotation or hip adductor strengthening exercises.

JOINT MOBILIZATION

Joint mobilization involves passive movement of a joint to relieve pain or restore mobility. Proper application requires knowledge of joint mechanics, normal range of motion, and proper technique.

Joint **mobilization** is one of the most commonly used manual therapy techniques in the treatment of restricted joint motion. **Manipulation** and mobilization are not new concepts. Hippocrates (460–355 B.C.) used these techniques in his medical practice and recorded various methods of manipulating bones and joints.

Through the years a variety of approaches to manipulation and mobilization have been developed. More recent schools of thought have been influenced by the teachings of manual therapists such as Geoffrey Maitland, Freddy Kaltenborn, James Cyriax, James Mennell, and Stanley Paris. Table 6.1 identifies the main distinctions of each of these manual therapists' approaches.

Table 6.1 Manual Therapy Schools of Thought	
Sources	**Key distinction**
James Cyriax	Uses selective tension techniques to identify faulty structures in the examination. Emphasizes the need for soft-tissue massage and frequently uses injection of muscle trigger points. Believes the disk is the primary source of low-back pain and uses nonspecific spinal techniques designed to move the disk to relieve nerve root pressure.
Freddy Kaltenborn	Believes the restoration of normal function is based on the restoration of normal arthrokinematics. The techniques incorporate the influence of muscle function and soft-tissue changes in the manifestation of the patient's loss of function. The techniques are eclectic and very specific.
Geoffrey Maitland	Uses primarily passive accessory movements to restore function after an extensive assessment based on information from the patient's subjective examination (history) and the evaluator's objective assessment. The movements are oscillations, the techniques are specific, and the goal is to relieve what he terms "reproducible signs."
James Mennell	Feels that "joint play" is key to normal joint function. Emphasizes the importance of the small accessory movements as necessary for full joint motion to occur. Techniques are more specific for the extremities than for the spine.
Stanley Paris	Incorporates both chiropractic and osteopathic orientations in his eclectic approach to normalization of arthrokinematics, especially joint play and component motions. As a general rule, the patient's pain is not used to guide treatment.

DEFINITION OF JOINT MOBILIZATION

Joint mobilization is on a continuum with manipulation. They both involve passive movement of a joint, but mobilization is under the patient's control in that voluntary contraction of a muscle will stop the movement. Manipulation is at such a speed that the patient is unable to stop the motion. Mobilization is frequently performed by sport rehabilitation specialists, but manipulation is not. Manipulation is most commonly performed in chiropractic applications, and is beyond the scope of this book.

JOINT MOTION

There are two types of joint motion: physiological and accessory. Physiological joint motion is movement that the patient can do voluntarily, such as flexion and abduction. Accessory motion is necessary for normal joint motion but cannot be voluntarily performed or controlled.

There are two types of accessory motion: joint play and component motion. Both component motion and joint play are necessary for full motion. Component motions are not capsular, but they accompany physiological motion. The rotation of the clavicle during shoulder flexion is an example of a component motion. Joint play occurs within the joint and is determined by the joint capsule's laxity. If you grasp and twist a finger, you can feel the joint play of the metacarpophalangeal joint.

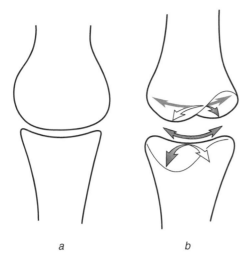

Figure 6.18 Joint surfaces of ovoid *(a)* and sellar joints *(b)*.

Figure 6.19 Roll: different points on one surface come in contact with different points on the second surface.

Figure 6.20 Slide: one point on a surface comes in contact with different points on a second surface.

Figure 6.21 Spin: a segment rotates about a stationary mechanical axis.

ARTHROKINEMATICS

Arthrokinematics refers to the motions between the bones that form a joint. There are five types of motion that occur within a joint: roll, slide, spin, compression, and distraction. These motions permit greater motion of a joint and can occur only with appropriate joint play. This concept is vital to understanding how joint mobilization works and how it can be applied.

Most joint surfaces are concave, convex, or both. Joints that have one concave and one convex surface are called *ovoid* (figure 6.18a). Joints that have a surface that is concave in one direction and convex in another with the opposing surface convex and concave in complementary directions are called *sellar* or *saddle joints* because of their similarity to a saddle (figure 6.18b). The shape of the joint determines its arthrokinematic motions.

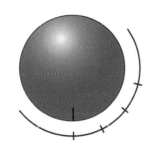

Roll

Roll occurs on **incongruent** surfaces when a new point of one surface meets a new point of the opposing surface (figure 6.19). Rolling occurs in combination with sliding or spinning in a normal joint. Roll occurs in the direction of bone movement.

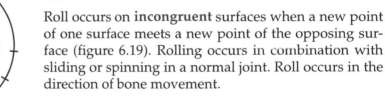

Slide

Slide occurs on congruent surfaces when one point of one surface contacts new points on the opposing surface (figure 6.20). Like rolling, sliding does not usually occur by itself in normal joints. When a passive mobilization technique is applied to produce a slide in a joint, the technique is referred to as a glide. The more congruent a joint is, the better it responds to gliding mobilization techniques to gain mobility.

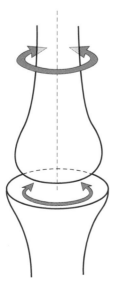

Spin

Spin occurs when one bone rotates around a stationary axis (figure 6.21). Like rolling and sliding, spin does not occur by itself during normal joint motion.

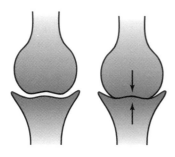

■ **Figure 6.22**   Compression.

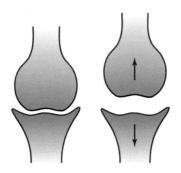

■ **Figure 6.23**   Distraction.

Compression

Compression is a decrease in the space between two joint surfaces (figure 6.22). Compression adds stability to a joint and is a normal reaction of a joint to muscle contraction. Some compression occurs during a roll on the side in the direction of the motion.

Distraction

Distraction of a joint occurs when the two surfaces are pulled apart (figure 6.23). A gentle distraction can relieve pain in a tender joint. Distraction is often used in combination with joint accessory mobilization techniques to further stretch the capsule.

CONCAVE AND CONVEX RULES

Knowing which type of joint is being treated and keeping in mind the concave and convex rules (figure 6.24) is basic to the application of correct mobilization techniques. In these rules, one joint surface is mobile, and the other is stable. The concave-convex rule states that concave joint surfaces slide in the same direction as the bone movement (figure 6.24). The convex-concave rule states that convex joint surfaces slide in the opposite direction of the bone movement. For example, if the thigh is stabilized to prevent the femur from moving at the knee, the tibia's concave joint surface slides posteriorly when the tibia moves posteriorly from extension to flexion. In contrast, if the glenoid is stabilized at the shoulder, the humerus's convex shoulder joint surface slides inferiorly as the arm is moved superiorly into abduction. In other words, if you want to increase knee flexion, your mobilization force on the tibia is in an anterior-to-posterior (AP) direction. If you want to increase knee extension, you apply a posterior-to-anterior (PA) mobilization force. On the other hand, when mobilizing the shoulder, if you want to increase shoulder flexion, you would apply an AP force.

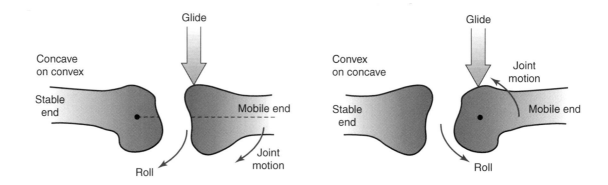

■ **Figure 6.24**   Rules for concave and convex joint surfaces. *(a)* Concave-convex rule: joint mobilization force is applied in same direction of bone motion. *(b)* Convex-concave rule: joint mobilization force is applied in the opposite direction of bone motion.

CAPSULAR PATTERNS OF MOTION

As discussed in chapter 5, all joints have expected, or normal, ranges of motion, and various causes can prevent normal motion. When loss of motion is caused by tightness within the joint capsule, specific characteristic changes are seen in the pattern of motion loss and are referred to as a **capsular pattern.** Table 6.2 indicates the capsular pattern for most joints. When you examine a joint's range of motion, knowing both the joint's normal degree of motion and the typical pattern of capsular restriction is necessary. When a capsular pattern is present, full joint motion will not be attained until the capsular tightness is addressed. A capsular pattern indicates that at least some of the loss of motion is due to tightness within the capsule and that joint mobilization should be included in the treatment program. A noncapsular pattern

Table 6.2 Capsular Patterns

Joints	Capsular pattern
Glenohumeral	External rotation is more limited than abduction. Abduction is more limited than flexion. Flexion is more limited than internal rotation.
Elbow	Flexion is more limited than extension. Supination and pronation are equally limited.
Wrist	Flexion and extension are equally limited. Pronation and supination are mildly limited at the distal radioulnar joint.
Finger	Abduction is more limited than adduction of the thumb CMC. Flexion is more limited than extension of the MCPs and IPs.
Hip	Internal rotation, abduction, and flexion are more limited than extension. Generally, no limitation of external rotation.
Knee	Flexion is more limited than extension.

Ankle
  Talocrural
  Subtalar
	Plantar flexion is more limited than dorsiflexion.
	Inversion is more limited than eversion.

Foot and toes
  1st MTP
  2nd–5th MTP
  IP joint
	Extension is more limited than flexion.
	Variable.
	Extension is more limited than flexion.

Lumbar spine	If a left facet is limited: Forward bending (FB) produces a deviation to the left. Side bending right (SBR) is limited. Side bending left (SBL) is unrestricted. Rotation left (RL) is limited. Rotation right (RR) is unrestricted.
Cervical spine	If a left facet is limited: FB produces some deviation to the left. SBR is unrestricted. SBL is comparatively unrestricted. RL is comparatively unrestricted. RR is most limited.

CMC = carpometacarpal; MCP = metacarpophalangeal; IP = interphalangeal; MTP = metatarsophalangeal.

indicates that structures other than the capsule are preventing normal motion and that joint mobilization will not significantly contribute to range-of-motion gains.

EFFECTS OF JOINT MOBILIZATION

As with many manual therapy techniques, the exact effects of joint mobilization are unknown, and many reported benefits are anecdotal with little objective evidence to identify their effects. Nonetheless, many clinicians report consistent, positive results from their treatments, so it is assumed within the allied health and medical world that some biochemical, biophysiological, or biomechanical benefits are produced by the techniques.

Neurophysiological Effects

Hertling and Kessler (1990) report that joint mobilization stimulates the joint's mechanoreceptors to decrease pain. Small-amplitude joint mobilization oscillations stimulate the mechanoreceptors that inhibit the transmission of nociceptive stimulation from the spinal cord and brain stem. Small-amplitude and mild joint mobilization oscillations also affect muscle spasm and muscle guarding. Inhibition of nociceptive stimulation results in relaxation.

Nutritional Effects

Distraction or small gliding movements can cause synovial fluid to move within the joint. The avascular articular cartilage within a joint depends on synovial fluid movement for its nutritional needs and nutrient-waste exchange. In edematous and painful joints, these movements can improve nutrient exchange to prevent deleterious effects of joint swelling and immobilization.

Mechanical Effects

More aggressive mobilization techniques can improve the mobility of hypomobile joints. Immobilized joints that have lost their normal range of motion develop collagenous adhesions and thickened connective tissue. Mobilization techniques that stretch collagen structures into their plastic range of deformation increase the tissue's mobility and improve the joint's motion. Mobilization not only stretches capsular tissues but also effectively loosens or breaks down adhesions to improve mobility (Kaltenborn 1980).

Cracking Noise

Occasionally, a mobilization or joint movement produces a cracking sound. When tension is produced in a synovial joint, increased pressure within the joint causes a vaporization of gas within the synovial fluid. When the gas is liberated as the gas bubble forms then collapses, the joint space expands. The collapse of the gas bubble causes the noise (Corrigan and Maitland 1989). Initial reports indicated that the gas formed was nitrogen, but it is now believed to be carbon dioxide.

Following this cracking, joint mobility often increases. This is believed to occur because of the expansion of the joint capsule from the increased pressure and the reflex relaxation of surrounding muscles through stimulation of inhibitory mechanoreceptors (Paris and Patla 1988). This increased joint mobility can be advantageous or disadvantageous. It is advantageous for hypomobile joints. For hypermobile joints, a reduction of muscle tone along with an increase in joint laxity can lead to increased joint stress and pain; the muscles reflexively tighten and cause additional discomfort. Although "cracking" one's back or neck may offer temporary relief, Paris and Patla (1988) believe that such joint cracking may increase the risk of disk injury. When cracking occurs repeatedly in the spine, the joints become unstable. Conversely, when it occurs repeatedly in the extremities, as when cracking the knuckles, the joint capsule eventually becomes thickened and increases the joint's stiffness.

APPLICATION OF JOINT MOBILIZATION

Before you apply joint mobilization, you must identify the forces and excursions that can and should occur as well as what is considered "normal" for a joint and the individual. These issues are discussed in the following sections.

Grades of Movement

Movements used in joint mobilization are divided into four grades, indicated I, II, III, and IV. Manipulation uses grade V. The grading is based on the amplitude of the movement and where within the available range of motion the force is applied. Grades I and IV are small-amplitude movements performed at the beginning and end of the range, respectively. Grades II and III are large-amplitude movements. Grade II movement does not reach the limits of the range, whereas grade III movement is performed up to the limit of the available range. These grades overlap somewhat, as seen in figure 6.25. Grade V is the manipulation grade and is usually small in amplitude and beyond the end range of a restricted joint.

I Figure 6.25
Grades of movement in a normal and a restricted joint: Grades I and II do not reach the limits of movement. Grades III and IV do reach the limits of movement. Grades I and IV are small amplitude, while grades II and III are large amplitude.

Adapted, by permission, from G. Maitland, 1991, *Peripheral manipulation*, 3rd ed. (Woburn, MA: Butterworth-Heinemann).

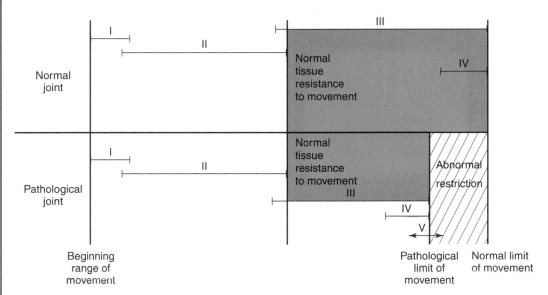

The amount of motion within each grade is relative to the specific joint and to the available motion within that joint. For example, a normal glenohumeral joint has larger grade I, II, III, and IV movements than a severely restricted glenohumeral joint and certainly larger movements than a metacarpophalangeal joint.

Grades I and II are generally used to relieve pain in joints. Oscillations in these grades stimulate joint mechanoreceptors to inhibit nociceptive feedback into the joints. These grades often are also used before and after treatment with grades III and IV, beforehand to relax the joint and afterward to relieve discomfort that the more aggressive grades may have caused.

Grades III and IV are used to gain motion within the joint. These grades stretch the capsule and connective-tissue structures that limit joint mobility. They can be uncomfortable but are not necessarily so.

Oscillatory motions are most often used with the various grades of movement. Sustained joint-play motions can also be used. The sustained techniques involve only three grades: I, II, and III. Their grade definitions are slightly different from those of oscillatory motions: Grade II goes to the end point of resistance, and grade III is essentially a stretch of the joint, going toward a normal joint's limit (figure 6.26). The techniques discussed here use the oscillatory motions, since they are the most common.

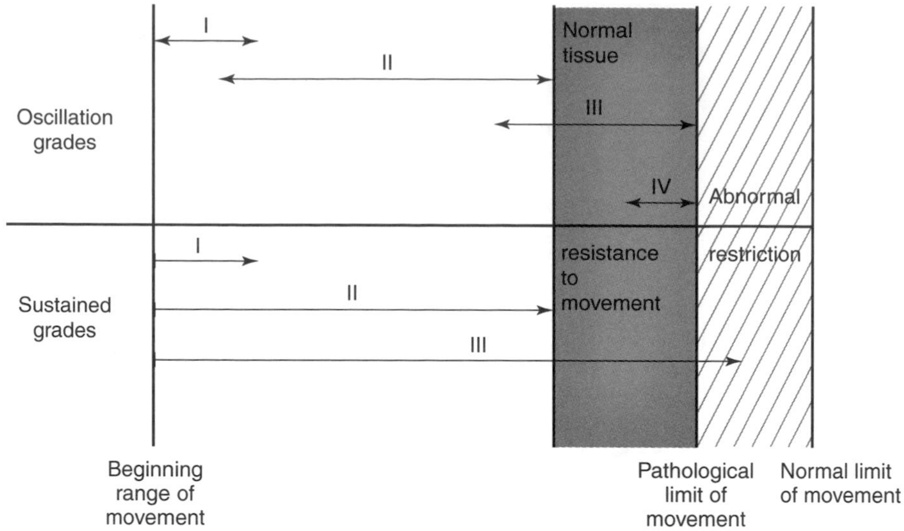

Figure 6.26 Sustained versus oscillation mobilization.

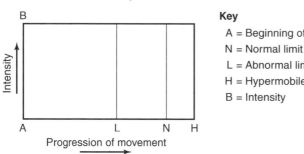

Figure 6.27 Movement diagram.

Key
A = Beginning of movement
N = Normal limit of ROM
L = Abnormal limit of ROM
H = Hypermobile range
B = Intensity

Movement Diagram

A movement diagram is a visual aid that can sometimes be helpful in determining which mobilization grade to use in a treatment. Either physiological or accessory movements can be diagrammed. A movement diagram is shown in figure 6.27. **AN** is the normal range of motion of a joint; **A** is the beginning of motion, and **N** is the normal limit of a motion. **L** is the abnormal limit of motion. **H** indicates a joint's hypermobile range. **B** is the intensity of a treatment technique.

You mark on the movement diagram where the patient reports pain. **P** in figure 6.28 represents where within the range of motion the patient reports pain and the intensity of the pain; P_1 indicates where the pain starts, and P_2 the intensity of pain at the end of motion. R_1 indicates where you first feel resistance during a passive movement of the joint, and R_2 is the intensity of the resistance at the end of the motion. If the patient has pain at rest, the **P** curve begins at **A** and is placed at a height on the vertical scale that corresponds to the intensity of pain reported by the patient. If the pain is mild, the mark is placed low on the **AB** line; if pain is moderate, the mark is placed higher (figure 6.28b). If the patient reports the start of pain at 50% of possible motion, P_1 is placed at the midpoint of the **AL** line (figure 6.28a). If the pain occurs gradually but progressively over the length of the motion, a gradually sloping upward line is drawn, but if pain begins suddenly and quickly intensifies, a steep line is used.

To determine where **R** is drawn, you passively move the joint through its available range and indicate on the graph where the start of the restriction can be palpated. If the restriction begins abruptly and inhibits motion, a steep, rapidly climbing line is drawn. If restriction is more gradual, a line with a gentler slope is drawn.

Once you complete a movement diagram, you can easily assess the treatment needs and determine whether to attend to the patient's pain or joint restriction first. If the pain is not significant, you may choose to treat the restriction first, but if pain appears more intense and increases more quickly than resistance on the movement diagram, pain should be relieved before restriction is treated.

Until you understand joint mobilization techniques and grades and develop the skill to palpate and evaluate pain and resistance, it is a good idea to draw a movement diagram on paper or in your head. It will help you determine what you need to treat first and what grades of mobilization are most appropriate.

(a) Pain occurs at 50% of the motion and intensifies quickly.

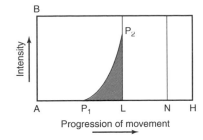

(b) Pain occurs at a moderate intensity at rest, but changes little throughout the motion.

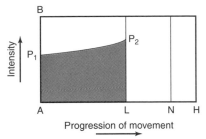

(c) Resistance is felt about 2/3 through available motion and is moderate by the end of the motion.

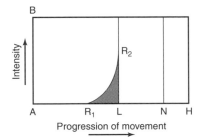

(d) Resistance occurs early in the motion and steadily increases throughout the motion.

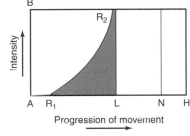

(e) Resistance is more significant than pain. Resistance occurs early and steadily increases, whereas pain is minor toward the end of the motion.

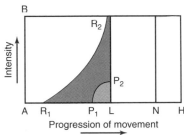

Key
A = Beginning of movement
B = Intensity
H = Hypermobile range
L = Abnormal limit of ROM
N = Normal limit of ROM

■ **Figure 6.28** Pain and resistance on movement diagrams.

Normal Joint Mobility

Determining normal and abnormal joint mobility requires practice and familiarity with the patient. Because joint mobilization is a manual therapy, you must develop your sense of touch so that you can detect what is normal for any particular joint. This can be done only through practice on normal subjects. Once normal mobility is identified, abnormal mobility is easier to recognize. Mobility that is normal for a glenohumeral joint is not normal for a wrist joint.

Normal mobility also varies for different populations and is determined by factors such as age, disease, sport, and position in a sport. For example, a 40-year-old man will not have the same normal lumbar spine mobility as his 15-year-old son has. Even though they may both have normal vertebral mobility, what is considered normal for the father is not normal for the son. Age plays a role in determining normal joint mobility.

Athletes from different sports also demonstrate various degrees of normal joint mobility. For this reason, it is important to compare the joint being treated with the contralateral side to assist in determining normal mobility for that individual. For example, a baseball pitcher may have a hypermobile glenohumeral joint when compared with a football lineman. A ballet dancer may have a hypermobile hip compared with a shot-putter. You must consider the specific needs and demands of a sport and even of a position within the sport when determining an individual's normal joint mobility.

Close-Packed and Loose-Packed Positions

The relative position of the joint surfaces must be considered prior to applying joint mobilization techniques. In a **close-packed position**, the joint surfaces are most congruent with each other. The convex surface of one bone is in complete congruence with the opposing concave surface of the other bone. The ligaments and capsule are taut, and the joint surfaces cannot be easily separated with traction. Joints are not initially mobilized in a close-packed position, but this position can be used to stabilize an adjacent joint before applying mobilization forces to another joint. For example, if you want to mobilize a proximal interphalangeal joint, the metacarpophalangeal joint can be positioned in full flexion, the close-packed position, to stabilize the proximal segment.

A **loose-packed position** is any position that is not close packed. The articular surfaces are not totally congruent, and some portions of the capsule are lax. Examinations and early mobilization techniques should both be performed with a joint in its maximum loose-packed position. This position is often referred to as a joint's resting position. See table 6.3 for a list of loose-packed and close-packed positions for the joints. As a general rule, extremes of joint motion are close-packed positions, and midrange positions are loose-packed positions.

Table 6.3 Loose-Packed and Close-Packed Joint Positions

Joints	Loose packed	Close packed
Fingers		
Metacarpophalangeal	20° flexion	1: Full opposition 2–5: Full flexion
Interphalangeal	20° flexion	Full extension
Wrist	0°	Full flexion
Elbow		
Humeroulnar	70° elbow flexion with 10° supination	Full extension
Humeroradial	Full elbow extension with full supination	Midflexion with midpronation
Radioulnar	70° elbow flexion with 35° supination	Full pronation or full supination
Glenohumeral	55° flexion with 20°–30° horizontal abduction	Full abduction with full external rotation
Hip	30° flexion, 30° abduction with slight external rotation	Full extension, internal rotation, and abduction
Knee		
Tibiofemoral	20°–25° flexion	Full extension with external tibial rotation
Patellofemoral	Full knee extension	Knee flexion
Ankle and midfoot		
Talocrural	10° plantar flexion	Full dorsiflexion
Subtalar and midtarsal	Midrange of inversion and eversion	Full inversion
Forefoot and toes		
Metatarsophalangeal 1	20° dorsiflexion	Full dorsiflexion
Metatarsophalangeal 2–5	20° plantar flexion	
Interphalangeal	20° plantar flexion	

Rules for Application

Before applying mobilization techniques, you should understand the following rules and use them as guidelines for all joint mobilization treatments:

1. The patient should be relaxed.

2. Before application, explain to the patient the purpose of the treatment and what sensations to expect.

3. Joint physiological and accessory mobility are assessed before and after the treatment. It may be necessary to check accessory mobility at various points within the physiological range.

4. Compare the joint to be treated with the contralateral joint to determine what is normal for the patient.

5. Determine treatment goals before treatment.

6. Grades I and II are used to relieve pain. Grades III and IV are used to increase mobility.

7. Stop the treatment if it is too painful for the patient.

8. Initial mobilization is performed in a loose-packed position.

9. One segment, usually the proximal joint segment, is stabilized, while the other is mobilized.

10. Your hands should be as close to the joint as possible.

11. The larger the surface area of contact, the more comfortable is the force application for the patient. When you use the entire hand, the fingers should be together, and as much of the finger and palm surface as possible should contact the patient's extremity.

12. Always use good body mechanics, and use gravity to assist the mobilization technique whenever possible.

13. The direction of the mobilization force is either parallel or perpendicular to the treatment plane. The treatment plane lies on the concave articulating surface, perpendicular to a line from the center of the convex articulating surface (figure 6.29). Traction is applied perpendicular to the treatment plane, and gliding is applied parallel to it. The treatment plane can change with a change in a joint's position. Carefully determine the joint's treatment plane before application.

14. Always apply the concave-convex and convex-concave rules when determining in which direction to apply the mobilization force.

15. Emphasize one plane of motion at a time, although more than one plane may be treated in a session.

16. The patient's response determines the selection of oscillating or sustained techniques. Oscillation is used more often than sustained techniques for pain relief. Gains in range of motion can be achieved by either oscillation or sustained techniques.

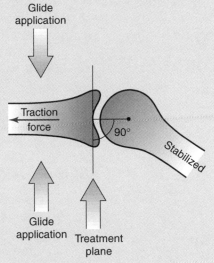

▌Figure 6.29 Direction of force application. Treatment of plane is either perpendicular or parallel to the treatment plane.

17. The patient's comfort and tolerance determine the speed and duration of treatment. Oscillation techniques should be applied smoothly and regularly at the rate of two to three oscillations per second and should be repeated for 1 to 2 min for pain and 20 to 60 s for tightness. Sustained techniques are applied for only about 10 s in painful joints and repeated several times between bouts of rest. For tightness, sustained techniques are held for 10 to 30 s, depending on the patient's tolerance, and repeated three to five times.

18. Begin and end mobilization treatments for increasing range of motion with grade I or II distraction oscillations to facilitate relaxation at the start of treatment and relieve pain following treatment.

19. Progression is individually determined by the patient's response to the treatment. You must evaluate the patient's response to treatment in terms of pain, changes in joint mobility and range of motion, and the patient's psychological reaction to determine whether changes in the mobilization techniques are warranted. Progression can involve increasing the length of the treatment, increasing the grade if treating a hypomobile joint, or changing the joint to a less loosely packed position.

20. Mobilization techniques should be accompanied by therapeutic exercise to reinforce the gains made with the treatment. The goal of treatment is to make positive changes in pathological conditions, so therapeutic exercises, such as flexibility or strengthening exercises, are most often indicated.

INDICATIONS

There are two main indications for the use of joint mobilization techniques. The first is joint pain. Grade I and II oscillations are used to relieve pain. The other indication is a hypomobile joint, which is determined by a capsular pattern of joint motion and less mobility than the contralateral joint.

PRECAUTIONS AND CONTRAINDICATIONS

Absolute contraindications to joint mobilization include malignancy, tuberculosis, osteomyelitis, osteoporosis, fracture, ligamentous rupture, and herniated disks with nerve compression. Joint effusion is a contraindication, since the capsule is already swollen from the extra fluid in the joint. Grade I and II mobilizations may be used to relieve pain, but grade III and IV techniques should be avoided. Relative contraindications, which are determined by the sport rehabilitation specialist's skills and expertise, or precautions include osteoarthritis, pregnancy, flu, total joint replacement, severe scoliosis, poor general health, and a patient's inability to relax. Precautions should also be taken when treating hypermobile joints using the pain-relieving grades. If you doubt whether to use joint mobilization, err on the side of caution and refrain from its use.

NEURAL MOBILIZATION

Neural mobilization should be used with extreme caution and only as a last resort when other treatment techniques have failed.

Of all the manual therapy techniques, neural mobilization is the most dangerous and must be used with care and precision. The sport rehabilitation specialist must not take its use lightly. Neural mobilization is discussed here so that you can be aware of its proper use and possible consequences.

FASCIAL CONNECTION

Like the myofascial system, the neural system is continuous throughout the body. It too is surrounded with fascia and can be affected by direct and indirect injuries to fascia and adjacent tissues. The effects of neural injury, like those of fascial injury, can be referred to distant areas. The referred pain of neural injuries is different from myofascial pain referral patterns, however.

AFFERENT SYSTEM

Referred pain from nerve-tissue injury follows the neural pathways and is described as tingling or burning. It can also jump from one area to another or progress along a neural pathway. The type of pain the patient reports is related to the nerve fiber carrying the impulse. Peripheral afferent nerve fibers that carry painful signals are called nociceptive fibers. The stimuli that activate pain fibers include mechanical forces, chemical irritants, and hot or cold temperatures. The A-delta and C fibers respond to pain stimuli that result in a pain-reflex withdrawal. They are myelinated afferent fibers that are excited by a mild mechanical stimulus. The A-alpha afferents are high-threshold mechanoreceptors that can also respond to temperature stimuli. The A-delta fibers are stimulated in sudden injuries, such as an ankle or knee sprain. About 75% of peripheral pain receptors are C fibers and respond to both mechanical and chemical stimuli. They can also spark the release of histamine through their excitation of mast cells and action as vasodilators. An insect bite, for example, can cause this activity. C fibers are also stimulated by swelling and stiffness and cause the aching sensation that occurs with these conditions. C fibers and A-delta fibers both respond to inflammation.

Once these fibers enter the dorsal horn of the spinal cord, many connections to both inhibitory and excitatory neurons are possible. The impulse can travel up the spinal cord to the thalamus and cortex. Stimulation of the cortex registers conscious pain sensation. Stimulation of the midbrain produces an inhibitory response through the release of endogenous analgesics (pain relievers that the body produces). Normal neural tissue does not refer pain at rest or during normal movement or activity. Pathological conditions, however, can produce referral patterns both proximally and distally from the site of pathology. This pain-referral pattern is referred to by Butler (1994) as **pathoneurodynamics.** The source of pathoneurodynamics can be either intraneural or extraneural, coming from injury either to the nerve itself or to the surrounding tissue that interacts with the nerve. In either situation, the physiology and mechanics of the nerve can be disrupted.

SUSCEPTIBLE SITES

Given that the nervous system, like the fascia system, is in intimate contact with other tissues throughout the body, it makes sense that when an area suffers an injury, neural tissue may also be affected. Certain nerves are susceptible to injury because of their location or pathway. Butler (1991) has identified these five susceptible sites:

1. In soft tissue or bony tunnels. A good example of this is the median nerve as it passes through the carpal tunnel at the wrist.

2. Abrupt neural branches, particularly in areas where the nerve's ability to move within the surrounding structures is limited. For example, the common plantar digital nerve in the web space between the third and fourth toes has limited movement, is formed from an abrupt junction of the lateral and medial plantar nerves, and is a common site for Morton's neuroma.

3. In areas where the nerves are relatively fixed. The common peroneal nerve as it traverses around the fibular head is an example of a relatively fixed nerve with little mobility.

4. High-friction areas where nerves are close to unyielding interfaces. Two examples are the nerves passing through the plantar fascia in the foot and the brachial plexus passing over the first rib.

5. Tension points, such as the tibial nerve in the popliteal fossa, where abnormal stress can be placed on the nerve.

PREVIOUS TRAUMA

Previous trauma can predispose an area to neural symptoms later. Like all other tissue, nervous tissue is surrounded by layers of fascia that serve to support and supply nutrients to the nerves. If a nerve is injured, it undergoes the healing process discussed in chapter 2. Scar tissue can be produced by the nerve, its surrounding fascia, and the other structures involved in the injury. The result can be a binding of the nerve that can affect its neurobiomechanics and neurophysiology.

Even an injury not directly involving neural tissue can affect the nervous system. Locally damaged blood vessels and ensuing edema can cause neural changes. The nervous system is very dependent on a continuous blood flow for survival and for functioning. Although the nervous system constitutes only 2% of the body's mass, it uses 20% of the circulating blood's oxygen supply (Dommisse 1975). Because nerve tissue has no means of storing reserves, if the blood supply is interrupted, damage to the nerve tissue can result from a lack of adequate oxygen and nutrients.

Nerve tissue damage secondary to either edema or vascular insufficiency results in fibrosis. A tethering effect on the nerve by the restriction of the scar tissue can reduce the flexibility and mobility of the neural tissue. Ultimately, symptoms of abnormal neural tension can occur in locations along the nervous system other than the site of injury. According to Butler (1991), this transpires because the mechanical alterations in one nerve location can alter tissue tension throughout the nervous system, impaired neural stimulation at one site can affect the entire neuron, mechanical changes from an injury are accompanied by vascular changes, and an abnormal nerve impulse can cause abnormal neural firing elsewhere in the nervous system.

DOUBLE-CRUSH SYNDROME

The condition in which an injury at one site produces signs and symptoms at another site is sometimes referred to as the **double-crush syndrome** or phenomenon

(Upton and McComas 1973). An example of this is carpal tunnel syndrome. In some cases of carpal tunnel syndrome, the cause is actually a neural lesion in the cervical spine. This should be ruled out, especially in cases of bilateral carpal tunnel syndrome. In patients who have a history of cervical injury and present with complaints of elbow or wrist pain bilaterally or unilaterally, a double-crush syndrome should be ruled out. Likewise, if a patient complains of bilateral shinsplints or foot pain, you should investigate prior low back injury and suspect a possible central lesion. Multiple-crush syndromes can be seen in patients who report more than one area of pain. For example, a patient who has a history of neck injury and reports midthoracic, elbow, and wrist pain should be evaluated for a multiple-crush phenomenon.

The term *crush* is a misnomer, since the injury is not necessarily a crush injury. The syndrome is actually caused by scarring and fibrosis, restricted blood flow, alterations in neural stimulation, or some combination of these. This pathology progressively increases pressure and friction on the nerve until symptoms of pain distal to the site of origin occur.

SYMPTOM PROFILE

Although a patient may use many adjectives to describe neural pain, it is often described as a deep, burning, aching, or heavy sensation. It can occur along the nerve's pathway, jump from one area to another, and clump around joints or tension areas. It can be constant or intermittent, although a constant pain is more indicative of inflammation and compressive pathology. Sometimes the pain is worse at night, and sometimes it is worse at the end of the day.

Pain that occurs because of local neural ischemia is described as sharp or knifelike. Ischemia-related pain lessens with easy motion and worsens with overuse. Sometimes an inflammation can cause a sharp pain, but it is generally an ache at the end of the day with stiffness in the morning or after prolonged inactivity. An inflammation-based pain feels better with gentle activity and worse with rest.

A good history of injuries and evaluation of the location and patterns of pain can help detect the source of the patient's pain. The following types of pain should be evaluated for neural origins: pain that occurs in susceptible neural-tissue areas, such as the carpal tunnel and fibular head; symptoms that do not match the common pain patterns; and pain that follows a dermatome, or sensory-nerve distribution.

TREATMENT

Treatment can be either direct or indirect. Direct treatment techniques are the same as those used in evaluation of neural tissue. Indirect treatment techniques can be as simple as changing posture and often involve altering a soft-tissue structure, which affects the nerve. A hamstring stretch can affect the sciatic nerve, and a cervical stretch can affect the brachial plexus.

There are several different direct neural mobilization techniques. Only a few of the more common ones are discussed here. Before these techniques are discussed, however, you should understand that neural mobilization is not a common treatment and should be used only as a last resort. Any of the neural techniques can easily injure the patient, so extreme caution must always be used in deciding whether and when to apply the technique and in applying the treatment. It is impossible to overstate this point. Even the most experienced sport rehabilitation specialists use neural mobilization only after all other modes of treatment have failed and only when benefit to the patient from its application is strongly indicated. It is used always with extreme caution, because it can further injure the patient. Precautions and contraindications are discussed later in this chapter. Neural mobilization techniques should be used only when the sport rehabilitation specialist knows the pattern of application and the expected outcome of the treatment.

TECHNIQUES

Seven neural tension tests are commonly used: one for the spine, three for the lower extremity, and three for the upper extremity. The spine test is passive neck flexion (PNF). The lower-extremity tests include straight-leg raise (SLR), slump test, and prone knee bend (PKB). The upper-limb tension tests are identified as ULTT1, 2a, 2b, and 3. The lower-extremity tests assess the sciatic and femoral nerves, while the upper-extremity tests assess the median, median, radial, and ulnar nerves, respectively. These test procedures are also used as treatment techniques. You must accurately apply the mobilization technique and assess for symptoms, responses, range of motion, and resistance before and after the treatment. All these techniques can be applied either proximally to distally or vice versa. The direction of application may produce varying results, depending on the location and cause of the irritation or restriction. The positions described here are described in detail by Butler (1991). His text and courses are recommended for readers who have an interest in pursuing neural mobilization techniques.

Passive Neck Flexion

PNF can be used by itself to assess spine disorders or along with the lower-limb or upper-limb tests. PNF can be performed with the patient sitting or lying supine. In the supine position, the patient lies supine without a pillow. The patient initiates the motion by lifting his or her head off the table (figure 6.30). The sport rehabilitation specialist places his or her hands under the head to support it and moves the neck into flexion while the patient remains relaxed.

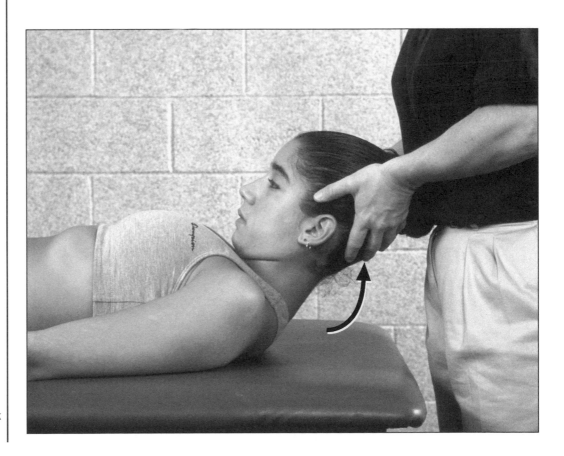

∎ Figure 6.30 In passive neck flexion the patient's head is supported as the neck is passively flexed.

Straight-Leg Raise

Straight-leg raise (SLR) is sometimes referred to as Leseague's test or Lazarevic's test. The patient lies supine without a pillow, and the sport rehabilitation specialist places one hand on the foot and the other on the quadriceps just proximal to the patella. The leg is lifted by the hand on the Achilles, while the hand on the quadriceps keeps the knee from bending. If enough flexibility is present, the heel may be placed on the sport rehabilitation specialist's shoulder (figure 6.31). Neural tension may be increased in the SLR with the addition of ankle dorsiflexion, ankle plantar flexion with inversion, hip adduction, hip internal rotation, or passive neck flexion, individually or in combination.

Prone Knee Bend

Prone knee bend (PKB) is similar to a quadriceps stretch. With the patient prone and his or her head turned to the side being treated, the sport rehabilitation specialist grasps the lower leg above the ankle and flexes the knee to move the heel toward the buttock while maintaining slight hip extension (figure 6.32). PKB is used to treat anterior thigh and groin pain.

Slump Test

The slump test should not be used on patients who have an irritable disorder. With the patient sitting on a table in a slumped or sagging position and his or her hands behind the low back, the sport rehabilitation specialist applies pressure to the shoulders to bow the spine without changing the hip position. The patient then brings the chin down to the chest, and the sport rehabilitation specialist applies slight overpressure to the head (figure 6.33a). The patient then extends one knee and follows this motion with ankle dorsiflexion while keeping the knee extended (figure 6.33b). Neck flexion pressure is released slowly. This technique must be applied with extreme caution; it is used as a test, not a treatment, because of its forceful application. It is used to assess the response of the nervous system to treatment. If the patient reports results before the entire technique is applied, it is not necessary to go through the full procedure. This procedure is not recommended for patients with a suspected disk injury.

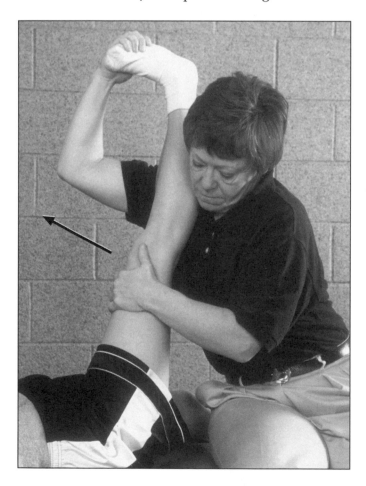

Figure 6.31 In the straight-leg raise tension is applied to the sciatic nerve. With the knee straight, additional neural stress can be applied with ankle dorsiflexion, hip adduction and internal rotation, and neck flexion.

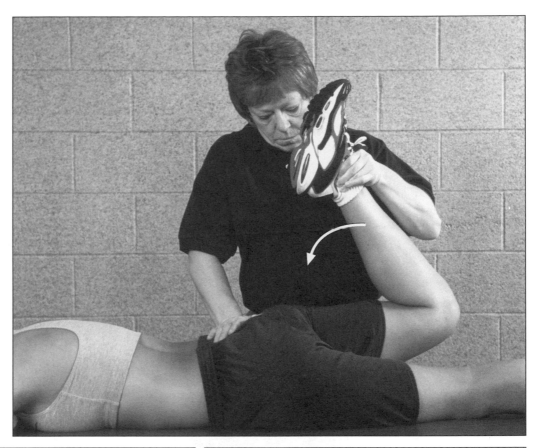

■ **Figure 6.32** Prone knee bend: tension is applied to the femoral nerve with passive hip extension and knee flexion.

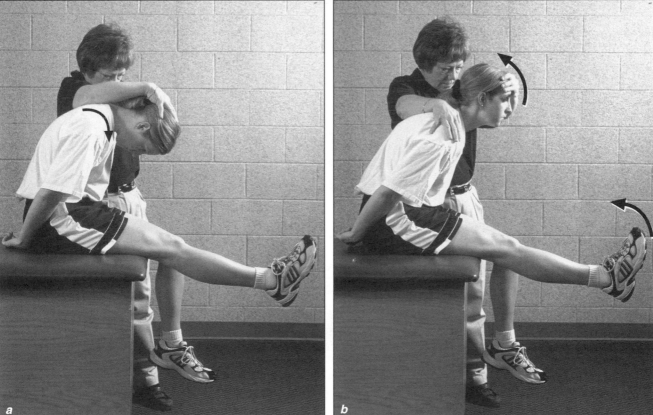

a

b

■ **Figure 6.33** Slump test: The shoulders are passively pushed downward to bow the spine and the chin is brought to the chest. While in this position, one knee is extended with the ankle dorsiflexed. Maintaining the leg position, the neck pressure is slowly released.

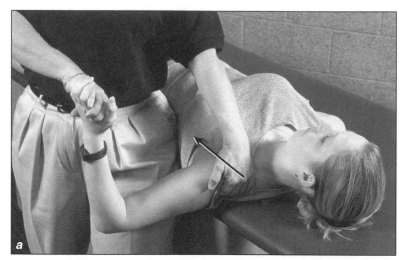

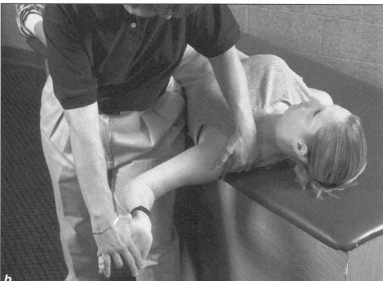

Upper-Limb Tension Test 1

ULTT1 is also called the brachial plexus tension test or Elvey's test. It is used to test the median nerve and to treat symptoms in the thoracic spine, neck, and arm. The patient should have full range of motion of the entire upper extremity and neck and should not have an irritable disorder. The patient lies supine; if treating the left upper extremity, you hold the patient's left hand with your right and place the patient's left upper arm along your left thigh. Place your left hand on top of the patient's shoulder and apply a stabilization force on the shoulder girdle to prevent elevation throughout the treatment (figure 6.34a). Then abduct the patient's arm to about 110° while keeping it in contact with your thigh (figure 6.34b). Externally rotate the patient's shoulder, then supinate the forearm, and extend the wrist, thumb and fingers, and elbow, in that order. The patient then flexes the neck laterally away from the left side (figure 6.34c).

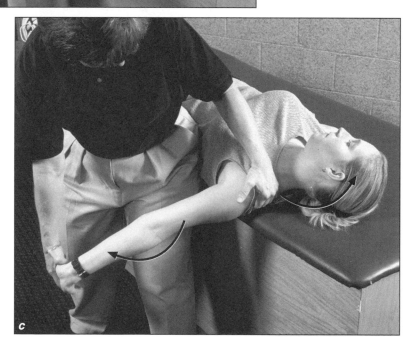

■ **Figure 6.34** Upper-limb tension test 1 for the median nerve.

Upper-Limb Tension Test 2a

Because shoulder girdle depression has such a significant impact on the brachial plexus, this position was developed by Butler (1991), who feels that ULTT2a is a more effective position than ULTT1. If the left arm is being treated, the patient lies on a slight diagonal on the table, with the head toward the left side and the left scapula off the table. You stand at the top of the patient's shoulder with your right thigh against the patient's shoulder. Your right hand holds the patient's elbow and the left hand crosses over to hold the wrist. Your thigh depresses the patient's shoulder girdle (figure 6.35a). Bring the patient's arm to about 10° of shoulder abduction, extend the elbow, and externally rotate the arm. Slide your right hand down to the patient's hand and extend the patient's wrist, fingers, and thumb (figure 6.35b).

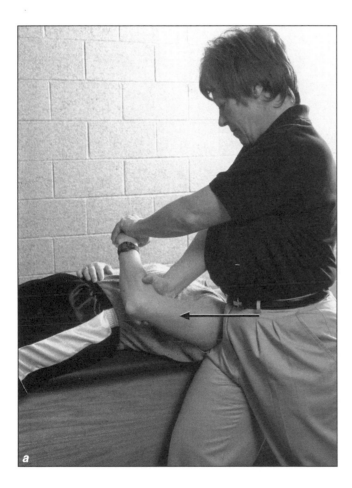 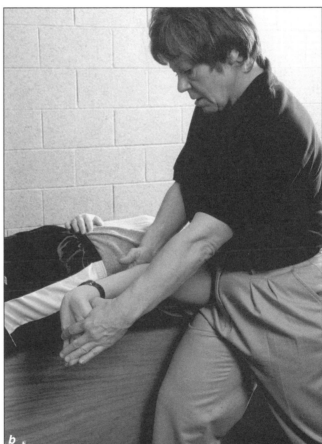

∎ **Figure 6.35** Upper-limb tension test 2a of the median nerve.

Upper-Limb Tension Test 2b

ULTT2b tests the radial nerve and is used to treat cervical, thoracic, and upper-extremity disorders, especially those involving the radial nerve. The patient and sport rehabilitation specialist are positioned as for ULTT2a. The hand placement, shoulder girdle position, and elbow extension are the same (figure 6.36a). You then internally rotate the patient's shoulder, pronate the forearm, and after moving your left hand to the patient's hand, flex and ulnarly deviate the patient's wrist and flex the patient's fingers and thumb (figure 6.36b).

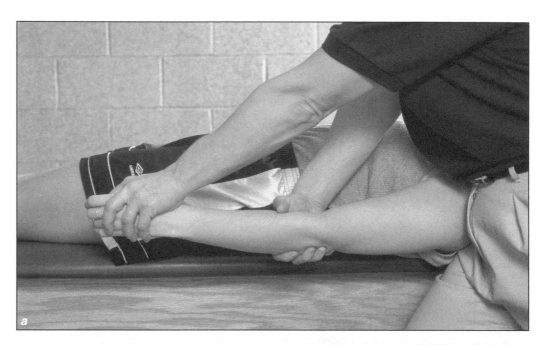

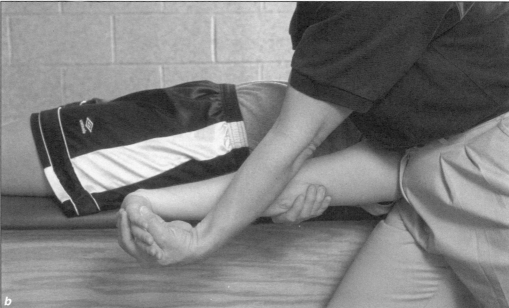

■ Figure 6.36　Upper-limb tension test 2b for the radial nerve.

Upper-Limb Tension Test 3

ULTT3 is used to test the ulnar nerve and to treat ulnar-nerve restrictions. The patient and sport rehabilitation specialist begin in the position described for ULTT1, with the patient's right shoulder girdle depressed and the patient's right arm resting on your right thigh (figure 6.37a). Externally rotate the patient's shoulder, then abduct the shoulder, flex the elbow, extend the wrist, and extend the fourth and fifth fingers (figure 6.37b). The patient can additionally flex the neck laterally away from the arm being treated.

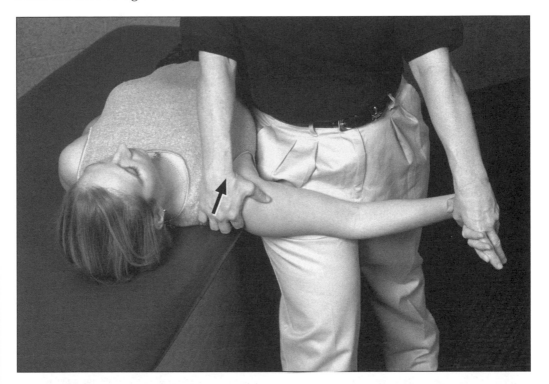

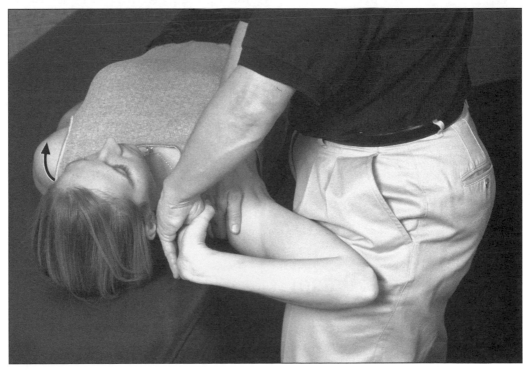

■ **Figure 6.37** Upper-limb tension test 3 of the ulnar nerve.

APPLICATION

Tension tests should be performed before all neural mobilization treatments to determine the appropriate force to apply during treatment. Pretreatment and post-treatment tension tests should be used to assess the patient's symptom response and the resistance of the tissue. Symptom responses include pain, numbness, and tingling; the sport rehabilitation specialist must know when and where in the motion these symptoms may occur to avoid them during the treatment. Identifying where tissue resistance occurs determines the extent of application for the mobilization technique and helps the specialist evaluate the results of the treatment.

Extreme caution must be employed when using neural mobilization to treat irritable conditions that affect neurophysiology. Unless the sport rehabilitation specialist has taken postgraduate courses on this topic, he or she should refrain from using neural mobilization on irritable conditions.

Caution also should be taken when using neural mobilization techniques to treat nonirritable conditions. These conditions are likely to have pathomechanical causes and secondary fibrosis, connective-tissue adhesions, and restriction of normal tissue mobility. Neural mobilization techniques to treat these conditions enter into the resistance range of grade III and IV motions, but pain should still be avoided. As a rule, grade III motions produce less pain than grade IV.

Throughout the treatment the patient's symptoms must be monitored. Initial treatment should not cause or increase symptoms. A constant dull ache and sensations of pins and needles should be avoided. The patient should be relaxed throughout the treatment.

The duration, amplitude, and number of repetitions can be changed as the treatment progresses and the patient responds positively to treatment. A sequence of slow oscillations can last 20 to 30 s, followed by a reassessment of the patient's condition. A sustained movement should be released if symptoms occur and should last no longer than 10 s even without symptoms. Sustained movement and oscillations can be repeated a number of times as the treatment progresses so that the treatment lasts for several minutes. The amplitude can be increased until some symptoms are produced, although the minimal force needed to achieve a positive response is all that is necessary. Complementary techniques, including muscle energy, myofascial mobilization, cross-friction massage, and neural self-mobilization, can also be added.

SELF-MOBILIZATION

If neural mobilization techniques provide positive results, it may be beneficial for the patient to perform self-treatment techniques. Along with these techniques, the patient's program should include therapeutic exercises and corrective techniques that can resolve the problem's precipitating factors.

Self-mobilization techniques for the lower limbs are easier to apply than those for the upper limbs. One of the more difficult tasks in self-mobilization of the upper limb is maintaining scapular depression during the activity. Specific instructions on correct application and proper sequencing must be given to the patient to ensure the best results. It is important that the patient demonstrate proper execution of the technique to the sport rehabilitation specialist before he or she attempts the technique without supervision. Figure 6.38 demonstrates lower- and upper-limb tension techniques.

PRECAUTIONS

Again, neural mobilization techniques should be applied only as a last resort after other treatment techniques have been unsuccessful. These techniques should be used only with extreme caution and continual feedback from the patient about the area's response to the treatment. Reproduction of painful symptoms should be avoided,

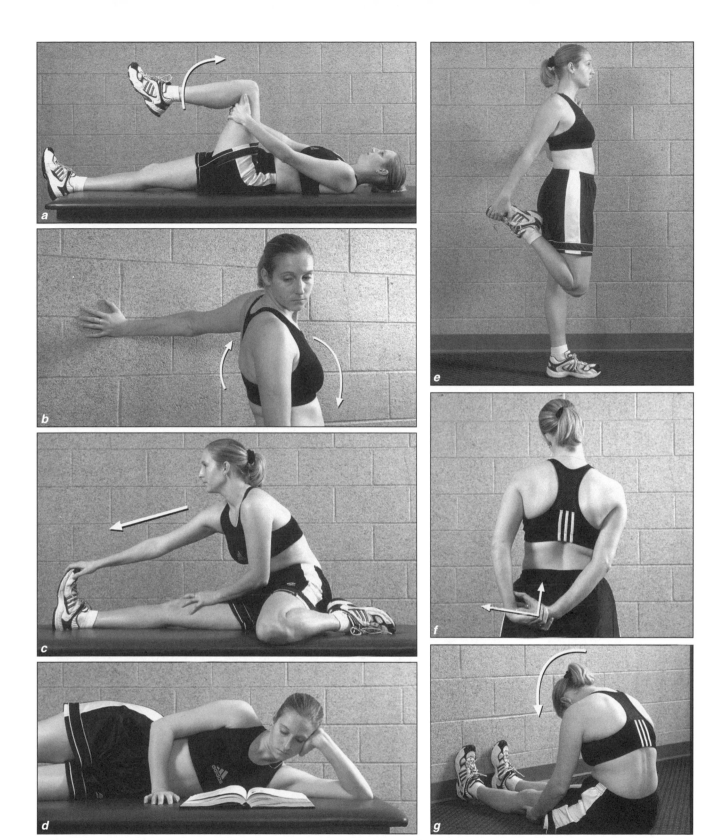

■ **Figure 6.38** Self-mobilization. *(a)* Sciatic nerve stretch: Patient lies supine with one leg flexed at the hip and hands clasped behind the thigh. In this position, the lower leg is raised into a straight-leg position. *(b)* Brachial plexus stretch (median nerve): Patient places the hand on the wall at shoulder level with the elbow straight. Maintaining the hand flat on the wall, the patient rolls away from the hand. *(c)* Combined straight-leg raise and prone knee bend stretch: Patient assumes a seated hurdler's stretch position with one leg flexed behind and the other extended in front. The patient reaches forward toward the foot. *(d)* Ulnar nerve stretch: Sidelying, the patient supports the head with the hand. The elbow is flexed and elevated above the shoulder. *(e)* Femoral nerve stretch: In standing, the patient flexes the knee and grasps the foot behind the buttock. *(f)* Radial nerve stretch: With both hands behind the back and the elbows straight, the uninvolved hands grasps the involved hand and passively moves the wrist into extension and pulls the arm across the body. *(g)* Slump: With feet positioned in neutral against a wall, the patient sits with knees extended and slumps the shoulders, moving the chin to the chest.

especially numbness and tingling sensations. The slump test and the upper-limb tension tests are complex maneuvers that can involve many structures and therefore require consistent care and discretion. It is much easier to irritate upper-limb nerves than lower-limb nerves, because the upper-limb nerves are smaller and traverse more complicated paths around bones and through muscles than those of the lower limbs.

A worsening disorder, indicated by increased symptoms, is an indication to stop the technique. The sport rehabilitation specialist should always apply treatment carefully and err on the side of caution if he or she has any doubts about the treatment.

Diabetes, AIDS, and other systemic diseases can weaken the nervous system. Extra care should be taken when applying neural mobilization techniques to patients with these conditions.

Whereas the circulatory system closely follows the nervous system throughout the body, care should be taken with individuals who have circulatory system disturbances. If a nerve is mobilized, the circulatory structure next to it is also mobilized.

CONTRAINDICATIONS

Contraindications to neural mobilization include malignancies of the nervous system or vertebral column, acute inflammatory infections, areas of instability, and spinal cord injuries. Suspected disk lesions, cauda equina lesions (suggested by changes in bowel or bladder function or changes in perineal sensations), dizziness related to vertebral artery insufficiencies, and any central nervous system disorder, such as spina bifida or multiple sclerosis are also contraindications. Worsening neurological signs are another important contraindication.

SUMMARY

1. *Discuss the three techniques of massage and their indications, precautions, and contraindications.* The primary massage techniques used in sports medicine include effleurage, or stroking; petrissage, or kneading; and friction. They are used to relieve pain, relax muscles, reduce swelling, and mobilize adherent scar tissue. Massage should be avoided in the presence of infection, malignancies, skin diseases, blood clots, and any irritations or lesions that may spread with direct contact. Precautions include clean hands and body surface to be treated, explaining the procedure before application, removing jewelry that may interfere with the application, using warm hands and massage medium, and draping the body part appropriately.

2. *Explain the progression of myofascial restriction after an injury.* Myofascial restriction occurs following an injury as scar tissue is formed and adhesions occur between the newly formed tissue and adjacent structures. Immobilization following an injury can also lead to myofascial restriction and loss of tissue mobility.

3. *Discuss the techniques for myofascial release.* The primary techniques for myofascial release include J-stroke, oscillation, wringing, stripping, and arm or leg pull.

4. *Explain the theory of the mechanism of myofascial trigger points.* The theory of myofascial trigger points is that a damaged sarcoplasmic reticulum interferes with normal muscle fiber activity. The calcium of the damaged sarcoplasmic reticulum stimulates the sarcomere to produce a sustained contraction as long as ATP is present. The sustained contraction no longer needs an action potential to continue, as long as the calcium and ATP are present together. Ischemic-causing substances also make afferent nerve endings hyperirritable to mediate referred pain, autonomic response, and motor-neuron response.

5. *Discuss the ice-stretch trigger point release theory.* According to the gate theory of pain, the sudden, brief application of cold inhibits the pain-spasm cycle and provides muscle relaxation and pain relief, especially when accompanied by a stretch.

6. *Explain the concave-convex and convex-concave rules.* Joint mobilization techniques are based on these rules. The concave-convex rule states that concave joint surfaces slide in the same direction as the bone movement, and the convex-concave rule states that convex joint surfaces slide in the opposite direction of the bone movement.

7. *Define joint mobilization grades of movement.* Movements in joint mobilization are divided into four grades. Grade I is small-amplitude movement in the beginning range of motion, grade II is large-amplitude movement in the middle of the nonrestricted range of motion, grade III is large-amplitude movement to the restricted range of motion, and grade IV is small-amplitude movement to the restricted range of motion.

8. *Discuss the direction of glide and traction in relation to the treatment plane.* Glide movements during mobilization should be parallel to the treatment plane, and traction is perpendicular to the treatment plane.

9. *Explain the double-crush syndrome.* A double-crush syndrome occurs when an injury at one site produces signs and symptoms at another site, so although a patient reports pain at one area, the actual injury is in another area. For example, patients with neck injuries commonly report pain in the arm.

10. *Discuss the dangers of neural mobilization.* Neural mobilization is used very carefully and only as a last resort. Incorrect use can result in nerve injury.

11. *Describe one neural self-mobilization technique for the upper extremity and one for the lower extremity.* Extreme care must be taken with any neural mobilization technique. Examples of neural self-mobilization techniques include the prone knee bend for the femoral nerve, the straight-leg raise for the sciatic nerve, and side lying on the elbow with the hand on the face for the ulnar nerve.

CRITICAL THINKING QUESTIONS

1. What problem would you suspect if, during a myofascial release treatment, a patient began to sweat and became pale? What steps would you take to relieve the symptoms? Why might this occur?

2. A patient you are treating for a shoulder injury has range-of-motion measurements of 120° flexion, 90° abduction, and 40° external rotation. What techniques would you use to improve range of motion? Why? If the patient's motion was 120° flexion, 125° abduction, and 70° external rotation, what techniques would you use to improve motion? Why?

3. A patient who had surgery on his ankle three months ago has severe joint and soft-tissue restriction of all motions. There is more loss of plantar flexion than of dorsiflexion, and the soft tissue around the ankle feels very stiff. What techniques would you use to improve motion and why? Which techniques would you emphasize the most and why?

4. If you give a patient a straight-leg-raise exercise to stretch the hamstrings and she complains of calf pain when performing it, what would you instruct the patient to do? What are the possible causes of the athlete's complaints, and what precautions should you take?

5. A patient complains of shoulder-blade pain with some arm movements and has headaches. What are the possible causes of the patient's complaints? What treatments would you initiate, and why would you select those techniques? Would you give the patient any home program, and if so, what would it include?

6. If you were the certified athletic trainer in the scenario described at the beginning of this chapter, what techniques would you use to relieve the soft-tissue adhesions of Sara's forearm? What home activities would you give her to increase soft-tissue mobility on her own?

REFERENCES

Beard, G., and E.C. Wood. 1969. *Massage principles and techniques.* Philadelphia: Saunders.

Butler, D.S. 1991. *Mobilization of the nervous system.* New York: Churchill Livingstone.

Butler, D.S. 1994. *Mobilization of the nervous system. Level II. 1996/97 course handbook.* Marina Del Rey, CA: Neuro Orthopedic Institute.

Corrigan, B., and G.D. Maitland. 1989. *Practical orthopedic medicine.* Boston: Butterworth.

Cyriax, J.H. 1977. *Textbook of orthopedic medicine.* Vol. 2, *Treatment by manipulation, massage and injection.* Baltimore: Williams & Wilkins.

Dommisse, G.F. 1975. Morphological aspects of the lumbar spine and lumbosacral region. *Orthopedic Clinics of North America* 6:163–175.

Greenman, P.E. 1996. *Principles of manual medicine.* Baltimore: Williams & Wilkins.

Hertling, D., and R.M. Kessler. 1990. *Management of common musculoskeletal disorders: Physical therapy principles and methods.* 2nd ed. Philadelphia: Lippincott.

Kaltenborn, F.M. 1980. *Mobilization of the extremity joints.* Oslo: Olaf Norlis Bokhandel.

Manheim, C.J. 1994. *The myofascial release manual.* 2nd ed. Thorofare, NJ: Slack.

Melzak, R. 1973. *The puzzle of pain.* New York: Basic Books.

Paris, S.V., and C. Patla. 1988. *E1 course notes: Extremity dysfunction and manipulation.* St. Augustine, FL: Patris.

Simons, D.G. 1981. Myofascial trigger points: A need for understanding. *Archives of Physical Medicine and Rehabilitation* 62:97–99.

Sutton, G.S., and M.R. Bartel. 1994. Soft-tissue mobilization techniques for the hand therapist. *Journal of Hand Therapy* 7:185–192.

Travell, J. 1976. Myofascial trigger points: Clinical view. In *Advances in pain research and therapy,* vol. 1, ed. J.J. Bonica and D. Albe-Fessard. New York: Raven Press.

Travell, J.G., and D.G. Simons. 1983. *Myofascial pain and dysfunction: The trigger point manual.* Vol. 1. Baltimore: Williams & Wilkins.

Travell, J.G., and D.G. Simons. 1992. *Myofascial pain and dysfunction: The trigger point manual.* Vol. 2. Baltimore: Williams & Wilkins.

Upton, A.R.M., and A.J. McComas. 1973. The double crush in nerve entrapment syndromes. *Lancet* 2:359–362.

SUGGESTED READING

Åstrand, P.O., and K. Rodahl. 1977. *Textbook of work physiology.* New York: McGraw-Hill.

Breig, A. 1978. *Adverse mechanical tension in the nervous system.* Stockholm: Almqvist & Wiksell.

Grieve, G.P. 1984. *Mobilisation of the spine.* New York: Churchill Livingstone.

Kenneally, M., Rubenach, H. , and R. Elvey. 1988. The upper limb tension test: The SLR of the arm. In *Physical therapy of the cervical and thoracic spine,* ed. R. Grant. New York: Churchill Livingstone.

Lee, D. 1986. Principles and practice of muscle energy and functional techniques. In *Modern manual therapy of the vertebral column,* ed. G. Grieves. New York: Churchill Livingstone.

Mackinnon, S.E. 1992. Double and multiple crush syndromes. *Hand Clinics* 8:369.

Rubin, D. 1981. Myofascial trigger point syndromes: An approach to management. *Archives of Physical Medicine and Rehabilitation* 62:107–110.

Wood, E.C., and P.D. Becker. 1981. *Beard's massage.* Philadelphia: Saunders.

CHAPTER SEVEN

Muscle Strength and Endurance

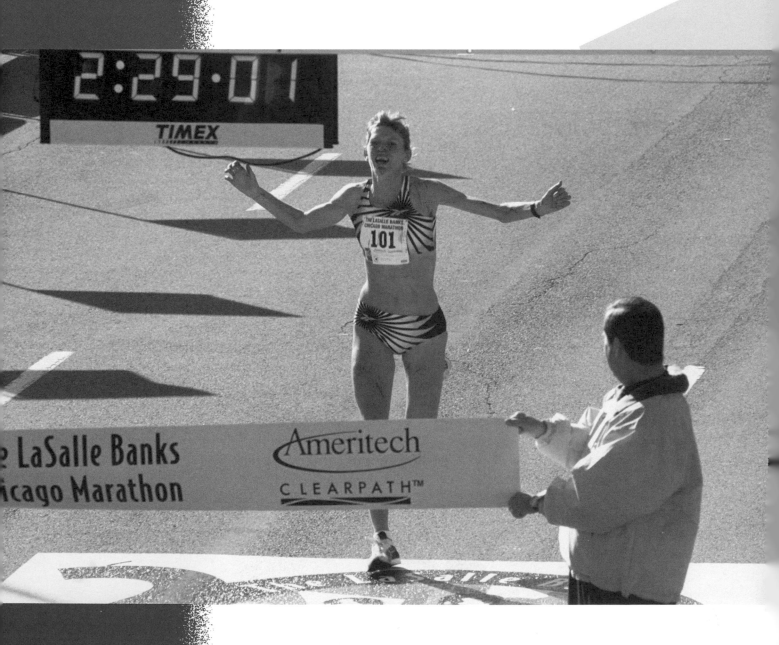

OBJECTIVES

After completing this chapter, you should be able to do the following:

1. Describe the sarcolemma and its function in muscle activity.

2. Identify the elements of a motor unit.

3. Explain how an action potential is transmitted.

4. Explain the differences between fast-twitch and slow-twitch muscle fibers.

5. Discuss the relationship between muscle strength, endurance, and power.

6. Identify the various types of dynamic activity.

7. Discuss the differences between open and closed kinetic chain activity.

8. Identify the various grades of manual muscle testing.

9. Discuss the grades of muscle activity.

10. List the PNF techniques commonly used in sports medicine and their purposes.

11. Identify four principles of strengthening exercises.

Now that Pam Roberts, certified athletic trainer for the local high school, has achieved good range of motion in Sam's knee, she is ready to begin a more aggressive strengthening program. Early in the season, Sam injured his knee during basketball practice. He underwent rehabilitation but continued to have difficulties with the knee throughout the season. Three weeks ago he underwent an arthroscopy for a partial meniscectomy.

Pam wants Sam to progress in a good rehabilitation program with effective, efficient, and appropriate strengthening exercises, but she's having difficulty deciding what equipment to use. Fortunately, the high school's booster club has been very generous to her athletic training program and has furnished her athletic training facility with a nice variety of rehabilitation equipment. She wants to do a combination of open and closed kinetic chain activities. Until now she has used manual resistance and body-weight resistance to provide strengthening activities, but at this point in Sam's program, more resistance would be beneficial.

If a little knowledge is dangerous, where is the man who has so much as to be out of danger?

Thomas Henry Huxley, English biologist and writer,
On Elemental Instruction in Physiology 1877

Thomas Huxley's words are worth considering as you begin reading about a topic that you may think you already know well. Even if you possess a good deal of knowledge, you cannot assume you will know best how to apply that knowledge. As you read this chapter, you will discover that much about muscle strength is yet to be learned. This text does not come close to presenting the body of knowledge available; however, the discussion covers the importance of muscle strength, the methods of achieving it, and the ways in which sport rehabilitation specialists can maximize muscle strength and endurance development in a therapeutic exercise program for injured athletes.

As you read this chapter, keep in mind that many of the concepts presented are not black and white but shades of gray. There is not necessarily a single answer for even simple questions such as "What is the best number of repetitions for increasing muscle endurance?" The "best" answer will emerge through your ability to combine the knowledge you obtain from this text with your own observation skills and common sense. This combination will enable you to determine your own "best" answers about what strengthening program will be most effective for a particular patient.

One can never have too much knowledge. Knowledge leads to understanding, understanding leads to appreciation, appreciation leads to respect, and respect leads to appropriate application. The greater your understanding of the "whys" and "hows," the less dangerous will be your application of the knowledge you possess.

Accordingly, then, the chapter begins with physiological and biomechanical information to help you achieve a true understanding of the rationale for techniques. The progression will provide you with additional skills so that you can design and build your own therapeutic exercise program for any patient, regardless of any obstacles or complications associated with the patient's injury profile.

MUSCLE STRUCTURE AND FUNCTION

The motor units in muscle consist of the nerve, or motor neuron, and muscle fibers. Within the fibers are small contractile elements called sarcomeres, and within the sarcomere are filaments called actin and myosin. Muscle function involves various processes that occur when a motor unit is stimulated by an excitatory impulse.

Before you can learn how to affect strength and muscle endurance, you must have an understanding of muscle structure and function. Such awareness serves as a foundation for understanding how strength changes occur, why certain techniques are applied, and how most effectively to provide an appropriate strength program.

STRUCTURE

Previous chapters have addressed the intimate relationship between connective tissue and other tissue throughout the body. Muscle also contains layers of connective tissue. The outer connective-tissue layer covering the entire muscle is the **epimysium;** the layer covering muscle fascicles or groups of fibers is called the **perimysium;** and the connective-tissue layer covering each muscle fiber is the **endomysium.** The endomysium is continuous with the muscle fiber's membrane, the **sarcolemma.** This macrostructure of muscle is shown in figure 7.1.

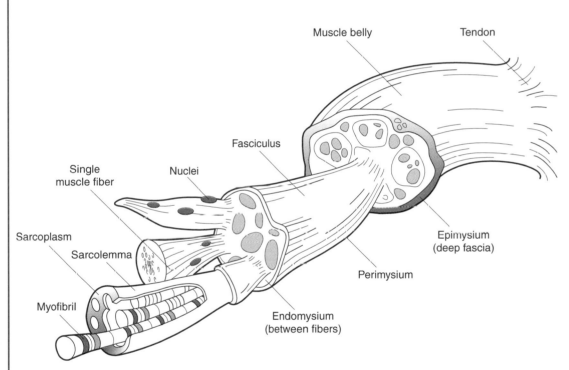

▌Figure 7.1   Muscle structure.

As mentioned in previous chapters, a **motor unit** is composed of the nerve, or motor neuron, and the muscle fibers that it innervates (figure 7.2). The number of motor units in any muscle depends on the size and the function of that muscle. For example, in a small muscle that performs primarily finely tuned activities, such as the intrinsic muscles of the hand, the ratio of muscle fibers to neurons is small. Larger muscles used primarily for gross motor activities, such as the gastrocnemius, have a much higher ratio of muscle fibers to neurons. Table 7.1 provides some examples of average numbers of muscle fibers in motor units of various muscles.

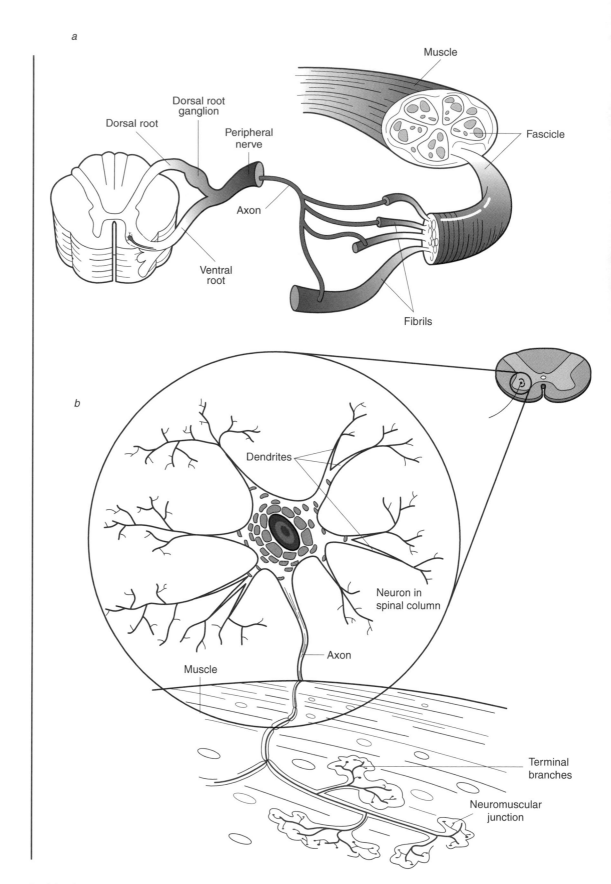

▌Figure 7.2   Motor unit: *(a)* schematic drawing of the components of a motor unit—the anterior horn cell, its axon and terminating branches, and the muscle fibers it innervates; *(b)* one neuron from the spinal cord with its axon extending into the muscle. The number of muscle fibers a single motor unit innervates can range from a few to several thousand (Johnson and Wiechers 1982).

Table 7.1 Average Number of Muscle Fibers in a Motor Unit in Different Skeletal Muscles	
Muscles	**Muscle fibers/motor unit**
Biceps brachii	750
Brachioradialis	> 410
Opponens pollicis	595
Platysma	25
Tensor tympani	8
Medial gastrocnemius	~ 1600–1900
Tibialis anterior	~ 560–660

Adapted from Enoka 1995.

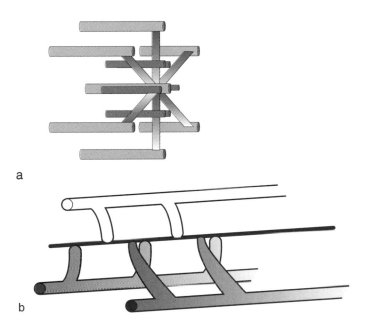

■ Figure 7.3   Filament arrangements: *(a)* cross-sectional view, *(b)* longitudinal view. Note hexagonal arrangement of thin filaments around thick filaments; triangular arrangement of thick filaments.

The **sarcomere** is the smallest contractile element of a muscle fiber. The **extrafusal fibers,** or myofibrils, contained within the sarcomere are called **actin** and **myosin.** Myosin fibers are the thicker filaments—with diameters about 1/10,000 that of a hair strand (16 nm)—and are surrounded in a hexagonal pattern by smaller actin filaments. A three-dimensional model shows that the myosin filaments form a triangular pattern in relationship to each other—so in a sarcomere there are six actin filaments around each myosin filament and three myosin filaments around one actin filament (figure 7.3).

Within a sarcomere, the actin and myosin are arranged longitudinally from Z-disk to Z-disk, where the actin filaments are anchored on either end of the sarcomere. The myosin filaments are in the equatorial center of the sarcomere and anchored with each other at the M-bridge in the center of the H-zone (figure 7.4). The A-band contains myosin and actin filaments, whereas the I-band contains only actin filaments. Because of the myosin filaments the A-band is darker; the combination of the A-band and the I-band gives skeletal muscle its striped appearance—hence the name, striated muscle.

FUNCTION

When a motor unit is stimulated by an excitatory impulse called an **action potential,** the myosin cross-bridges flex and pull the actin filaments toward the center of the sarcomere. During this process the H-band becomes smaller and the Z-disks are stretched toward the sarcomere's equatorial center to produce a shortening of the sarcomere. The theory that describes this process is called the sliding-filament theory.

When the sarcomere is lengthened, the H-zone gets larger; when it shortens, the H-zone gets smaller. During lengthening and shortening of the sarcomere, the length of the filaments does not change. Only the relative sizes of the areas of the sarcomere that do not contain myosin (I-band) or actin (H-zone) change (figure 7.5).

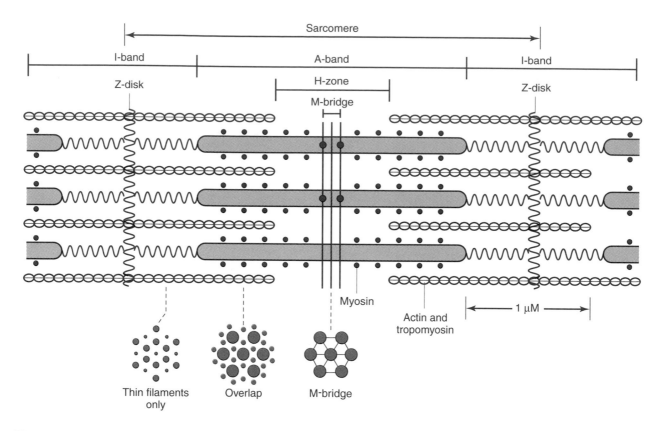

■ Figure 7.4 Longitudinal *(top)* and cross-sectional *(bottom)* diagrams showing the principal elements of the sarcomeric cytoskeleton *(black)* and the thick and thin filaments *(blue)* forming the contractile apparatus.

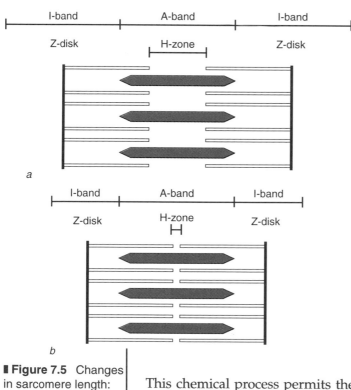

■ Figure 7.5 Changes in sarcomere length: (*a*) on stretch, (*b*) shortened.

The biochemical process that causes this shortening is rather complex and occurs instantaneously. There are two tubular systems vital to the activity of the sarcomere. The **sarcoplasmic reticulum** is an internal tubule system that is arranged parallel to and surrounds the sarcomere in a fishnet mesh arrangement and that terminates near the Z-disks. The transverse tubule (T-tubule) system extends into the inner aspects of the fiber to encircle the myofibrils and also runs perpendicular to the sarcoplasmic reticulum. The T-tubules terminate near the Z-disks between two sarcoplasmic reticulum tubules in a triad arrangement (figure 7.6). The sarcoplasmic reticulum stores calcium ions that are released when an action potential is released from the afferent nerve. The calcium ions are released from the sarcoplasmic reticulum and sent through the T-tubules to the Z-disks. The calcium ions then bind to the **troponin,** a protein located at regular intervals along the actin filament. This in turn causes a shift in **tropomyosin,** another protein that runs along the actin filament. This chemical process permits the head of the myosin cross-bridges to attach more readily to the actin and cause a shortening of the sarcomere (figure 7.7).

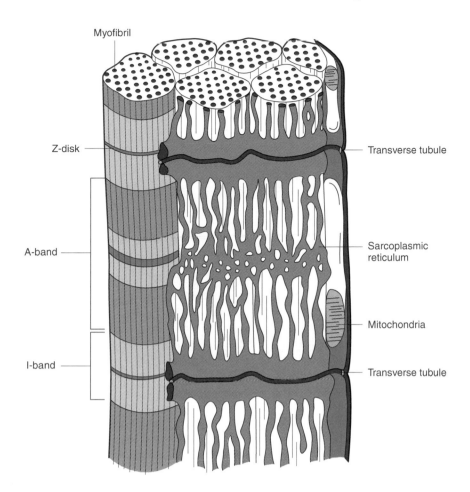

▌ Figure 7.6   Tubule system.

The cross-bridges contain an enzyme, myosin **ATPase,** which is a catalyst that breaks down the **adenosine triphosphate (ATP)** into **adenosine diphosphate (ADP)** and phosphate for energy production. This is the energy source for the sarcomere activity. As long as calcium ions are present and ATP hydrolysis occurs to permit the cross-bridges to recock, the activity can continue. As long as calcium ions are available and energy production through ATP conversion can cause the cycle of cross-bridge attachment-release-recocking to occur, muscle activity is sustained. On the other hand, if calcium ions are recaptured in the sarcoplasmic reticulum or ATP production and conversion cannot be continued, the muscle relaxes.

Because the positively charged calcium is stored in the sarcoplasmic reticulum and not the actin, during muscle inactivity the actin and myosin are not bound by cross-bridges. At rest, they are separated from each other because the negatively charged ATP is bound to the myosin filament's cross-bridges and the actin filaments are also negative. When an excitatory impulse is sent to release the calcium ions, the calcium ions bind with the ATP on the myosin filaments' cross-bridges and neutralize the ATP's negative charge. Since the myosin remains negatively charged, the actin now binds with the myosin. When the cross-bridges fold in toward the trunk of the myosin, the ATP comes into contact with the myosin's ATPase. When this enzyme breaks down the ATP, the actin and myosin break contact as the ATP becomes negatively charged once again. Through a variety of energy systems, the ADP that is released from ATP breakdown is reformed again into ATP. If an excitatory stimulus continues, this cycle is repeated.

The sarcoplasmic reticulum also contains **mitochondria.** Mitochondria are the most metabolically active part of the sarcomere because they contain the substances needed for metabolism. They store the glycogen used for energy production. They also

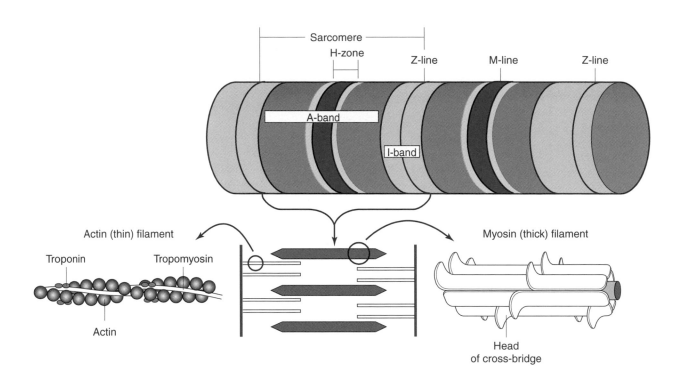

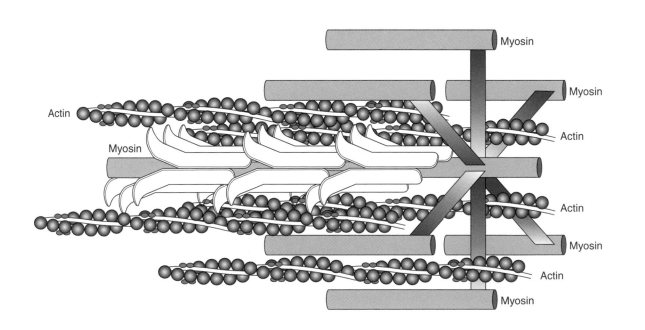

Figure 7.7 Cross-bridges.

Adapted from National Strength and Conditioning Association 2000.

contain the enzyme that is used to metabolize lactic acid for energy to form ATP. The more mitochondria present in the sarcoplasmic reticulum, the more active the muscle.

One motor unit can innervate several muscle fibers in a muscle. These fibers are spaced throughout the muscle and are not necessarily in proximity to one another. Because the lengths of the nerve's end plates vary according to the distance between the motor point and the muscle fiber that the nerve stimulates, the impulse does not reach all of the muscle fibers at the same time. This causes an asynchronous firing of the muscle fibers. This asynchronous firing of a single motor unit produces a smooth muscle contraction.

NEUROMUSCULAR PHYSIOLOGY

The physiological properties of skeletal muscle include irritability, contractility, viscosity, extensibility and elasticity, fatigue, and summation.

As mentioned in the preceding chapter, many sensory receptors provide input to the central nervous system and can influence the neuromuscular system. Figure 7.8 indicates that various sensory receptors on the skin—including the free nerve endings that perceive pain and temperature, the Meissner's corpuscles that receive light touch sensation, and the pacinian corpuscles that perceive pressure sensation—all transmit afferent impulses to the central nervous system. These impulses can be interpreted at various levels within the central nervous system, including the spinal cord, brain stem, cerebellum, and cerebral cortex. Once received and interpreted, a response is transmitted down the spinal cord through appropriate spinal pathways to the anterior horn and along efferent nerves to the motor structures that will respond to the impulses they receive.

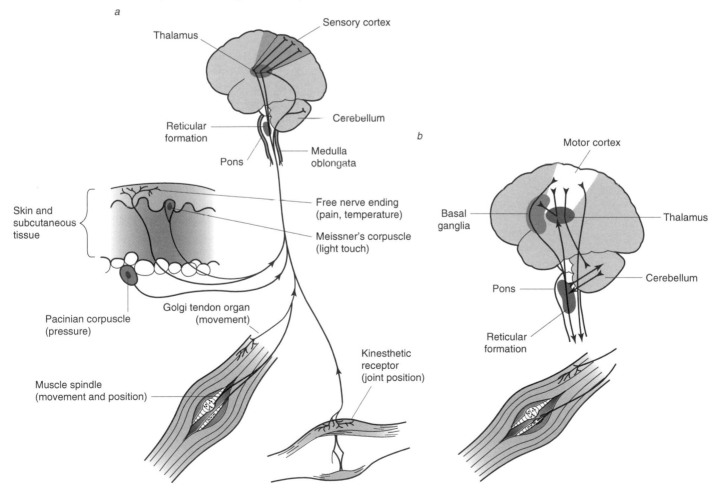

▌ Figure 7.8 Neural pathways: *(a)* sensory; *(b)* motor.

When an impulse is strong enough to produce an action potential, the motor neuron fires and all of the muscle fibers that it supplies respond; this is in accordance with the **all-or-none principle**. Within the muscle itself, a few or many motor units can be facilitated to fire at one time. As a rule, the more motor units recruited, the stronger the muscle's response. The stimulation of an electrical impulse, an action potential, is carried along the motor neuron to the neuromuscular junction. At this junction the action potential causes the release of a chemical, acetylcholine, which in turn stimulates the sarcolemma to release its calcium ions, beginning the muscle activity just described. When this occurs once, the result is a muscle twitch.

RESTING POTENTIAL

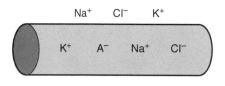

Figure 7.9 Resting membrane potential.

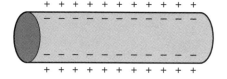

Figure 7.10 Arrangement of charges on the membrane of an axon.

The wall of a nerve or muscle cell membrane has a **resting potential.** There are positive and negative ions in the intracellular and extracellular fluids of the nerve and muscle cell membranes. The extracellular fluid contains many sodium (positive) and chloride (negative) ions. Inside the cell are many potassium (positive) ions, protein molecules (A^-), and some chloride (negative) ions (figure 7.9). This distribution of ions produces a resting potential of the cell. If a microelectrode is placed on the inside and outside of a cell, it will show that an axon's intracellular fluid is 70 to 90 mV. This is represented by figure 7.10, which demonstrates the interior negative charge and exterior positive charge of the cell membrane. There is a natural tendency to attempt to attain an equilibrium of the ions. The task of keeping the balance of ion concentration in check—because the potassium tends to "want" to leak out of the cell and sodium to leak into it—is the responsibility of the sodium-potassium pump. This constant level of activity produces a net resting membrane potential average of approximately –85 mV.

When an excitation impulse occurs, a change in the electrical charge along the cell membrane occurs and produces an action potential. The membrane potential goes from negative to positive and quickly returns to negative once the impulse has passed. This process, which takes probably no longer than .5 ms (Clarke 1975), is much like throwing a rock into water and producing one wave. The rock serves as the initial stimulus, and the wave is the depolarizing impulse that is sent along a nerve axon or muscle fiber, creating a brief change and then returning the water to its original calm. The process continues until the wave hits the shore, its final destination.

PHYSIOLOGICAL PROPERTIES

Skeletal muscle physiological characteristics are unique to skeletal muscle and are vital for the normal functioning of this type of muscle. It is important to know how a muscle works at its cellular level in order to fully appreciate how it responds to demands we place on it during therapeutic exercise. It is also important to know the normal responses of muscle so that when an injury occurs, you are able to recognize what alterations in therapeutic exercises will provide appropriate demands but not aggravate a muscle injury. The following sections provide a brief look at some of the physiological properties.

Irritability

The amount of stimulation required to initiate the response of a muscle fiber is determined by the **irritability** of the motor unit. Irritability is a physiological property of skeletal muscle. To cause a response, a minimum amount of stimulation—called a **threshold stimulation**—is necessary. A subthreshold stimulation level causes no muscle activity. If the stimulus is above the threshold level, the response is greater because either more motor units are affected or the duration of discharge of impulses along one motor unit is increased.

If a muscle fiber is stimulated for about 1 ms (Brown 1980), the membrane depolarizes and is unable to be immediately restimulated. This is called the **absolute refractory period**. In other words, a muscle fiber cannot respond to two stimuli that are less than .001 s apart. There is a **relative refractory period** when the membrane becomes partially repolarized and can respond if the stimulus is greater than the normal threshold level.

The **refractory period** includes a latent period during which there is a momentary cessation of activity as the area is prepared to fire. The latent period not only occurs in the electrical phase of contraction, but is also seen in the energy production and mechanical results of the response as shown in figure 7.11. Once the depolarization of the membrane occurs, the energy changes are facilitated and the mechanical response of the muscle is produced.

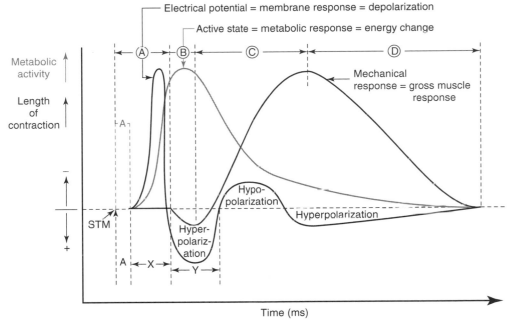

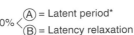

Electrical potential

A = latent period*
A + X = absolute refractory period = depolarization
• cannot respond to additional stimuli

Y = relative refractory period
• start of repolarization
• responds to ↑ stimuli

Depolarization = Na⁺ is pumped into cell

Latent period = From point of stimulation to point of *first measurable* response

Active state

A = Latent period*
• peak is at the beginning of mm contraction
• begins *very* soon after depolarization of electrical potential
• involves a long metabolic recovery period
• is at ¹/₂ of its maximum capacity before the muscle reaches maximum contraction

Mechanical response

Ⓐ = Latent period*
Ⓑ = Latency relaxation
• cross-bridges are released just before shortening
• will not be seen unle fiber is under tensior

Ⓒ = Contraction = 20%
Ⓓ = Relaxation = 70%

▌ Figure 7.11 Time relationship of electrical, chemical, and mechanical responses in a simple muscle twitch.

Contractility

After depolarization, the mechanical response is the contraction. This is the second physiological property of skeletal muscle—simply the ability to contract. In a muscle fiber it is a simple twitch response. One contraction, or twitch response, occurs for each stimulus. If a muscle is to sustain a contraction, multiple succeeding stimuli must be produced. The **contraction phase** of a mechanical response follows a 10% latency period and occurs through the next 20% of the cycle. As seen in figure 7.11, the mechanical response is delayed longer than the electrical potential and metabolic response because of the series elastic component of the muscle fiber.

Viscosity

Viscosity is the internal resistance that limits the rate of muscle contraction. The general rule is that the faster the rate of muscle contraction, the greater the internal resistance and the less the external force that can be exerted. At faster speeds, more force is required to lift the same weight. Water provides a good example of viscosity. If you put your arm under water, you will find that moving your hand slowly through the water is relatively easy. But if you move your hand as fast as you can, you'll notice that you need much more strength.

This is an important property to recall when you are instructing a patient in a therapeutic exercise program. For example, if you want a wrestler with an injured ankle to lift 22.5 kg (50 lb) in a slow heel-raise exercise, you should not expect him to be able to lift the same weight in a faster heel-raise exercise and perform as many repetitions as he can at the slower speed, using the same control and range of motion.

Extensibility and Elasticity

A muscle's individual fibers follow Hooke's law: Stress applied to a stretch of a body is proportional to the strain (change in length) that is produced as long as the elasticity limit of the body is not exceeded. Because of the fiber's elastic components, when a stretch is applied, there is some return to the fiber's original length; but because the fiber also contains plastic elements, there is some change in length if the force applied is of sufficient magnitude or duration. These principles are discussed in chapter 5.

As a muscle is stretched, it becomes more **extensible** because its connective tissue is heated and stretched with the activity. On the other hand, if a part is inactive, it gets stiff. The connective tissue around joints gel rather than remaining fluid, and motion becomes restricted (Kottke 1982). If an area has reached this state and is stiff, overstretching it can cause tearing of capillaries and connective tissue. This stiffness can be overcome by active exercise. Active exercise before stretching helps to increase the muscle's temperature, reduce its viscosity, and relieve the stiffness. Overall, a stretch is more effective if done after a warm-up of active exercise.

Contracture

Contracture is a failure of relaxation of a muscle. Relaxation is a normal metabolic process of a muscle following contraction. Many believe that the onset of fatigue causes both a decrease in the ability to produce an initial maximal contraction output and a decrease in the ability to reach a maximum relaxation level. One theoretical explanation is a lactic acid buildup in the muscle as demonstrated in figure 7.12. As the muscle fatigues, the resting length shortens.

Contracture is one reason for the importance of stretching after exercise. As the muscle fatigues with ac-

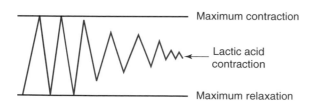

■ Figure 7.12 Contracture.

tivity, the fibers shorten and do not resume their normal resting length. One theory is that over a period of time, the gross muscle loses flexibility if stretches are not performed to regain the normal resting length of the fibers.

Contracture is also the reason you should have the patient perform more-strenuous and more-demanding therapeutic exercises early in the day's rehabilitation session. As the patient fatigues and the muscle fibers' resting lengths decrease, the muscle's ability to perform the activity correctly becomes limited, so the risk of injury increases. The more difficult and challenging activities should be performed early in the day's session to ensure good results.

It is important not to confuse muscle contracture with an orthopedic contracture, which is a connective-tissue shortening that causes a reduced range of motion. Nor should you confuse contracture with a **muscle spasm,** which is a prolonged reflex muscle contraction.

Fatigue

The property of **fatigue** is closely related to contracture. Fatigue can result either from exhaustion of a muscle with prolonged activity or from failure of the circulatory system to provide the necessary nutrients to continue muscle activity. One agent responsible for local muscle fatigue fatigue is **lactic acid.** A by-product of muscle activity, lactic acid increases after intense or prolonged muscle contraction because there is not enough oxygen available to oxidize the lactic acid. In a resting muscle, the quantity of lactic acid is 0.5 to 2.2 mmol/kg of muscle, but in a muscle that is exercised to exhaustion, the lactic acid level is 25 mmol/kg of muscle (Stone and Conley 1994). Lactic acid is measured as small amounts leak from the muscles into the blood. As activity increases, the amount in the blood increases and is used as an index for calculating how vigorously the patient is working. Lactic acid buildup is associated with muscle tiredness and pain. The ability to tolerate increased levels of lactic acid varies from one person to another and is to some extent a determining factor in endurance. Endurance training does not change the levels of lactic acid buildup, but it can make the patient more tolerant of the pain produced by the lactic acid.

Lactate levels are influenced by the intensity of the activity, the exercise duration, the state of training, initial glycogen levels, and muscle fiber type (Stone and Conley 1994). The type II, fast-twitch fibers produce lactic acid at a higher rate than the type I, slow-twitch fibers. High-intensity activities such as sprints and weight lifting produce higher levels of lactic acid than low-intensity prolonged activities such as distance running and aerobic exercises. Individuals who are conditioned tolerate higher levels of lactate than untrained individuals.

If you are working with a patient who has become severely deconditioned because of prolonged inactivity, you need to keep this factor in mind, especially in the early sessions of the therapeutic exercise program when the deconditioning may be more severe. The patient's ability to tolerate exercise intensity changes in severe deconditioning, so earlier exercise sessions require more rest periods than later sessions.

The muscle's circulation is impeded more with sustained isometric activity than with either isotonic or brief isometric activity. The sustained activity of the muscle restricts blood so that fatigue occurs more quickly than with other types of muscle activity. You need to consider this when designing a therapeutic exercise program. The section "Relationship Between Muscle Strength and Muscle Endurance" deals more extensively with recovery from fatigue.

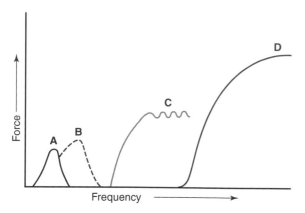

Figure 7.13 Twitch, twitch summation, tetanus, and tetany of a motor unit: **A**, single twitch; **B**, force resulting from summation of two twitches; **C**, tetanus; **D**, tetany, sometimes called a fused tetanus.

Reprinted, by permission, from National Strength and Conditioning Association, 2000, *Essentials of strength training and conditioning*, 2nd ed., edited by T.R. Baechle and R.W. Earle (Champaign, IL: Human Kinetics), 17.

Summation

If a second twitch is produced before a muscle fiber completely relaxes, a greater force is produced. This phenomenon, known as **summation of forces,** is similar to what occurs when a moving car is hit from behind—the car will move forward with a greater force than it did before it was hit. If a series of stimuli is delivered to the muscle fiber at a rapid frequency, the muscle fiber produces a **tetany**, a sustained maximal contraction (figure 7.13). While tetany is a sustained muscular contraction, a **tetanus** is an intermittent contraction that is noted by a fibrillating tremor (figure 7.13, **C**). An asynchronous discharge of several motor units produces a smooth mechanical contraction of a muscle.

FAST- AND SLOW-TWITCH FIBERS

The fast-twitch and slow-twitch fibers of skeletal muscle differ in appearance, metabolic capabilities, and contraction characteristics.

Skeletal muscle is composed of **fast-twitch** and **slow-twitch fibers.** The ratio of these fibers varies within the individual from muscle to muscle, and from individual to individual for the same muscle. In other words, one sprinter may have more fast-twitch fibers in the quadriceps than another sprinter does, and may have more fast-twitch fibers in the quadriceps than in the hamstrings. The ratio is determined by genetics and muscle demands. Whether or not a fiber can convert from one fiber type to another is an unresolved question; but a muscle that is considered an antigravity muscle, such as the soleus, tends to have more slow-twitch fibers than a muscle that is used more for locomotion and fast or powerful movements, such as the quadriceps, which has a combination of fast- and slow-twitch fibers.

The two fiber types have different appearances, metabolic capacities, and contraction characteristics. Their names are based on their relative speed of activity. The slow-twitch fibers, sometimes referred to as type I fibers or slow oxidative fibers, are darker and take about 110 ms to reach their peak tension when stimulated (figure 7.14). The fast-twitch fibers, sometimes called type II fibers or fast oxidative fibers, are lighter in color and reach their maximum tension approximately 50 ms after being stimulated (Wilmore and Costill 1999) (figure 7.15). The slow-twitch fibers have a slower-acting myosin ATPase, and the fast-twitch fibers have a

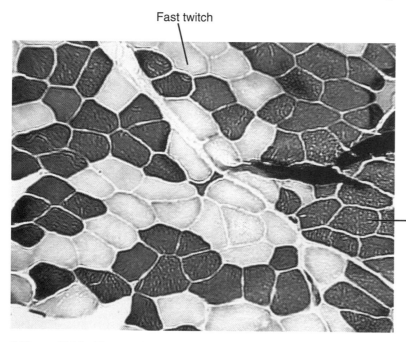

Fast twitch

Slow twitch

Figure 7.14 Fast- and slow-twitch fibers.
Reprinted from Wilmore and Costill 1999.

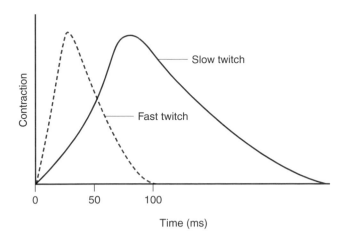

Figure 7.15 Contraction-relaxation curves for fast-twitch (FT) and slow-twitch (ST) skeletal muscle fibers.

faster-acting myosin ATPase, so the ATP is converted more quickly to produce energy faster for the fast-twitch fibers than for the slow-twitch fibers. The fast-twitch fibers also have a more extensive sarcoplasmic reticulum, allowing a more efficient delivery of calcium ions to permit a quicker fiber response to stimulation. The slow-twitch fibers have a greater quantity of mitochondria, more myoglobin, and more glycogen stores, so they are better equipped for prolonged or sustained activity (table 7.2).

Fast-twitch fibers are divided into three subclassifications: type IIa, IIb, and IIc. Very little is known about type IIc. These fibers are found in very small quantities in muscles, approximately 1% to 3% on average. Type IIa and type IIb fibers are approximately equal in quantity in an average muscle (Wilmore and Costill 1999). Although the differences between these fast-twitch fibers are not yet understood, the type IIa fibers are more often recruited during muscle activity than the other type II fibers. The type IIb fibers require a greater stimulus to fire, so they are not recruited in low- or medium-intensity activities, but are used in high-intensity activities such as the 100-m swim.

The slow-twitch fibers have more mitochondria than the fast-twitch fibers. Since mitochondria are the primary energy-storage facilities for the cells, they give the fibers a greater potential to produce a greater oxidative capacity. The higher mitochondria count and related increased myoglobin and blood supply account for the cells' red color. With a greater energy source available, the slow-twitch fibers are able to sustain activity for a longer time than the fast-twitch fibers. For this reason they are considered endurance fibers and are the fibers primarily responsible for a patient's ability to perform low-intensity endurance activities such as a marathon.

Fast-twitch fibers have fewer mitochondria and less ability to sustain activity. Their activity is anaerobic, so they fatigue quickly. However, they are capable of

Table 7.2 Type I and Type II Muscle Fibers

Characteristics	Type I	Type II
Speed	Slowest	Fastest
Axon size	Smaller	Larger
Color	Red	White
Conduction velocity	Slow: 110 ms	Fast: 50 ms
Fatigue resistance	Greatest	Least
Recruitment threshold	Lower	Higher
Firing rates	Lower minimum and maximum	Higher minimum and maximum
Myosin ATPase	Slow acting	Fast acting
Mitochondria	Greater number	Smaller number
Activity	Endurance	Brief bursts

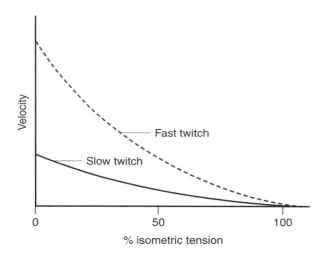

Figure 7.16   Force-velocity curves for fast-twitch (FT) and slow-twitch (ST) skeletal muscle fibers.

producing a more powerful output and are responsible for high-power, short-term activities such as a 400-m sprint (figure 7.16). A factor that allows fast-twitch fibers to produce stronger forces is the fast-twitch motor unit's higher content of muscle fibers in comparison to a slow-twitch motor unit. The greater number of responding muscle fibers causes a greater force production.

MUSCLE STRENGTH, POWER, AND ENDURANCE

Muscle strength is the maximum force a muscle can exert, and power is strength over a distance for a specific time. Endurance is the ability to prolong an activity. Exercises for muscle strength and endurance lie on a continuum from low to high repetitions with high to low resistance.

Before discussing how to improve muscle function, it is necessary to identify the components involved.

MUSCLE STRENGTH

Strength is the maximum force that a muscle or muscle group can exert. In healthy patients it is usually measured in 1-RM, the one-repetition maximum. A 1 RM is the weight that a muscle or muscle group can lift for only one repetition. If a patient can perform only one repetition of a forearm curl with 20.5 kg (45 lb), that is his 1 RM, or strength, for the forearm curl. A patient who can lift 22.5 kg (50 lb) for 1 RM in a forearm curl has twice the strength of a patient who has a 1 RM of 11.3 kg (25 lb).

POWER

Power is strength that is applied over a distance for a specific amount of time. Power is involved in most athletic events and is strength incorporated with speed. The volleyball player who can leg press 180 kg (400 lb) in half the time it takes a basketball player to lift the same weight has twice the power of the basketball player. Power is represented mathematically by the formula in the shaded box.

$$P = \frac{F \times D}{T}$$

P = Power   D = Distance
F = Force   T = Time

You may recall from chapter 3 that work is force × distance. In essence, power is work performed over time. Power increases either through performance of the same amount of work in less time or through an increase in the amount of work performed in the same amount of time.

Speed, however, depends on coordination, efficiency of movement, and timing (Stamford 1985). These elements are developed later in the therapeutic exercise program than strength because, to some extent, they depend on the patient's strength. Since power involves the element of speed, ways of improving power are discussed in chapter 9.

MUSCLE ENDURANCE

Muscle endurance is the ability of a muscle or a muscle group to perform repeated contractions against a less-than-maximal load. A muscle's endurance, or ability to prolong activity, depends on the status of the energy systems available and the forces resisted. With advanced conditioning levels, circulatory and local metabolic exchanges improve. The greater the forces resisted, the more quickly fatigue occurs. If a patient's 1 RM on a bench press is 136 kg (300 lb), the patient will be able to lift 68 kg (150 lb) for more repetitions before fatiguing than if the patient lifts 113 kg (250 lb).

RELATIONSHIP BETWEEN MUSCLE STRENGTH AND MUSCLE ENDURANCE

Muscle strength and muscle endurance can be placed on a continuum of exercise. High-intensity, low-repetition exercises, at one end of the continuum, emphasize primarily strength gains. Low-intensity, high-repetition exercises, at the other end of the continuum, produce primarily muscle endurance gains. Much research has focused on exactly where the dividing line is between muscle strength gains and muscle endurance gains.

High-intensity exercises that are performed for 3 to 9 repetitions appear to best emphasize strength (Berger 1962). A high-intensity exercise is defined as one that is at least 90% of the 1 RM (Wathen 1994). Low-intensity exercises performed for 20 or more repetitions at an intensity of 70% of the 1 RM emphasize primarily muscle endurance improvement. Exercises that are moderate intensity—at 70% to 90% of the 1 RM—and are performed for 6 to 12 repetitions provide gains in both strength and muscle endurance, although not as much as when either strength or muscle endurance is emphasized individually. Most researchers have found that in order to produce strength gains, an exercise must provide resistance levels of at least 66% of the muscle's maximum. Endurance gains are made by increasing strength through high-resistance, low-repetition exercises, but not as effectively as by increasing the repetitions of an exercise. Conversely, some strength gains are achieved with high-repetition exercises, but not as well as with high-resistive, low-repetition exercises. As a general recommendation, if your primary emphasis is strength, perform no more than 10 repetitions; but if your goal is primarily endurance increases, repetitions above 15 to 20 are advised. The closer the exercise resistance is to the maximum resistance, the fewer repetitions performed in the exercise; the further from the maximum resistance the exercise resistance is, the more repetitions the patient is able to perform. The relationship between muscle strength and muscle endurance, relative to the repetitions used to make gains in each of the parameters, is seen in figure 7.17.

Two to three sets of exercises are recommended for optimal strength gains (Knuttgen 1976). Working a muscle optimally and to fatigue requires a recovery period between sets. Several studies have addressed the relationship between fatigue and recovery of muscles, both in isometric and in isotonic activities. The recovery following fatigue from isotonic exercise is slower than that from isometric exercise, but the recovery curves have similarities. As seen in figure 7.18, the recovery rate is rapid within the first 30 to 90 s. The rate of recovery then declines slightly over the next couple of minutes before making another rate change to a very gradual return to full recovery that takes place over a longer time period. The exact time of recovery

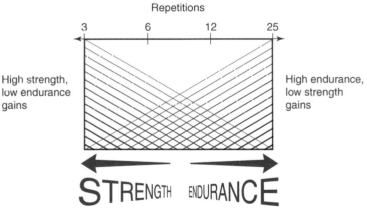

Repetitions

High strength, low endurance gains

High endurance, low strength gains

STRENGTH ENDURANCE

▌ **Figure 7.17** Relationship between muscle strength and endurance. Greater strength gains are achieved with lower repetitions and higher resistance, whereas greater endurance gains are achieved with higher repetitions and lower resistance.

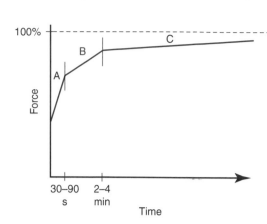

Key

A = Initial rapid recovery
B = Less rapid but still quick recovery
C = Prolonged time to full recovery

A + B = Metabolic waste removal
C = Reserves replacement

■ **Figure 7.18** Recovery following fatigue.

depends on the study design and the type of exercise investigated, but all researchers have found a similar curve for the recovery pattern. When the activity is isokinetic, it takes approximately 4 min for a muscle to recover to 90% to 95% of its initial torque levels following an exercise bout to fatigue (Sinacore, Bander, and Delitto 1994). Recovery from isometric and isotonic exercises to fatigue occurs most rapidly in the first minute—58% and 72%, respectively. After the first minute, the recovery from isometric activity occurs at about a 35% faster rate than from isotonic activity (Clarke 1971). In all of these types of exercise recovery, there is an initial burst of recovery within 30 to 90 s. This is followed by a slightly slower but still rapid recovery. In the final phase of recovery, it takes more than 40 min for the muscle to return to prefatigue-strength levels. On the basis of his findings, Lind (1959) extrapolated the probability that it would take more than 90 min for a muscle to fully recover.

Because of these differing recovery rates, a presumption has been that there are different recovery systems that lead to the muscle's overall recovery following exercise to fatigue (Lind 1959). The initial rapid recovery is thought to occur because of the removal of lactic acid and other buildup of metabolites that took place during the activity. The slower recovery may involve replacement of the muscle's metabolic reserves that were depleted during the activity.

These fatigue recovery findings have an impact on your therapeutic exercise program design. For example, if you are treating a hockey player with a quadriceps strain and he or she performs a leg press to fatigue, you should allow a $\frac{1}{2}$- to 1-min recovery before the next exercise set. If you are using an isokinetic machine to rehabilitate the quadriceps, the recovery time should be 2 to 4 min. With the use of isometric exercises, the rest between sets should be about 1 min.

Sometimes it is not possible to employ high-intensity exercises even though strength gains are needed. This situation is common, especially in early stages of therapeutic exercise when the patient's pain limits the resistance tolerated. In such cases, it helps to remember that the patient can still achieve strength gains using low-resistance, high-repetition exercises. For example, if a gymnast develops a patellar tendinitis and is unable to tolerate much weight during a leg press, he or she can use less weight and lift it for more repetitions to build the needed quadriceps strength. Later in the program as the quadriceps' strength improves, the patient can use higher-resistance and lower-repetition exercises.

The number of repetitions a patient performs depends on several factors, including the patient's pain tolerance, the phase of the healing process, and the demands on the patient after return to competition. For example, a football defensive lineman's therapeutic exercise program is primarily strength based; a soccer player's program involves endurance exercises; and a basketball player—whose sport demands both strength and endurance—will have a program that includes both strength and endurance exercises. If a patient begins a therapeutic exercise program one week after surgery, the resistance exercises are mild so as not to cause undue stress on newly forming tissue.

High-resistance, low-repetition exercises cause an increase in **hypertrophy** of the fast-twitch, type II muscle fibers. Moderate-resistance, higher-repetition exercises produce a more general increase in hypertrophy by affecting the size of both type I and type II fibers.

As a sport rehabilitation specialist, you must possess knowledge of injuries and sport performance requirements and must use good judgment to determine what level of resistance exercises to incorporate into the patient's therapeutic exercise program. Appreciating the patient's injury and having a sound knowledge of strengthening activities provide a good basis for making those judgments.

FORCE PRODUCTION

Muscle force production is determined by the angle of the joint, the size of the muscle and its fiber arrangement, the speed of contraction, and the muscle fibers that are activated.

Some of the concepts in this section were introduced in chapter 3, but they are worth a brief review here. Putting together all the factors that determine strength output of a muscle not only helps clarify the concepts discussed in chapter 3, but also enables you to more fully appreciate the therapeutic exercises that can improve a patient's strength.

Muscle strength is determined by the angle of the joint, the length of the muscle and the sarcomere, the size and fiber arrangement of the muscle, the speed of contraction, and the number and type of muscle fibers activated. Let's look at each of these factors briefly.

JOINT ANGLE

As you recall from chapter 3, joint movement is the result of a muscle's pull on the joint. The amount of force directed toward causing rotation of the joint (movement) and the amount of force directed at compression or distraction of the joint (stability or instability) are determined by the angle of the joint and the vector forces that are produced. Since movement around a joint is rotational, the force is called **torque.** Torque is determined by the amount of applied force and the length of the lever arm: $T = F \times D$ (torque = force times distance). As the joint moves through its motion, the lever-arm length changes, causing a change in the muscle's torque. For example, when a patient performs a biceps curl, as the elbow moves from 90° flexion to 125° flexion, the lever arms of the resistance and the biceps shorten. Since the lever arm of the resistance (weight) undergoes a greater change than the lever arm of the biceps, the weight gets easier to lift by the time the patient has completed the full motion, as seen in figure 7.19. In terms of joint angle, the greatest force production occurs when the tendon's lever arm is at its greatest length.

a

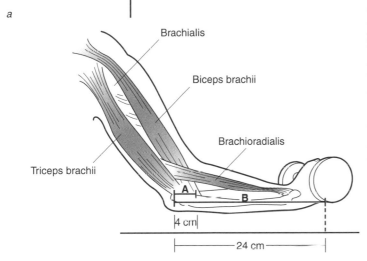

b

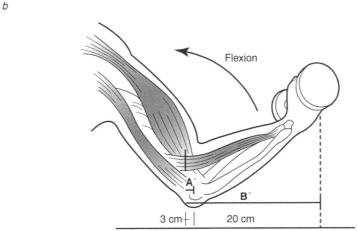

■ **Figure 7.19** Change in biceps lever-arm length **(A to A´)** and change in resistance lever-arm length **(B to B´)** with different joint angles.

LENGTH-TENSION

A muscle's strength production involves both active and passive elements. The active component is the motor unit; the passive component is the connective tissue surrounding the whole muscle, its fascicles, and its fibers. A muscle's ability to actively shorten lessens as the length of the muscle diminishes to about 50% of its resting length. In going from resting, or full, length to 50% of its resting length, the muscle uses only its active component. At a muscle's shortest position, all of the cross-bridges between the fibers' actin and myosin filaments are used up. If, however, the muscle is lengthened before it shortens, its passive component, the connective-tissue element, becomes taut and produces an additional resistive force because of its elasticity. The optimal length of a muscle for producing increased strength—because of the combined release of elastic energy from the passive elements and the actin-myosin cross-bridging from the active elements—is slightly beyond its resting length (figure 7.20). Stretching the muscle beyond that point further separates the actin and myosin to cause less cross-bridging, so that less force, rather than more, is produced.

When it is desirable to achieve a maximum force from a muscle, it is advantageous to produce a quick stretch of the muscle to use its elastic energy component. This factor is frequently utilized in activities such as proprioceptive neuromuscular facilitation and plyometric exercises, both of which are discussed later.

The length-tension factor requires additional consideration for multijoint muscles. The performance of a muscle that crosses more than one joint is profoundly affected by the position of both joints. For example, if you are working with a patient's injured knee and want to obtain a maximal contraction from the hamstrings, the beginning position for placing the hamstrings on stretch is with the hip in flexion and the knee in extension. If the exercise is performed with the patient prone, the hip is extended and the hamstring is already in a partially shortened position. In this position, it is impossible to apply a pre-exercise stretch to the hamstring muscle.

MUSCLE SIZE AND FIBER ARRANGEMENT

Muscle fibers are arranged in series or in parallel with each other. Those muscles with series arrangements are longer muscles that are able to produce a greater shortening velocity. The muscles with parallel fiber arrangement have a larger cross-sectional area and are able to produce a greater force. As a simplified example, if a muscle is composed of three muscle fibers that are placed end to end and these are stimulated to contract simultaneously, the muscle will shorten three times as much as a muscle with one fiber (figure 7.21). The muscle with the three fibers in a side-by-side (parallel) arrangement, however, will produce a contraction three times as powerful as a muscle with one fiber.

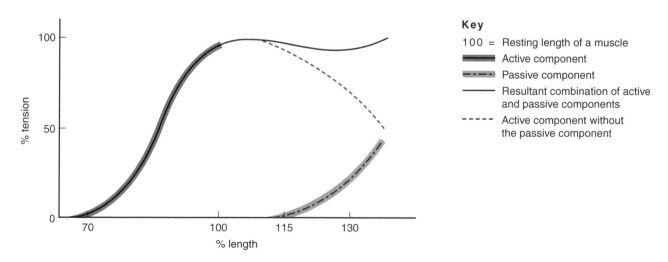

Key
100 = Resting length of a muscle
▬▬▬ Active component
▬ ▪ ▬ ▪ Passive component
──── Resultant combination of active and passive components
- - - - Active component without the passive component

∎ Figure 7.20 Length-tension factor: Because of the active and passive muscle-tissue elements, a muscle produces its greatest strength slightly beyond its resting length.

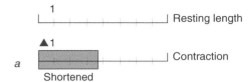

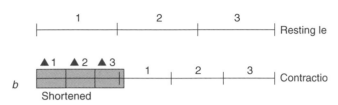

■ **Figure 7.21**   Series fiber arrangement: *(a)* one fiber, *(b)* three fibers in series.

There is a direct correlation between a muscle's cross-sectional size and its strength. The cross section is the width of the muscle taken at an angle perpendicular to the length of the fiber. The cross section is greater when muscle fibers are arranged at angles to the axis of the muscle. Because of its featherlike appearance, this is called a pennate arrangement. The more pennates in a muscle, the greater the cross section. Those muscles with pennates tend to be force-producing muscles, not shortening-velocity muscles. Whereas the sartorius is an example of a shortening-velocity muscle, the gastrocnemius is an example of a multipennate muscle. The angle of pennation of any specific muscle varies from one person to another. Hunter (1994) believes that even if two people have the same size muscle, the angle of pennation may be a factor in the differences between their strength and speed.

SPEED OF CONTRACTION

When a muscle shortens, the force produced is inversely proportional to the velocity of shortening. Billeter and Hoppeler (1992) assume that this occurs because there are fewer cross-bridges between actin and myosin filaments with a higher velocity shorten-ing. For example, a patient who lifts 22.5 kg (50 lb) quickly finds that same weight relatively easy to lift when performing the activity more slowly.

When a muscle lengthens, the force is directly proportional to the velocity of movement. For example, when using a lengthening activity in therapeutic exercise, the patient is able to tolerate more resistance than with muscle-shortening activities. A variety of studies have addressed the relationship between force production and muscle length. One study (Hortobagy and Katch 1990) showed that force production using a muscle-lengthening activity is 120% to 160% more than with a muscle-shortening activity. Other investigators (Wilmore and Costill 1999) believe that this figure is close to 130%.

NUMBER AND TYPE OF MUSCLE FIBERS

As mentioned earlier, larger muscles are able to produce more force than smaller muscles. Fast-twitch fibers are able to produce more force than slow-twitch fibers because there are more muscle fibers in each motor unit of the fast-twitch fibers. If you are rehabilitating two patients with knee injuries and similar-sized quadriceps, the patient with more fast-twitch fibers is able to produce a stronger output of the quadriceps than the patient with fewer fast-twitch fibers in the quads. For this reason, it is fruitless to compare one patient to another and expect the two to be able to perform equally even if they are the same size and have similar injuries.

TYPES OF MUSCLE ACTIVITY

Muscles perform several types of activity: Static activity occurs when there is tension but no change in the muscle's length; dynamic activity occurs when there is a change in the muscle's length; and isokinetic activity is a particular type of dynamic activity.

Although some authors refer to the types of muscle activity as muscle contraction, it is not entirely accurate. Contraction implies a shortening of the muscle, but as you will see, a muscle does not always shorten when it acts. Therefore "muscle contraction" is referred to here as *muscle activity or movement*. There are two types of muscle activity, static and dynamic. **Static activity** is also called **isometric. Dynamic activity** is divided into **isotonic** and **isokinetic.** Isotonic activity is further divided into **concentric** and **eccentric** movements.

STATIC ACTIVITY

Static, or isometric, activity is produced when muscle tension is created without a change in the muscle's length. Static activity is used not only in therapeutic exercise but also in daily activities and sport participation. Trunk muscles act statically to provide a stable base for arm and leg movements. The shoulder acts as a stabilizer when a patient moves the elbow and hand. The advantage of isometrics is that this type of activity can strengthen a muscle without imposing undue stress on injured or surgically repaired structures. For example, in situations such as a recent fracture or a rotator cuff repair in which movement is restricted or limited, isometrics can begin early in the therapeutic exercise program until full motion is indicated. Isometrics can also be used when the muscle is too weak to offer sufficient resistance against gravity or other outside forces. The disadvantage of isometrics is that strength gains are isolated to no more than 20° within the angle at which the isometric is performed. It is important to remember to caution the patient to avoid a **Valsalva maneuver** during isometric exercises. This occurs when the patient holds his or her breath, causing an increase in intrathoracic pressure. This can in turn impede venous return to the right atrium, leading to an increase in peripheral venous pressure (increasing blood pressure) and reducing cardiac output because of lowered cardiac volume. If you see patients holding their breaths during exercise, remind them to breathe in order to avoid the Valsalva maneuver risk.

If a maximal effort is exerted in an isometric exercise, tension within the muscle progressively decreases because of fatigue. At 5 s the tension is 75% of the tension exerted at the start of the isometric activity. By 10 s, the strength drops to 50% of the original tension (figure 7.22). Because of this fatigue factor, no one has the ability to produce a sustained maximal contraction. An example of this is when you assist in carrying a stretcher with an injured athlete on it. As the upper-extremity muscles that are performing the isometric activity of grasping the stretcher begin to fatigue, the muscles start to burn, and the transport team has to stop because someone will request a rest if it takes more than a few minutes to carry the patient.

This concept is important to remember when a patient performs isometric exercises in a therapeutic exercise program. It is unnecessary for a maximal isometric activity to be performed for more than 5 to 10 s at a time; 6 s is the recommended duration for one maximal isometric exercise (Hettinger and Müller 1953). The number of repetitions and frequency of exercise throughout the day depend on the condition of the muscle, the ability of the body part to move, and the phase of the healing process.

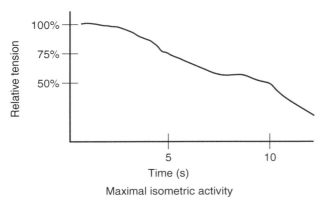

Figure 7.22 Maximal isometric force production.

Strength gains are achievable if the muscle's effort is 66% to 100% of its maximum output. Efforts at 35% to 66% of maximal isometric output produce some gains in strength, but the increase is slow. Most daily activities, apart from sport activities, produce periodic tensions of 20% to 35% of maximum. This level of output maintains strength. If a muscle is immobilized and rendered inactive, there may be a loss of strength of 8% a week (MacDougall et al. 1980) to 5% a day (Muller 1970).

Keep in mind that it takes about one week to increase strength by 5% (MacDougall et al. 1980) to 12% (Muller 1970). These numbers may vary from one study to another because of the different protocols researchers use, but all the data make a similar point: The rate of strength lost is much quicker than the rate of strength regained. One can see that it may take up to a week to recover the strength lost in one day of inactivity. This realization highlights how important it is to keep a muscle active if activity is causing no deleterious effects. If a patient must keep an injured part immobilized, isometric exercises can become very important in retarding atrophy and weakness.

DYNAMIC ACTIVITY

The term *dynamic* in relation to activity implies a change in the position of a muscle. Dynamic activity is further defined by the specific types of activity that occur.

Isotonic Activity

Isotonic activity is dynamic in that it entails a change in the muscle's length. If the muscle shortens, the activity is called *concentric*. If the muscle lengthens, the activity is called *eccentric*. Although you can isolate muscle activity to produce either concentric or eccentric motion, most sport and daily activities involve the use of both concentric and eccentric actions. For example, lifting a weight in an elbow curl is a concentric action, and lowering the weight is an eccentric action. Likewise, jumping for a basketball rebound is a concentric action that is preceded and followed by an eccentric action.

An eccentric action can produce about 30% more force than a concentric action (Wilmore and Costill 1999). For example, if an 18-kg (40-lb) weight can be lifted in a curl exercise concentrically, the same muscle can lift 23.5 kg (52 lb) eccentrically when the arm is lowered. It is believed that the muscle's noncontractile elements provide the additional forces during eccentric activity that permit increased muscle loading.

Concentric and eccentric action contrast in several other ways. Although it takes more energy to perform a concentric action, there does not seem to be any difference in strength gains between the two types of exercise. As the speed of a concentric activity increases, the muscle's ability to produce force decreases. The opposite is true for eccentric exercises: As speed increases with eccentric exercise, the force increases initially, then eventually levels off or decreases. The differences in speed and force production of concentric and eccentric activity are demonstrated in figure 7.23.

There is also a greater likelihood of delayed-onset muscle soreness with eccentric exercise. Although the research is not conclusive, some believe that this is the result of a combination of damage occurring to muscle membranes and a secondary inflammatory reaction within the muscle (Wilmore and Costill 1999).

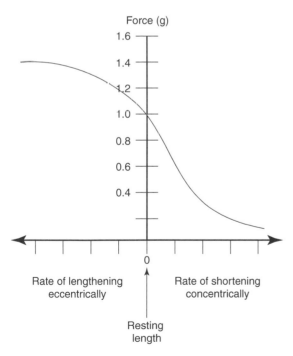

Figure 7.23 Concentric-eccentric force-length relationship.

Adapted from Åstrand and Rodahl 1986.

You can prevent this delayed-onset muscle soreness by taking a few precautionary steps when executing a therapeutic exercise program incorporating eccentric exercise. One way is to avoid eccentric exercises early on when the muscles are particularly weak. Another way is start at a lower level of intensity and gradually increase the intensity as the patient is able to tolerate higher-level exercises. Delayed-onset muscle soreness is generally less of a problem as the patient becomes stronger and becomes accustomed to higher levels of exercise intensity. The occurrence of delayed-onset muscle soreness does not necessarily mean you should limit therapeutic exercise in subsequent sessions, but you should realize that the patient may not be able to offer as great an effort if delayed-onset muscle soreness is present. You should make a decision regarding the use of eccentric exercises in advance and determine whether risking a reduced-intensity session the next treatment day outweighs the benefits of providing eccentric exercises and risking muscle soreness. This is an individual determination that you should base on the patient's tolerance and motivation, the goals for therapeutic exercise, the level of healing, and the patient's current strength status.

The term *isotonic* means "having the same tension." It is, in fact, inaccurate, because the amount of tension produced by the muscle varies throughout the range of motion. The amount of tension produced depends on lever arms and the physiological principles previously discussed. The greatest amount of tension created in an isotonic activity is actually the force that the muscle or muscle group can produce at its weakest position in the motion. For example, if a patient lifts 18 kg (40 lb) in an elbow curl, that weight is the maximum the elbow flexors can exert at their weakest point. If the patient performs the exercise while standing, the weakest point occurs when gravity is at its greatest, which is when the elbow is at 90° flexion. The muscle group can lift more than 18 kg at the beginning of the motion and at the end of the motion as gravity's lever-arm length shortens. It can also lift more in the beginning of the motion, where the muscles are at their greatest physiological length, than it can at the end of the motion when they are at a physiological disadvantage. Because the elbow flexors can lift no more than 18 kg at 90°, the maximum weight the patient can lift if he or she wants to go through the full range of motion is 18 kg. By the same token, because the weight feels relatively lighter in the beginning and at the end of the motion, the patient is able to lift the weight at a faster speed during those parts of the motion. As the weight becomes more difficult to move around the 90° range of motion, the patient's movement slows down.

Isokinetic Activity

Isokinetic activity is a type of dynamic activity in that it involves motion. It differs from isotonic activity, however, in that the velocity is controlled and maintained at a specific speed of movement. Isokinetic means "having the same motion" and refers to the unchanging speed of movement that occurs during these activities. Whereas the speed of motion remains constant, the amount of resistance provided to the muscle varies as the muscle goes through the range. To return to the example of the elbow curl, if the exercise is isokinetic the patient's elbow moves through its motion at a uniform speed, but maintaining that uniform speed requires varying the amount of resistance. In that part of the motion where an isotonic exercise would be easy, the resistance in an isokinetic exercise is greater; and where the isotonic exercise would be normally more difficult, the resistance offered isokinetically is less in order to accommodate the varying strength of the muscle group as it goes through a constant motion. It is assumed in isokinetics that the patient provides a maximal output throughout the exercise. Isokinetics is sometimes called **accommodating resistance** exercise because of the change in resistance given throughout a range of motion. Today's equipment makes it possible to perform isokinetic activities isometrically, eccentrically, and concentrically. Although isokinetics was very popular during the 1970s and 1980s, closed kinetic chain activities are the current trend.

OPEN AND CLOSED KINETIC CHAIN ACTIVITY

The differences between open and closed kinetic chain activities relate to whether or not the distal segment moves freely in space (open) or does not (closed).

A kinetic chain is a series of rigid arms linked by movable joints. This is a mechanical description of the body. **Open kinetic chain** and **closed kinetic chain** within the body are identified in terms of the distal segment of the extremity, the hand or foot. The kinetic chain is open when the distal segment moves freely in space. Kicking and throwing a ball are open kinetic chain activities. A kinetic chain is closed when the distal segment is weight bearing and the body moves over the hand or foot. Running and the pommel horse event in gymnastics are closed kinetic chain activities. Generally, open kinetic chain athletic activities produce high-velocity motions such as throwing a ball or swinging the lower leg during running; closed kinetic chain activities are functional activities that place lesser shear forces on the joints, so they are safer to use earlier in a therapeutic exercise program.

Both open and closed kinetic chain systems involve a relationship between one joint and the others within the chain. This is important to remember in therapeutic exercise, because if you ignore the other joints within the chain when rehabilitating an injured joint, success of the program will be elusive. Function of one joint is not exclusive: The function of one joint determines the function of the other joints within the chain. Abnormal stresses applied to an injured joint are absorbed by other structures within the chain and have the potential to cause additional problems if those stresses are not tolerated by those other areas. For example, if a baseball pitcher has a weak shoulder and is unable to keep the arm elevated correctly during the pitch, he or she may develop elbow pain because of the additional stress transmitted by the abnormal force application transmitted from the shoulder.

Most lower-extremity activities in sport are closed kinetic chain events. They can involve isometric, concentric, and eccentric activities. Closed kinetic chain exercises can be used to improve strength, power, stability, balance, coordination, and agility and are capable of generating large forces but relatively low velocities of movement. Lower-extremity closed kinetic chain activities are functional in that they occur in normal activities from walking and standing to running and jumping. In a closed kinetic chain, no link within the chain can move independently of the others; all are affected by movement of one segment. For this reason, the inadequacies of a weak link in the chain can be compensated for by other links within the chain, but additional stresses are generally applied to those other links. When upper or lower extremities are weight bearing, they function in a closed kinetic chain.

Open kinetic chain activities are also used in daily activities and in sport. Examples of open kinetic chain activities are kicking, throwing, and lifting lower-body weights in a seated position, as in performing knee extensions. Even part of the running or walking cycle involves an open kinetic chain activity. In an open kinetic chain, any link in the chain is free to move independently of the other links. Generally, the forces generated by an open kinetic chain are small but the velocities are large. Body parts that operate in an open kinetic chain are non-weight bearing.

Open and closed kinetic chain activities are produced in both upper and lower extremities (figure 7.24). But different stresses are applied to the body by the two types of activities. The differences in stresses occur because the motion is different. In open kinetic chain activity, the proximal segment initiates the movement for the distal segment. For example, the shoulder motion initiates the movement at the hand. In closed kinetic chain activity, there is compression of the joints, and stabilization occurs because of coactivation of opposing muscle groups. In a squat, the hamstrings activate to counteract knee flexion movement while the quadriceps work eccentrically. The

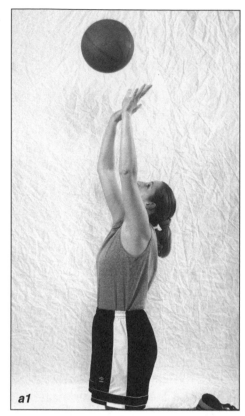

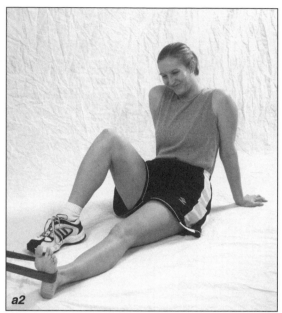

Figure 7.24 Open (*a*) and closed (*b*) kinetic chain activities for the upper (*a1, b1*) and lower (*a2, b2*) extremities.

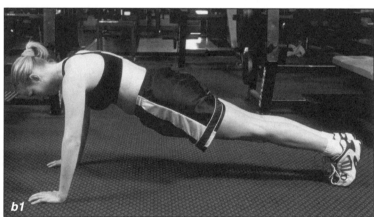

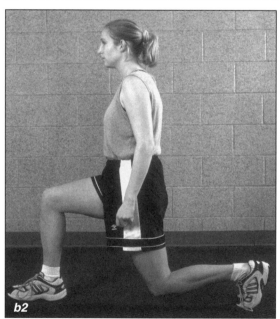

result is stabilization of the knee through simultaneous activity of opposing muscle groups.

Continuing to look at the knee, in open kinetic chain knee flexion, only the hamstrings are working. In open kinetic chain knee extension, the quadriceps are isolated. This exercise increases the moment force of the leg as it goes from flexion to extension. Moment force is the product of the amount of force (weight of the leg) and the perpendicular distance from the joint to the distal end of the limb (lever arm). In other words, as the leg is brought into extension, the work required to lift the lower limb increases because the moment arm of the resistive force increases. This not only requires more strength as the leg reaches terminal extension, but in an open kinetic chain the knee suffers a high shear force with an active contraction of the quadriceps as the knee goes from flexion to extension, especially during the last 30°. This shear force results from the anterior translation of the tibia as it is pulled by the quadriceps tendon. In a closed kinetic chain, the shear force is counteracted by a co-contraction of the hamstring. The end result is reduced stress on the knee during terminal extension, especially the anterior cruciate ligament, and increased stability of the joint through the simultaneous contraction of the hamstrings and quadriceps in a closed kinetic chain exercise.

Although closed kinetic chain exercises are more functional than open ones, in situations when the patient is non-weight bearing it may be necessary to use open kinetic chain exercises. The advantage of open kinetic chain activities in this situation is that strengthening activities need not be delayed until weight bearing is permitted. Open kinetic chain exercises also isolate muscles that are weak, so that correct emphasis can be placed on weaker muscles. One precaution in the use of closed kinetic chain exercises is that because more than one muscle group is used, substitution of stronger muscles rather than correct use of weaker muscles is always a possible pattern and should be corrected when observed. A therapeutic exercise program should include a combination of open and closed kinetic chain exercises for optimal results.

EVALUATING MUSCLE STRENGTH

Sport rehabilitation specialists evaluate the strength of muscles with various types of machines or through manual muscle testing.

Chapter 3 addressed the idea that joint motion is produced by the muscles applying force in an arc of motion. The amount of tension a muscle produces is determined by its lever-arm length and its angle of pull. In functional situations you do not need to calculate the amount of force produced, but you should have an idea of the relative strength of the muscle.

EVALUATION EQUIPMENT

Strength can be objectively determined in a variety of ways. Isokinetic devices, to be considered later, can evaluate isokinetic strength; cable tensiometers can measure isometric strength; and free weights or weight machines can be used to measure 1 RM maximum isotonic strength (figure 7.25).

Instruments that measure strength of specific areas or muscle groups are also available. For example, the grip dynamometer and the pinch dynamometer (figure 7.26) measure grip and finger pinch strength, respectively.

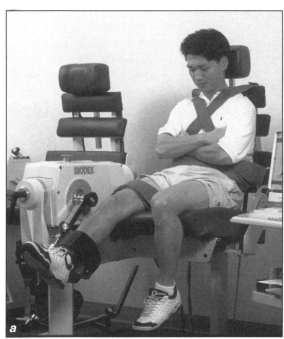 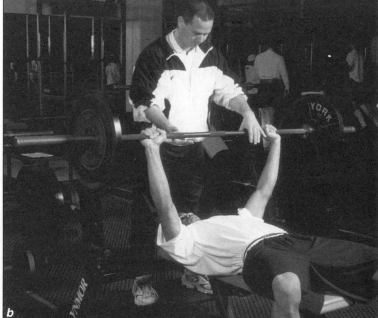

■ **Figure 7.25**   Strength evaluation: *(a)* isokinetic testing, *(b)* 1RM.

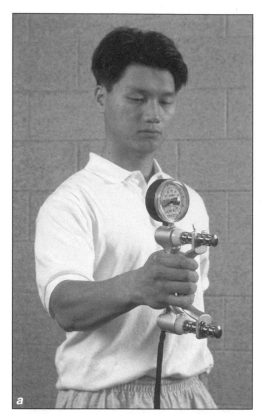

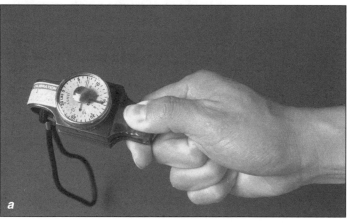

■ **Figure 7.26** Special test equipment: *(a)* grip dynamometer measures hand-grip strength, *(b)* pinch dynamometer masures finger-pinch strength.

MANUAL MUSCLE TEST

Not everyone has an isokinetic machine or cable tensiometers, however, and establishing a 1 RM for an injured extremity may not be appropriate. The 1 RM is an isotonic measure used most often in normal patients; 1 RM is not often used in assessment of strength in therapeutic exercise because it imposes too much stress on an injured part and may aggravate the injury.

The more universal, efficient, and readily available method of evaluating strength is the manual muscle test. The basis of this test is assessment of the muscle's ability to move a joint through its normal range of motion in as isolated a manner as possible. Depending on the muscle's strength, gravity is eliminated, or is used by itself, or is used in conjunction with an outside manual force applied by the sport rehabilitation specialist. The strength of the muscle is graded from 0 to 5. Sometimes verbal grades, ranging from no function to normal, are given instead of the numerical grades.

The manual muscle test was developed and first used by a New York physician, Robert Lovett, in 1912. Lovett later collaborated with a physiologist, Dr. E.G. Martin, and published the tests in 1916. These first tests used the verbal scoring system. During the 1920s and into the 1950s, others further refined and redefined Lovett's manual muscle test. The polio epidemic during the 1950s played a major role in the evolution and use of manual muscle testing and grading. In 1946 a committee of the National Foundation for Infantile Paralysis developed the revised manual muscle test standards that are commonly used today. In 1961 Smith, Iddings, Spencer, and Harrington provided a numerical index and added + and – to the grades (Daniels and Worthingham 1972). These grades are summarized and defined in table 7.3.

Since the development of these grades, it has become common practice to further define the scoring through the use of plus and minus signs. Just as with school grades, the +/– system in muscle grading defines the gray areas into which scores sometimes fall. For example, a deltoid that offers minimal resistance to antigravity with resistance is less than a grade 4 and more than a grade 3, so the sport rehabilitation specialist grades it as 4–. The grade is recorded as 4–/5, indicating that the strength of the muscle is 4– on a 5-point scale. If a muscle has some motion against gravity but not full range of motion, the sport rehabilitation specialist may give it a 3–/5 grade. If it has full motion in a gravity-eliminated position and is able to tolerate some resistance in this position but still is unable to go through a full range of motion in an antigravity position, its grade is 2+/5.

When the sport rehabilitation specialist provides manual resistance to a muscle, the position most commonly used for the resistance in grade 4 and 5 muscle tests is an antigravity position with the muscle at the end of its range. Before a resistance is given to a muscle, the muscle actively moves the joint through its full range of motion. If that is successful, the sport rehabilitation specialist then applies manual resistance to determine the strength grade. Resistance can also be applied through the full range of motion or at various positions to determine strength. If testing positions are different from the standard positions, this should be noted on the record.

Table 7.3	Muscle Strength Grades			
% Normal strength	**Number grade**	**Letter grade**	**Descriptive grade**	**Definition**
100%	5	N	Normal	Full range of motion against gravity and is able to tolerate full manual resistance to movement.
75%	4	G	Good	Full range of motion against gravity and is able to tolerate some, but not full, resistance.
50%	3	F	Fair	Full range of motion against gravity but is unable to tolerate additional resistance.
25%	2	P	Poor	Full range of motion with gravity eliminated. It is unable to go through a full range of motion in an antigravity position. It may be able to tolerate some resistance when gravity is eliminated.
10%	1	T	Trace	Has evidence of slight contractility, but no joint motion occurs. A flicker of tension in tendon or muscle may be seen or palpated, but the joint does not move.
0%	0		Zero	There is no evidence of contractility of the muscle. Facilitation produces no observable voluntary response in the muscle.

When applying a resistance force, you should exert the pressure in a direction that is opposite to the muscle's line of pull, providing stabilization if needed to permit isolated testing of the specific muscle or groups you are evaluating. Give the resistance on or near the joint distal to the joint being tested. Avoid placing your hand on the belly of the muscle being tested. Give the resistance gradually, building it up as you see that the patient is able to accept more resistance until you have determined the maximal resistance tolerated. Provide the maximum resistance possible to obtain an accurate result: If the muscle is able to tolerate more resistance than you have provided, the score may be inaccurate. Compare to the opposite side to determine what is "normal" for the patient. What is "normal" for a golfer may not be "normal" for a football lineman; what is "normal" for a recreational sprinter may not be "normal" for a competitive sprinter.

If a muscle is unable to perform a movement through its full range of motion in an antigravity position, it is placed in a gravity-eliminated test position to determine whether it has at least grade 2/5 strength. If full motion in an antigravity position is possible, resistance can be provided in this position to determine whether a 2+/5 strength is present. Figure 7.27 presents examples of strength testing of the hip, knee, ankle, shoulder, elbow, and wrist muscles.

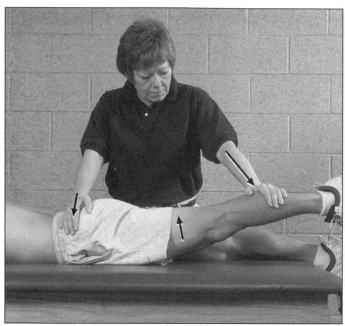

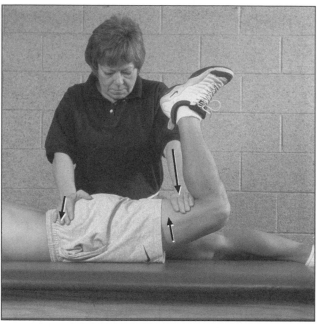

(a) Grade 4 and 5 test for hip extension with gluteus maximus and hamstrings. Note stabilization of hip to prevent pelvic rolling or hip flexion.

(b) Grade 4 and 5 test for hip extension with isolation of gluteus maximus. Stabilization of hip and pelvis is necessary to isolate hip extension motion.

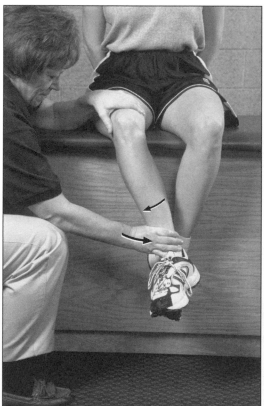

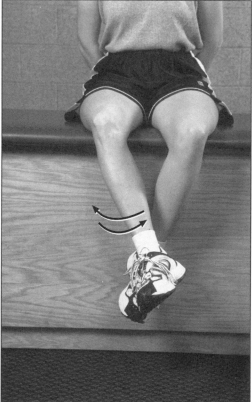

(c) Grades 4 and 5 test for hip internal rotators: while stabilizing the thigh, resistance is applied to the lower leg against internal rotation movement.

(d) Grade 3 test for hip internal rotators: patient should not lower the knee or roll the pelvis as the hip is moved through external rotation.

▌Figure 7.27
Manual muscle tests.

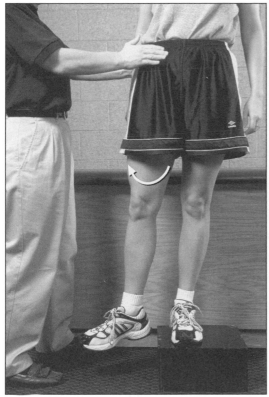

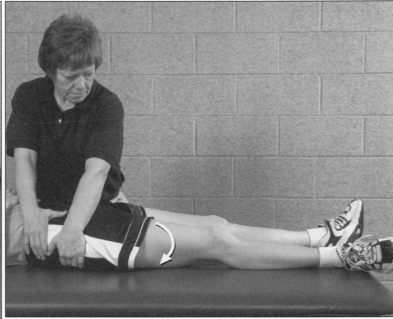

(f) Grade 1 test for hip external rotation: hip external rotators are palpated as the patient performs the movement. The upper hand stabilizes the pelvis.

(e) Grade 2 test for hip external rotation: as the patient moves the hip through a full range of motion, the pelvis is stabilized to isolate movement.

(g) Grade 4 and 5 test for hip adduction: resistance is applied to the thigh during movement into adduction while avoiding hip flexion or rotation substitution.

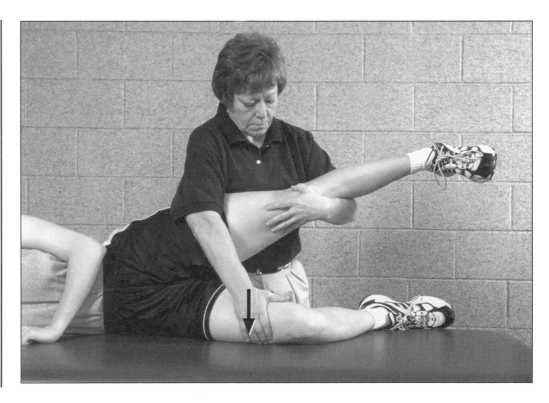

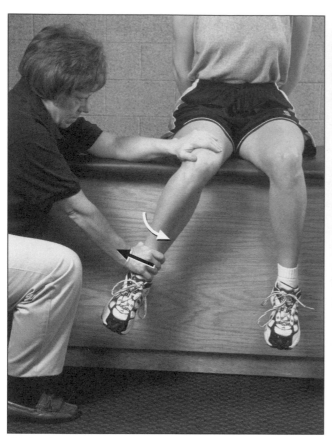 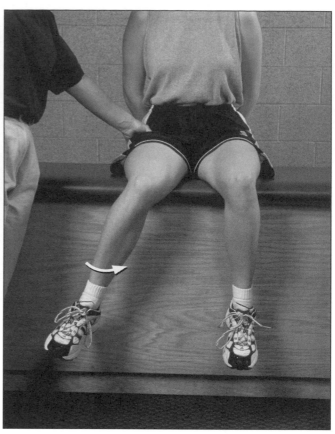

(h) Grade 4 and 5 test for hip external rotation: the thigh is stabilized while resistance is applied to the lower leg against hip external rotation movement.

(i) Grade 3 test for hip external rotation: while stabilizing the pelvis, the hip is moved through a full range of external rotation.

(j) Grade 1 and 2 test for hip adduction: while stabilizing the pelvis and palpating the hip adductors, movement into adduction is attempted. Watch for hip rotation or flexion substitution.

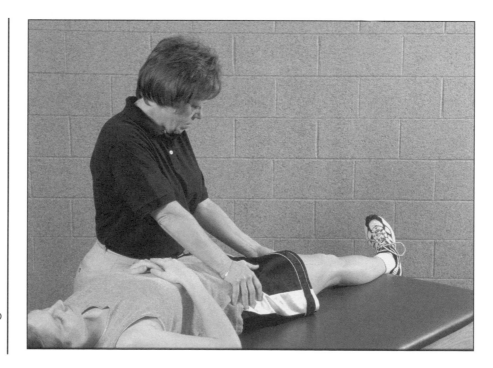

■ **Figure 7.27** *(continued)*

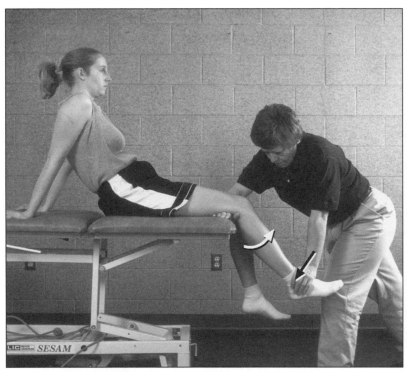

(k) Grade 4 and 5 test for knee extension: with one forearm under the thigh to elevate the thigh and protect it against the table surface, resistance is provided against knee extension motion.

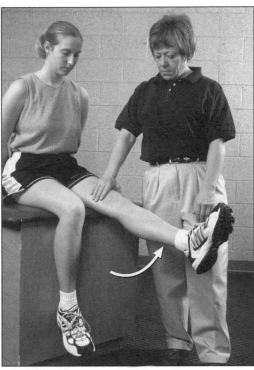

(l) Grade 3 test for knee extension: while the thigh is stabilized, the knee is extended through a full range of motion without resistance.

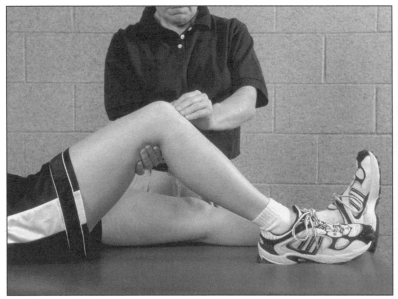

(m) Grade 1 test for knee extension: with the quadriceps on stretch in knee flexion, the quadriceps tendon is palpated as the knee is actively extended.

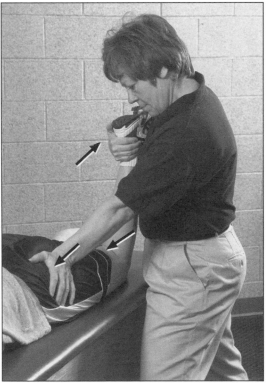

(n) Grade 4 and 5 test for knee flexion: with the hip and pelvis stabilized, resistance at the ankle is provided to knee flexion. Resistance to lower-leg rotation can be simultaneously provided to isolate medial and lateral hamstrings.

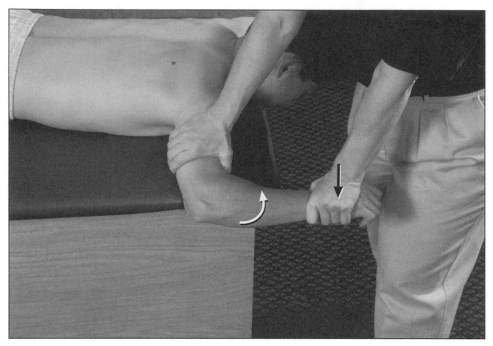

(o) Grade 4 and 5 test for shoulder external rotators: while stabilizing the arm, downward resistance is applied at the forearm.

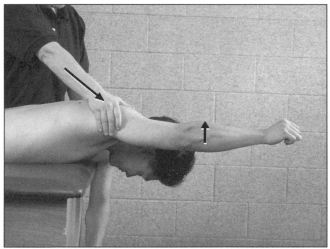

(p) Grade 4 and 5 test for lower trapezius.

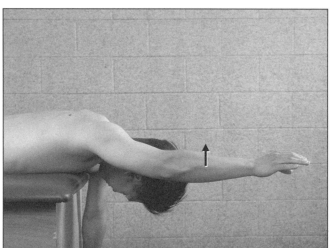

(q) Grade 3 for lower trapezius.

❚ **Figure 7.27**
(continued)

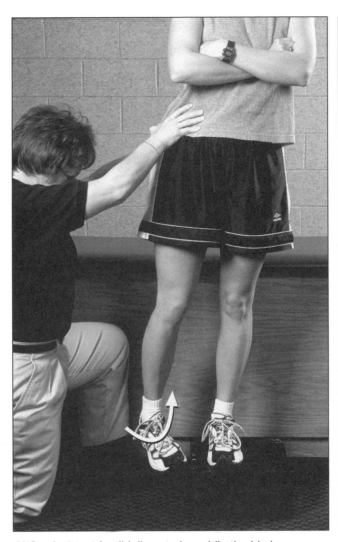

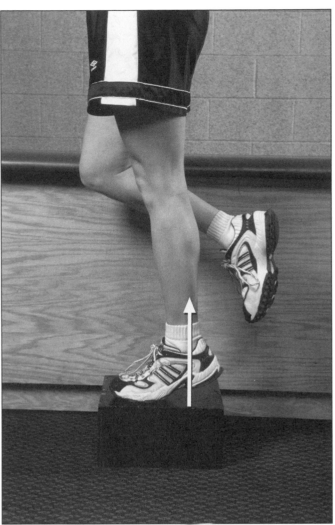

(r) Grade 3 test for tibialis anterior: while the hip is stabilized, the foot is moved into dorsiflexion and inversion through a full range of motion. The test may be performed in sitting or standing.

(s) Grade 4 and 5 test for plantar flexion: full heel elevation should occur 20 times for normal strength. Watch for body rocking and knee flexion substitutions.

A thorough presentation of strength-testing positions and techniques for all grades of movement is available in various muscle-testing textbooks. Two suggestions are *Muscles, Testing and Function*, 4th ed. (Kendall 1993) and *Muscle Testing: Techniques of Manual Examination*, 3rd. ed. (Daniels and Worthingham 1972).

On rare occasions you may encounter a patient who does not offer a smooth resistance during the muscle strength test. The resistance is a series of catch-and-release tensions of the muscle as it goes through its range of motion. Called a **cogwheel resistance**, this response occurs in individuals who are not producing a maximal effort. Reasons for the response may include fear, pain, and malingering. When you see this form of resistance you should be aware that it is not a normal response, but rather a voluntary response that produces an inaccurate test result.

GRADATIONS OF MUSCLE ACTIVITY

Muscles perform various gradations of muscle activity; from the least active to the most active, these are passive range of motion, active assistive range of motion, active range of motion, and resisted range of motion.

Just as there are grades of muscle strength, there are grades of muscle activity. The kind of muscle activity possible is determined by the muscle's strength.

PASSIVE RANGE OF MOTION

Passive range of motion (PROM) is an activity that requires no active work on the part of the muscle. The motion is produced by an outside force, either a machine or another person. The intent is to maintain range of motion in situations in which either the muscle is incapable of moving voluntarily or it is desirable that the muscle not perform actively. Continuous passive motion machines, discussed in chapter 4, are sometimes used after surgery when motion is beneficial but active motion is not possible because of limitations such as pain, swelling, or spasm or because restriction of muscle activity is desirable. The sport rehabilitation specialist can also perform PROM by moving the extremity through its motion without the patient's assistance.

ACTIVE ASSISTIVE RANGE OF MOTION

Active assistive range of motion (AAROM) is performed either when the muscle is incapable of producing the full motion without assistance, or when it is desirable for the individual to perform limited voluntary activity with assistance from an outside source to achieve the objective of the exercise. For example, if a patient has undergone reconstructive surgery on the shoulder, it may be desirable for him or her to perform actively through part of the motion, but not in the portions of the motion that may impose risk of shear stress or possible detachment of recently repaired tendons. Or a patient who has incurred a hamstring strain may not have full range of knee flexion because of weakness of the hamstrings. The hamstring is able to perform the motion through part of the range, but requires assistance from the sport rehabilitation specialist to complete the motion.

ACTIVE RANGE OF MOTION

Active range of motion (AROM) occurs when the patient is able to produce full range of motion of the segment, with no assistance. No resistance is applied. These types of exercises are also sometimes referred to as range-of-motion (ROM) exercises. Following surgery, the physician may permit a patient to perform full AROM exercises but may not want any outside resistance to be applied. These exercises are performed to maintain or increase range of motion and help prevent atrophy of the muscles involved in the motion.

RESISTED RANGE OF MOTION

Resisted range of motion (RROM) falls into the broad category of dynamic exercises. Motion with resistance applied to the muscles is permitted. These types of exercise are commonly referred to as strengthening exercises or progressive resistive exercises. A later section of this chapter introduces the variety of progressive resistive exercise programs used in the rehabilitation of sport injuries.

STRENGTH EQUIPMENT

The primary methods of increasing strength include use of body weight, rubber tubing and bands, free weights, and isotonic and isokinetic machines. Each has its own advantages and disadvantages.

Many types of equipment are available to provide strength gains in both rehabilitation and conditioning programs. Most equipment can be used for both purposes. Cost varies greatly also—from very little to several thousand dollars. What you decide to use in your therapeutic exercise programs depends on your familiarity with the equipment, availability, and the specific needs of the injured patients. Regardless of the amount or kind of equipment you have, you can design a very comprehensive, progressive, and appropriate therapeutic exercise program for every patient you treat. Your imagination and knowledge are ultimately the determining factors in the quality of the program you create.

The following sections deal with the most common items of equipment available on the market. Most are items you will become familiar with before you complete your curriculum.

MANUAL RESISTANCE

Manual-resistance equipment is the least-expensive therapeutic exercise equipment. The only requirement is you. Manual-resistance exercise is an active exercise in which the sport rehabilitation specialist applies the force for producing either static or dynamic muscle activity. Manual resistance can be applied isometrically if movement is not desirable, if pain occurs with motion, or if the patient's muscle has a specific area of weakness within a range of motion.

Manual resistance can also be applied concentrically or eccentrically, through part of the motion or the full motion. It can be applied in a straight plane of movement or in a more functional diagonal plane.

Technique

Once you have assessed strength and identified deficiencies, you can determine how much resistance to apply during the exercise and whether you will need to provide additional special considerations such as an isometric activity at any point in the range of motion.

Before performing the exercise, the sport rehabilitation specialist explains to the patient the exercise, the sensations to be expected, the number of repetitions or qualifications for the duration of the exercise, and any necessary precautions. For example, I sometimes tell the patient that the goal is 15 repetitions or state that we will continue the exercise until "one of us gets tired, or I start to sweat." If I want to deliver an isometric in the middle range, I tell the patient ahead of time to prepare him or her that at that point the motion will stop but the exercise will continue. As part of preparation it is also a good idea to take the extremity passively through the range of motion in the desired plane to let the patient know exactly what is expected during the exercise.

The resistance should be applied in a manner that permits the patient to perform the desired motion smoothly. The motion should not be jerky or uncontrolled. During the activity, the patient should produce a maximal effort and continue to breathe throughout. Occasionally, as already mentioned, a verbal reminder to breathe is necessary to prevent a Valsalva maneuver.

The sport rehabilitation specialist should watch carefully to see that substitution and unwanted movement patterns do not occur. It is important to correct the patient's motion if there is any substitution so the exercise is properly performed and facilitation of the appropriate muscle occurs.

Just as with manual muscle testing, the force application should be near the joint distal to the joint being moved. If you cannot control the resisted movement because the patient's muscle is stronger than you are, as can be the case when you apply manual resistance to the hip, you can apply the resistance even more distally, at the ankle rather than the knee; this is permissible only if pain is not produced at the knee when the force is applied at the proximal ankle. The more distal application gives you a longer lever arm so that you need to do less work to offer the same amount of resistance to the hip. You can apply the same technique to shoulder exercises; in this case you offer resistance at the proximal wrist, instead of at the elbow, but only if no pain occurs at the elbow. The exercise should be pain free and should offer enough resistance to produce the desired results.

Advantages

As already suggested, the greatest advantage of manual resistance is that it requires no equipment. It is also a good way to establish rapport with the patient, because a hands-on technique usually results in the patient's developing trust and confidence in the sport rehabilitation specialist. This often leads to a greater desire to work harder. It also gives you immediate feedback about the patient's progress. You assess the changes and improvements each time you perform the exercises, and you can make immediate changes according to the patient's response to a specific exercise. If the patient gets stronger each day, you can immediately increase the resistance or repetitions. The ability to modify the speed of the exercise within a set, the ability to change from concentric to eccentric activity or to include both as appropriate, and the ability to incorporate isometric resistance into the weaker points of the motion are all unique to manual exercises. A progression of exercises is easily incorporated into a therapeutic exercise program either through increasing the manual resistance or through increasing the number of repetitions in a set.

Disadvantages

There are some unique disadvantages to the use of manual resistance. Because it requires one-on-one work with the patient, this method may be more time consuming than others and may not easily fit a situation that necessitates working with several patients at one time.

Another disadvantage is that manual resistance does not provide an objective measure for changes in strength. As a subjective method, it relies on performance by the same sport rehabilitation specialist to reflect the changes on a daily or periodic basis.

In addition, if the sport rehabilitation specialist is not sensitive to the amount of force he or she is applying, judgment about the amount of force and about subsequent changes in the patient's condition may not be dependable. If you are more fatigued than usual on a given day, you may provide less force than on other days; without good awareness of how you feel you may incorrectly perceive a significant increase in the patient's strength.

BODY WEIGHT

Exercise using body weight also requires no equipment. The patient's own body weight provides the resistance. A variety of exercises for the upper and lower extremities and the trunk can be used, along with progressions, to offer an adequate system of therapeutic exercises.

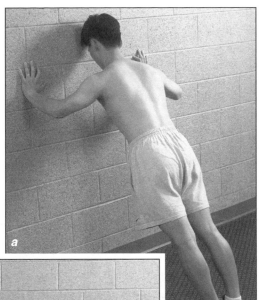

Technique

You can provide a progression by increasing the amount of body weight used in an exercise, by prolonging the time of the exercise, or by increasing the number of repetitions or sets. For example, if a patient has weak scapular rotators, a progression of increasing the amount of body weight for a push-up exercise starts with a wall push-up, as seen in figure 7.28a. The patient can progress from the wall to an incline, perhaps in a position with the hands on the back of a chair or a countertop (figure 7.28b), and then with the hands on a chair seat (figure 7.28c). An even more advanced position is a modified push-up. As strength improves, the patient changes to a regular push-up position (figure 7.28d). If additional resistance is desirable, the patient can move

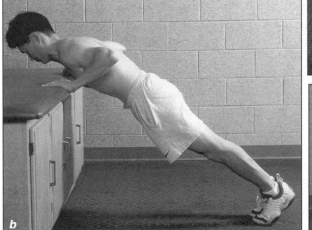

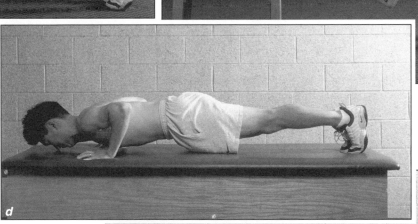

▌Figure 7.28 Body-weight resistance push-up progression: The easiest push-up is performed using a wall (a). Progression then moves to an incline (b) and (c), to the floor (d), to an inverted position (e). The positions shown in figures b–d increase difficulty by increasing the lever-arm length of the body. The position shown in figure e increases the difficulty by forcing the arms to bear more of the body's weight.

to a decline push-up in which the feet are higher than the hands (figure 7.28e). The most advanced push-up is a handstand push-up. This is one example of a progression from easy to most difficult, providing the patient with a body-weight resistance exercise.

Examples of additional progressions include increasing the number of repetitions and/or sets the patient must perform, having the patient perform an isometric at the middle or end of the motion, and increasing the time of the hold as strength increases. A change of speed also changes the effort of the exercise.

You must impress on patients that performing an exercise through a full range of motion is necessary for maximal benefit. Partial range-of-motion execution provides for strength gains only in the portion of the motion being exercised. In the beginning, the patient should do the exercises slowly and in a controlled manner so that he or she executes them correctly without substitution of activity by the wrong muscle. As strength and control improve, the speed of the exercise may increase to more correctly mimic functional activities.

It is also important to instruct the patient in correct execution of the exercise, providing information about common substitution patterns to avoid. This helps to minimize incorrect technique and to produce better results.

Once the patient has demonstrated the correct technique, he or she can perform the exercises without your assistance. This builds a sense of independence and control over the therapeutic exercise program and requires the patient to demonstrate initiative.

It is sometimes beneficial to give patients handouts illustrating these exercises. Such information serves as a reminder of correct exercise execution and also helps the patient comply with the therapeutic exercise program.

Advantages

The most obvious advantage of body-weight resistance exercises is that they require no equipment. They can be performed anywhere, whether the patient is in the clinic, in the athletic weight room, at home, or on the road. A related advantage is that there is no expense, although handouts aimed at improving compliance may add minimal costs.

Another plus is that once the patient can perform the exercises correctly and continue them independently, treatment sessions can focus on other activities that may require the expertise of the sport rehabilitation specialist.

Many weight-resistive exercises, such as the standing squat, are actually functional activities. They can be used as a progression of activities that naturally lead to those functional activities performed in the patient's sport.

Disadvantages

A disadvantage of body-weight exercises is that if the patient is performing them independently, there is no guarantee that he or she is doing them correctly or even doing them at all. On the other hand, it is not difficult to tell whether or not gains are being made outside the treatment sessions. If there are gains, chances are that the patient is complying; and, obviously, the converse is just as true.

Occasionally, a patient is unable to tolerate body-weight resistance exercises either because the area is too weak or because performing them is too painful. In this situation, it is better to begin with activities that provide less body-weight resistance—such as a wall push-up, or even independent isometrics—and entail tensing the muscle without additional resistance. Once strength has improved, body-weight resistance activities can be incorporated.

Some areas of the body lend themselves better than others to body-weight resistance and progressive exercises using body weight. For example, the fingers and wrists are difficult to exercise with body resistance, especially in the beginning when the patient may not be able to perform an activity such as fingertip push-ups.

RUBBER TUBING AND BANDS

Rubber tubing and bands provide dynamic resistance exercises. They are packaged in large and small rolls, so strips can be cut to varying lengths; they also come in a range of resistance levels indicated by color coding. Although various companies market the bands, the most familiar spectrum corresponding to resistance levels from lightest to heaviest is tan, yellow, red, green, blue, black, silver (gray), and gold (butterscotch). The color-coding scheme for tubing is similar.

Technique

Rubber tubing and bands can be used both in straight-plane exercises and in functional patterns. Depending on the specific activity, the patient may use his or her own body to secure the band, or may use an object such as a door or table leg to secure it.

The bands and tubing can be used to mimic exercises performed with other equipment that is available in the clinic but not available for the patient at home. For this reason, tubing and bands are useful for home exercises.

Because of the variety of types of exercises that one can perform with tubing and bands, it is difficult to discuss specific application techniques. You should give the patient general guidelines, however, before providing bands or tubing to use for independent exercise. You should instruct the patient to perform the exercise slowly and in a controlled manner so the targeted muscles are used correctly. Going through a full range of motion is necessary for developing strength throughout the muscle's range. In addition, the area being exercised must be stabilized to ensure correct performance. Inadequate stabilization causes substitution and exercise of the wrong muscles.

To determine which color band or tubing to use, you will perform a manual muscle test on the appropriate muscle. Trial and error may be necessary, but after the test you should be able to narrow down the choice of colors. You have selected the appropriate color when the patient can perform the activity through an appropriate range of motion for the desired number of repetitions and feels that the muscle has been at least moderately exercised.

Once again, to ensure better compliance, it is advisable to give patients handouts that include drawings or photos along with providing oral explanations of the exercise. As mentioned in chapter 1, studies show consistently that if an individual receives both written and oral instructions, the likelihood of correct performance of the exercise and of compliance increases significantly.

Advantages

The cost of rubber tubing and bands is relatively low. In some clinics, it may be possible to recoup the costs by billing the patient or the patient's insurance company. These items are easy to transport, because they weigh little and are not bulky, so patients can take them home or can easily pack them into suitcases and exercise almost anywhere.

Since exercises using bands or tubing are easily converted to home exercises, they need not be repeated in the treatment sessions. Treatment time can then be better spent on other activities that require the expertise of the sport rehabilitation specialist. This allows the patient to gain a sense of responsibility, independence, and control over the injury.

The color coding for the bands and tubing offers an easy-to-implement system of progression. As the patient's strength increases, you can provide additional colors to achieve greater resistance with the same exercise. Additional instruction is not necessary, because the exercise itself is the same.

Exercises that mimic functional motions can be used with the tubing and bands. This provides for strength gains in functional patterns. This method is especially convenient for upper-extremity muscle groups that may not easily lend themselves to body-weight resistance and other exercise systems.

Disadvantages

Since the patient does rubber-tubing and band exercises independently, you do not have control over compliance. It is the responsibility of the patient to perform the exercises. This can be an advantage or a disadvantage, depending on the patient's attitude, dependability, and motivation.

Another disadvantage is that as the band or tubing stretches during the exercise, the resistance increases, causing more resistance to the muscle as it reaches its weaker point in the motion. The resistance is then greater at the end than at the beginning of the motion when the muscle was at a stronger physiological length. So although the band offers resistance to the muscle, the resistance does not coincide with the muscle's ability to produce force.

If the clinic cannot recoup the cost of bands and tubing, the expense can add up quickly. The heavier bands are more expensive than the lighter bands, so as a patient's strength increases, the cost of distributing the bands and tubing also increases. If a facility provides tubing and bands for patients but is unable to recoup the costs, additional budget allowances are necessary.

Although it is possible to design exercises for the hip and knee using bands and tubing, the greater number of exercises using these items involve the upper extremities. Figure 7.29 provides examples of some rubber band exercises for the upper- and lower-extremity muscles.

FREE WEIGHTS

When most people think of strengthening, they think of free weights. Free weights include cuff weights, barbells, and dumbbells. They come in a variety of sizes and styles. The weight is either attached to the body part or held by the patient during the exercises. Cuff weights typically cannot be changed in size. Some can be modified by the addition of preset weighted tubes or packets that are placed in a pocket on the cuff. The cuffs can be attached to ankles or wrists.

Some dumbbells and barbells are adjustable: various weights can be placed on the bar and are secured with collars. Other dumbbells and barbells are fixed and their weight cannot be changed. *Dumbbells* refers to weights that

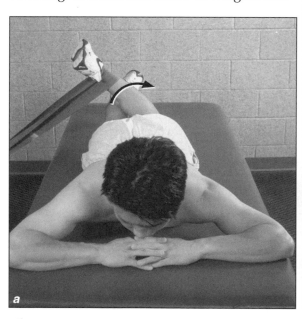
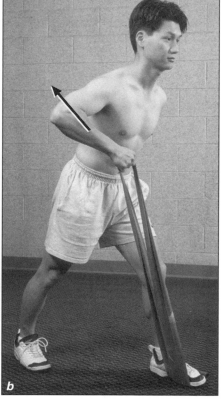

❚ **Figure 7.29** Rubber band exercises: *(a)* hip internal rotator resistive exercise, *(b)* shoulder horizontal extension (or bent-over row) exercise.

are used in one hand, are usually smaller, and are either fixed weights or adjustable. *Barbells* refers to a larger free-weight system that requires using both hands. Barbells are used for lower- and upper-body strengthening. The bars vary in length from 1.5 m to 2.1 m (5–7 ft). A bar that has become popular in the past several years for conditioning and later-stage rehabilitation is the standard Olympic bar, which weighs 20.5 kg (45 lb) and is about 2.2 m (87 in.) long. The collars used to secure the weight plates to an Olympic bar weigh 2.25 kg (5 lb) each. The sleeves on which the plates are mounted are larger than more conventional plates and rotate so that the plates do not stick to the bar when it is lifted. The plates are also larger in diameter than the traditional plates so that a patient who drops the bar is not crushed or otherwise injured by the weight.

Technique

As with any exercise, proper instruction in execution is necessary in order to achieve appropriate strengthening without substitution of activity by incorrect muscles. It may be helpful, especially in the beginning, to have the patient use a relatively light weight so that he or she can achieve the correct technique and learn what muscle should be performing the activity. Stabilization of the part being exercised is necessary and is more difficult with free weights than with machine weights. Once you are confident that the patient is able to perform the exercise correctly and understands the proper procedure, you can provide a more appropriate exercise resistance.

The patient should have control of the weight throughout the full range of motion. A complete range of motion during the exercise is necessary to provide for strength gains throughout the motion. The patient should perform the activity in a slow, controlled manner. As the muscle's strength improves and more functional activities are appropriate, the speed of the motion may increase, depending on the goals of the exercise.

Free-weight exercises are more difficult to perform than machine-weight exercises, because while the weight is being lifted it must also be controlled. The exercising extremity must stabilize itself with the added weight and control the weight simultaneously. This requires work not only of the specific muscle being exercised, but also of the surrounding muscles.

One selects the exercise weight according to the strength of the muscle being exercised, while also considering the repetition and set goals. The weight should be heavy enough to challenge the patient yet light enough to allow him or her to accomplish the goals.

What determines the position in which the patient performs the exercise is the point in the motion where the greatest resistance is desired. For example, in an elbow curl, the greatest resistance in standing occurs when the elbow is at 90°. If the patient performs the exercise in supine, the greatest resistance is in the beginning of the exercise when the elbow begins to go into flexion from full extension. If a cuff weight is attached to a patient's ankle for a hamstring curl exercise, the maximum resistance occurs in the beginning of knee flexion if the patient is lying prone, but it occurs at 90° knee flexion if the exercise is performed in standing. This is so because the maximum resistance is determined by the relationship between the pull of gravity on the weight and the position of the segment being exercised. When the pull of gravity is perpendicular to the lever arm, the resistance is at its greatest. The sport rehabilitation specialist must determine where in the motion to place the primary emphasis for strength before selecting the proper position for the exercise.

When a muscle's position changes to attain a maximum resistance at a different angle, the stresses to the muscle change. If, for example, a patient has been performing an elbow curl with 4.5 kg (10 lb) in a supine position, when the patient changes to a sitting position the weight tolerance will be different. The maximum stress is now applied at the middle of the motion rather than at the beginning, and the muscles may not have the strength to lift 4.5 kg by the time the elbow moves to 90°. One must consider this when determining the patient's exercise position.

A pulley system is a form of free-weight system. A pulley board or other unit includes a cable to which a weight is attached and at least one, or most often two, pulleys. The pulleys are often adjustable to provide more variety in exercise positions. The position of the pulley and rope determines where in the range of motion the greatest resistance is provided to the muscle. This occurs when the line of the rope from the pulley to the extremity is at a 90° angle to the extremity. Figure 7.30 demonstrates this concept.

Again, you can change the maximum resistance by changing the angle of the force. In this case, the angle of the force is determined not by gravity but by the pulley position. These lever-arm concepts are presented in chapter 3.

The equipment should be secured before the patient is allowed to lift the weight. This means checking that the collars are secure so that they will not fall off during lifting. If the patient is using cuff weights, the straps should be in good shape and secured so that the weight will not fall off when the patient begins to move the extremity.

The amount of weight lifted must be adjusted as the patient's strength improves. Once strength improves, the weight's proportional resistance is reduced. The exercise becomes easier, and changes in strength do not occur unless the weight increases. You must periodically re-evaluate strength in order to determine whether or not the patient is ready for a resistance increase.

Advantages

With free weights, the amount of resistance offered to the patient is not limited by the sport rehabilitation specialist's strength. This is the most obvious advantage of free weights over manual resistance.

There is a variety of free-weight equipment on the market today, ranging from the plain, simple, and inexpensive to the complex, "gadgetized," and expensive. Selection depends on budget, space, needs, preference, and ability to use the equipment.

Free weights can be used in a number of ways to increase muscle strength, and they can be used in different positions to provide maximum resistance at varying angles. This can add variety to the therapeutic exercise program.

Another benefit is that free weights make it is easy to determine quantitative measures of strength and of improvement in strength. This gives the sport rehabilitation specialist an evaluative tool and provides the patient with an automatic motivating factor. The sport

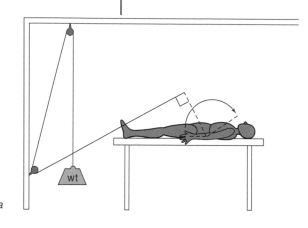

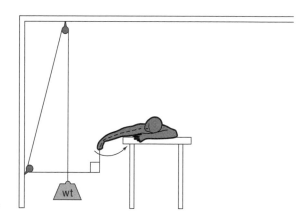

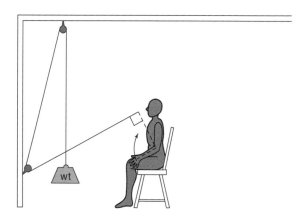

■ **Figure 7.30**   Different pulley angles for an elbow flexor strength exercise: *(a)* supine, *(b)* prone, *(c)* seated. Maximum resistance occurs when angle of pulley cable to the arm is 90°.

rehabilitation specialist can document objective improvements when the patient's weights change. The patient is motivated to increase the amount of weight lifted and feels a sense of accomplishment when achieving weight goals.

The cuff weights can be used in a functional activity when attached to the wrist or ankle. For example, an injured soccer player can add resistance kicking during activity by attaching a weight cuff to the ankle.

Disadvantages

The greatest disadvantage of free weights is safety, which you must always consider when using this equipment. The risk of injury if the weight is too great or is not used properly is a consistent danger. The patient should be instructed to use the weights correctly and to return them to their proper place when finished with the exercise. A patient cannot control a weight that is too heavy. In this situation the patient may drop the weight or strain a muscle.

Because lifting free weights is an isotonic activity, the amount of weight lifted is no greater than that which the muscle is able to lift at the weakest part of its motion. The amount of resistance changes as the lever-arm length changes, so the weight does not remain constant throughout the motion.

Finally, lifting weights can be boring. Patients who are bored are less likely to work as hard during the exercise. It is also more difficult to become motivated if the exercise is not interesting, and compliance may be more difficult.

ISOTONIC MACHINES

In addition to free weights, a variety of machines can be used for isotonic exercises. Some have a fixed lever system that offers different amounts of resistance. Changes in resistance occur differently, depending on the machine. The most commonly used machines provide altered resistance with weights, resistance bands, or hydraulic pressure. This category of equipment includes a long list of machines made by many companies. A list of generic examples includes hydraulic devices, multiple-station units, individual freestanding stations, and rubber-cord resistive machines.

Isotonic machines provide a constant load during an exercise. As with free weights, the load lifted is whatever the muscle at its weakest point is able to manage.

The design of some machines is such that one can control the allowable range of motion by placing a weight key at different positions on the weight's arm. This can change the excursion of the exercise and the weight lifted. For example, you can change a range-of-motion excursion on a bench-press machine by first elevating the bench-press arm and then inserting the key at the desired weight load.

Because the weights of these machines vary, they also allow performance of isometric exercises. To use the machine this way, you place the weight key at a weight that is too heavy for the patient to lift, or lock the lever so that movement is not possible.

Other simple isotonic "machines" fall into this category because they offer isotonic activity against a mechanical resistance. This group includes a large variety of equipment such as the N-K table (named after its two designers R.B. Noland and F.A. Kuckhoff), hand putty, and grip exercisers.

Technique

As always, instruction in proper use of the equipment and proper execution of the exercise is necessary. You should not assume that patients are able to perform an exercise correctly merely because they state that they have done the exercise before. Patients often either perform an exercise incorrectly or, because of weakness, use the wrong muscles to perform an exercise that was easy before they were injured. You should first demonstrate the exercise for the patient and then have the patient do the exercise while you observe for correct execution.

It is important to watch the speed of the exercise to observe for and caution against muscle substitution. Educate the patient regarding the proper speed and performance. This is especially important if you intend to have the patient perform the exercises independently later in the program. Changes in speed can occur with strength advances. As indicated with other exercises, the patient should perform a full range of motion.

Advantages

The greatest advantage in the use of isotonic machines is safety. The weight is guided and controlled by the machine, so the chances of injury resulting from the weight's dropping or the patient's losing control of the machine are very slim.

The multiple-station units allow many patients to work simultaneously. You can easily establish a circuit program on the machine so that either one patient or several can exercise at one time.

Once the exercises have been established, the patient can exercise without assistance. The sport rehabilitation specialist can perform periodic reevaluation with increases in repetitions, sets, or weights. The treatment time can then be used for other, more directed activities.

It is easy to establish an exercise progression on the machine by changing the numbers of repetitions or sets, the speed of the exercise, or the resistance. Changing these parameters can also add some variety to a therapeutic exercise program.

Weight machines most often have either a specific weight indication or an arbitrary number indication on the plates. This permits an objective measure of improvement. Quantifying gains introduces a motivating factor and is an objective measure of progress for both the patient and the sport rehabilitation specialist.

Some pieces of equipment are not expensive; some can even be hand made and modified to fit specific clinic or individual needs. For example, a wrist exerciser can be made from a weight disk, dowel, and rope.

Disadvantages

Some of the disadvantages of isotonic machines are the same as for free weights. One is that the muscle's weakest point determines the maximum weight that can be lifted.

Using equipment can be boring. It may be difficult to motivate patients to perform daily exercises on the machines.

Additionally, some isotonic machines are very expensive and require considerable facility space. This is particularly true for the individual freestanding machines. The multi-unit machines may require less space, but they are also expensive, and many still require a relatively large space for installation and operation.

ISOKINETIC MACHINES

Isokinetic exercise machines have been available since the early 1970s. They were very popular during the 1970s and 1980s. Several manufacturers produced isokinetic equipment during the 1980s. Today, emphasis has moved away from isokinetic equipment, and the demand has dwindled drastically. Today, there are only two manufacturers—Biodex (Biodex Corporation, Shirley, NY) and Cybex (Henley Health Care, Cybex Medical Division, Sugarland, TX). The Biodex is shown in figure 7.31.

Isokinetic machines offer resistance at a constant speed, so the amount of resistance varies through the range of motion. This is sometimes referred to as *accommodating resistance*. To produce a constant speed, the machine offers a matching resistance when the patient attempts to push the arm of the machine as hard as possible. For an isokinetic exercise to produce the desired results, the patient must resist the machine with maximal muscle activity.

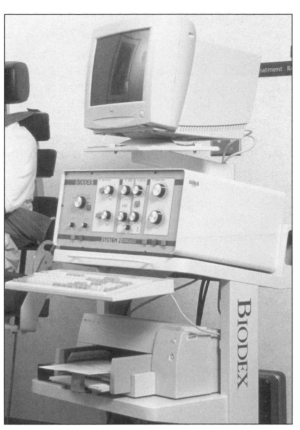

∎ Figure 7.31
Isokinetic machine.

Technique

The machines today offer resistance concentrically, eccentrically, and isometrically. The type of exercise used depends on the settings established on the machine by the sport rehabilitation specialist. The settings are determined according to the specific goals and the type of exercise the sport rehabilitation specialist decides is the best method of achieving those goals.

The speed of the isokinetic machine is preset before the exercise begins. Settings range from very slow (less than 30°/s) to very fast (over 300°/s). Even at the fastest settings, the speeds do not mimic the speeds of motion during functional activities. For example, throwing a ball results in forearm speeds greater than 9000°/s (Braatz and Gogia 1987). Even normal walking produces a swing-through-phase speed of about 48 kph (30 mph). One of the early claims of isokinetic advocates was that the isokinetic machines could mimic functional speeds; now that we can measure true joint speeds we know that this is not the case.

It is necessary to instruct the patient in proper execution on the equipment. The exercise sensation is not necessarily one that the patient has experienced before, since other equipment provides a variation in resistance and speed whereas isokinetic equipment forces the patient's speed to remain constant throughout the motion.

Isokinetic equipment can be used at submaximal levels. This is particularly important if the patient's injury is recent or if the patient has too much pain to permit a maximal-resistance output. It is important to explain to the patient the goal of the exercise if that goal is less-than-maximal output.

The equipment should be properly set before the exercise begins. Isokinetic machines can be placed in a variety of positions to be used on a variety of joints. Proper alignment of the machine's joint is necessary to avoid placing undue torque on the patient's joint. Correct machine lever-arm length should also be determined before the beginning of exercise.

Instructions should include precautions about avoiding pain during the exercise and eliminating substitution by other muscle groups. Stabilization straps should be applied to ensure minimum substitution. If the patient experiences pain, changes in the exercise parameter settings are indicated.

Advantages

Isokinetic equipment provides a constant-speed, accommodating-resistance exercise to produce a maximum muscle resistance throughout the range of motion.

The machines can be used for maximal and submaximal muscle output. Less-than-maximal output can be controlled to permit exercise without increasing injury. Likewise, use of a maximal muscle output can provide increased stress to the muscle as the healing and muscle's tolerance improve.

Diagonal patterns can be performed on the equipment to produce a more functional form of exercise. This can assist the muscles in relearning functional activities.

The machine produces measurable and reproducible results and can be used for testing as well as exercising. The machine's computer records the muscle's output throughout the range of motion and can correlate the strength with a specific degree within the motion.

The computer's visual readings provide immediate feedback to the patient and to the sport rehabilitation specialist. Goals can also be indicated on the screen. This information serves to motivate the patient as a goal is established and results of efforts toward it can be seen. The sport rehabilitation specialist also receives immediate information about the patient's effort, areas of weakness through the range of motion, and points at which there should be greater emphasis in other therapeutic exercises.

Comparison of records between one session and another also provides feedback on progress. Maintaining a record reveals concrete and objective changes in the patient's progress.

The machine's speeds can be varied, so a patient can exercise at slower or faster speeds to work on fast-twitch and slow-twitch muscles in the same session. Exercises can be used to improve strength, muscle endurance, coordination, and speed of movement.

Disadvantages

Isokinetic machines have two primary disadvantages. One is cost: An isokinetic machine, with the equipment and computer, costs over $40,000. Many facilities find this price prohibitive. The other clear disadvantage is that the exercises are primarily open kinetic chain exercises. This makes them often nonfunctional, especially for the lower extremity.

Another disadvantage is that in performing evaluations, the sport rehabilitation specialist must remain consistent with respect to speed, settings, and positions from one session to another in order to obtain consistent results. Changing anything during the activity, even the motivating commands, can alter the results.

Some sport rehabilitation specialists find the setup of the machine and the need to change its position and pieces of equipment too complicated and too time consuming to be practical. This is the case especially if the machine is used infrequently.

Isokinetic computers can offer a great deal of information on the patient's performance. This can be an advantage or a disadvantage. It can be advantageous if the sport rehabilitation specialist understands the information and its significance for the therapeutic exercise program. It is disadvantageous, however, if he or she does not understand the data and does not take time to learn their significance. In this case, the sport rehabilitation specialist may be frustrated and intimidated by the information and instead of using the machine, discard it as impractical.

If many patients are using the machine for therapeutic exercise, they may need to wait their turns. One patient may use the machine for several bouts of exercise or for various positions. This takes time and can prohibit its use by others for extended periods. In situations in which a sport rehabilitation specialist has limited time to spend with a patient, this may not be a piece of equipment that is available at the right time or convenient to use.

OTHER EQUIPMENT

Other accommodating-resistance machines provide variable resistance through the range of motion. One type of equipment, familiar in gyms, is known as Nautilus (Nautilus, Deland, FL)—so named because its cam resembles the cross section of the shell of the sea mollusk nautilus. Machines of this type offer a variable resistance through a cam system. The cam allows the lever-arm length of the machine to change so that the amount of resistance changes. These changes are supposed to coincide with the change in the muscle's lever arm, so that as the muscle's strength changes, a concomitant change in the resistance is offered to it by the machine; however, because these machines are not designed for all body sizes, the machine's resistance may not match the individual's muscle-length changes through its range of motion.

Smaller men and many women may find that the machines do not accommodate their lever-arm lengths. In these cases, using the machines may cause injury.

Other machines and exercise equipment are available for strengthening. Some of these devices are mentioned in other chapters in connection with such topics as proprioception. Nautilus and other machines may not be indicated for therapeutic exercise use, especially in the earlier stages of rehabilitation. The sport rehabilitation specialist must understand the functions, the weight minimums and increments, and the way in which each machine operates before determining whether or not a piece of equipment is appropriate for a patient's use. The patient's abilities, healing phase, size, injury limitations, and restrictions are all factors to consider before advocating the use of any machine.

PROPRIOCEPTIVE NEUROMUSCULAR FACILITATION

Exercise techniques based on proprioceptive neuromuscular facilitation use impulses from the afferent receptors in various parts of the body to stimulate the desired motion. One such technique, reversal of antagonists, is common in sport rehabilitation because it mimics daily and sport performance activities.

Sherrington, a neurophysiologist, provided the basic concepts that were used by Herman Kabat, MD, during the late 1940s and early 1950s to develop **proprioceptive neuromuscular facilitation (PNF)** exercise techniques. The underlying significance of this technique was in the use of combinations of primitive movement patterns performed with a maximum amount of resistance applied throughout the range of motion. The techniques were originally found to be useful in the treatment of neuromuscular disorders, but over time they have also proven beneficial for application to orthopedic disorders. Proprioceptive neuromuscular facilitation has been helpful in restoring flexibility, strength, and coordination of injured muscles and joints.

FACILITATION

It is in this sense—restoration—that sport rehabilitation specialists use PNF today. Proprioceptive neuromuscular facilitation incorporates the inhibitory and excitatory impulses from the afferent receptors of skin, muscle, tendon, verbal, and auditory neurons that facilitate a response from the motor neurons, resulting in a desired action. For example, the sport rehabilitation specialist's hands on the patient's leg provide a stimulus from the skin receptors; a stretch force applied by the sport rehabilitation specialist on the muscle stimulates the muscle spindle and Golgi tendon organs; the patient's ability to see where the leg is going stimulates the patient's oculomotor system to produce the desired motion pattern; and the verbal cueing and guidance of the sport rehabilitation specialist during the activity stimulate the patient's auditory receptors to send messages to increase or decrease muscle activity.

Each of these afferent stimuli can influence the motor response. To see the significance of this point, you can easily perform a couple of simple tests. With a patient lying supine, place one hand on the hamstring and one hand on the quadriceps. Ask the patient to resist you in a straight-leg raise, and judge the amount of resistance the patient provides. Now place your hands only on the quadriceps and have the patient repeat the resisted movement. You should experience greater resistance with both of your hands on the quadriceps surface and less resistance with one hand on the hamstrings and one on the quadriceps. With tactile input of both surfaces, the afferent stimulation is a mixed one, producing both facilitation in and inhibition to the anterior muscles. When both hands are on the same surface, facilitation to the muscles performing the action is provided without inhibition from sensory nerves of the hamstring surface.

A quick stretch provided in a PNF movement immediately before the exercise produces a stretch reflex from stimulation of the muscle spindles and Golgi tendon organs. This causes increased response from the muscle.

Taking the patient's leg passively through the activity before performing the actual exercise gives the patient the visual feedback to realize the direction and pattern that the leg should traverse. If you do not do this before the exercise, you will find not only that the patient is confused about what to do, but also that the output of the muscle is significantly less. The more confidence the patient has about being able to perform the pattern correctly, the stronger the motion will be.

Verbal input is used commonly in athletic events. We do it when we cheer a team or player during competition. When we want a patient to perform an exercise at a maximal output, we use verbal cues to encourage him or her to do the most work possible. Verbal cues in PNF provide the same stimulus. They are also necessary for permitting the patient to correctly perform the pattern of activity desired. Cueing with brief, well-timed words and phrases facilitates an improved muscle response.

PATTERNS OF MOVEMENT

The premise underlying PNF is that central nervous system stimulation produces mass movement patterns, not straight-plane movements. Natural motion does not occur in straight planes but in mass movement patterns that incorporate a diagonal motion in combination with a spiral movement. In other words, all major parts of the body move in patterns that have three components. These diagonal patterns include the components of flexion and extension. Because the patterns are diagonal, they also include motions either toward and across the midline (adduction) or away and across the midline (abduction). Rotation is the third component of PNF patterns. Figure 7.32 demonstrates these components. Although PNF can be used for the trunk as well as the extremities, discussion of PNF here is limited to the upper and lower extremities, since these are the areas primarily treated in sports medicine with PNF.

The movement patterns are referred to as D1 and D2. D1 flexion and D1 extension patterns are moving into flexion and into extension, respectively. D2 patterns are divided in the same way.

This is easier to remember if you recall that in the upper extremity, external rotation always goes with flexion, and in the lower extremity, external rotation always goes with adduction. For example, in the upper extremity as the shoulder goes from extension to flexion it always externally rotates whether the movement is adducted or abducted (figure 7.33a). So when the arm goes into extension, the shoulder internally rotates, and the varying motion is either adduction in a D1 pattern or abduction in a D2 pattern.

Because external rotation accompanies adduction in the lower extremity, when the hip is moved into flexion the movement also includes external rotation when it is adducted and internal rotation when it is abducted (figure 7.33b). On the other hand, when the hip moves into extension, it also has external rotation if it is adducted (D2) and internal rotation if it is abducted (D1).

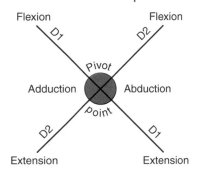

▌Figure 7.32 PNF patterns: Neural motion occurs in diagonal planes of component motions.

▌Figure 7.33 (a) External rotation is associated with flexion while internal rotation is associated with extension in the upper extremities. (b) In the lower extremities, adduction and external rotation occur together as do abduction and internal rotation.

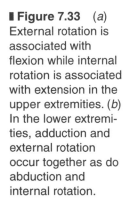
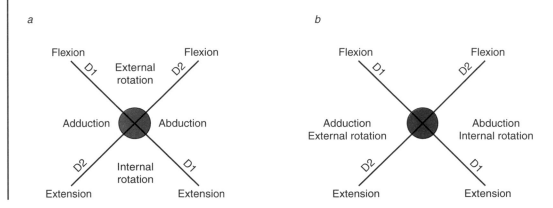

When you think about it, these are natural patterns that you see every day in sport and daily activities. For example, when throwing a ball overhand, the arm starts in abduction, flexion, and external rotation. As the ball is thrown, the follow-through ends with the arm in an extension, adduction, and internal-rotation position. Kicking a soccer ball also demonstrates the PNF pattern: As the ball is kicked the leg moves from extension, abduction, and internal rotation to a follow-through position of flexion, adduction, and external rotation. When you sit in a relaxed position with your feet up and hands behind your head, the shoulder is in flexion, abduction, and external rotation, and your legs are extended in front of you, crossed, and in adduction and external rotation.

If you remember these natural positions, the patterns of movement for the part of the extremity beyond the shoulder and hip should make sense. Figures 7.34 and 7.35 diagram and illustrate the positions of the other joints.

In each position, the joints go from one extreme to the other by the time the movement is complete. For example, if the patient begins with the shoulder extended, abducted, and internally rotated, the elbow extended, the forearm pronated, the wrist ulnarly extended, and the fingers and thumb extended, the end position will be the D1 flexion position—in shoulder flexion, adduction, and external rotation, elbow flexion, forearm supination, wrist radially flexed, and fingers and thumb flexed and adducted. Note that the elbow and the knee can be moved from flexion to extension or extension to flexion with any of the patterns. The position the elbow or knee is in at the end of the motion is the opposite of its position at the beginning of the movement.

Essentially, all that has been written about PNF in recent years has been based on the works of Knott and Voss (1968). The patterns of movement, techniques, and principles most commonly used today center on the information these authors have provided to the medical community. For the best results, they advocate the use of basic principles in the application of PNF.

PRINCIPLES

The principles of application incorporate the physiological facilitation and inhibition responses of the body to stimuli. Effective use of these responses produces an optimum result. The primary principles of application are the following:

1. *The sport rehabilitation specialist's hand placement is important for providing appropriate facilitation of the deep-touch and pressure receptors.* The hands should be placed on the surface side toward which the extremity is to move to stimulate those muscles. For example, if the patient's hip is moving into extension, the knee is flexing, and the foot is plantar flexing, the hamstrings and plantar foot should be the points of contact.

Manual contact using appropriately applied pressure also helps guide the patient's extremity in the correct direction. The contact should be firm and reassuring, not painful or hesitant.

2. *Verbal cues are given in a moderate tone if the patient is providing a maximal output.* If additional force is desired, a stronger, sharp verbal command is given. The wording should be one- or two-word phrases, simple and meaningful. For example, "push" or "pull," "hold" or "relax," and "rotate" or "across" are all simple commands that give the patient easy-to-understand, clear instructions. The commands should be timed correctly in relation to the activity.

3. *The technique should not be painful.* Pain will produce a reflex withdrawal and cause an inhibition of activity rather than a facilitation.

4. *Proper instruction in the PNF pattern before the start of exercise is important if the muscles are to receive optimal facilitation.* The patient should receive simple instructions

Joint	D1 flexion	D2 flexion
Shoulder:	Flexion	Flexion
	External rotation	External rotation
	Adduction	Abduction
Forearm:	Supination	Supination
Wrist:	Radial flexion	Radial extension
Fingers:	Flexion	Extension

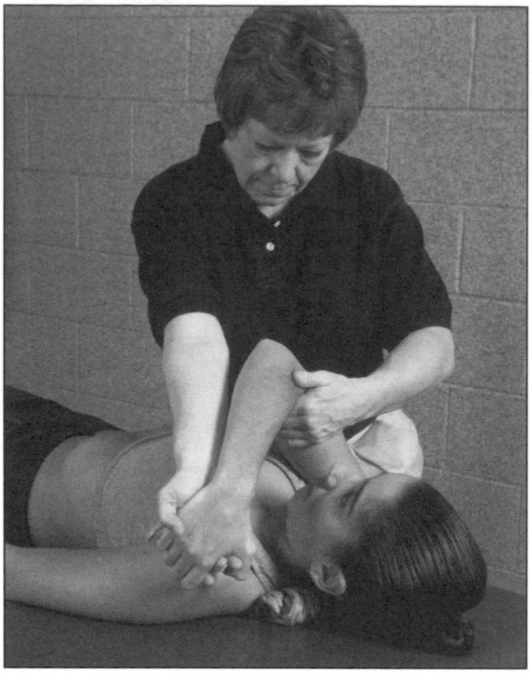

D1 flexion

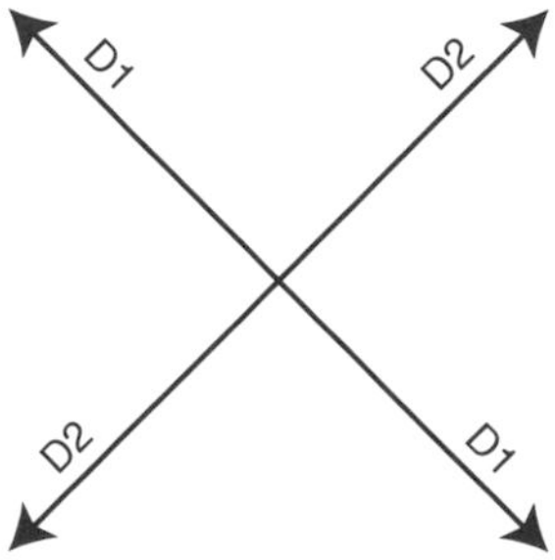

Joint	D2 extension	D1 extension
Shoulder:	Extension	Extension
	Internal rotation	Internal rotation
	Adduction	Abduction
Forearm:	Pronation	Pronation
Wrist:	Ulnar flexion	Ulnar extension
Fingers:	Flexion	Extension

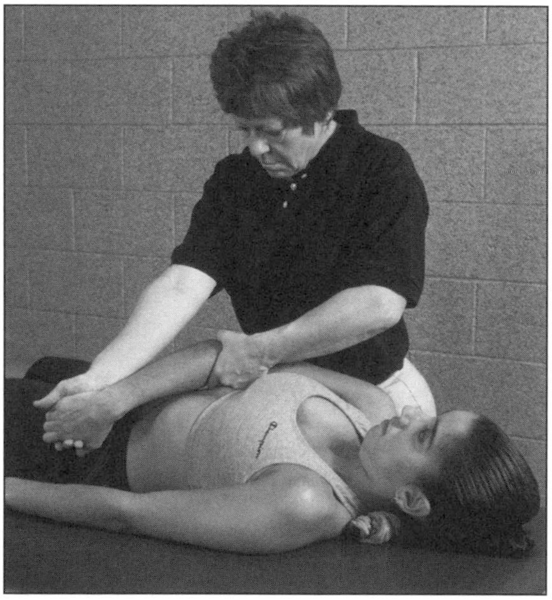

D2 extension

Figure 7.34 Upper-extremity PNF patterns.

that include the sequencing of activities, the diagonal pattern, and appropriate speed of activity. If the patient knows before execution what is expected and understands the exercise, the patient is better able to perform the activity and elicit a stronger response from the muscle. The visual stimulation of seeing the movement before performance of the exercise provides additional feedback for the patient's increased facilitation of the muscles.

5. *Rotation is an important component of the diagonal motion.* It begins distally and progresses toward the proximal muscle groups as the patient continues through the

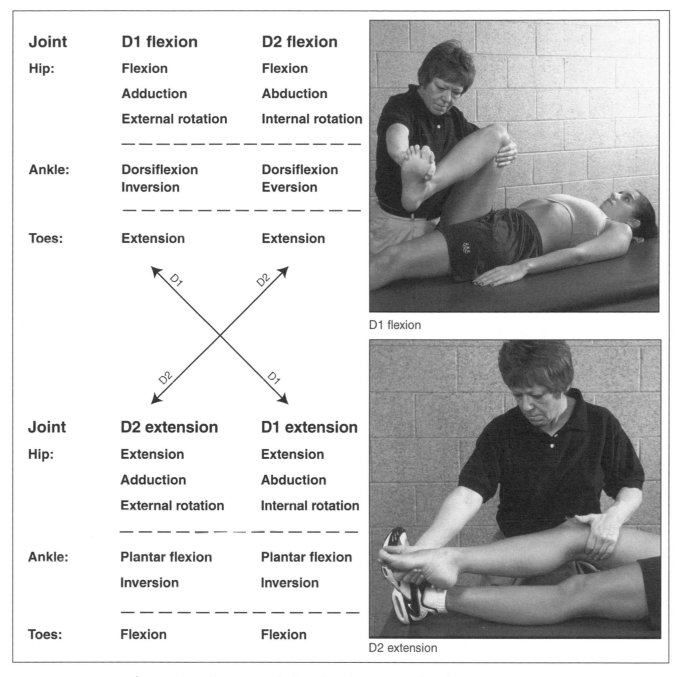

Joint	D1 flexion	D2 flexion
Hip:	Flexion	Flexion
	Adduction	Abduction
	External rotation	Internal rotation
Ankle:	Dorsiflexion	Dorsiflexion
	Inversion	Eversion
Toes:	Extension	Extension

D1 flexion

Joint	D2 extension	D1 extension
Hip:	Extension	Extension
	Adduction	Abduction
	External rotation	Internal rotation
Ankle:	Plantar flexion	Plantar flexion
	Inversion	Inversion
Toes:	Flexion	Flexion

D2 extension

❚ **Figure 7.35** Lower-extremity PNF patterns.

motion. Proper verbal cueing for correct distal-to-proximal movement assists the patient in proper execution of the exercise.

6. *Providing traction to separate the joint surfaces or approximation to compress the joint surfaces stimulates the joint's proprioceptive nerve endings.* As a general rule, traction is used in the pulling motions and approximation is used in the pushing motions. If a joint is very irritable, traction or approximation may aggravate it; one must use caution and good judgment before applying this technique.

7. *A quick stretch applied immediately before the beginning of the movement pattern uses the stretch reflex to facilitate the muscle into a stronger initial response.* In some injuries, a stretch may be contraindicated. Once again, caution and good judgment are needed before a quick stretch is applied.

8. *The motions are performed precisely and through a smooth range of motion.* The movement is not jerky. Isometric contractions should build until maximal output from the

patient's muscle is achieved. No motion is produced by an isometric activity, and the sport rehabilitation specialist does not break the isometric hold.

9. *The sport rehabilitation specialist must use good body mechanics.* Application of manual resistance in PNF techniques requires that the sport rehabilitation specialist use his or her own body efficiently and safely and conserve energy. Proper body mechanics makes this possible.

TECHNIQUES

Stretching techniques of PNF, including hold-relax, contract-relax, and slow reversal-hold-relax, are discussed in chapter 5. The techniques used for strengthening are repeated contractions, rhythmic initiation, slow reversal, slow reversal-hold, and rhythmic stabilization.

Repeated contractions is a technique used with very weak muscles or with muscles that have specific areas of weakness within their range of motion. Repeated isotonic activity of the weak muscle is performed until fatigue occurs. In more advanced procedures, an isometric activity in the weaker portion of the motion can be incorporated with the isotonic movement.

Rhythmic initiation is used to increase a muscle's ability to initiate movement. It includes voluntary relaxation, passive movement, and repeated isotonic activity of the agonistic muscles. This technique is used to help an individual initiate movement in situations of diseases of the neuromuscular system such as Parkinson's, and is rarely advantageous for sport rehabilitation.

The techniques involving reversal of antagonists are the ones most commonly used in sport rehabilitation. They most mimic normal activity because they incorporate the use of first one muscle group and then its opposing muscle group, much as daily activities and sport performance activities do.

Slow reversal is a reversal-of-antagonists technique that provides a maximum resistance from the sport rehabilitation specialist throughout a range of motion. This is followed by resistance to the opposite motion. For example, the sport rehabilitation specialist applies resistance to the upper-extremity D1 pattern going into flexion. At the completion of the agonistic movement, the sport rehabilitation specialist reverses hand positions on the patient's arm to provide resistance to D1 going into extension against the antagonists. In the slow reversal-hold technique, the procedure is the same except that an isometric hold is performed at the end of the motion.

Rhythmic stabilization uses isometric activity of agonists and antagonists. The sport rehabilitation specialist offers resistance that does not break the isometric activity of the antagonist and then offers resistance to isometric activity of the agonist. This produces a co-contraction to improve stabilization. The technique is repeated several times without movement of the extremity. It can be repeated at several points within the range of motion.

These techniques can be applied individually or in combination. Their use is determined by the patient's deficiencies and needs.

STRENGTHENING PRINCIPLES

The sport rehabilitation specialist should be deliberate about when in a program to start strengthening exercises and should follow the principles of specificity, no pain, attainable goals, and progressive overload.

When do strengthening exercises begin in a therapeutic exercise program? The answer depends on the severity of the injury, the tissue injured, the physician's preference, and the patient's tolerance. Once a therapeutic exercise program starts, strengthening exercises at some level should begin. At first they may be no more than isometrics or exercises that concentrate on areas adjacent to the injured site. Chapter 2 addresses the importance of rest and the importance of activity. The sport rehabilitation specialist makes a careful judgment and considers the variable factors to determine when the strengthening exercises should occur and how intense they should be.

The sport rehabilitation specialist should have a sound reason for using any strengthening exercise in a patient's therapeutic exercise program. Use of many exercises that have the same goal and that work the same muscle may be a waste of time unless the specific goal is to increase muscle endurance and provide variety to prevent boredom. The sport rehabilitation specialist should design a therapeutic exercise program specific to the needs of the patient as determined by analysis of the patient's deficiencies and knowledge of the demands of the patient's sport. A strengthening program may emphasize primarily strength or muscle endurance or a combination of these.

Progression of a patient in a therapeutic exercise program is individually determined. Each patient is different. Expectations based on other patients' progression or the sport rehabilitation specialist's hopes are unrealistic and unfair. You should continually evaluate the patient during the treatment program so that you can accurately determine the response to treatment and maintain an optimal course of treatment.

A strengthening program is designed according to four principles. The acronym **SNAP** stands for the primary concerns in the establishment of any strengthening program:

Specific exercises
No pain
Attainable goals
Progressive overload

Let's look at each of these issues individually.

SPECIFIC EXERCISES

A therapeutic exercise program should contain specific exercises to achieve the long-term goal, the patient's return to sport performance. This concept is often referred to as the **SAID** principle: Specific Adaptations to Imposed Demands (Wallis and Logan 1964). This means that the muscle will adapt and perform according to the demands placed on it. For example, if a patient lifts low weights for high repetitions, the muscle will gain endurance. If a patient wants to gain strength, exercises should be close to his or her 1 RM and consist of less than six repetitions. The SAID principle also means that exercises should mimic stresses placed on a muscle during functional activities to produce appropriate strength gains. If a patient's sport calls for sustained activity, such as holding a pike position on the parallel bars in gymnastics, then the strength exercises for that patient should include isometric hip flexor and abdominal exercises. If the patient's sport is soccer, which does not demand sustained movements, the therapeutic exercise program for that patient requires more isotonic endurance- and power-related activities.

Since a muscle's greatest recovery occurs in the first 30 to 90 s following exercise to exhaustion, the design of the therapeutic exercise program should take this into account (figure 7.36). As a muscle continues an activity, the maximal output declines as fatigue becomes more of a factor with progressive repetitions. Exercise sets should include a rest period of 30 to 60 s between each set. A rule of thumb is a 1:1 ratio between the time it takes to perform the exercise and the rest time. Later in the program the patient may need more or less rest, depending on the intensity of the exercise and the demands of the patient's sport.

a

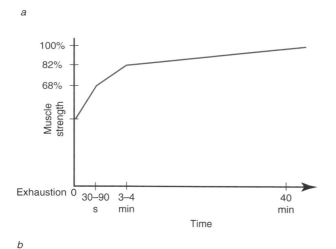

b

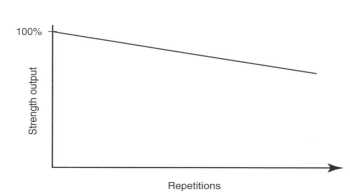

■ Figure 7.36 Effects of fatigue on strength and recovery: *(a)* recovery from fatigue, *(b)* maximal output declines with fatigue from repetitious activity.

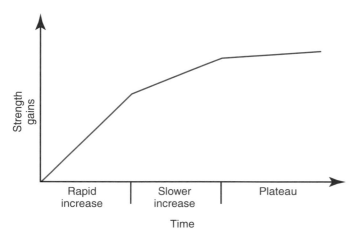

■ Figure 7.37 Rate of strength gains in a rehabilitation program.

In the early stages of a therapeutic exercise program, rapid gains in strength are commonly seen in a debilitated or deconditioned muscle. This occurs during the first three to five weeks of a therapeutic exercise program without a change in the muscle's atrophy (Moritani and deVries 1979). Many believe that these initial strength gains are primarily the result of neural adaptations within the muscle's neuromuscular system.

Reflex inhibition of the muscle occurs with injury or inactivity. Immediate weakness is present after surgery as well. These sudden declines in strength are attributable to decreased neural activity. Because neural adaptations occur quickly with injury, it is postulated that they are also affected with attempts to restore the injured part.

Strength is determined by both muscle fiber and neural control. The initial rapid gains in strength are attributed to improved neuromuscular recruitment, efficiency, coordination, and motor unit re-education. Many researchers believe that improved neural activation results in an increased activation of synergists with a better coordination and co-contraction of the synergists, an inhibition of the antagonists, and improved activation ability and sensitivity to facilitation of the prime movers. A learning factor also affects the neural element of muscle activity.

Although evidence to date appears to be anecdotal only, clinical observation has indicated that the rate of strength gains decreases as a therapeutic exercise program advances in time and duration (Houglum 1977) (figure 7.37). Once the neural components have been retrained, the gains are primarily made through muscle fiber hypertrophy. The greatest gains in strength occur in the early stages of a therapeutic exercise program—presenting the probability that neural changes are more significant than muscle size changes, especially in rehabilitation. Primary hypertrophic changes occur more commonly in patients who have lifted weights over a longer period of time or who use drugs to enhance hypertrophy.

In the early stages of a therapeutic exercise program, especially in cases in which muscle inactivity has been prolonged, the initial exercise efforts should emphasize facilitation of the neural elements of the atrophied muscle. In addition to active exercise, electrical stimulation to assist in the facilitation of these neural pathways and in facilitation of proper muscle response may expedite recovery.

Refer to Denegar's (2000) text, *Therapeutic Modalities for Athletic Injuries*, in the Athletic Training Education Series, for specifics on the application of electrical stimulation for muscle facilitation.

If a therapeutic exercise program following severe injury or surgery is prolonged, you can observe the cycle of rapid increase, slower increase, and plateau. These changes can occur over one cycle or more than one cycle. The pattern is individually determined and not predictable. If the patient reaches a plateau early in the program before achieving goals, you should explain that this is not unusual and that gains will come if the patient persists in the program. This situation can be difficult for the patient, since it may seem that no amount of effort produces gains. Patience and perseverance are key to maintaining a good motivation level during this time. Sometimes the psychological lift of having a day off from the therex program can have a rejuvenating effect.

NO PAIN

There should be no pain during strengthening exercises. Delayed pain or postexercise pain should be avoided. Postexercise pain accompanied by postexercise edema is an indication that the exercises have been too severe. It is advisable to reduce the severity of the exercise or even postpone the application of a strengthening exercise if you observe these symptoms. Pain produces a reflex withdrawal of muscle activity so that the muscle will not achieve an optimal output. Progression of strengthening exercises should be gradual and within the patient's tolerance. If you increase resistance too much too quickly, the patient's body may experience an inflammatory response. Increased edema and pain are key signs of inflammation.

ATTAINABLE GOALS

Goals for the patient should be challenging but attainable. This means that it should be possible for the patient to move the selected weight for the required number of repetitions and sets and to perform the specific exercise. Most patients are goal-oriented and are determined to achieve any goal set for them, by themselves or by others. If goals are not achievable, the unrealistic expectations placed on the patient will serve only to frustrate both you and the patient. If you discover during the course of the exercise routine that you have set too high a goal, it is best to adjust the goal. Occasionally you may need to adjust goals according to the patient's response to the previous exercise session. This is more often the case early in the rehabilitation program when you may not yet know the patient's abilities, motivation level, and response to treatments. Realistic expectations are the key to a good therapeutic exercise session.

PROGRESSIVE OVERLOAD

Providing a **progressive overload** of exercises is key to muscle strengthening. To continue to produce strength gains, the load must be progressively greater. This concept is sometimes referred to as the **overload principle:** As a muscle's strength increases, the muscle must be overloaded. For example, if a biceps can lift 8 kg, it must lift more resistance than 8 kg in order to achieve increased strength. If the muscle lifts 8 kg repeatedly from one exercise session to the next, its strength will be maintained but will not increase. The weight must be greater than 8 kg, but still be possible to lift, in order to produce strength gains.

When it is not possible to actively exercise the injured area, **cross-training** can produce strength gains. Cross-training occurs when the contralateral part is exercised, resulting in strength gains on the opposite extremity. This form of training, sometimes also referred to as *cross-education,* has been around since the 1800s and has been used with varying degrees of success. The results depend primarily on the amount of resistance provided to the exercising extremity: The greater the effort of the extremity, the greater the results. This is a useful technique that you can apply in therapeutic exercise programs when the patient's injured area is restricted, perhaps because it is in a cast or splint, and exercise of the part is limited.

EXERCISE PROGRESSION

Several commonly used progressive overload systems are available. Each sport rehabilitation specialist combines knowledge of these systems with his or her own experience to select or design a system that will work best for each patient.

A progressive overload can be applied using various systems of progression. Several programs have been advocated by a number of professionals over the years and have been used rather widely in sports medicine.

DeLorme and Watkins (1948) provided a system that would serve as a basis of progressive strengthening for many years. They used 10 RM as a maximum strength. They advocated the use of three bouts, or sets, of exercise, 10 repetitions each: The first set is at 50% of maximum, the second set at 75% of maximum, and the final set at 100% of the 10 RM (table 7.4).

Zinovieff, a physician who worked at England's United Oxford Hospitals, published a revision of the DeLorme program that he named the Oxford Technique (1951). Zinovieff found that with the DeLorme system his patients were too fatigued to complete the final set of 10 RM exercises. He suggested reversing the system, starting with the 10 RM on the first set of 10 repetitions and progressively reducing to 75% and then 50% on each successive set of 10 repetitions (table 7.5).

A number of authors have advanced a variety of other resistive exercise progressions. One of the more frequently used systems is the **DAPRE** (**D**aily **A**djusted **P**rogressive **R**esistive **E**xercise) technique (Knight 1985). This is a complex system of daily exercise (six days a week) progression that meets the individual's ability to tolerate increased resistance. Table 7.6 illustrates the establishment of an RM and number of repetitions along with the determination of the next session's exercise weight.

The essential element of DAPRE is that on the third and fourth sets of exercise, the patient performs as many repetitions as possible. The number of repetitions the individual can perform on the third set determines the amount of weight to be added for the fourth set of the day as well as for the next treatment session.

Table 7.4	DeLorme and Watkins Strength Progression	
Set	**Repetitions**	**Weight**
1	10	50% of 10 RM
2	10	75% of 10 RM
3	10	100% of 10 RM

Table 7.5	Oxford Technique of Strength Progression	
Set	**Repetitions**	**Weight**
1	10	100% of 10 RM
2	10	75% of 10 RM
3	10	50% of 10 RM

Table 7.6 DAPRE System of Strength Progression

Technique

Set	Repetitions	Weight
1	10	50% of working weight
2	6	75% of working weight
3	As many as possible	100% of working weight
4	As many as possible	Adjusted from 3rd set*

*See Adjustment guidelines below

Adjustment guidelines

Number of repetitions performed during prior set	4th-set weight adjustment based on 3rd set	Next-day weight adjustment based on 4th set
0–2	↓ wt; redo set	↓ wt; redo set
3–4	↓ by 0–5 lb	Keep the same
5–7	Keep the same	↑ by 5–10 lb
8–12	↑ by 5–10 lb	↑ by 5–15 lb
13 or more	↑ by 10–15 lb	↑ by 10–20 lb

The number of repetitions performed on the third set determines the weight used on the fourth set. The next treatment day's starting weight is determined by the number of repetitions performed on the fourth set of the previous treatment.

Based on Knight 1985.

The intent of the program is to have the patient perform as many repetitions during the set as possible. The goal is 5 to 7 repetitions. If the patient does 8 to 12 repetitions, the weight change is minimal; but if the patient performs 15 to 20 repetitions, the weight change is significantly larger. This program continues until the strength of the injured part is within 10% of the strength of the noninjured counterpart. At that time the emphasis shifts to other deficiencies such as muscle endurance or coordination, and the DAPRE program is continued twice a week to maintain strength.

Most certified athletic trainers develop an exercise routine that seems to work best for them in achieving progression of a patient's strength. In the early stages of strengthening, the program I prefer has the patient lifting a weight that can be controlled for 6 to 15 repetitions for two sets. That weight is continued, with the patient's attempting to perform as many repetitions as possible, until he or she is able to perform the exercise successfully for three sets of 20 to 25 repetitions each. At this point the weight increases and the patient reduces the number of repetitions. It is important, though, for the patient to perform as many repetitions as possible during each exercise session. The number of sets and repetitions depends on the demands of the patient's sport. Once the patient has achieved the desired base-strength level, the number of sets, the number of repetitions, or the speed of the exercise changes to meet the patient's sport demands.

As mentioned earlier in this chapter, Wathen (1994) advocates the use of three to six repetitions for strength gains, repeated for about three sets. Figure 7.38 shows the relative gains in muscle strength and endurance with varying numbers of repetitions.

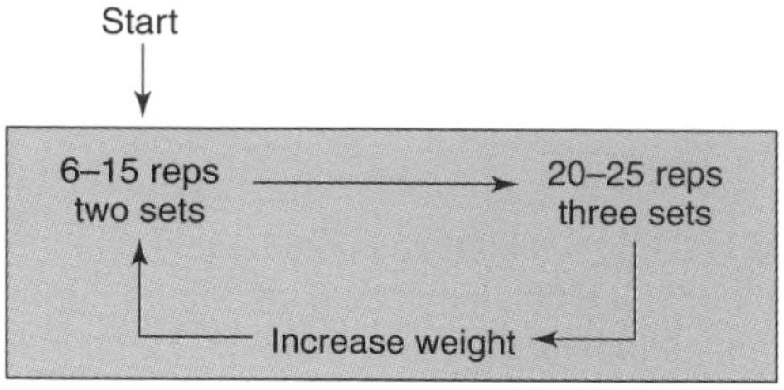

Start

6–15 reps
two sets $\longrightarrow$ 20–25 reps
three sets

Increase weight

■ **Figure 7.38** Houglum progression.

The program that the sport rehabilitation specialist chooses depends on individual preferences, on his or her judgment about which program would benefit the patient most, and on time availability. All the programs we have considered have been shown to be beneficial for making strength gains. As you gain experience over time with many patients who have varied therapeutic exercise needs, you will find a system that seems to work best for you. Until then, I recommend that you keep an open mind, try different programs, and investigate the systems presented here as well as others to see what produces the best results for you. Whether you use an existing program or design one yourself, the key element for success is that it must be progressive; it must continue to stress the patient's muscles for continuing improvement toward the specific rehabilitation goals. Experienced professionals often adjust programs according to what produces the best results.

SUMMARY

1. *Describe the sarcomere and its function in muscle activity.*

   The contractile element of a muscle fiber is the sarcomere. Actin and myosin filaments and their relationship to each other via cross-bridges determine the length of the sarcomere and its activity status. A complex system of biochemical processes and the stimulation of an action potential produces muscle activity through the release of calcium and ATP to cause a sliding of actin and myosin over each other, shortening the sarcomere's length.

2. *Identify the elements of a motor unit.*

   A motor unit consists of a number of muscle fibers and the nerve that innervates the fibers. When stimulated, a motor unit behaves according to the all-or-none law in that all muscle fibers of the motor unit contract.

3. *Explain how an action potential is transmitted.*

   The sarcoplasmic reticulum releases calcium to the muscle fibers through its T-tubules to the Z-disks where the calcium binds to the troponin on the actin filaments. This causes the tropomyosin on the actin filaments to shift and allow the head of the myosin cross-bridges to attach to the actin, shortening the sarcomere. The ATPase on the cross-bridges breaks down ATP for energy to allow the cross-bridges to recock and continue muscle activity. As long as calcium is present, the activity can continue.

4. *Explain the differences between fast-twitch and slow-twitch muscle fibers.*

   Compared to fast-twitch or type II fibers, the slow-twitch, type I fibers are smaller, are red, have a slower conduction velocity, fatigue more quickly, have a lower recruitment threshold, have lower minimum and maximum firing rates, have slower-acting myosin ATPase, have a greater number of mitochondria, and function in endurance activities rather than in rapid, brief bursts of activity.

5. *Discuss the relationship between muscle strength, endurance, and power.*

   Muscle function includes strength, endurance, and power. Athletic activity involves all these factors to different degrees, depending on its specific demands. Muscle strength and endurance are closely related. Strength is the ability to produce force, and endurance is the ability to produce less forceful activities over a longer period of time; power is the strength output related to time.

6. *Identify the various types of dynamic activity.*

   Dynamic activity includes muscle tension with movement. Dynamic activity is divided into isotonic and isokinetic activity. Isotonic activity is further divided into concentric and eccentric activity.

7. *Discuss the differences between open and closed kinetic chain activity.*

   Open kinetic chain activity occurs when the distal aspect of the limb is not fixed; closed kinetic chain activity occurs when the distal aspect is fixed or anchored.

8. *Identify the various grades of manual muscle testing.*

   Muscle strength is rated from 5 (normal) to 0 (no function). A grade 4 muscle is one that offers some resistance beyond gravity but not normal resistance; a grade 3 muscle is able to lift the limb against gravity but unable to offer any additional strength; a grade 2 muscle is one that is able to move the limb through a full range of motion in a gravity-eliminated position; and a grade 1 muscle provides some voluntary activity but is unable to move the segment through a range of motion.

9. *Discuss the grades of muscle activity.*

   Passive motion is performed by an outside force without voluntary muscle activity; active assistive motion is motion that occurs through a combination of voluntary and assistive mechanisms; active motion occurs without the aid of any outside mechanism; and resistive motion occurs through a range of motion within which resistance to that motion is present.

10. *List the PNF techniques commonly used in sports medicine and their purposes.*

    Repeated contractions, rhythmic initiation, slow reversal, slow reversal-hold, and rhythmic stabilization are the PNF techniques most commonly used for strengthening. The techniques used to gain motion include hold-relax, contract-relax, and slow reversal-hold-relax.

11. *Identify four principles of strengthening exercises.*

    Development of a therapeutic exercise program must include consideration of SNAP guidelines: specific exercise, no pain, attainable goals, and progressive overload.

CRITICAL THINKING QUESTIONS

1. If you provide manual resistance to a patient's shoulder flexors, will the position in which the patient has been placed make any difference? Why or why not?

2. What steps could you take to improve performance if a patient were unable to perform a straight-leg raise without assistance because of weakness? How would your selection improve the patient's performance? How would it enable the patient to perform a straight-leg raise independently?

3. Explain four techniques that you could use to change the resistance without changing the amount of weight in a shoulder flexion exercise.

4. For a patient who has weakness in the quads, explain three progressive open kinetic chain and three progressive closed kinetic chain exercises you could use to strengthen the quads. What, if anything, would determine whether you started with the open or closed kinetic chain exercises?

5. If a patient were unable to bear weight on the lower extremity, not because of medical restriction but because of apprehension, what progression of activities would you select so that the patient could progress to weight bearing? What obstacles would you have to overcome for the patient to gain confidence that the leg would support him or her?

6. Is a patient able to lift a heavier dumbbell in elbow flexion in a seated or supine position? Where in the motion is the weight the most difficult for the patient to lift? Why? Is it a good idea to have the patient perform an elbow curl in both positions? Why? What other elbow-curl exercise would be an adequate substitute for a dumbbell exercise?

7. List six progressive exercises that you would give Sam in the chapter's opening scenario. What is your justification for each exercise, and what are your criteria for progression?

REFERENCES

Berger, R.A. 1962. Optimal repetitions for the development of strength. *Research Quarterly* 33:334–338.

Billeter, H., and H. Hoppeler. 1992. Muscular basis of strength. In *Strength and power in sport,* ed. P.V. Komi. Boston: Blackwell Scientific.

Braatz, J.H., and P.P. Gogia. 1987. The mechanics of pitching. *Journal of Orthopedic and Sports Physical Therapy* 9:56–69.

Brown, D.R. 1980. *Neurosciences for allied health therapies.* St. Louis: Mosby.

Clarke, D.H. 1971. The influence on muscular fatigue patterns of the intercontraction rest interval. *Medicine and Science in Sports* 3:83–88.

Clarke, D.H. 1975. *Exercise physiology.* Englewood Cliffs, NJ: Prentice-Hall.

Daniels, L., and C. Worthingham. 1972. *Muscle testing: Techniques of manual examination,* 3rd ed. Philadelphia: Saunders.

DeLorme, T.L., and A.L. Watkins. 1948. Technics of progressive resistance exercise. *Archives of Physical Medicine* 29:263–273.

Denegar, C. 2000. *Therapeutic modalities for athletic injuries.* Champaign, IL: Human Kinetics.

Enoka, R.M. 1995. Morphological features and activation patterns of motor units. *Journal of Clinical Neurophysiology* 12: 538–559.

Hettinger, T., and E. Müller. 1953. Muscle strength and muscle training. *Arbeits Physiology* 15:111–126.

Houglum, P. 1977. The modality of therapeutic exercise: Objectives and principles. *Athletic Training* 12:42–45.

Hortobagy, T., and F.I. Katch. 1990. Eccentric and concentric torque-velocity relationships during arm flexion and extension. *European Journal of Applied Physiology* 60:395–401.

Hunter, G.R. 1994. Muscle physiology. In *Essentials of strength training and conditioning,* ed. T.R. Baechle. Champaign, IL: Human Kinetics.

Johnson, E.W., and D. Wiechers. 1982. Electrodiagnosis. In *Krugen's handbook of physical medicine and rehabilitation,* 3rd ed., ed. F.J. Kottke, G.K. Stillwell, and J.F. Lehmann. Philadelphia: WB Saunders.

Kendall, F.P. 1993. *Muscles, testing and function*, 4th ed. Baltimore: Williams & Wilkins.

Knight, K.L. 1985. Guidelines for rehabilitation of sports injuries. *Clinics in Sports Medicine* 4:405–416.

Knott, M., and D.E. Voss. 1968. *Proprioceptive neuromuscular facilitation.* New York: Harper & Row.

Knuttgen, H.G. 1976. Development of muscular strength and endurance. In *Neuromuscular mechanisms for therapeutic and conditioning exercises,* ed. H.G. Knuttgen. Baltimore: University Park Press.

Kottke, F.J. 1982. Therapeutic exercise to maintain mobility. In *Krusen's handbook of physical medicine and rehabilitation,* ed. F.J. Kottke, G.K. Stillwell, and J.F. Lehmann. Philadelphia: Saunders.

Lind, A.R. 1959. Muscle fatigue and recovery from fatigue induced by sustained contractions. *Journal of Physiology (London)* 147:162–171.

MacDougall, J.D., Elder, G.C.B., Sale, D.G., Moroz, J.R., and J.R. Sutton. 1980. Effect of training and immobilization on human muscle fibers. *European Journal of Applied Physiology* 43:25–34.

Moritani, T., and H.A. deVries. 1979. Neural factors versus hypertrophy in the time course of muscle strength gain. *American Journal of Physical Medicine* 58:115–130.

Muller, E.A. 1970. Influence of training and of inactivity on muscle strength. *Archives in Physical Medicine and Rehabilitation* 51:449–462.

Sinacore, D.R., Bander, B.L., and A. Delitto. 1994. Recovery from a 1-minute bout of fatiguing exercise: Characteristics, reliability, and responsiveness. *Physical Therapy* 74:234–244.

Stamford, B. 1985. The difference between strength and power. *Physician and Sportsmedicine* 13:155.

Stone, M.H., and M.S. Conley. 1994. Bioenergetics. In *Essentials of strength training and conditioning,* ed. T.R. Bacchle. Champaign, IL: Human Kinetics.

Wallis, E.L., and G.A. Logan. 1964. *Figure improvement and body conditioning through exercise.* Englewood Cliffs, NJ: Prentice-Hall.

Wathen, D. 1994. Load assignment. In *Essentials of strength training and conditioning,* ed. T.R. Baechle. Champaign, IL: Human Kinetics.

Wilmore, J.H., and D.C. Costill. 1999. *Physiology of sport and exercise.* 2nd ed. Champaign, IL: Human Kinetics.

Zinovieff, A.N. 1951. Heavy-resistance exercises. The "Oxford Technique." *British Journal of Physical Medicine* 14:129–132.

CHAPTER EIGHT

The ABCs of Proprioception

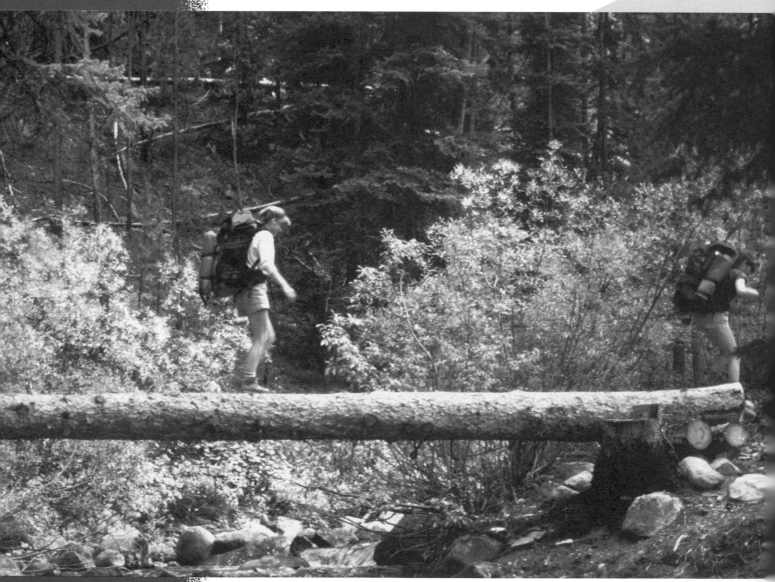

© Michael Olenick.

OBJECTIVES

After completing this chapter, you should be able to do the following:

1. List the afferent receptors involved in proprioception.

2. Identify the CNS sites that relay proprioceptive information to the motor system.

3. Discuss the ABCs of proprioception.

4. Identify the systems that control balance.

5. Describe the components involved in coordination.

6. Explain a progression of proprioceptive exercises for the lower or upper extremity.

Proprioception has always been a topic of interest for certified athletic trainer, Drew Andrews. Even as a student in college, any topic related to the neurophysiology of proprioception fascinated him. He understood the interrelationship between balance, coordination, and agility, and was fascinated by how they must all work together to allow simple to complex motions, from standing and walking to highly skilled sport activities.

Drew had started Michelle, the school's star pentathlete, on simple agility activities early in her hip rehabilitation program, but now she was ready to begin more intensive agility and sport-specific activities. Before she came into the athletic training room for her program this afternoon, Drew would design an agility program that would progress her to a full and successful return to her sport.

Strength grows stronger by being tried.

Seneca, *Ad Lucilium*, c. 186 B.C.

As we saw in the preceding chapter, Seneca's words are wise: Strength does increase when a progressive program is applied in therapeutic exercise. Once an injured athlete has the strength to control the body, the therapeutic exercise program emphasizes exercises to regain lost agility, balance, and coordination. In part, agility, balance, and coordination are determined by flexibility, strength, and endurance—which is why these must improve before a patient can expect to have agility, balance, and coordination. If a muscle is too weak to move a body part, it cannot be expected to control the movement of that part. Likewise, an extremity must have the flexibility and muscle endurance necessary to allow it to function and meet the demands of athletic activity. If a muscle has limited flexibility so that it lacks the full motion required for an activity, or if a muscle is unable to work long enough to perform an activity accurately, the muscle will be unable to coordinate the segment properly for that activity.

Agility, **B**alance, and **C**oordination are also controlled by what are collectively referred to as proprioceptors (figure 8.1)—which is why this chapter refers to the **ABCs of proprioception. Proprioception** is fundamental to correct performance, and correct athletic performance requires good agility, balance, and coordination. In other words, proprioceptors play a vital neurosensory role in the patient's motor skills and are a key factor in the ability to perform sport tasks with dexterity, mastery, and proficiency. It is certainly necessary for the patient to have good flexibility as well as muscle endurance and strength in order to perform well, but proprioception is crucial if the patient is to execute any athletic skill with accuracy, consistency, and precision. To know how to influence proprioception in athletic performance, we must first understand what proprioceptors are and how they affect athletic skill.

Proprioception is the body's ability to transmit position sense, interpret the information, and respond consciously or unconsciously to stimulation through appropriate execution of posture and movement. Neuromuscular control of proprioception is produced by the input received from receptors within skin, joints, muscles, and tendons. These proprioceptors play an important role in the maintenance of posture, the conscious and

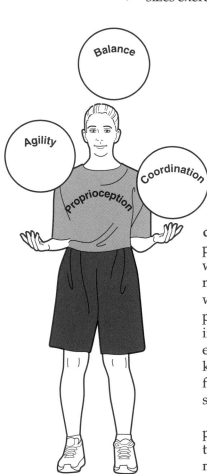

Figure 8.1 Components of proprioception.

unconscious awareness of joint position, and the production of motion. Proprioception is what allows us to know what position our fingers are in without looking at them. It is what maintains our balance when we stand. It is what enables us to write smoothly. It is what enables us to jump, run, and throw. It is what permits us to change our delivery when we miss the goal on a jump, to move from an asphalt to a gravel surface, and to correct the overshoot of our target with our throw. Although we must first have the flexibility, muscle strength, and endurance to be able to perform these activities, it is proprioception that gives us the agility to change the direction of movement quickly and efficiently, the balance to maintain our stability, and the coordination to produce the activity correctly and consistently.

Proprioceptors are afferent nerves that receive and send impulses from stimuli within skin, muscles, joints, and tendons to the **central nervous system** (CNS). Some of these impulses transmit information regarding the tension of a muscle and the relative position of a body part to control muscular activity. Some of these proprioceptive elements, such as Golgi tendon organs and muscle spindles, have been discussed in previous chapters. Other afferent elements also provide input to the CNS and determine a patient's performance ability.

An individual's agility, balance, and coordination are determined by the reception, interpretation, and response that are initiated by proprioceptors. Proprioceptors can be classified according to their location. A brief look at these elements will enhance your ability to develop appropriate therapeutic exercise programs for injured athletes.

NEUROPHYSIOLOGY OF PROPRIOCEPTION

The major categories of proprioceptors are cutaneous receptors, muscle and tendon receptors, and joint receptors. To varying degrees, they all influence proprioception.

The proprioceptors are located in the skin, muscles, tendons, and joints. There are several different receptors that have unique abilities to respond to different stimuli (figure 8.2).

CUTANEOUS RECEPTORS

Isolation of skin and subcutaneous proprioceptive **afferent receptors** has been primarily confined to investigations of the hand. The receptors in the skin are fast-adapting afferents, slow-adapting I afferents, and slow-adapting II afferents. The fast-adapting afferents are responsible for vibration sense, and the slow-adapting I and slow-adapting II afferents are responsible for sensory perceptions such as skin stretching. Most believe that these receptors do not play a major role in proprioception. Evidence suggests that they provide cues regarding skin stretching and fingertip touching but do not have a major impact on joint proprioception (Grigg 1994).

Rapidly adapting receptors produce a rapid burst of impulses that is quickly eroded. These receptors detect sudden changes in speed and movement such as acceleration and deceleration. On the other hand, slowly adapting receptors produce a constant maintenance level of stimulation. They are responsible for providing information regarding joint and limb position and slow changes in position.

MUSCLE AND TENDON RECEPTORS

The **muscle spindles** and **Golgi tendon organs (GTOs)** are the primary afferent receptors of muscles and tendons. These sensory structures are discussed in chapter 7. They are complicated structures that produce complex neuromuscular responses not only from the muscles and tendons where they are located, but also in the corresponding **antagonistic** and **synergistic** muscles. The GTO detects tension within a

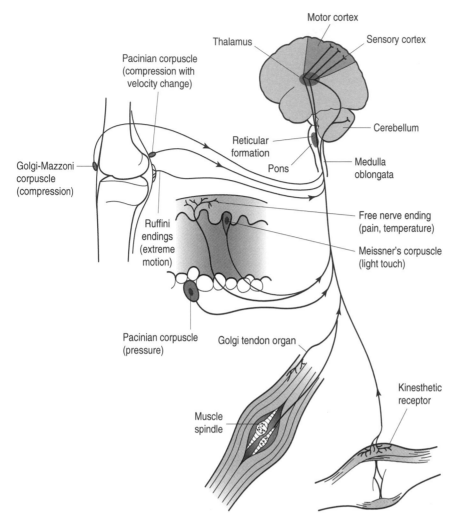

muscle and responds to both the contraction and the stretching of a muscle. Its afferent stimulation produces muscle relaxation. The muscle spindle, on the other hand, responds to the stretch of a muscle. Its afferent stimulation causes a contraction of the muscle. Stimulation of these structures also causes facilitation to opposing muscles and to synergists to assist in accomplishing the desired movement. The GTO and muscle spindle are able to determine joint position because of their muscle-length sensitivity. This capability also allows them to act as limb stabilizers.

JOINT RECEPTORS

A variety of afferent receptors that primarily lie within the connective tissue of a joint's capsule and surrounding ligaments and influence proprioception. They are divided into fiber type Groups II, III, and IV. Group II afferents are large-diameter axons that have high-speed conduction and Group III and IV afferents are thinly myelinated or nonmyelinated, small-diameter axons that have slower conduction of stimuli. The small-diameter nerves do not conduct as fast as the large-diameter nerves because they are not myelinated and/or their size offers more resistance to conduction than the larger diameter fibers.

The large-diameter myelinated afferents are called Group II afferents. There are two types of nerve endings in this group, Ruffini endings and pacinian corpuscles. Both types are located in the joint capsule. Although the two types are sensitive to different stimuli, they both measure joint motion. The Ruffini endings, located in the joint capsule on the flexion side of the joint, are slowly adapting and respond more to loads on the surrounding connective tissue than to displacement of that connective tissue. These receptors are stimulated by extreme joint motion when the capsule is stressed in extension with rotation. They are thought to be limit-detectors and protectors of unstable joints.

Pacinian corpuscles lie throughout the capsule, joint, and periarticular structures. Because they are rapidly adapting receptors, they are thought to be compression sensitive, especially during high-velocity changes when the joint accelerates or decelerates as it moves into its limits of motion.

Another afferent nerve ending, Golgi-Mazzoni corpuscles, are located in joint capsules. They are stimulated by joint compression but not by joint motion. Any weight-bearing activity stimulates these slowly adapting receptors. They do not appear to play a role in proprioception except in identification of joint compression.

■ Figure 8.2   Proprioceptive afferent receptors.

The small-diameter nonmyelinated axons are divided into Group III and Group IV afferents. Group IV afferents are C fibers and Group III afferents are small-diameter A fibers. These are grouped together because they are both pain receptors and are called free nerve endings because of the appearance of their nerve terminals. Located throughout soft tissue and articular structures, these are **nociceptors** that are stimulated by pain and inflammation when a joint is placed in an end position. They do not play a role in proprioception, but can evoke a flexion response to cause a joint to unload and thereby protect it.

OTHER RECEPTORS

Ligaments also contain receptors. Although receptors have been identified in the knee and shoulder, the most thoroughly investigated ligament receptors are those in the knee's anterior cruciate ligament. These receptors are generally not active in the middle ranges of movement but become stimulated when the ligament is stressed. When stimulated by ligament tension, they produce an inhibitory response of the **agonistic** muscles.

As important as it is to realize that many different afferent receptors in many structures are affected by joint movement, it is also important to understand that they do not work independently (Strasmann and van der Wal et al. 1990). There are afferent nerves that collaborate with each other throughout the body. The afferent nerves in a locale work together to produce a complete picture of joint position and joint motion for the CNS so that it can process and interpret the input and produce an accurate response. To make this easier to understand, think about what it would be like to try to correct a baseball pitcher's delivery if you watched only the pitcher's hand. You could not accurately identify necessary changes in the delivery unless you had the complete picture of the pitcher's performance—by watching the entire delivery and analyzing all of the joint movements and positions. Similarly, the CNS cannot determine the position of an extremity unless it receives input from all sensory, motor, and joint receptors.

CENTRAL NERVOUS SYSTEM PROPRIOCEPTOR SITES

After the afferent nerves send their input to the CNS, the body's motor response depends on which of three CNS sites has received the impulse—the spinal cord, the brain stem, or the cerebral cortex.

Once the afferent nerves have sent their input to the CNS, the body's motor response is determined by the location within the CNS that interprets the stimuli and initiates the efferent reaction. There are three areas within the CNS that will react to the stimuli: **spinal cord, brain stem,** and **cerebral cortex.**

SPINAL CORD

If an impulse goes from a dorsal root afferent nerve either to an **internuncial** connecting nerve or directly to an efferent nerve in the spinal cord, and then immediately out the ventral root to the muscle, it is called a **spinal reflex.** This is a response in its simplest form. The reflexes that do not use an internuncial neuron produce a more rapid response than those that use an internuncial nerve. This is because of the additional time it takes to transmit from one nerve to another. The fewer the connections, the more rapid the reflex response. These proprioceptive reflexes are often used to protect an area through muscle splinting or rapid withdrawal motion. For example, a joint that is under ex-cessive stress can be protected by the activation of the muscle's reflex flexion response to suddenly reduce the load on a joint. Reflexes are also used to provide joint stability, especially when there is a sudden change of direction or position. The joint proprioceptors, the muscle spindles, and GTOs all work together

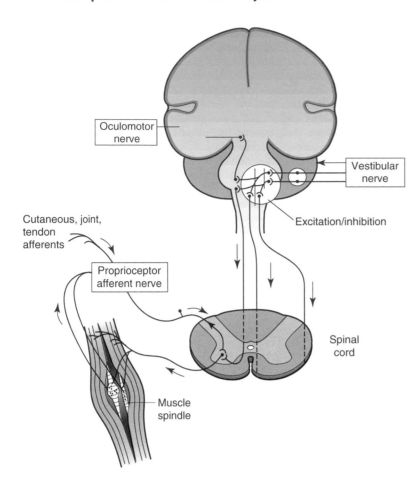

Oculomotor nerve

Vestibular nerve

Excitation/inhibition

Cutaneous, joint, tendon afferents

Proprioceptor afferent nerve

Spinal cord

Muscle spindle

▌ Figure 8.3 Balance pathways include oculomotor, vestibular, and proprioceptor pathways. These three neural pathways for balance provide inhibitory and excitatory stimulation to affect the body's motor response.

to produce a reflex response that provides the joint with stability to prevent injury.

BRAIN STEM

The brain stem is the primary proprioceptive correlation center. The proprioceptors relay information via interneurons in the spinal cord that connect to ascending pathways to the brain stem to maintain desired position or posture (figure 8.3). The brain stem also receives input from other areas such as the eye's visual afferent centers and the ear's vestibular afferent centers to assist in maintaining balance reflexively. The brain stem then sends excitatory or inhibitory efferent stimulation to produce an appropriate response. We will consider the importance of these sensory systems in the section "Balance."

CEREBRAL CORTEX

Sensory pathways travel to the cortex of the **cerebrum** (figure 8.3). This is the highest level of the brain and the location of conscious movement—the center of volitional control of movement. It is here that correct movement is learned and consciously controlled before it becomes an automatic response. To understand this process, think about how you learned to type. When you were first learning, you were very conscious of what your fingers were doing and where they were on the keyboard. Now, after several years of typing, you do not have to think about what you are doing because the activity has become automatic. You make fewer mistakes and perform the activity faster than you did as a beginning typist. This is what occurs with any activity that is practiced repeatedly; conscious performance becomes automatic performance, and cognitive awareness of the activity is not required.

The ABCs of proprioception include simple and complex functions. This is relative, though, since even the simplest function involves complex neuromuscular connections. Agility, balance, and coordination are all interrelated and so impact each other. This is the case simply because they have similar roots, the body's proprioceptors. These functions are discussed here in order of their complexity, beginning with the simplest and progressing to the more highly challenging functions.

BALANCE

Balance involves three systems—the vestibular system, the oculomotor system, and the proprioceptive system. The sport rehabilitation specialist can perform simple tests to evaluate balance.

Balance is fundamental to most activities. Balance is required to perform a simple activity such as standing. Correct athletic performance requires the maintenance of balance. An athlete who does not have good balance is in danger of injury. If balance is not restored following an injury, the risk of reinjury significantly increases.

Balance is the body's ability to maintain equilibrium by controlling the body's center of gravity over its base of support. Balance is important in both static and dynamic activities. Standing and sitting are static balance activities. Examples of dynamic balance activities include walking, running, and dancing.

Balance is influenced by strength and by input from the CNS. It is because strength influences balance that strength is emphasized before proprioception in a therapeutic exercise program. As already mentioned, the brain stem receives sensory input from the vestibular system, the visual system, and the proprioceptors (figure 8.4). The combination of input from the ears, eyes, and proprioceptors is crucial to maintaining good balance and posture. If you have ever had an inner ear infection, you may remember the difficulty you had in maintaining balance. A simple test to highlight the importance of visual input for balance is to stand on one foot with your eyes open and then close your eyes. You will discover that without the visual input, it is more difficult to maintain balance. So, too, when proprioceptors are damaged following surgery or injury, balance can be impaired.

Other factors can influence balance, but they depend on the visual, auditory, and proprioceptive systems. For example, a patient's ability to focus on the task at hand is basic to the cognitive portion of the proprioceptive system, and a patient's ability to perform skills on different playing surfaces is directly related to the proprioceptive system.

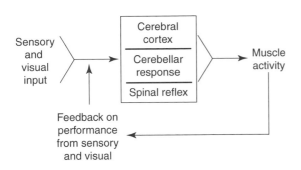

I Figure 8.4 Feedback system for coordination.

VESTIBULAR SYSTEM

The **vestibular system** within the inner ear is responsible for sending messages to the CNS regarding vertical and horizontal position and motion. The vestibular system includes three semicircular canals within the inner ear that detect changes in position and aid the body in maintaining an upright posture, and also two sacs. One sac, the saccule, regulates equilibrium; the other, the utricle, senses forward-backward head motion. Both sacs respond to gravity and are sensitive to head and body motions. The inner ear provides a vestibular ocular reflex. This allows the eyes to remain steady when the body is in motion. This reflexive attempt to keep the eyes steady during body motion is called **nystagmus**.

OCULOMOTOR SYSTEM

Vision assists in providing feedback about the relative position of the body in space. This feedback system is referred to as the **oculomotor system.** As already noted, with your eyes closed it is more difficult to maintain good balance than with your eyes open. If you dive under water with your eyes closed or are in water in which vision is impaired, you can get disoriented and not know whether you are upright relative to the water's surface and bottom. If you sit in an environment that contains a lot of activity, the oculomotor and vestibular systems work together to determine whether you or the environment is moving. Sometimes the feedback is not interpreted correctly and you have a sense of moving when, in fact, you are staying still and it is the environment that is moving. This may occur when your car is stopped at a light but the car next to you is moving forward—you may have a sense that you are moving backward.

Patients who must perform activities requiring rapid change of position, such as ice skaters, gymnasts, or dancers, must learn to disregard the visual input in order not to get dizzy. The vestibular system provides rapid feedback about the change in position that occurs in these athletic events, but the athlete uses the technique of visual fixation, focusing on one object and disregarding other moving objects, in order to prevent dizziness and loss of balance.

PROPRIOCEPTIVE SYSTEM

The proprioceptive system is sometimes referred to as the **somatosensory system.** We have already discussed the importance of a good proprioceptive system for balance. When proprioceptor nerves are damaged in injuries, the system's ability to function is impaired. Joint proprioceptors in the knee and ankle are commonly injured in sport, resulting in a reduction of balance and an increase in reaction time. If their function is not restored, the patient risks reinjury and impaired performance.

Balance must be restored and exercises must be included as part of the therapeutic exercise program if the injured athlete is to have good stability and safety during performance. There are exercises that begin at a basic level and progress to more complex, functional activities as the patient's balance improves. These specific exercises and functional activities are discussed in later chapters.

BALANCE EVALUATION

There are simple tests to determine a patient's balance deficiencies. The difficulty of these tests changes as the patient's performance level improves, proceeding from static to dynamic and from simple to more complex. The simplest test is the **Romberg test,** in which the patient stands with feet together and eyes closed. No loss of balance is a normal response. Most patients should be able to perform this test without difficulty. A slightly more difficult test is the stork stand, in which the patient stands only on the injured leg. The patient should be able to maintain this position for 30 s without touching the other foot to the floor or using hand support. If the patient is able to perform this test satisfactorily, you can use another test that is slightly more difficult, a stork stand with the eyes closed. The patient should also be able to perform this activity for 30 s. Difficulty with any of these static tests indicates a balance deficit and needs to be addressed in the therapeutic exercise program.

COORDINATION

The components of coordination include perception of activity, feedback, performance adjustment, and repetition. Development of coordination involves progression of activities from simple to more complex, as well as repetition.

Coordination is another proprioceptive function fundamental to athletic activities. **Coordination** is the complex process by which a smooth pattern of activity is produced through a combination of muscles acting together with appropriate intensity and timing. Several muscles are involved in a coordinated activity. These muscles are connected by a complex neurological network of sensory receptors, internuncial neurons, ascending and descending corticospinal pathways, and efferent receptors. Some muscles are stimulated to provide an activity while others are inhibited to permit the activity, and still others are stimulated to provide synergistic or stabilizing responses to permit the desired motion to occur. Each muscle must provide an accurate response both in timing and in intensity in order for the activity to be coordinated. If a muscle is too weak to provide the appropriate response, the activity will be uncoordinated and undesirable. For example, if a volleyball player does not have an appropriate amount of strength in the scapular rotators, the arm is not in the correct position to hit and place the ball accurately. A soccer player who has weak hip abductors on the standing leg does not have the stability needed for holding the body firm and providing the base necessary to kick the ball well enough with the opposite leg. An archer does not have accuracy in shooting without the strength in the deltoids to control the weight of the bow or the pull on the string.

If muscles are weak, they must work harder to achieve a specific output of activity. This causes an irradiation of stimulation, called **overflow,** to other muscle groups. We see this in a simple activity such as opening a jar. If the cover comes off with little effort, minimal activity of the hand and arm is required. However, if the cover is stuck and more effort is needed, the arm muscles tighten, the grip gets stronger, the jaw muscles contract, and the entire body tenses as we attempt to open the jar. Likewise, when the muscle is performing an activity but is not strong enough to provide the appropriate motion, it tries as hard as it can to perform the activity and in so doing stimulates otherwise inactive muscles to assist. This overflow causes an undesired motion. For this reason, it is important to have the patient achieve strength gains before you include coordination activities in a therapeutic exercise program.

COORDINATION COMPONENTS

There are specific requirements for coordinated movement. Let's briefly look at them so that the logical progression of therapeutic exercises for improved coordination becomes clear.

Activity Perception

Probably the most basic of all elements within coordination is the awareness of **volitional** muscle activity. An awareness of joint position and movement is fundamental to the ability to perform activity. Proprioceptors are key to this awareness. Vision is also important, for it gives the patient feedback about the result of the activity: Has the activity been performed as desired? Vision slows down the response to activity, but especially in the beginning when a new activity is being learned and motor patterns are being established, vision is important to the development of accuracy of motion.

Feedback

The learning process involved in the development of coordinated movement is similar to programming a computer. An activity is performed; the CNS evaluates the quality of the performance; the body sends information to the CNS to make adjustments for undesired activity; and the activity is repeated with the adjustments made. The proprioceptors are the most important elements in this feedback process. The sensory afferents send information to the cerebrum where awareness of the activity is received, to the **cerebellum** where automatic adjustment of muscle position and length is made, and to the spinal cord for reflex adjustments (figure 8.4). Upper-center information is then relayed to the brain stem where it is integrated with other input and sent back down the spinal cord to provide an adjusted performance.

Repetition

As the activity becomes more accurate with repetition and adjustments, the performance becomes more consistent. To think about this we could use an analogy from cross-country skiing. The more the tracks on a trail are used, the deeper they get and the easier it becomes to stay within them. Deviation from the tracks becomes less likely the more the trail is used.

Repetition is a requirement for development of accuracy and coordination. As the activity is repeated, the effort decreases and there is less chance of overflow to the wrong muscles. Eventually, an activity **engram** that can be repeated precisely and accurately is developed. An engram is an effect or performance that is impressed upon the CNS through repetition. At this point the coordinated activity becomes automatic and is no longer a conscious process.

Inhibition

In the development of coordination it is important to inhibit undesired muscle activity. **Inhibition** cannot be trained directly (Kottke 1982). It must be facilitated by precise, slow, and controlled activity until the engram is developed and the patient can increase speed without producing unwanted muscle responses. In the early developmental stages of coordination the activity should not be so difficult that the patient's performance causes an overflow and unwanted muscle responses. Given that early coordination requires cognitive awareness and conscious correction, it is best that the patient not be distracted with too many activities. Such distractions will lead to imprecise patterns of movement because the patient will not be able to concentrate adequately on any one activity. It is better to alternate attention if the situation calls for performance of more than one activity at a time.

Inhibition is part of the computer-like adjustment process that eventually results in coordinated activity. The patient should start with low-level, basic activity to eliminate the overflow to other pathways until a coordinated pattern is established. As the desired motion becomes an engram, the activity can become more difficult, because the capacity to inhibit undesired activity becomes greater with improved coordination.

COORDINATION DEVELOPMENT

Precision of motion, speed of motion, and strength are fundamental to coordination in sport activities. As previously mentioned, once strength is achieved, coordination development through repetition of activity is crucial. The patient needs to have activities that are simple in the beginning and that become more complex as skill progresses. In the beginning, simple static exercises may be enough of a challenge. Coordination development progresses from static activities to dynamic activities. For example, once the patient is able to stork stand on an unstable surface such as a foam roller or trampoline, he or she can begin dynamic activities such as balance-board and jumping activities for the lower extremities or ball tossing at a target for the upper extremities.

Progression of coordination starts with simple activities and moves to more complex ones. Increasing the speed of the activity, increasing the force, and increasing the complexity are all ways to advance the difficulty of coordination exercises. All co-ordination activities require repetition. This means that any coordination exercise in a therapeutic exercise program should include many repetitions. This is especially important as the exercises progress to resemble the patient's sport activities.

Accuracy of performance is vital to coordination development. The sport rehabilitation specialist must be cognizant of this when the patient is performing therapeutic exercises. Once the patient begins to fatigue and coordination becomes less accurate, the activity should be discontinued. Continued execution of uncoordinated motions will engram undesired movement. This is also an important consideration with regard to the placement of coordination exercises within a therapeutic exercise session. The patient should perform coordination activities early in the session when fatigue is not as much of a factor as it will be toward the end.

AGILITY

Agility is an advanced skill that is built on flexibility, strength, and power first, followed by coordination and balance.

Agility is the ability to control the direction of a body or segment during rapid movement. Athletic agility requires a number of qualities: flexibility, strength, power, speed, balance, and coordination. It involves rapid change of direction and sudden stopping and starting.

Most sports require agility of the lower extremities. A football receiver must be able to cut suddenly to the left or right to evade a defensive player; a soccer forward must zigzag down the field to move the ball around an opponent; and a basketball player must sprint down the court and then suddenly stop to perform a jump shot. Upper-extremity agility is required of a piano player who moves the fingers rapidly across the keyboard, a water polo player who attempts to fake out an opponent and then score a goal, the hockey goalie who suddenly blocks a shot with his hands, and the racquetball player who moves quickly from a backhand to a forehand shot.

Agility is a highly advanced skill that requires a base of flexibility, strength, and power. Adequate flexibility provides a base for speed and power. Since power is needed for agility and power is force times distance divided by time (F × D/T), one increases power by increasing the distance through which the body part moves. Greater flexibility produces greater power. Power is important because the greater the power, the more quickly a patient is able to move.

Strength is also a component of agility. A patient who has good strength can control the inertia that forceful movement creates. If a 90-kg (200-lb) patient is unable to control his weight during movement, the movement will be of no value. Strength is a controlling factor in a patient's maneuverability.

In order to be effective, speed must be accompanied by coordination. Coordination, as we have seen, is important for proper execution of an activity.

As with coordination activities, therapeutic exercise for agility should begin with simple exercises and progress to more complex activities as skill level improves. The ultimate goal of agility exercises is for the patient to become able to perform all agility activities involved in that patient's sport. Execution of simple activities, including simple drills, is used in the early stages of agility exercises. These activities are usually components of an athletic skill and are performed at slower-than-normal speeds. As the patient improves, the activity becomes more complex and the speed more closely resembles that of normal sport participation.

Activities that can test a patient's agility should resemble the patient's sport activities. It is your responsibility as a sport rehabilitation specialist to understand the demands of the patient's sport and the patient's position within the sport so you can provide appropriate agility exercises. For example, agility activities for a basketball player should include exercises such as lateral line running, figure-8 cone running, sudden-stop activities, and running backward. Agility exercises for a volleyball player may include sprint running forward and backward with sudden direction changes, lateral running drills, and run-and-stop-jump activities. Performance of these activities is graded by speed of the activity, ability to suddenly change direction, ability to use the injured and noninjured leg equally in all directions, and smoothness of execution.

THERAPEUTIC EXERCISE FOR PROPRIOCEPTION

Therapeutic exercises for developing balance, coordination, and agility follow exercises for flexibility and strength gains. Exercises for the lower and the upper extremities progress from simple to complex and emphasize accuracy through repetition.

Agility, balance, and coordination are parameters that naturally follow flexibility and strength within a therapeutic exercise program. It is often not possible to distinguish which exercises develop balance and which exercises develop agility except at the extreme ranges of the exercise spectrum. This is because balance and agility are often intimately related and can be difficult to distinguish except in very basic exercises that are elementary static balance activities and the more complex preparticipation agility exercises. What becomes difficult is distinguishing the exercises that are more complex than static balance and less complex than preparticipation agility exercises. Exercises that develop dynamic balance, improve coordination, and enhance early agility are not as easily categorized because they may involve any combination of agility, balance, and coordinaiton.

There is a general progression of exercises for proprioception that is important whether you are working with upper- or lower-extremity injuries. Proprioception exercises should be a routine part of a therapeutic exercise program.

GENERAL CONCEPTS

Some concepts related to exercise for proprioception have already been introduced but are important enough to be repeated. Balance is achieved first, followed by coordination, and finally agility. The order is important because agility depends on coordination and coordination depends on balance. Balance exercises start with static activities and progresses to dynamic activities as balance improves.

All exercises for proprioception progress from simple to complex. Simple exercises include activities in which the patient has only one or two items of concentration. Simple exercises also include activities that require only enough muscle activity to produce the desired result without overflow to unwanted muscles. Simple exercises involve activities performed slowly and deliberately in controlled situations and environments. Distractions should be avoided when a high level of concentration is required of the patient.

Progression from simple to complex occurs only after the patient has mastered the simple exercise. You can make the activity more complex by having the patient perform the simple activity at a faster pace or by requiring a more powerful output with control. Progression from simple to more complex can also include exercises requiring the patient to perform more than one task simultaneously. A task can become more complex when one of the feedback mechanisms is restricted, as when the patient performs the simple activity with eyes closed. Progression to exercises that mimic sport participation occurs as soon as the patient's abilities allow.

A goal in proprioceptive exercises is to have the patient perform the activity accurately. To encourage this, the difficult proprioceptive activities should come early in the therapeutic exercise session rather than later; when the patient is more fatigued, coordination is more difficult.

Repetition is always necessary for performance accuracy. Repetition is successful only if the patient is able to improve execution with repeated attempts. The sport rehabilitation specialist must carefully observe the patient for signs of fatigue to prevent inaccurate engrams from developing.

LOWER-EXTREMITY PROGRESSION

Although specific exercises are addressed in part IV as specific therapeutic exercise programs for the various areas of the body, a brief description of proprioceptive programs is presented here.

Static balance activities begin with the stork stand with eyes open. The patient stands on the foot of the involved leg with arms at sides. The goal is to stork stand for 30 s without touching the elevated foot to the floor. If a patient has difficulty with the stork stand, he or she can begin with stance in a tandem position with the toe of one foot touching the heel of the foot in front of it (figure 8.5a); this is more difficult with the injured leg in the back position. Without using arms to balance, the patient stands in this position 30 s with eyes open. The patient can progress to standing in a tandem position for 30 s with eyes closed. After accomplishing stork standing with eyes open for 30 s (figure 8.5b), the patient performs it with the eyes closed for 30 s. Balance activities progress from stork standing with eyes closed to stork standing on an unstable surface such as a minitrampoline or $\frac{1}{2}$ foam roller, eyes open and eyes closed (figure 8.5c).

You can also create increased difficulty in stork standing by having the patient perform a distracting activity such as playing catch. This can become even more challenging if the ball is weighted.

The patient can also perform static balance activities in a sport-specific position. For example, a gymnast can perform the stork stand on a balance beam or with the hip in external rotation. A tennis player can perform static balance activities on the balls of the feet with hip and knee flexion. A wrestler can perform static balance activities on the unstable surface of a mat.

After having mastered static balance, the patient progresses to dynamic balance. These activities include sport-specific demands such as running, lateral movements, and backward movements. More advanced dynamic activities include jumping, cutting, twisting, and pivoting. They begin as low-level activities, performed at a slow

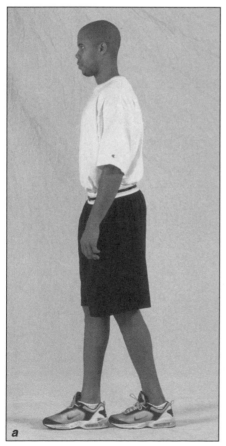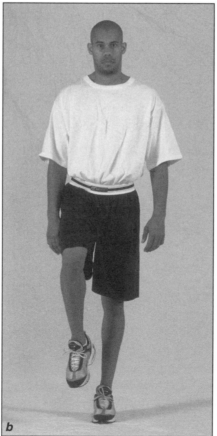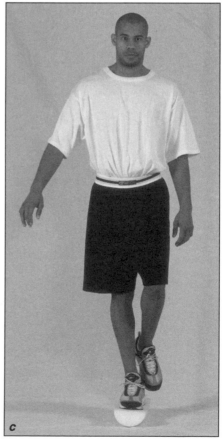

Figure 8.5 Static balance progression: *(a)* tandem stance balance, *(b)* stork stand balance, *(c)* stork stand on $\frac{1}{2}$ foam roller.

speed with balance and control, and progress to faster speeds. Some activities, such as jumping, can begin with the use of both legs but then progress to unilateral activities as the patient gains skill and confidence in execution. Plyometrics can be incorporated into the later stages of proprioceptive exercises within a therapeutic program. Plyometrics is a specialized system of exercises used only in the final stages of a program when the patient has good strength, flexibility, and control. Plyometrics are discussed in chapter 9.

In the final stages of these dynamic movements, the exercises are advanced to mimic specific sport situations. These exercises represent the true agility activities required of the patient in sport participation. You must know the component activities and understand the stresses applied in the sport to be able to design this part of the therapeutic exercise program. These activities fine-tune the patient's agility skills and restore the patient's confidence in his or her ability to return to the sport. Many of these activities are called functional exercises and are discussed in chapter 10.

The use of braces, sleeves, and tape to enhance proprioception of ankle and knee injuries is still a matter of some dispute. There is evidence that proprioception input from skin and subcutaneous sensory receptors assists in perception of motion (Lephart et al. 1992). There is also evidence that proprioceptive function is improved with bracing (Iqbal et al. 1994). Other information indicates that the benefit of joint support is inversely proportional to the proprioceptive ability of the joint (Perlan, Frank, and Fick 1995). The proprioceptive influence of these devices on functional activities is controversial. Most studies on proprioception and kinesthesia have been able to demonstrate an improved awareness of the patient as to joint position or joint sense, but no evidence demonstrates that joint stability is enhanced during functional activities with use of such devices (Barrack, Lund, and Skinner 1994). They may provide adequate skin sensory input to give the injured athlete a sense of security so that sport performance can improve.

Without any strong evidence to support or discourage the use of braces and sleeves, you must decide about using them on an individual basis. If the patient feels more confident and better able to perform athletic activities, these devices may provide sufficient psychological benefit to warrant application.

UPPER-EXTREMITY PROGRESSION

Although most lower-extremity sport activities are closed chain activities, upper-extremity activities are both open and closed chain. The patient's sport requirements in relation to open or closed chain activities will determine the thrust of the proprioceptive exercises to be used in the therapeutic exercise program. A well-rounded program should include both open and closed kinetic chain activities, but end-program emphasis is determined by the demands of the particular sport. For example, a pitcher's demands are open kinetic chain, so the majority of proprioceptive exercises for a pitcher should be of this type. A gymnast performs open and closed kinetic chain activities and thus should do a combination of open and closed kinetic chain proprioceptive exercises; but a patient on a crew team performs closed kinetic chain activities, so the program for this patient should include primarily closed kinetic chain exercises.

Initial open kinetic chain proprioceptive exercises can include proprioceptive neuromuscular facilitation rhythmic stabilization. Rhythmic stabilization can progress to closed kinetic chain exercises. In a closed kinetic chain, the exercise can progress from co-contraction without movement, to movement on a stable surface, to movement on an unstable surface. For example, the patient can either be positioned on a Swiss ball and move his or her body with the hands on the floor, or be positioned with hands on the ball and the body supported on a table (figure 8.6). The activity can start with bilateral support and then advance to use of only the involved arm.

1. Patient lies prone on a Swiss ball with feet off the floor. Patient begins with both hands on the floor then raises the uninvolved arm to balance for 30 s (figure 8.6a).

2. Patient lies prone on a table with lower extremities on the table and hands on the Swiss ball. The Swiss ball is rolled outward and the position is held for 30 s (figure 8.6b).

3. Progressions for both exercises can include the patient's moving the ball using only the arms to propel the ball forward and backward and from side to side.

4. Further progression can include resistance to movement, for example on a Fitter or with manual resistance (figure 8.7).

Active and passive repositioning can be useful for early proprioceptive gains. Passive repositioning occurs when the sport rehabilitation specialist passively moves the patient's uninvolved upper extremity into a position and the patient then moves the injured upper extremity into the same position. This activity can progress from eyes open to eyes closed. When a mistake occurs, the patient visually compares to correct the position and repeats the exercise.

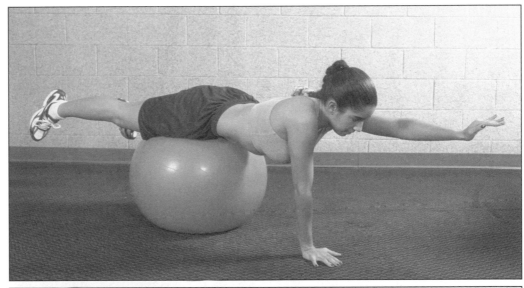

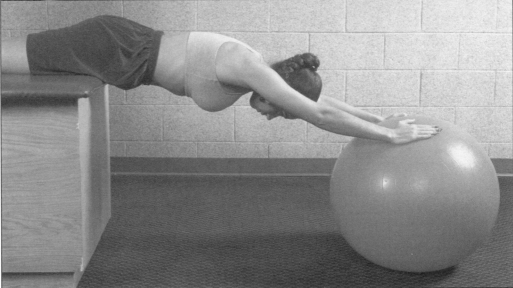

■ **Figure 8.6** Proprioception exercises for the upper extremity on the Swiss ball: *(a)* patient is supported by Swiss ball only, *(b)* patient is supported by a table and a Swiss ball.

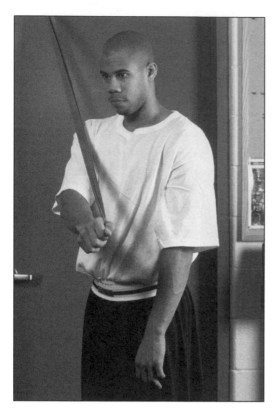

Figure 8.7 Resisted proprioceptive exercise.

In active repositioning, the sport rehabilitation specialist moves the injured arm into a position and then returns it to the starting position. With eyes closed, the patient then reproduces the position the arm was placed in.

Both these activities can be performed in straight-plane and in functional positions. The best response will be achieved in functional positions near the end of the joint's range of motion.

Functional exercises can be easily incorporated into an upper-extremity program. Proprioceptive neuromuscular facilitation exercises using manual resistance, machines, and tubing provide for strength and proprioceptive gains. Proprioceptive exercises start slowly and increase in speed as the patient is able to maintain control of the arm throughout the activity.

Plyometric exercises for agility can also be used for the upper extremity. Plyometric exercises for the upper extremities can include the use of body resistance and medicine balls as discussed in chapter 9.

As with lower-extremity functional exercises, upper-extremity agility exercises should be designed with knowledge of the requirements of the patient's specific sport. For example, functional exercises for a throwing-sport patient should progress from throwing activities that initially include short distances and easy throwing, to longer distances with an increase in speed, and finally a full-speed throw for functional distances.

SUMMARY

1. *List the afferent receptors involved in proprioception.*

   Proprioception, an important part of therapeutic exercise programs, is determined by the input of several afferent receptors in skin, muscle, tendon, joints, and other areas.

2. *Identify the CNS sites that relay proprioceptive information to the motor system.*

   The afferent receptors transmit information to one of three CNS sites: the spinal cord, the brain stem, or the cerebral cortex. The most rapid reflexes involve quick transmission and response from the spinal cord. The slower responses are sent from the cerebral cortex where conscious execution of the response is initiated.

3. *Discuss the ABCs of proprioception.*

   The ABCs of proprioception are agility, balance, and coordination. Balance is fundamental to coordination and agility. A patient must have good balance, coordination, and agility to fully meet the demands of his or her sport. Specific exercises are used to restore these functions. These exercises can be initiated early in a program with simple activities and progressed to more complex activities as the patient advances in the therapeutic exercise program.

4. *Identify the systems that control balance.*

   Balance is influenced by three systems, the vestibular, oculomotor, and proprioceptive systems. These all provide input to the CNS to maintain both static and dynamic balance.

5. *Describe the components involved in coordination.*

Coordination includes the process of perceiving an activity, getting feedback from the CNS about the result of the activity, and correcting the activity through a series of repetitions and alterations until the activity is performed correctly and without the need for cerebral cortex input.

6. *Explain a progression of proprioceptive exercises for the lower or upper extremity.*

Therapeutic exercise for proprioception progresses from easy to difficult, from static to dynamic, from slow to fast, and from simple to complex. As a sport rehabilitation specialist you must understand the complexity and requirements of the patient's sport in order to include appropriate proprioceptive exercises that will eventually permit the patient to return to full sport participation.

CRITICAL THINKING QUESTIONS

1. If a patient stands on one leg with eyes shut, which balance system is eliminated? How can the other two balance systems be eliminated in a stork-stand activity?

2. Would you expect a patient with an ankle sprain to have difficulty balancing on one leg? Why? List three progressive exercises that you could use to improve balance. What would be your criteria for advancement from one exercise to the next?

3. Coordination exercises are more effectively performed in a therapeutic exercise program before the patient becomes fatigued. Why is this? Would when, during the day's program, new coordination exercises were introduced make any difference in performance? Why?

4. Identify three criteria that should be met before a patient advances from balance to coordination activities, and from coordination to agility activities. You should be able to explain to the patient why you are setting these criteria.

5. List three agility exercises you would provide Michelle on her first day of agility training in the chapter's opening scenario. Provide two progressions for each exercise and your criteria for each progression.

REFERENCES

Barrack, R.L., Lund, P.J, and H.B. Skinner. 1994. Knee joint proprioception revisited. *Journal of Sport Rehabilitation* 3:18–42.

Grigg, P. 1994. Peripheral neural mechanisms in proprioception. *Journal of Sport Rehabilitation* 3:2–17.

Iqbal, S., Schwellnus, M.P., Noakes, T., and C. Lombard. 1994. A fivefold reduction in the incidence of recurrent ankle sprains in soccer players using the Sport-Stirrup orthosis. *American Journal of Sports Medicine* 22:601–606.

Kottke, F.J. 1982. Therapeutic exercise to develop neuromuscular coordination. In *Krusen's handbook of physical medicine and rehabilitation,* ed. F.J. Kottke, G.K. Stillwell, and J.F. Lehmann. Philadelphia: Saunders.

Lephart, S.M., Kocher, M.S., Fu, F.H., Borsa, P.A., and C.D. Harner. 1992. Proprioception following ACL reconstruction. *Journal of Sport Rehabilitation* 1:188–196.

Perlan, R., Frank, C., and G. Fick. 1995. The effect of elastic bandages on human knee proprioception in the uninjured population. *American Journal of Sports Medicine* 23:251–255.

Strasmann, T., van der Wal, J.C., Halata, Z., and J. Drukker. 1990. Functional topography and ultrastructure of periarticular mechanoreceptors in the lateral elbow region of the rat. *Acta Anatomy* 138:1–14.

CHAPTER NINE

Plyometrics

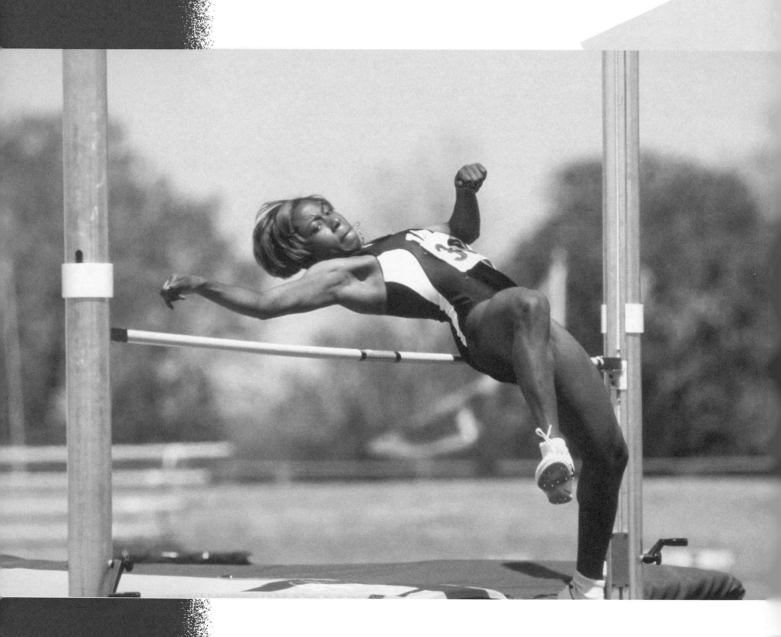

OBJECTIVES

After completing this chapter, you should be able to do the following:

1. Identify the mechanical and neurological components of the neuromuscular principles involved in plyometrics.

2. Describe the factors involved in plyometric program design.

3. List three considerations for plyometric program execution.

4. List the precautions and contraindications for plyometrics.

5. Outline a progression of four plyometric exercises for either a lower- or an upper-extremity program.

Certified athletic trainer Matthew Fischer has been recently hired by the local sports medicine clinic to head up its plyometric rehabilitation program. Once patients are sufficiently re-habilitated, Matthew establishes the final phase of their sport rehabilitation program, the plyometric phase. Matthew comes to the clinic with extensive experience and is well qualified to design and manage such a program to advance patients in this final portion of their rehabilitation.

Matthew's most recent patient is his most challenging patient to date. Adam is a 70-year-old gold medal track patient who competes in the senior Olympics and has the endorsement of several companies. Adam strained his hamstrings several weeks ago and is now nearing the end of his rehabilitation program. Although Adam is energetic and enthusiastic, he also has a history of other lower-extremity injuries and underwent cardiac bypass surgery eight years ago. The cardiac surgery and his postoperative recovery were what originally piqued his interest in track.

Matthew sees Adam as an exciting challenge and is looking forward to designing a plyometric program to enable Adam to fully return to his competitive level of participation.

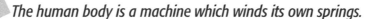

The human body is a machine which winds its own springs.

Julien Offray de La Mettrie, *L'Homme machine*

The human body is indeed a machine. A finely tuned machine of an athlete's body is able to wind its springs to produce results that include running fast, jumping high, and throwing far, and doing all of these activities with grace, skill, speed, and efficiency. These athletic skills are the combined result of natural talent and proper training. An injured athlete possesses the same inherent talent he or she has always had, but the effects of training diminish with injury and inactivity. The capacity to perform athletic skills at preinjury levels must be restored through therapeutic exercise and retraining before the patient is able to return safely to sport competition.

The patient's "machine" is not ready for competition until the patient can meet the demands of the sport and can demonstrate preinjury-level athletic performance. This means being able to execute activities with strength, power, and explosiveness. These activities include rapid starts and stops, quick changes in direction, and sudden reversals from acceleration to deceleration—all performed automatically, economically, and efficiently. Execution of activities of this magnitude requires a relearning of the neuromuscular system.

The relearning process utilizes what is commonly referred to as **plyometrics**. Plyometrics not only is a precursor to functional activities, but also can include specific functional sport activities. Plyometrics is the use of a quick movement of eccentric activity followed by a burst of concentric activity to produce a desired powerful output of the muscle. In other words, a plyometric exercise is one that facilitates a muscle to produce a maximum strength output as quickly as possible. It is a brief, explosive exercise. Power production is the ultimate goal in plyometrics. You will recall from previous discussions that power is force times distance divided by time (F × D/T). The quicker the time, the greater the power. For example, if a patient weighing 80 kg (176 lb) jumps .6 m (2 ft) in the air and takes 1 s to perform the activity, he produces 360 ft-lb of power (180 × 2 ÷ 1). If, however, he is able to jump the same distance in half the time, he will produce 720 ft-lb of power (180 × 2 ÷ .5).

Power is calculated as force divided by distance, over a given amount of time:

$$P = F \times D/T$$

The term *plyometrics* was not used until 1975 when an American track and field coach, Fred Wilt, originated the term (Chu 1992). Its Greek origins are *plio* and *metric*, which mean "more" and "measure," respectively. Before Wilt coined the term, plyometrics was referred to as "jump training." Although plyometric activities have been used since people first ran and jumped, plyometrics became popular in the late 1960s when people attributed the high-performance abilities of Olympic athletes from the Eastern European countries to the jump-training exercises used by their coaches.

NEUROMUSCULAR PRINCIPLES

Plyometrics works on the basis of specific mechanical and neurological components of the neuromuscular system. The mechanical components are contractile and noncontractile elements; the neurological components are the muscle spindles and the Golgi tendon organs.

The theory of how plyometrics works is based on information about the neuromuscular system and its response to stress. Many of these principles have been discussed in previous chapters. Putting these principles into practical application in plyometrics helps the sport rehabilitation specialist understand the "whys" and "hows" of incorporating plyometrics into a therapeutic exercise program.

Plyometrics involves the technique of first lengthening, then shortening the muscle to produce an increased power output. This is referred to as **stretch-shortening** exercise. The stretch-shortening exercise is based on the stretch-shortening principles, which in turn are based on knowledge of the mechanical and neurological components of the neuromuscular system.

MECHANICAL COMPONENTS

The mechanical components can be divided into contractile elements and noncontractile elements. Both are important elements that play a role in plyometrics and will be briefly presented here.

Contractile Elements

The **contractile elements** (CC) are the myofibrils. As discussed in chapter 7, the myofibrils contain the sarcomeres, the contractile element of the muscle. Muscle is the only structure in the body that actively shortens or lengthens to cause motion. The contractile elements of the muscular system control the noncontractile elements.

Noncontractile Elements

The noncontractile elements or components include the muscle's tendons and the connective tissue surrounding the muscle and its fibers. The noncontractile elements are divided according to their arrangement and include a **series elastic component** (SEC) and a **parallel elastic component** (PEC). The tendons, sheath, and sarcolemma are the primary structures that make up the SEC, and the muscle's connective tissue composes the PEC (Dean 1988).

Interaction of the Series Elastic Component, Parallel Elastic Component, and Contractile Component

When a muscle actively shortens, the component responsible for the muscle's ability to move the extremity or resist a force is the CC. As the muscle continues to shorten, a stretch is applied to the SEC.

When a muscle actively lengthens as in an eccentric activity, the components responsible for producing the force are the CC, SEC, and PEC. The SEC and PEC offer resistance to the movement as the muscle is elongated. The CC controls the speed and quality of the movement. When a muscle elongates, the contribution of the passive component force makes it unnecessary for the active component to produce the same total force as was produced during the shortening activity. To use a theoretical example, if a force of 4.5 kg (10 lb) is needed to lift a weight during a shortening activity, the active components must produce all 4.5 kg of force in order for the weight to be lifted. If the same weight is moved during a lengthening activity, only 3 kg (7 lb) of force needs to be produced by the active component, because 1.3 kg (3 lb) is produced by the passive components. The muscle works less to produce the same force during the lengthening activity. Although the exact differences in eccentric and concentric forces vary depending on the muscle groups investigated, this example demonstrates that less active force is required by the muscle during eccentric activity than during concentric activity. (The numbers used in the example should not be interpreted as precise.) Whereas less work is required from active components during eccentric exercise, less energy is used during eccentric exercises—so if equal active muscle force is generated in concentric and eccentric activity, greater overall force will be produced during eccentric activity.

As discussed in chapter 7, force production is different for concentric and eccentric activity (figure 9.1). At faster speeds of eccentric activity, a muscle is able to produce greater forces than at lower speeds, but the opposite is true for concentric activity. The importance of this principle will become apparent later in the discussion of specific plyometrics.

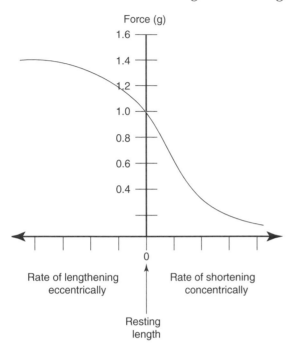

■ Figure 9.1   Concentric-eccentric force-production relationship.

Adapted from Åstrand and Rodahl 1986.

NEUROLOGICAL COMPONENTS

The proprioceptors that play important roles in plyometrics are the muscle spindles and Golgi tendon organs (GTOs). The muscle spindle is stimulated by sudden changes in the muscle's length, as during an eccentric movement. It produces a stretch, or **myotatic reflex,** to facilitate a muscle shortening. The **stretch reflex** is the most basic sensorimotor response system because it does not involve an internuncial neuron, but instead goes directly from the afferent sensory nerve (muscle spindle) to the spinal cord where it makes contact with the efferent motor neuron to permit a rapid response by the muscle. Because no additional nerves are involved in the relay process, the stretch reflex is one of the fastest reflexes in the body. It is also referred to as a **monosynaptic response** because only one synapse is involved.

The GTOs play an inhibitory role in muscle activity. As the muscle shortens, the GTOs are stimulated to send impulses to the spinal cord that relay, via an internuncial neuron, facilitation to limit muscle force production. Because of the internuncial neuron, this reflex is slightly slower than the muscle spindle reflex.

It is believed that during plyometric training, the GTO excitatory level is increased so that more stimulation is necessary to facilitate a response from the GTO, and this allows for an increased tolerance for additional stretch loads in the muscle (Wilk et al. 1993). As the stretch loads are better tolerated, there may be the ability to create a stronger stretch reflex that would result in additional power during the concentric phase of motion (Lundin 1985).

PLYOMETRIC FORCE PRODUCTION

Working together, the components of the mechanical and neurological systems that operate in plyometric activities increase strength and power output.

Force production during plyometric activity is facilitated through the mechanical and neurological systems that have been described. Combined, these produce the desired results of increased strength and power for athletic activity. The noncontractile, elastic elements are important in force production of stretch-shortening exercises. A simplified example of the way noncontractile elements work is a rubber band model: If the rubber band is stretched and then released, it shortens rapidly. The more it is stretched, the greater its force when the stretch is released. This is so because the greater the stretch, the greater the quantity of stored (potential) elastic energy there is within the rubber band. When the stretch is released, the stored elastic energy converts to kinetic energy to produce the rubber band's recoil.

Plyometric exercises provide for an increased output of power during concentric activity. This has to do with transfer of the elastic energy that is produced during eccentric activity immediately prior to concentric activity. In a muscle that moves eccentrically, the load that is produced in the muscle during its lengthening is stored as elastic energy in the noncontractile elements. As the muscle moves from eccentric to concentric activity, the elastic energy is released and assists in producing the force during the concentric action. It is believed that a muscle's increased power during plyometric exercise training may be the result of a combination of an increased level of muscle elasticity and the adaptations that occur in the neurological components (Wilk et al. 1993).

Another important factor in increased strength and power output is development of neuromuscular responses to the stresses applied. Raising the threshold of the GTOs permits a greater stretch of the muscle to provide for greater concentric activity. If a muscle is able to go through a greater range of motion, the ability to produce greater forces is improved. For example, the patient who squats to only 60° of knee flexion does not jump as high as when he or she squats to 110° of knee flexion prior to takeoff. Greater forces can be produced when greater lengthening prior to concentric activity is permitted.

Another factor in improved performance with plyometric activity is the improved neuromuscular coordination. As speed increases and the activity is performed more accurately, the strength to perform the activity is improved. Energy and movement are not wasted on ineffective activity. Neuromuscular training involves development of the engram as discussed in chapter 7. Better coordination permits greater power production since the activity can be performed more efficiently and in less time.

When speed and coordination of activity are improved, greater power can be produced, as follows from the force-velocity relationship of increased strength with increased speed during eccentric activity (figure 9.1). The greater the eccentric activity, the greater the concentric response will be; and the less time it takes a patient to perform an activity, the more power the patient will produce.

PLYOMETRIC EXERCISE PHASES

Plyometric activities occur in three distinct phases. In the eccentric phase the muscle is prestretched; in the amortization phase it makes a transition to the third, or concentric phase; and in the concentric phase it produces the powerful outcome.

Plyometric exercises can be divided into three phases: the eccentric phase, the amortization phase, and the concentric phase. All three phases are important to plyometric performance. The eccentric phase prepares the muscle, the amortization phase transitions the muscle, and the concentric phase is the outcome.

ECCENTRIC PHASE

The eccentric phase occurs when the muscle is prestretched as it actively lengthens. The slack is taken out of the muscle, and its elastic components are put on stretch. This is the preparatory phase that "sets" the muscle as the individual gets ready to perform the activity. This phase utilizes muscle spindle facilitation so that the quality of the response is determined by the rate of the stretch. The muscle's activity directly correlates with the quantity of the stimulation: the greater the stimulation, the greater the muscle's response. The eccentric phase is the most important phase of plyometric activity because it increases the stimulation to provide for this increased muscle response.

The muscle spindle responds better to a rapid stretch and accommodates to a slow one. For this reason, the rate of the stretch is a more important factor than the amount of stretch. If a muscle lengthens quickly, it is able to produce more tension than if it is forced to elongate slowly (Koutedakis 1989). The best results occur when the eccentric phase is performed quickly and through a partial range of motion.

AMORTIZATION PHASE

The eccentric phase is followed immediately by the **amortization** phase, which is simply defined as the amount of time it takes to move from eccentric to concentric motion. This phase should be quick. If too much time is spent here, the elastic energy is dissipated as heat and is wasted. A prolonged amortization phase also inhibits the stretch reflex. The concentric motion that results when the amortization is slow is weaker than intended. The amortization phase is the transition phase. The quicker the transition from eccentric to concentric activity, the more forceful the movement will be. The force produced is a result of the combination of the stretch reflex and the elastic energy released. The force produced is also influenced by the amount of time it takes to transit from eccentric to concentric activity. The time and force produced are inversely proportional to each other: the more time the transition takes, the less force is produced.

CONCENTRIC PHASE

The final phase, the concentric phase, is the result of the combined eccentric and amortization phases. The concentric phase is the outcome phase. If the eccentric activity has been quick and the amortization has occurred rapidly, the concentric phase will produce the desired powerful outcome (table 9.1).

If these phases are performed precisely, the end result should be an increased force production with a greater speed. Over time, with practice and neurological facilitation, this speed-strength production becomes more efficient because the plyometric exercises lead to an improved synchronous activity of motor units and an earlier recruitment of the motor units. Plyometrics bridges the gap between strength and explosive power by integrating the mechanical and neurological factors that influence these sport performance elements (Wilt 1975).

Table 9.1 Plyometric Phases

Phase		Activity
1	Eccentric	Preparation
2	Amortization	Transition
3	Concentric	Outcome

PRE-PLYOMETRIC CONSIDERATIONS

Patients must have certain levels of strength, flexibility, and proprioception in order to participate safely in plyometric exercises.

Development of power is important in most sports; it is an important element of basketball, volleyball, gymnastics, track and field, baseball, softball, and skating, for example. Since power is crucial for sport performance and plyometrics promotes power development, plyometric exercises should be included in the therapeutic exercise programs of patients who are returning to sport. Before plyometrics can become part of a therapeutic exercise program, however, specific parameters must be present, because plyometrics places great demands on the body.

STRENGTH

Strength is basic to plyometric exercises. The patient should have enough strength to adequately control the activity. As the difficulty of the plyometric exercise increases, the patient needs to have even greater strength. One can minimize the potential for overuse injuries from plyometric activities with good pre-plyometric strength levels.

A greater strength provides for a better output during the plyometric exercise. Again, if $F \times D/T = P$, then the greater the force, the greater the power. Additionally, if a muscle has a greater cross section because of its hypertrophy following strengthening, it will have greater elastic elements to provide additional eccentric strength. Minimum strength requirement recommendations for plyometric exercises vary and depend on the severity of the plyometric exercise. For more severe lower-extremity plyometric exercises, the recommendation is that the patient be able to perform a squat with 60% of body weight for five repetitions within 5 s (Chu 1998). Less intense plyometric exercises such as skipping or hopping can begin earlier. Logic, common sense, and a knowledge of the patient's strength and the stresses applied with any exercise are required of the sport rehabilitation specialist who is determining the use of plyometric exercises.

FLEXIBILITY

Flexibility is another pre-plyometric exercise requirement. As mentioned earlier, greater flexibility permits a greater lengthening of the muscle. A greater lengthening provides for a better eccentric phase that will lead to better concentric activity. A muscle that lacks good flexibility is unable to generate the forces for optimal plyometric results. The muscle is also at risk for injury because the reduced flexibility leads to a diminished level of force absorption, needed especially for impact and deceleration stresses. For example, the patient who is able to flex his knee to only 60° will be unable to absorb the forces imposed on him when he jumps from a 40 cm (16 in.) box; but the patient who is able to fully flex her knees can absorb the impact stresses much more effectively to prevent the forces from being transmitted up the extremity.

PROPRIOCEPTION

Another pre-plyometric consideration is the ABCs of proprioception as discussed in chapter 8. The patient must have agility, balance, and coordination to control the rapid and forceful movements in plyometric activities. The amount of control required depends on the complexity and severity of the plyometric activity. For example, a plyometric activity such as jumping rope is not as complex or as severe as the plyometric activity of bounding with vertical jumps. Although both activities require agility, balance, and coordination, the patient's abilities are more challenged with the bounding and vertical jump activities. For this reason it makes sense not to include even simple plyometric exercises in a therapeutic exercise program until the patient is able to perform some of the basic static and dynamic ABC activities discussed in chapter 8.

Because flexibility, strength, and proprioceptive elements are prerequisites to plyometric exercises, the progression of a therapeutic exercise program is important. As noted in chapter 1, each component is built on the previous one and serves as a foundation for the next one. Likewise, there are progressions within each parameter. Plyometrics is no different from any other type of exercise we have considered and must move in a progression from the simplest to the more difficult.

PLYOMETRIC PROGRAM DESIGN

A plyometrics progression for a sport rehabilitation program uses a number of variables: intensity, volume, recovery, and frequency.

A plyometric program is designed to improve the patient's overall coordination, efficiency, speed, and power output in preparation for sport participation. Most sports require high power outputs and involve repetitive stretch-shortening muscle activity. Plyometric activities are the bridge between therapeutic exercise and functional performance. These exercises utilize the components of flexibility, strength, and proprioceptive elements that the patient developed in earlier exercise sessions and put these components to functional use through the further development of power, speed, coordination, and efficiency of movement. Whereas many plyometric exercises mimic functional sport skills, others serve as building blocks for progression from simple activities to functional skills.

Just as a patient with a 4/5 grade muscle strength cannot be expected to lift the same weights as a patient with a 5/5 grade muscle strength, a patient should not be expected to perform high-level plyometric exercises when beginning plyometric activities within the therapeutic exercise program. A progression is crucial to avoid injury and provide a successful outcome. The progression is from general exercises to more sport-specific activities, from simple to complex, and from low-stress to high-stress activities.

One can use a number of variables to provide a plyometric exercise progression: intensity, volume, recovery, and frequency.

INTENSITY

Intensity is the degree, extent, or magnitude of effort applied during an exercise or activity. In strengthening, it is the amount of weight used; in flexibility, it is the force applied to the stretch; in proprioception, it is the complexity of the agility, balance, or coordination activity. In plyometrics it is the stress of the activity. You can change stress in plyometrics by using weights during the activity, increasing the height of the vertical jump, increasing the distance of the horizontal jump or the throw, increasing the weight of the medicine ball, or increasing the speed of the activity. You can also increase stress by changing the complexity of the exercise. For example, hopping with one leg is more stressful than hopping with two legs, and hopping side to side is more stressful than hopping in place.

VOLUME

Volume is the total quantity of work performed during one session. Volume in lower-extremity plyometric exercises is measured in total number of foot contacts for jumping activities and in distance for bounding activities during the session. Volume in the upper extremity and in medicine-ball exercises is measured in the total number of repetitions and sets. Selection of the volume of plyometrics depends on the intensity and goals of the session.

Although no guidelines have been established for therapeutic exercise, for normal athletic conditioning the lower-extremity guidelines for beginners at low intensity levels are 60 to 100 foot contacts (Chu 1998). The sport rehabilitation specialist must have knowledge of the patient's ability and of the stresses applied by the activity, and must combine this knowledge with observation of the patient's performance quality, in order to determine the appropriate volume of plyometric exercises for the therapeutic exercise session.

RECOVERY

Recovery is the amount of rest time between sets or exercise groupings. The amount of rest time determines whether the plyometric exercises will be more effective in improving power or improving muscular endurance. The less rest time between exercise sets, the more the emphasis is on endurance; but longer rest times will provide for more improvement in power. As a general guideline, rest periods of 45 to 60 s between sets or exercise groupings promote power increases (Chu 1989). This translates to a work-to-rest ratio of 1:5 to 1:10 (Chu 1998). For example, if an exercise set takes 5 s to perform, the recovery could be 25 to 50 s. If the exercise set takes 10 s to perform, the recovery could be 50 to 100 s.

If muscle endurance is a goal with plyometric exercise, the recovery time between exercise sets is less; the general guideline is 10 to 15 s. This amount of rest time does not allow an optimal recovery of the muscle, so muscle endurance improves.

Plyometric exercises can also be used to develop aerobic conditioning through use of a circuit program in which the patient performs various exercise groupings for 12 to 20 min with less than a 2 s rest between the exercises. A circuit program can develop aerobic, power, and muscle endurance levels.

FREQUENCY

Another variable is the frequency with which plyometric activities are used in a therapeutic exercise program. Frequency depends on the exercise intensity and the patient's tolerance and ability to recover. As a rule of thumb you should allow at least 48 h between plyometric exercise sessions. The research is very unclear about the time it takes healthy patients to recover from plyometric exercise, and is essentially nonexistent on frequency of plyometrics in therapeutic exercise programs. Your judgment, common sense, and knowledge of stresses and the patient's abilities are key to determining frequency during an individual patient's program.

PLYOMETRIC PROGRAM CONSIDERATIONS

A number of special considerations must enter into the decision whether and how to use plyometrics within a patient's therapeutic exercise program. Plyometrics is appropriate for patients with certain characteristics and not others. Plyometric activities require particular types of surfaces and footwear. Other considerations involve progression and goals for this type of exercise.

Because plyometric activities are generally more intense than other types of exercises, one must consider several special issues regarding their application in therapeutic exercise programs. If the patient has satisfied the pre-plyometric considerations and has the flexibility, strength, and proprioceptive elements required for plyometric activities, he or she must also meet other criteria in order to participate safely. In addition, plyometric exercises must be performed on an appropriate surface, and progression and goals must be determined appropriately.

AGE

Although most children use plyometric activities in their everyday activities such as running, jumping, hopping, and skipping, one must use plyometrics carefully with children and youth from ages 8 to 13. Plyometric activities for prepubescent and early-pubescent patients should remain at low volume and low intensity. As an example, jumping with both feet and without the use of boxes or weights is low-intensity jumping. Children are at higher risk than older individuals for injury with plyometrics because their central nervous systems are not mature and their GTO activation threshold is lower than in adults. The proprioceptive feedback mechanism is unable to provide necessary safeguards against the high stresses of plyometrics. Muscles and bones of prepubescent patients are also not strong enough to tolerate the moderate and high stresses of more advanced plyometric exercises (Gambetta 1986). Because of variability in physical maturity, it may be a safe rule of thumb to restrict patients under age 16 from participating in moderate- to high-intensity plyometrics.

BODY WEIGHT

The design of a plyometric program must take into account the patient's weight. Patients weighing 100 kg (220 lb) or more are not able to participate in the same plyometric exercises as lighter patients (Allerheiligen and Rogers 1995). The stresses imposed on tendons and joints may be too great for safe participation by these patients in higher-intensity plyometric activities. For example, a 113-kg (250-lb) patient may perform single-leg hops for only half the distance that a 68-kg (150-lb) patient can. The intensity of plyometric exercises for heavier patients should be selected cautiously.

COMPETITIVE LEVEL

Patients involved in competitive sports are more appropriate candidates for moderate- and high-level plyometric exercises than those in recreational activities are. The competitive patient has more advanced performance goals than the recreational patient and typically has more intense sport participation requirements. Although therapeutic exercise programs for all patients should include some level of plyometric exercises, only the competitive patients require higher-intensity plyometric activities.

SURFACE

The best surfaces for plyometric lower-extremity activities are those that have "give" to them. Although it can be indoors or outdoors, the surface should be one that yields to absorb some of the impact stress of the plyometric activity. Ideal surfaces include spring-loaded floors, Resilite mats, and grass. Harder surfaces such as asphalt, concrete, and carpet or rubber over concrete should be avoided. Although the surface should be able to absorb some of the impact forces produced during the activity, it should not be so yielding that it reduces the elastic recoil, the crucial element of plyometric activity. If the surface prevents sufficient amortization and impedes the individual's concentric phase, the surface is probably too soft. For the higher-stress plyometric activities, this becomes a key consideration.

FOOTWEAR

Shoes that offer good support and provide some cushion for shock absorption are the best shoes to wear for plyometrics. A shoe can offer too much absorption and thus be too spongy, causing instability instead of providing stability in landing. If this is the case, the individual may report a sense of instability or an inability to properly execute the exercise, or you may be able to observe instability at the foot landing or takeoff during the exercises. Shoes should be in good condition, should not be excessively worn, should be tied properly, and should fit well.

PROPER TECHNIQUE

Technique is probably the most important among the special considerations. Foot position is an essential factor in jumping activities. The patient should land on the midfoot and then roll forward to push off from the balls of the feet (Gambetta 1986). The patient should not land on the balls of the feet or the heel, since these techniques increase the impact forces and thereby increase stress applied at the foot, ankle, and knee. The midfoot landing also allows a shorter amortization time so that a more powerful concentric motion can occur.

The trunk should remain upright with a straight back so that summation of forces from the back, abdominals, and arms can be utilized. The arms can contribute 10% of the force of the plyometric jump, so both timing of activities and posture are important factors (Gambetta 1986). Keeping the back straight will avoid back injuries and permit this transmission of forces.

The quality of the execution is important. As a sport rehabilitation specialist you must carefully observe the patient's quality of performance. As the patient fatigues, performance quality declines. This can result in two problems: risk of injury and development of an improper engram. It is important to know the proper exercise technique and to observe the patient's performance closely so that you can discontinue the exercise when performance begins to deteriorate.

PROGRESSION

A gradual progression from simple to difficult, from few to more, and from general to specific is vital to avoid injury in plyometric activities. The patient's body must be allowed time to adapt to the new stress levels in order to avoid overstress injuries. As we have seen, there are a variety of ways to implement progression into a program. Changing the intensity, reducing the rest, and increasing the duration of the activity will all provide for a progression.

GOALS

The program's goals are individually determined by the patient and the demands of the patient's sport. The specific exercises within the program are determined by the sport-specific requirements of each patient. For example, a long jumper will have a different plyometric jumping program than a basketball player, and a volleyball player will have a different jumping program than a wrestler. You must understand the stresses, skills, and demands of the patient's sport so that you can incorporate appropriate plyometric exercises into the therapeutic exercise program at the proper time.

You should assess the patient's plyometric performance at certain times during the therapeutic exercise program. Any time you initiate a plyometric activity, you should take initial measurements of the patient's performance. For example, in a standing jump, you should measure the jump height the first time the patient attempts the jump. As the patient progresses through the program, more intensive plyometric activities are introduced. Each time the patient performs a new activity, you should record initial values of the performance and establish new goals. Additional measurements can be taken either at specific intervals, such as every week, or when the patient is ready to advance to a more difficult activity. These recordings help the sport rehabilitation specialist maintain objective measures of improvement. They also provide additional motivation and goals for the patient.

PRECAUTIONS AND CONTRAINDICATIONS

Precautions concerning the use of plyometrics relate to the time the patient spends on these activities and to vulnerability to post-exercise soreness. There are also a few frank contraindications to the use of plyometrics in a therapeutic exercise program.

As you realize, there are precautions for any therapeutic exercise program. Because plyometric activities can be vigorous, you must consider additional precautions before deciding to incorporate them into an individual's therapeutic exercise program. In addition, you must be aware of several clear contraindications to plyometric activity.

Precautions

• **Time.** Because plyometric activities place such high stresses on the body, they should not be performed for extended periods of time. They also should be performed in the early part of the therapeutic exercise session before the patient becomes fatigued and his or her strength, flexibility, and coordination are less than optimal. The time to perform the plyometric activities is after the warm-up but before fatigue increases and with it the risk of injury.

• **Postexercise delayed-onset muscle soreness.** It is important to caution the patient that because plyometric activities are more strenuous than other exercises, he or she may experience postexercise soreness. Delayed-onset soreness is common especially at the time plyometric exercises are introduced into the program or when the intensity changes.

Contraindications

• **Acute inflammation.** Plyometric exercises should be avoided in acute inflammatory conditions. The intensity of these exercises can increase the inflammation.

• **Postoperative conditions.** Persons with immediate postoperative conditions should not engage in plyometric exercise. The tissues are unable to tolerate the stress of such exercises and are highly vulnerable to injury.

• **Instability.** Gross joint instability, until strength is sufficient to control the joint, is a contraindication. Strength is a prerequisite to any plyometric exercise. Strength permits the control necessary for safe and effective plyometric exercise execution.

EQUIPMENT

Some plyometric exercises require no equipment, and others use a variety of items that are easy to obtain or to construct.

Equipment for plyometric activities need not be elaborate or expensive. In fact, most plyometric exercises require little or no equipment. In the following sections we review some of the most commonly used items.

CONES

Plastic barrier or traffic cones are used as jump obstacles or for sprint activities. Their plasticity makes them safe for patients to land on. These cones come in various sizes from 20 to 60 cm (8 to 24 in.) (figure 9.2).

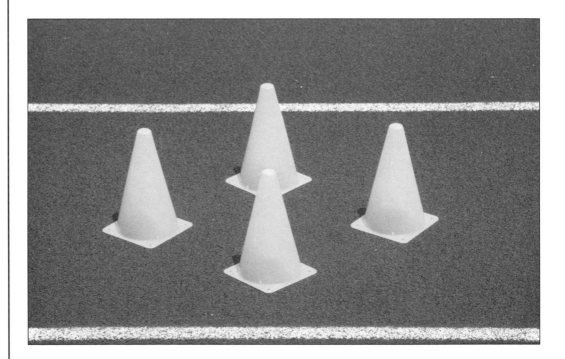

∎ **Figure 9.2** Plyometric cones.

BOXES

Boxes come in a variety of heights, ranging from 15 to 106 cm (6 to 42 in.), and various designs. The top should have a nonslip surface. The lower boxes are used for less intense activities and the higher ones for more intense activities (figure 9.3).

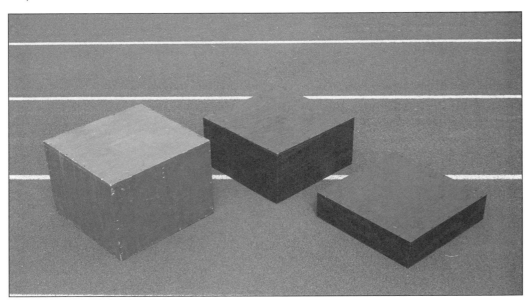

■ **Figure 9.3**   Plyometric boxes.

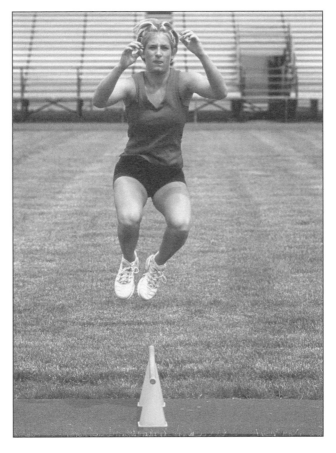

HURDLES

Hurdles are used for more advanced plyometric exercises. Some are adjustable within ranges of 15 to 100 cm (6 to 40 in.). A low hurdle can be easily constructed from two cones and a dowel (figure 9.4).

■ **Figure 9.4**
Plyometric hurdle constructed from cones and a dowel.

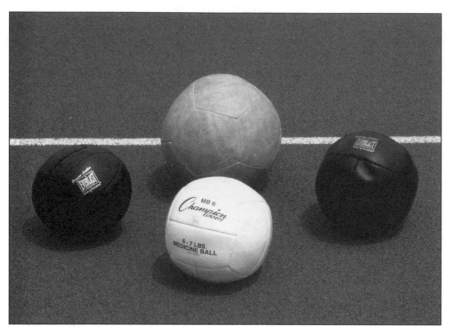

■ Figure 9.5
Medicine balls.

MEDICINE BALLS

Medicine balls are useful in plyometric activities for the upper extremities and trunk, and also provide additional resistance for lower-extremity plyometrics. They come in a variety of sizes, weights, and surfaces. The leather-covered balls are limited to indoor use because moisture shortens the life of the cover. Balls should be of a manageable size and should have a surface that permits the patient to maintain an adequate grasp. If one-hand activities are required for the exercise, the ball should have a diameter that will accommodate the patient's hand (figure 9.5).

OTHER EQUIPMENT

A variety of other equipment can be used for various plyometric activities. Jump ropes, stairs, and barriers are examples of items that are usually readily available. Their specific use depends on the goals of the exercise and the imagination of the sport rehabilitation specialist.

LOWER-EXTREMITY PLYOMETRICS

Lower-extremity plyometric exercises use various types of jumps, as well as bounding and box drills, in various combinations to provide a progression of intensities.

Once the patient has the prerequisite strength, flexibility, and coordination, and the tissues have healed sufficiently to tolerate the stress of such activity without incurring damage or additional inflammation, plyometric exercises can become a part of the therapeutic exercise program.

PROGRESSION

A lower-extremity plyometric exercise progression involves six types of exercises: jumps-in-place, standing jumps, multiple jumps and hops, bounding, box drills, and depth jumps (Chu 1998).

Jumps-in-Place

Jumps-in-place are repeated jumps that begin and end in the same place. They can range in intensity from low to high. The low-intensity jumps are good activities for developing a brief amortization phase. The specific goal, to develop a short amortization phase with a rapid rebound, often serves to develop the patient's jump technique. Jump-in-place exercises should relate to the patient's sport. For example, a two-foot ankle hop is suitable for a basketball player, and a hip-twist ankle hop is well suited to a skier. As the patient progresses, he or she can perform more difficult jumps-in-place or can advance to another type of jump exercise.

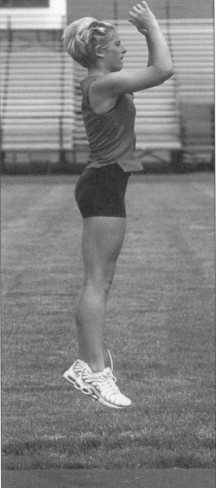

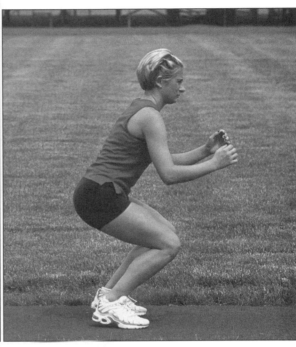

Two-Foot Ankle Hop

Have the patient jump in place using only the ankles. The patient should jump as high as possible. The knees will bend, but only slightly (figure 9.6a). This exercise is particularly good for patients who play basketball.

■ Figure 9.6 Jump-in-place plyometric exercises: *(a)* two-foot ankle hop, *(b)* hip-twist ankle hop.

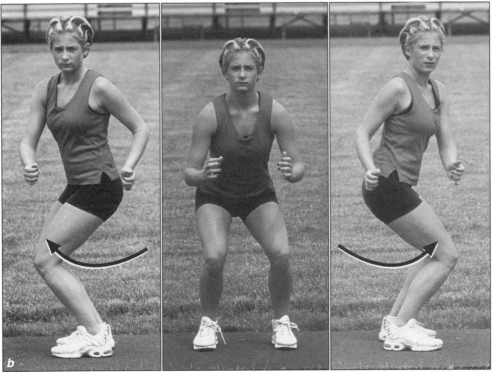

Hip-Twist Ankle Hop

Have the patient, with feet together, jump and twist 90° to the left, return to start position, and then repeat to the right. The patient should twist from the hips, not the knees (figure 9.6b). This exercise is particularly good for patients who ski.

Standing Jumps

Standing jumps are single jumps that emphasize a maximal effort with motion occurring either vertically or horizontally. Recovery between each attempt is necessary for a maximal effort each time. A progression of this type of jump could consist, for example, of beginning with a standing long jump, progressing to a jump over a cone, and advancing to a standing long jump with a sprint. Standing jumps can go forward or laterally and can involve barriers. Patients can combine standing jumps with multiple jumps, running, or sprinting in different directions.

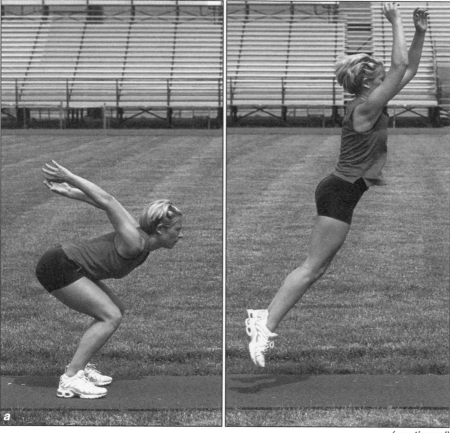

Standing Long Jump

The patient's feet are shoulder-width apart. Have him or her explode from semi-squat position to jump as far forward as possible. The patient should use arms to assist (figure 9.7a). This exercise is particularly good for patients who swim or participate in track.

(continued)

■ **Figure 9.7**   Example of a standing jump progression: *(a)* standing long jump, *(b)* standing jump over barrier, *(c)* standing long jump with sprint.

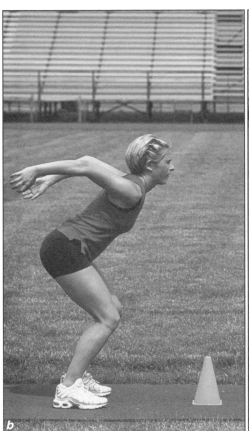

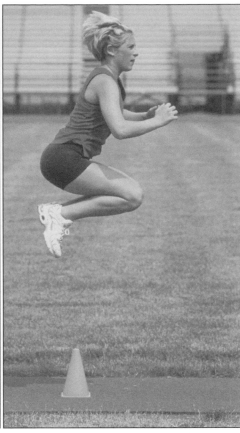

Standing Jump Over Barrier

Have the patient, with feet shoulder-width apart, jump upward and over cone, landing on both feet simultaneously. The patient should keep hips over knees and feet (figure 9.7b). You can add cones from 0.9 to 1.8 m (3–6 ft) apart for multiple jumps. This exercise is particularly good for patients who are figure skaters or basketball players.

Standing Long Jump With Sprint

Using arms to assist, the patient should jump as far forward as possible. Immediately after landing, have him or her sprint forward as fast as possible for 10 m (figure 9.7c). Add sprints to left and right for additional activities (figure 9.7c). This exercise is particularly good for patients who play hockey, participate in track, or play football.

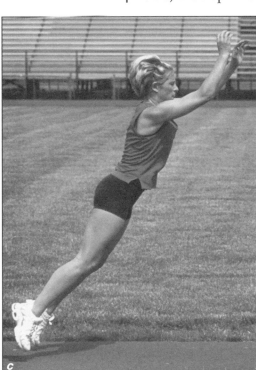

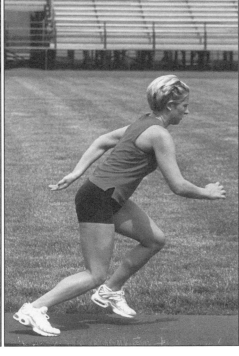

▌Figure 9.7   *(continued)*

Multiple Jumps and Hops

Multiple hops and jumps combine the skills of jumps-in-place and standing jumps. The patient attempts to jump maximally and repeats the jumps without resting. The total distance in each set of exercises is usually kept under 30 m (Chu 1998). The jumps can be performed with one or two legs, in a straight line or in multiple directions, with or without barriers. A front cone hop is an example of a simple multiple-hop exercise. The single-leg hop and a series of stadium-step hops are examples of more difficult multiple hops.

Single-Leg Hops

Have the patient jump from left leg, propelling as far upward and forward as possible, using arm movement to assist, then landing on the same leg. The patient should use forward movement of the right non-weight-bearing leg to propel forward for the next jump, landing on right leg. Remind the patient to keep hips and knees directly over the landing foot (figure 9.8a).

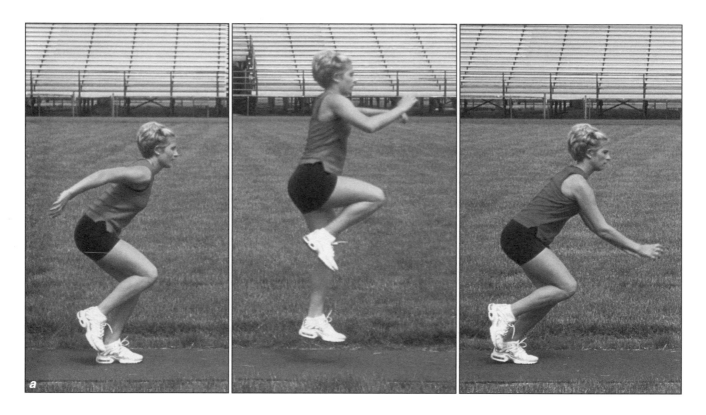

▌Figure 9.8   Examples of multiple jumps or hops: *(a)* single-leg hops, *(b)* stadium hops.

Refer to examples of plyometric jumping exercises for the lower extremities in Don Chu's *Jumping into Plyometrics*, second edition (1998). It is advisable for you refer to this book for additional suggestions for plyometric exercises and progression programs.

Stadium Hops

Have the patient jump one step at a time using both legs. The movement should be rapid, light, and continuous up the stairs, without stops or hesitation. The patient can progress to taking two steps at a time or using one leg and alternating (figure 9.8b). This exercise, as well as the single-leg hops on the previous page, is particularly good for patients who wrestle or play hockey.

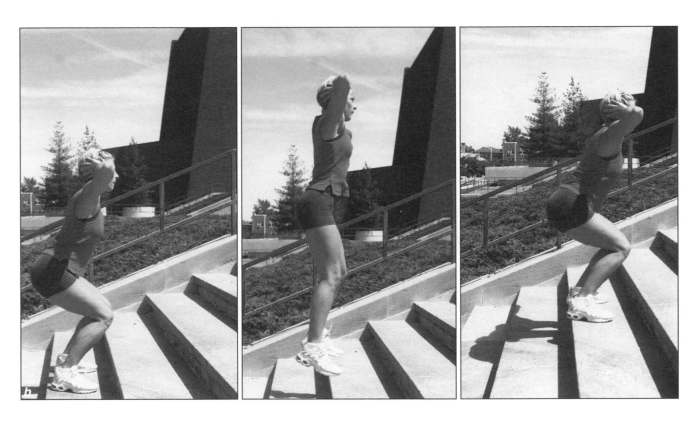

▮ **Figure 9.8**   *(continued)*

Bounding

Bounding exercises are an exaggeration of the running stride. They are used to improve stride length and speed. These exercises are most commonly used for patients in track and field events. Distances usually exceed 30 m (Chu 1998). A simple bounding exercise is skipping; an advanced bounding exercise is single-leg bounding. Skipping and bounding are explosive activities with the patient exploding quickly from landing and jumping upward and forward.

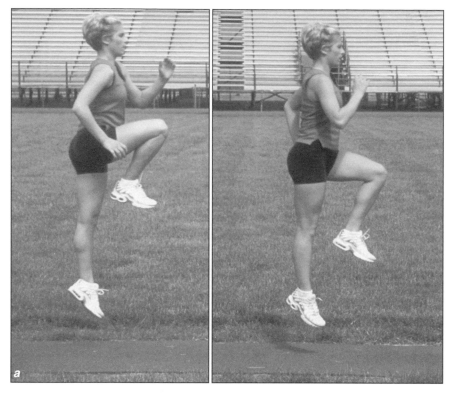

Skipping

Have the patient lift the right leg with knee bent 90° while also lifting left arm with elbow bent 90°. Then the patient should alternate with opposite extremities (figure 9.9a).

▌Figure 9.9 Examples of simple and more difficult bounding exercises: *(a)* skipping, *(b)* bounding.

Single-Leg Bounding

While on the right leg, the patient should move forward and upward as far as possible by using the momentum of the left leg and both arms to propel forward, landing on the right leg. Have the patient continue the forward and upward movement, this time landing on left leg (figure 9.9b).

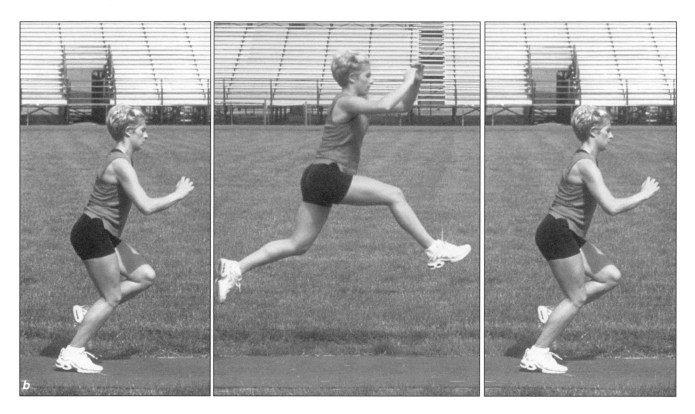

∎ **Figure 9.9**   *(continued)*

Box Jumps

Box drills involve the more advanced skills required for multiple jumps and hops because they include jumps and hops onto and off boxes of varying heights. These exercises can be low or high intensity, depending on the box height. They use both vertical and horizontal jumps. Examples of box jumps are shown in figure 9.10.

Front Box Jump

Begin with a box about 30 cm (12 in.) high. Jump onto the box with both feet. Step down and repeat. Can increase difficulty by increasing the box height or using one leg, alternating left and right (figure 9.10a).

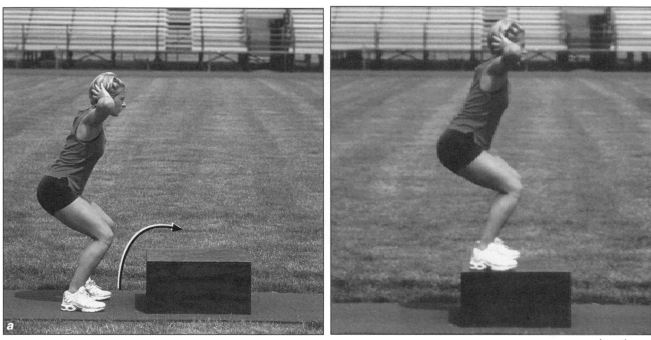

(continued)

■ **Figure 9.10**   Examples of box jumps: *(a)* front box jump, *(b)* pyramiding box jumps.

Pyramiding Box Hops

Place up to five boxes of increasing height about 0.6 to 0.9 m (2–3 ft) apart in a line. Jump onto the first box, onto the floor on the other side, and then onto the next box, repeating to the end of the row. Use the arms to assist in the motion (figure 9.10b).

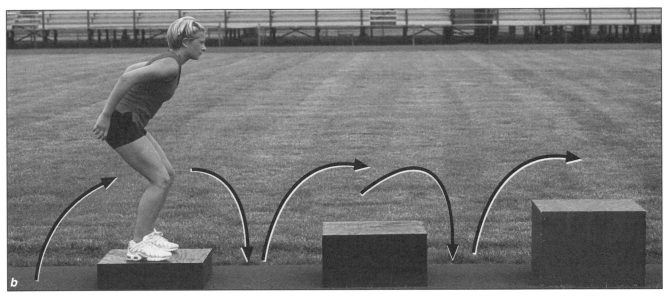

■ **Figure 9.10** *(continued)*

Depth Jumps

Depth jumps are the most aggressive plyometric exercises. They are box jumps of greater intensity in that the patient is challenged by his or her own weight and the acceleration of gravity. The motion in depth jumps includes stepping off a box, dropping to the ground, and then rebounding immediately upward. These are intensive exercises that the patient must perform with caution. Jumping off the box is avoided in these exercises because a jump will increase the distance to the floor and significantly increase the stresses applied to the patient.

An example of progression using depth jumps consists of starting from a simple depth jump in which the patient steps down from a box and jumps vertically, using both feet, and advancing to a much more difficult depth jump—a single-leg depth jump in which the patient lands on one foot and jumps as high as possible from the one leg.

A more challenging progression can include using a higher box or using more than one box and jumping onto the second box from the ground.

Depth Jump

Have the patient step off a 30-cm (12-in.) box, landing on the floor with both feet. As rapidly as possible, the patient should jump upward as high as possible, using the arms to reach upward (figure 9.11a).

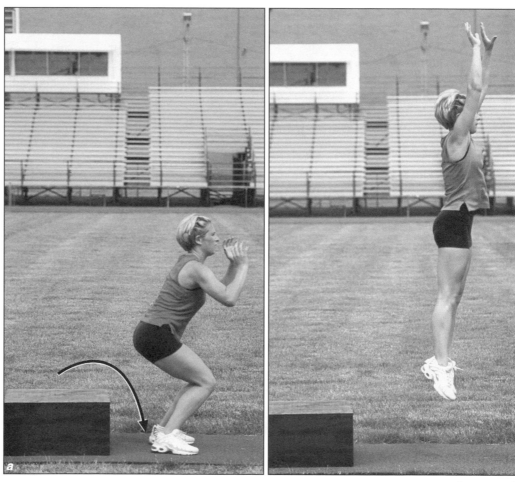

■ **Figure 9.11**
Examples of depth jumps: *(a)* depth jump, *(b)* single-leg depth jump.

(continued)

Single-Leg Depth Jump

Have the patient step off a 30-cm box, landing on the left leg only. The patient should spring upward as high as possible from the left leg. Then have him or her repeat the exercise with the right leg (figure 9.11b).

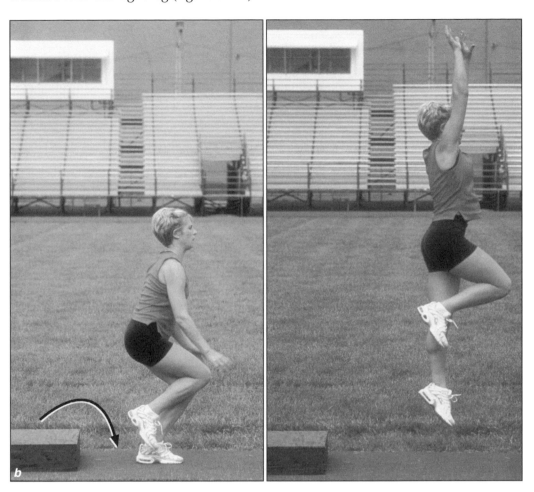

■ Figure 9.11
(continued)

Box Height

You must select a box height for depth jumps carefully. If the height is too great, the risk of injury increases. A height that is too great also requires the muscles to absorb the impact of the drop, and the time required to absorb the force makes the amortization time too long to be effective.

Chu (1998) recommends determining a box height for depth jumps using the following procedure. The patient performs a standard jump-and-reach test, and the target point the patient achieves is marked. The patient then performs a depth jump from a 45-cm (18-in.) box and attempts to reach for the same point as attained on the test. If the mark is attained, the box height increases by 15-cm (6-in.) increments until the patient is unable to achieve the target point. The first box at which the patient is unable to achieve the target point is the depth-jump box height. If the patient cannot reach the target point from the 45-cm box, either the box should be lowered or the patient should not perform the activity until he or she has achieved greater strength.

SELECTION

Although all the types of plyometric exercises provide a progression of difficulty from low to high intensity, you must analyze the exercise to determine its relative intensity. For example, a high-level standing jump may be more intense than a moderate-level box jump.

The selection of exercise for a patient's program depends on the demands of the patient's sport and the level of participation of that patient. For example, you may give one patient appropriate plyometric exercises with varying intensities of multiple jumps and hops; another patient may be more appropriately stressed with box jumps and depth jumps. Two patients in the same sport, one at a recreational level and the other at an intercollegiate competitive level, have different requirements because of the different competitive demands. This is a prime consideration in exercise selection.

UPPER-EXTREMITY AND TRUNK PLYOMETRICS

Plyometrics for the upper extremity and the trunk use tossing and throwing activities with medicine balls.

We will consider upper-extremity and trunk exercises together, because many of the upper-extremity exercises with medicine balls strongly influence the trunk muscles and vice versa. Some exercises are specific to either the upper extremity or the trunk, as indicated. Because the trunk plays a vital role in stabilization during upper-extremity activities, the strength of the muscle groups in the trunk is important to the strength of the upper extremity, and the trunk muscles are active during upper-extremity activities.

Plyometrics for the upper extremity and trunk have essentially the same considerations as those for the lower extremity. The exercises should be specific to the sport demands of the patient, should provide a progression of difficulty so that there is a challenge and the patient makes the desired gains, and should be performed with controlled speed of movement.

You can provide progression by changing the intensity. This can be done by changing the weights of the medicine balls, the speed of the activity, and the distance the medicine balls are passed. Passing medicine balls includes tossing and throwing. Tossing is defined as passing a ball a short distance with the arm below 90° of shoulder flexion; throwing is defined as passing the ball a long distance with the arm above 90° of flexion (Chu 1989).

Passing exercises can be performed with either a partner or a rebounder—a trampoline inclined so that it permits return of the ball to the patient (figure 9.12).

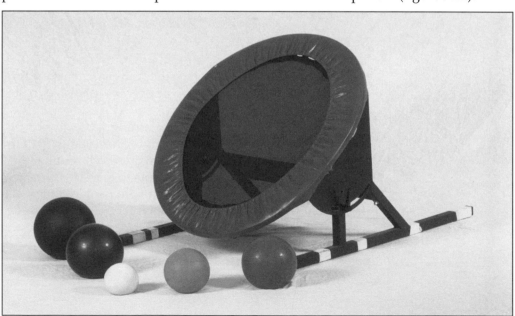

▌Figure 9.12
Rebounder and medicine balls.

Figure 9.13 provides examples of medicine-ball plyometric exercises for the upper extremities and trunk. The chest-pass photo shows the patient executing a chest pass from a distance of about 3 m (10 ft), using the forward movement of the legs to co-incide with the snap of the ball. Follow-through should continue until the arms are fully extended in front of the body and the backs of the hands face each other. In the overhead throw, once again the patient uses leg movement to coincide with arm motion so that as the ball is released from behind the head, the patient moves from the back to the front leg. Follow-through is with the arms straight, upward, and forward. During both activities, the trunk muscles are kept in a taut position and the back is held straight to allow force from the legs to be transmitted through the trunk to the arms.

As with lower-extremity plyometrics, upper-extremity and trunk plyometrics should be specific to the patient's needs. They should provide specific challenges that will permit the patient to make gains in the areas most challenged by the patient's sport. The SAID principle is as important in plyometric exercises as it is in strength exercises. As was mentioned in chapter 7, the SAID principle is an acronym for **S**pecific **A**daptations to **I**mposed **D**emands and refers to the body's ability to adapt to stresses applied through exercise.

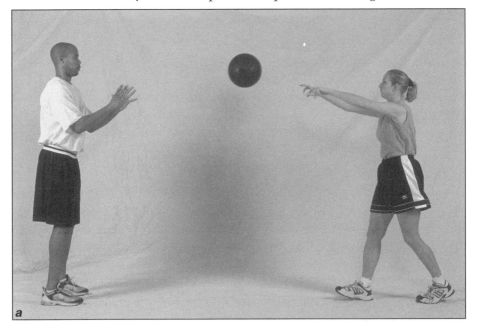

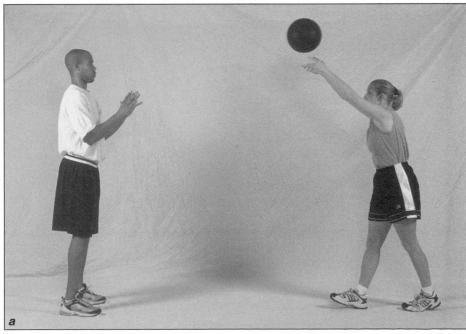

■ **Figure 9.13** Upper-extremity and trunk plyometrics: *(a)* chest pass, *(b)* overhead throw.

SUMMARY

1. *Identify the mechanical and neurological components of the neuromuscular principles involved in plyometrics.*

   Plyometrics involves the technique of first lengthening, then shortening the muscle to produce an increased power output. This type of exercise is based on the stretch-shortening principles. It is believed that a muscle's increased power during plyometric exercise training may result from a combination of an increased level of muscle elasticity and the adaptations that occur in the muscle spindle and GTO.

2. *Describe the factors involved in plyometric program design.*

   Every plyometric exercise includes three aspects—the lengthening or eccentric phase, the amortization phase, and the contracting or concentric phase. The lengthening phase prepares the muscles for the rapid change, or amortization, and allows for a greater contraction to produce greater results.

3. *List three considerations for plyometric program execution.*

   When designing a plyometric program, one must consider the patient's physical condition and the sport's demands. Specifically, the patient should have adequate flexibility, strength, and proprioception before beginning a plyometric program. Special considerations also include factors such as the patient's age, weight, level of competition, footwear, the surface, proper technique, progression, and goals.

4. *List the precautions and contraindications for plyometrics.*

   Precautions include factors such as the amount of time involved in plyometrics and the possibility of delayed-onset muscle soreness postexercise. Contraindications include an acute inflammation, postoperative conditions, and instability.

5. *Outline a progression of four plyometric exercises for either a lower- or an upper-extremity program.*

   An example of a lower-extremity plyometric exercise progression for a basketball player might include beginning with a two-foot ankle hop and progressing to a single-foot ankle hop, side-to-side hops, standing jump-and-reach, long jump with lateral sprint, and box depth jumps.

CRITICAL THINKING QUESTIONS

1. If a plyometric jump is not executed quickly from the eccentric to the concentric phase, the patient is unable to jump as high during the concentric phase. What could the reasons be? What can be done if a patient does not understand the concept of a rapid change from eccentric to concentric and insists on pausing between the two phases? What cues or instructions can you provide to improve performance?

2. A patient with an ankle sprain is now ready for plyometric exercises. What are the criteria that he or she has to meet before these exercises can be added to the therapeutic exercise program?

3. A gymnast with a wrist sprain is ready for plyometric activities before returning to functional activities. Identify three plyometric activities that would prepare him or her for functional activities. What would your criteria be for progression from plyometric to functional activities?

4. The head certified athletic trainer of the college where you are working has asked you to write a sheet of instructions that the certified athletic trainers will hand out to patients before they begin the plyometric phase of their rehabilitation programs. What instructions will you include on the sheet? What precautions will you list? Are there any criteria that you will include for determining whether a patient is eligible for a plyometric program?

5. In the chapter's opening scenario, what precautions is Matthew concerned about with Adam? What first-day plyometric activities would you recommend that Matthew have Adam perform, and what should Matthew look for when Adam performs them? How would you determine when Adam can progress in his plyometric program?

REFERENCES

Allerheiligen, B., and R. Rogers. 1995. Plyometrics program design. *Strength and Conditioning* 17:26–31.

Chu, D. 1989. *Plyometric exercises with medicine balls.* Livermore, CA: Bittersweet.

Chu, D. 1998. *Jumping into plyometrics,* 2d ed. Champaign, IL: Human Kinetics.

Dean, E. 1988. Physiology and therapeutic implications of negative work. *Physical Therapy,* 68:233-237.

Gambetta, V. 1986. In Roundtable discussion: Blelik, E., Chu, D.A., Costello, F., Gambetta, V., Lundin, P., Rogers, R., Santos, J., and F. Wilt. Practical considerations for utilizing plyometrics. Part 1. *National Strength Coaches Association Journal* 8:14–22.

Koutedakis, Y. 1989. Muscle elasticity—plyometrics: Some physiological and practical considerations. *Journal of Applied Research in Coaching and Athletics* 4:35–49.

Lundin, P. 1985. A review of plyometric training. *National Strength Coaches Association Journal* 7:69–74.

Wilk, K.E., Voight, M.L., Keirns, M.A., Gambetta, V., Andrews, J.R., and C.J. Dillman. 1993. *Journal of Orthopedic and Sports Physical Therapy* 17:225–239.7

Wilt, F. 1975. Plyometrics. What it is—how it works. *Athletic Journal* 55:76–90.

CHAPTER TEN

Functional Exercise

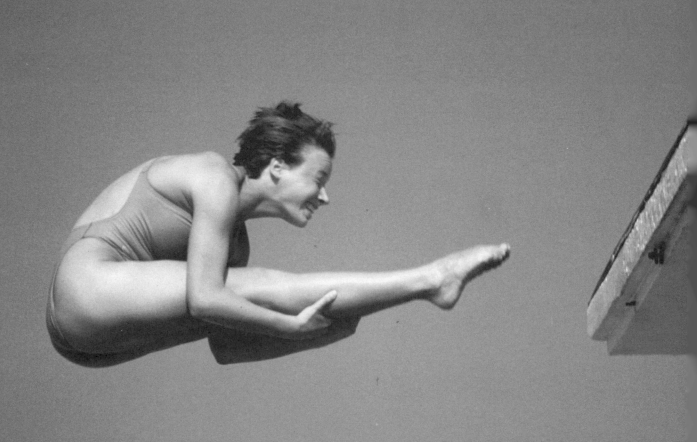

OBJECTIVES

After completing this chapter, you should be able to do the following:

1. Explain the difference between functional exercise and functional testing.

2. Identify the contributions of functional exercise to a therapeutic exercise program.

3. Discuss the differences between basic and advanced functional activities.

4. List factors that can be varied in a progression of functional activities.

5. Identify precautions for functional exercises.

6. Outline a sample of functional progression for either the lower or upper extremity.

Catherine Pierce is a certified athletic trainer working with the college's tennis team. At the end of last season, Tom, the star singles player, underwent a shoulder capsular shift repair. He has progressed well through his rehabilitation program and is now ready to begin the process of returning to functional activities. It has been several months since Tom has swung a tennis racket, and he has a lot of apprehension about whether he will be able to return to competition. Catherine is confident that he will do well once he has completed the functional rehabilitation phase of his program.

For the past few weeks Catherine has had Tom get used to holding a tennis racket by having him bounce a ball on the ground and in the air with his elbow near his side. Now it is time for Tom to begin ground strokes. Catherine has outlined the progression of the program she has designed for Tom, informing him that the program will move at his own pace and allow him and his shoulder to become accustomed to one level before advancing to the next level. Tom has confidence in Catherine's ability and judgment because she has done an excellent job of bringing him this far along in his rehabilitation program. He knows that if she feels he can do an activity, he probably can do it.

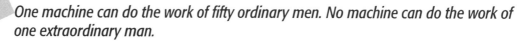

One machine can do the work of fifty ordinary men. No machine can do the work of one extraordinary man.

Elbert Hubbard, *The Philistine*

This chapter addresses an important but often forgotten aspect of therapeutic exercise: functional activities. Too frequently the injured athlete's program focuses on restoring flexibility, strength, power, and endurance, and the specific sport demands are forgotten. During the later stages of the therapeutic exercise program it becomes important to prepare the injured athlete to withstand the specific stresses of his or her sport and meet the skill demands of the sport; it is also essential for the patient to have confidence that he or she can return to full participation.

Most healthy athletes want to perform at exceptional levels, to be the extraordinary athlete. The presence of that preinjury attitude is critical if an injured athlete is to return successfully to sport participation. To restore that attitude, the sport rehabilitation specialist must include functional activities in the therapeutic exercise program. Functional activities are exercises that mimic the stresses, demands, and skills of the sport.

The sport rehabilitation specialist must understand and appreciate not only the patient's sport but also his or her position within that sport. Offensive and defensive football players encounter different stresses and demands, just as the defensive lineman and defensive halfback position requirements are different. A volleyball setter and a volleyball hitter have different needs; a softball pitcher and a softball outfielder experience different stresses. The sport reha-bilitation specialist should know the injured athlete's specific sport requirements and also know how to incorporate those requirements into the therapeutic exercise program.

Once the basic parameters of flexibility, strength, endurance, and proprioception have been achieved, specific exercises mimicking sport skills should be incorporated into the program. This will restore the injured athlete's confidence in his or her sport performance ability and will also provide an avenue for renewing the skills lost following the injury.

DEFINITIONS, FOUNDATIONS, AND GOALS

Functional exercise within a therapeutic exercise program encompasses exercise and evaluation. The goals of functional exercise are to attain full functional level of performance, restore the patient's confidence, and return the patient to sport participation.

Before we can discuss specific functional programs and activities, we must understand what functional exercises and evaluations are, as well what their basis and goals are. Once you realize how a therapeutic exercise program progresses to its functional exercise portion, it will become clear when and how to apply functional exercises to this final phase.

DEFINITIONS

Functional exercise actually has two components in a therapeutic exercise program: exercise and evaluation. **Functional exercises** are activities that move an injured athlete toward a safe return to sport participation as soon as is feasible. These activities include exercises and skill drills in a progressive sequence that allows the patient to use the gains from one exercise to advance to the next level of exercise or skill drills.

Functional evaluation is performed throughout the program. **Functional evaluation** is an assessment of the patient's ability to perform an exercise or skill drill safely and accurately before he or she is allowed to advance to the next level. The final functional evaluation takes place before the patient returns to sport participation. In order to safely advance to each therapeutic exercise level, the patient must pass the functional tests. The functional tests vary according to the patient's level within the therapeutic exercise program. Examples of these tests are discussed later.

GOALS

Functional exercise has four goals. The first goal is to attain full functional levels of flexibility, strength, endurance, and coordination. The second is to achieve full functional ability so that normal speed, power, control, and agility are restored. The third goal of functional exercise is to restore the injured athlete's self-confidence in his or her own sport performance as well as confidence in the injured body segment. The final goal is to return the injured athlete to sport participation safely and efficiently at a level at least equivalent to that of preinjury performance.

The first and second goals are achieved through the therapeutic exercise program for basic and advanced functional activities. These are discussed in the next section. The third goal is achieved through the advancement of functional exercises and the success the injured athlete experiences at each level. Success builds self-confidence, and failure makes self-confidence elusive; so it is important that the sport rehabilitation specialist provides exercise goals that are challenging yet achievable. Both being injured and being unable to participate in sport often cause an injured athlete to become unsure of his or her sport performance skill. Not participating also leads to loss of some of the skills that were so natural before the injury. To reestablish in the patient a preinjury level of self-confidence in his or her athletic skills, it is necessary to incorporate into the therapeutic exercise program a progression of specific exercises that mimic the skill requirements of that person's sport.

The final goal is achieved when all the other goals have been met. This goal is the end result and the primary goal of any therapeutic exercise program. To achieve it, the sport rehabilitation specialist must include both basic and advanced functional activities in the therapeutic exercise program. A final functional evaluation takes place before the injured athlete returns to full sport participation, but it is the injured athlete's ability to participate successfully in the sport that is the final test of a therapeutic exercise program.

CONTRIBUTIONS TO THERAPEUTIC EXERCISE

Functional exercises contribute to the total rehabilitation process by imposing unique combinations of stresses on the injured athlete according to the individual's sport and position within the sport.

Functional exercises are a part of the total rehabilitation process. In that sense, they make a vital and unique contribution to the preparation and return to competition of the injured athlete. They must place unique combinations of stresses on the injured athlete to produce unique results. The following sections deal with eight of these demands and the corresponding results.

NORMAL MOTION

Functional exercises are designed to reproduce the specific motions of the injured athlete's sport. They are individually designed for each sport and for the position the injured athlete plays so that they mimic the normal activity that the patient will perform upon returning. Normal activity requires normal motion. If normal motion is lacking, the injured athlete places undue stress on areas that must compensate for needed motion, and these areas are at risk for additional injury. For example, if a tennis player does not have the normal shoulder flexion and external rotation needed for serving, he or she may develop a low back injury by hyperextending the lumbar spine to hit the ball overhead.

MULTIFACETED MUSCLE ACTIVITY

Several different types of strengthening activities are used in functional exercises. They commonly include a mixture of isometric, concentric, and eccentric activities, because most functional activities include these types of movements. The muscle must have the strength, coordination, and control to change from one type of movement to another quickly and to produce the summation of forces effectively. Even in the simple activity of running, the lower-extremity muscles undergo a rapid change of concentric and eccentric activity in their roles as accelerators, decelerators, and stabilizers during different parts of the running cycle.

MULTIPLANAR MOTION
AND MULTIPLE MUSCLE-GROUP PERFORMANCE

Functional activities are not performed in straight-plane movements. They involve the simultaneous use of many planes including rotational, frontal and horizontal planes. They also include the use of many muscle groups that are recruited at one time to produce the desired activity. Functional exercises must mimic these functional activities by incorporating many muscle groups working in multiple planes.

Multiplanar motion is performed in a coordinated manner through the simultaneous facilitation and inhibition of many muscles. Even an activity like throwing a ball not only involves the shoulder, elbow, wrist, and hand muscles but also requires coordinated multiplanar motions from trunk and lower-extremity muscle groups.

STABILIZATION AND ACCELERATION CHANGES

Functional motion requires that some muscles work to stabilize a part while other muscles work to either accelerate or decelerate or to change from stabilization to acceleration or deceleration quickly. If functional exercises are to mimic sport activities, muscles must be trained to perform these fluid functional changes that are part of even basic sport activities. To use the example of a throw, the trunk must be stabilized if the shoulder is to have a platform to propel the ball from. Even in an activity such as walking, the hip and lower leg muscles stabilize and limit lateral movement as the body is propelled forward.

PROPRIOCEPTIVE STIMULATION

Proprioception is the awareness of body movement and position. As discussed in chapter 8, proprioception is vital to sport performance. Proprioceptive skills, basic and advanced, must be fine-tuned and must be prepared to meet the demands of the sport the patient will be returning to. Performance of functional exercises requires the use of proprioception, and improvement of the patient's functional performance directly correlates to his or her proprioceptive development.

AGILITY AND POWER DEVELOPMENT

Agility and power are key requirements for most sports. Agility is necessary in order for the basketball player to dribble the ball downcourt, for the volleyball player to dive and pass the ball to the setter, and for the hurdler to time each jump correctly. Power allows the sprinter to reach the finish line before the other competitors, the football defensive lineman to sack the quarterback, and the crew team to sprint to the end of the race. Agility and power are required in a gymnast's floor exercise routine, an ice skater's triple-lutz jump, and a water polo player's scoring a goal. Agility and power must improve as the patient increases his or her ability to perform functional activities. Progressive functional exercises steadily stress and, therefore, increase the patient's ability to perform at an agility and power level sufficient for appropriate skill execution within the sport and at the patient's level of competition.

SKILL DEVELOPMENT

Functional exercises—from the basic exercises to the more advanced—have as their goal the injured athlete's return to sport participation. The advanced functional exercises used in the later stages of rehabilitation are specifically designed with this goal in mind. These functional exercises mimic the sport activities and place the same demands on the injured athlete that he or she will encounter when returning to participation. The specific skills needed to perform the rehabilitation exercises are the same skills that are needed to perform within the sport.

CONFIDENCE DEVELOPMENT

As the patient succeeds in performing those functional exercises that mimic the demands of the sport, confidence returns. By the time the patient is ready to resume sport participation, he or she has demonstrated an ability to perform the skills that participation requires. This gives the individual the self-confidence to perform without hesitation and also to meet the demands of the sport with confidence in the injured part.

BASIC FUNCTIONAL ACTIVITIES

The basic functional exercises that begin an injured athlete's therapeutic exercise program follow a progression to build the foundation for improvement in more specific skill activities.

In a good therapeutic exercise program, functional exercise and functional evaluation take place from the very beginning. The program starts with exercises for achieving basic parameter goals such as flexibility, strength, endurance, and proprioception. To some extent, these can be considered functional exercises because they are used to attain a goal that is necessary for functional performance. For example, in order to jump hurdles, a runner has to gain a functional degree of flexibility in the hamstrings. In order to compete, a wrestler must have full functional flexibility in the shoulders. A pitcher needs functional muscle endurance to pitch a game. A gymnast must be able to stork stand on the ground before he or she can stand on a balance beam.

Basic functional exercises have been discussed in previous chapters. At this point, the progression and sequence of the exercises should seem logical to you. Exercises for flexibility, strength, endurance, and proprioception follow a logical sequence. Each parameter requires a coherent progression of exercises that provides increasing stress as the area adjusts to and becomes able to tolerate greater stresses because of improvements already made.

Your functional evaluation tools utilize objective criteria. For example, gains in range of motion are evaluated by goniometry, and strength gains are evaluated by manual muscle testing or the use of objective tools such as isokinetic equipment or grip dynamometers. Once you have determined that a patient has reached specific goals, you advance the individual to the next goal. For example, once the patient has achieved 105° of knee flexion, he or she may exercise on a stationary bike. Once the injured athlete is able to perform two sets of 15 repetitions of a biceps curl, you may either increase the weight or increase the repetitions. A patient should be able to stork stand on the ground before stork standing on an uneven surface. These are examples of functional progression of basic parameters.

ADVANCED FUNCTIONAL ACTIVITIES

Advanced functional exercises build on fundamental skill functions that the injured athlete has already achieved and often include plyometrics and specific skill drills.

Functional progression of advanced parameters involves more specific skill activities. A patient must start with fundamental skill functions and progress to advanced skill functions after having mastered some of the basic skills. Advanced functional activities include plyometrics and specific skill-drill exercises. In addition to flexibility, strength, muscle endurance, and proprioception, they require the more advanced skills of agility, speed, power, and control. Depending on the requirements of the advanced skill, some advanced functional exercises can be started earlier in the program while the patient is still working to achieve proficiency of basic skill execution. For example, the patient can start basic coordination exercises such as bouncing a basketball before he or she has achieved full range of motion or full strength.

As with the evaluation of functional performance of basic exercises, evaluation of advanced functional exercises involves periodic assessment and a logical progression. The injured athlete should have good static and dynamic balance before performing plyometric exercises. He or she should be able to perform plyometric exercises before specific skill activities are incorporated into the therapeutic exercise program. These are all logical, commonsense concepts. The skill of the sport rehabilitation specialist is a factor in determining exactly when the progressions should occur and what they should be. This skill is based on knowledge about tissue healing; knowledge of the influences of the stresses applied by various exercises and activities; observation of the patient's reaction to the stresses; knowledge of an exercise sequence; and knowledge of the specific demands, skills, and requirements of the injured athlete's sport and position within that sport. The sport rehabilitation specialist's skill is also based on good judgment and common sense about how much stress to apply and when during the therapeutic exercise program to apply that stress.

Because the earlier chapters have addressed the progression of basic functional exercise and evaluation, this chapter focuses on progression of advanced functional exercise and evaluation.

ADVANCED FUNCTIONAL-EXERCISE PROGRESSION

Advanced functional exercises focus on the parameters of force and intensity, speed, distance, complexity, and support. Stresses are increased gradually and progressively according to the patient's ability to handle them, as well as other individual factors.

You may have noticed that some proprioceptive parameters are included in basic functional exercises and that agility is in the advanced functional exercises category. This is because proprioception is a transition parameter. Because of the wide range of complexity of proprioception, one of its simplest efferent results, balance, becomes a basic functional activity. Agility, however, requires a great deal of skill and is considered a more advanced functional activity.

Some basic functional exercises actually mimic advanced functional activities in that they are performed during specific sport activity. Examples of basic functional activities in various sports are stork standing in ice skating, standing on the unstable surface of the edge of a diving board, and walking on a gymnastic balance beam.

These examples of basic functional activities serve only as a reminder that it is sometimes difficult to draw the line between basic and advanced activities. It is a good idea to remember this as you think about progression of advanced functional exercises. You will also notice that some of the topics discussed here are similar to those presented in previous chapters on progression of exercises. The reason is that the same progression principles hold true, whether the topic is strength, plyometrics, or functional activity.

As with any progression in a therapeutic exercise program, the increase should be gradual in order to allow the body time to adjust to new levels of stress, should provide a continual overload stimulation to improve performance, and should involve systematic adjustments in parameters that influence the desired end of the progression—the ultimate return of the patient to competition. These parameters include force, speed, distance, complexity, and support.

FORCE AND INTENSITY

Force and intensity are the amount of resistance that an activity provides. Forces and intensities vary in type depending on the specific activity and the outcome desired. The intent is to provide an overload in accordance with the SAID principle that has been described in chapter 7. The force or intensity starts light and increases as the injured athlete is able to tolerate increased loads. For example, in an upper-extremity functional exercise such as a volleyball pass, the patient may begin with a medicine-ball exercise using a 0.9-kg (2-lb) ball and increase to 1.8 kg (4 lb), then 2.7 kg (6 lb), and so on until the appropriate medicine-ball weight is achieved.

SPEED

Speed is the rate of a functional exercise. In the beginning, the speed is slower so that the injured athlete can master correct execution of the exercise. As skill improves, the speed requirement increases. For example, an injured track athlete may begin running at half-normal speed for a specific distance but then increase the speed as his or her ability to handle increased stresses improves. In an upper-extremity exercise such as throwing, the patient may begin throwing at one-quarter to one-half normal speed and increase the speed of the throw as technique execution improves.

Specific speeds for initial functional exercises are individually established and are determined by a variety of factors. These factors include the length of time the patient has been out of full sport participation, the severity of the injury, the individual's competitive level, preinjury distances, motivation level, and goals for return to participation. As a rule of thumb, initial functional exercise speed may be one quarter to one half the normal or preinjury speed and progress to three-quarter speed and then to full speed. This is a very general rule, however, and you must always take into consideration the individual patient's condition and abilities, as well as the demands of the exercise.

DISTANCE

Distances for functional activities range from short to long. The greater the distance, the greater the requirements of the activity. In the lower extremity, increasing distance may include increasing the patient's running distance or jumping distance. In the upper extremity it may include throwing or hitting a ball farther or swimming farther.

As in determining functional exercise speeds, one sets specific distances in initial functional exercises individually and according to the factors already discussed.

A general guideline, though not a hard-and-fast rule, is to start with no more than one quarter to one half the preinjury distance. Initial distance, however, may be significantly less for a patient such as a marathoner who has been out of competition for four months and had a preinjury running distance of 16 km (10 miles) per workout, or for an outfielder who must throw a ball 55 m (180 ft). The sport rehabilitation specialist uses his or her best judgment and knowledge of healing and athletic demands to determine the most appropriate distances for initial functional exercises. It is better to underestimate than to overestimate the injured athlete's ability to withstand stresses. You can avoid aggravation of an injury when you underestimate but provoke it when you overestimate.

COMPLEXITY

Complexity of a functional exercise refers to how involved the activity is and how challenging it can be. Functional exercises progress from simple to complex. Each level of progression places more demands on the patient's ability and skill. For example, in the lower extremity, a jumping progression may begin with a simple standing jump activity and progress to multiple jumps-in-place, to a forward or backward jump, and to multiple forward or backward jumps. Upper-extremity functional exercises may begin with a simple activity such as bouncing a tennis ball into the air from the racket, and then progress to a forehand stroke, to a backhand stroke, to a combination of backhand and forehand strokes against a backboard, and to a combination of backhand and forehand strokes against another player across a net.

You can also increase complexity by having the patient perform a simple exercise and then progress to performing a number of simple exercises at one time. For example, a stork stand with eyes open becomes more complex when you have the patient catch a ground ball while stork standing. The progression continues when you have the patient catch the ground ball while stork standing on an uneven surface.

The sport rehabilitation specialist determines on an individual basis how complex the initial functional exercise should be and how quickly the complexity should increase. You must consider the factors already outlined and make the best judgment. Remember, it is always better to err on the side of caution when advancing the patient so that progression continues consistently forward, without regression.

SUPPORT

Support refers to the number of extremities that are bearing weight during the activity. In simple standing, support is bilateral; in a stork stand, support is unilateral. Unilateral stance is more difficult than bilateral stance. Jumping on one leg is a progression from performing the same activity on two legs. Throwing a ball with one hand overhead is more difficult than throwing a ball with two hands overhead; performing a push-up with one hand is more difficult than performing it with two hands.

The type of exercise is what determines whether the level of activity is basic or advanced. Once the activity begins to mimic a specific sport activity or is a component of a sport activity, it is considered an advanced functional exercise. The progression of advanced functional exercises follows the same principles as for other types of exercises. For example, a common functional exercise progression for an injured track athlete may including starting with running a mile run at half speed, increasing distance or intensity until the patient has attained near-normal levels, and then increasing to three-quarter speed with the patient maintaining the previously achieved intensity and distance. Once normal speed and distance on level ground are achieved, hill work may proceed.

Throughout the progression, the exercises should be difficult enough to challenge the patient without causing failure. For this reason, the judgment and evaluative skills of the sport rehabilitation specialist are crucial in the decisions about the nature and pace of the progression of functional exercises. As the patient nears the end of the therapeutic exercise program and realizes that return to sport participation is near, he or she must have self-confidence in performance ability, as well as confidence in the injured part, in order to be able to return to competition without hesitation or doubts. A progression of functional exercise to the final stages of advanced functional activities—essentially skill activities that mimic sport participation—must be severe enough to impose demands on the patient but simultaneously build the necessary self-assurance.

There may be several functional exercises that the patient is performing in one therapeutic exercise session. Some exercises may be at different demand levels than others. For example, one exercise may be at half-speed while another is at three-quarter speed. The session may include a simple exercise and also one that is much more complex. Selection of the level of each exercise is based on the injured athlete's ability to execute each specific functional exercise.

PRECAUTIONS

Because advanced functional activities increasingly challenge the patient's abilities, it is important to observe several important precautions within this part of the sport rehabilitation program. The patient must understand the exercise and avoid pain; the sport rehabilitation specialist must be aware of the patient's healing process and of his or her confidence and tolerance levels.

Advanced functional exercises are more complex, more challenging, and more rigorous than the basic functional exercises. This is generally so because more planes of motion, more muscle groups, more complex and simultaneous movements, and more agility are required for correct execution. Because of the increased demands such activities impose, there are also precautions that one must respect in assigning advanced therapeutic exercises to a patient.

EXPLAIN THE EXERCISE TO THE INJURED ATHLETE

Before executing the exercise, the patient should be made aware of how to perform the exercise, what its goals are, and what positions or movements to avoid. For example, the sport rehabilitation specialist demonstrates or else explains a stork stand on a trampoline by telling the patient that the eyes should remain open, that the arms are kept at the sides, and that the position should be maintained for 30 s. During execution, cues are given to correct the performance. The cues should be constructive and should include specific suggestions about how to improve the execution. Having the patient perform the exercise on the good side first may provide the individual with an impression of the correct performance. This is particularly helpful if the sport rehabilitation specialist tells the patient to note how the leg muscles feel when standing on the good leg and then try to attain the same feeling when standing on the injured leg. Instructing the injured athlete to tighten the gluteals and thighs may help to enhance stability.

AVOID PAIN AND SWELLING

Residual pain and swelling, especially on the following day or evening, should be avoided. Any increase in pain or swelling indicates that the exercise level is too severe for the injured area. If this occurs, the patient should return to the previous level of exercise until the injured part is able to tolerate additional stress.

Any time a patient advances in a program, the sport rehabilitation specialist should observe for increases in pain and edema and instruct the patient to report any symptoms.

UNDERSTAND TISSUE INTEGRITY

The sport rehabilitation specialist must be aware of the healing sequence and the time required for a specific tissue to complete the healing process. He or she must consider the tissue's structural integrity and understand the amount of stress involved in each specific functional exercise before including any functional activity in the therapeutic exercise program.

KNOW THE PATIENT'S CONFIDENCE LEVEL

Performance of functional exercises requires the patient's confidence in his or her ability to perform the activity and in the ability of the injured part to tolerate the stress of the activity. If the patient mentally or emotionally is not prepared to handle a particular functional exercise, you should start with a less stressful, less complex activity that the person feels able to perform before advancing to more complex, more stressful exercises.

BE AWARE OF PROGRESSION TOLERANCE

Advanced functional exercises are introduced at lower-than-normal speed, intensity, and difficulty. Increases in these parameters are made one at a time until the exercise is at normal functional performance levels. The body must be allowed to adapt to increased levels of functional exercises before additional changes are made. This will ensure that the patient's confidence can increase and that tissue overload is not excessive, thereby preventing additional injury.

FUNCTIONAL EVALUATION

Step-by-step evaluation determines when the patient should advance to the next stage in the functional exercise program. The final functional evaluation, whose purpose is to determine whether the patient is ready to return to sport participation, is highly individualized.

Evaluation of function is an ongoing process. Throughout the therapeutic exercise program the sport rehabilitation specialist evaluates the patient's ability to perform both basic and advanced functional exercises. Advances in the program take place only after the patient is able to successfully perform to expected levels at each evaluation step. With the stork stand, for example, you do not have the patient progress until he or she is able to stork stand with eyes open for 30 s. Once the patient passes that evaluation, the next phase of balance proceeds—but not until then. Then the patient may stork stand on an uneven surface or on the ground with eyes closed. Which specific exercise to use next depends on the demands of the patient's sport.

The final functional evaluation occurs before the injured athlete is allowed to return to full sport participation. At this time the functional evaluation is highly individualized and is based on the specific demands of the patient's sport and position. The patient's performance in the evaluation determines his or her readiness to return to sport participation. Final functional evaluation includes highly specific drills and tests the person's sport skill. These functional evaluations should be as objective as possible and mimic the individual's sport as much as possible. For a gymnast, the functional evaluation may include dismounts, tumbling skills, or apparatus skills. For a basketball player, the functional evaluation includes dribbling, shooting, cutting, or passing drills. For a football defensive lineman, the functional evaluation includes assessment of skills such as blocking, lateral or forward movements, agility, or quick changes of direction. Because specific functional activities vary greatly from sport to sport and from position to position within a sport, you must be familiar with the sport requirements for the patient. You may need to obtain the coach's help in defining functional exercises and tests for some sports or positions. It is the goal of the final functional evaluation, however, to demonstrate to the patient, the medical team, and the coach that the individual is able and ready to withstand the stresses of full sport participation.

The functional tests for determining readiness to return to full participation must fulfill certain criteria, some of which have been previously mentioned. One criterion is that the evaluation tool should be as objective as possible. The test should be repeatable so that it can be used both in initial evaluation and in final evaluation to measure changes and assess whether or not the patient has achieved the appropriate goals. The functional tests should provide useful information to the patient, coach, and medical team about the progress and status of the patient's performance. They should also be able to show whether or not the functional exercise program is providing the advancement of parameters necessary for return to participation.

In the final functional evaluation, your observation and assessment of the patient's performance is critical. Any sport activity should be performed without hesitation, and the use of each extremity should be appropriate, with no favoring of the injured limb. The injured athlete should move quickly, stabilize appropriately, and demonstrate self-confidence with all maneuvers. On the basis of the athlete's performance, you should be unable to identify which extremity has been injured.

A LOWER-EXTREMITY FUNCTIONAL PROGRESSION

A progression for lower-extremity function may begin with non-weight-bearing exercise and proceed to stork-standing exercises, dynamic movement activities such as lunges and jogging, and running activities. Lower-extremity functional testing should reflect the patient's sport activity as much as possible and should be as objective as possible.

This section presents functional exercises for the lower extremity and then describes functional testing that could be included as part of the assessment before the injured athlete is allowed to return to full sport activity.

FUNCTIONAL EXERCISES

Any functional exercise should be preceded by a simple warm-up activity. Simple functional exercises for the lower extremity can begin relatively early with a non-weight-bearing exercise such as proprioceptive neuromuscular facilitation. Partial weight-bearing use of the BAPS board can also begin early in the therapeutic exercise program. As the patient becomes weight bearing, he or she can start to do stork standing, first with eyes open and then with eyes closed. This activity can progress from the floor to a BAPS board (figure 10.1), trampoline, $1/2$ foam roller, or balance board (figure 10.2) and then to combining the balance activity with another activity such as ball catching. Stork-standing activities will then progress to dynamic movement activities such as lunges, step-ups and step-downs, walking, and jogging. Running activities begin with a forward jog on a flat surface, progress to increased speed and distances, and then move on to lateral runs and cuts and sudden changes in direction. In figure 10.3a, the patient pushes forward from the left foot to the right foot and then moves laterally to the left foot before retracing the steps to the starting position, moving from one position to the next as quickly as possible. Figure 10.3b shows W-sprints requiring the patient to sprint forward to the first marked spot or cone, then backpedal to the second marker, and then sprint forward to the next, repeating the series as illustrated to completion of the exercise. Figure 10.3c shows a figure-8 run, which uses markers or cones around which the patient runs in a figure-8 pattern. The exercise in figure 10.3d is similar to the W-sprint except that the patient runs straight ahead, pivots on the right outside leg to cut sharply to the left, runs straight ahead for a designated distance, and pivots on the left outside leg to cut sharply to the right until the end of the course. Each of these exercises can become more difficult if you require either a faster pace or smaller distances between the sudden motion changes.

Figure 10.4 shows examples of jumping exercises. In the jumping exercise in figure 10.4a, the patient faces a

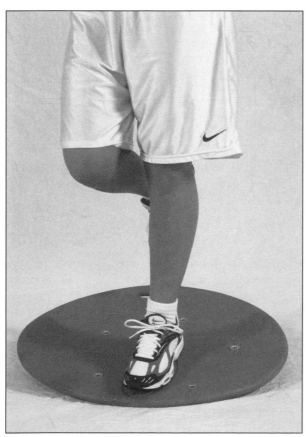

▌Figure 10.1   BAPS board.

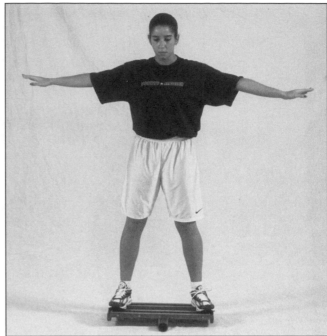

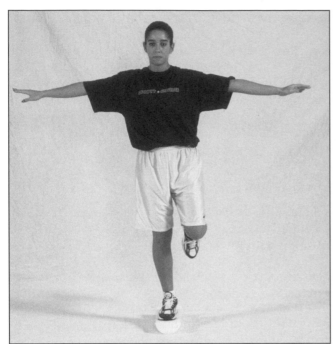

■ **Figure 10.2**   Balance activities: *(a)* stork stand on ¹/₂ foam roller, *(b)* balance board.

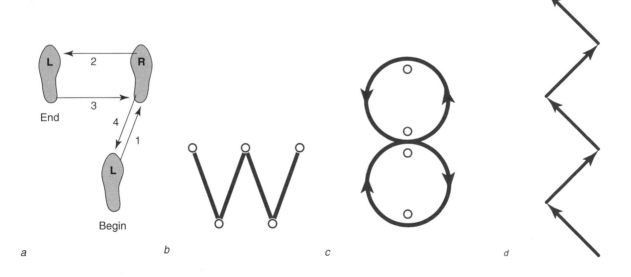

■ **Figure 10.3**   Agility drills, running: *(a)* 90° lunge, *(b)* W-sprint course, *(c)* figure-8 course, *(d)* Z-course (zigzag).

platform, places one foot on top of the platform, and then jumps as high as possible, switching foot placement so that the opposite foot ends up on the platform. This is a continuous and rapid jump-and-switch maneuver for a specified time or number of repetitions. A lateral jump is displayed in figure 10.4b; here the patient jumps from side to side over a ball or other object, attempting to stay within the cones. Difficulty can be increased by spreading the outside cones and having the injured athlete jump over the ball and toward the cones, or by placing a number of balls and cones in a line and having the person perform a series of lateral jumps in both directions.

A progression of jumping activities includes starting with jumping forward on a flat surface, then progressing to jumping backward and jumping laterally, first with both legs and then with only the involved leg. Jumping then can progress to box

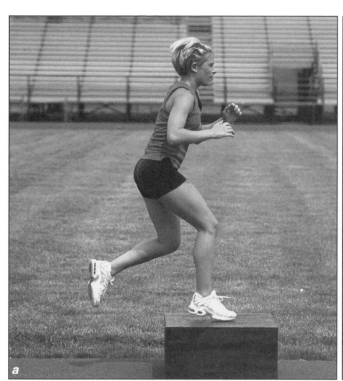 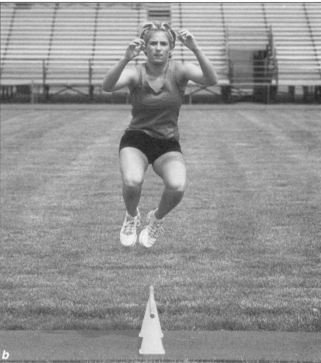

▌Figure 10.4   Agility drills: jumping.

jumps, starting with low boxes and advancing to higher ones. Progressions for these lower-extremity and running activities are presented in figures 10.5 and 10.6.

Specific exercises are determined by the patient's sport demands. As much as possible, running and jumping exercises should mimic the activities that the injured athlete will be performing once he or she returns to sport participation.

FUNCTIONAL TESTING

Several different tests for lower-extremity function can be used. The tests chosen should reflect the patient's sport activities as accurately as possible and should be as objective as possible. To measure gains in performance, you should use the same test to evaluate performance at the time the patient begins the functional exercise and before he or she returns to sport participation.

Lower-extremity tests can be classified as running tests for time and distance, jumping tests for height and distance, and agility tests. The running tests can be sprints or can be timed long-distance runs, depending on the sport requirements.

Jumping tests can include a standing vertical jump, a step-and-jump, a repeated jump for distance, and a single jump for distance. A volleyball player's jump test is more functional if it is either a standing or a step-and-jump test, whereas a field athlete's test is more functional if it is a multiple or run-and-jump-for-distance test.

Agility tests use cariocas, zigzag runs, figure-8 runs, shuttle runs, and box runs, to name a few. Whatever activities are selected, the distances, angles, and sizes of the turns and circles should be the same on the pretest as on the posttest for accurate comparisons. Goals should also be predetermined. The specifics of these goals may be defined either with reference to established norms or by the team coach who uses the exercises for team guidelines.

Example of Balance and Agility Progression Program

1. Beginning level
   a. Double-weight support for balance: static
      1) Stand with eyes closed, feet together
      2) Stand in tandem-stance position
         — eyes open
         — eyes closed
   b. Single-weight support for balance: static
      1) Stork stand with eyes open, 30 s
      2) Stork stand with eyes closed, 30 s
      3) Stork stand with eyes open on unstable surface
         — trampoline
         — $^1/_2$ foam roller
      4) Stork stand with eyes closed on unstable surface
         — trampoline
         — $^1/_2$ foam roller
      5) Stork stand with complex activity
         — Stork stand on ground while playing catch
            – sport ball
            – medicine ball
         — Stork stand on uneven surface while playing catch
            – sport ball
            – medicine ball
2. Intermediate level: dynamic activities
   c. Two-leg support: balance board, wobble board
   d. One-leg support: trampoline jumping
   e. One-leg support: hopping
   f. Treadmill retrowalking
   g. BAPS board
   h. Fitter
   i. Step-up exercises
3. Advanced level
   j. Running activities (start at reduced speeds and distances, and progressively advance to normal speeds and distances)
   k. Jumping activities (bilateral support)
      1) Lateral jumping
      2) Forward-backward jumping
      3) Command jumping
   l. Hopping activities (unilateral support)
      1) Lateral hopping
      2) Forward-backward hopping
      3) Command hopping
   m. Cariocas
   n. Plyometric box jumping
4. Precompetition level
   o. Sport-specific running, jumping, cutting activities at full speed
   p. Normal sport-specific drills
   q. Resumption of sport participation

Note: Jumping and hopping activities may start as exercises performed in place, but then can progress to line, target, and zigzag jumping and hopping exercises.

▮ Figure 10.5 Example of balance and agility progression program.

Example of Lower-Extremity Functional Exercise Progression

1. Non-weight-bearing exercises

   • Proprioceptive neuromuscular facilitation
   • Joint reposition sense activities
2. Partial weight-bearing exercises
   • Pool exercises
   • BAPS board
   • Stationary bike
3. Full weight-bearing exercises
   • Lunges
     — partial depth
     — full depth
   • Running
     — running on level surface 50% maximum speed, $\frac{1}{4}$ normal distance
     — running on level surface 75% maximum speed, $\frac{1}{4}$ normal distance
     — running on level surface 100% maximum speed, $\frac{1}{4}$ normal distance
     — running on level surface 100% maximum speed, $\frac{1}{2}$ normal distance
     — running on level surface 100% maximum speed, full normal distance
     — running on incline surface 75% maximum speed, $\frac{1}{2}$ normal distance
     — running on incline surface 75% maximum speed, $\frac{3}{4}$ normal distance
     — running on incline surface 75% maximum speed, full normal distance
     — running on incline surface 100% maximum speed, full normal distance
   • Sprinting
     — sprinting on level surface 50% maximum speed, $\frac{1}{4}$ normal distance
     — sprinting on level surface 75% maximum speed, $\frac{1}{4}$ normal distance
     — sprinting on level surface 100% maximum speed, $\frac{1}{4}$ normal distance
     — sprinting on level surface 100% maximum speed, $\frac{1}{2}$ normal distance
     — sprinting on level surface 100% maximum speed, $\frac{3}{4}$ normal distance
     — sprinting on level surface 100% maximum speed, normal distance
   • Jumping/Hopping
     — jumping rope, both feet
     — jumping rope, one foot
     — jumping lines, both feet forward, backward
     — jumping lines, one foot forward, backward
     — jumping lines, both feet zigzag forward, backward
     — jumping lines, one foot, zigzag forward, backward
     — box jumps, 6-in. boxes, two feet, forward
     — box jumps, 6-in. boxes, two feet, sideways
     — box jumps, 6-in. boxes, one foot, forward
     — box jumps, 6-in. boxes, one foot, sideways
     — box jumps of increasing heights with sequences above repeated
   • Agility
     — cariocas, 50% speed, both to left and to right
     — cariocas, 75% speed, both to left and to right
     — cariocas, 100% speed, both to left and to right
     — circle-8s with same sequence as cariocas, starting with large circles and reducing the size to tight circles
     — zigzag sprints with same sequence as cariocas
     — command drills with sudden changes in direction of any agility exercise on command

   Note: Any of these exercises can be made more difficult by increasing distance or number of sets, or using weights with the exercise.

∎ **Figure 10.6** Example of lower-extremity functional exercise progression.

AN UPPER-EXTREMITY FUNCTIONAL PROGRESSION

As with lower-extremity functional exercise, upper-extremity functional activities should resemble the activities of the patient's sport. Functional testing for the upper extremity varies greatly because use of the upper extremity differs markedly from one sport to another.

As in the discussion of the exercise program for the lower extremity, this section describes functional exercises and functional assessment for the upper extremity.

FUNCTIONAL EXERCISE

Like lower-extremity functional work, upper-extremity functional exercises may begin early in the program with proprioceptive neuromuscular facilitation (figure 10.7) and manual resistance to scapular stabilization activities. And again, upper-extremity exercises should be preceded by warm-up activities. Partial weight-bearing activities on a Swiss ball can sometimes be used early in the program as well. Closed kinetic chain activities such as weight-bearing exercises, first on a stable surface and then on an unstable surface, can be used once full weight bearing is permissible. Patient is in a push-up position with hands on BAPS board or wobble board. Both hands are on the board while the patient moves the board. In a push-up position, patient can start with two arms and advance to one, while the hands move side to side by bouncing. In a push-up position, the patient moves the Fitter platform side to side. All push-up positions can progress from a modified push-up position on hands and knees to a full push-up position on hands and feet. The injured athlete must attain scapular muscle strength, rotator cuff strength, and large shoulder muscle and other upper-extremity strength gains, along with proper range of motion, before beginning specific functional sport exercises. Having achieved proper stabilization, strength, range of motion, and control, the patient can progress to specific functional exercises such as throwing, golf exercises, tennis exercises, or swimming exercises. A progression of throwing begins with shortened distances for reduced speed and with power throwing at reduced repetitions; it advances to increased distances, numbers of throws, and severity of throws. See figure 10.8 for an example of a throwing progression.

A golf progression may begin with the putter and short irons for putting and chipping activities and progress to longer irons, fuller swings, and then to the woods with a full swing. With each club the swing begins as a partial swing and increases to a full swing as the patient gains progressive control of the club. Repetitions also increase as the patient's endurance improves. See figure 10.9 for a sample golf progression.

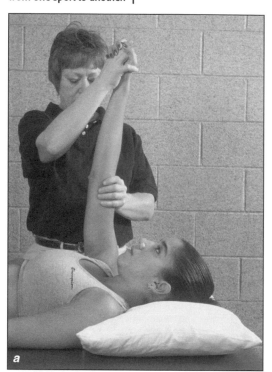

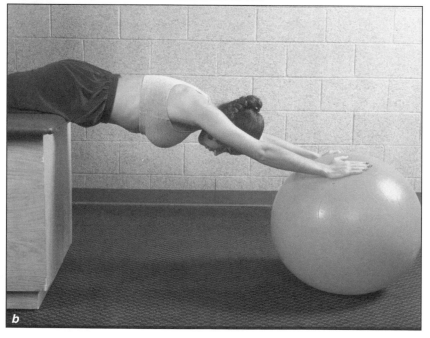

∎ **Figure 10.7** Functional exercise progression for the upper extremity: *(a)* open kinetic chain, *(b)* closed kinetic chain.

Baseball/Softball Throwing Progression Program

1. Beginning level
   a. 40–45-ft distance
      50% normal speed
      30 throws, 2 sets
   b. 40–45-ft distance
      50% normal speed
      30 throws, 4 sets
   c. 40–45-ft distance
      75% normal speed
      30 throws, 3 sets
   d. 40–45-ft distance
      75% normal speed
      30 throws, 5 sets
   e. 60-ft distance
      75% normal speed
      30 throws, 3–4 sets
   f. 60-ft distance
      75% normal speed
      30 throws, 5 sets

2. Intermediate level
   g. 60-ft distance
      100% normal speed
      30 throws, 3–4 sets
   h. 100-ft distance
      75% normal speed
      30 throws, 3–4 sets
   i. 100-ft distance
      75% normal speed
      30 throws, 5 sets
   j. 100-ft distance
      100% normal speed
      30 throws, 3–4 sets
   k. 100-ft distance
      100% normal speed
      30 throws, 5 sets
   l. 150-ft distance
      75% normal speed
      30 throws, 3–4 sets
   m. 150-ft distance
      75% normal speed
      30 throws, 5 sets
   n. 150-ft distance
      100% normal speed
      30 throws, 5 sets

3. Advanced level
   o. 180-ft distance
      75% normal speed
      30 throws, 3 sets
   p. 180-ft distance
      75% normal speed
      30 throws, 5 sets
   q. 180-ft distance
      100% normal speed
      30 throws, 3 sets
   r. 180-ft distance
      100% normal speed
      30 throws, 5 sets

4. Precompetition level
   s. Throw off mound
      100% normal speed
      30 throws, 3–4 sets
   t. Throw off mound
      100% normal speed
      30 throws, 5 sets

Note: All throwing sessions begin with a warm-up and end with a cool-down. Warm-up and cool-down throws are performed as light, arcing tosses. A rest of at least 3 to 5 min between sets is allowed. If the patient experiences pain with an increase to the next level, he or she should return to the previous level for another session. If the patient is not a pitcher, throwing progression follows the same routine as listed, but the distances vary according to the sport (e.g., discus, javelin, football) and are determined by the distances and weights used within the sport.

▌**Figure 10.8** Example of baseball or softball throwing progression program.

Golf Progression Program

1. Beginning level
   a. Putts and chips
      20 putts, varying distances
      10 chips
   b. Putts and chips
      20 putts, varying distances
      20 chips
   c. Putts and chips
      20 putts, 3 sets
      20 chips, 2 sets
   d. Putts and chips
      20 putts, 3 sets
      20 chips, 3 sets

2. Intermediate level
   e. Short irons, no more than three clubs
      partial swing, 1 × 20 each
   f. Short irons, no more than three clubs
      partial swing, 2 × 20 each
   g. Short irons, no more than three clubs
      partial swing, 3 × 20 each
   h. Short irons, no more than two clubs
      full swing, 1 × 20 each
   i. Short irons, no more than two clubs
      full swing, 2 × 20 each
   j. Short irons, no more than two clubs
      full swing, 3 × 20 each

   k. Long irons, no more than three clubs
      partial swing, 1 × 20 each
   l. Long irons, no more than three clubs
      partial swing, 2 × 20 each
   m. Long irons, no more than three clubs
      full swing, 2 × 20 each
   n. Long irons
      full swing, 3 × 25 each
   o. All irons
      full swing, 1 × 20 each

3. Advanced level
   p. Woods
      partial swing, 2 × 20 each
   q. Woods
      full swing, 2 × 20 each
   r. Woods and irons
      full swing, 1 × 20–25 each

4. Preparticipation level
   s. Par-three course
   t. Nine-hole course
   u. Return to regular play

Note: All sessions begin with a warm-up and end with a cool-down. A rest of at least 3 to 5 min between sets is allowed. If the patient experiences pain with an increase to the next level, he or she should return to the previous level for another session.

■ **Figure 10.9** Example of golf progression program.

We have already briefly looked at a progression of tennis functional exercises. A simple stabilization exercise such as bouncing the ball on the floor with the racket can begin once the scapular stabilizers and rotator cuff are able to maintain proper control. This activity can advance to bouncing the ball in the air with the racquet. More advanced exercises progress from a forehand to a backhand to overhead and serve strokes. See figure 10.10 for a general outline of progression.

A swimmer's progression may begin with the use of a stroke for a short distance or with alternating strokes for short distances and performing the stroke for no more than half-normal speed. Distances and speed increase as tolerated. See if you can develop an example of a swimmer's progressive program using these guidelines.

Tennis Progression Program

1. Ball bounce
   Bounce the tennis ball on the racket into the air. Start by grasping the racket on the neck and advance to the handle.
   a. 50 bounces with a palm-down grip
   b. 50 bounces with a palm-up grip
   c. 50 bounces alternating between palm down and palm up

2. Forehand strokes
   Forehand strokes only against a backboard or wall
   d. 50% power: 5×10
   e. 75% power: 3×20
   f. 100% power 3×40

3. Backhand strokes
   Backhand strokes only against a backboard or wall
   g. 50% power: 5×10
   h. 75% power: 3×20
   i. 100% power: 3×40

4. Alternate strokes
   Alternate between backhand and forehand strokes against a wall or backboard
   j. 75% power: 5×15
   k. 100% power: 3×30
   l. 100% power: 4×40

5. Overhead serve
   Overhead serve against a wall or backboard
   m. 50% power: 5×10
   n. 75% power: 3×20
   o. 100% power: 3×40

6. Game
   p. Play one set of tennis
   q. Play two sets of tennis
   r. Play three sets of tennis
   s. Play full game of tennis

Note: All sessions begin with a warm-up and end with a cool-down. The patient should attempt to hit a specific target or targets on the backboard or wall. If the patient experiences pain with advancement to the next level, he or she should return to the previous level for the next 2 to 3 sessions before returning to the next level.

▌**Figure 10.10**   Example of tennis progression program.

I want to emphasize that the progressive functional exercise programs presented here are only examples. Specific exercise progressions vary depending on the patient's needs, abilities, level of competition, length of time away from the sport, and degree of injury. The programs described in this chapter offer only general guidelines and are a means of demonstrating how to progress and change parameters of a functional exercise program.

FUNCTIONAL TESTING

It is more difficult to evaluate the upper extremity and obtain objective and measurable criteria than in the lower extremity. This is because of the variety of uses of the upper extremity in sport activities. If a speed gun is available, it is relatively simple to measure the speed of a patient's throw. However, if you do not have a speed gun or the patient's sport does not involve throwing, measuring functional skill objectively is more difficult.

Functional goals are individually determined and based on the patient's preinjury performance. For a golfer, it may be his or her score on 18 holes of golf. For the swimmer, it may be the ability to perform a specific swim event within the same time he or she had in preinjury performances. For the tennis player, measurement using a speed gun for a serve is simple, but evaluating participation performance may be more difficult. Establishing goals such as hitting a specific target across the net on a given number of consecutive forehand and backhand shots, and using that number for pretest and posttest performance guidelines, may be a way of establishing an objective measure. When establishing any goal in this manner, it is important for you to consult with the coach to arrive at realistic and achievable goals.

RETURNING THE PATIENT TO FULL PARTICIPATION

Four criteria are used to determine that the patient has completed the sport rehabilitation program and is ready to return to sport participation. These relate to the status of the injury itself and to the patient's functional levels, sport-specific skills, and degree of confidence.

Once the therapeutic exercise program, including advanced functional exercises, has been completed and the patient is ready to return to full participation, specific criteria must be fulfilled before the individual is actually allowed to return. The entire therapeutic exercise program has been designed and administered by the sport rehabilitation specialist for this very goal. The true test of the success of the program comes with the patient's return to his or her sport.

In order for that to happen, the patient must meet four specific criteria:

1. The acute signs and symptoms of the injury have resolved, and no pain or edema is present.

2. The patient is able to demonstrate full range of motion; normal strength, muscle endurance, and cardiovascular endurance; and appropriate proprioception, agility, and coordination in relation to the required sport skills.

3. The patient is able to perform any and all sport activities at least as well as he or she could before the injury. As has been mentioned, you should be unable to identify the area that has been injured if the patient is performing the activities appropriately.

4. The patient has the confidence in both his or her own ability and the ability of the injured area to perform, without any hesitation or doubt, or any modification of performance or mechanics.

If these criteria are met and the patient is able to pass all functional evaluation tests, the sport rehabilitation specialist has accomplished the goals established at the start of the therapeutic exercise program.

SUMMARY

1. *Explain the difference between functional exercises and functional testing.*

   Functional exercises are used in a therapeutic exercise program from its early stages to its final stages. The early stages utilize functional exercises designed primarily to restore basic parameters such as flexibility, strength, endurance, and balance. In the later stages, more advanced functional activities gradually push the patient to the final level of functional activities, those that mimic sport participation. Functional testing uses activities or drills that are specific to the patient's sport demands and activities to mimic the maneuvers and movements that will be required when the patient returns to sport participation. This testing assesses whether the patient is ready to return to full participation.

2. *Identify the contributions of functional exercise to a therapeutic exercise program.*

   Functional exercises are used to ready the patient physically for the stress and demands of his or her sport and to prepare the patient mentally. The effects of successful execution of functional activities come through the patient's discovery that the injured segment is able to withstand the stresses of his or her sport.

3. *Discuss the differences between basic and advanced functional activities.*

   Basic exercises begin early in the therapeutic exercise program to assist in achieving flexibility, strength, endurance, and proprioception. Advanced exercises, however, include specific skill activities that more closely resemble or even duplicate the demands of sport activity on the patient and the rehabilitated segment.

4. *List factors that can be varied in a progression of functional activities.*

   Functional exercises proceed from slow to fast, simple to complex, low force to high force, short distance to long distance, and bilateral support to unilateral support. A progression of functional exercises includes a steady change to allow for SAID principle advancement. Functional exercises include some characteristics unique to functional exercises and some characteristics common to most exercises.

5. *Identify precautions for functional exercises.*

   Some precautions are those discussed in prior chapters and include explaining the exercise to the patient, avoiding pain and swelling, considering tissue integrity when designing exercises, knowing the patient's confidence level, and being aware of the patient's progression tolerance.

6. *Outline a sample of functional progression for either the lower or upper extremity.*

   The specific progression and selection of exercises depend on the patient's sport and position within the sport, especially as he or she nears the final stages of the program. A lower-extremity program may include a progression from non-weight-bearing use of the BAPS board that can start early in the therapeutic exercise program. As the patient becomes weight bearing, stork standing first with eyes open and then with eyes closed can begin. A progression of this activity can go from using the floor to using either a trampoline or a $1/2$ foam roll or balance board to combining the activity with another activity such as ball catching. Stork-standing activities can then progress to dynamic movement activities such as lunges, step-ups and step-downs, walking, and jogging. Running activities begin with a forward jog on a flat surface, proceed to increased speed and distances, and then to lateral runs and cuts and sudden changes in direction.

CRITICAL THINKING QUESTIONS

1. On the basis of the scenario at the beginning of this chapter, what would you do to improve Tom's confidence in his tennis abilities? What activities would you have him do on the first day of his functional program? List three levels of progression and give your criteria for advancement. When would you have him start overhead activities and serves?

2. When would you decide that Tom is able to return to full participation? What would your criteria be for this, and why have you set these criteria?

3. A volleyball player who injured his knee and who has completed the rehabilitation program up to the functional activities level is very anxious to return to full sport participation. You estimate that it will be another week before he has successfully completed the functional activities portion of the program. What will your first day's activities include, and how will you establish a progression of activities? What are your criteria for each level of progression? What specific activities must he be able to perform before he may resume full volleyball participation?

4. A cross country competitor is now ready for functional activities. She has been running short distances of no more than 2 min without difficulty. What distance, speed, and terrain progression will you give her over the course of the next two weeks? Write up a two-week progression of functional activities that will move her to full sport participation.

SUGGESTED READING

Cordova, M.L., and C.W. Armstrong. 1996. Reliability of ground reaction forces during a vertical jump: Implications for functional strength assessment. *Journal of Athletic Training* 31:342–345.

Kegerreis, S. 1983. The construction and implementation of functional progressions as a component of athletic rehabilitation. *Journal of Orthopedic and Sports Physical Therapy* 5:14–19.

Kegerreis, S., Malone, T., and J. McCarroll. 1984. Functional progressions: An aid to athletic rehabilitation. *Physician and Sportsmedicine* 12:67–71.

Kegerreis, S., and T. Wetherald. 1987. The utilization of functional progressions in the rehabilitation of injured wrestlers. *Athletic Training* 22:32–35.

Keskula, D.R., Duncan, J.B., Davis, V.L., and P.W. Finley. 1996. Functional outcome measures for knee dysfunction assessment. *Journal of Athletic Training* 31:105–110.

Lephart, S.M., Perrin, D.H., Fu, F.H., and K. Minger. 1991. Functional performance tests for the anterior cruciate ligament insufficient athlete. *Athletic Training* 26:44–50.

Tippett, S.R., and M.L. Voight. 1995. *Functional progressions for sports rehabilitation.* Champaign, IL: Human Kinetics.

PART THREE

General Therapeutic Exercise Applications

The essence of thought, as the essence of life, is growth.

Oscar Wilde, *The Artist as Critic:*
Critical Writings of Oscar Wilde, edited by Richard Ellman, 1969

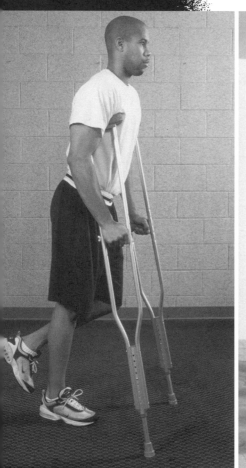
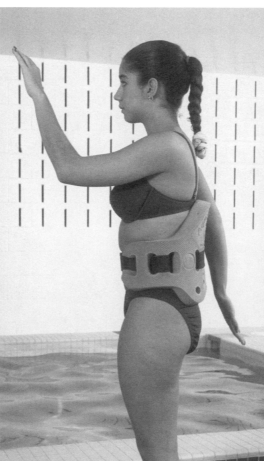
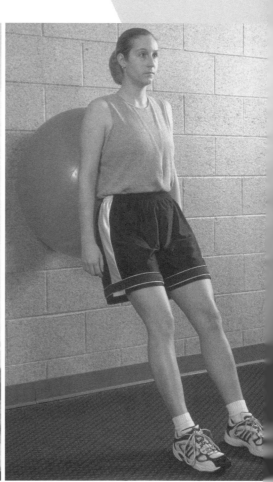

As you progress through this text, you should continue to grow in your knowledge of therapeutic exercise and your appreciation of the complexity, expanse, and intricacy of the information that a sport rehabilitation specialist must possess. In reading part I, you obtained information vital to an understanding of the material in part II. Now that you have a basic knowledge of the physical and physiological concepts that underlie the principles of therapeutic exercise, we can investigate some general applications of this information. The remaining parts of this book, parts III and IV, will use the foundation established in these earlier chapters to provide you with the guidelines in the remaining chapters. These guidelines will allow you to develop and build a sound therapeutic exercise program for the patients you will encounter as an allied health professional.

Part III deals with general concepts that are important in themselves but also serve as the final foundational elements for the knowledge in part IV. Part III presents information on topics such as posture, body mechanics, and ambulation with and without aids. It also presents information on general therapeutic exercise programs that can be used with most injuries and for most body segments.

Chapter 11 presents information about posture and body mechanics. It is not unusual to find that posture abnormalities, the ways that people use the body in physical activity, and muscle imbalances are key to an injury or are the reason an injury does not respond readily to therapeutic exercise procedures. Learning about posture, body mechanics, and body awareness will help you become more knowledgeable about often undetected sources of injury.

Chapter 12 presents an overview of normal walking and running. This is followed by information on ambulation with assistive devices as well as correct methods of applying the devices to an individual. You will also read about how to instruct the patient in the correct use of assistive devices, a critical topic for ambulation safety.

The next two chapters include information on commonly incorporated therapeutic programs using aquatics and aquatic equipment (**chapter 13**) and foam rollers and Swiss balls (**chapter 14**). Increasingly, therapeutic exercises include these items, so they are included as part of the total picture of therapeutic exercise.

The final chapter in part III, **chapter 15**, deals with therapeutic exercise for tendinitis. Tendinitis can affect several different parts of the body. Although it would have been possible to discuss tendinitis in part IV, which covers therapeutic exercise of specific body parts, I have chosen to devote a separate chapter to tendinitis. Tendinitis is a complex problem that can nag a patient for extended periods of time and delay resumption of full sport participation. Specific activities and procedures can alleviate the problem. Considering the uniqueness of tendinitis in comparison to acute athletic injuries, I have given special attention to the relevant principles, concepts, and precautions and to recent developments in the treatment of tendinitis.

Once you have completed part III, the remaining section, part IV, should simply be a matter of putting all the information gathered from parts I, II, and III together to create your own therapeutic exercise program. As you proceed through part III, continue to use your deductive reasoning skills, the knowledge that you have acquired from the previous chapters, and your common sense to see if you can anticipate the information presented in each chapter of part III. Although some of the material will be new, much of it will be based on what you have already learned.

CHAPTER ELEVEN

Posture and Body Mechanics

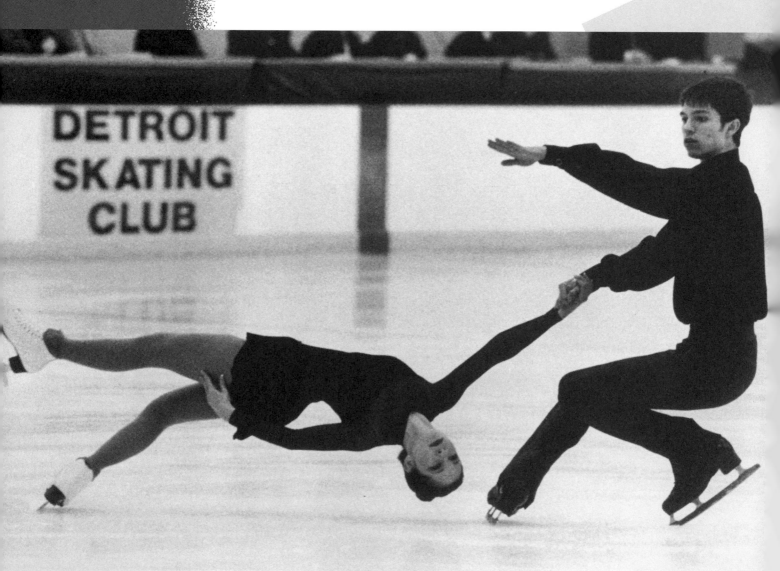

DETROIT
SKATING
CLUB

© Jim West.

OBJECTIVES

After completing this chapter, you should be able to do the following:

1. Identify the primary elements of proper alignment in standing from an anterior, posterior, and side view.

2. Discuss common postural faults and describe their causes.

3. Outline corrective exercises for common postural faults.

4. Explain the importance of good posture and proper body mechanics in athletics.

5. List the basic principles of good body mechanics.

6. Discuss an example of the use of proper body mechanics by the sport rehabilitation specialist during a treatment program.

7. Explain the differences and similarities between the Feldenkrais Method and the Alexander Technique.

Benjamin Klein is the certified athletic trainer who was hired by the local furniture-manufacturing company to rehabilitate the company's injured employees. Benjamin has provided the employees with in-service training on proper lifting mechanics, and injuries have decreased as a result. Nonetheless, some injuries still occur.

His most recent patient, Russell, is about to begin functional activities before returning to his workstation at full duty. Russell injured his back about three weeks ago when he lifted a box incorrectly. At the time of the initial evaluation, Benjamin noticed that Russell's posture in both sitting and standing was poor, so he corrected the patient's posture very early in the program. The postural changes that Russell has made have improved his condition considerably. Benjamin wants to be sure that another injury does not occur, so he will instruct Russell how to lift properly before allowing him to return to full duty.

Teachers open the door, but you must enter by yourself.

Chinese proverb

This chapter opens the door on the topic of posture and body mechanics. Now that you have become familiar with basic concepts and therapeutic exercise program parameters, it is time to see how they can be applied. Part III begins with this chapter on posture and body mechanics because these factors can affect performance and increase injury risk. If you are to improve an individual's posture or body mechanics, you must first identify what is normal. This chapter deals with normal standing and sitting posture, common causes and effects of pathological posture, and correct body mechanics. Body mechanics, as discussed here, relates to daily activities, to sport activities, and also to the activities that you as a sport rehabilitation specialist perform during your treatment sessions with patients. Two of the more commonly used body-awareness techniques will also be introduced.

Once you have developed an appreciation for proper posture and correct body mechanics, it will become easier for you to evaluate injuries, especially chronic injuries, and develop the appropriate therapeutic exercise programs. Use of proper posture for you as the sport rehabilitation specialist is important if you are to conserve energy, prevent injuries for yourself, and provide efficient and effective manual therapy and manual-resistance applications.

POSTURE

Posture, or the relative alignment of various body segments, includes standing alignment and sitting alignment. Anterior, posterior, and lateral views show whether alignment of the various segments of the body is normal.

Posture is the relative alignment of the various body segments with one another. When a person has good posture, the body's alignment is balanced so that stress applied to the body segments is minimal. When a person has poor posture, the body's alignment is out of balance, causing exaggerated stresses to various body segments. Over time this continual stress, even at relatively low levels, causes anatomical adaptations. These changes alter the individual's ability to perform and affect the body's overall efficiency.

Although people seldom stand still, static standing posture is used as the reference for posture evaluation. Static posture can reveal abnormalities in relative balance and alignment of body parts that can affect structure and function. Before we can discuss improper posture, we must identify normal posture.

CORRECT STANDING ALIGNMENT

Standing posture is assessed in three planes: sagittal, frontal, and transverse. A plumb line is used as a point of reference. This term is derived from the Latin word, *plumbum,* meaning "lead." A **plumb line** is a string with a weight (formerly a lead weight, but any weight object will do) at the end. When suspended, the string forms a vertical line. The patient stands behind the plumb line as posture is assessed.

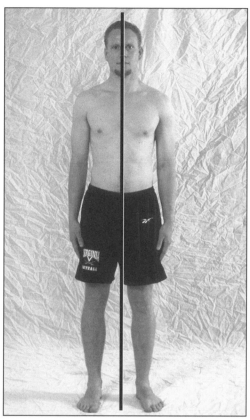

Anterior View

From the anterior, or front, view, the plumb line bisects the body into symmetrical left and right sides (figure 11.1). The patient should stand so that the feet are equidistant from the plumb line. The arms should be relaxed with the palms of the hands facing the sides of the thighs. In this position, the line should bisect the nose and mouth and run through the central portion of the sternum, umbilicus, and pubic bones. The earlobes should be level with one another, as should the shoulders, fingertip ends, nipples, iliac crests, patellae, and medial malleoli. The patellae should point straight ahead with the feet straight or turned slightly outward. The knees and ankles are in line with each other, with the knees angled neither inward nor outward.

∎ **Figure 11.1** Frontal posture view.

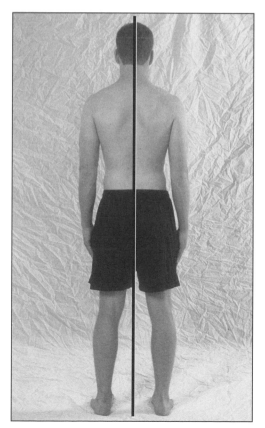

Posterior View

The posterior, or back, view should demonstrate alignment similar to that observed from the front (figure 11.2). The plumb line should bisect the head and follow the spinous processes from the cervical through the lumbar spine. The earlobes, shoulders, scapulae, hips, posterior superior iliac spine, gluteal fold, posterior knee creases, and medial malleoli should appear level left to right. The scapulae should lie against the rib cage between the second and seventh ribs and about 5 cm (2 in.) from the spinous processes. The calcaneus should be straight and the calcaneal tendon perpendicular to the floor. Trunk muscles should appear balanced, with symmetrical development. The shoulders should be positioned down and relaxed. Body weight should appear equally distributed over the two feet.

∎ **Figure 11.2** Posterior posture view.

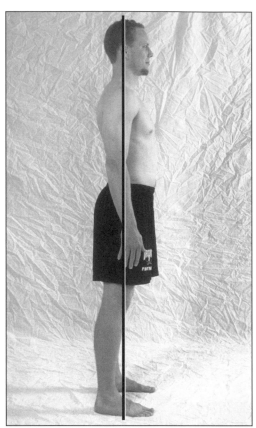

❚ Figure 11.3 Lateral posture view.

Lateral View

From a lateral or side view, the patient stands with the plumb line slightly anterior to the lateral malleolus (figure 11.3). When the patient is positioned with the plumb line referenced at the ankle, observe the lateral alignment from the head down. The plumb line should pass through the external auditory meatus, the earlobe, the bodies of the cervical vertebrae, the center of the shoulder joint, and the greater trochanter. The plumb line should run midway between the back and chest and the back and abdomen, slightly posterior to the hip joint, and slightly anterior to the center of the knee just behind the patella. A horizontal line should connect the anterior superior iliac spine (ASIS) and posterior superior iliac spine (PSIS). The patient should remain relaxed with the body's weight balanced between the heel and the forefoot. The knees are straight but not locked. The chin is slightly tucked, and the chest is held slightly up and forward. There is a mild curve inward of the low back and neck regions.

CORRECT SITTING ALIGNMENT

As in standing, correct sitting posture places the minimum amount of stress on the body. Students in high school and college and many individuals in the work force spend much of their day in chairs. Incorrect sitting posture can aggravate an injury and, in prolonged sitting situations, can lead to injury.

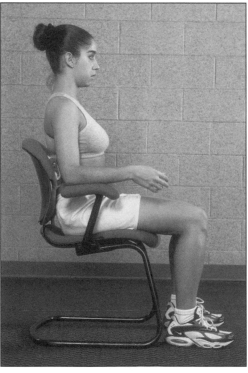

❚ Figure 11.4 Correct sitting posture with lumbar-roll support.

In a correct alignment, the chair seat height must allow the individual's feet to rest comfortably on the floor with the knees and hips at 90°. The chair seat depth should be such that the edge of the seat does not press against the back of the individual's knees. The chair back should support the lumbar and thoracic spine and come to the lower border of the scapulae. A lumbar roll will contour to the curve of the lumbar spine and can provide additional low back support. Higher-backed executive chairs should provide full thoracic support and permit the person to lean back comfortably. If the chair has arms, they should be at a level that provides for shoulder relaxation and permits the forearms to rest comfortably with the elbows at 90° (figure 11.4).

If the person is sitting at a desk, the chair height should be such that the person's forearms rest comfortably on the desk without hunching the shoulders up or down. If the chair height must be increased to achieve a correct position, a footrest may be necessary to maintain 90° knee and hip positions and still keep the feet flat on the floor. When the individual is using a computer keyboard, the forearms are at 90° or slightly more, and the wrists are in a neutral position with the fingers resting on the keyboard.

All sitting postures should provide for good spinal alignment and normal spinal curves. The head should not be too far forward or the shoulders rounded forward.

PATHOLOGICAL ALIGNMENT

Unfortunately, over time most people develop bad posture habits. The best posture can be observed in young children. Toddlers who are learning to stand and walk have good body alignment and move with straight posture. It is only as we get older that we develop bad habits that eventually lead to poor posture.

Good posture allows the individual to use his or her body efficiently and effectively. Bad posture, however, places abnormal stresses on the body and increases the demands during performance (Kendall, McCreary, and Provance 1993). Over time, bad posture habits develop, causing shortening of some structures and lengthening of opposing structures with secondary weakness of both shortened and lengthened structures. This change in strength with a change in relative muscle length is discussed in chapter 7 within the context of length-tension relationships. These changes can impair the individual's efficiency of movement. Inefficient movement burdens an already stressed area during performance, and over time, can cause injury. For this reason, the sport rehabilitation specialist should have an awareness of the common pathological postures. This knowledge can help the sport rehabilitation specialist develop an appropriate corrective therapeutic exercise program.

Abnormal alignment is usually recorded in terms of relativity. Rather than precise measurement, terms such as "mild," "moderate," and "severe" are used to identify and grade abnormal alignment. For example, a swimmer may have a mild forward-head posture, or a gymnast may have a severe lumbar lordosis.

Pelvis and Lumbar Area

Common posture faults in the pelvis and lumbar area include excessive lumbar lordosis, flat lumbar spine, and scoliosis. Scoliosis is discussed in the section "Thoracic Area." Often associated with a lumbar lordosis or flat lumbar spine is anterior pelvic tilt or posterior pelvic tilt, respectively.

A normal lumbar curve is slightly lordotic, but an excessive lumbar curve places undue stress on the lumbar spine and other segments (figure 11.5). An excessive **lumbar lordosis,** also referred to as "swayback," is accompanied by an anterior pelvic tilt in which the ASIS is rotated down in relation to the PSIS. It can be caused by tight hip flexors pulling on the lumbar spine and by weak low back extensors and abdominal muscles, especially lower abdominals. Over time, this abnormal postural alignment can result in tightness of lumbar fas-

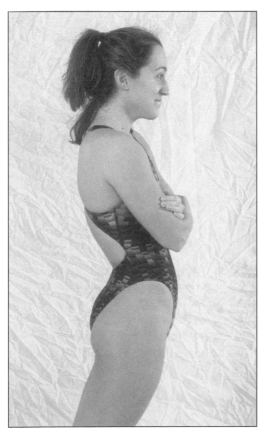

■ **Figure 11.5** Lumbar lordosis.

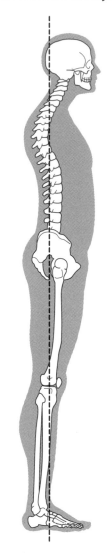

cia, increased stress to the anterior longitudinal ligament of the spine, narrowing of the vertebral disk spaces that will cause a narrowing of the intervertebral foramen, and approximation of the vertebral articular facets. These changes can result in nerve root compression, sciatica, joint inflammation, and degenerative disk and vertebral changes.

In a flat lumbar spine, lumbar lordosis is reduced and there is a posterior pelvic tilt so that the PSIS is lower than the ASIS (figure 11.6). Abnormal hip extensor and rectus abdominis tightness is counterbalanced by weak hip flexors and lumbar extensor muscles. This posture reduces the lumbar spine's ability to absorb impact forces and increases the stress of the spine's posterior longitudinal ligament.

❙ Figure 11.6 Flat lumbar spine.

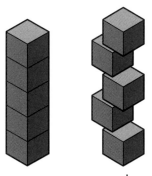

❙ Figure 11.7 Building-block alignment.

Thoracic Area

When you align building blocks, you find that if one block is not placed directly on top of the one below, the next block must be placed askew to compensate for the one that was poorly placed (figure 11.7). The body likewise compensates for malalignments by adjusting positions of adjacent structures in an attempt to keep the body balanced.

Therefore, in the thoracic region, the area can be excessively rounded or excessively flat, depending on the positions of the lumbar segments. It is common to see a **thoracic kyphosis,** or excessive rounding of the thoracic area (figure 11.8), in response to a lumbar lordosis. Chest muscles, including the intercostals, pectoralis major and minor, serratus anterior, and latissimus dorsi, are usually tight and are counterbalanced by weak thoracic erector spinae, rhomboids, and trapezius muscles. A thoracic kyphosis is typically associated with a round-shoulder posture. The scapulae can also be more than the normal 5 cm (2 in.) from the vertebrae.

A kyphotic posture can lead to **thoracic outlet syndrome,** which is discussed in chapter 16. Secondary cervical problems can result from excessive pressure placed on the cervical area by malalignment of the

❙ Figure 11.8 Kyphosis.

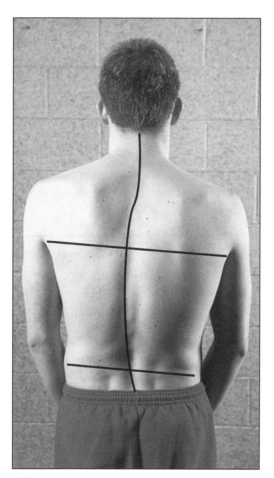

■ **Figure 11.9** Mild scoliosis. Notice the uneven hips, unequal arm hang, and unequal shoulder and scapula heights.

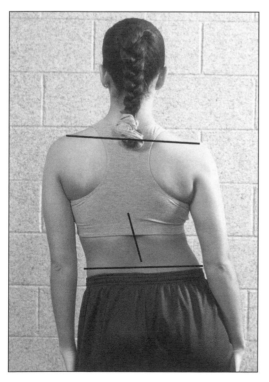

thoracic spine. People such as swimmers who place high demands on rhomboid and trapezius muscle groups can experience fatigue in these groups because of their lengthened and weakened status.

A flattening of the upper back, or a reduction of the thoracic curve, is not as common as a kyphotic posture. This flattening is characterized by an exaggerated attention posture that includes depressed scapulae and flat neck; it results in tightness in the thoracic erector spinae and scapular retractors with secondary weakness of the scapular protractors and anterior thoracic muscles. This posture can also lead to thoracic outlet syndrome because of the increased compression it produces between the first rib and clavicle.

Scoliosis is commonly seen in the thoracic or lumbar spine or in both areas. **Scoliosis** is a lateral curve of the normally straight spine and is classified as either a C-curve or an S-curve. A C-curve is usually indicated as either right or left according to its direction of convexity. A C-curve with a compensating secondary curve is called an S-curve (figure 11.9). In an attempt to keep the head level, the body compensates for a C-curve by developing a counterbalancing lesser lateral curve that results in an S-curve configuration. Scoliosis usually also includes a rotation of the vertebrae. If this occurs in the thoracic spine, an asymmetry of rib position can be observed from an anterior or posterior view, with one side of the rib cage more anterior than the contralateral side. If leg-length differences are the source of the scoliosis, the pelvic landmarks may not be level. Shoulders are often not level in scoliosis as well.

Common causes for scoliosis are congenital deformities of the spine, leg-length differences, and long-term unilateral activities. Tennis players, among others involved in physical activity, often may develop a scoliosis because of their participation in a unilaterally demanding sport. Tight structures are found on the side of the concavity, while weaker structures are on the convex side of the scoliosis curve.

Scoliosis can cause muscle fatigue and increased ligamentous stress on the convex side because of weakness of those structures. Impingement of nerve roots with secondary nerve root pain can be seen on the concave side. If the scoliosis is caused by a leg-length discrepancy, the longer leg commonly has a lower longitudinal arch to compensate for the leg-length difference.

A scoliosis should not be confused with a lateral shift of the thoracic or lumbar spine. A shift is present when the pelvis and shoulders do not lie in the same frontal plane. Either the pelvis or the shoulders are shifted to the left or right of the midline of the body (figure 11.10). This shift can be caused by muscle spasm or pain from an impinged nerve root as the body attempts to move away from the source of pain. It is usually a temporary condition that is relieved when the cause is eliminated.

■ **Figure 11.10** Lateral shift. Notice the even hips with a shift of the trunk to the left. Hips and shoulders are not in alignment.

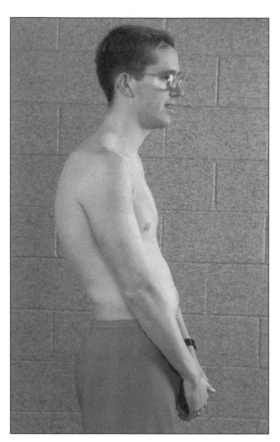

▌Figure 11.11
Cervical lordosis,
thoracic kyphosis,
and lumbar lordosis.

Head and Cervical Area

In response to the abnormal lumbar and thoracic alignment, the cervical spine develops a compensatory alignment. Most commonly, a forward positioning of the head occurs through either a flattening of the cervical curve or an exaggeration of the normal cervical lordosis. A **cervical lordosis** includes an increased flexion of the lower cervical and an increased extension of the upper cervical spine (figure 11.11).

Weakness in the lower cervical and upper thoracic erector spinae and anterior neck muscles is overpowered by tightness in cervical muscles including the levator scapulae, sternocleidomastoid, scalenes, suboccipitals, and upper trapezii. This imbalance encourages and perpetuates the abnormal cervical posture.

Many problems can result from prolonged poor cervical posture. Both the weak and the tight muscles can experience fatigue. The exaggerated cervical position can also increase cervical disk pressure, add irritation to cervical facet joints, increase nerve root pressure, and impinge on neurovascular bundles to increase the risk of thoracic outlet syndrome. Prolonged abnormal positioning also increases the stresses applied to the cervical spine's posterior and anterior longitudinal ligaments. Scholastic and collegiate athletes who spend their days in the classroom often sit with their elbows on the desk and their chins in their hands, and people in the work force spend their days at a computer sitting in a rounded-back and forward-head position; these positions exaggerate the cervical lordotic posture that places increased stress on the cervical spine. Prolonged posterior longitudinal ligament stress is marked by the formation of a "dowager's hump" at the base of the cervical spine in persons who have had long-term forward-head posture. In addition, temporomandibular joint stress can be exaggerated by abnormal cervical posture and lead to temporomandibular joint disorders.

Lower Extremities

Lower-extremity malalignment can begin in the feet, knees, or hips and often affects other structures along the closed kinetic chain. Common postural faults in the lower extremities include excessive flexion or extension, excessive abduction or adduction, and excessive internal or external rotation. The normal angle between the femoral neck and the femoral shaft in adults is 120° to 125° (figure 11.12). This angle is larger in infants and children, decreasing from 150° in a newborn to 133° in a teenager until it reaches 120° to 125° during the adult years. An abnormally larger angle is referred to as **coxa valga,** and a smaller angle is called **coxa vara.** As the neck-shaft angle increases with a coxa valga, there is an apparent lengthening of the limb. The opposite is true with a coxa vara, in which the

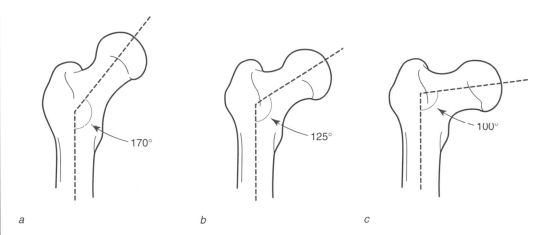

a   b   c

Figure 11.12
Femoral neck-shaft angles: *(a)* coxa valga causes increased femoral-joint pressure, *(b)* normal position, *(c)* coxa vara produces increased stress on femoral neck.

limb shortens as the neck-shaft angle decreases. People with coxa valga have a higher propensity for eventual hip-joint arthritis, whereas those with coxa vara are more prone to femoral neck fractures.

There is a normal relative forward projection of the femoral neck relative to the femoral condyles in the transverse plane of the femur. This angle decreases with age. A newborn's femoral neck-condyle angle is around 30° whereas in adults it is 8° to 15° (figure 11.13). **Anteversion,** an increased angle, results in greater hip internal rotation and causes squinting patellae and toeing-in during standing. A decreased angle, called **retroversion,** produces greater hip external rotation, and in standing the feet rotate outward. Anteversion decreases hip stability and places the hip at risk for dislocation, whereas retroversion increases the joint's stability.

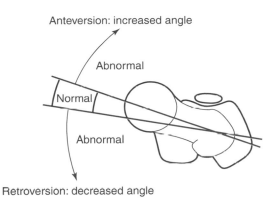

Figure 11.13 Relative position of the femoral neck and femoral condyles. Normal anteversion in an adult is 8° to 15°.

The normal sagittal alignment of the femur and tibia at the knee is straight; an angling of the knees toward each another is called **genu valgus** or **genu valgum.** A bowing outward of the knees is called **genu varus** or **genu varum** (figure 11.14). These malalignments have a variety of causes. If they occur on one side, leg-length discrepancy may be the cause. Quadriceps weakness can genu valgus. Valgus deformities can be the source of excessive foot pronation, and varus deformities can be related to high arches.

In normal standing, the patellae should face forward with the feet positioned forward or slightly outward. The condition in which the patellae face toward each other is referred to as **squinting patellae** and may be related to either medial hip rotation, hip anteversion, medial tibial rotation, or lateral rotation of the feet (figure 11.15). The condition in which the patellae face outward in relation to each other is referred to as **frog's eye** or **grasshopper eye.** This condition is often the result of lateral hip rotation or lateral tibial rotation, and the feet often face inward in a pigeon-toed fashion.

In a side view, the knee is straight but not locked. If the line of gravity falls in front of the knee, the knee is hyperextended, a condition referred to as **genu recurvatum** (figure 11.16). Excessive stress is placed on the knee's ligamentous structures

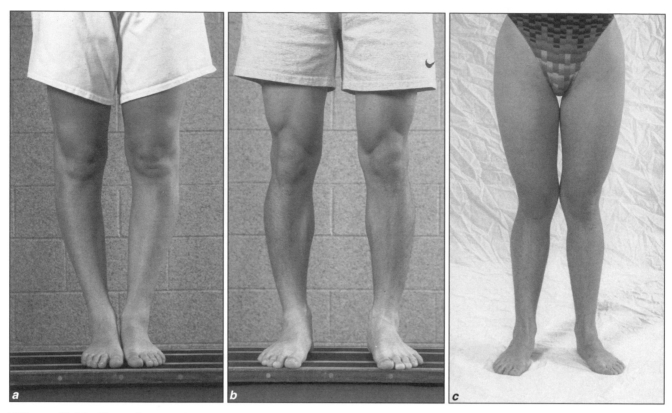

Figure 11.14 Knee alignment in the sagittal plane: *(a)* genu varus, *(b)* normal, *(c)* genus valgus.

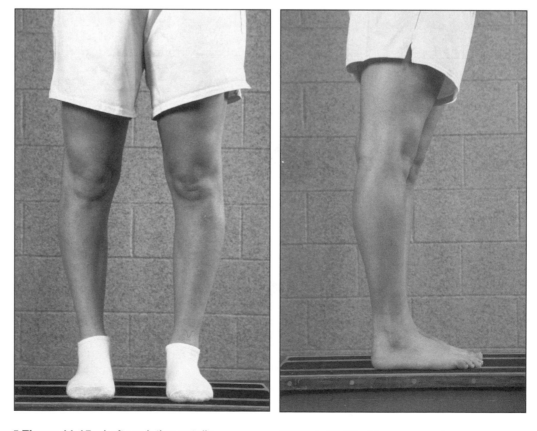

Figure 11.15 Left squinting patella.

Figure 11.16 Genu recurvatum.

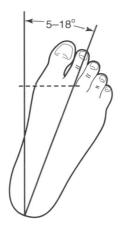

Figure 11.17
Normal adult foot
position in weight
bearing.

in this position. Genu recurvatum is commonly accompanied by excessive lumbar lordosis and anterior pelvic rotation.

Tibial torsion is present when the lower leg appears rotated in relation to the thigh. This is most evident when one looks at the positions of the patellae in relation to the positions of the feet. In an adult, the feet normally face approximately 12° to 18° from the sagittal axis of the body. In youth, this angle can be as small as 5° (figure 11.17). Excessive tibial torsion is usually lateral and is correlated with squinting patellae. To measure tibial torsion, place the patient in supine with the patellae facing directly upward. A line bisecting the medial and lateral malleoli creates an angle with the plane of the tabletop; this is the tibial torsion measurement (figure 11.18). Normal values are 15° to 18°. Excessive lateral tibial torsion can increase patellofemoral stresses and lead to increased patellofemoral stress, instability, and fat-pad entrapment.

Medial tibial torsion is associated with genu varum, and lateral tibial torsion is associated with genu valgum. These conditions can become apparent with habitual use of poor sitting postures, especially in children, as seen in figure 11.19.

Foot position can influence knee and hip positions, and the converse is also true. One determines medial longitudinal arch height by drawing a line from the bottom of the medial malleolus to the weight-bearing surface of the first metatarsophalangeal joint. In both weight bearing and non-weight bearing, the navicular tuberosity should be on the line (figure 11.20). If the navicular tuberosity falls below the line, the arch is abnormally low; and if it falls above the line, the arch is abnormally high. A high arch is referred to as **pes cavus**. A low arch, **pes planus**, is often associated with excessive foot pronation and calcaneal eversion and can be accompanied by genu valgum

Figure 11.18 With the patella facing the ceiling, a line between the medial and lateral malleolus forms an angle with a line parallel to the tabletop for identifying the individual's tibial torsion.

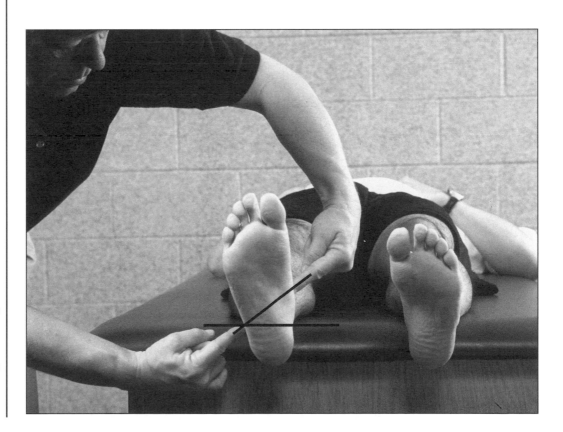

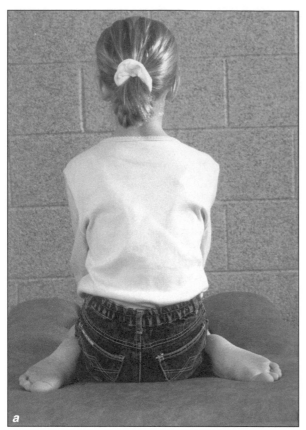 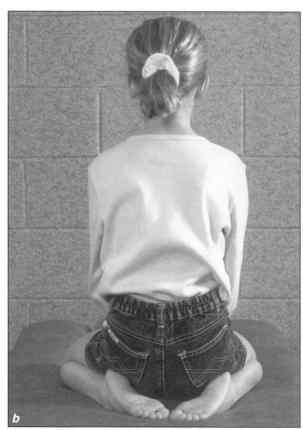

■ Figure 11.19 Poor sitting posture for knees: (a) encourages lateral tibial torsion, (b) encourages medial tibial torsion.

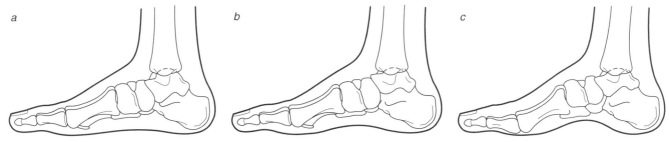

■ Figure 11.20 Arch positions: (a) pes planus, (b) normal alignment, (c) pes cavus.
Adapted from Richardson and Iglarsh 1994.

and/or femoral anteversion. A pes planus is hypermobile, allowing for excessive rearfoot and forefoot motion during gait. This type of foot structure may not have the stability to create a strong base, and it places excessive stresses on soft-tissue structures and adjacent joints as the patient attempts to perform sport activities. The greater the hypermobility, the greater the loss of stability. Increased stress on foot and ankle structures can lead to injuries, including plantar fasciitis, hallux valgus, and Achilles tendinitis.

Calcaneal eversion with increased forefoot pronation can be identified from a posterior view of the ankle. In this position, the Achilles tendon appears to be at less than a 90° angle to the floor, and the calcaneus is in an everted position (figure 11.21).

Pes cavus, a higher-than-normal arch, is associated with a more rigid foot structure and produces less mobility of the joints within the rearfoot and forefoot. This type of foot has less ability to absorb stress than a foot with a normal arch position

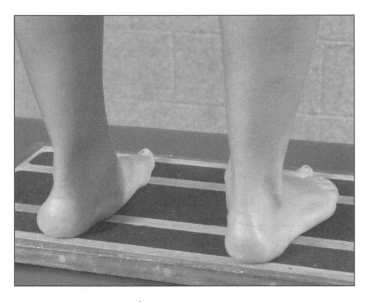

Figure 11.21 Pronation. Notice the everted position of the left calcaneous.

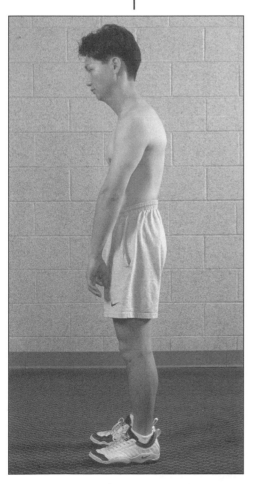

and is more prone to stress fractures. With reduced flexibility and associated diminution of stress-absorption capacity, increased stress is imposed on the joints of the foot. A high arch is often associated with hammertoes or claw toes and can be related to femoral retroversion.

Toe positions are normally in a straight line. A positioning of the great toe toward the other toes is called **hallux valgus.** A common cause is hypermobility of the foot. Over time, this additional stress on the first metatarsophalangeal joint causes it to become deformed (figure 11.22).

Toes that become flexed or extended at the metatarsophalangeal joints or the interphalangeal joints are known as claw toe and hammertoe deformities, respectively. **Claw toes** are extended at

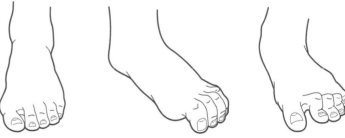

a   b   c

Figure 11.22 Toe deformities: *(a)* hallux valgus, *(b)* claw toes, *(c)* hammertoes.

Parts b and c reprinted from Richardson and Iglarsh 1994.

the metatarsophalangeal joints and flexed at the proximal and distal interphalangeal joints; **hammertoes** are extended at the metatarsophalangeal joints, flexed at the proximal interphalangeal joint, and extended at the distal interphalangeal joint. These conditions are usually accompanied by a high longitudinal arch and a rigid foot. Corns and calluses on the toes develop secondary to abnormal pressures as the elevated portion of the toes rubs against the inside of the shoe.

Upper Extremities

The primary area affected by bad posture in the upper extremity is the shoulders. If a person has a poor thoracic posture with rounded shoulders, the scapulae protract forward and downward around the rib cage. This positioning presents itself as an anterior rounding of the glenohumeral joint, and the dorsal hands will face forward and rest on the anterior thigh rather than on the lateral thigh as they should (figure 11.23). This can lead to glenohumeral impingement, weakness of the scapular rotators, and tightness of anterior shoulder girdle muscles. These soft-tissue changes can cause inefficient use of the shoulder for upper-extremity activities in sport and can place the individual at risk for upper-extremity injuries.

Figure 11.23 Upper-extremity posture deviation.

MUSCLE IMBALANCES

Improper posture is often perpetuated by muscle imbalances. Causes of muscle imbalance include overuse, loss of motion or flexibility in a muscle or muscle group, postural deviations, and injuries. It is necessary to determine the muscle imbalances involved before correcting postural deviations.

Muscle imbalances often impact posture. To correct posture, the sport rehabilitation specialist must be able to identify the muscle imbalances that perpetuate the patient's improper posture.

CAUSES

Poor posture results from an abnormal relationship between the forces that act on an area. Normal posture occurs when there is a balance of forces acting on bones and joints. Normal posture permits an efficient and effective use of the body to produce the desired motions.

When a body is in bad posture, the joints and muscles are already under stress, and activity increases that level of stress. In bad posture, muscles must work harder to produce desired motions and are not as efficient or as effective. Bad posture can also restrict muscles from performing optimally. For example, a freestyle swimmer with rounded shoulders has difficulty getting enough external rotation and abduction on the recovery phase of the stroke, so either hand entry into the water is premature or the swimmer has to compensate with an exaggerated body roll. The swimmer will also suffer an impingement injury of the shoulder because the scapula does not upwardly rotate and retract as it should. If this swimmer were to come to you with a rotator-cuff tendinitis and you did not correct the posture and muscle imbalances, your treatment success would be short-lived, for episodes of the injury would recur.

Sometimes pain in an area is the result of poor posture or muscle imbalances in another area. The site of pain is not always the source of the problem. For example, a gymnast who complains of back pain and has a lumbar lordosis may in fact be having back pain because of hip-flexor tightness, not a back injury. The hip flexors place abnormal stress on the lumbar vertebrae because tight hip flexors pull on the lumbar vertebrae, increasing low back stress and making the area more susceptible to injury. The gymnast's back pain could also be related to hyperextended knees, which will tend to pull the pelvis forward, increasing lumbar lordosis. When combined with weak abdominals, especially weak lower abdominals, these factors can contribute significantly to low back pain.

Commonly, the source of muscle imbalance is a loss of motion or flexibility in a muscle or muscle group, as well as lengthening and weakness from prolonged or sustained stretch of the opposing muscle or muscle group. If a muscle is shortened, its opposing muscle must be lengthened to compensate. It is this reciprocal activity that allows us to feed ourselves, walk, and perform most activities; when one muscle shortens, the opposing muscle lengthens to allow the activity. For example, when you perform a biceps curl, the biceps shorten and the triceps lengthen; or when you bend your knee, the hamstrings shorten and the quadriceps lengthen. When a lengthened or shortened position is sustained, a muscle's resting length changes over time. The sustained shortening of one muscle causes a loss of flexibility and strength, and the sustained lengthening of the opposite muscle causes a loss of strength and tone. One can compare the results of sustained lengthening to what occurs when a weight is hung on the end of a rubber band and left that way for a period of time. When the weight is removed, the rubber band has less tone than before, and less spring. So, too, a muscle that is positionally lengthened loses its spring and becomes weaker. If a patient performed only flexibility exercises to restore balance, the imbalance, caused by tightness of one muscle and weakness of its opposing muscle, would overpower the effects of stretching and would continue to encourage the imbalanced posture.

Some sports are more likely to cause postural deviations than others. Participants in sports that emphasize muscle activity on anterior more than on posterior body regions, such as swimming and boxing, are more likely than other athletes to develop postural deviations. Unilateral activities such as racket sports encourage muscle imbalance from left to right and can cause such postural deviations as scoliosis.

As the body ages, postural deviations become more pronounced. A mild forward-head posture in a young adult becomes a moderate forward-head posture in the middle-aged adult and becomes even more severe as the individual ages. As the muscle naturally weakens with age, it has increasing difficulty opposing tight structures, so pathological postures become even more apparent with aging—further increasing joint and muscle stresses.

Muscle imbalance can also result from joint abnormalities. These abnormalities run the spectrum from hyermobility to hypomobility. When joints are hypermobile, displaying an excessive amount of motion, the muscles must work harder to provide joint stability. This is true for a joint that is uniplanar or multiplanar. Joints that lack normal mobility—hypomobile joints—have less-than-normal motion and place additional stresses on muscles and joints. These conditions can also add stresses to other body segments. For example, the individual who has foot-joint hypermobility with excessive pronation may develop patellar tendinitis. This may be secondary to additional stresses on the patellar tendon when its insertion is rotated medially with the internal tibial rotation that occurs during prolonged pronation.

Injuries can also cause muscle imbalances. Scar-tissue adhesions following a ligament injury can cause the joint to become hypomobile, especially if the joint was immobilized immediately after the injury. The deleterious effects of immobilization are discussed in chapter 2. If the joint is not immobilized, ligamentous laxity can occur, making the joint hypermobile.

Another cause of imbalances is muscle strains. If the injured muscle is not properly rehabilitated, its normal strength is not regained. If adhesions within the muscle occur, the site can become tight, limiting flexibility and causing increased stress to the site or adjacent sites.

TREATMENT

It becomes important in any injury evaluation to assess the patient's posture and look for muscle imbalances that either may have contributed to the injury or may result from the injury. You should also look at the total body, not merely the injured site, because postural deviations from other locations may be responsible for the injury.

It is important to correct postural deviations not only to address the patient's current injury but also to prevent recurrence. As has been mentioned, if a postural deviation is either the source of an injury or a contributing factor, you must correct the postural deviation as part of the rehabilitation program in order to prevent recurrence of the injury. If you do not, the chance is good that the injury will become chronic.

In correcting postural deviations, the sport rehabilitation specialist must first identify the structure that has become tight and the opposing structure that has become overstretched. He or she can then give the patient exercises to correct the muscle imbalance—that is, to lengthen the short or tight structures and strengthen the opposing weak or lengthened structures. For example, if the freestyle swimmer's posture is a rounded-shoulder position, examination will show that the anterior chest muscles are tight; the downward scapular rotators are tight; and the upper back muscles, scapular retractors, and upward scapular rotator groups are weak and lengthened. The treatment program should include lengthening activities for muscles including the pectoralis minor, anterior deltoid, and pectoralis major and strengthening activities for muscles such as the lower trapezius, middle trapezius, and posterior deltoid. It should also include activities that will recruit and retrain muscles to produce the desired activity in a normal fashion. It is useful to provide reminders that will facilitate correct postural alignment—for example, a visual cue such as a colored dot on the face of the patient's watch or on a fingernail can be used to remind the patient to think about and correct his or her posture. An example of a more extreme reminder is tape applied between the shoulder blades to help the patient remember to keep the shoulders in correct alignment.

Conscious correction of posture is necessary for bad posture to improve. The patient must become aware of the abnormal posture and then make a deliberate effort to alter the habitual posture; otherwise, posture does not change. As the patient continues to improve muscle balance through proper exercises and to correct bad postural position, and maintains a proper posture more and more frequently, the posture eventually will improve.

It is more difficult in the initial stages than it will be later for the patient to change posture, for two primary reasons. The first one is habit. Habit, whether good or bad, is easy and comfortable and thus difficult for anyone to change. The second reason is the relationship between the weak and tight muscles. The tight muscles overpower the weak and lengthened muscles, making it difficult for the patient to maintain a proper posture when attempting correction. But as the muscle imbalance is reduced, the task becomes easier. Conscious effort is vitally important throughout the process if the patient is to achieve the ultimate goal of improved postural alignment.

POSTURE- AND MUSCLE IMBALANCE-RELATED INJURIES

To make it easier to understand the process, let's look at a couple of examples of injuries and their relationship to improper posture and muscle imbalance.

Lower Extremity

Iliotibial band (ITB) friction syndrome is a common problem in injured athletes, particularly in runners. The pain occurs along the ITB and is typically located along the superior-lateral aspect of the knee or toward the hip. The patient reports that the pain worsens with hill running. The examination reveals a tight ITB, and the patient stands with the leg in more internal rotation than normal. Muscle testing demonstrates weakness of the quadriceps and hip external rotators, and probably weakness of the gluteus maximus as well. Examination of the soft tissue along the ITB reveals tenderness to palpation in areas of soft-tissue thickness.

Treatment includes softening the ITB-restrictive areas with deep friction massage techniques, as well as lengthening the tight ITB and strengthening the lengthened, weak gluteus maximus, hip external rotators, and quadriceps muscles. Instructions to the patient include conscious positional correction, that is, keeping the leg in only slight external rotation alignment when standing or walking. The use of a modality, such as heat, prior to friction massage allows for better massage results by making the soft tissue more pliable.

Upper Extremity

A common upper-extremity problem in patients who participate in upper-extremity sports such as tennis, golf, swimming, and gymnastics is shoulder impingement. This often appears as rotator-cuff tendinitis, and the patient complains of pain with movements such as shoulder elevation, putting the hand behind the back, and resisted activities. He or she experiences pain through the middle arc of shoulder range of motion, and the impingement test produces a positive sign. The rotator-cuff tendons are tender to palpation at their insertion on the greater tubercle. Examination of muscles reveals tightness of the pectoralis minor, anterior deltoid, latissimus, and pectoralis major. The rhomboids and levator scapulae may also be tight. Weakness is apparent in the lower and middle trapezii, infraspinatus, and teres minor. The capsule may have areas of restriction. The scapulae may not rotate fully into an upward and retracted position because of weakness of the upward rotators and tightness of the downward rotators.

Effective treatment of this condition must include correcting the faulty posture, strengthening weak muscles, and stretching tight muscles. Balance between muscle length and strength of opposing muscle groups is the goal that will lead to reduced impingement in the shoulder. It is important to make the patient aware of the proper posture of the shoulder and thoracic area so that he or she can work at improving posture and alignment. Exercises should include stretching of the anterior capsule, pectoralis minor, pectoralis major, and latissimus. Strengthening exercises should include appropriate exercises for the lower and middle trapezius muscles, the infraspinatus, and teres minor. Restoring the balance between scapular upward and downward rotators, protractors and retractors, and elevators and depressors must be part of the rehabilitation program for resolution of postural defects and muscle imbalances to occur. Because weakness with lengthening of the posterior muscles is one of the sources of shoulder impingement, retraining the depressors, retractors, and upward rotators to provide the appropriate movement of the scapula during shoulder movement is vital to reducing impingement of the rotator cuff.

A Challenging Example

Let's look at one more example and outline an appropriate program. A basketball player comes to you with complaints of pain around the patella, especially when jumping for a rebound. During the day he also has pain going down stairs, and in the weight room he has pain on the leg extension and squat machines. When he stands in front of you, the patellae face forward and the feet are laterally rotated. In weight bearing, the longitudinal arches are low. When he performs a step-down exercise, you notice that he lacks full control of the knee and that there is a slight knee wobble medially to laterally as he lowers himself. Range-of-motion testing shows tightness of the ITB, but range of motion of the knee is normal. Strength testing indicates weakness of the vastus medialis oblique (VMO), and you can see some atrophy of the VMO compared to that in the contralateral knee. With the patient in long sitting, the patella is positioned with the medial side higher than the lateral side. When he contracts the quadriceps, you observe that the patella tracks superiorly and laterally. What is the cause of this individual's pain, and what treatment plan would you provide for him? Think for a moment before you read on, and identify the types of corrective exercises and the progression you would recommend to resolve this problem.

The cause of the patient's pain is a malalignment and maltracking of the patella. This in turn is caused by a combination of weakness of the VMO, tightness of the ITB, and malalignment of the feet. Lower-than-normal arches can result in a tibial torsion to increase stresses on the patella. You should check hip rotation to eliminate tightness of the medial rotators; because the ITB is tight, this is a strong possibility. The patella is not tracking normally because of weakness of the VMO and tightness of the ITB overpowering the VMO pull. There may also be an imbalance between the vastus lateralis and the VMO that adds to the lateral tracking. Tightness of the ITB can also be responsible for the lateral tilt of the patella.

Treatment for this patient should include stretching exercises for the hip and ITB and progressive strengthening exercises for the VMO, such as terminal knee-extension exercises, squats, step exercises, and lunges; these exercises should be pain free and should increase in intensity, repetitions, and number of sets as the patient's strength increases. Taping the patella to correct for alignment will also reduce the pain. If inspection of the feet reveals excessive pronation, taping the arch and limiting rearfoot motion may be beneficial.

The exercises you select should be designed to increase flexibility of the tight muscles and increase strength of the weak muscles to provide for a restoration of balance between muscles. If modalities are the only treatment technique used or if strength is the only type of exercise included, the rehabilitation program will not succeed in relieving the patient's complaints and permitting a full and successful return to sport participation.

BODY MECHANICS

Proper body mechanics is fundamental to proper posture. Important principles include keeping the spine straight, lowering the center of gravity, and keeping the base of support broad. Patients need to perform daily activities using correct body mechanics, and the sport rehabilitation specialist should also pay attention to his or her own body mechanics.

Body mechanics is related to posture in that proper body mechanics is easier to maintain with good posture. **Body mechanics** refers to the way the body is positioned and used during activity. Incorrect body mechanics increases stresses placed on various body segments, but correct body mechanics makes the most effective use of the body's forces and lever systems. Body mechanics is briefly discussed here because an awareness of good body mechanics is important to the sport rehabilitation specialist from both a personal and a treatment perspective. From a personal perspective, use of proper body mechanics makes you more efficient in the application of manual therapy and exercises. It conserves your energy and makes the most effective use of your body.

From a treatment perspective, a knowledge of correct body mechanics in the execution of specific sport activities allows you as a sport rehabilitation specialist to provide the patient with proper exercises. Such exercises will enhance the patient's sport performance and include corrective techniques to further prepare the individual for returning to competition.

BASIC PRINCIPLES

A few basic concepts are important to remember regardless of the activity that is being performed. The first principle is that the spine should remain straight. A "straight spine" is one that has the natural curves with the pelvis in neutral. A straight spine has a slight lumbar lordosis, thoracic kyphosis, and cervical lordosis. In this position, each vertebra is in correct alignment with the adjacent vertebrae (figure 11.24). Pelvic neutral is present when the pelvis is in a midposition between an anterior and a posterior pelvic tilt. In this position the stress on the pelvis is minimal, and the vertebrae should be balanced. This position is sometimes referred to as **neutral spine** or **pelvic neutral.**

Maintaining a neutral spine is important if forces from the lower extremities are to be properly transmitted to the trunk and upper extremities. It is easier to understand this concept if you think of the legs, trunk, and arms as three connected sections. When the sections are all rigid, forces are transferred easily; but if the middle section, the spine, is a spring rather than a rigid structure, it is more difficult to transfer forces from one section to another. When the middle segment is not rigid, the forces produced in the lower segment are dissipated and the upper bar, the arms, must develop their own forces—a far more difficult and strenuous method of delivering force for desired activity.

For this reason, it is important for athletes to have a straight back during activities, especially those activities that require force transmission. For example, a football lineman squats with the back straight to utilize the driving force from the legs; the weightlifter keeps the back straight in a squat to transfer the lifting force from the legs to the arms; the golfer's back is straight so that the summation of forces from

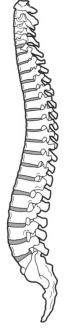

■ **Figure 11.24**
Proper spinal alignment is a "straight spine".

the legs and trunk can drive the ball down the fairway. The sport rehabilitation specialist must also maintain a straight back so the power of the legs, not the arms, delivers the manual resistance for therapeutic exercises.

If the back is not kept straight, transfer of forces from the lower extremities to the trunk and upper extremities is not possible. To see the significance of this, have a friend bend over from the waist so that his or her back is not straight, and then push on the shoulders in an attempt to propel the person off balance. Now have your friend bend at the hips and keep the back straight as you again attempt to push his or her body off balance. You will find that with the back straight, the power of the legs will provide for increased stability and better resistance to outside forces.

When lowering the body to sit, or to lift an object, the back should remain straight so less stress is applied to the spine. It is not enough just to bend the knees. The knees must bend, but the hips are also pushed back while the chest is kept up. If the hips are not pushed back, the bend occurs in the back, not the hips, and the lower back will round, losing the back's proper alignment. If the chest is lowered, the spine will round and lose its proper straight position (figure 11.25b).

Lowering the center of gravity increases the body's stability. This is important if resistance to outside forces is needed. For example, if you push your friend while he or she is standing fully upright, it will be easier for you to move the person than if he or she squats down to reduce the body's center of gravity. This is one reason linemen in football or rugby get into a squat position.

Broadening the base of support is another method of providing increased stability. If your friend stands with feet together, it is much easier to push him or her off balance than if the feet are positioned apart. A broader base of support produces a larger area for the center of gravity to move within before balance is lost. When you move an object, a broad base of support will increase your stability.

Another principle of good body mechanics is to stand in the direction of force application. This allows the use of force transfer from the legs. For example, when you throw a ball forward, your feet should be in a backward-forward straddle. This permits transfer of forces from the back leg to the front leg as your trunk is rotated and your arm is brought through the throwing motion. To see this concept, throw a ball with your feet in a side-by-side stance and then with your feet in a backward-forward

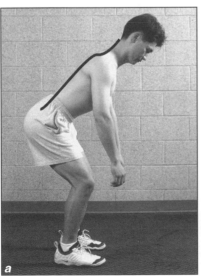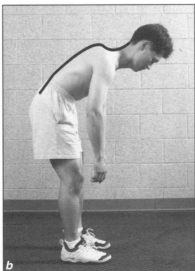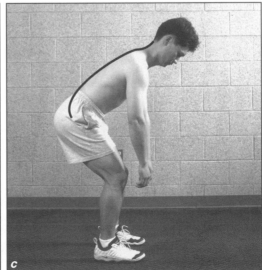

▌Figure 11.25 Keeping back straight when bending: *(a)* knees and hips flexed, hips pushed backward, lumbar curve maintained, chest is held up; *(b)* leg and lower back positions are maintained properly, but head and chest are lowered; *(c)* leg and chest positions are maintained, but lumbar curve is lost and hips are not pushed backward.

straddle stance. You will find that the ball goes farther with the straddle stance. If it is necessary to transfer an object or exert a force from one side of the body to the other, the best stance is a side-by-side stance with the feet in line with the shoulders. For example, if you are resisting a patient's straight-leg raise with the patient supine on the table, your stance should be side by side as you face the table. This way, as the patient raises his or her leg, your weight can transfer from the leg you have positioned next to the patient's foot (lower) to the one you have positioned next to the patient's hip (upper). You will be able to use a body-weight shift from your lower to your upper leg as the center of gravity of the patient's leg moves in that direction.

Abdominal strength is important for force transfer from the lower to the upper extremities. Strong abdominals provide the support needed to keep the back straight, help to diffuse the forces applied to the back, and assist in the transfer of forces from the legs to the arms. Arm and leg movement must be assisted by stabilization of the spine for the arms and legs to produce the desired activity. You can see this if you have someone resist your shoulder flexion-to-extension movement. You should feel your abdominals tighten as you extend the arm against his or her resistance. You should also feel the abdominals tighten when hip flexion is resisted. An injured athlete's therapeutic exercise program should include abdominal strengthening exercises.

THE PATIENT'S DAILY ACTIVITIES

Performing daily activities using correct body mechanics is important because it conserves energy, makes for efficient and effective use of the body, and reduces stress on the back and other segments. Knowledge of these techniques enables you to instruct patients, especially those with back injuries, in minimizing stress to the injured area.

Every day, patients lift and carry objects such as book bags, backpacks, athletic gear, and athletic bags. The way an object is lifted depends on its size and weight. It is important to test the weight of the object before it is lifted. If an object is heavy, the proper way to lift it is front on. This includes facing the object, standing as close to the object as possible, and standing so that when the back is straight and the person is flexed at the hips and knees, the arms fall directly over the object. As the individual bends the knees to lift the object, the knees should never be lower than the hips. Placing the knees below the level of the hips imposes a great deal of stress on the knee's meniscus. Additional lowering of the body is achieved by pushing the hips backward, bending the knee as far as possible but keeping the knee higher than the hip, and keeping the chest up and the back straight. With the abdominals tightened, the person lifts the object by straightening the legs while moving into a standing position (figure 11.26). The object should be kept close to the body to reduce its force (force equals weight times distance). The farther away from the body the object is, the more force is required to lift it.

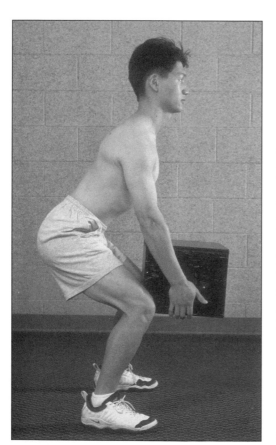

▌Figure 11.26   Proper lifting technique.

the legs and trunk can drive the ball down the fairway. The sport rehabilitation specialist must also maintain a straight back so the power of the legs, not the arms, delivers the manual resistance for therapeutic exercises.

If the back is not kept straight, transfer of forces from the lower extremities to the trunk and upper extremities is not possible. To see the significance of this, have a friend bend over from the waist so that his or her back is not straight, and then push on the shoulders in an attempt to propel the person off balance. Now have your friend bend at the hips and keep the back straight as you again attempt to push his or her body off balance. You will find that with the back straight, the power of the legs will provide for increased stability and better resistance to outside forces.

When lowering the body to sit, or to lift an object, the back should remain straight so less stress is applied to the spine. It is not enough just to bend the knees. The knees must bend, but the hips are also pushed back while the chest is kept up. If the hips are not pushed back, the bend occurs in the back, not the hips, and the lower back will round, losing the back's proper alignment. If the chest is lowered, the spine will round and lose its proper straight position (figure 11.25b).

Lowering the center of gravity increases the body's stability. This is important if resistance to outside forces is needed. For example, if you push your friend while he or she is standing fully upright, it will be easier for you to move the person than if he or she squats down to reduce the body's center of gravity. This is one reason linemen in football or rugby get into a squat position.

Broadening the base of support is another method of providing increased stability. If your friend stands with feet together, it is much easier to push him or her off balance than if the feet are positioned apart. A broader base of support produces a larger area for the center of gravity to move within before balance is lost. When you move an object, a broad base of support will increase your stability.

Another principle of good body mechanics is to stand in the direction of force application. This allows the use of force transfer from the legs. For example, when you throw a ball forward, your feet should be in a backward-forward straddle. This permits transfer of forces from the back leg to the front leg as your trunk is rotated and your arm is brought through the throwing motion. To see this concept, throw a ball with your feet in a side-by-side stance and then with your feet in a backward-forward

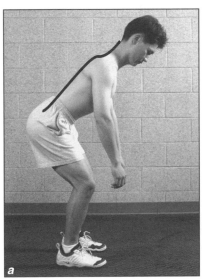
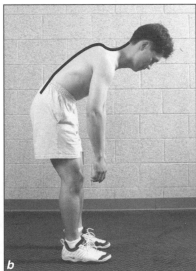
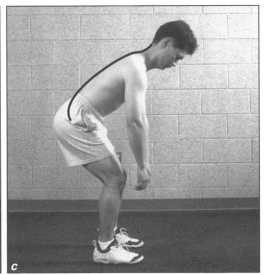

Figure 11.25 Keeping back straight when bending: *(a)* knees and hips flexed, hips pushed backward, lumbar curve maintained, chest is held up; *(b)* leg and lower back positions are maintained properly, but head and chest are lowered; *(c)* leg and chest positions are maintained, but lumbar curve is lost and hips are not pushed backward.

straddle stance. You will find that the ball goes farther with the straddle stance. If it is necessary to transfer an object or exert a force from one side of the body to the other, the best stance is a side-by-side stance with the feet in line with the shoulders. For example, if you are resisting a patient's straight-leg raise with the patient supine on the table, your stance should be side by side as you face the table. This way, as the patient raises his or her leg, your weight can transfer from the leg you have positioned next to the patient's foot (lower) to the one you have positioned next to the patient's hip (upper). You will be able to use a body-weight shift from your lower to your upper leg as the center of gravity of the patient's leg moves in that direction.

Abdominal strength is important for force transfer from the lower to the upper extremities. Strong abdominals provide the support needed to keep the back straight, help to diffuse the forces applied to the back, and assist in the transfer of forces from the legs to the arms. Arm and leg movement must be assisted by stabilization of the spine for the arms and legs to produce the desired activity. You can see this if you have someone resist your shoulder flexion-to-extension movement. You should feel your abdominals tighten as you extend the arm against his or her resistance. You should also feel the abdominals tighten when hip flexion is resisted. An injured athlete's therapeutic exercise program should include abdominal strengthening exercises.

THE PATIENT'S DAILY ACTIVITIES

Performing daily activities using correct body mechanics is important because it conserves energy, makes for efficient and effective use of the body, and reduces stress on the back and other segments. Knowledge of these techniques enables you to instruct patients, especially those with back injuries, in minimizing stress to the injured area.

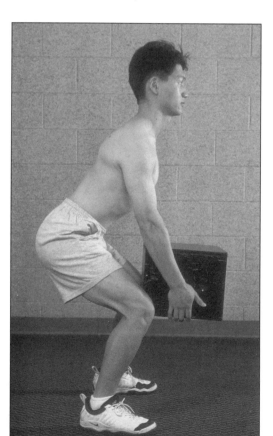

Every day, patients lift and carry objects such as book bags, backpacks, athletic gear, and athletic bags. The way an object is lifted depends on its size and weight. It is important to test the weight of the object before it is lifted. If an object is heavy, the proper way to lift it is front on. This includes facing the object, standing as close to the object as possible, and standing so that when the back is straight and the person is flexed at the hips and knees, the arms fall directly over the object. As the individual bends the knees to lift the object, the knees should never be lower than the hips. Placing the knees below the level of the hips imposes a great deal of stress on the knee's meniscus. Additional lowering of the body is achieved by pushing the hips backward, bending the knee as far as possible but keeping the knee higher than the hip, and keeping the chest up and the back straight. With the abdominals tightened, the person lifts the object by straightening the legs while moving into a standing position (figure 11.26). The object should be kept close to the body to reduce its force (force equals weight times distance). The farther away from the body the object is, the more force is required to lift it.

❚ Figure 11.26 Proper lifting technique.

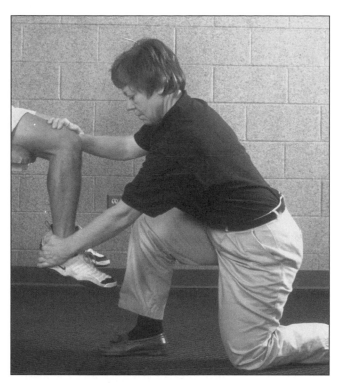

minimize risk of injury and maximize body forces. This is true for the athlete during sport participation, for the sport rehabilitation specialist during execution of therapeutic exercises, and for everyone in daily activities.

❚ Figure 11.31 Rehabilitation specialist with proper body mechanics.

BODY-AWARENESS PROGRAMS

Body-awareness programs, which focus on self-improvement through awareness of movement patterns and abilities, include the Feldenkrais Method and the Alexander Technique.

Over the years, many programs have been developed to improve body awareness through body movement. Two of these programs are introduced here. The intent is to familiarize you with the various kinds of approaches that body-awareness programs use. The two basic premises common to all these programs is that the techniques produce self-improvement through increased body awareness and that a strong body-mind interaction exists that determines an individual's movement patterns and abilities. The whole body, not just the area of pain or dysfunction, is addressed. Some athletes use these programs to enhance their athletic skill and performance. Others find the programs useful in treating injuries that impede normal body function.

FELDENKRAIS METHOD

Moshe Feldenkrais (1904–1984) was a Russian-born Israeli who obtained a doctorate in physics from the Sorbonne in Paris. He held a black belt in judo and was a recognized judo instructor. An old soccer injury of the knee became painful and crippling in Feldenkrais's later years. Physicians were unable to provide a satisfactory medical treatment, so he taught himself medicine, anatomy, therapeutic exercise, and body mechanics. His mechanical and electrical engineering background was an asset as he developed what became known as the Feldenkrais Method. He taught himself to walk pain free using this method. By the 1950s he had given up his career as a research scientist and had begun to devote his work to teaching and using the Feldenkrais Method.

Dr. Feldenkrais believed that an individual develops inefficient movement patterns for a variety of reasons—that cultural influences, illness, injury, and other factors

For more information about the Feldenkrais method, see the Feldenkrais Guild of North America's Web site at **www.feldenkrais.com**.

can cause limited movement leading to inhibition of normal movement ability. In the Feldenkrais Method, movement patterns and habits are assessed before a treatment program is initiated. Feldenkrais believed that a person's unconscious pattern of movement is influenced by several factors, including several factors, including the unconscious sensorimotor relationship that affects muscles and joints and their associated motor skills and abilities; the individual's perception of balance, space, and gravity; self-image; and kinesthetic awareness. His approach for changing these components to improve movement involves engaging the whole person in the treatment regimen, promoting self-esteem, and improving learning skills.

Pain is avoided in the Feldenkrais Method. Pain encourages the unfavorable muscle movement patterns that the person has established. Movement is usually performed slowly through an easy direction of motion. Slow and easy movement allows the individual to become sensitive to motions and positions, allows muscle relaxation, and permits a change of position through a new and more correct movement pattern.

As the individual progresses, the movements become more advanced in their complexity, speed, size, and trajectory of motion. This process permits an increased awareness of kinesthesia and coordination and causes a decrease in pain.

The Feldenkrais Method encompasses two approaches to this somatically based re-education. One is "Awareness through Movement" and the other is "Functional Integration." Awareness through Movement includes the use of active motion either with the individual or with a group. In 45- to 60-min sessions the instructor guides patients through a series of active movements using imagery and focused attention. Through the guidance, the patients become aware of their somatic reception and the influence it has on their movement. Imagery and visualization help them to develop this awareness and movement perception. The goal is for patients to become aware of their bodies and how their bodies move, of the relationship between one segment and another during movement, and of the influences that affect their movement.

The lessons often include developmental movements such as rolling, crawling, and standing up. They also include somatic awareness, visualization, and imagery for functions such as posture, breathing, and simple movements. The exercises are not vigorous but rather are explorations of the somatopsychic connections that increase self-awareness and facilitate an assessment of sensory-based movement. The movements often start as very small motions with emphasis on ease of movement, comfort, and development of an awareness of the way the muscles and bones are integrated with the individual's somatosensory system and personality. Small movements progress to more complex, larger, and faster ones until the movements are functional and can be put to daily use. Imagery and verbal suggestion guide the patient toward incorporating the new movement patterns into daily activity.

Functional Integration uses individualized sessions designed to meet the person's specific needs to improve movement. As with Awareness through Movement, Functional Integration is a learning-based method of improving movement efficiency, coordination, awareness, and self-control. Movement awareness and response are facilitated through the use of touch, imagery, repetition, and guidance. A new awareness and perception of movement are created and integrated into the individual's motions through the instructor's guidance, much as one dance partner is guided by the other, until the new neuromuscular patterns become ingrained and translate into a change in the injured patient's active performance.

An Example of the Feldenkrais Method

As an example of the Feldenkrais Method, a simple 2-min activity experiment from Alon (1990) is reprinted here. It is designed to improve and refine an individual's ability to look up. Take a couple of minutes to go through it and note any changes you experience. To perform the activity, go through the following steps:

In a sitting position, raise your head upward and try to see the ceiling. Make a note how this movement works for you. At what point in your reach do you have a feeling of difficulty? What happens to your breathing? Now, shift your attention to the feet. Take off one shoe and extend that foot forward, as far as you can; the sole stays flat on the floor. Begin to slowly flex your toes downward, dragging them along the floor closer to your heel. In this position, lift the ball of the foot from the floor and decrease the angle of bending in the ankle. All this time, the heel is still anchored to the floor. This is an unusual combination of movements involving the foot. Allow the foot to return to its comfortable place on the floor, and repeat the whole sequence several times.

In the next step, place your foot in full contact with the floor again, but this time bend the toes upward, raising them into the air while the ball of the foot stays on the ground. Alternate several times between the two movements, from bent ankle to outstretched ankle, with the heel planted all the time on the floor. The toes point to the floor when the foot comes up, and they are turned to the ceiling when the ball of the foot rests on the floor. See if you can reduce the amount of effort which you invest in bending the ankle and the toes. Notice that to design a strange arrangement which is perhaps totally new to you, you have to use a device other than direct physical power. Identify within yourself this quality of listening and clarification—it is this quality which makes the difference between exercise and learning.

Now, bring the foot back to its usual place, and again lift your head so as to look at the ceiling. Has your scan of the ceiling now been made a bit easier than it was earlier?

The Feldenkrais Method is a complex system that takes time to learn. There are several classifications of Feldenkrais-trained professionals. Awareness-through-movement Feldenkrais teachers must have a minimum of 2 years of instruction; Feldenkrais practitioners have a minimum of 4 years of instruction; assistant trainers have a minimum of 7 years of activity; and trainers must have at least 11 years in the area. The Feldenkrais Guild in Albany, Oregon, is the accrediting body for the Feldenkrais Method.

ALEXANDER TECHNIQUE

Frederick M. Alexander (1869–1955) was an Australian-born actor who owned his own theater company and performed readings of Shakespeare. Before the invention of microphones, voice projection was vital to an actor's livelihood. After many fruitless attempts by physicians to cure the projection difficulty that Alexander had, he discovered that his problem lay in his body posture and movement. He discovered how faulty posture, incorrect movement patterns, and inefficient movement could affect health, movement, and body function. He eventually abandoned his theatrical career and studied the human body and techniques to improve its efficiency of movement. In the early 1900s he moved from Australia to England, where he taught his techniques.

Alexander discovered that posture is complex and that it involves not just sitting or standing straight, but also supporting and balancing against gravity during all daily activities. Children, he noticed, have good posture and good mechanics; but as people become older, the stresses and strains of life increase muscle tension and affect posture, as well as the way they use the body. Alexander believed that daily stresses over time cause increased muscle tension. This increased tension causes

For more information about the Alexander Technique, see **http://alexandertechnique.com**, **www.life.uiuc.edu/jeff/alextech.html**, or **www.ati-net.com**.

people to use their bodies inefficiently and ineffectively, eventually leading to injury and poor performance. For this reason, Alexander advocated unlearning, rather than learning. He felt that once we discarded the old, incorrect way of performing activities, the body would move naturally and easily.

The Alexander Technique involves the self-examination of functions such as posture, breathing, balance, and coordination. It is an educational process that includes an increased perception of kinesthesia and balance, self-awareness, and natural, stress-free movement. The Alexander Technique is also used to improve functional activities for fine-arts performers and athletes. As an individual's awareness, kinesthesia, and performance improve, pain is relieved and movement becomes more efficient.

The Alexander Technique includes first becoming aware of and releasing the tension that has become habitual over many years of improper movement; it then focuses on re-education to new ways of standing, sitting, and moving that are easier, more efficient, and less stressful to the body. The final phase of the technique includes development of new ways of handling the stresses encountered in daily living so that unnecessary muscle tension does not return. Changing behavior is vital to creating an effective and permanent alteration in body movement. Alexander's method of body awareness, re-education, and self-awareness is designed to allow the individual to make choices that ultimately influence movement. His intent was to create a re-education process that provides a stronger awareness of inner and outer self.

Alexander discovered that the body works as a whole, not in parts. He saw that a painful body part may be influenced by another area that may be the actual site of the pain or dysfunction. He also discovered that an individual produces the same reaction repeatedly until the abnormal motion becomes habitual and feels natural, even though it is abnormal. To correct these problems, he inhibited old motions, encouraged new and more correct motions, and had the individual repeat the corrected motions until the new task became natural. He would use light touch, verbal cueing, and self-awareness techniques until the individual did not need the touch and verbal cueing to perform the task correctly.

Alexander Technique sessions usually last 30 to 60 min and involve group classes or individual lessons. These lessons are a cooperative effort between the participant and the instructor. As the participant receives feedback, he or she gradually feels a lightening sensation. Normally, no more than about eight sessions are needed.

Alexander thought that there were two levels of control or "direction," primary and secondary. The primary control, according to Alexander, stems from the core of the body—the head, neck, and back. If freedom of this primary direction is not managed first, secondary control is not possible. Alexander's primary directions include release of neck, head, and back tension. Releasing the neck is necessary before releasing the tension in the head, and both those sites must be released before the back tension can be released.

Once the primary directions have been applied, the secondary directions can follow. These directions are more numerous and involve the extremities. Depending on where tension is, the secondary release areas may include the shoulders, hip, hands, knees, or other sites. For example, to release tension in the feet, the individual may be instructed to think of the feet spreading onto the ground as the toes lengthen. To release the tension in the upper chest, the person may be instructed to allow the shoulders to release away from one another.

The Alexander technique is one of thought rather than of action. It emphasizes the individual's thinking of the release rather than actually performing the activity. Attempting to produce the action often increases muscle tension instead of relieving it. The individual must practice following the directions several times so that he or she becomes very familiar with them and can feel a change in control. Awareness of actions and performance makes one better able to control those actions and change performance.

Alexander Technique instructors must obtain a minimum of 1600 h or three years of experience and education before they can become certified. The American Center for the Alexander Technique is headquartered in New York City.

It will be helpful to consider a couple of athletic activities and incorporate into them the Alexander Technique of improved awareness and conscious correction with assistance. The common activity of running requires an inefficient expenditure of energy if it is not performed correctly. The Alexander Technique teacher uses gentle touch and verbal instructions to correct the runner's movements until the runner is able to perform the technique using self-awareness and self-correction.

The Alexander Technique as used in soccer can also be used to improve kicking technique. The Alexander Technique teacher can provide instruction to permit the soccer player to release unwanted muscle tension, become aware of muscle activity, and correct the kicking technique to permit a more effective and efficient movement.

An Alexander Technique Experiment

Try this sample experiment reprinted from Barlow (1977) on yourself:

Lie down on the floor with a book under your head, your hips and knees bent with your feet flat on the floor. Find a quiet place so you won't be disturbed, and don't succumb to additional stimuli such as wriggling, scratching, and irrelevant thought patterns.

Think, "neck release, head forward and up." As you give this sequence thought, at first you won't "realize" what the direction means, but as you continue you will begin to associate it with an awareness you've had in the past. By "awareness" is meant that what should be a normal sense of "being in yourself," as opposed to the state of mind-body split that is so often present in adults. While you are still preserving by direction this awareness of the head and neck—an awareness in which your verbal order [of the words and directions] will be part and parcel of the actual perception as the organizing component of it—add on the verbal direction, "lengthen and widen your back." Your lessons will already have made you familiar with the meaning of this phrase, and it is likely that fresh meaning and fresh simplification will accrue as you run over the sequence to yourself. For example, you may realize that the whole of the back is lengthening in one unit instead of thinking of the upper back as separate from the lower back; or perhaps you may suddenly notice that widening of the back includes releasing the shoulder blade and upper arm. At this point, your interest in the new realization may have caused you to "lose" the head direction, and it will be necessary to reinforce it before returning to the lengthening and widening direction.

The process of adding together the direction to the head and the direction to the back may take several minutes or even longer; indeed, if it seems to take less time, you almost certainly have been making a muscular change by direct movement, instead of sticking to realizing the meaning of the orders. Remember that in this process we do not move our bodies in the same way as when we pick up an external object, a brush or pen or pail. To move our forearm is not the same as to move a spoon. Moving ourselves and bits of ourselves—as opposed to moving external objects—is always a question of allowing movement to take place, rather than of [making movement take place by] picking up and putting down somewhere else. Allowing the movement, say, of an arm will involve a total general awareness of the body; the active process involved in this particular movement is small compared with the active process of awareness that is going on in the whole of the body all of the time. Similarly, a movement of standing up after sitting down—a movement which involves mainly a leg adjustment—does not require only the leg activity, but primarily a maintenance of the awareness of the rest of the body while allowing the necessary leg movement to take place.

SUMMARY

1. *Identify the primary elements of proper alignment in standing from an anterior, posterior, and side view.*

   In an anterior position, a plumb line should bisect the nose and mouth and should run through the central portion of the sternum, umbilicus, and pubic bones. The earlobes should be level with one another, as should the shoulders, fingertip ends, nipples, iliac crests, patellae, and medial malleoli. The patellae should point straight ahead, with the feet straight or turned slightly outward. The knees and ankles are in line with each other with the knees angled neither inward nor outward in relation to each other.

   From a side view, the plumb line should pass through the external auditory meatus, the earlobe, the bodies of the cervical vertebrae, the center of the shoulder joint, and the greater trochanter. The plumb line should run midway between the back and chest and between the back and abdomen, slightly posterior to the hip joint, and slightly anterior to the center of the knee just behind the patella. A horizontal line should connect the ASIS and PSIS. The patient should remain relaxed with the body's weight balanced between the heel and the forefoot. The knees are straight but not locked. The chin is slightly tucked and the chest is held slightly up and forward. There is a mild curve inward of the low back and neck regions.

   In the posterior view, a plumb line should bisect the head and should follow the spinous processes from the cervical through the lumbar spine. The earlobes, shoulders, scapulae, hips, PSIS, gluteal fold, posterior knee creases, and medial malleoli should appear level left to right. The scapulae should lie against the rib cage between the second and seventh ribs and about 5 cm (2 in.) from the spinous processes. The calcaneus should be straight, and the calcaneal tendon should be perpendicular to the floor. Trunk muscles should appear balanced, with symmetrical development. The shoulders should be positioned down and relaxed. Body weight should appear equally distributed over both feet.

2. *Discuss common postural faults and describe their causes.*

   A muscle strength imbalance or shortening of a muscle or group can cause common postural faults. These changes usually occur over time and can cause any number of postural changes, depending on the specific area. Some examples of common postural faults include anterior-posterior or lateral spinal deformities such as scoliosis, lordosis, and kyphosis; hip anteversion and retroversion; winking or frog-eye patellae, genu recurvatum; genu and ankle varus and valgus; pes cavus and pes planus; and hammertoes, claw toes, and bunions.

3. *Outline corrective exercises for common postural faults.*

   Once the cause of the fault has been determined, corrective exercises are used to reduce or relieve the fault. In many instances, strengthening of weak muscles combined with stretching of tight structures is fundamental and vital to correction, especially the strengthening of the weak muscles. In addition, the individual must make a conscious effort to correct postural faults in order to stop poor habits and establish new, correct ones.

4. *Explain the importance of good posture and proper body mechanics in athletics.*

   Good posture is vital to good execution of sport activity because it improves efficiency and reduces the risk of injury. Imbalances that occur because of poor posture and mechanics place the body at risk of injury because of already increased stresses on structures. One area must compensate for the deficiencies in another area, causing the body to perform less efficiently and effectively.

5. *List the basic principles of good body mechanics.*

   Maintain a "straight" spine so that forces from the legs can be transferred upward; reduce the height of the center of gravity for increased stability; widen the base of support for more stability; stand in the direction of movement or force application; and maintain good strength in the abdominals and lower-extremity muscles.

6. *Discuss an example of the use of proper body mechanics by the sport rehabilitation specialist during a treatment program.*

When providing manual resistance, the sport rehabilitation specialist stands close to the patient, uses leg strength to deliver the manual resistance, keeps the back straight, and stands with the feet in the direction of the resisted movement.

7. *Explain the differences and similarities between the Feldenkrais Method and the Alexander Technique.*

Both methods are based on correction of the dysfunctional somatic feedback system and use of self-awareness, re-education, and repetition as part of the correction process. The Feldenkrais Method improves movement through changing awareness of movement; it engages the entire person in the treatment program by promoting self-esteem and improving learning skills. The Alexander Technique emphasizes the unlearning of old and improper habits and establishing new habits based on self-evaluation and increased perception of kinesthesia and natural movement.

CRITICAL THINKING QUESTIONS

1. You are working in an industrial clinic where back injuries are frequent. In an effort to be more efficient, you design a handout for these back patients that will include instructions for proper lifting and sitting. What items will you include in the handout? Will you include any precautions? What about general information on back anatomy and mechanics? Why would you or would you not include this information?

2. A shoulder patient you are treating has poor upper back and cervical posture. You feel that this is complicating the shoulder injury and that you must correct the patient's posture before you can effectively impact the shoulder. How can the thoracic and cervical posture affect the shoulder? What will you do to improve this posture? What cues and instructions will you provide the patient?

3. The secretary for your department spends most of her day at the computer and on the phone. She is complaining about upper back and neck pain and has asked you to help her. On what areas will your assessment be focused? What is the probable cause for her complaints, and what can she do to alleviate the problem?

4. A patient with plantar fasciitis has some postural deviations in the lower extremities. In addition to excessively pronated feet, she also has tibial torsion and squinting patellae. What other deviations in the hips would you expect, given these abnormalities?

5. Based on the opening scenario for this chapter, what instructions would you give Russell on proper lifting mechanics? What precise lifting instructions would you give him? What types of lifting activities would you include in his program?

6. When you are providing lower-extremity proprioceptive neuromuscular facilitation to a patient who is lying on the table, what correct body mechanics would you use? What would be the position for your base of support? How would you transfer your body weight? Where would your body be positioned to offer the best resistance on hip extension? On hip flexion?

REFERENCES

Alon, R. 1990. *Mindful spontaneity: Moving in tune with nature: Lessons in the Feldenkrais Method.* New York: Harper & Row.

Barlow, W. 1977. *The Alexander Technique.* New York: Knopf.

Kendall, F.P., McCreary, E.K., and P.G. Provance. 1993. *Muscles: Testing and function.* 4th ed. Baltimore: Williams & Wilkins.

SUGGESTED READING

Daniels, L., and C. Worthingham. 1977. *Therapeutic exercise for body alignment and function.* Philadelphia: Saunders.

CHAPTER TWELVE

Ambulation and Ambulation Aids

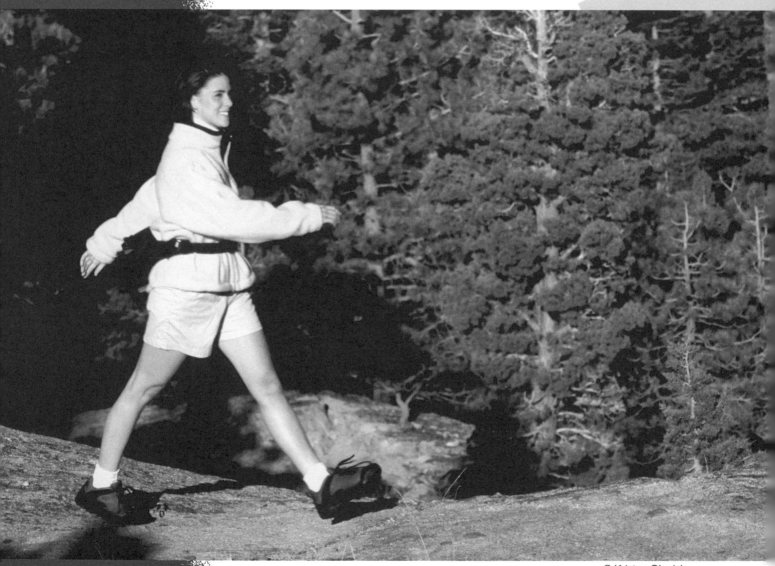

OBJECTIVES

After completing this chapter, you should be able to do the following:

1. Discuss the general concepts of gait.

2. Identify the range-of-motion changes during the gait cycle.

3. Explain the muscle activity involved in ambulation.

4. Describe the general mechanical differences between walking and running.

5. Discuss one abnormal gait commonly seen following an athletic injury.

6. Outline the various types of gait with assistive devices.

7. Explain the technique involved in stair climbing with assistive devices.

8. Identify the safety measures involved in ambulating with assistive devices.

When Mary Ann, a competitive, 38-year-old soccer player, first injured her ankle, she was unable to walk on it. The second-degree sprain was conservatively treated with a cast for two weeks and then placed in a splint for four weeks. By the time Tony Valencia, certified athletic trainer, saw Mary Ann, she was out of the splint and off crutches but was still not able to walk normally. Tony analyzed her gait to evaluate for deficiencies in range of motion and strength before performing specific motion and strength tests. Because she was not walking normally, he did not have her run, but he knew that one day he would analyze her running gait as well.

Since Mary Ann was still limping severely, he instructed her in how to walk with a cane. She didn't want to use crutches any longer, but saw the cane as a compromise until she could walk normally without it. Tony was careful to provide her with precautions about using the cane and would not allow her to use it on her own until she demonstrated proper use on the floor, carpet, and stairs.

You can observe a lot just by watching.

Yogi Berra, baseball player, manager, and philosopher

This chapter deals with the mechanics of walking and running and the use of assistive devices for ambulation. Analysis of the way a patient walks or runs requires observation by the sport rehabilitation specialist. Watching how he or she moves during ambulation, from the feet all the way up to the shoulders, can yield important information. To know whether or not a patient ambulates normally, you must understand what normal gait is. Before you can instruct a patient in how to use assistive devices during ambulation, you must first understand the mechanics of those assistive devices and the desired gait with the devices.

Ambulation is a normal activity that we perform every day without thinking about it, about what it involves, or about how we do it. We just do it. When an injury prevents normal ambulation, the activity becomes difficult and energy consuming. It no longer is something we take for granted and no longer is automatic.

This chapter introduces the mechanics of walking and addresses the differences between walking and running. We will consider normal ambulation and then the use of assistive devices in ambulation. Topics include the mechanics of assistive device applications, various types of gaits with different types of assistive devices on different surfaces, and methods of selecting assistive devices for the patient.

NORMAL GAIT

Elements of gait include the gait cycle, the center-of-gravity pathway, gait kinematics, gait kinetics, and ground reaction forces. Lower-extremity injuries can lead to abnormalities of these elements and are reflected in the patient's pathological gait.

Ambulation, or walking, is the locomotion method we use to move our body from one place to another. The way we walk is called gait. Although each person's gait is slightly different from everyone else's, all normal gaits have basic similarities. In fact, considering how many body types and sizes there are among human beings, it is surprising how little normal gait differs from one person to the next. Major differences commonly result from postural variations, weaknesses, structural abnormalities, and soft-tissue length alterations, some of which are discussed in chapter 11. Knowledge of normal gait is essential to the sport rehabilitation specialist so that he or she can correct abnormal gait following injury and understand the use of assistive devices.

GAIT CYCLE

One **gait cycle** is the time from the point at which the heel of one foot touches the ground to the time it touches the ground again. A gait cycle is divided into two phases, the stance phase and the swing phase. The **stance phase** occurs when the foot is in contact with the floor and the extremity is bearing partial or total body weight. The stance phase is subdivided into three parts. **Heel strike** occurs when the heel first comes in contact with the floor. **Foot flat,** as the term implies, occurs when the foot is flat on the floor. The **midstance** phase occurs when the foot is directly under the body's weight and the entire foot is in contact with the floor. Because the body weight is transferred entirely to the one supporting leg and the other leg is in the middle of its swing phase, this is also referred to as **single-leg support**. **Heel-off** occurs when the weight begins to transfer to the front of the foot, and the heel is lifted off the floor. Partial weight remains on the extremity as the other extremity is in contact with the floor again. **Toe-off** occurs when the foot comes off the floor and the swing phase begins. This is also referred to as *push-off,* since the extremity now propels the body forward and the leg continues into the second phase of gait.

The second phase, **swing phase**, occurs when the foot is not in contact with the floor and no weight is borne on the extremity. The swing phase begins with toe-off and is divided into early-, mid-, and late-swing phases. Immediately after toe-off, the leg begins its early swing, or **acceleration,** as momentum is increased in its non-weight-bearing propulsion forward. The middle portion of the swing phase is called **swing-through.** The leg continues its swing-through until just before heel strike when it goes through the late swing, or **deceleration,** to slow its forward propulsion, make a smooth contact with the floor, and begin a new gait cycle. Alternative terminology can also be used and is often seen in research reports on gait. With this nomenclature, the heel strike with the floor is termed **initial contact,** and as the foot progresses to increased weight bearing, it goes from initial contact to **loading response** (foot flat), then **midstance** (single-leg support). In this terminology, heel-off is referred to as **terminal stance** and progresses to **preswing** (toe-off). The swing phase begins with toe-off and is divided into **initial swing** (early swing/acceleration), **midswing** (swing-through), and **terminal swing** (late swing/deceleration). Some researchers and clinicians prefer this terminology because there are more divisions, and the terms provide for greater consistency in reporting analysis and results.

Clinicians vary in the terminology they use. Clinicians' choice of terminology for gait analysis most often depends on the method they were taught and on what is most intuitive for them. Both groups of terms are presented here so you can become familiar with each. The alternative terms are used interchangeably throughout this text.

If one gait cycle from the beginning of stance phase to the end of swing phase is 100%, stance phase is approximately 60% of the gait cycle. Within the stance, heel strike to foot flat covers 0% to 12% of the gait cycle; midstance occurs over the next 12% to 30%; heel-off begins at 30% and continues until toe-off at the start of the swing cycle (figure 12.1). The remaining 40% of the gait cycle occurs during the swing phase. As speed of the gait increases, the percentages between the stance and swing phases become more equal. In running, the percentage becomes greater for the swing phase than for the stance phase.

During the first and last 10% of stance in walking, the body is supported by both lower extremities (Ounpuu 1994). This occurs at the beginning of the stance phase during heel strike for one leg and at the end of the stance phase, just before toe-off, for the other. This form of support is referred to as **double-limb support.** When one leg is in its swing phase, the body is supported by only one leg; this is referred to as single-limb support.

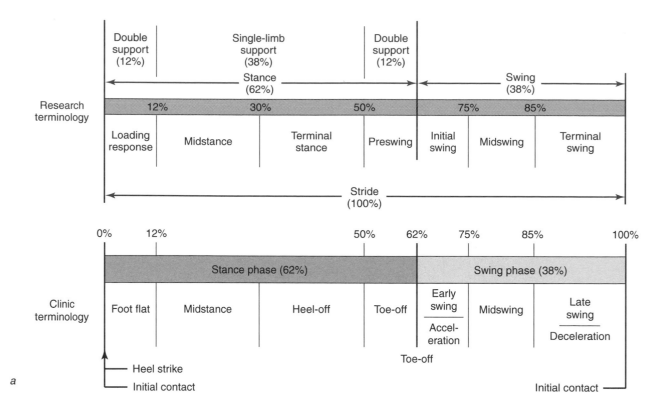

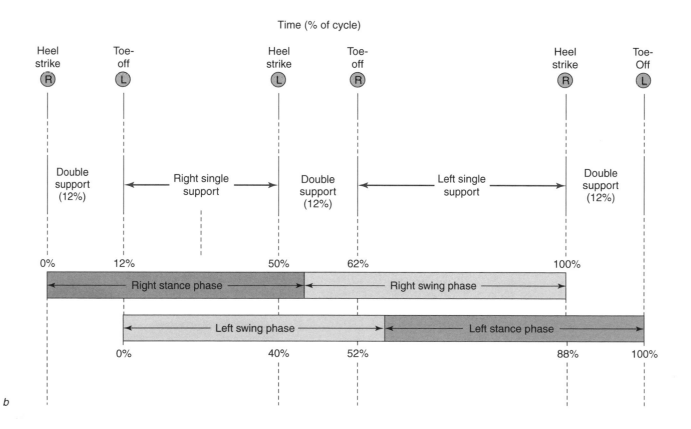

Figure 12.1 Gait cycle: (*a*) single-leg gait cycle, (*b*) double-leg gait cycle.

CENTER-OF-GRAVITY PATHWAY

During ambulation, the body's center of gravity is propelled forward. Its position also changes because of the associated changes in position of the joints and extremities during ambulation. Before we can understand the changes that occur and their importance, we must clarify some terms.

Stride length is the distance from heel strike of one foot to heel strike of the same foot in one gait cycle. **Step length** is the distance from heel strike of one foot to heel strike of the other foot in one gait cycle. Although stride length depends on the individual's height, an average stride length is 156 cm (61 in.) (Lehmann 1982).

The body's side-to-side movement as weight is shifted from one lower extremity to the other is called **stride width** (figure 12.2). It is the distance between the midline of one foot at mid-stance and the midline of the other foot at mid-stance. Stride width also has individual determining factors such as body size and weight, but the average stride width is 8 cm (about 3 in.) (Lehmann 1982).

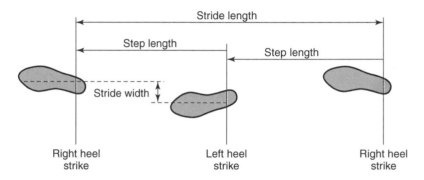

▌Figure 12.2 Stride length and stride width.

There is large variation in the rate at which individuals walk. Reports of normal walking speed range from just under 60 strides per minute (Murray et al. 1964) to 101 to 122 steps per minute (Winter 1987). As cadence increases to jogging, running, and sprinting speeds, stance and swing phases are directly influenced. We will consider the mechanics of running in the section "Normal Running Gait" later in this chapter.

As the body is propelled forward, it attempts to create motion that is as efficient as possible. Keeping the center-of-gravity movement to a minimum is the means of achieving efficiency of movement. Short of the lower extremities' being wheels instead of legs, a multijoint system is the best way to propel the body forward efficiently. Although with a wheel system the body would move very efficiently over flat surfaces, movement over uneven surfaces would become quite difficult. Using a number of joints from the pelvis to the foot, the body minimizes center-of-gravity pathway changes by changing the position of the joints as the body moves, and also allows for adjustment to varying types of surfaces and terrain.

In order for propulsion of the body to be smooth and efficient, the body must produce enough force to move forward but also control the movement and momentum so that the body remains stable as its positions change; it must also absorb the impact shock of moving weight from one leg to the other. All these capabilities must be present and must be controlled if movement is to be efficient and effective. Loss of one of the contributing factors can result in poor quality of movement, high energy requirements, or injury.

Since the body does not move on wheels, its bipedal system's most efficient method of transport is a sinusoidal motion. The body's center of gravity moves in a wavelike fashion and thereby conserves energy and reduces impact forces (figure 12.3). The body accomplishes a sinusoidal motion during locomotion through six determinant motions in different joints.

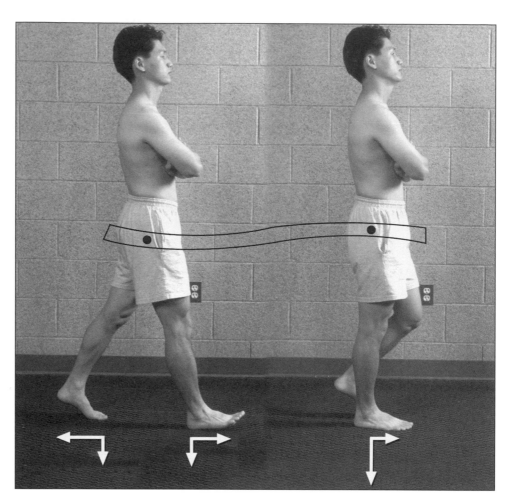

■ **Figure 12.3** Sinusoidal motion.

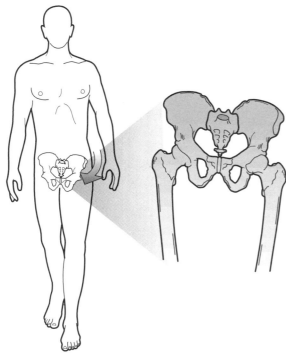

■ **Figure 12.4** Pelvic rotation causes an increase in the length of the leg's stride to reduce the center of gravity's vertical displacement.

Pelvic Rotation

Pelvic rotation occurs around a horizontal axis in the transverse plane. As one leg swings forward, the pelvis rotates forward to increase the length of the leg's stride. The pelvis attains its maximum rotation on one side, 4°, at the point of double-leg support. With lengthening of the leg, the center of gravity is prevented from dropping lower than it otherwise would (figure 12.4). This motion reduces the center-of-gravity movement by $^3/_8$. The pelvis rotates 4° on the opposite side as that leg rotates forward during the same process. The total pelvic rotation is 8°, or 4° on each side.

Pelvic Tilt

During midstance the pelvis tilts downward from the stance leg so that the hip on the swing-leg side is lower than that on the stance-leg side (figure 12.5). This movement is controlled by the hip abductors of the stance leg. Because the center of gravity is midway between the hips, it is lowered when the swing leg is lowered. This movement depresses the center of gravity during midstance by 5° and decreases the vertical displacement of the center of gravity by $\frac{3}{16}$.

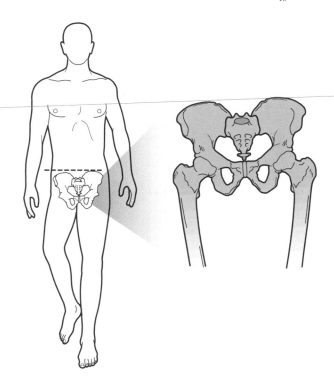

❚ Figure 12.5 Pelvic tilt decreases vertical displacement of the center of gravity.

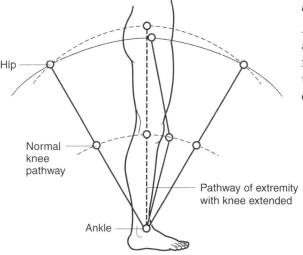

Knee Flexion at Midstance

At heel strike the knee is in extension, but immediately afterward it begins to flex until it flexes to 15° by midstance (figure 12.6). This knee flexion reduces the center of gravity's vertical excursion by $\frac{7}{16}$ when it is at its highest point of the sinusoidal curve.

❚ Figure 12.6 Knee flexion at midstance decreases vertical displacement of the center of gravity at midstance.

Ankle Motion

The center of gravity of the ankle joint is lowest at heel strike and toe-off and highest at midstance. This is the opposite of what happens with the knee joint, as seen in figure 12.7. These combined motions help to reduce the vertical excursion of the center of gravity and smooth out its sinusoidal curve.

The combined effects of pelvic rotation, pelvic tilt, and knee and ankle motions during stance are responsible for reducing excursion of the center of gravity by 2.5 cm (1 in.) so that the overall vertical displacement is less than 5 cm. This becomes significant in terms of energy expenditure. The less movement, the less energy expended.

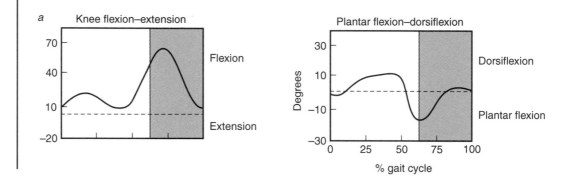

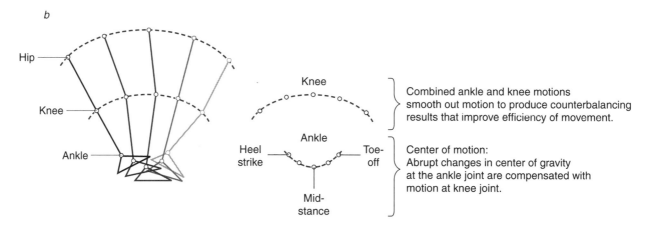

■ Figure 12.7 Knee and ankle motions in gait. The opposite motions occuring at the ankle and knee reduce vertical excursion of the center of gravity.

Lateral Motion of Pelvis

In order for a person to stand with stability, the center of gravity must be over the base of support, the feet. When we stand on two feet, the center of gravity is between the feet. For standing on one leg, the center of gravity must shift so that it is over the supporting leg. If the thighs were arranged in a parallel fashion, a maximum shift of 15 cm (6 in.) of the pelvis would be needed to transfer the center of gravity from one supporting leg to the other during single-limb support (figure 12.8). Because the femurs are not straight but adducted, placing the knees in a valgus position, the lateral shift required of the pelvis in moving from one leg to the other is 4.3 cm (1.7 in.) for an adult. This lateral sway of less than 5 cm (2 in.) is also a sinusoidal curve, making the movement from one leg to the other during gait as smooth as possible.

The maximal position of the sinusoidal curve occurs left to right during midstance of each leg and at the midline during double-limb support. The height of the sinusoidal curve in vertical displacement also occurs during midstance of each leg and is at its lowest point during double-limb support.

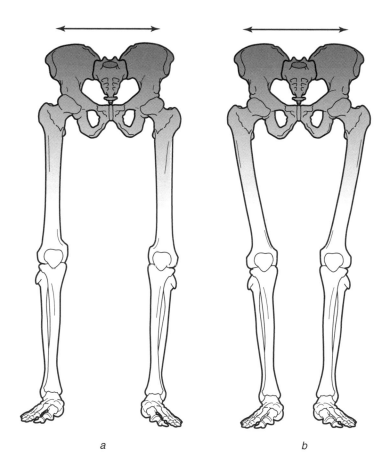

a *b*

■ **Figure 12.8** Hip and knee alignment in lateral pelvic shift. Adducted thigh alignment reduces lateral sway during gait. *(a)* If thighs were parallel, it would require a lateral movement of 15 cm during ambulation. *(b)* Normal hip angulation minimizes lateral pelvic motion during ambulation to less than 5 cm.

GAIT KINEMATICS

The sinusoidal curves of motion that occur during ambulation are caused by changes in the joints' range of motion. Some of these changes are not large but are important for smooth, energy-efficient motion. Movement occurs in the sagittal, coronal, and transverse planes. If movement in one plane is restricted, smooth gait will not occur. Therefore the sport rehabilitation specialist needs to understand the sequence, degree, and timing of joint motion so that if deficiencies exist, he or she can correct them.

Trunk and Upper Extremities

Throughout all cycles of normal gait, the trunk is held in an erect and neutral position. This is necessary to maintain the center of gravity over the base of support. Trunk movement is coordinated with pelvic movement so that as the pelvis rotates in one direction, the trunk rotates in the opposite direction (figure 12.9). The swing of the arms assists the trunk in its rotation, so trunk muscle activity and energy requirements for trunk movement are reduced. This coordination of movement between the pelvis and trunk aids in making the gait smooth, stable, and efficient.

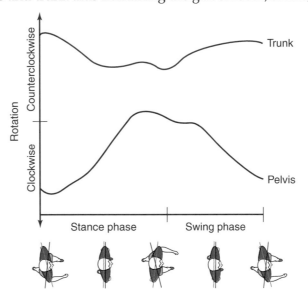

■ **Figure 12.9** Trunk and pelvic rotation.

Modified, by permission, from M.P. Murray, A.B. Drought, and R.C. Kory, 1964, "Walking patterns of normal men," *Journal of Bone and Joint Surgery* 46-A: 335, fig. 10.

Pelvis

Pelvis movement is defined in terms of the movement of the iliac crest. Forward motion of the iliac crest produces an anterior pelvic tilt, and backward motion produces a posterior pelvic tilt. Pelvis motion in the coronal, sagittal, and transverse planes is seen in the graphs in figure 12.10.

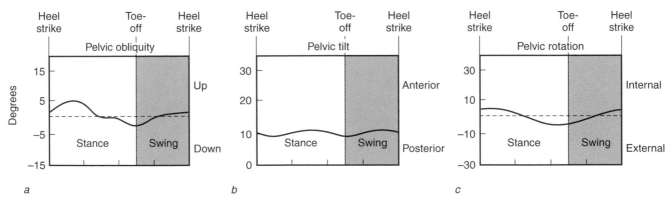

■ **Figure 12.10** Pelvic motion in (a) coronal plane, (b) sagittal plane, (c) transverse plane. Pelvic motion is a triplanar event during ambulation.

Heel Strike to Midstance

As the heel hits the ground at heel strike, the pelvis remains level and is in a 5° forwardly rotated position in the sagittal plane; as the body progresses toward midstance, the pelvis reduces its anterior tilt. In the coronal plane it is elevated 4° at heel strike and begins to drop after initial contact has been made. As the leg goes from heel strike to midstance, the pelvis internally rotates 4°.

Midstance to Toe-Off

By the time the leg is reaching the end of stance phase, the pelvis has moved into a posterior rotation position of about 5°. In a coronal plane during midstance to toe-off, the pelvis continues to drop until it reaches a total of 8° of lateral movement. During the final moments of stance phase, the pelvis rotates externally, 8° from the initial position of 4° internal rotation to an ending stance position of 4° external rotation.

Early Swing

In early swing, the pelvis is level and in a posterior rotation of 5° moving toward anterior rotation. In the coronal plane it begins to move from a downward to an elevated position. Rotation in the transverse plane is gradual from 4° of external rotation to 4° of internal rotation by late swing.

Late Swing

The pelvis continues to be level throughout the gait cycle, moving in the sagittal plane from an anterior position at the middle of the swing phase to a posterior position by the end of late swing. Coronal plane movement continues from its maximum downward position during early swing on its way toward an elevated position such that it is slightly elevated by the end of swing. Rotation also continues to progress in an internal direction as swing phase is terminated.

Total motions of the pelvis during a gait cycle are 4° of anterior-posterior tilt, 8° of lateral tilt, and 8° of rotation.

Hip

Hip motion also occurs in three planes of movement: the coronal, sagittal, and transverse planes (figure 12.11).

Heel Strike to Midstance

At heel strike the hip is in 30° of flexion, slight adduction of 2° to 6°, and near-neutral rotation at 5°. As the leg advances in the stance phase, the hip becomes less flexed, becomes less adducted, and goes from slight internal rotation to slight external rotation.

Midstance to Toe-Off

In the last half of the stance phase, the hip goes from 10° of extension at heel-off to 5° extension at the time of toe-off. The hip is at neutral in the coronal plane at heel-off and goes into 4° of abduction at toe-off. After midstance the hip moves from internal

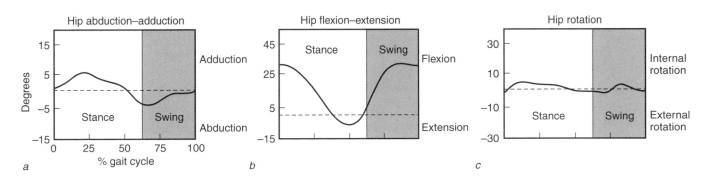

▌Figure 12.11 Hip motion in the (a) coronal plane, (b) sagittal plane, (c) transverse plane. Hip motion is triplanar with the greatest movement occurring in the sagittal plane and the least occurring in the transverse plane.

rotation to neutral at heel-off until it reaches 4° of external rotation at toe-off. Part of the apparent hip extension that occurs from midstance to toe-off is actually the result of a posterior rotation of the pelvis.

Early Swing

In its initial swing, the hip flexes to 20°, has reached its maximum abduction of an average of 5°, and continues to have slight external rotation.

Late Swing

Frontal plane movement continues to advance to 30° just before the end of swing. Coronal plane movement continues to advance from maximal abduction just after the start of early swing toward the midline until a neutral position is achieved just before heel strike. Transverse plane movement oscillates from internal to neutral to external rotation then back to slight internal rotation just before heel strike.

Total hip motions occurring during the gait cycle include 43° in the sagittal plane from flexion to extension, 13° of abduction-adduction in the coronal plane, and 8° of rotation in the transverse plane.

Knee

The knee performs the greatest amount of motion during the swing phase of the gait cycle. Rotation of the knee occurs through the gait cycle and is probably affected by a combination of tibial rotation and hip rotation working synchronously.

Heel Strike to Midstance

At heel strike the knee is in or close to full extension. The tibia is externally rotated 8° to 10°. As weight acceptance on the leg increases, the knee is flexed to 15° and tibial rotation begins to occur in an internal direction (figure 12.12).

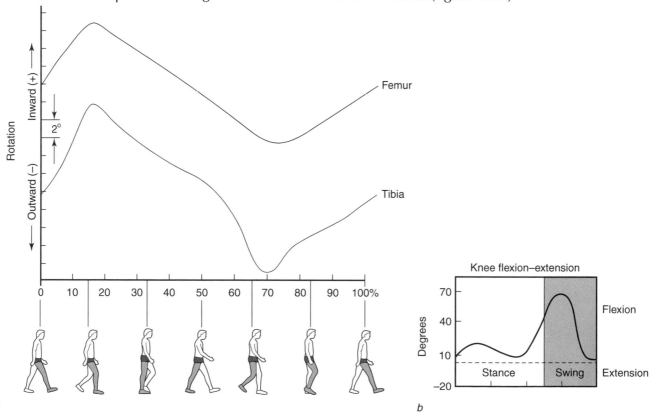

■ **Figure 12.12** Knee motion: *(a)* maximum inward rotation of hip and knee occur prior to midstance, and maximum external rotation occurs at the end of stance and into early swing phase; *(b)* maximum knee extension occurs after midstance, whereas maximum knee flexion occurs in swing phase.

Midstance to Toe-Off

By the time the leg reaches midstance, the knee has achieved its maximum degree of flexion in the stance phase and begins to move into full extension at heel-off. After achievement of maximal tibial internal rotation just before midstance, a return to external rotation occurs during the later half of stance until maximal external rotation is achieved immediately before toe-off. Immediately before toe-off, the knee is passively flexed to 35° by the active movement of the ankle as it goes into plantar flexion and forces the knee to flex.

Early Swing

The knee continues to progress to a maximum of 60° of flexion; this occurs so that the foot clears the ground during the swing phase. In the body's attempt to conserve energy, foot clearance from the floor during swing is a mere 0.87 cm (.3 in.) (Rodgers 1988), just a few millimeters. That distance leaves little room for error from fatigue or restricted motion. The tibia begins moving from the maximum externally rotated position that it was in at toe-off toward inward rotation, although it continues to be positioned in external rotation throughout swing.

Late Swing

After achieving 60° of flexion in the first half of swing, the knee moves progressively and steadily toward extension until it is at 0° just before heel strike. Total knee range of motion in the sagittal plane is 60°, and tibial rotation is 18°. Maximum knee flexion during the stance phase occurs during midstance, and maximum knee flexion during the swing phase occurs during midswing. Maximum knee internal rotation occurs between heel strike and midstance in what researchers call the loading response, and maximum external rotation occurs at toe-off.

Ankle

The ankle and foot work together during gait and provide for needed balance as the body moves over uneven ground. The ankle joint is responsible for forward motion and stability, and the foot joints are responsible for medial and lateral adjustments. The foot and ankle are fairly complex structures and are highly variable in structure and function from one individual to the next. As with other measurements indicated here, the values given are averages.

Heel Strike to Midstance

At heel strike, the ankle and toes are in neutral (figure 12.13). As weight is borne on the leg, the ankle moves into 15° of plantar flexion before midstance. The subtalar joint moves into pronation to accept the forces of impact. The toes remain in a neutral position through midstance. Once the leg moves into midstance, the ankle moves into 10° of dorsiflexion. This 10° permits a smooth glide of the limb as the body moves over its support. A lesser amount of motion causes the body to lurch as it moves into midstance. Once heel strike occurs, the calcaneus everts to cause subtalar pronation. This pronation permits the midtarsal area to remain flexible and to adapt to varying terrains. Pronation also allows the foot to act as a shock absorber. The subtalar joint remains in pronation until just before midstance when it begins to supinate. The longitudinal arch passively lengthens from heel strike until it reaches its maximum length at midstance. At heel strike the foot makes contact with the ground on the posterior aspect of the heel slightly lateral to the midline. As the body moves forward and more weight is borne on the leg, the weight is transmitted to the front of the heel in the midtarsal foot area.

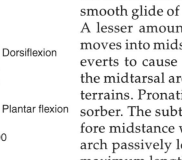

I Figure 12.13 Ankle motion.

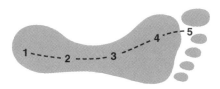

Key

1 = Initial contact
(heel strike)

2 = Loading response
(foot flat)

3 = Midstance

4 = Terminal stance
(heel-off)

5 = Preswing
(toe-off)

▌**Figure 12.14**
Weight transmission during walking: Initial contact at heel strike occurs in the posterior-lateral heel and advances forward on the foot through the stance phase. At midstance the body's weight is just behind the metatarsal heads and at toe-off the weight is primarily over the first and second metatarsal heads.

Midstance to Toe-Off

Following midstance, the ankle moves quickly from 10° of dorsiflexion to about 20° of plantar flexion by the time of toe-off. The calcaneus inverts and causes the subtalar joint to move into supination so the foot will become stable for propulsion at toe-off. The longitudinal arch begins to shorten, and the metatarsophalangeal joints extend to 30° after midstance until reaching their maximum extension of about 60° at toe-off. The interphalangeal joints remain in neutral throughout the stance and swing phases of gait. As stance progresses, the body's weight is advanced forward on the foot (figure 12.14). At midstance it is located just behind the metatarsal heads, and at toe-off the weight is primarily over the first and second metatarsophalangeal joints.

Early Swing

Once toe-off occurs, the ankle begins a dorsiflexion movement until it reaches a neutral position. By the time of middle swing, the ankle and toes are in a neutral position.

Late Swing

The ankle and toes remain close to neutral throughout the remaining part of swing phase. The subtalar joint remains in pronation through the swing phase.

Total movement from plantar flexion to dorsiflexion in the sagittal plane is 30°. A great deal of motion in the lower extremities occurs during one stride. Figure 12.15 presents a summary of the joints' motions during ambulation. The motion is usually rapid, and some motions are difficult to detect visually without a video camera or similar device that can slow the motion so visual detection is possible. If visual recording devices are not available, it is useful to have the patient walk on a treadmill at a comfortable pace while you observe the gait from anterior, lateral, and posterior views. It is best to take an overall perspective first and notice any gross abnormalities in stride-length differences, stride width, and cadence. The next focus is on individual segments and any abnormalities in the patient's joint movements. These may include pelvic obliquity, premature heel-off or toe-off, knee position during various phases of gait, and calcaneal position during weight bearing. It makes little difference if your segmental observations begin proximally or distally, but whatever routine you select is best performed consistently in the same manner so you don't overlook any segment.

GAIT KINETICS

Movements that occur during ambulation are the result of forces acting on the body. These forces include primarily those produced by the muscles, ground reaction forces, gravity, and momentum.

The muscles function in gait to produce acceleration, deceleration, and stabilization. Acceleration is needed to propel the body or segment forward to produce motion. Acceleration is generally the result of the muscle's concentric activity. Deceleration is used to slow down momentum of the segment or body to produce a smooth and controlled motion during ambulation. Deceleration is most commonly produced by the eccentric activity of muscles. Muscles that act as stabilizers are used as guy wires to hold a segment stable during movement. Stabilization is frequently produced by isometric activity. Some muscles are used at some times during gait as accelerators and at other times as decelerators. Other muscles are used primarily for stabilization of the body or segment.

Obviously, not all muscles are being used all the time during gait. The cyclic activity of a muscle in gait allows for periods of rest for a muscle. The muscles used during gait perform brief periods of peak activity followed or preceded by less activity or

Normal Gait

	Stance 60%					Swing 40%		
	Heel strike	Foot flat	Midstance	Heel-off	Toe-off	Early swing	Midswing	Late swing
Trunk	Erect Neutral	Erect Neutral	Erect Neutral	Erect Neutral	Erect Neutral	Erect Neutral	Erect Neutral	Erect Neutral
Pelvis	Level Forward rotation	Level 5° forward rotation Upward lateral rotation	Level Neutral rotation	Level 5° posterior rotation Downward lateral rotation	Level Posterior rotation Downward lateral rotation	Level Posterior rotation moving forward Lateral position is down	Level Neutral lateral rotation moving up	Level 5° forward rotation
Hip	30° flexion Slight adduction Neutral rotation	30° flexion Slight adduction Slight rotation	Extends Slight adduction Slight internal rotation	10° hyper-extension Slight abduction	Neutral Extension Slight internal rotation	20° flexion External rotation	Flexing External rotation	30° flexion Mild external rotation going to internal rotation
Knee	Full extension Tibia in external rotation	15° flexion Tibia in internal rotation	Moves toward extension	Full extension	35° flexion	Cont. to 60° flexion Tibial external rotation	Begin to move to 30° flexion Tibial external rotation	Cont. to extend
Ankle	Neutral	15° plantar flexion Pronation	10° dorsi-flexion Starts to supinate	Moving into plantar flexion Supinating	20° plantar flexion	Moving to neutral	Neutral	Neutral
Toes	Neutral	Neutral	Neutral	MTP: 30° extension IP: Neutral	MTP: 60° extension IP: Neutral	Neutral	Neutral	Neutral

(continued)

❚ **Figure 12.15** Summary of kinetics and kinematics for the hip, knee, and ankle in the sagittal plane through the gait cycle. Movement is a smoothly flowing change of range of motion in each joint throughout the gait cycle.

Hip

Initial contact/Heel strike	Loading response/Foot flat	Midstance/Single-leg support	Terminal stance/Heel-off	Preswing/Toe-off	Initial/Early swing	Midswing/Swing-through	Terminal/Late swing
0%	0–15%	15–40%	40–50%	50–60%	60–75%	75–85%	85–100%
ROM Flexion 30° neutral abduction, adduction rotation	30° flexion	Full extension	10° hyper-extension	Neutral extension	20° flexion	Flexion from 20° to 30°	30° flexion
Muscle activity Gluteus maximus, medius, tensor fascia lata, and hamstrings	Gluteus maximus, gluteus medius, tensor fascia lata, and hamstrings	Gluteus medius, tensor fascia lata	Hip flexors to prevent further extension	Hip flexors to initiate swing	Hip flexors	Hip flexors	Hamstrings to decelerate hip

Knee

Initial contact/Heel strike	Loading response/Foot flat	Midstance/Single-leg support	Terminal stance/Heel-off	Preswing/Toe-off	Initial/Early swing	Midswing/Swing-through	Terminal/Late swing
0%	0–15%	15–40%	40–50%	50–60%	60–75%	75–85%	85–100%
ROM Full extension	15° flexion	Moving toward full extension	Full extension	35° flexion	60° flexion	From 60° to 30° flexion	Extension to 0°
Muscle activity Quadriceps	Highest point of quadriceps activity Hamstrings active as hip extensors	Quadriceps first half of midstance Once knee is extended, quadriceps silent	None	None	Short head of biceps, sartorius, gracilis	None	Quadriceps and hamstrings decelerate the lower extremity

Ankle

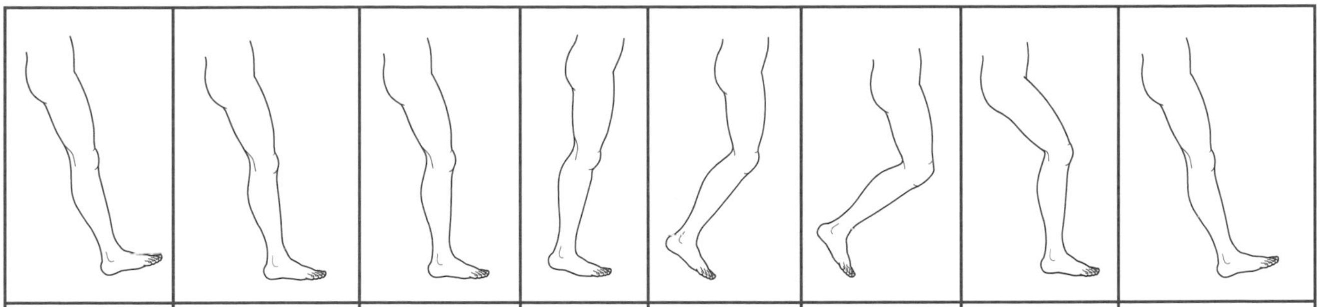

Initial contact/ Heel strike	Loading response/ Foot flat	Midstance/ Single-leg support	Terminal stance/ Heel-off	Preswing/ Toe-off	Initial/ Early swing	Midswing/ Swing-through	Terminal/ Late swing
0%	0–15%	15–40%	40–50%	50–60%	60–75%	75–85%	85–100%
ROM Neutral	15° plantar flexion	Neutral to 10° dorsi-flexion	Heel-off Prior to heel contact, opposite foot Moving into plantar flexion	20° plantar flexion	10° plantar flexion moving to neutral	Neutral	Neutral
Muscle activity Dorsiflexors maintain neutral position	Dorsiflexors control amount of plantar flexion, prevent foot slap	Plantar flexors control advance of tibia	Plantar flexors control tibia, restrict dorsiflexion	Dorsiflexors begin activity	Dorsiflexors active for toe clearance	Dorsiflexors maintain neutral position	Dorsiflexors maintain neutral position

Figure 12.15   *(continued)*

periods of rest give the muscle enough recovery time so that an activity such as walking can continue for extended durations if necessary. Because walking is the means by which we move our body from one location to another, it matters quite a bit that locomotion does not require continuous muscle activity.

The greatest energy requirement of muscles is present during the stance phase; less energy is required during the swing phase. The times of the greatest amount of muscle activity are in the first 10% of the stance phase and the last 10% of the swing phase. Periods of relative inactivity occur during midstance and the swing phase. The times of greatest muscle activity are during periods of acceleration and deceleration. The swing phase is a relatively quiet time in relation to muscle activity because the momentum produced during the final stages of stance carries the leg forward. As the muscles prepare the leg for heel strike during the final stages of swing, their activity increases.

Let's take a brief look at the specific muscles that produce ambulation. Once you know what muscles are important for gait, it becomes easier to establish corrective gait-training and therapeutic exercises for gait deficiencies after an athletic injury.

An easy way to look at muscles for gait is to divide them into categories according to their function. These categories include shock absorbers, stabilizers, accelerators, and decelerators. Some categories overlap because, for example, shock absorption requires deceleration. It is helpful to further divide categories according to the various body segments the muscles influence. Refer to figure 12.16 for a summary of the muscle activity described in the following sections.

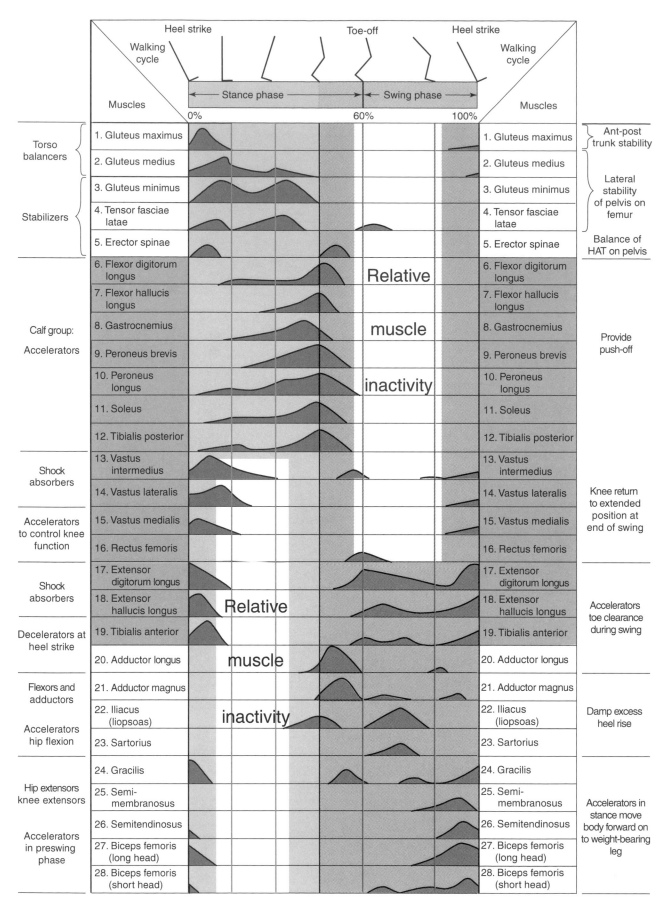

Figure 12.16 Muscle activity during gait.

*Peaks indicate periods of highest activity on each graph.

Adapted from Perry, J., *Gait analysis: Normal and pathological function,* 1992, with permission from SLACK Incorporated.

Shock Absorbers

During the first 15% of stance from heel strike to foot flat, the quadriceps are working as shock absorbers to reduce impact forces. They do this by eccentrically flexing the knee. At heel-strike impact, the foot extensors—also working eccentrically as shock absorbers—prevent the foot from slapping down onto the ground. The quadriceps group decelerate knee flexion and control the amount of knee flexion that occurs during the first 15% of the gait cycle. At the instant the heel makes contact with the floor, the foot dorsiflexors are at their peak output as they work to keep the forefoot off the floor; they then immediately act to control the lowering of the foot to the floor, functioning as a decelerator and shock absorber so that the movement is smooth.

Stabilizers

The hip extensors and torso muscles act as stabilizers to maintain the trunk in an erect position as the weight is transferred from one leg to the other, preventing excessive side tilting of the pelvis or trunk. The gluteus maximus stabilizes the spine to prevent a forward lean of the trunk during weight bearing and weight transfer from left to right; the gluteus medius, gluteus minimus, and tensor fascia lata stabilize the pelvis laterally on the femur; and the erector spinae muscles balance the head, arms, and trunk on the pelvis. These groups reach their peak levels of activity during the beginning and late stages of stance as the weight is transferred from one leg to the other. The tensor fascia lata also works during the early swing phase to stabilize the pelvis and prevent a lateral tilt.

Accelerators

Accelerators in the lower leg and thigh have peak outputs at various times during gait. The posterior calf accelerators have their peak activity during the end of stance phase as they accelerate the lower leg forward, providing for a push-off to produce an accelerated passive momentum of the leg during the swing phase. The posterior calf muscles begin activity during the middle portion of the weight-bearing phase as they provide control and balance during weight bearing. This is especially true of the lateral muscles, the ankle inverters and everters. Since the peroneals and tibialis posterior work through the majority of the weight-bearing phase, it is easy to appreciate how tendinitis may develop if their workload is increased because of poor foot mechanics as seen in an excessive pronator.

During swing, the foot and toe dorsiflexors are working to lift the foot and toes to clear the floor and prepare the foot for the right position at heel strike.

The thigh accelerators work primarily in the early and middle stages of swing to increase hip flexion to clear the foot from the ground. They also adduct the thigh to keep it close to the support leg and reduce the energy requirements for holding the trunk erect during single-leg stance on the other leg.

Decelerators

During swing phase, the hamstrings work as decelerators of the knee to slow the swing of the lower leg so that heel strike occurs smoothly. The hamstrings also act as accelerators in the very early portion of the stance phase to bring the body forward onto the weight-bearing leg.

Note that the shock-absorbing activity of the quadriceps group, mentioned earlier, is also categorized as a decelerating activity. Shock absorption is provided through the deceleration of the muscles. This is also true for the dorsiflexors during the early portion of the stance phase.

GROUND REACTION FORCES

Ground reaction forces are the forces exerted between the body and the ground during ambulation. Since the foot hits the ground at an angle, there is a combination of vector forces. One is a shearing force that is parallel to the ground, and the other is a vertical force that is perpendicular to the ground. The shear forces occur in fore-aft and lateral-medial directions. At heel strike the fore-aft shear force is a forward force, and during push-off it is a backward force. If you step on ice and lose your footing as your heel hits the ground, the forward force causes your leg to move forward. The reverse is true if you lose your footing during push-off; your foot moves backward.

Shortening stride length reduces fore-aft shear forces but increases vertical forces (figure 12.17). This is why it is safer to walk on ice with a shortened stride length: There is less forward force to slip the foot forward on heel strike and less backward force to slip the foot backward during push-off.

Fore-aft, or anteroposterior, forces are indicative of the deceleration forces that slow the body during heel strike and the acceleration forces that speed up the body before toe-off. The medial-lateral shear force is predominantly a medial shear force through heel strike; it moves to a lateral shear force as weight is transferred to the front of the foot. The medial-lateral shear forces are indicative of how the body weight is being transferred from side to side.

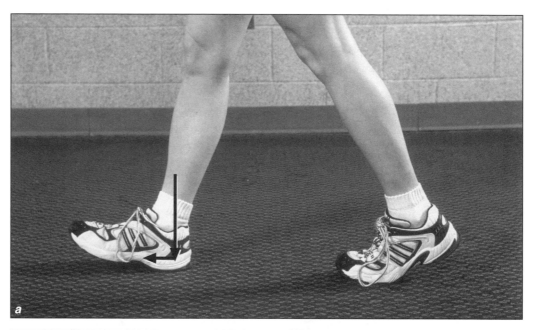

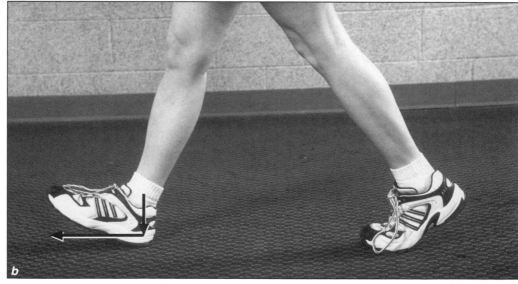

❙ Figure 12.17 Shortened stride reduces fore-aft shear force. *(a)* Shortened stride produces a greater perpendicular force vector than fore-aft force vector. *(b)* A longer stride produces a greater fore-aft force vector than perpendicular force vector.

Vertical forces applied to the foot during weight bearing are the effects of the body's weight. The amount of vertical force varies through the gait cycle and reflects shock absorption and deceleration during heel strike and acceleration as the body prepares to push off and move into the swing phase. The greatest vertical force occurs during push-off as the body is accelerating to propel itself forward and off the ground. Vertical forces are at minimal levels when the body weight is shared with the other lower extremity during double-limb support (figure 12.18).

Awareness of ground reaction forces is important in assessment of gait and athletic injury. Some of the greatest forces applied to the foot occur during acceleration. This can be crucial information when you are treating a patient who is a runner or a jumper or who participates in any sport in which ground reaction forces impact performance. For example, a pitcher who is experiencing first metatarsophalangeal joint pain will have difficulty during ball release and will require treatment of the toe, since ground reaction forces applied to the painful joint significantly impact the follow-through.

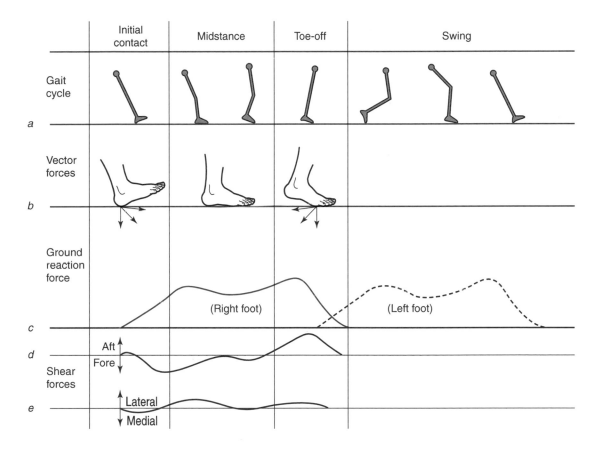

∎ Figure 12.18 Ground reaction forces in walking.

Adapted, by permission, from D.E. Klopsteg and P.D. Wilson, 1954, *Human limbs and their substitutes* (New York: McGraw-Hill). Courtesy of the National Academy of Sciences, Washington, DC.

PATHOLOGICAL GAIT

Pathological gait is a reflection of injury, weakness, loss of flexibility, pain, or bad habits. As with normal gait, observation of pathological gait begins with an overview assessment and proceeds with segmental assessment.

When a segment does not move as it should during ambulation because of injury, weakness, loss of flexibility, pain, or bad habit, a pathological gait results. The body attempts to continue to ambulate, but it must make adjustments to accommodate for the loss of normal function. This places stress on other segments and promotes weakness, and if the situation continues it can cause additional injury. Here we consider a few typical pathological gaits that result from athletic injuries.

When assessing gait, you should have the patient walk while you observe the entire body's movements. First, gain an overview and note any obvious abnormalities that would indicate the need for a more detailed assessment of any area. Part of the overview assessment includes observation of stride length, stride width, cadence, trunk lean, and arm swing. The arms normally swing in time with the opposite lower extremity. An unequal arm swing may indicate either a leg-length discrepancy or tissue shortening on one side. After this, the observation proceeds either from proximal segments down or from distal segments up. Head position, shoulder position, shoulder movement relative to pelvis movement, knee alignment, and foot and heel positions during stance are evaluated from anterior and posterior views. Side-view assessment includes observations of knee position at heel strike, midstance, and heel-off; head, trunk, and hip alignment; swing-through motion of the lower extremity; arm swing; pelvis motion; and timing of heel strike, heel-off, and toe-off. You should evaluate any observed segmental deviation for possible causes. Following are some common gait deviations seen in athletic injuries.

GLUTEUS MEDIUS GAIT

If an athlete sustains an injury that necessitates prolonged non-weight bearing on an extremity, or if he or she directly injures the hip, the gluteus medius can become weak. Once the patient resumes full weight bearing, the gluteus medius is too weak to maintain a level pelvis during single-leg stance. What is typically seen is a drop of the pelvis on the uninvolved side, from heel strike on the involved side through to heel strike on the uninvolved side. This is referred to as a **Trendelenburg, or gluteus medius, gait.** Sometimes the patient swings the opposite shoulder and trunk forward while standing on the uninvolved leg.

When the gluteus medius is weak, the pelvis drops on the opposite, non-weight-bearing side because it does not have the muscular support it needs for stability. To compensate for this, a patient may move the trunk laterally over the weak hip. This forces the erector spinae and quadratus lumborum of the opposite side to contract and lift the pelvis.

QUADRICEPS GAIT

Surgery or severe injury to the knee or quadriceps can leave the quadriceps very weak and unable to function properly during ambulation. Even after strengthening the quadriceps, the patient can continue to ambulate with a pathological gait because of bad habits established during ambulation when the muscle was too weak to be used properly. With a quadriceps gait, the patient keeps the knee extended at heel strike and through the stance phase. If the quadriceps is very weak, a lurch immediately after heel strike will occur as the individual forces the femur backward and the hip forward to passively lock the knee. The hip extensors then stabilize the knee to keep it locked after heel strike.

ANKLE TIGHTNESS

If an athlete sustains an ankle sprain and subsequently suffers a reduced range of motion in dorsiflexion, a pathological gait develops. During midstance when the ankle should move suddenly from plantar flexion to dorsiflexion, the person lurches forward over the foot, experiences increased knee extension, and moves quickly toward heel-off in an attempt to shorten the time requirement for dorsiflexion. There may be a rapid movement from heel strike to foot flat if the ankle does not have dorsiflexion to 0°, and the patient may either hike the involved hip upward or increase knee flexion in an attempt to clear the toes from the floor during the swing phase.

PAINFUL KNEE

When an athlete incurs an injury and ambulates with pain, you can observe a typical, obvious pathological gait. The patient attempts to reduce the time spent on the painful extremity and minimize the stresses placed on it during gait. The stride is shortened and asymmetrical; heel strike is replaced by direct movement to foot flat or initial contact on the distal foot to minimize impact stress; knee flexion during midstance is usually exaggerated if the knee has increased edema; and the knee motion is minimized during the swing phase. To compensate for the lack of motion during the swing phase the patient either hikes the hip up, goes on the toes during midstance of the uninvolved leg, or uses a circumduction swing, all in an attempt to clear the foot from the floor.

NORMAL RUNNING GAIT

Running gait differs from walking gait in several major ways—stride length and rate, joint motions, ground reaction forces, and kinetics.

Running and walking differ, just as running differs at different speeds. Running differs from walking in that the stance phase is shortened, the swing phase is lengthened, there is no time of double support, and there is a nonsupport phase in which neither leg is weight bearing. The nonsupport phase in a running stride, also referred to as the **double float** phase, occurs during the early-portion initial swing of one leg and the end of terminal swing for the other leg (figure 12.19). Since gait characteristics also change with a change in running speed, categories of running must be defined.

A variety of factors affect running mechanics, including speed, age, somatotype, fatigue, surface, footwear, and skill level. Researchers who compare running speeds vary considerably in their categorizations. In one study, for example, slow runners are defined as those who run 4 m/s (4.4 yd/s), or are able to run a mile in 6:42 (6 min, 42 s). A fast runner is defined as one who runs 8 m/s (8.7 yd/s) or 91 m (100 yd) in

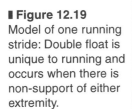

■ Figure 12.19
Model of one running stride: Double float is unique to running and occurs when there is non-support of either extremity.

Adapted from Ounpuu 1994.

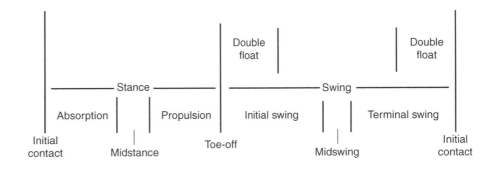

11.4 s. A sprinter is able to run 10 m/s or 100 yd in 9.1 s (Dillman 1975). In another study, a runner is defined as someone moving at 19.3 kph (12 mph; slightly less than a 5-min mile), and a sprinter is one who is able to run 27.6 kph (17.1 mph; 109 m in 12.2 s) (Mann and Hagy 1980). Whereas the average walking speed is approximately 1.4 m/s (1.5 yd/s), ranges in running speeds vary from 2 to 5.5 times the speed of walking (Perry 1990). These variations make analysis and comparison of results difficult at best.

In most instances, terminology used for walking is the same as for running. A few additional terms are used for running, however. Step length is defined in the same way as stride length: the distance from heel strike of one foot to the next heel strike of the same foot. Because runners do not always impact the ground at the heel, initial contact is called foot strike rather than heel strike. Cycle time, or stride time, is the amount of time it takes to perform one step length. Stride rate is the inverse of stride time. As mentioned previously, the nonsupport phase is the time when there is no weight bearing. The stance phase is sometimes referred to as the support phase for consistency with the term "nonsupport phase."

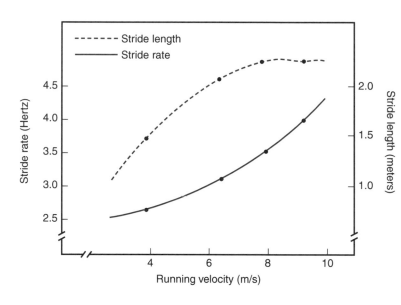

STRIDE LENGTH AND STRIDE RATE

Although researchers differ in their definitions of running speeds, the information available on running yields several basic observations. Stride length and cadence increase with an increase in velocity. Cycle time decreases with an increase in speed. After about 7 m/s (7.6 yd/s), stride length does not increase remarkably, but stride rate does (figure 12.20).

▌Figure 12.20   Stride length and running speed.

Adapted, by permission, from K.R. Williams, 1985, "The biomechanics of running." In *Exercise and sport sciences reviews,* vol. 13, edited by R.L. Terjung (Baltimore: Williams & Wilkins), 389–441. Copyright 1985 by W.B. Saunders Company.

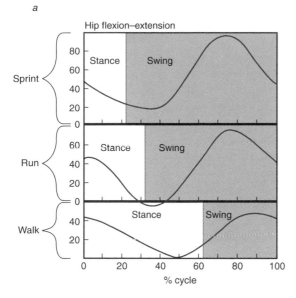

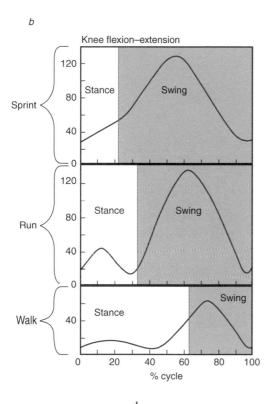

JOINT MOTIONS

Generally, as speed increases, the body tends to move its center of gravity lower by increasing the degree of hip flexion, knee flexion, and ankle dorsiflexion during the early stages of the stance phase.

The thigh increases its flexion prior to heel strike with increases in speed, but thigh position changes little with speed variations during weight bearing. Overall, hip motion increases as speed increases (figure 12.21).

The knee motion changes with changes in speed. There are greater degrees of knee flexion and there is less extension with greater speeds. During sprinting, the knee does not extend; it continues through the gait cycle in varying degrees of flexion. Some evidence indicates that at higher speeds the trend is toward extension at toe-off, although full extension is not achieved (Williams 1985). During the swing phase, knee flexion has been recorded at more than 120° (Williams 1985). Increased knee flexion provides for additional shock absorption, but it also requires greater quadriceps output. This topic is discussed later in the section "Kinetics."

Ankle plantar flexion at toe-off has been recorded in ranges between 59° and 75° (Williams 1985). Which part of the foot makes initial contact with the ground depends on the angles of the hip, knee, and ankle. Runners most often land on the midfoot. As a general rule, faster runners tend to land at the midfoot, and slower runners land at the rearfoot (Williams 1985).

Although an erect trunk is thought to be the best position for running form, most reports indicate that runners use a forward trunk lean throughout the running cycle (Williams 1985). The amount of trunk lean increases from 4° to 7° in runners at speeds up to 7 m/s (7.7 yd/s) and to 11.6° in sprinters running at 9.2 m/s (10.06 yd/s).

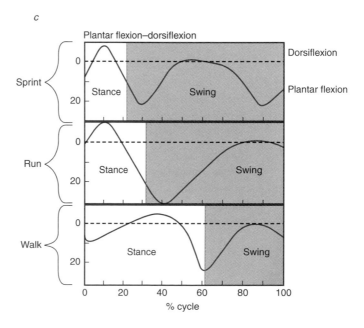

▌Figure 12.21
Range of motion during running. As locomotion speed increases, the swing phase (nonsupport phase) time increases and joint range of motion changes.

Adapted from Mann and Hagy 1980.

GROUND REACTION FORCES

As speeds increase, ground reaction forces also increase. In running and walking, ground reaction forces reach two peaks. The first is at impact during initial contact. This peak, which occurs very quickly with running impact, is referred to as the impact peak. The second peak occurs during the last half of support and is referred to as an action peak because of the muscles' influences on it during the acceleration prior to toe-off (figure 12.22).

Vertical impact forces encountered during running are mathematically combined with joint positions to determine joint moments. Joint moments are the stresses applied to the joints. During running, the knee encounters flexor moments 7.7 times greater than those encountered during walking. The hip and ankle flexion demands during running are double those during walking (Perry 1990).

Body weight, surfaces, shoes, speed, and where on the foot the runner lands all influence the impact peak forces. Softer surfaces can eliminate the impact peak. A good running shoe has a lower impact peak than a poorly constructed shoe. Runners who land on the midfoot or forefoot have a significantly reduced impact peak compared to those landing on the rearfoot; and rearfoot landers have a single peak whereas midfoot landers generally have a biphasic peak impact. Faster runners have greater ground reaction forces than slower runners.

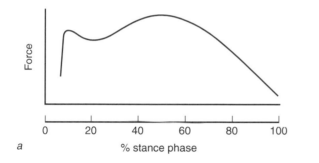
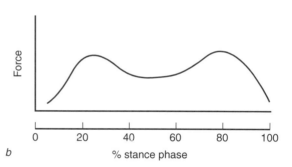

▌Figure 12.22 The impact ground reaction force in running occurs very quickly. (*a*) Running, (*b*) walking.

Adapted from Ounpuu 1994.

KINETICS

Specific activity varies greatly, depending on running speeds and on the investigation, but a general conclusion is that muscle activity increases with increased running speeds, as seen in figure 12.23.

Hip

There is an increase in hamstring activity from heel strike and throughout stance as the hamstring assists concentrically in hip extension. The semimembranosus particularly is at an advantage for providing hip extensor force since it is 1.4 times larger than the biceps femoris (Perry 1990). The hamstrings also play a concentric and stabilizing role during trunk lean. The rectus femoris too is more active at foot strike, but this activity diminishes by the end of support. The rectus femoris is also active during hip flexion in the early swing phase. The hamstrings and hip extensors in the late-swing leg act eccentrically to slow hip flexion and prepare the leg for the support phase.

a

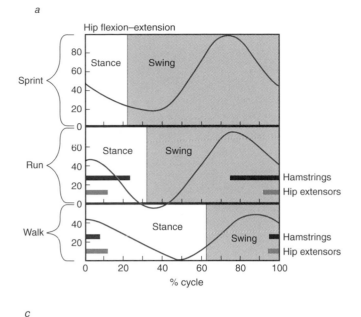

b

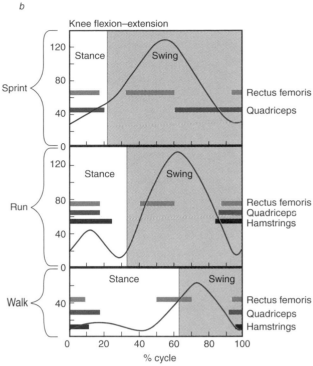

c

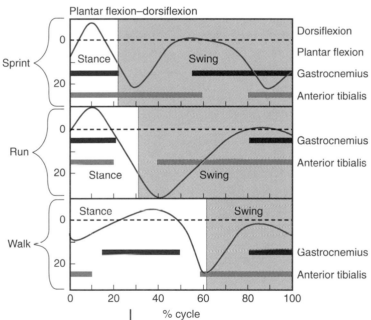

■ **Figure 12.23**
Muscle activity with range of motion during walk, run, and sprint.

Adapted from Mann and Hagy 1980.

Knee

The quadriceps, especially the vastus lateralis and vastus medialis, are extremely active at foot strike; they continue to be active along with the rectus femoris during the early portion of support. High demands are placed on the quadriceps muscles during most of the stance phase. Their activity diminishes as the leg continues to the end of support, but increases again just prior to foot strike in preparation for its impact-loading response. As running speeds increase, the amount of time the quadriceps are active in both the stance and swing phases increases.

The hamstrings begin their aggressive activity to prepare the knee in the last half of swing phase for landing in stance phase. The hamstrings continue their activity halfway through stance and may be an active restraint against anterior tibial shear. During the last half of stance the hamstrings and quadriceps are in co-contraction, presumably for additional knee support.

Ankle

At foot strike the tibialis anterior and triceps surae group co-contract to stabilize the foot at impact. The contraction of the posterior muscle group through most of the stance phase may provide tibial stability for improved quadriceps function. If the runner's foot strike is at the heel, the tibialis anterior immediately eccentrically contracts to control foot pronation. The triceps surae concentrically contracts to provide thrust for propulsion of the body into the nonsupport phase. This is especially true for faster speeds (Williams 1985).

MECHANICS OF AMBULATION WITH ASSISTIVE DEVICES

The sport rehabilitation specialist should understand several issues regarding the use of assistive devices for ambulation. These include proper fitting, correct gait patterns, proper use on various types of surfaces, and safety instructions and precautions.

Now that you have an understanding of normal gait mechanics, you will more easily appreciate the intricacies of ambulation with assistive devices. Assistive devices are used either to provide additional stability during ambulation or to reduce or eliminate weight bearing on a lower extremity. They can permit the patient to walk safely and unassisted by others. As a general rule, assistive devices are used during weight bearing if the patient is unable to walk normally. The purpose is to prevent the added stresses of abnormal gait from causing additional injury.

FITTING

Before a patient can use any assistive device, the device must be properly fitted to the individual's height. Axillary, or underarm, crutches are measured with the crutch tips flat on the ground and approximately 15 cm (6 in.) lateral to and 15 cm in front of the foot (figure 12.24). There should be a two- to three-finger space between the top of the axillary pad and the patient's axilla. The handgrip should be at a level such that there is a 20° to 30° bend in the elbow with the crutch at the correct length as the patient stands with the crutches 15 cm laterally and 15 cm anterior to the feet.

Forearm crutches are adjusted so that the handgrip is at the level of the greater trochanter and the forearm cuff is just distal to the elbow. This should provide for about a 30° elbow bend during weight bearing. Cane measurements are made with the arm in a relaxed resting position at the side and the cane next to the leg. The top of the cane handle should be at wrist level.

GAIT PATTERNS

A basic concept in the use of assistive devices is to keep the center of balance within the base of support. A person is more stable with the use of assistive devices because the base of support is increased (figure 12.25). Gait patterns are generally designated according to the number of support points in contact with the floor. These contacts include the assistive devices and the feet.

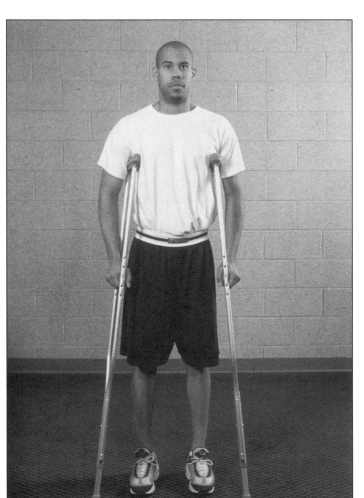

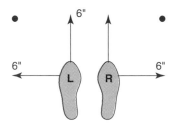

b

■ **Figure 12.24**   With the crutches 15 cm (6 in.) lateral and anterior to the feet, and the shoulders relaxed, proper crutch height should allow two to three fingers between the axilla and axillary pad. Elbows should be flexed 20° to 30°.

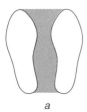

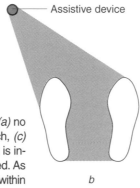

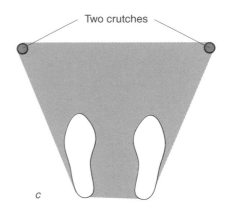

Assistive device

Two crutches

■ Figure 12.25 Base of support with *(a)* no assistive devices, *(b)* one cane or crutch, *(c)* two crutches. The base of support area is increased when assistive devices are used. As long as the patient's center of gravity falls within the base of support, the patient is stable.

a

b

c

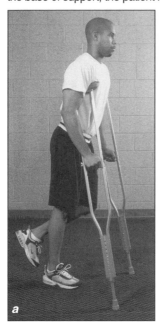

a

Three-Point Gait

A three-point gait is so termed because there are three points of contact with the floor—two made by the assistive device and one made by the foot. This gait is used when the patient is unable to bear weight on one extremity. It is also called a right (or left) non-weight-bearing gait. In young, healthy athletes who have been injured, underarm crutches are the most frequently used assistive devices. Forearm crutches or a walker can also be used in a three-point gait.

In a three-point gait, while remaining non-weight bearing on one leg, the patient advances the crutches simultaneously in front of the body along with the non-weight-bearing leg; he or she then bears weight on the crutch handles and lifts the weight-bearing leg to move it either to or in front of the crutches (figure 12.26).

A gait in which the individual swings the weight-bearing leg to the crutches is called a swing-to gait. If the weight-bearing leg is advanced far enough to land in front of the crutches, the gait is a swing-through gait. The swing-through gait requires more balance and confidence than the swing-to gait does. A patient who is hesitant about using the crutches uses a swing-to gait initially; as the individual gains confidence and it is safe to do so, he or she advances to a swing-through gait. The swing-through gait is faster than the swing-to gait, but requires more balance and control.

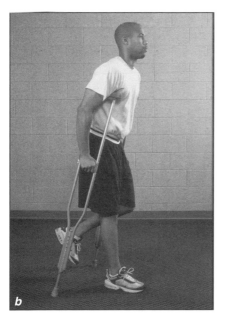

Swing-to

b

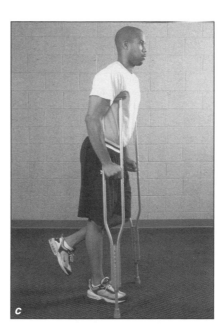

Swing-through

c

■ Figure 12.26 In a three-point gait, the patient places the crutches in front of the body *(a)* and advances the weight-bearing leg either to the crutches *(b)* or in front of the crutches *(c)*. Weight is borne entirely by the hands during the swing-to or swing-through phase of this gait.

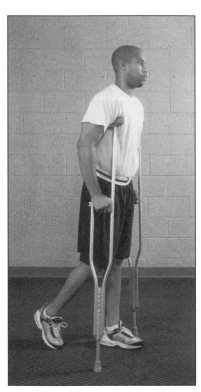

Four-Point Gait

A four-point gait is used when partial weight bearing is allowed on the involved extremity. The injured leg continues to move with the crutches, but some body weight is placed on the injured extremity. The amount of weight permitted is dictated by the patient's pain or the physician. In this gait, the crutches and involved leg advance simultaneously. Partial body weight is placed on the extremity, and the remaining weight is placed on the hands (figure 12.27). The uninvolved leg is then advanced forward in a normal stride, passing the opposite leg as it swings through.

A modification of the four-point gait is seen in nonathletes who use crutches for assistance with bilateral lower-extremity involvement. This involves using one crutch with each lower extremity. The most stable method, although the slowest, is advancing the left crutch with the right leg and the right crutch with the left leg. This type of four-point gait is not common in the athletic population when only one extremity is involved.

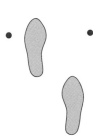

■ **Figure 12.27**   A four-point gait is used when partial weight bearing is permitted. The crutches are used with the involved extremity with partial weight on the crutches and partial weight on the lower extremity.

Single Support

When a single device, either a cane or a crutch, is used, it is placed in the hand on the side opposite to the leg injury. Single devices are used primarily for stability, not weight-bearing support, because only about 25% of the body's weight can be borne on a cane or on one crutch (Lehmann 1982).

Single support is essentially a second-class lever system. It is designed to be efficient, and minimal force from the upper extremity is required to produce the desired effect of support for the involved leg. The injured lower extremity's hip is the fulcrum from which the cane or crutch leverage is applied. The head, arms, and trunk (HAT) are the resistance force that are positioned between the fulcrum and the cane or crutch (figure 12.28). If the cane or crutch were placed in the hand on the same side as the injured leg, they would provide no assistance for weight distribution, and the patient would have to lurch over the outside of the involved leg to place the HAT weight between the cane and the injured leg.

In a single-support gait, the cane or crutch moves with the injured leg so that the two advance together. As the patient bears weight on the injured leg and advances the uninvolved leg forward, some weight is also applied to the single-support device. This gait is used when minimal support for balance is required or when the patient is able to bear weight on the extremity but displays an abnormal gait because of pain, loss of motion, or weakness.

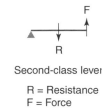

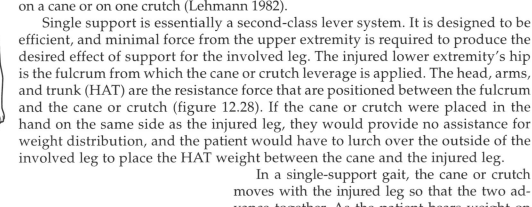

Key
1 = Lever-arm length of body weight
2 = Lever-arm length of cane support

Second-class lever

R = Resistance
F = Force

■ **Figure 12.28**   Ambulation with single support.

ASSISTIVE DEVICES ON VARIOUS SURFACES

The patient will be ambulating with assistive devices on varying surfaces such as stairs and ramps, so he or she needs to receive instruction before being allowed to use the assistive devices without supervision. Risk of injury and falling is significant until you have determined that the patient is safe.

Stairs

When ambulating where there is a railing, the patient should use it. A railing is more secure than crutches and will provide more safety going up and down stairs. If the person is using two crutches, both are placed in the same hand, the one away from the railing.

Stair climbing involves two basic concepts. One is that the uninvolved leg advances up the stairs first and the involved leg advances down the stairs first. This can be confusing, so you can use a simple reminder. "The good go up to heaven and the bad go down to hell," is a reminder that most patients find easy to recall.

The second concept is that the assistive device always goes with the involved leg. In other words, the crutches go on the same step as the injured extremity. For example, when descending stairs, the patient grasps the railing with one hand and holds both crutches in the opposite hand (figure 12.29a). The crutches advance down a step (figure 12.29b); then the involved extremity is lowered to the same step (figure 12.29c). The patient bears weight on the arms and involved leg, if weight bearing is permitted, and then lowers the uninvolved leg to the same step. For ascending steps the process is the reverse; the uninvolved leg is advanced first (figure 12.29d), and then the crutches and involved leg are raised to the same step.

If the stairs do not have a railing, the patient must use the crutches in both hands in lieu of a railing. This is less safe and requires more concentration, especially in the first few attempts; but navigation is feasible according to the same concepts as with a railing. Curbs are essentially stairs without railings and are managed the same way.

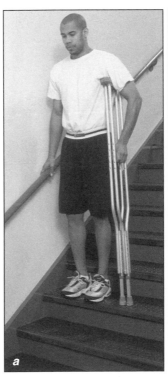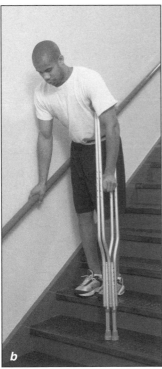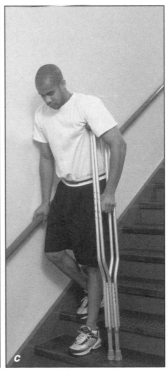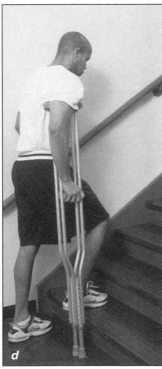

■ **Figure 12.29**   To ambulate on stairs with crutches: *(a)* Use the rail if one is present and place both crutches in one hand. *(b)* Advance the crutches to the lower step and move the rail hand to keep the hands even. *(c)* Lower the body to the step, bearing weight on the hands as the involved leg is lowered before the uninvolved leg. *(d)* When going up stairs, the uninvolved leg leads, and the crutches remain on the lower step with the involved leg until the uninvolved leg is secure on the higher step.

Ramps

Ramps may have varying degrees of incline, but the principle for ambulating on them with assistive devices is the same in any case. The most important concept on ramps is that, as with stairs, the crutches and involved leg are kept together. The other important concept is that the individual needs to take shorter steps going up and down for the sake of safety. The tendency is to take larger steps going down a ramp, but this can be dangerous and lead to falls. The patient should also remember to maintain an upright posture going down ramps since the natural pattern is to lean forward. This can lead to falling, but a reminder to take shorter steps can reduce this risk.

Transfers

Getting up and down from a chair when one is using assistive devices can be treacherous. Using the correct technique will ensure greater safety. If using crutches, the individual places both crutches in one hand, holding the handgrips with the hand, and places the crutches in a vertical position near the chair but in front of it and to its side. The other hand is placed on the arm of the chair or on the seat if there are no chair arms. The patient pushes from the crutch handgrips and chair simultaneously to gain assistance in standing. He or she then places a crutch under each arm before proceeding. This technique is used with two crutches, one crutch, or a cane.

SAFETY INSTRUCTIONS AND PRECAUTIONS

Walking with assistive devices can be energy consuming and poses a risk of falling, especially if the activity is performed incorrectly or with faulty equipment. Precautions should be taken at the outset to minimize these factors.

Equipment

Crutch tips, handgrips, and axillary pads should be inspected to make sure that they are not worn or damaged. Lack of tread on a crutch or cane tip can cause the assistive device to slip when weight is applied to it. Cracked or damaged handgrips and axillary pads can cause the pads to become loosened during use and put the patient at risk of falling.

If the crutches are adjusted with screws, the screws should be secured and in working order. Wing nuts should be firmly in place.

Environmental Factors

Throw rugs are among the environmental factors that pose a risk to people using assistive devices. The patient must take care not to trip when walking on rugs of this type. Removing them until the person is able to ambulate without the assistive device may be the safest thing to do.

Extra caution must be taken in rain, ice, or snow. A slippery surface increases the patient's risk for falling. Instructions to ambulate more slowly and use smaller steps should be given. If the crutches are advanced too far forward, the fore-aft shear force, discussed earlier, has a greater forward than downward component, causing the crutch to slip forward and putting the person at risk for falling.

To avoid someone's accidentally tripping over or kicking the assistive device, the patient should keep the crutches or cane to his or her side rather than in front, but not so far out as to present an obstacle for another person. An exaggerated outward position also places too much pressure on the patient's sides if axillary crutches are being used. The devices should be advanced far enough forward to provide for an economical gait but not so far as to endanger the patient's balance and increase the risk of falling.

Axillary Crutches

The patient should be instructed in proper use of axillary crutches. The purpose of the axillary pads is not to allow the patient to rest the axilla but rather to serve as a cushion against the lateral chest wall so that the crutches do not slip out from under the arms. Resting the axillas on these pads poses a risk of radial nerve damage from pressure on the nerve as it runs through the axilla. The patient's weight should be borne through the hands, not the axillae.

SUMMARY

1. *Discuss the general concepts of gait.*

   The gait cycle is divided into two phases, stance and swing. The stance phase is divided into initial contact, or heel strike; foot flat; midstance; heel-off, or terminal stance; and preswing, or toe-off. The swing phase is divided into initial, or early swing; midswing; and terminal swing. In normal walking, the stance phase constitutes about 60% of the gait cycle. Double support occurs during loading response and preswing.

2. *Identify the range-of-motion changes during the gait cycle.*

   At initial contact, the hip is at 30° flexion, the knee is at full extension, and the ankle is in neutral. By midstance the hip is extending, the knee has moved from 15° flexion toward extension, and the ankle has moved from 15° plantar flexion to 10° dorsiflexion. At toe-off the hip has moved from 10° extension to neutral, the knee is in 35° flexion, and the ankle is in 20° plantar flexion. During swing, the hip moves from 20° to 30° flexion, the knee moves into 60° flexion and progresses to full extension, and the ankle remains in neutral.

3. *Explain the muscle activity involved in ambulation.*

   Muscles are divided into groups: shock absorbers, accelerators, decelerators, and stabilizers. Muscles act in cyclic fashion, with the greatest activity occurring during early and late stance and early and late swing as muscles prepare to change activity.

4. *Describe the general mechanical differences between walking and running.*

   In running there is a double-float portion in the gait cycle during which the body is not supported by either lower extremity. The stance phase is divided into initial contact, midstance, and toe-off. The swing phase becomes longer than the stance phase, the stride length increases in a curvilinear fashion in relation to running speed, and ranges of motion for all joints increase with increased running speeds.

5. *Discuss one abnormal gait commonly seen following an athletic injury.*

   Prolonged knee extension is an example of a common gait following knee injury and subsequent quadriceps weakness. It occurs because the quadriceps lack control of the knee, and keeping the knee locked prevents the knee from buckling during weight bearing.

6. *Outline the various types of gait with assistive devices.*

   A three-point gait is used with two crutches when weight bearing on the involved extremity is prohibited. A swing-to or swing-through gait can be used with a three-point gait. A four-point gait is used when partial weight bearing on the involved extremity is permitted. The involved extremity is placed between two crutches; some weight is borne by the crutches and some by the extremity. When a cane or single crutch is used, it is placed in the hand opposite the involved extremity, and weight is simultaneously borne by the involved extremity and the cane.

7. *Explain the technique involved in stair climbing with assistive devices.*

When going up stairs, the patient places the uninvolved extremity on the upper stair, places weight on the crutches or the crutches and handrail, and hops up. Going down stairs, the individual places the involved extremity and crutches on the lower stair before lowering the uninvolved leg.

8. *Identify the safety measures involved in ambulating with assistive devices.*

The assistive device should be adjusted for proper fit; crutch tips, pads, and grips should be inspected for wear before use. Proper instruction in the use of assistive devices on various surfaces and in proper transfer techniques should be provided before the patient is permitted independent use. Instructions should cover use on slippery surfaces, avoiding axillary pressure with crutches, and proper weight bearing on the involved extremity. Scatter rugs should be removed from the patient's environment, and the person should receive instruction about keeping the assistive device close to the body to avoid tripping or falling.

CRITICAL THINKING QUESTIONS

1. If the patient you are treating has limited range of motion in dorsiflexion and plantar flexion, what kind of gait deviation would you expect to see? How would it alter the timing of the knee and ankle motions? Would the patient have normal knee motion during weight bearing? If not, why not? What possible substitutions might the patient use to compensate for the loss of ankle motion?

2. If a patient has weak quads, there will be full knee extension during midstance. Why will this occur? What must be done before normal knee flexion during midstance occurs?

3. If hip flexors are tight, what changes in gait will occur? What changes in pelvic rotation can occur? Will tight hip flexors cause an apparent short-leg syndrome? Why?

4. If the hip abductors are weak, what type of abnormal gait would you expect to see? Identify what can be used to correct this type of gait, and explain the mechanics of how the correction works.

5. You are developing a handout for instructions on gait with crutches. Assuming that the instructions will be for conditions that are non-weight bearing on one extremity, what instructions will you include? What precautions will you include? What surfaces will you deal with in your instructions?

6. Based on the chapter's opening scenario, what instructions should Tony give Mary Ann for ambulation with a cane? What precautions should he also include? What criteria should he use to determine when Mary Ann can begin running?

REFERENCES

Dillman, C.J. 1975. Kinematic analyses of running. In *Exercise and Sport Sciences Reviews*, ed. J.H. Wilmore and J.F. Keogh. New York: Academic Press.

Klopsteg, D.E. and P.D. Wilson. 1954. *Human limbs and their substitutes.* New York: McGraw-Hill.

Lehmann, J.F. 1982. Gait analysis: Diagnosis and management. In *Krusen's handbook of physical medicine and rehabilitation,* ed. F.J. Kottke, G.K. Stillwell, and J.F. Lehmann. Philadelphia: Saunders.

Mann, R.A., and J. Hagy. 1980. Biomechanics of walking, running, and sprinting. *American Journal of Sports Medicine* 8:345–350.

Murray, M.P., Drought, A.B., and R.C. Kory. 1964. Walking patterns of normal men. *Journal of Bone and Joint Surgery* 46-A:335–360.

Ounpuu, S. 1994. The biomechanics of walking and running. *Clinics in Sports Medicine* 13:843–862.

Perry, J. 1990. Gait analysis in sports medicine. *Instructional Course Lectures* 39:319–324.

Rodgers, M.M. 1988. Dynamic biomechanics of the normal foot and ankle during walking and running. *Physical Therapy* 68:1822–1830.

Williams, K.R. 1985. The biomechanics of running. In *Exercise and Sport Sciences Reviews,* ed. R.L. Terjung, 13:389–441.

Winter, D.A. 1987. *The biomechanics and motor control of human gait.* Waterloo, ON, Canada: University of Waterloo Press.

CHAPTER THIRTEEN

Aquatic Therapeutic Exercise

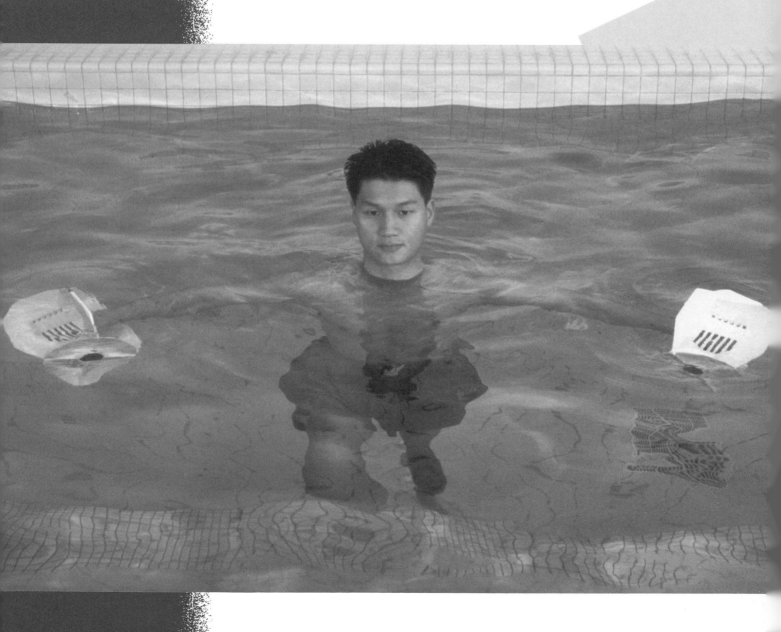

OBJECTIVES

After completing this chapter, you should be able to do the following:

1. Identify and discuss the physical properties of water that affect the ability to exercise in water.

2. Define and explain the difference between assistive and resistive aquatic equipment and give examples of each.

3. List precautions and contraindications for aquatic exercise.

4. Identify three advantages of aquatic therapeutic exercise.

5. List three aquatic exercises for each body segment and identify their purposes.

Before Amanda Decker became a certified athletic trainer she had been a swimming instructor at the local beaches during the summer. She was well aware of the physical properties of water and of ways it can be used to either assist a body in water or resist it. In her current job as aquatic rehabilitation specialist at the city's largest sports medicine facility, she felt her position was a perfect match for her since it combined her sports medicine knowledge with her love for the water.

Amanda's patients had various kinds of injuries and were at different levels within their rehabilitation programs. Amanda enjoyed this situation because it allowed her to make use of the various pieces of exercise equipment and the various water properties. With some patients she used the water to eliminate weight bearing for ease of lower-extremity activities. With others she used the water to resist movement in strengthening activities. Still other people were in the water to stress their cardiovascular systems. Some weight-bearing patients were in shallow water so that they would encounter greater weight-bearing forces, while others were in the deeper end for activities that were less weight bearing. Some patients could use water dumbbells for resistance activities, whereas others were challenged simply by the water's drag and viscosity. Several of the patients were just beginning their rehabilitation work and using the water to gain motion, while others were in the final phases, letting the water provide them with an aggressive program of activities.

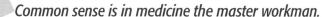

Common sense is in medicine the master workman.

Peter Mere Latham, 1789–1875,
General Remarks on the Practice of Medicine

Common sense in the application of knowledge is what makes a skillful clinician. It also is a key to good judgment. Decisions about what therapeutic exercises to apply, when to use them, and how best to deliver them are based on a healthy mixture of knowledge and common sense.

This chapter includes information that you will apply in a systematic, appropriate manner on the basis of your newly gained knowledge of exercise and your common sense. General concepts and principles of aquatic exercise are introduced first. On this foundation, examples of exercises for the trunk, lower extremities, and upper extremities are then presented.

Water-based treatment has been in existence for a long time. The ancient Greeks and Romans used water therapeutically. The development of whirlpools and Hubbard tanks promoted the use of water in the early 1900s. Recently there has been a resurgence of interest in aquatic therapy, emphasizing its use in exercise rather than its more traditional effects. This chapter addresses the therapeutic exercise use of aquatic therapy rather than its use as a thermal modality.

For additional information on aquatic modalities, refer to *Therapeutic Modalities for Athletic Injuries* by Craig Denegar (2000).

Aquatic therapeutic exercise is the application of therapeutic exercise that takes place in water. Exercise in water is advantageous when the patient is unable to perform land-based exercises, allowing the individual to begin exercises sooner than would otherwise be possible. It also provides a means of exercise while the patient is non-weight bearing on an injured lower extremity. Aquatic therapeutic exercise (aquatic therex) can offer the patient a total exercise program that includes activities for cardiovascular conditioning, flexibility, strength, and muscle endurance. It can be instituted early in a rehabilitation program and can continue past the time when the patient is able to perform land-based exercises.

PHYSICAL PROPERTIES AND PRINCIPLES OF WATER

Several major physical properties of water, including specific gravity, buoyancy, center of buoyancy, and hydro-dynamics, affect the way people exercise in water.

An understanding of how water affects the body's ability to move and exercise is necessary before one can apply water exercises. Although some of these properties can be specifically determined by formulas, we will not focus on the precise mathematical applications here. It is important only to appreciate that one can acquire an understanding of the impact of these properties on the body exercising in water by gaining a thorough knowledge of these mathematical formulas.

SPECIFIC GRAVITY

Specific gravity is also called **relative density**. It refers to the density of an object relative to that of water. It is, then, a ratio of an object's weight to the weight of an equal volume of water. The specific gravity of water is 1. If an object has a specific gravity greater than 1, it will sink in water since its relative weight per volume is more than that of water. If an object has a specific gravity of less than 1, it will float in water. If the object's specific gravity is 1, it will float just below the water's surface.

Specific gravity for the human body varies from one individual to another and can also vary from one body segment to another within the same individual. The individual's specific gravity depends on the body's composition of lean and fat mass and the distribution of body fat. The specific gravity of fat is 0.8, that of bone is 1.5 to 2.0, and that of lean muscle is 1.0 (Hay 1978). The average range of specific gravity for the human body is 0.95 to 0.97 (Davis and Harrison 1988). Since the specific gravity of the average human body is less than 1, people will most often float. As a general rule, women have more body fat than men, so women float better than men. A lean, muscular person may have a specific gravity of 1.10; an obese individual may have a specific gravity of 0.93 (Edlich et al. 1987). These wide variations in individual specific gravities lead to a wide range of abilities to float. Patients who are more muscular and have less fat mass may have a difficult time floating and may require flotation devices during aquatic therex.

BUOYANCY

Archimedes' principle of buoyancy states that a body partially or fully immersed in a fluid will experience an upward thrust of that fluid that is equal to the weight of the fluid the body displaces. Buoyancy and specific gravity are closely related in that a body with a specific gravity of less than 1 will float because the weight of the water it displaces is less than the weight of the full body. For example, if a person has a specific gravity of 0.95, 95% of the body will be submerged and 5% of the body will float above the water's surface. The amount of water displaced is 95% of the body weight. Specific-gravity values, in essence, indicate the amount of the body that floats and the amount that is submerged; and the weight of the body or part of the body submerged is equal to the weight of the water it displaces.

CENTER OF BUOYANCY

Center of buoyancy is the center of gravity of the displaced fluid and the point at which the buoyant force acts on the body. In water, two opposing forces act on the body. Buoyancy is the upward force, and gravity is the downward force. Each has a center point of balance. When a floating body is in equilibrium, the center of buoyancy and the center of gravity are in vertical alignment with each other (figure 13.1).

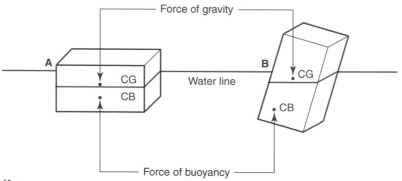

Key
CG = Center of gravity
CB = Center of buoyancy
  A = Body in equilibrium with CB and CG in vertical alignment
  B = Body out of equilibrium with CB and CG out of alignment

■ **Figure 13.1**   When the center of bouyancy and the center of balance are not in vertical alignment, a person must actively work to keep from rolling in the water.

Reprinted from Bates and Hanson 1996.

In this position, the body is balanced. If the center of buoyancy and the center of gravity are not in a vertical relationship to each other, the body is out of equilibrium and will tend to roll or turn. For example, if you place a kickboard between your knees, the center of buoyancy will cause your lower extremities to float upward.

HYDRODYNAMICS

Movement through water is governed by the fluid's resistance to movement, the size and shape of the object moving, and the speed of the object. Some of the factors that impact a body's movement through fluid are interrelated.

Viscosity

Viscosity is the resistance to movement within a fluid that is caused by the friction of the fluid's molecules. Additional factors include physical properties such as cohesion (the attraction of water molecules to adjacent water molecules), adhesion (the attraction of water molecules to the individual's body), and surface tension (the attraction of water molecules on the surface to each other). Movement within the water is resisted by the adhesion and cohesion of water molecules to the person in the water and to other water molecules, respectively. Surface tension provides a resistance when an individual attempts to break the water's surface with the body or a body segment.

Drag

Drag is the water's resistance to a body that is moving through it. There are three types of drag: form drag, wave drag, and frictional drag (Koury 1996).

Form Drag

Form drag is the resistance that an object encounters in a fluid and is determined by the object's size and shape. A larger object has more drag than a smaller object. A broad-shaped object has more drag than a streamlined object. Form drag is directly related to turbulence. The greater the form drag, the greater the turbulence. Turbulence causes an area of low-pressure behind the object that tends to pull the object backward (figure 13.2).

A streamlined object moving through water produces a laminar flow—a smooth movement of water that causes a minimal amount of resistance to movement. There is less form drag because of less turbulence. The water molecules all travel at the same speed past the body. Friction of the fluid is minimal because the water molecules separate easily, moving smoothly behind the object.

On the other hand, a broad-shaped object produces a turbulent flow as it moves through the water. The object has more form drag because of the greater turbulence created behind it. The layers of the water move irregularly as they run into the object and rush to move past and behind it. This causes a circular movement of the water layers as they rejoin behind the

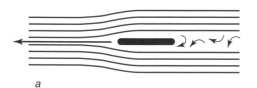

a

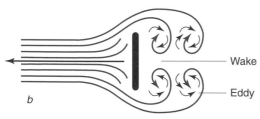

b

— Wake

— Eddy

■ **Figure 13.2**   Form drag: *(a)* laminar flow *(b)* turbulent flow. Form drag is caused by turbulence behind an object moving through a fluid.

Reprinted from Bates and Hanson 1996.

object. This circular motion of water layers pulling against the moving object is called an **eddy**. As a consequence of the disturbance caused by the eddy, a wake or trail is left in the water (seen as either bubbles behind the body or white water, depending on the amount of turbulence created).

Form drag can be used in an aquatic therex program as a means of altering resistance to exercises. A change in the position of the body or body segment can increase or decrease form drag. For example, moving the arm horizontally in the water with the palm down causes less form drag than with the hand in a vertical position. Shortening or lengthening the body's extremity decreases or increases the form drag, respectively, since the longer lever arm pushes more water than a shorter one. Adding equipment such as hand paddles increases the surface area of the hand, and other equipment such as long paddles increases the lever-arm length; both provide additional form drag to increase the resistance of an exercise.

Wave Drag

Wave drag is the water's resistance as a result of turbulence. The greater the speed of an object, the greater the wave drag. Wave drag is reduced if movement remains under water. The amount of water wake is an indication of wave drag. Swimming pools often have a splash gutter around the periphery to reduce wave drag for swimmers.

Exercises performed in calm water produce less resistance than those performed in turbulent water. The individual can create wave drag during an exercise by changing positions frequently and rapidly. Increasing the speed of an exercise also increases the wave drag that the exercise causes. For example, walking in water provides the body with 5 to 6 times the resistance that walking in air does. Running water, however, increases the resistance to more than 40 times that of air (McWaters 1988).

Frictional Drag

Frictional drag is the result of water's surface tension. This is not a factor in therapeutic exercise, but it becomes an important element for the competitive swimmer. Frictional drag can add crucial milliseconds to a race time, and swimmers can reduce it by shaving body hair before competition. Recently, custom-made bodysuits constructed from unique, new fibers have been designed to reduce frictional drag.

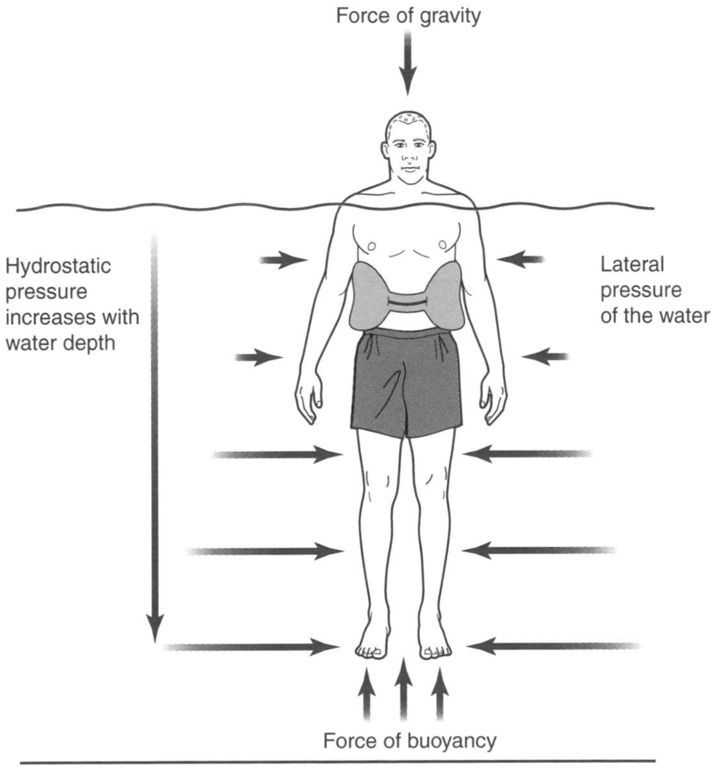

HYDROSTATIC PRESSURE

Pascal's law states that pressure from a fluid is exerted equally on all surfaces of an immersed object at any given depth (figure 13.3). The more deeply the object is immersed, the greater the pressure it encounters. Atmospheric pressure at the surface is 14.7 psi. For every foot of submersion, water pressure increases by 0.43 psi (Edlich et al. 1987). Hydro-static pressure can positively affect edema both by reducing edema postinjury and by allowing exercise without the risk of increasing edema.

WEIGHT BEARING IN WATER

Since buoyancy and gravity are opposing forces on a body in water, the more deeply the body is submerged in water, the less weight is borne by the lower extremities (figure 13.4). Because a

Force of gravity

Hydrostatic pressure increases with water depth

Lateral pressure of the water

Force of buoyancy

Figure 13.3 Pascal's law

Adapted from Bates and Hanson 1996.

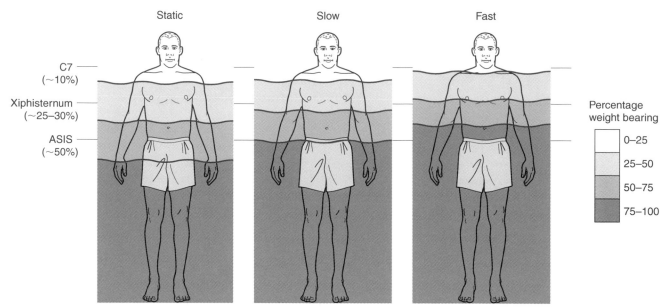

■ **Figure 13.4**   Weight bearing in water.

Reprinted, by permission, from R.A. Harrison, M. Hillman, and S. Bulstrode, 1992, "Loading of the lower limb when walking partially immersed: Implications for clinical practice," *Physiotherapy* 78(3): 164–167. Copyright 1992 by Chartered Society of Physiotherapy.

male's center of gravity is lower than a female's, the specific percentage of body weight borne at different depths varies slightly from female to male. For example, with the body immersed to the xyphoid process, females bear 28% of their weight whereas males bear 35% of their weight (Thein and Brody 1998).

These percentages are useful information, especially in the early stages of rehabilitation. For example, an injured basketball player who is partial weight bearing to 50% on the left lower extremity can perform therapeutic exercises for the left leg in water that is at hip level. As the patient is permitted to bear more weight on the leg, he or she can perform the exercises in shallower water.

Changing walking speed in the water changes the weight-bearing forces in the water (Harrison, Hillman, and Bulstrode 1992). Generally, the faster a person walks in the water, the higher the weight-bearing percentages. For example, if you walk at a slow pace, you must walk in water that is at a level below the axilla in order to be 50% weight bearing. If you walk at a fast rate, 50% weight bearing occurs in water above the axilla level.

EQUIPMENT

Major categories of aquatic equipment include safety equipment and exercise equipment. Equipment for exercising in the water comprises many types of assistive devices, which help to stabilize or support the patient in the pool, and resistive devices that increase the difficulty of an exercise.

In recent years, more and more manufacturers have been producing more types and varieties of aquatic exercise equipment. Aquatic equipment can be divided into safety equipment and exercise equipment. Exercise equipment is used and classified as assistive or resistive.

SAFETY EQUIPMENT

The specific safety equipment required at a pool depends on the size of the pool and on state regulations. Safety equipment includes various rescue equipment such as ring buoys, the shepherd's crook, and rescue tubes. Ring buoys are useful in towing and in-water rescues; the shepherd's crook is used for rescue of victims from the side of the pool. A rescue tube has an attached tow rope and can support one or more persons. It is flexible enough to wrap around a body.

Spine boards should be among the items of safety equipment at a pool (figure 13.5). These are made of wood, plastic, or fiberglass and have neck and head straps and/or supports. Transport litters or stretchers should be readily available.

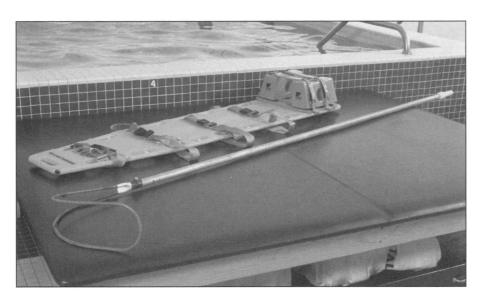

■ Figure 13.5 Safety equipment. A shephard's crook or other retrieval equipment and a spine board should be readily available.

Secondary safety equipment should include a basic first-aid kit. In addition to the routine first-aid items, the kit should contain items such as rubber gloves, earplugs, nose plugs, and waterproof bandages.

EXERCISE EQUIPMENT

Exercise equipment most often comprises items that are portable but may also include installed or fixed equipment. Rails and benches are examples of fixed equipment. Portable items may range from simple kickboards to elaborate in-water gym equipment. The selection of specific items depends on the budget and on the sophistication of the pool exercises incorporated into a rehabilitation routine.

Assistive Devices

Assistive exercise equipment helps to stabilize or support the patient in a desired position while in the water; this may be upright, supine, or prone. Flotation devices are used to maintain buoyancy in these positions. They can also serve to assist in the motion of an exercise and often are used to provide additional motion of a joint. The following sections deal with some of the more commonly used devices.

Flotation Cuffs

Flotation cuffs are worn on the upper arms or on the ankles to provide buoyancy for the arms or legs (figure 13.6). When used on the ankles, they can facilitate gait activities or provide buoyancy for range-of-motion activities.

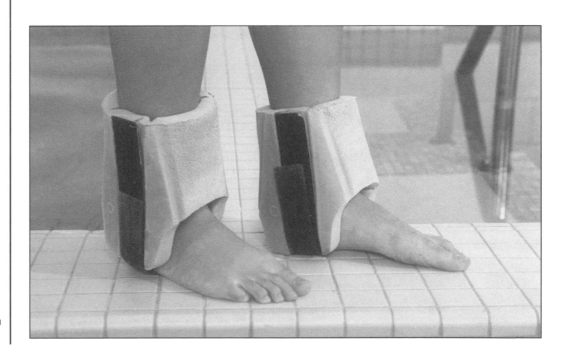

■ Figure 13.6 Flotation cuffs.

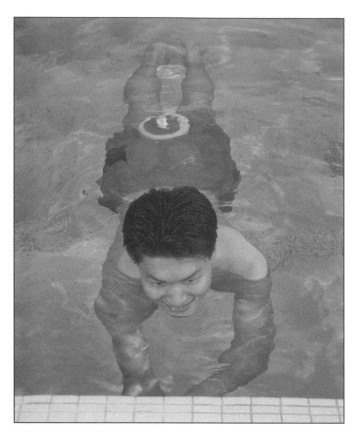

I Figure 13.7   Pull buoy.

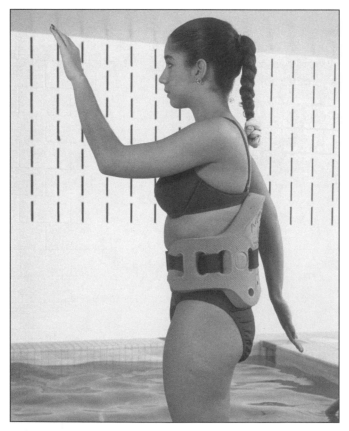

I Figure 13.8   Flotation belt.

Pull Buoys

Pull buoys are usually Styrofoam devices that are held between the thighs to provide flotation for the legs and lower body during arm exercises (figure 13.7).

Vests and Belts

Vests and belts are used to maintain buoyancy for the trunk during deep-water arm or leg exercises. They are also used for deep-water running and prone- or supine-position exercises (figure 13.8). They should fit comfortably and snugly so they do not ride up. They should also fit well enough not to impede arm or leg movement.

Kickboards

Kickboards provide buoyancy for the arms, legs, head, or trunk. They are available in soft or hard materials and can be used in a vertical, supine, or prone position. They can be used on the water's surface or under the water (figure 13.9). A disadvantage of using kickboards with the arms is that prolonged positioning can cause shoulder fatigue.

Water Dumbbells

Water dumbbells resemble regular dumbbells; but they are made of Styrofoam, and the bar is padded (figure 13.10). The dumbbell can be placed under the axillas or under the knees to provide buoyancy. Dumbbells offer buoyancy to the arms without adding to the stress of the shoulders the way kickboards can. The bars come in different lengths: The shorter lengths are used under the axilla or held in each hand, and the longer lengths are used under the knees or held with both hands.

Other Buoyancy Equipment

Other buoyancy equipment encompasses items such as inner tubes, water mattresses, ski belts, and cervical float collars. Facilities with restricted budgets may use empty plastic gallon containers as flotation devices.

Resistive Devices

Resistive devices can advance the difficulty of an exercise to increase muscle strength or endurance. They increase exercise difficulty by increasing a body segment's surface area, requiring increased speed of movement, or adding buoyancy or weight.

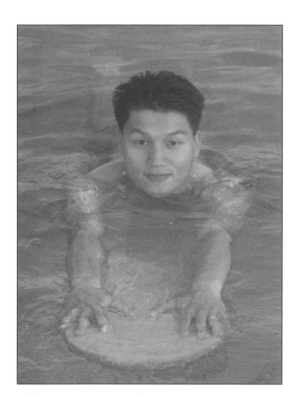

Lower Extremity
Lower-extremity resistive devices are designed to increase resistance to lower-extremity movement. They do this by either increasing the friction during ambulation in the water or increasing the form or wave drag of the lower extremity.

Water shoes are used when the patient is in shallow water and able to touch the bottom of the pool. They are not used during swimming or kicking. They increase the weight of the lower extremity and increase the lower leg's drag in the water. Their rubberized soles make them good for providing traction during walking, running, or jumping activities. The surface of the sole results in an increase in friction to increase resistance as well as providing stability during these activities.

Fins, which come in a variety of styles and lengths, increase resistance because of the increase in drag they produce. The shorter fins are more appropriate for patients with limited ankle range of motion. Shorter fins are more manageable in the water, offer less resistance than longer fins, and allow the patient to perform a more normal kick while swimming. Any fin that is used should fit the patient well and not pinch, as pinching can cause blisters or cramping.

Boots covering the feet and ankles increase form and/or wave drag during the exercise (figure 13.11). Extension panels on the front or sides of the boot cause turbulence of the water during movement to increase the extremity's form and wave drag. Boots can be used for exercise or during walking or running activities to increase difficulty.

Upper Extremity
Upper-extremity resistive devices, like those for the lower extremity, are designed to increase extremity resistance by increasing form or wave drag or turbulence.

Webbed gloves are the least-resistive devices for the arms. They can be used earlier in the aquatic exercise program than some of the other devices. The gloves are made of Lycra, nylon, or neoprene, so they are soft and pliable. They thus permit the patient to

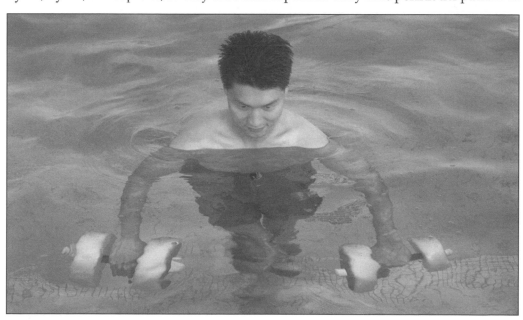

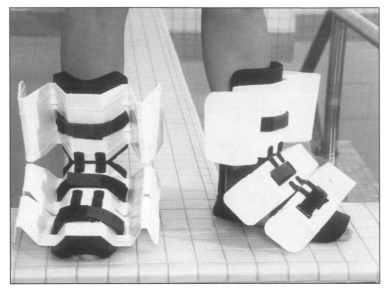

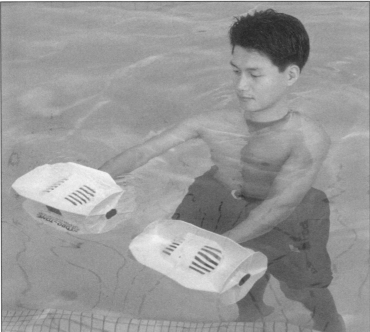

close or open the hand to reduce or increase the water resistance during an exercise.

Paddles either are handheld or are attached to the hand with straps. They come in a variety of sizes and shapes. The larger the size, the more resistance the paddles produce by increasing form and wave drag. Some paddles look like dumbbells except that they are flat and their disks can be open-vented or close-vented to reduce or increase resistance. Typically made of rigid plastic, paddles offer more resistance than gloves.

Bells provide greater resistance to the arms than the other devices and so are appropriate in the later stages of an aquatic exercise program. Like the boots, they offer resistance by providing turbulence and form and wave drag. They are similar in structure to the boots (figure 13.11) and have either side panels or hollow cores.

Cardiovascular Devices

Cardiovascular devices are available either as separate aquatic containers or as treadmills that can be immersed in swimming pools. The separate containers offer resistance by providing turbulence against an individual who is walking. These devices are costly, but they may be an aquatic exercise solution for facilities without swimming pools. They do require substantial space and some maintenance but obviously not as much as a regular swimming pool.

▌**Figure 13.11** Boots and bells.

INDICATIONS, ADVANTAGES, PRECAUTIONS, AND CONTRAINDICATIONS

One major advantage of aquatic therex, among others, is that exercise in the water is feasible for patients who are not yet weight bearing. Precautions and contraindications relate to the use of medications, various medical conditions, and illness.

Although aquatic exercise has the advantage that it can begin early in a rehabilitation program when other forms of exercises are contraindicated, aquatic exercise is not for everyone. Before deciding to use an aquatic therapeutic exercise program, the sport rehabilitation specialist must be aware of the indications, as well as the limitations and dangers, of this type of system.

INDICATIONS

An aquatic therapeutic exercise program is indicated when the patient has many of the typical signs and symptoms associated with sport injuries. These include pain, edema, muscle spasm, loss of motion, weakness, limited endurance, or restricted weight-bearing status. Aquatic exercise can also serve as a method of maintaining cardiovascular conditioning or normal status of the uninvolved extremities.

ADVANTAGES

The indications lead naturally to advantages of the use of aquatic exercises. This type of exercise can be particularly beneficial when the patient is non-weight bearing on the injured extremity. While the patient may be restricted in activities on dry land, he or she may perform a wide range of activities in the water. The warmth of the water causes a relaxation of muscles. The buoyancy reduces joint compressive forces to allow movement and positioning with reduced pain. The warmth of the water also reduces pain sensation by bombarding the sensory system with temperature input and decreasing the painful noxious input that travels the same pathways. This relief of spasm and reduction of pain assists in breaking down the pain-spasm injury cycle discussed in chapter 2.

Reduction of joint compressive forces and relaxation of muscles permit better movement of the injured area. Buoyancy equipment can help even further in reducing stress to the area's muscles and permit greater ease of movement. Reduction of gravitational forces on the body allows activity when weight bearing is not permissible. Walking in water with reduced weight bearing makes it possible for muscles to function properly for the gait sequence. This encourages the maintenance of muscle tone and balance. Weight bearing can be progressive if the patient walks in water of decreasing depths; the lower the water level, the greater the weight bearing.

Instituting exercises early helps the patient maintain or develop a healthy attitude, promotes body awareness and balance, and stresses newly forming tissue without overstressing it. Improved circulation in the injured site increases the exchange of nutrients and metabolites to advance the healing process. Movement in water can often relieve or reduce pain due to immobilization or edema. If pain and edema can be reduced to affect the pain-injury cycle, the healing rate may be accelerated so that recovery occurs more readily.

The patient's ability to begin exercises sooner also helps to prevent the deconditioning that can play a part in delaying the return to sport participation.

PRECAUTIONS

As with any exercise, the sport rehabilitation specialist must be aware of precautions and must take special care to administer the aquatic rehabilitation program with these in mind. In the presence of any doubt or question about the patient's ability to perform an aquatic program, it is essential to consult the physician in advance.

Fear of the Water

A patient's fear of water often calls for encouragement and patience. It is advisable to use a vest, even in shallow water, for reassurance. The patient should begin in shallower water if the injury permits. As a sport rehabilitation specialist you may have to give the patient assistance and physical support through a hands-on approach, especially until he or she becomes more comfortable in the water. Any patient who experiences an excessive fear of the water should not be forced into an aquatic exercise program.

Medications

Some medications that affect heart rate, blood pressure, or respiration, or any other medication that may alter cardiorespiratory function, may impact the patient's ability to exercise in the water. The sport rehabilitation specialist should check with the patient's physician or pharmacist before permitting the individual in the water.

Ear Infections

If the patient has a tendency toward chronic ear infections, he or she should apply proper protective ear devices before entering the water. Exercises should be designed so that the head is kept above the water to reduce the risk of an infection.

Specific Conditions

Patients with certain systemic or compromising diseases such as diabetes, cardiovascular disease, or seizure disorders should be carefully monitored while in the water. If the person is sensitive to the pool chemicals, it is essential to observe for unwanted side effects.

No patient should ever be in the pool alone, even if he or she is a good swimmer. Someone should always accompany patients during aquatic exercise.

CONTRAINDICATIONS

Under certain conditions or in certain situations, patients should not be allowed in the pool for aquatic therapeutic exercises. These are absolute contraindications that, if ignored, could lead to serious consequences.

Illness

A patient who has a contagious infection and is at risk of transmitting the infection to others should not be allowed in the water.

A severe cold or the flu warrants keeping the patient out of the water until he or she has recovered. Any urinary tract infection should be resolved before the patient is allowed in the water. If the patient has a temperature of 100° F, aquatic exercise must be postponed. Not only is the temperature a problem in that it indicates an illness; it may rise further because of the temperature of the water and the exercise.

Open Wounds

Open wounds should be healed before a patient is allowed into the pool. After surgery, the healing time is usually about seven days. However, if any portion of the surgical scar is open, the patient should remain out of the water.

Other Medical Conditions

Some conditions are not usually found in the athletic population but need to be mentioned as a point of information. Conditions that are absolute contraindications for an individual's participation in an aquatic exercise program include tracheostomy, severe kidney disease, presence of a nasogastric tube, fecal incontinence, radiation treatments within the past three months, and a history of uncontrolled seizures.

AQUATIC THERAPEUTIC EXERCISE PRINCIPLES AND GUIDELINES

The sport rehabilitation specialist moves the patient through a sequence of water-based exercises in accordance with the principles of progression for other forms of exercise.

As with therapeutic exercises on land, aquatic therapeutic exercises follow a system of progression. They begin with range-of-motion and flexibility exercises, progress to strength and endurance exercises, and then advance to coordination and agility activities before the patient begins doing sport-specific functional activities. It is also recommended that an exercise session begin with a warm-up and end with a cool-down.

The length of the warm-up depends on the temperature of the water. Therapeutic pools used exclusively for exercise are often set at 92° to 98° F (33–37° C). Swimming pools are set at a lower temperature, 80° to 85° F (27–30° C). The cooler the pool temperature, the longer the warm-up should be.

A cool-down is particularly important if the exercise session has included cardio-vascular activities. Cool-down activities can include walking, easy treading water, or sculling in deep or shallow water. It is important to remind the patient to rehydrate following exercises in the pool. Because of the warm water temperature, the patient will perspire and not realize it.

PRINCIPLES RELATED TO WATER PROPERTIES

The sport rehabilitation specialist determines the primary portion of the aquatic exercise session on the basis of specific findings, and gears the session toward correcting the deficiencies observed. The same principles of advancement are used for aquatic exercises as for dryland exercises.

Additionally, because of the properties of water discussed earlier, other factors enter into the selection of specific exercises. These include hydrostatic pressure, drag and turbulence, and buoyancy.

Hydrostatic pressure can affect the edema of a segment. It is more advantageous to exercise a swollen extremity in deep water than in shallower water because of the greater hydrostatic pressure at greater depths.

A longer lever arm increases form drag. The straighter the arm, the greater the resistance. It is best to start with a shorter lever arm and progress to longer ones as strength improves. You can make additional changes in lever-arm length by changing the position of the resistive equipment. The farther away from the body's core the resistance is, the greater it is.

Resistance can be provided for a segment using the properties of water. Increasing the speed of the activity causes increased resistance to movement. Moving objects toward the surface of the water, increasing the surface area by using the equipment discussed earlier, and using floats can all increase water resistance to provide for additional strength gains. Exercising in differing depths of water will also change the weight bearing and resistance.

Buoyancy can make an exercise easier or more difficult, depending on the relative position of the center of buoyancy and center of gravity. Buoyancy becomes a greater factor for the body in deeper water.

AQUATIC EXERCISE PROGRESSION

Although we have noted that an aquatic therex program can serve to maintain cardiovascular conditioning and status of the uninvolved extremities, we will not consider such exercises in detail. The emphasis here is on the injured segment. Keep in mind that cardiovascular activities are generally performed in the deep water unless in-water treadmills are used. Deep-water cardiovascular exercises include activities such as running, treading water, and swimming. If it is desirable to exercise the uninjured extremities, the more advanced exercises that are presented later in this chapter can be used.

Early-Phase Exercises

The early portion of an aquatic therex program includes gait-training activities in appropriate-depth water, range-of-motion exercises, and perhaps early strengthening activities, if these are indicated and tolerated. Gait training emphasizes the correct manner of ambulation, proper posture, and good balance. The sport rehabilitation specialist should rely on knowledge of proper posture and proper gait timing and sequencing as discussed in chapters 11 and 12 to assist and instruct the patient in correct posture and gait techniques. The goals in this phase are to achieve normal gait in water and restore normal range of motion.

It is beneficial to use buoyancy equipment in range-of-motion exercises. Buoyancy equipment allows the extremity to come to the water's surface, where range-of-motion gains are easiest to achieve. At the surface, the drag is kept to a minimum, so movement is made with less effort. Resistance exercises in the beginning are low level and are provided without resistive devices. Use of the body segment's own drag in the water is sufficient in the early stage of strengthening activities. Speed of movement is kept slow initially so that less resistance is offered by the water. Koury (1996) recommends limiting initial bouts of resistance exercises to one to two sets of 10 to 15 repetitions, but the specific numbers of sets and repetitions are individually determined and based on the patient's level of fitness, tolerance, and ability and on the program goals. Either increasing the repetitions or increasing the sets makes the exercise progressive. Which of the two methods to use is specifically determined by the individual's tolerance, sport, rate of healing, and fitness level.

Middle-Phase Exercises

As the patient progresses, restoration of muscle strength and endurance—the goal of the middle phase—receives more emphasis.

Viscosity-producing drag and buoyancy-permitting motion are now used to provide resistance to increase strength. Speed of motion and lever-arm length are other variables that change the resistance. Deeper water offers additional resistance because it increases pressure on the extremity and increases stability requirements.

Progression with resistive equipment includes starting with short objects and progressing to longer objects. Using lower-profile objects is less difficult than exercising with higher-profile objects. The more drag an object provides, either because it increases the water's resistance or because its profile is made larger, the greater the resistance. The more turbulence the object produces, the greater the resistance. The farther along the extremity the object is placed, the greater the resistance it offers. Each of these ways of increasing resistance creates an additional level of difficulty.

You can also increase the intensity of an exercise by increasing the repetitions or sets. This will help improve endurance more than strength, but there will also be strength gains at a lower rate. This principle is discussed in chapter 7.

Advanced-Phase Exercises

The later stages of the aquatic therex program present a progression toward achieving the goal, normal restoration of the ABCs of proprioception—agility, balance, and coordination. This prepares the patient to withstand the stresses that will be applied during land-based activities.

Gait-training activities can now include walking at a faster pace or running, side-stepping, cariocas, and retrograde walking. Hopping, jumping, squatting, and other sudden changes in direction are also appropriate in this phase. Coordination exercises with eyes open and eyes closed can be included as well.

Strength activities can continue to increase in intensity if the sport rehabilitation specialist uses more aggressive resistive equipment, increases the speed, requires more than one activity simultaneously, increases repetitions and sets, or changes the shape or size of the resistive equipment.

Land-based exercises may have started during this phase or during the middle stage. Whether or not the aquatic therex program continues depends on the patient's interest in the program, the sport rehabilitation specialist's preference, rehabilitation goals, and equipment and pool availability.

End-Phase Exercises

If a patient continues in the pool for therapeutic exercises, this is the final stage of aquatic-based exercises. Because of involvement of land exercises, aquatic exercises constitute a fraction of the time of the total therapeutic exercise program; however, some patients may prefer to continue in the water because of satisfaction they receive from their workout. The goal in this phase is to prepare the patient for the specific demands of his or her sport.

Activities during this phase mimic the skill demands of the patient's sport; include aggressive coordination, agility, and speed activities; and reinforce performance of specific sport skills using proper posture. High-demand activities can include plyometrics such as box jumping drills and bench stepping. Sport-specific activities can include the use of equipment such as a golf club, tennis racket, or baseball bat in the water.

Progression Guidelines

Progression requires close observation by the sport rehabilitation specialist and accurate reporting by the patient to the specialist. You should observe the patient's response to the exercise program and the quality of performance. If the patient is able to perform the required exercises correctly, swiftly, and without difficulty, he or she should advance to the next level of difficulty. You must also assess the patient's range of motion, strength, and balance in order to note improvements or changes. This assessment is based on both observation and specific objective testing.

The patient must communicate to the sport rehabilitation specialist any increases in pain or swelling or other symptoms following an exercise session. In the absence of any increase, he or she can progress to the next level.

It is essential to advance the patient at a rate that will provide for a continued overload, but not so quickly that his or her body is unable to adapt to the stresses and incurs an injury.

DEEP-WATER EXERCISE

Important benefits of exercise in deep water include the absence of weight bearing and the lack of impact forces on the body of the patient.

Even patients who are unable to swim can exercise in deep water. Because of its advantages, deep-water exercise warrants special attention in this chapter. We will look briefly at the benefits of this type of exercise.

The most obvious benefit of deep-water exercise is that it involves no weight bearing and no impact forces on the body. This is particularly important if the patient wants to exercise but either is unable to tolerate impact forces or needs to remain non-weight bearing. For example, a basketball player who has patellar tendinitis that is sufficiently intense to restrict ground running may be able to tolerate running in deep water. This activity can help keep the individual's cardiovascular fitness level and strength intact during the rehabilitation process. A runner with a stress fracture is another example of a patient who can benefit from deep-water running.

Since gravity is opposed by buoyancy in deep water, the forces of gravity on a submersed body are minimal. If weights are applied to the ankles, a slight traction force is produced by the force of gravity and the counterbalance force of buoyancy. This can be important for a patient who has low back pain secondary to either facet irritation or intervertebral disk compression.

Deep-water exercises are essentially concentric. Trauma to inflamed tendons, muscles, or bones is reduced without eccentric activity, yet good strengthening can be provided with deep-water exercises.

Some Recommendations for Optimal Benefits

During deep-water exercises, the body should remain in good alignment to keep stresses reduced and to use muscles effectively. The head should be out of the water and in proper alignment with the rest of the body. There should be no forward positioning of the neck or upward positioning of the chin to produce an excessive cervical lordosis. The lumbar and thoracic spine should be in correct alignment as discussed in chapter 11 in relation to proper standing posture (figure 13.12). Buoyancy vests or belts help the patient maintain a good postural alignment in deep water. If the spine is not in a neutral position, the center of gravity and the center of buoyancy are not in a vertical alignment. It becomes more difficult for the patient to maintain a vertical position in deep water when the spine is not in good alignment.

To keep the spine in a good alignment, the patient should attempt to keep the chest lifted and to maintain some tension in the abdominals and gluteals. This preserves good spinal alignment in the water just as it does on land.

Arm activity during deep-water exercises should occur from the shoulders, not the elbows. The arms, as in land running, are used in a pumping activity, with initiation of the activity occurring at the shoulders.

As in ground running, hip flexion and extension coincide with knee flexion and extension. The ankle goes into plantar flexion during leg extension motion and into dorsiflexion as the hip moves into flexion.

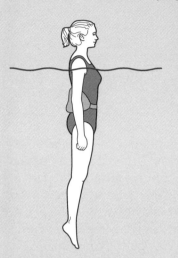

▌Figure 13.12   Correct vertical alignment.

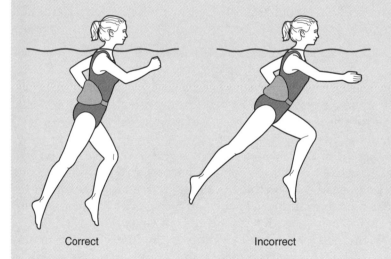

Correct   Incorrect

▌Figure 13.13   Position for deep-water running

Throughout deep-water running, the spine remains in neutral with a slight forward bend (figure 13.13). The movement through the water is produced by the extremities, not the trunk. It is necessary for the trunk muscles, the abdominals and the back extensors, to act as stabilizers of the trunk as the body is propelled through the water by the arms and legs.

AQUATIC THERAPEUTIC EXERCISES

Many water-based therapeutic exercises are similar to exercises that patients do on dry land. As with dryland exercise, most aquatic exercises for the spine and the lower and upper extremities can be made more demanding to provide a progression.

The sections that follow present a variety of aquatic exercises for the spine, the lower extremities, and the upper extremities. First, though, a few special points relevant to water-based exercise deserve mention. The first concerns refraction in water and its effect on observation. When light rays move from the air through water, they bend as a result of the lower density of water compared to that of the air. This bending of the light rays makes the bottom of the pool appear closer to the surface than it actually is. It also makes the submerged portion of the patient's body appear distorted (figure 13.14). The submerged body segments appear to be flexed at a different angle than the body segments that are not in the water. This can make it difficult

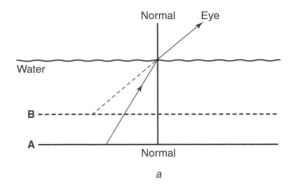

a

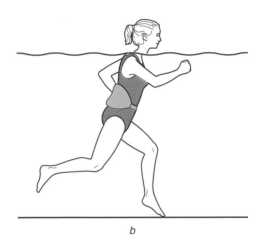

b

Figure 13.14 Refraction of light causes rays reflected from the true bottom of the pool **A** to appear at a false bottom **B** *(a)*. Refraction can create illusions in alignment of body segments *(b)*.

for someone standing at poolside to accurately judge the position of the body or body segment. At times it may be necessary for the sport rehabilitation specialist to get into the water with the patient to make sure the positioning is correct, especially if the patient has difficulty with propriocep-tion and is unable to align him- or herself correctly without tactile guidance.

The patient should wear a vest or ski belt while performing deep-water exercises. The use of fins can make deep-water exercises more difficult, so goals of the exercise should be determined before the decision to use them is made.

Another point relates to exercises in shallow water. It is advisable for a patient exercising with the feet on the bottom of the pool to wear aquatic shoes. These will enhance balance and provide friction resistance, as well as protecting the patient's feet from abrasions.

The exercises described here are intended only as suggestions and are presented in a progressive series. The discussion is far from all-inclusive. Indeed, the range of possible exercises is limited only by the patient's abilities and your imagination and knowledge. If you know the goals of an aquatic therex program, understand the injury limitations, know the patient's abilities, and have an appreciation of the water's physical properties, you can incorporate any appropriate exercise into the aquatic therex program that your ingenuity allows.

A final point is that you should determine the depth of the water for the exercise according to the patient's confidence in the water, weight-bearing status, and the goal of the exercise.

Some of the exercises are presented, along with their purposes, in the following sections. For many of the strengthening exercises, however, the discussion does not specify which muscles the activity is designed to strengthen. Using your knowledge of kinetics and aquatic principles, attempt to identify the muscles each exercise is intended for.

EXERCISES FOR THE SPINE

An important concept to remember about aquatic spine exercises is that the patient should maintain a neutral spine in all activities. This keeps the vertebrae in good alignment, places minimal stress on the spine, and uses the spine and trunk most efficiently, effectively, and correctly. If the patient is unable to maintain a proper spinal alignment during an exercise, the intensity, complexity, or demand level should be decreased and the patient should concentrate on a lower-level exercise until he or she has mastered spinal alignment at that level. If an individual has difficulty identifying correct spinal alignment with even the basic exercises, it may be necessary for the sport rehabilitation specialist to get into the pool and use tactile stimulation to provide sensory feedback. This feedback will help the patient identify and maintain correct neutral spine alignment.

You will see that many of the exercises described here are similar to dryland exercises. When patients perform them in warm water, the activity is often easier and more comfortable.

Spine Exercises in Shallow Water

The following sections describe only a few of many exercises that could be suggested for the spine. They begin with the cervical spine and move to the pelvis.

Neck Stretches

To stretch the lateral neck, the patient side-bends the neck to the left while holding the right arm down and across the front of the body, as seen in figure 13.15a. Reverse neck and arm position to stretch the left lateral neck. Figure 13.15b shows an alternative stretch in which the left hand is over the head. In this position, the patient provides a gentle stretch with the left arm while keeping the opposite arm behind the back. In the neck flexion stretch in figure 13.15c, the patient places both hands on the back of the head and performs a gentle stretch forward as the chin is tucked toward the chest. The levator scapula stretch (13.15d) is similar to that seen in figure 13.15b except that the neck is rotated slightly.

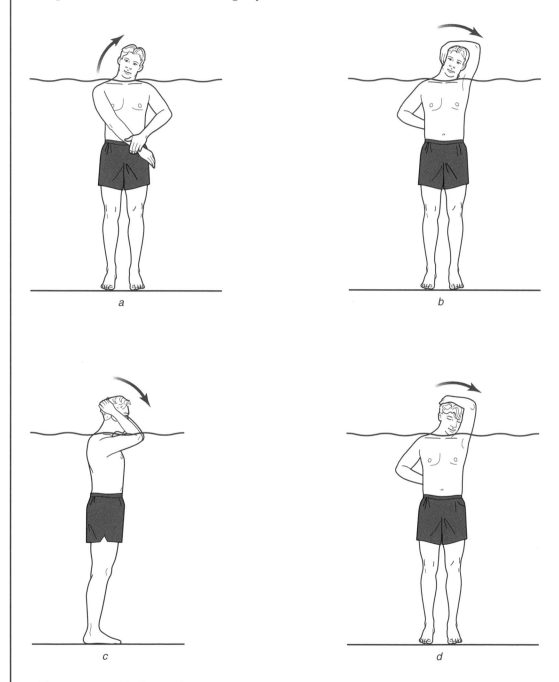

▮ Figure 13.15 Neck stretches, shallow water: *(a)* active lateral neck stretch, *(b)* stretch to right lateral neck with assistance of left arm, *(c)* stretch to posterior neck muscles using weight of both arms to assist, *(d)* right levator scapula stretch.

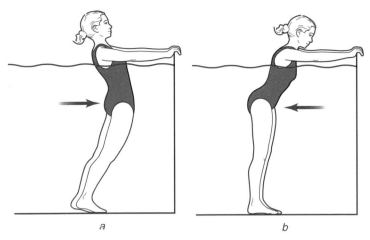

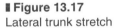

Figure 13.16 Spine flexion (a) and extension (b).

Spine Flexion-Extension

Standing with hands on the pool wall and feet shoulder-width apart, the patient keeps the arms straight throughout the exercise (figure 13.16). The hips are pressed forward toward the wall, then backward. During the move forward, the chest is lifted upward; when moving backward, the patient attempts to make the spine rounded.

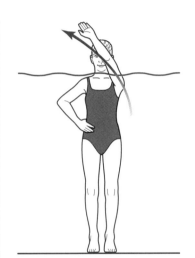

Figure 13.17
Lateral trunk stretch

Lateral Stretch

With the feet shoulder-width apart, the patient raises one arm overhead and reaches upward and across the body (figure 13.17).

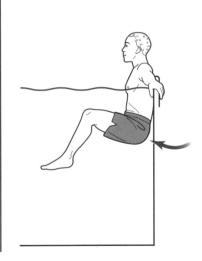

Figure 13.18
Pelvic roll.

Pelvic Roll

With the back against the pool wall, the patient supports him- or herself by holding on to the edge of the pool as seen in figure 13.18. With the lumbar spine kept flat against the pool wall and the abdominals tight, the legs are lifted until the knees and hips are at 90°. In this position, the patient slowly lifts the pelvis off the wall by tightening the lower abdominals. The pelvis is rolled back to the wall before the legs are lowered.

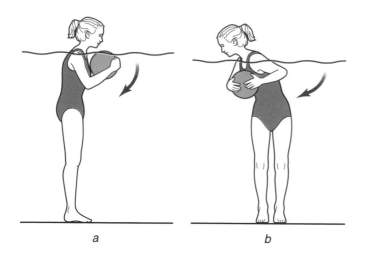

a   *b*

Standing Crunch

The patient stands with a flotation device or a ball against the chest (figure 13.19). The abdominals are contracted to flex the spine, and the position is held for at least 5 to 10 s. A pelvic tilt should be maintained throughout the exercise. This exercise can be modified to include rotational crunches as seen in figure 13.19b. The trunk is rotated about 10° to one side before the crunch is performed. The motion is repeated to the opposite side.

▌**Figure 13.19** Standing crunches *(a)* and rotational crunches *(b)*.

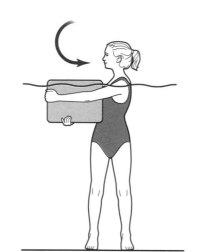

▌**Figure 13.20** Trunk rotation.

Trunk Rotation

In a neutral standing position, the patient rests the arms on a kickboard that is floating in the water. Slowly and in a controlled manner, he or she rotates to one side and then to the other (figure 13.20). The motion should remain pain free throughout. If pain is present, the motion should be restricted to a pain-free range. The exercise can be advanced through increasing the surface area of the resistance device.

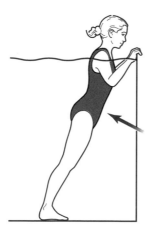

▌**Figure 13.21** Wall push-off.

Wall Push-Offs

The wall push-off strengthens the thoracic spine. Standing away from and facing the pool wall, the patient keeps the spine straight and does not bend at the hips or the back during the exercise (figure 13.21). The feet are kept in the same position throughout the exercise. The patient begins the exercise with the hands on the pool wall and the arms straight. He or she then leans forward and bends the arms until the chest comes close to the pool wall, and finally pushes away from the wall until the arms are straight.

Pull-Downs

With the feet shoulder-width apart, the knees slightly bent to relieve stress to the low back, and the spine in neutral, the patient moves arm bells from in front of the body downward toward the sides (figure 13. 22). The elbows are kept in flexion and the spine in neutral throughout the motion.

Spine Exercises in Deep Water

The patient must have good trunk control in order to perform the spine exercises. An individual who has difficulty with the exercise should perform it in waist-high or chest-high water first.

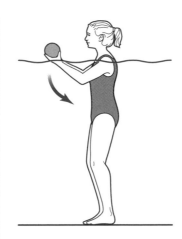

Figure 13.22   Pull-down.

Double-Leg Lift

With flotation devices in the hands or under the arms, the patient maintains a neutral spine as he or she lifts the legs to a 90° hip flexion position with the knees extended (figure 13.23). The abdominals must remain tight throughout the exercise. If it is too difficult for the patient to maintain a neutral spine position during this exercise, have the person either begin with a single-leg lift or bend the knees so that the hips and knees are at 90° at the top of the motion.

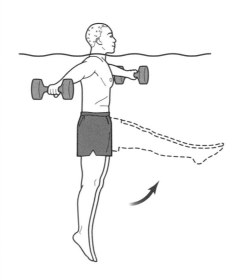

Figure 13.23
Double-leg lift.

Trunk Rotations

Using a flotation tube, the patient maintains a vertical position in the water (figure 13.24). The hips and knees are flexed, and the oblique muscles are used to rotate the hips first in one direction and then to the opposite side. The exercise is more demanding if the legs are fully extended.

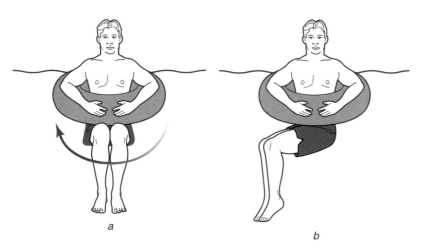

a   b

Figure 13.24   Trunk rotations.

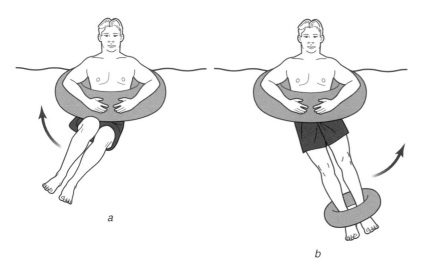

Lateral Flexion

Using a flotation tube or other flotation device, the patient flexes the hips and knees to 90° (figure 13.25a). He or she maintains this position while lifting the left hip laterally toward the left ribs and then lifting the right hip laterally toward the right ribs. The back should not twist or arch during this exercise. You can make this exercise more difficult by having the patient supine in the water with a flotation device at the waist and a small flotation tube or bells at the feet (13.25b).

▍Figure 13.25   Lateral flexion *(a)* and added resistance with flotation device at feet *(b)*.

EXERCISES FOR THE LOWER EXTREMITIES

Exercises in this section begin with the simpler exercises in shallow water and advance to deep-water exercises. Keep in mind that the patient may progress to some deep-water activities while still needing to continue with some shallow-water activities. The primary determinants of the time to move from shallow to deep water are your assessment of the patient's ability to perform an exercise, the goals, and the patient's comfort in water.

Ambulation and Balance Activities in Shallow Water

The following are examples of shallow-water exercises. You can increase difficulty by increasing the depth of the water in which the patient performs the activity. As previously discussed, the patient should maintain control of the body throughout each exercise.

1. **Forward walking.** This is useful as a gait-training exercise. Encourage the patient to maintain a correct gait pattern, as outlined in chapter 12, while in the water. Look for correct trunk stability. In the beginning, if necessary, the patient may use buoy lines or may walk along the side of the pool for balance.

2. **Backward walking.** This exercise works particularly on the extensor muscles of the trunk and legs. It is good for balance and coordination as well. Emphasize normal stride backward with a good toe-to-heel pattern, normal and equal stride length, and proper weight shifting. The patient should maintain proper trunk alignment.

3. **Toe walking.** The patient walks on his or her toes. This exercise is good for strength and proprioception.

4. **Heel walking.** The patient walks on the heels. This is a strengthening exercise for the dorsiflexors and a proprioceptive exercise as well.

5. **Single-leg balance.** The patient stands on the involved leg and moves the other leg forward to hold that position for 30 s (figure 13.26). To advance this exercise, you can have the patient stand on the involved leg while moving the uninvolved leg forward and backward or sideways. This exercise focuses on static balance improvement.

6. **Lunges.** The patient performs a forward lunge by taking a large step forward and then bringing the back leg up to meet the front leg. This activity is good for increasing strength and range of motion of the hip and knee. Good trunk alignment is necessary throughout the exercise. The patient can also do backward lunges and side lunges to increase hip extension and hip abduction, respectively. These exercises are good for balance and strength as well.

7. **Grapevine.** The grapevine is also referred to as a carioca or braid step. The patient first steps to the side with the first leg, then in back (crossing behind the first leg) with the second leg, out to the side again with the first leg, then in front (crossing in front of the first leg) with the second leg. This exercise is good for improving proprioception through improving coordination and balance.

8. **Running.** Analogously to walking in the water, water running should imitate the technique of land running as much as possible. The patient should use the arms to keep an upright posture and should avoid the tendency to lean forward. Running forward, running backward, and cutting can all be performed in shallow water as a prelude to land running.

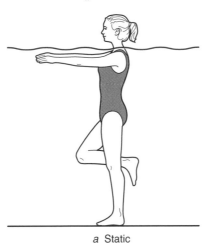

a Static

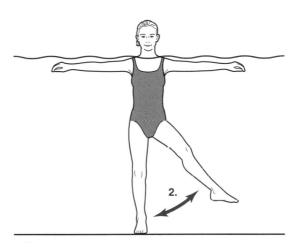

▌Figure 13.26
Single-leg balance, shallow water. The trunk should remain stable and erect throughout the exercise, with tension maintained in abdominal and gluteal muscles.

b With contralateral leg movement

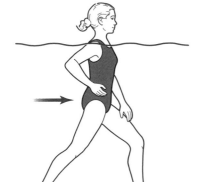

Hip Exercises in Shallow Water

Good trunk stability is important during all of the following hip exercises. You should instruct the patient to maintain vertical trunk alignment and to maintain tension in the abdominals to assist in this activity.

1. **Hip extension.** This activity can be used to stretch the hip flexors and strengthen the hip extensors (figure 13.27). The patient stands in a backward-forward straddle position with the involved leg behind. The spine is kept in a neutral position throughout the exercise. Keeping the abdominals tense will help ensure a correct spinal alignment. The involved knee is kept straight and the hip is pushed forward while the heel stays on the floor. The gluteals are tightened during the exercise.

▌Figure 13.27   Hip extension, shallow water.

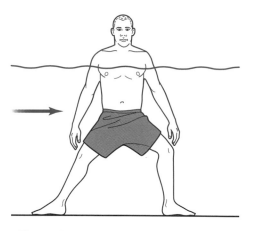

Figure 13.28 Hip abductor stretch, shallow water.

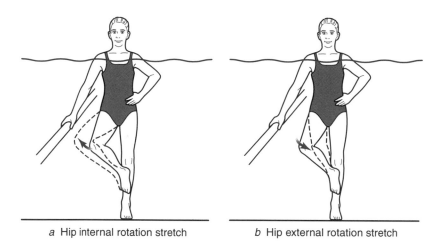

a Hip internal rotation stretch

b Hip external rotation stretch

Figure 13.29 Hip rotation, shallow water.

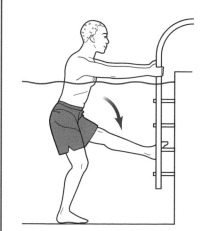

Figure 13.30 Hamstring stretch.

2. **Hip adductor stretch.** In this activity for stretching the hip adductors, the patient stands in a side-straddle position (figure 13.28). The uninvolved knee is bent as the weight is shifted to that side. The involved knee is kept straight, and the trunk is kept in an upright position.

3. **Hip internal-external rotation.** These exercises can be used to stretch one group as they strengthen the opposing muscle group. The patient may need to hold on to the pool wall or rail. The knee and hip of the involved leg are flexed, with the sole of the foot on the shin of the opposite leg (figure 13.29). The knee of the involved leg is then rotated outward as far as possible to stretch the internal rotators. To stretch the external rotators, the knee is moved inward toward the opposite leg. The trunk should remain in neutral throughout the exercise, and the pelvis should not rotate.

4. **Figure-8s.** This alternative to the rotation exercise just described offers resistance more than increases in range of motion. The patient draws figure-8s in the water with the entire leg, initiating the movement from the hip, not the knee or ankle. Progressions from this exercise can include proprioceptive neuromuscular facilitation patterns in the water and breaststroke kicking.

Knee Exercises in Shallow Water

The first two knee exercises in the following list are flexibility exercises; the others are strengthening exercises. The initial strengthening exercises should use only the limb as the source of resistance. As the patient's strength and control improve, you can add drag equipment to the activity or can have the patient perform the exercise faster as long as he or she maintains control of the limb.

1. **Quadriceps stretch.** This stretch is similar to the land exercise in which the patient grasps the ankle of the involved leg, which is positioned behind, and attempts to pull the foot toward the buttock. The knee should remain pointing downward, and the trunk should remain in a neutral position.

2. **Hamstring stretch.** The patient places the involved foot on the pool wall or on a step. The knee is slightly bent, and as the stretch is applied, the knee is extended (figure 13.30). Good trunk alignment is maintained throughout the exercise.

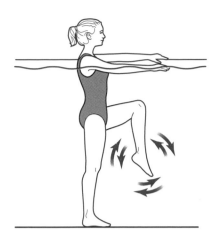

■ **Figure 13.31** Single-leg bicycle.

3. **Single-leg bicycle.** The patient flexes and extends the involved hip and knee in a cycling pattern while holding on to the side of the pool (figure 13.31). The trunk remains in neutral and does not move. This exercise is more difficult if the patient performs it without holding on to the side of the pool.

4. **Squats.** With the feet shoulder-width distance apart, the patient slowly bends the knees until the thighs are almost parallel to the pool floor. The spine should remain in a neutral position throughout the exercise. You can make this exercise more difficult by having the patient perform it without holding on to the side of the pool or perform it only on the involved leg. In a further progression, the patient performs a jump squat so that he or she lifts off the pool floor.

5. **Step-ups.** The involved leg is placed on the top of a box or platform. The patient steps onto the box by lifting his or her body upward, using the knee and hip muscles (figure 13.32). The trunk remains in a neutral position throughout. The patient should avoid trunk lean. This exercise can be performed with the patient standing in front of, behind, or at the side of the box for reverse step-ups, forward step-ups, or lateral step-ups, respectively.

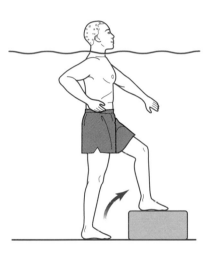

■ **Figure 13.32** Step-up, shallow water.

Ankle Exercises in Shallow Water

The ankle exercises outlined here are similar to those frequently performed on land, but the water is an ideal place to begin these exercises when weight bearing on the extremity is limited. In these situations, the patient begins in deeper water and progresses to shallower water as more weight bearing is permitted.

1. **Gastrocnemius-soleus stretch.** The patient stands facing the pool wall and places the involved leg behind him or her and the uninvolved leg in front. The heel of the involved leg is kept in contact with the pool floor; the knee is kept straight; and the body weight is moved forward onto the hands and front leg. This stretches the gastrocnemius. For stretching the soleus, the leg is brought forward slightly; the involved knee is bent; and the heel is kept on the pool floor as the weight is moved forward.

2. **Heel raises.** To perform this activity the patient may need initially to hold on to the side of the pool for stability. The patient slowly rises up onto the toes while the knees remain straight. The body should not lean or move forward. This exercise becomes more difficult if the injured athlete does not hold on to the side of the pool. It is also more difficult if he or she stands only on the involved leg or moves to shallower water.

3. **Ankle walking.** The patient walks on the toes, on the heels, on the inside of the feet, and on the outside of the feet. Progressions include increasing the stride length, increasing the speed, moving to shallower water, and using resistive equipment.

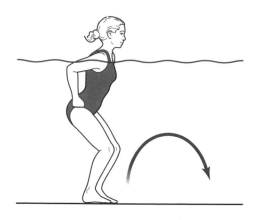

■ **Figure 13.33**
Hoppping, shallow water.

4. **Hopping.** The patient jumps forward, using the arms to assist but keeping the spine in neutral (figure 13.33). The knees should bend to absorb the impact forces. Progression of this exercise includes going from using both legs to one-legged hops, moving to shallower water, increasing the repetitions or sets, and increasing the speed.

Ambulation Activities in Deep Water

The following activities are appropriate when weight bearing is restricted. Cycling and running in deep water can also serve as cardiovascular activities, as well as lower-extremity exercises.

1. **Stride walking.** Stride walking is the use of exaggerated strides that are initiated from the hips. The spine should remain in neutral during the exercise.

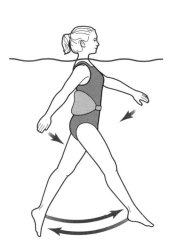

2. **Cycling.** Cycling is performed with the patient in a vertical position. The patient mimics a bicycle motion with exaggerated hip and knee movement. The motion can be either forward or backward.

3. **Running.** Running in deep water, as with walking activities, is a good exercise for patients who must remain non-weight bearing. Running in deep water can include jogging or sprinting. The form is as close to dryland running as possible. The trunk should remain in neutral throughout the running phase.

4. **Cross-country skiing.** The patient performs a reciprocal motion of the arms and legs, similar to the cross-country skiing action, while maintaining a neutral spine position as seen in figure 13.34.

■ **Figure 13.34**
Deep-water cross-country skiing.

Hip Exercises in Deep Water

Deep-water exercises are more difficult than shallow-water exercises if only because the patient must also work to maintain an upright posture and stable trunk. Instructions to keep abdominal muscles tense and the chest elevated can be useful cues. Use of a flotation belt can assist the patient in the early phases of deep-water exercise.

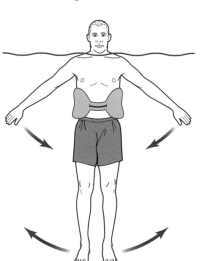

1. **Jumping jacks.** The elbows and knees are kept straight, and the spine is in neutral (figure 13.35). The arms begin in an abducted position. As the hips are abducted, the arms are adducted, and vice versa.

■ **Figure 13.35**
Jumping jacks, deep water.

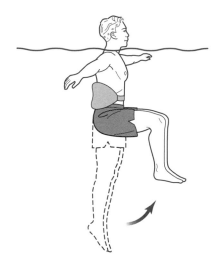

Figure 13.36 Double-knee lift, deep water.

2. **Double-knee lift.** The patient lifts both legs together, bringing the knees toward the chest while the spine remains in neutral (figure 13.36).

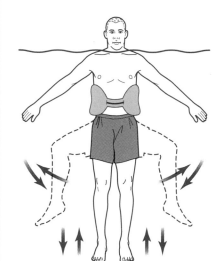

Figure 13.37 Hip flexion with external rotation, deep water.

3. **Flexion with external rotation.** The patient is in a vertical position with the spine in neutral (figure 13.37). The legs are moved together, simultaneously into hip flexion and external rotation, and are then returned to the starting position.

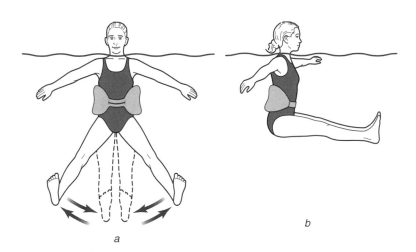

a

b

Figure 13.38 Hip abduction, deep water: (a) front view, (b) side view.

4. **Hip abduction.** In a vertical position, the patient keeps the knees straight and the spine in neutral. The hips are abducted at the same time and then returned to the starting position. This exercise is more difficult if the patient performs abduction with the hips first flexed to 90°, as seen in figure 13.38.

5. **Flutter kicking.** Flutter kicking on the back or on the stomach, with two legs or with one, is useful for the hip. Be sure that the patient initiates the movement from the hip, not the knee.

Knee Exercises in Deep Water

The knee exercises suggested here become more difficult if you have the patient perform them with both legs simultaneously or with resistance attached to the feet. Trunk and hip control should be maintained throughout the exercise.

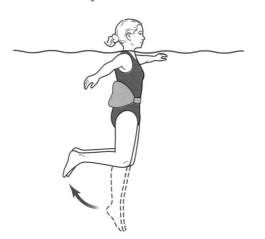

1. **Double-knee bend.** In a vertical position with the spine in neutral, the patient simultaneously flexes the knees while keeping them pointing directly downward (figure 13.39).

■ **Figure 13.39**
Double-knee bend, deep water.

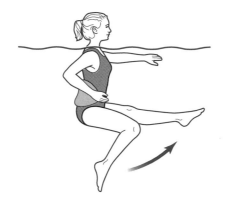

2. **Seated knee extensions.** With the hips flexed to 90° and the thighs together, the patient extends the involved knee to full extension (figure 13.40). A vertical position is maintained throughout. To make this exercise more difficult, have the patient extend both knees simultaneously.

■ **Figure 13.40**
Seated knee extension, deep water.

EXERCISES FOR THE UPPER EXTREMITIES

Keep in mind that just as with the lower-extremity exercises, the following exercises for the upper extremities do not constitute a complete list but are merely some suggested activities for use in therapeutic exercise. Although weight bearing is not the issue for the upper extremity that it is for the lower extremity, aquatic exercises can provide the patient with another way of rehabilitating the arm. Diversification of activities can help to maintain the patient's interest in the therapeutic exercise program, and the variety can be enjoyable for the sport rehabilitation specialist as well.

Shoulder Exercises in Shallow Water

Presentation of upper-extremity exercises will start with the shoulder and progress through the upper extremity, beginning with stretches and advancing to strengthening exercises.

1. **Pectoralis stretch.** In water above shoulder level, and with the arms elevated to shoulder level with elbows extended, the patient horizontally abducts the arms, squeezing the shoulder blades together. The palms should be facing upward.

2. **Capsule stretch.** With the involved arm at shoulder level, the patient grasps the elbow of the involved arm with the uninvolved hand and pulls the involved arm across the chest to stretch the posterior capsule (figure 13.41a). To stretch the anterior

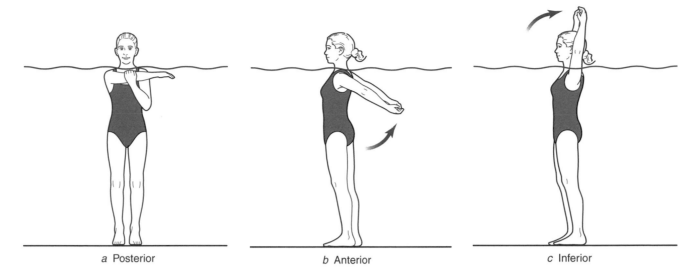

a Posterior   b Anterior   c Inferior

Figure 13.41 Capsule stretches.

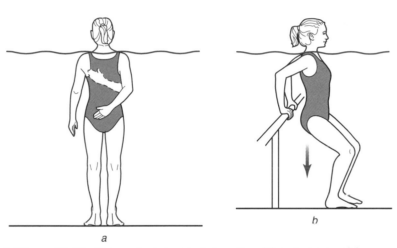

a

Figure 13.42 External rotator stretch, active (a) and passive (b).

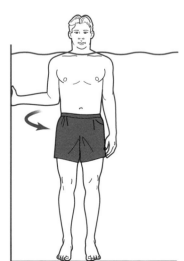

Figure 13.43
Internal rotator stretch.

capsule, the patient grasps the hands behind the back and attempts to lift the hands upward (figure 13.41b). Figure 13.41c demonstrates the inferior-capsule stretch with the patient's hands overhead. The back should not be arched or out of a neutral spine position for any of these stretches.

3. **External rotator stretch.** For this stretch of the external rotators, the patient places the involved hand on the low back (figure 13.42a). Keeping a neutral spine and erect posture, the patient bends the elbow and reaches upward as high as possible with the hand. In an alternative stretch, the patient grasps a bar or stair rung behind the back and attempts to bend the knees (figure 13.42b).

4. **Internal rotator stretch.** The patient stands with the involved side near the pool wall. The elbow is bent to 90° and the palm is on the wall (figure 13.43). The patient rotates the trunk away from the wall while keeping the hand in contact with the wall surface and the elbow at his or her side. This exercise stretches the internal rotators.

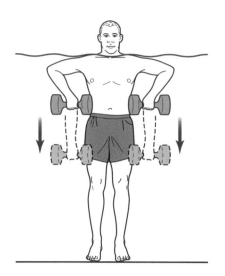

■ Figure 13.44
Shoulder press-
down.

5. **Shoulder press-down.** This is a shoulder-strengthening exercise. Using dumbbells or another flotation device, the patient allows the arms to elevate under the water until the upper arms are at shoulder level and in an abducted position (figure 13.44). The patient then pushes the dumbbells downward until the elbows are extended.

6. **Shoulder abduction-adduction.** Using resistive devices and keeping the elbows straight, the patient abducts the arms until the hands are at shoulder level and then returns to the starting position. The trunk remains in a neutral position.

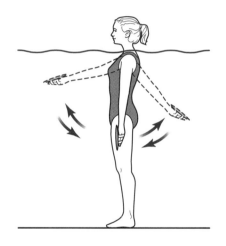

■ Figure 13.45
Shoulder flexion-
extension.

7. **Shoulder flexion-extension.** This exercise is similar to the preceding one, but the arm moves from flexion at shoulder level to hyperextension with the hand moving past the hips (figure 13.45).

8. **Horizontal abduction-adduction.** In this exercise the patient keeps the arms at shoulder level and the elbows straight. The spine is kept in neutral. With resistive devices in the hands, the patient moves the arms through horizontal abduction and horizontal adduction.

9. **Internal rotation-external rotation.** With the elbow at the side, the spine in neutral, and a resistive device attached to the hand, the patient moves the arm into external rotation and internal rotation. If only one direction is desired, on the return to the starting position the hand is rotated so that the hand's profile in the water is reduced.

Elbow Exercises in Shallow Water

Stretching exercises are often more comfortable when performed in water. The elbow can be particularly uncomfortable to stretch and may be better stretched in the pool than on land. Strength exercises can also be useful when performed in the pool. Consider the following activities:

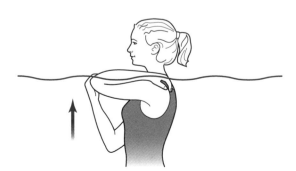

■ Figure 13.46
Elbow extensor
stretch.

1. **Elbow extensor stretch.** To increase the range of motion of the elbow in flexion, the patient bends the elbow as far as possible, and then applies additional force by using the uninvolved hand to increase the motion of the involved elbow (figure 13.46).

2. **Forearm curl.** Using a resistive device, the patient flexes the elbow as the shoulder is abducted and the arm is brought toward the water's surface. The shoulder and trunk should be maintained in a stable position throughout the exercise.

3. **Supination-pronation.** With the elbow at the side and bent to 90°, the patient holds on to a resistive device with the hand. The hand is slowly moved from a palm-up position through a full range of motion to a palm-down position, and then to the starting position, while the trunk and shoulder are maintained in stable positions.

4. **Elbow extension.** With the elbow kept at the side and a resistive device in the hand, the patient moves the elbow from a fully flexed to a fully extended position. The hand should remain in a palm-down position.

UPPER-EXTREMITY EXERCISES IN DEEP WATER

Because so many of the deep-water exercises for one upper-extremity joint also work the other joints, we will consider all the upper-extremity exercises together.

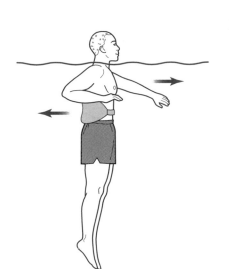

1. **Bent-arm pull.** With the body maintained in a vertical position, the patient keeps the arms at approximately shoulder level (figure 13.47). As one arm is brought back with the elbow bent, the other arm moves forward until the elbow is fully extended. This motion occurs in a reciprocal fashion.

■ **Figure 13.47** Bent-arm pull, deep water.

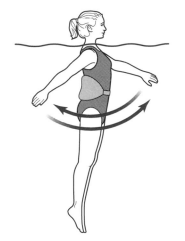

2. **Straight-arm pull.** With the body in a vertical position, the elbows kept straight, and the trunk stable and erect, the patient alternately swings the arms forward and then backward into hyperextension (figure 13.48). As the arm is brought forward, the hand faces upward; as the arm is brought backward, the hand faces downward.

■ **Figure 13.48** Straight-arm pull, deep water.

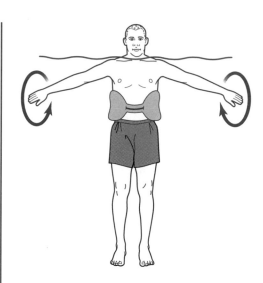

▌**Figure 13.49** Arm circles, deep water.

3. **Arm circles.** In a vertical position, the patient places the arms at shoulder level (figure 13.49). With the elbows kept straight, the arms are moved in circles, clockwise and counterclockwise. The resistance can be altered by changing the size of the circles, changing the speed of movement, or attaching resistive devices to the hands.

4. **Breaststroke.** With the body in a vertical position, the patient keeps the arms at shoulder level. The arms begin in a horizontally adducted position and are moved into full horizontal abduction as during a breaststroke.

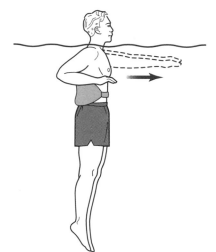

▌**Figure 13.50** Shoulder press, deep water.

5. **Shoulder press.** In a vertical position, the patient pushes both arms forward at shoulder level from the chest as in a shoulder-press exercise with weights (figure 13.50). To increase the resistance of this exercise, you can add resistive devices, increase speed, or increase the number of repetitions.

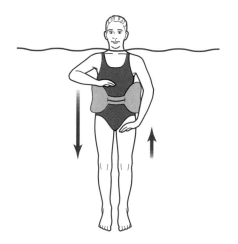

▌**Figure 13.51** Elbow press, deep water.

6. **Elbow press.** In a vertical position, the patient flexes and extends one elbow, alternating the motion with the opposite arm (figure 13.51). The movement occurs in an up-and-down motion in front of the body.

7. **Wave.** In a vertical position, the patient places the arms at shoulder level away from the sides. The elbows are kept straight throughout the exercise. The wrists are alternately flexed and extended through their full range of motion.

SUMMARY

1. *Identify and discuss the physical properties of water that affect the ability to exercise in water.*

   The physical properties of water, including specific gravity, buoyancy, center of buoyancy, and hydrodynamics, influence the way a patient is able to exercise in water. Water has a specific gravity of 1. If a body's specific gravity is less than 1, the body will float; but if the specific gravity is more than 1, the body will sink. Buoyancy occurs when the specific gravity is less than 1. In order for a body to remain upright while floating, the center of buoyancy must be in line with the center of gravity; otherwise the patient must work to maintain an upright position. Resistance to movement in water is called drag; the greater the drag, the more resistance there is. We can influence drag by increasing the speed of movement, turbulence, surface area being moved, and depth of the water.

2. *Define and explain the difference between assistive and resistive aquatic equipment and give examples of each.*

   Assistive devices in the water provide the body support to aid in buoyancy; examples are the kickboard and the flotation belt. Resistive equipment in the water increases the drag and makes it more difficult for a body to move; examples are paddles and boots.

3. *List precautions and contraindications for aquatic exercise.*

   The most common precaution relates to the patient's fear. Other precautions relate to certain medications that can compromise the patient's situation, to ear infections, and to certain medical conditions. A patient who has epilepsy, for example, may be endangered in a pool and must be closely observed. Contraindications include illness, open wounds, and medical conditions that may be dangerous for either the patient or others in the pool; in these cases the individual must not be allowed in the pool.

4. *Identify three advantages of aquatic therapeutic exercise.*

   Aquatic exercise can begin early in the therapeutic exercise program; patients with non-weight-bearing conditions can begin water exercises before land exercises. Aquatic therex can relax muscle spasm and pain, and provides for diversity and variety in the patient's rehabilitation program.

5. *List three aquatic exercises for each body segment and identify their purposes.*

   An example of a trunk exercise is the lateral stretch in shallow water, used to improve flexibility. An example of a lower-extremity exercise is step-ups in shallow water, which increase strength of the knee muscles, especially the quadriceps. An upper-extremity exercise is the shoulder press-down with water dumbbells, used to strengthen the shoulder depressors.

CRITICAL THINKING QUESTIONS

1. Why is it that some of the patients you place in the pool have no trouble floating while others must work to keep their heads above water? What principle does this phenomenon involve?

2. If the patient you are rehabilitating is non-weight bearing on an injured ankle but wants to perform cardiovascular activities in the pool, what program will you design for him? What water depth should he be in for resistive exercises?

3. The softball player with whom you have been working to rehabilitate her shoulder is fearful of going into the water. You would like to have her in the pool, since water activity would help increase her shoulder motion and strength. What would you do to encourage her to get into the pool and relieve her fears? What would be your initial exercises with her, and at what water depth would you place her?

4. You are using the pool to rehabilitate a gymnast with a hip strain until she has less pain with land activities. Her motion is good, but her strength is limited in all hip motions, especially abduction. List resistive exercises that you will include in her pool program, and provide a progression for each one.

5. Identify a simple core stabilization exercise that you would use for a patient with a recent back injury, and include a four-step progression for the exercise. What would your criteria be for advancement from one level to the next?

REFERENCES

Davis, B.C., and R.A. Harrison. 1988. *Hydrotherapy in practice.* New York: Churchill Livingstone.

Denegar, C. 2000. *Therapeutic modalities for athletic injuries.* Champaign, IL: Human Kinetics.

Edlich, R.F., Towler, M.A., Goitz, R.J., Wilder, R.P., Buschbacher, L.P., Morgan, R.F., and J.G. Thacker. 1987. Bioengineering principles of hydrotherapy. *Journal of Burn Care and Rehabilitation* 8:580–584.

Harrison, R.A., Hillman, M., and S. Bulstrode. 1992. Loading of the lower limb when walking partially immersed: Implications for clinical practice. *Physiotherapy* 78 (3):164–167.

Hay, J. 1978. *The biomechanics of sports techniques.* Englewood Cliffs, NJ: Prentice-Hall.

Koury, J.M. 1996. *Aquatic therapy programming.* Champaign, IL: Human Kinetics.

McWaters, G. 1988. *Deep water exercise for health and fitness.* Laguna Beach, CA: Publitech Editions.

Thein, J.M., and L.T. Brody. 1998. Aquatic-based rehabilitation and training for the elite athlete. *Journal of Orthopedic and Sports Physical Therapy* 27:32–41.

CHAPTER FOURTEEN

Swiss Balls and Foam Rollers

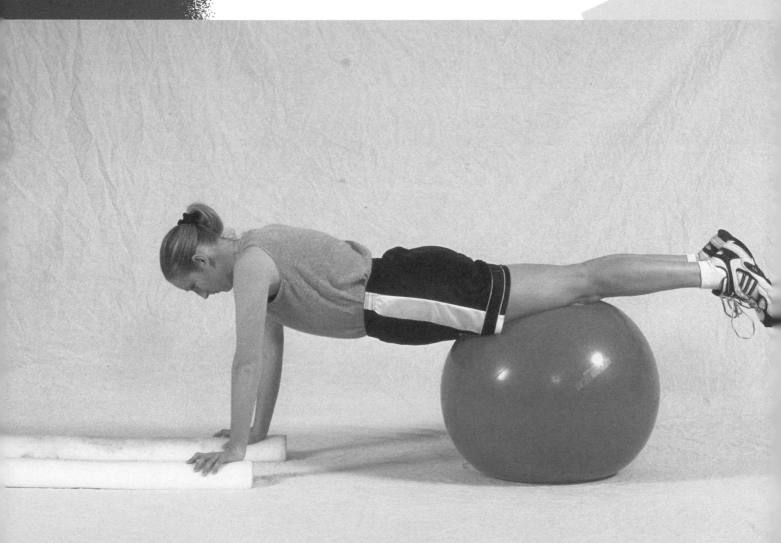

OBJECTIVES

After completing this chapter, you should be able to do the following:

1. Explain how Swiss balls and foam rollers can increase the challenge of a traditional exercise.

2. Identify the rehabilitation parameters that are benefited by the use of Swiss balls or foam rollers.

3. Discuss safety factors, precautions, and contraindications relating to the use of Swiss balls and foam rollers.

4. Explain how to properly fit a Swiss ball.

5. List one exercise each for the trunk, upper extremity, and lower extremity using a Swiss ball, and identify its purpose.

6. List one exercise each for the trunk, upper extremity, and lower extremity using foam rollers, and identify its purpose.

Of all the exercise equipment in the sports medicine facility where Tim Maxwell worked, he enjoyed the Swiss balls and foam rollers the most. He believed that these items could provide a challenging and interesting rehabilitation program for any of his patients. In his opinion, no other piece of equipment challenged the trunk muscles as well as the foam roller. Tim routinely placed all his patients on it, since not only back injuries, but also upper- and lower-extremity injuries, could benefit from the challenge of the foam roller.

As much as he liked foam-roller rehabilitation, Tim also liked the Swiss ball for its versatility in upper- and lower-extremity and trunk rehabilitation. Whenever possible, he liked to include both of these items in a patient's program. He would often provide patients with a Swiss ball and foam roller so that they could continue their rehabilitation programs at home.

The beauty of the foam roller and Swiss ball, Tim thought, was that the rehabilitation exercises could be easy or difficult; patients could perform them initially in the clinic and then progress to a home program; they weren't expensive; and they made what might otherwise be a boring weight program, fun and interesting for those patients he worked with who were physically active.

Life is change. Growth is optional.

Karen Kaiser Clark, author, speaker

Sports medicine and the treatment of athletic injuries have changed over the years. Many techniques we use today were unknown 20 years ago. Among the changes in therapeutic exercise techniques is the use of Swiss balls and foam rollers. These are both relatively new items in the orthopedic and sports medicine arena that are commonly used in therapeutic exercise programs today.

This chapter presents information about how to introduce Swiss balls and foam rollers into the sport rehabilitation program, techniques to use, and examples of exercises that patients can perform with them. We also consider indications, precautions, and contraindications that represent crucial guidelines for the use of Swiss balls and foam rollers in therapeutic exercise programs.

SWISS BALLS

Swiss balls can be used in a progression of exercise to challenge flexibility, strength, muscle endurance, balance, coordination, and joint- and body-position awareness. Ball size is chosen according to the patient's height. Safety factors include avoidance of bouncing in combination with spine movements and being aware of several contraindications.

The Swiss ball, a large vinyl ball, was developed by an Italian toy manufacturer and first produced in 1963 under the name Gymnastik, and later, Gymnic. Using the Bobath method, Dr. Elsbeth Köng, a Swiss pediatrician, and Mary Quinton, an English physiotherapist, developed pediatric neurological rehabilitation programs using Swiss balls. In the 1960s, Dr. Susan Klein-Vogelbach, a physical therapist in Switzerland, began using the Swiss balls as an instructional tool in classes for adult orthopedic and other medical problems.

The term **Swiss ball** refers to the large vinyl balls because U.S. physical therapists who introduced the balls in this country first saw them used in clinics in Switzerland (Posner-Mayer 1995). Although Swiss balls were introduced in the United States during the early 1970s, they did not begin to catch on until the late 1980s. Today, many facilities use them for a wide range of orthopedic activities, including spinal stabilization, upper- and lower-extremity strengthening and flexibility, balance and coordination, and body awareness.

SWISS-BALL CHALLENGES

Most patients enjoy exercising with balls. Balls provide a diversion from uninteresting and boring exercises. Swiss-ball activities can also be more challenging than regular exercises. The use of the Swiss ball in therapeutic exercises can stimulate interest, offer activity complexity, and motivate the patient to perform more diligently.

The Swiss ball can provide challenges within a variety of rehabilitation parameters. Swiss-ball exercises can increase flexibility, strength, muscle endurance, balance, coordination, and joint- and body-position awareness. They can be used for open and closed chain activities. They can provide for a progression of difficulty to continually challenge the patient as parameters improve. Swiss balls can be used throughout a therapeutic exercise program to offer the patient a number of stimulating activities.

A simple activity becomes more complex and challenging when it incorporates additional elements. For example, standing on the ground is a relatively simple activity for a patient, but standing on a boat that is moving through water, or standing on skis while moving downhill, is more challenging. Sitting on a chair at a desk requires little balance; sitting on a Swiss ball requires more balance. Lying on a table is no challenge, but lying prone on a Swiss ball with only one hand in contact with the ground requires effort.

Activity on a Swiss ball requires more effort because the surface is unstable—the instability challenges balance. Coordination is more difficult on a Swiss ball because more than one body segment and more than one system must participate at one time to maintain position or balance during an activity. Coordination is additionally tested if the patient is required to perform more than one activity while on the Swiss ball.

Body weight can be used in a variety of positions to offer resistance during activity. Using weights during exercises on the Swiss ball makes the exercise more stressful. The unstable surface requires a greater effort by the exercising muscles, as well as effort by a greater number of muscles, to perform the exercise. Increasing repetitions, sets, and difficulty of the exercises on the Swiss ball can each improve muscle endurance and strength.

Flexibility can also be improved on the Swiss ball. Many people find the ball a comfortable surface on which to perform stretching exercises. The Swiss ball can also provide a comfortable and relaxing gravity-assisted method of stretching (figure 14.1).

When the body performs an activity, it receives feedback on the accuracy and quality of the performance in the form of sensory information from visual, auditory, vestibular, and somatosensory systems. Adjustments in performance are made based on the feedback received and interpreted at various neural levels as discussed in chapter 8. Joint- and body-position awareness is facilitated in Swiss-ball exercises

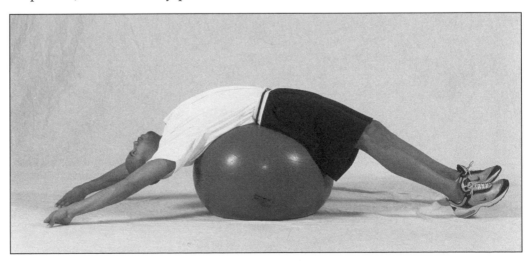

▌Figure 14.1
Gravity-assisted
Swiss-ball stretch.

because there is a continual change of position, and the body must adjust and adapt to those changes appropriately, while performing the activities correctly.

INCREASING SWISS-BALL CHALLENGES

Whether your goal is to increase strength, balance, or flexibility, there are several ways you can make Swiss-ball activities more challenging. The obvious modification is the addition of resistance equipment such as weights, rubber tubing, or bands or the use of manual resistance to increase strength gains.

Other modifications include decreasing the base of support. For example, if a patient is balancing on the ball with both hands on the floor, a narrower placement of the hands will make the activity more difficult. This activity becomes even more difficult if you have the patient perform it with only one hand on the ground, or perform movement on the ball while supporting the body with one hand on the floor (figure 14.2).

Increasing the lever-arm length makes the activity more difficult. For example, a push-up performed on the Swiss ball will increase in difficulty if the ball is moved from under the thighs to under the shins (figure 14.3).

Increasing the distance traveled is another way to make the exercise more difficult. Going through a greater range of motion requires recruitment of more muscle fibers, so the muscle must work harder. For example, the difficulty of a squat exercise with the Swiss ball is increased if the range of motion of the squat is increased (figure 14.4).

As with many other exercises, increasing the speed of movement and requiring the same amount of control as with the slower speed will increase the difficulty of the exercise on a Swiss ball.

EQUIPMENT AND EXERCISE AREA

There are currently several manufacturers of vinyl Swiss balls. Gymnic and Physioball are well-known Swiss-ball names. These balls are durable enough to withstand an individual's weight. The Gymnic ball will hold 454 kg (1000 lb), while the Physioball resists loads up to 299 kg (660 lb).

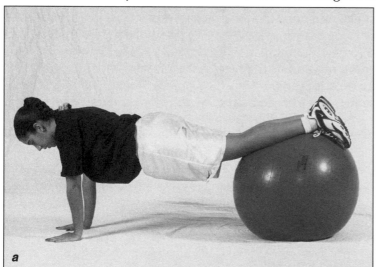

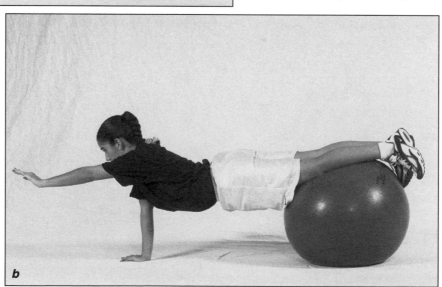

▌Figure 14.2 Reduced base of support from two arms (*a*) to one arm (*b*) on Swiss ball increases the activity's difficulty.

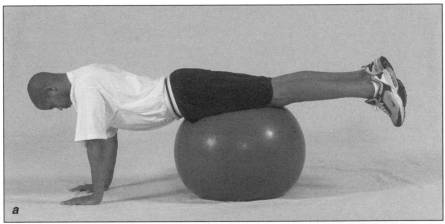

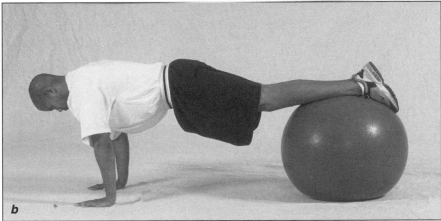

■ **Figure 14.3** Increased lever-arm length on Swiss ball increases the activity's difficulty. Ball is moved from the thighs *(a)* to the lower legs *(b)*.

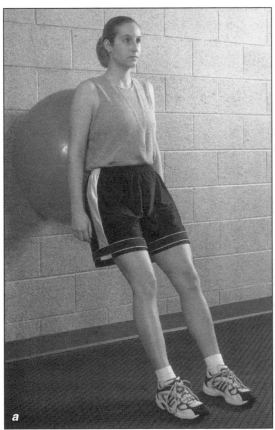 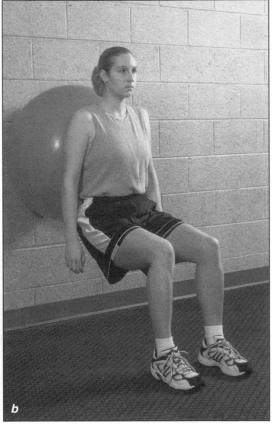

■ **Figure 14.4** Moving through a greater ROM on the Swiss ball requires greater muscle activity. *(a)* Slight squat motion, *(b)* full squat.

Swiss balls come in various sizes. A given company makes balls in different colors corresponding to different sizes; but because the colors vary among the companies, you should select balls according to size, not color. Ball size is indicated by diameter. The size to select for a particular patient is determined by the patient's height. Table 14.1 lists appropriate Swiss-ball sizes for individuals of varying heights. When the patient is sitting on the ball, the hips and knees should be at 90°. If the patient's height is between the heights listed in table 14.1, use the larger-sized ball and underinflate it to fit the patient.

Table 14.1   Swiss-Ball Sizes

Patient's height	Swiss-ball size (diameter)	
	cm	in.
Under 5 ft	45	18
5 ft to 5 ft 7 in.	55	$21\frac{1}{2}$
5 ft. 8 in. to 6 ft. 2 in.	65	25
6 ft 3 in. to 6 ft. 10 in.	75	$29\frac{1}{2}$
Over 6 ft 10 in.	85	$33\frac{1}{2}$

The floor surface should be firm and smooth but not slippery. Firm mats, linoleum, hardwood, and low-pile carpet are good surfaces. Surfaces should not be rough or uneven. Swiss balls should not be used outdoors because of the unevenness of the surface and because objects on the ground, such as pebbles or debris, can puncture them. The area where a patient exercises with a Swiss ball should be spacious enough to allow moving and rolling without danger of hitting furniture or other objects that could cause injury.

SAFETY FACTORS

The sport rehabilitation specialist should keep some safety factors in mind when beginning an exercise session that uses a Swiss ball. The patient's clothing should be free of objects such as belt buckles that may puncture the ball. The patient should wear rubber-soled shoes that provide traction. If the shoes are worn outside, the soles should be inspected for pebbles that could fall off and puncture the ball.

The patient's clothing should be proper athletic wear that allows freedom of movement. If the individual will be on the floor on the knees, he or she should wear sweatpants or warm-up pants that will protect the skin from abrasions. Pants of these types will also prevent the skin from sticking to the ball and reduce restriction of movement or skin discomfort.

When performing exercises on the Swiss ball, patients should not combine bouncing on the ball with bending and twisting or rotating the spine. This can cause injury to the spine. The exercises should be performed with control and not so quickly that the motions are incorrect.

The patient's hair should be restrained if necessary, so that it does not impede the exercise, hamper vision, or get in the way.

CONTRAINDICATIONS

Although contraindications are not commonly seen in the athletic population, the sport rehabilitation specialist should be aware of them. An individual who has a fear of using or falling off the ball, and who cannot be reassured, should not use the Swiss ball. Increased pain, dizziness, or any other undesirable symptom is an indication to stop the exercises. Any disease or injury that is contraindicated for specific exercises should be avoided. For example, using the feet to stabilize while sitting on the ball would be contraindicated when the patient is non-weight bearing on an injured knee.

Swiss-Ball Care

As mentioned earlier, the Swiss ball should not be used outdoors. A Swiss ball can be easily damaged by pebbles or other sharp or hard objects on the ground. The balls should be kept away from excessive or prolonged heat sources such as lamps, heat ducts, and direct sunlight.

Swiss balls should be inflated when at room temperature. They can be inflated with an air compressor, air-mattress pump, or gas-station air compressor or pump with a trigger nozzle attachment. A bicycle pump will not work well because of the large volume of air the ball requires—using a bicycle pump will simply take too long. A ball is maximally inflated when it is firm; but as already indicated, less-than-maximal inflation is appropriate when a patient's height requires a slightly smaller ball.

Warm, soapy water and a cloth are used to clean the ball. Abrasive or chemical cleaners may cause damage and should be avoided.

SWISS-BALL EXERCISES

Swiss-ball exercises can improve trunk stabilization, flexibility, and strength; there are also many Swiss-ball exercises for strengthening the upper and lower extremities. The upper-extremity exercises become more challenging if the Swiss ball is used in combination with such devices as rubber bands or tubing and weights.

Many Swiss-ball exercises are used for trunk stabilization, but a number of these can be used to strengthen the upper and lower extremities as well. The activities described here by no means represent all Swiss-ball exercises and are examples only. As with many other therapeutic exercises, specific Swiss-ball activities are limited only by the sport rehabilitation specialist's knowledge and imagination and the patient's restrictions.

TRUNK EXERCISES

For all Swiss-ball exercises, the patient should be instructed to maintain a pelvic-neutral posture throughout the activity. To maintain this position, the patient must know where his or her pelvic neutral is located and must keep some tension in the muscles controlling the position, especially the abdominals.

Bounce and Kick

This is a stabilization exercise. The patient sits on the ball in pelvic neutral. Without rotating the spine or hips, the patient bounces on the ball. While bouncing, he or she alternates kicking out one leg and then the other, one kick for each bounce (figure 14.5). This becomes more difficult if the patient simultaneously raises the opposite arm.

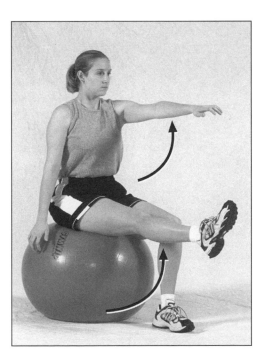

■ **Figure 14.5**
Bounce and kick.

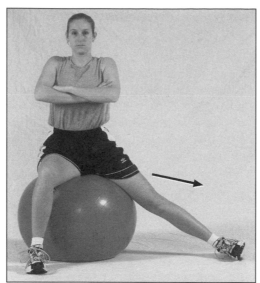

■ **Figure 14.6** Side foot reach.

Side Foot Reach

This is also a stabilization exercise. The patient sits on the ball in pelvic neutral. The arms are crossed (figure 14.6). As the patient bounces on the ball, he or she extends one leg out to the side and then brings it back to the starting position. Movements should coincide with the bounces. The opposite leg is then moved to the other side in similar fashion. This is more challenging if arm movements are added, with the same-side arm extending sideways simultaneously with the leg.

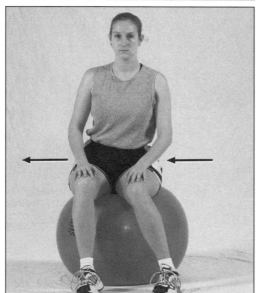

■ **Figure 14.7** Lateral glide to the right.

Lateral Glide

The lateral glide is for pelvic flexibility. The patient sits on the ball in pelvic neutral (figure 14.7). The pelvis is rolled out to one side and then the other, then returns to pelvic neutral. The patient uses the trunk muscles to perform the exercise, not the legs.

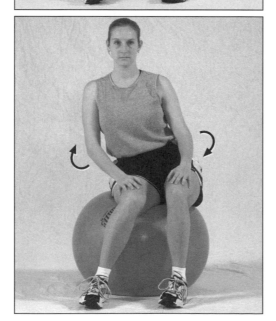

■ **Figure 14.8** Clockwise pelvic circles.

Pelvic Circles

This exercise is for pelvic flexibility. The patient sits on the ball in pelvic neutral and rotates the pelvis first clockwise and then counterclockwise (figure 14.8). The pelvic and trunk muscles are used to produce the motion, not the legs. The legs and shoulders should move minimally.

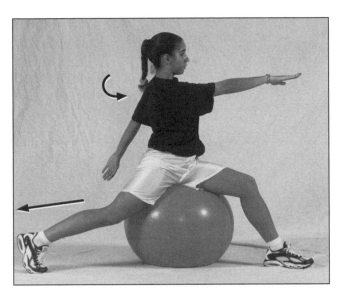

Figure 14.9 Trunk rotation in sitting.

Trunk Rotation in Sitting

This exercise is for trunk flexibility. The patient sits on the ball in pelvic neutral with the arms abducted to 90°. The trunk is rotated to the left, and the right arm reaches in the direction of the trunk rotation as the right leg is extended behind the person (figure 14.9). The patient returns to the starting position and repeats the motion to the right.

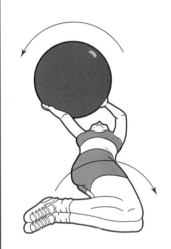

Figure 14.10 Trunk rotation in supine.

Trunk Rotation in Supine

This is a variation of the exercise just described. The patient lies supine on the floor with the knees and hips bent, holding the ball in the hands with the arms straight and directly overhead. Keeping the abdominals tight to stabilize the spine, the individual moves the ball to the right as the hips are rotated to the left (figure 14.10). The hip movement is initiated from the low back.

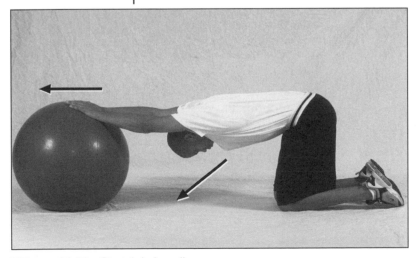

Figure 14.11 Stretch in kneeling.

Stretch in Kneeling

This stretch for the back can be used for the shoulders also. The patient kneels on the floor with his or her hands on the ball, which is in front of the person. The patient bows forward and lets the ball roll out (figure 14.11). The arms are straight as the patient attempts to lower the upper trunk toward the floor.

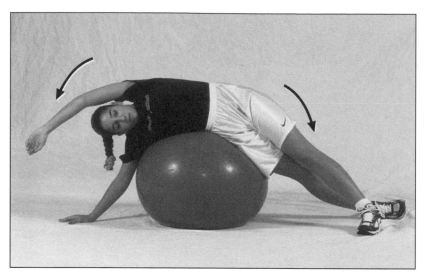

■ **Figure 14.12**   Lateral stretch.

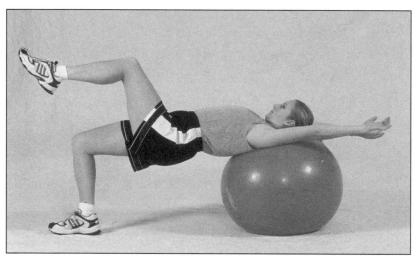

■ **Figure 14.13**   Supine leg lift.

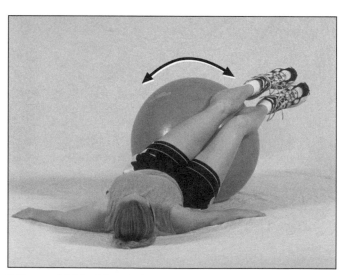

■ **Figure 14.14**   Hip rotation.

Lateral Stretch

This stretch is for the lateral trunk. The patient kneels beside the ball and lies sideways on the ball to touch the lower hand to the floor (figure 14.12). The upper arm is extended overhead.

Thoracic Stretch

The patient sits on the ball with the feet about shoulder-width apart. He or she then lies back on the ball as it rolls up the back until the buttocks are toward the floor and the shoulder blades are on the ball (figure 14.1). The patient then raises the arms overhead and pushes the ball backward with the legs so that the head moves closer to the floor and the knees are straight.

Supine Leg Lift

This exercise strengthens the back extensors. The patient sits on the ball and walks out until the head and shoulders are supported on the ball (figure 14.13). While the individual maintains pelvic neutral, he or she alternately lifts the legs off the floor in a marching sequence. There should be no rolling of the trunk or hips, and the pelvis should not drop. This becomes more difficult if done with the arms overhead.

Hip Rotation

This hip rotation exercise strengthens the oblique muscles. The patient lies in supine on the floor, with the lower legs on the ball and arms at the sides (figure 14.14). The individual rolls the knees from side to side as far as possible without falling off the ball. The abdominals, kept tightened, initiate the movement of the hips. The back should not arch, and the shoulders should remain on the floor throughout the exercise.

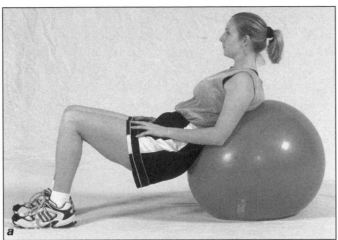

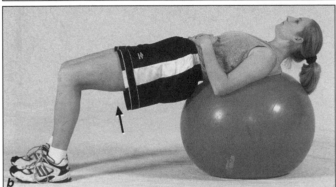

Bridging

This exercise, which strengthens the back extensors, can be performed in two positions. In one variation, the patient is positioned on the ball so that the shoulder blades are on the ball and the feet are on the floor about shoulder-width apart (figure 14.15, a and b). The pelvis is in neutral and the abdominals are tight as the patient lifts the buttocks and extends the hips. The movement is initiated at the buttocks, and the pelvis is kept in neutral throughout. This exercise is more challenging if the patient marches in place while maintaining pelvic neutral.

The other variation of the bridging exercise is with the patient lying supine on the floor and the feet on the Swiss ball. Keeping pelvic neutral, the individual lifts the hips off the floor as the buttocks and abdominals are tightened (figure 14.15c). You can make this exercise more difficult by having the patient alternate leg lifts off the ball (figure 14.15d). The exercise also becomes more challenging if you have the patient change the arm positions, from arms extended away from the body, to arms across the chest, to hands behind the head.

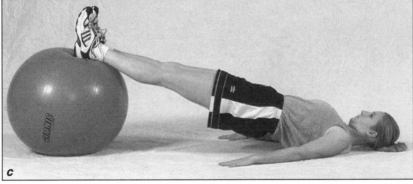

▌Figure 14.15
Bridging: *(a)* beginning position, *(b)* end position, *(c)* variation—isometric hold with feet on ball, *(d)* variation—alternate leg raise while maintaining trunk position.

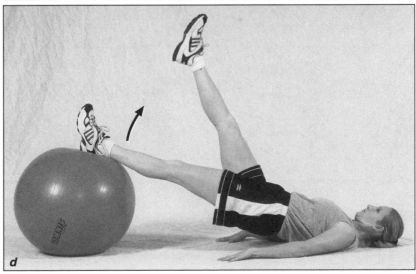

Back Extension in Prone

This exercise strengthens the back extensors. The patient lies prone on the ball; the ball is under the lower abdomen and pelvis, and the balls of the patient's feet are on the floor. The trunk is flexed forward with the pelvis in neutral (figure 14.16a). The patient lifts his or her trunk by squeezing the gluteals and the lower back paraspinal

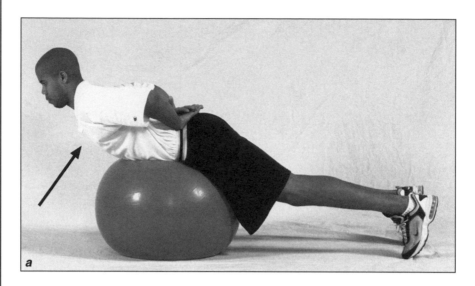

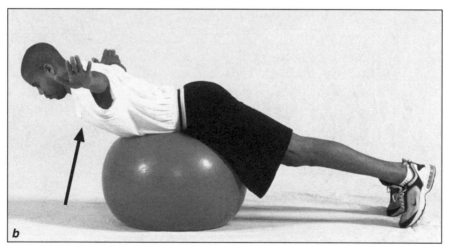

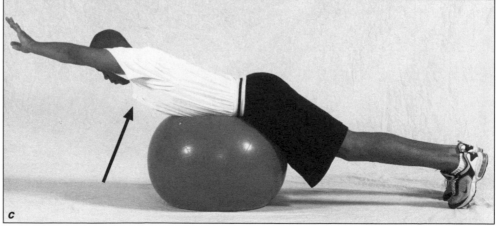

▌Figure 14.16 Back-extension progression. Changes in arm placement change the exercise's difficulty by moving the center of gravity.

(continued)

muscles. The arm positions change to increase the difficulty of the exercise, beginning with the hands behind the back and progressing so that the hands are out to the sides (figure 14.16b) and then overhead (figure 14.16c). To create an additional level of difficulty, the patient places his or her feet on a chair as seen in figure 14.16, d through f.

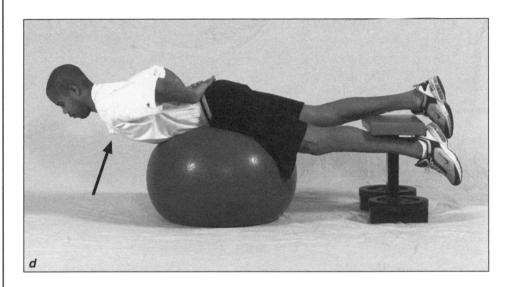

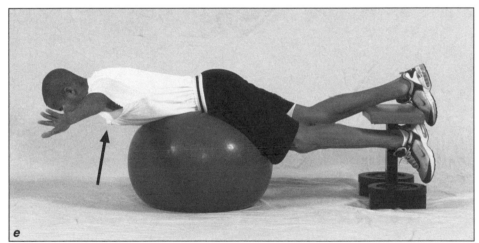

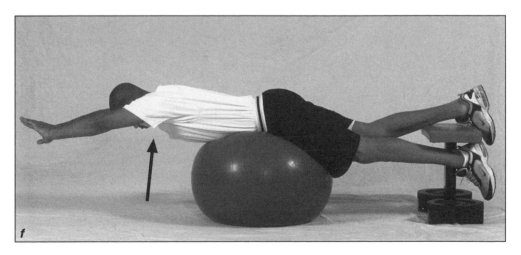

■ **Figure 14.16**
(continued)

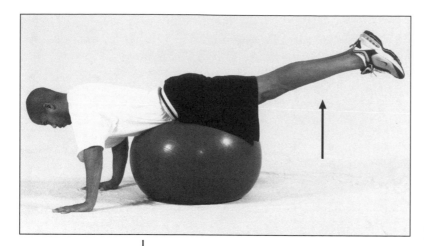

Prone Leg Lift

This leg lift strengthens the trunk extensors. The patient lies prone on the ball with the hands and the balls of the feet on the floor. The Swiss ball should be positioned under the lower abdomen and pelvis. The patient squeezes the buttocks to raise the legs, keeping the pelvis in neutral and the knees straight (figure 14.17).

❚ **Figure 14.17**   Prone leg lift.

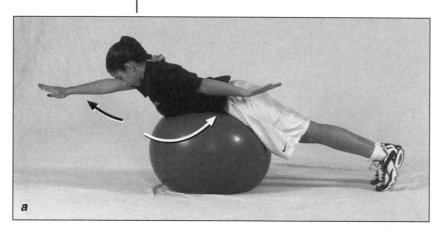

Swimming

This exercise strengthens the midback region. With the ball placed under the patient's stomach and the legs extended, with only the balls of the feet on the floor, the patient places one arm straight out in front and the other behind, by the hip (figure 14.18a). The patient maintains a neutral spine as the arms reverse positions (figure 14.18b). Weights can be added to increase the difficulty of the exercise.

❚ **Figure 14.18**
Swimming.

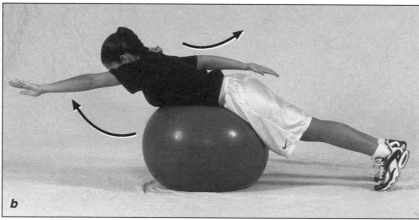

Seated Abdominal Strengthening

The patient sits on the Swiss ball in pelvic neutral. The feet are shoulder-width apart. Maintaining pelvic neutral, the person leans back on the ball, moving from the hips, not the spine (figure 14.19a). Changing the arm positions changes the difficulty of the exercise. The least-difficult variation is with the arms outstretched. As the arms move upward toward the head, the exercise increases in difficulty. The activity can stress the oblique muscles if the patient places the arms overhead and alternately lowers each arm to the opposite knee as seen in figure 14.19b.

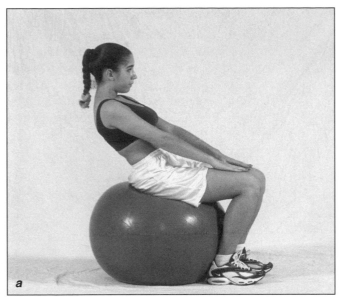
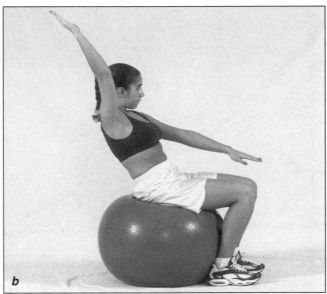

Figure 14.19 Seated abdominal strengthening: *(a)* with arms forward, *(b)* more difficult with alternating arms over head.

Ball Lift

The purpose of this exercise is to strengthen the lower abdominals. The patient lies on the back and maintains pelvic neutral. The ball is picked up between the ankles, and the hips are maintained at 90° flexion (figure 14.20a). With the lower abdominals kept tight, the knees are bent and straightened. The progression for this exercise is from moving the knees to lowering the legs toward the floor and straightening the knees as the legs are lowered (figure 14.20b). It is important that the lower abdominals remain tight throughout this exercise and that the lower back maintain contact with the floor.

To increase the difficulty, the patient rotates the legs, bringing one in front of the other and then reversing positions. Again, the pelvis should remain in neutral, and the lower spine remains in contact with the floor as seen in figure 14.20c.

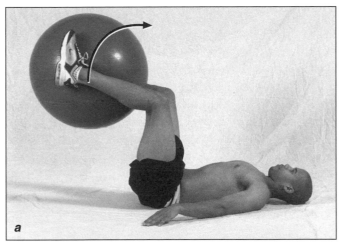
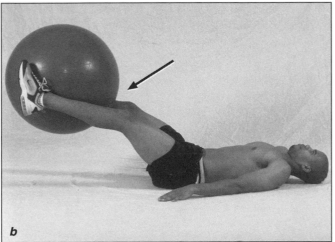
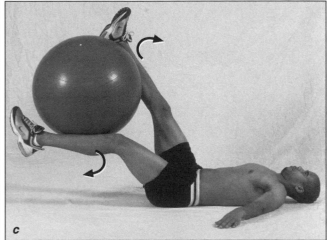

Figure 14.20 Ball lift: *(a)* hips are at 90° and knees are extended, *(b)* legs are lowered while back remains flat, *(c)* legs are rotated with spine in neutral.

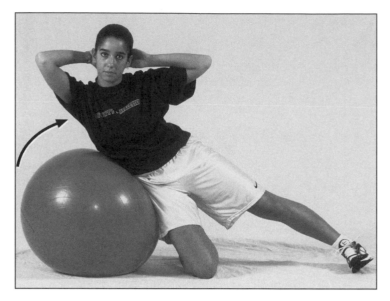

Side Sit-Ups

This sit-up strengthens the obliques. The patient kneels on the floor beside the ball. The individual then lies sideways on the ball, with the hip and trunk in contact with the ball and the upper leg outstretched (figure 14.21). The patient then lifts sideways off the ball.

▌**Figure 14.21**   Side sit-up.

Prone Walk-Out

This exercise strengthens the abdominals. The patient walks forward until the ball is at the shins and the arms support the weight of the trunk in a push-up position as shown in figure 14.22a. Pelvic neutral is maintained while this position is held on a timed basis.

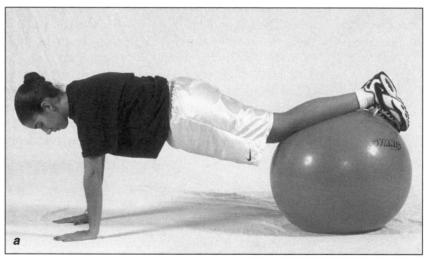

A variation of this exercise is to have the patient maintain pelvic neutral while bringing the knees up toward the chest (figure 14.22b). You can add difficulty by having the patient roll the ball to one side and then to the other so that the side of the thigh comes in contact with the ball while the legs remain in the position seen in figure 14.22b. This variation also exercises the oblique muscles.

▌**Figure 14.22**   Prone walk-out: *(a)* beginning position, *(b)* ending position. The ball can be rolled from side to side for an additional level of this exercise (see arrow).

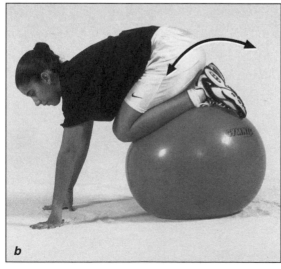

LOWER-EXTREMITY EXERCISES

Some of the trunk exercises also can be used for the lower extremities. A few additional exercises for the lower extremities are described here.

Reverse Squats

This squat strengthens quadriceps, calf, and gluteal muscles. The patient places the ball on the wall and leans into the ball such that the ball is at waist level (figure 14.23a). The patient remains on his or her toes throughout the exercise, and the feet are shoulder-width apart. The individual squats down to a comfortable level (figure 14.23b).

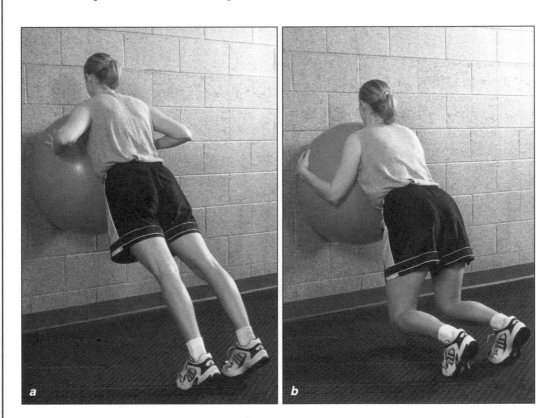

Figure 14.23
Reverse squats: *(a)* start position, *(b)* end position.

Side Leg Lift

This exercise strengthens hip abductors. The patient kneels and lies sideways on the ball in a position similar the side sit-up position shown in figure 14.21. The upper leg is lifted toward the ceiling with the knee straight and the leg in line with the trunk. The leg should not move into the flexion plane.

Half Squat

This exercise strengthens the quadriceps. The patient stands with the ball on the wall and with the ball placed in the low back. The feet are positioned shoulder-width apart, and far enough in front of the person so that when he or she squats, the knees do not bend more than 90° (figure 14.4). Additional knee flexion places too much stress on the patellofemoral joint. A patient who has knee pain during this exercise should place the feet farther out or reduce the depth of the squat.

Hamstring Curl

This exercise strengthens the hamstrings. The patient lies supine on the floor with his or her feet on the Swiss ball. The hips are kept off the floor so that the trunk and legs form a straight line, as illustrated in figure 14.16c. While maintaining a hip-elevated position, the patient bends the knees to move the ball closer to the hips, and then extends the knees to the starting position. A progression includes starting with the arms on the floor and then moving them to the chest and overhead. In another progression the patient first uses both legs, then crosses the uninvolved over the involved leg, and finally uses only the involved leg.

Side-Lying Ball Lift

This exercise strengthens the hip and trunk muscles. The patient lies on his or her side with the knees and hips extended; one arm is overhead, and the other is across the front for stabilization as shown in figure 14.24a. The ball is grasped between the lower legs, and the pelvis is maintained in neutral. Both legs are lifted off the floor as high as possible, with the legs and spine kept straight (figure 14.24b).

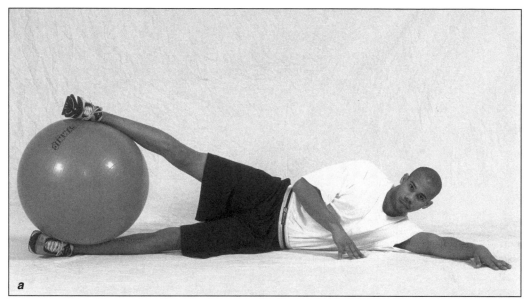

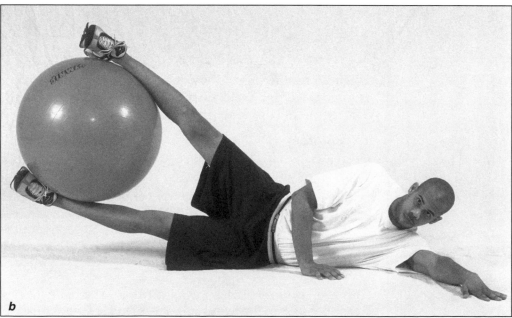

■ **Figure 14.24** Side-lying ball lift: *(a)* start position, *(b)* upward lateral movement of the legs.

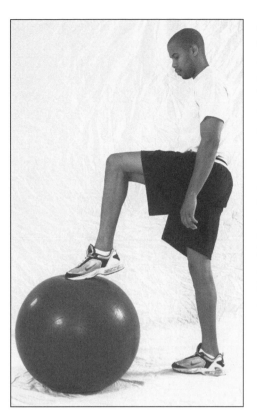

Figure 14.25 Ankle
motion exercise.

Ankle Motion Exercise

This is a balance exercise for the lower extremity. The patient stands in pelvic neutral with the uninjured foot on top of the ball; he or she then writes the alphabet with the uninjured foot, using the ball as a base of support (figure 14.25).

UPPER-EXTREMITY EXERCISES

As with the lower-extremity exercises, some of the upper-extremity exercises were described earlier in the section on trunk exercises. Although they are not mentioned here, many upper-extremity exercises using rubber tubing and rubber bands, as well as medicine-ball exercises, become more difficult when performed on the Swiss ball.

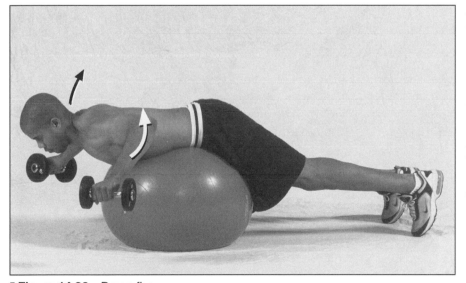

Figure 14.26   Prone flys.

Prone Flys

This exercise is used to strengthen scapular retractors. The patient lies prone on the Swiss ball with the ball under the lower abdomen or upper thighs. The legs are straight, with the balls of the feet in contact with the floor. The patient's arms are below the chest, and elbows are bent (figure 14.26). The patient lifts the elbows toward the ceiling and squeezes the shoulder blades together. Weight is used to provide resistance.

Triceps Extension

The patient is inclined or seated on the ball, with the ball supporting the low back or midback as illustrated in figure 14.16a. The abdominals are kept tight to maintain pelvic neutral. The arms are overhead with the elbows bent and hands behind the head. Keeping the arms above the head, the patient straightens the elbows.

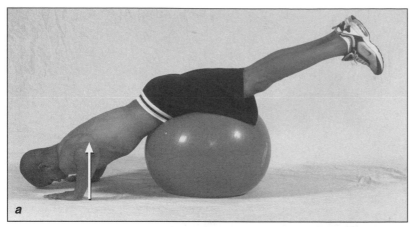

Push-Ups

The patient lies prone on the ball with hands on the floor and feet elevated. The ball is placed under the lower abdomen or pelvis (figure 14.27a). The patient performs a push-up, keeping good spinal alignment throughout the motion (figure 14.27b). Progressions of this exercise include placing the ball under the thighs, placing the ball under the lower legs (figure 14.27c), and performing the push-up with the hands on the ball and the feet on the floor (figure 14.27d).

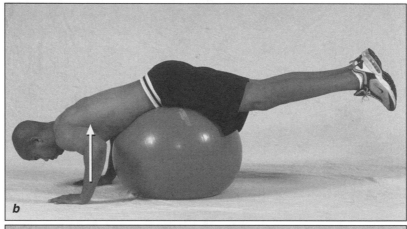

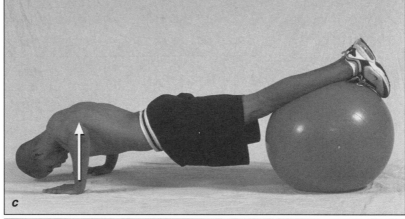

■ **Figure 14.27** Push-up progression: *(a)–(c)* progression is provided by increasing the lever-arm length, *(d)* progression is provided by using an unstable base for the arms.

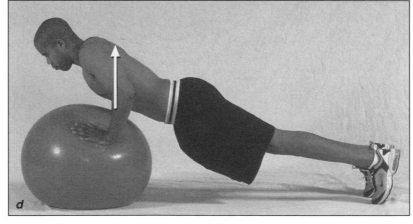

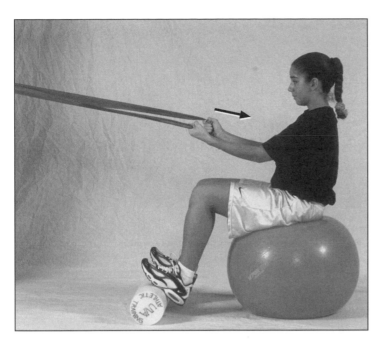

Scapular Retraction

This exercise uses the Swiss ball with rubber bands or tubing. The patient sits on the ball, with the feet on a foam roller for a more difficult exercise or on the floor for a less difficult exercise. While maintaining balance on the Swiss ball, the patient pulls the bands and squeezes the shoulder blades together, keeping the elbows below shoulder level (figure 14.28). Upper-extremity exercises using rubber tubing, medicine balls, and other equipment become more challenging with the use of the Swiss ball.

■ **Figure 14.28**   Scapular retraction.

FOAM ROLLERS

Foam rollers help to improve joint- and body-position awareness, balance, proprioception, flexibility, and strength. Precautions relate to various skin conditions and various types of hypermobility, and the sport rehabilitation specialist should keep in mind several contraindications.

Moshe Feldenkrais was one of the first to use rollers as a therapeutic tool. He used rollers in his Feldenkrais Method, discussed earlier in this text (chapter 11). Feldenkrais used wooden rollers until 1972, when he was introduced to **foam rollers** while in the United States.

In recent years, the use of foam rollers has become commonplace within rehabilitation in neurological, orthopedic, and sports medicine facilities. Several annual professional workshops and seminars in foam roller use take place across the country.

Foam rollers are used in therapeutic exercise to improve body awareness and joint-position sense, enhance balance and proprioception, aid in muscle re-education, and promote flexibility and strength. Because of its cylindrical shape, the foam roller provides little contact with the floor and moves quickly and easily; standing on the roller challenges the patient's balance reaction. As with the Swiss ball, the roller presents an unstable surface and thus a more challenging platform for performing what are normally easily managed activities. The use of foam rollers offers the patient a diversion from routine exercises and still accomplishes many of the same goals that more traditional exercises do. Rollers are relatively inexpensive and can be used in the treatment facility and at home.

FOAM-ROLLER DESIGN

Most foam rollers are made of Ethafoam, which is a polyethylene product; others are made of polyurethane. They all are cylindrical and come in a variety of lengths, circumferences, and densities. Diameters are 7.6, 10.0, and 15.2 cm (3, 4, and 6 in.). The lengths vary from 30 cm to about 180 cm (1–6 ft). Rollers can also be cut in half longitudinally with a bread knife to form a $^1/_2$ roll so one side is flat and the other is a half circle.

The Ethafoam rollers are dense rolls that can support up to 159 kg (350 lb). Because of their buoyancy, patients can also use them in aquatic therex programs. Their density makes them effective for use in soft-tissue and joint mobility exercises, and they are also firm enough for muscle strengthening. The Ethafoam rollers can also help to improve proprioception. The softer polyurethane rolls offer more stability. They can be more comfortable to lie on than the Ethafoam rollers, but they tend to lose their shape more quickly and become difficult to roll.

PRECAUTIONS AND CONTRAINDICATIONS

Before the sport rehabilitation specialist uses a foam roller, he or she must observe several precautions and must evaluate the patient for existing contraindications. If an individual has contusions, acne, or other skin disturbances, the sport rehabilitation specialist should observe for responses that aggravate the condition.

Patients experiencing temporary conditions of vertigo brought on by ear infections or other disorders should either postpone using a foam roller or should use the roller under careful supervision and be sure to perform slow, controlled, and adequately supported movements.

Hypermobility of joints, postpartum hypermobility, and acute fractures are conditions that require caution in the use of foam rolls. Performing some activities on a foam roller can aggravate these types of hypermobility.

A patient showing signs of nausea, light-headedness, pallor, or shortness of breath should be taken off the foam roller. The few outright contraindications for the use of foam rollers are commonsense ones. Any symptoms of increased pain, dizziness, nausea, or tinnitus are contraindications, as are full-weight-bearing restrictions on segments. Other contraindications not commonly seen in athletics include osteoporosis, connective-tissue disorders such as fibromyalgia and rheumatoid arthritis that are in a flare-up condition, current use of anticoagulant medication, and tumors.

FOAM-ROLLER EXERCISES

Patients can perform foam-roller exercises for the trunk, lower extremity, and upper extremity with or without other equipment such as Swiss balls and rubber tubing and bands.

As with the Swiss-ball exercises, the foam-roller exercises described here do not represent an entire program but rather serve only as examples. The exercises suggested may give you ideas for others. You can use foam rollers with equipment such as the Swiss ball, rubber tubing and bands, and other accessory equipment. The following exercises are presented according to body segment.

TRUNK EXERCISES

Some of the exercises described here for the trunk may also be used for upper and lower extremities. Some are stretching exercises, some are for strengthening, and others are self-massage techniques.

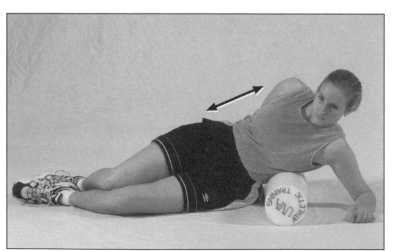

Quadratus Massage

This exercise relaxes the quadratus lumborum to increase range of motion. The patient lies on a horizontally positioned foam roller with the roller in the small of the back (figure 14.29). The individual rolls to his or her side and gently rolls back and forth to relax the quadratus.

∎ **Figure 14.29**   Quadratus massage.

Thoracic Massage

This exercise massages the thoracic area to relax muscles and improve range of motion. The patient lies supine on a foam roller positioned perpendicular to the line of the body. The roller is placed under the thoracic region (figure 14.30). The patient supports his or her head in both hands and keeps the buttocks lifted off the floor. He or she rolls gently up and down from the lower ribs upward to the shoulders.

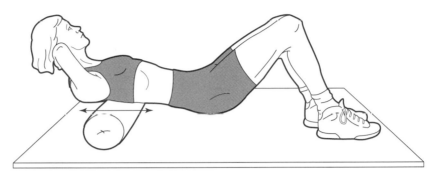

▌Figure 14.30
Thoracic massage.

Low Back Mobilization

The purpose of this exercise is to improve low back flexibility. The patient stands with feet shoulder-width apart; the foam roller is hooked under the elbows and across the low back. The patient arches the back into the roller.

Cat Stretch

This is a back-flexibility exercise using two foam rollers. The patient is in a kneeling quadruped position, with both knees on one roller and both hands on another roller. The patient arches the back up as high as possible by tightening the abdominals and then relaxes the back toward the floor.

Quadruped Balance

This exercise develops balance and pelvic stabilization. The patient kneels on one roller and places the hands on a second roller, as in the cat stretch just described. Keeping pelvic neutral throughout the exercise, the patient first lifts one leg and the opposite arm and then reverses the position (figure 14.31).

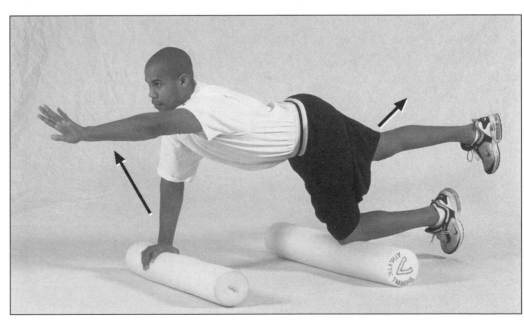

▌Figure 14.31
Quadruped balance using two foam rollers.

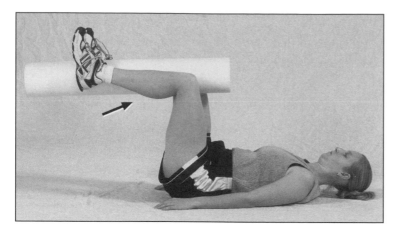

Supine Lower Abdominal Exercise

This exercise strengthens the lower abdominal muscles. The patient lies supine with the knees bent. The roller is placed between the knees (figure 14.32). The patient tightens the lower abdominals and lifts the knees toward the chest, keeping the back flat on the floor. The back should not arch at any time during this exercise.

■ **Figure 14.32**   Supine lower abdominal exercise.

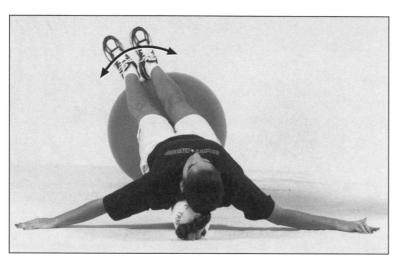

Supine Oblique Exercise

This exercise strengthens the obliques. The patient lies on the foam roller and places his or her feet on a Swiss ball (figure 14.33). While keeping the knees straight, the patient rolls the ball from side to side. The back should not arch.

■ **Figure 14.33**   Oblique exercise.

Abdominal Crunch

This exercise strengthens the abdominals. The patient takes a kneeling position; the roller is under both knees, and the hands are flat on the floor. The patient pulls the knees up toward the chest. This exercise becomes more difficult if the patient begins the exercise in a prone position (figure 14.34a) and moves to the same end position as in the easier exercise (figure 14.34b).

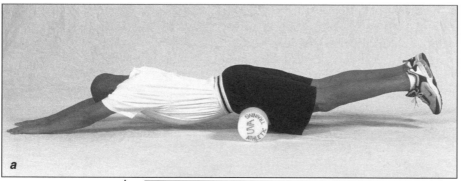

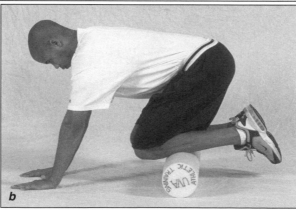

■ **Figure 14.34**   Abdominal crunch: *(a)* start position, *(b)* end position.

Rotational Crunch

This exercise strengthens the obliques. The patient lies prone on a Swiss ball with the thighs on the ball and each hand on a $^1/_2$ roller, flat side down (figure 14.35a). The patient brings the knees toward the chest and then rotates the hips, first to one side and then to the other, so that the bottom lateral thigh rests on the ball (figure 14.35b). A pelvic neutral position is maintained throughout the exercise. This exercise becomes more difficult with the $^1/_2$ rollers placed flat side up.

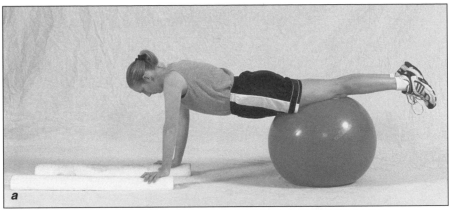

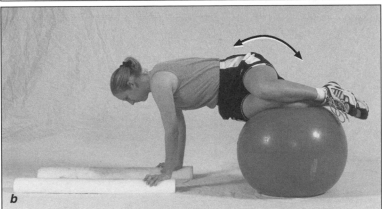

■ **Figure 14.35** Rotational crunch: *(a)* start position, *(b)* with knees up, patient rolls side to side from one hip to the other.

Bridging

This exercise strengthens hamstrings, hip extensors, and back extensors. The patient lies supine on the floor with the feet placed on a horizontally positioned foam roller (figure 14.36a). The patient lifts the hips upward and rolls the roller toward the buttocks. This activity becomes more difficult if the individual performs it with only one leg at a time (figure 14.36b). A pelvic neutral position should be maintained throughout.

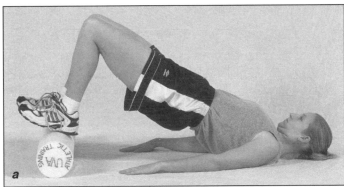

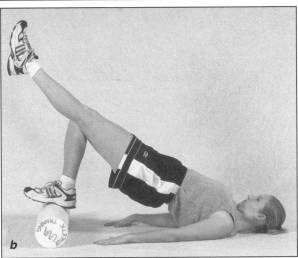

■ **Figure 14.36** Bridging: *(a)* start position, *(b)* end position.

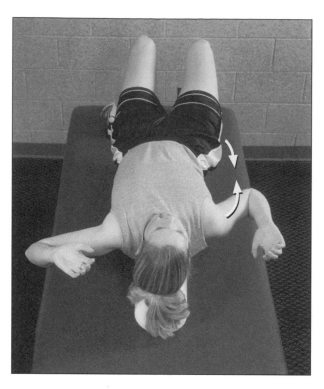

Quadratus Lumborum Strengthening

The patient lies supine longitudinally on the foam roller. The knees are bent and the feet flat on the floor. The shoulders and elbows are at 90° in a goalpost position. The patient brings the right elbow and the right rear pocket toward each other without changing the arm position and then repeats the movement to the opposite side (figure 14.37).

■ **Figure 14.37**
Quadratus lumborum strengthening.

LOWER-EXTREMITY EXERCISES

Foam roller activities for the lower extremities can include techniques for massage, flexibility, strengthening, and proprioception.

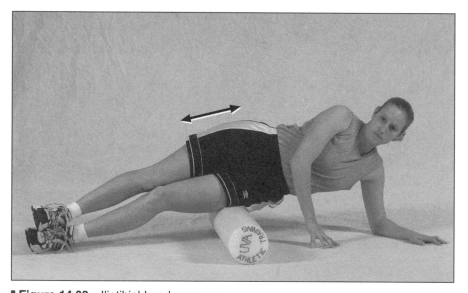

Iiotibial-Band Massage

This exercise massages the iliotibial band (ITB) to increase flexibility. The patient lies on his or her left side with the left elbow bent. The roller is placed under the left thigh, and the left leg is positioned under and in front of the right leg (figure 14.38). The patient gently moves the roller from the knee to the hip. The reverse position is used to massage the right ITB. Areas of tenderness will be areas of soft-tissue restriction. This massage should normally be comfortable.

■ **Figure 14.38** Iliotibial-band massage.

Quadriceps Massage

This exercise massages the quadriceps to increase flexibility. The patient lies on the floor with the roller in a horizontal position under and across the thighs. The individual then places his or her upper-body weight on the hands and pulls the body back and forth with the arms, allowing the roller to gently move up and down the thigh.

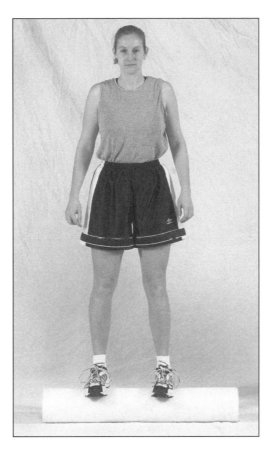

Figure 14.39
Standing balance.

Standing Balance

This exercise improves balance. The patient stands with both feet on a horizontally positioned foam roller (figure 14.39). To prevent falling, the patient needs to mount the roller using both hands to grasp a support structure, such as a table or spotters, and must become secure before letting go with the hands. It may be necessary for the sport rehabilitation specialist to assist with additional manual support in the initial attempts to balance. If this exercise is too difficult, the patient can begin by standing on one or two $^1/_2$ rollers with the flat side up, that is, by using either one $^1/_2$ roller for each foot or only one $^1/_2$ roller for both feet. You can make this exercise more difficult by having the patient stand only on one leg. Standing in a forward-backward tandem position on the roller is also more advanced.

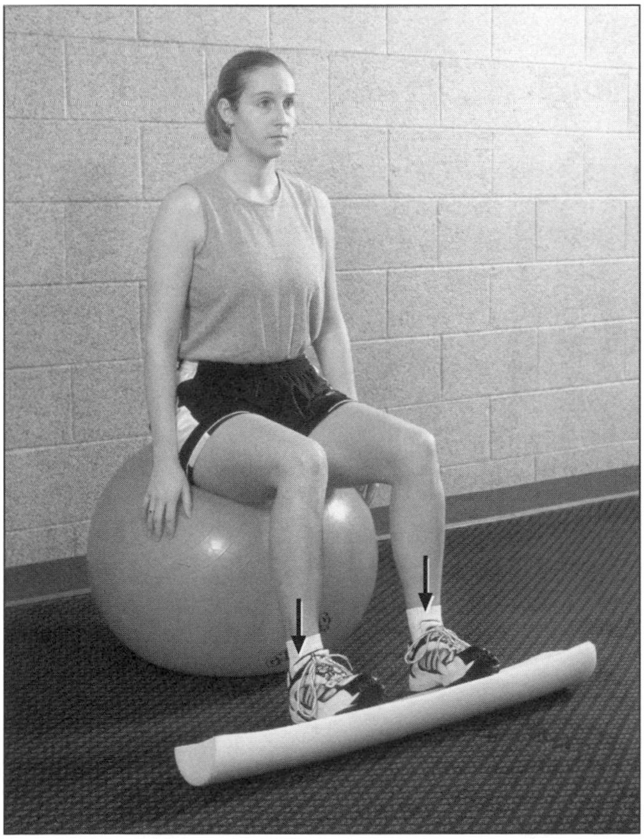

Anterior Tibialis Stretch

The patient kneels on the floor. The foam roller is on the ground behind the body and crosswise with the body. The tops of the distal feet are placed on top of the roller. The patient then leans back to sit on his or her heels while keeping the distal feet on the roller.

Gastrocnemius Stretch

The patient stands on the flat portion of a $^1/_2$ roller, with the balls of the feet on the roller and the heels on the floor. The knees are straight but not locked, and the body leans forward slightly while the patient uses the arms for balance and support.

Soleus Stretch

The patient sits in a chair and places the balls of the feet on a $^1/_2$ roller, flat side up (figure 14.40). He or she then pushes the heels to the floor.

Figure 14.40   Sitting soleus stretch.

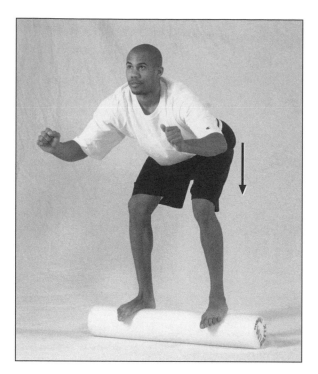

Squats

The patient stands on the roller, with the roller in a horizontal position and the feet about shoulder-width apart. The patient squats and raises the arms in front to maintain balance (figure 14.41). This is an advanced exercise that requires good balance and postural control. The patient may need stabilizing assistance from a spotter or need to use one hand on a stable object until balance is maintained.

▌Figure 14.41
Squats.

UPPER-EXTREMITY EXERCISES

Upper-extremity exercises on the foam roller can begin early in a therapeutic exercise program in the form of flexibility exercises and then progress to open and closed kinetic chain activities as the patient improves.

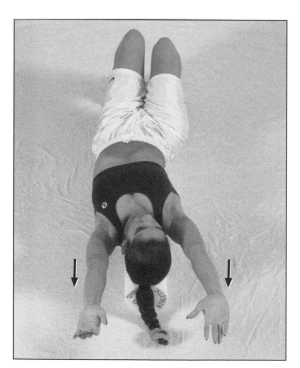

Arm Stretches

The patient lies supine longitudinally on the roller with the knees bent and feet flat on the floor. The patient then moves the arms 90° away from the body, then 135°, and then overhead (figure 14.42). During each of these movements he or she attempts to pull the arms to the floor.

Push-Ups

The patient kneels on the floor, places the hands shoulder-width apart on the roller, and then performs a push-up. With the hands on the roller, the progression for this exercise is from the modified position on the knees, to the regular position, to a position in which another roller is placed under the knees, and finally to a position in which the additional roller is placed under the shins.

▌Figure 14.42 Arm stretches.

Resistive Band Exercises in Standing

Isolated or combined movement patterns using rubber tubing or bands can be performed on foam rollers. The beginning-level exercise is performed on $^1/_2$ rollers with the flat side up (figure 14.43), and the more advanced exercise is performed with the patient's standing on a full foam roller.

Resistive Band Bench Press in Supine

The patient lies in a supine hook-lying position with the knees bent and the feet flat on the floor. The resistive band is secured under the roller at chest level. The patient pushes the hand toward the ceiling until the elbow is in full extension. This exercise can be performed either with one arm or with both (figure 14.44).

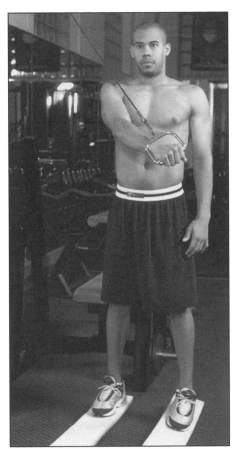

Figure 14.43 Resistive band exercise in standing.

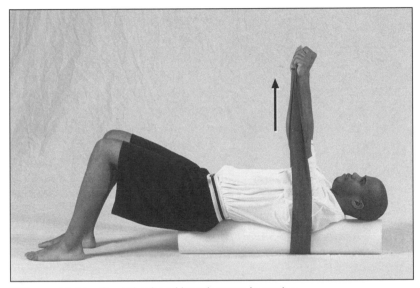

Figure 14.44 Resistive band bench press in supine.

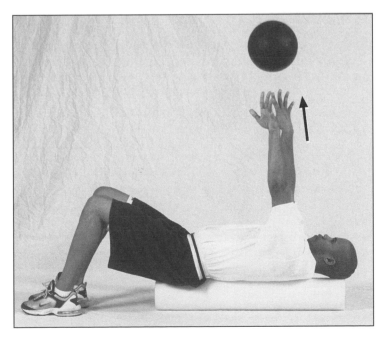

Ball Toss in Supine

The patient lies in a supine hook-lying position on the roller with the knees bent and feet flat on the floor. He or she then tosses a ball, either a Swiss ball or a medicine ball, toward the ceiling (figure 14.45).

Triceps Press

The patient sits on the floor with the legs straight out in front. One roller is placed under the ankles, and a small roller is placed on each side of the body near the hips. The patient places his or her hands on the rollers next to the hips and presses down to straighten the elbows and lift the buttocks off the floor. The shoulders should depress the scapulae as much as possible.

Figure 14.45 Ball toss in supine.

SUMMARY

1. *Explain how Swiss balls and foam rollers can increase the challenge of a traditional exercise.*

   Swiss balls and foam rollers provide an unstable surface for an exercise. They can be used for open and closed chain activities. They can provide a progression of difficulty to continually challenge the patient as parameters improve. Swiss balls can be used throughout a therapeutic exercise program to offer a number of stimulating challenges to the patient.

2. *Identify the rehabilitation parameters that are benefited by the use of Swiss balls or foam rollers.*

   Flexibility, strength, muscle endurance, balance, coordination, and joint- and body-position awareness are all stressed with Swiss ball and foam roller activities.

3. *Discuss safety factors, precautions, and contraindications relating to the use of Swiss balls and foam rollers.*

   For safety, the patient's clothing should be proper athletic wear to allow freedom of movement and should be free of objects such as belt buckles; shoes should have rubber soles to provide traction; bouncing on the ball should not be combined with bending and twisting or rotating of the spine; long hair should be restrained; and exercises should be performed with control and not too quickly. Precautions for the sport rehabilitation specialist to observe include carefully explaining and demonstrating the exercise before having the patient attempt it, taking proper care of the equipment, fitting the ball correctly, and not using the equipment if you have any doubt about an patient's ability to handle it. Contraindications include fear of falling off the ball or roller, use of any medication that poses a danger, and complaints of increased pain or dizziness.

4. *Explain how to properly fit a Swiss ball.*

   With the patient sitting on the ball and the feet flat on the floor, the hips and knees should be at 90°.

5. *List one exercise each for the trunk, upper extremity, and lower extremity using a Swiss ball, and identify its purpose.*

   A bridge is an exercise for strengthening the back extensors; hip rotations in supine are used to gain flexibility and strength of the hip muscles; and a push-up with the feet on the ball can serve as an early upper-extremity strengthening exercise.

6. *List one exercise each for the trunk, upper extremity, and lower extremity using foam rollers, and identify its purpose.*

   Lying on the foam roller and lowering the knees from the chest is a lower abdominal strengthening exercise; lying sideways on the roller and rolling the lateral thigh along the foam roller is a massage technique for the ITB; and lying with the foam roller down the spine with the arms out to the side is a stretch for the anterior shoulder.

CRITICAL THINKING QUESTIONS

1. Because the Swiss ball can be used early in rehabilitation, you decide to use it in stabilization exercises for weak scapular muscles. Identify three low-level stabilization exercises that would incorporate the Swiss ball. What would be a more rigorous Swiss-ball stabilization exercise? Identify a Swiss-ball exercise that can also be used for the trunk.

2. You have decided to give a Swiss ball to a patient with a back injury. You feel that she is now ready to continue the Swiss-ball exercises on her own at home. You want to limit the number of exercises to 10 so that the patient will be more likely to perform all of them. Identify no more than 10 exercises that you would give this patient, and justify each one.

3. A patient wants to buy a Swiss ball to use at home during the semester break but does not know what size to buy. What guidance would you give him?

4. A patient with weak abdominals is going home for the summer and wants to take with her either a Swiss ball or foam roller, but not both. Which one would you advise her to take with her and why? List four exercises on the piece of equipment you have selected for her to take.

REFERENCE

Posner-Mayer, J. 1995. *Swiss ball applications for orthopedic and sports medicine.* Denver: Ball Dynamics International.

SUGGESTED READING

Craeger, C.C. 1996. *Therapeutic exercises using foam rollers.* Berthoud, CO: Executive Physical Therapy.

Institute of Physical Art. 1991. *Integrating function: The foam roll approach.* Steamboat Springs, CO: Author.

CHAPTER FIFTEEN

Therapeutic Exercise for Tendinitis

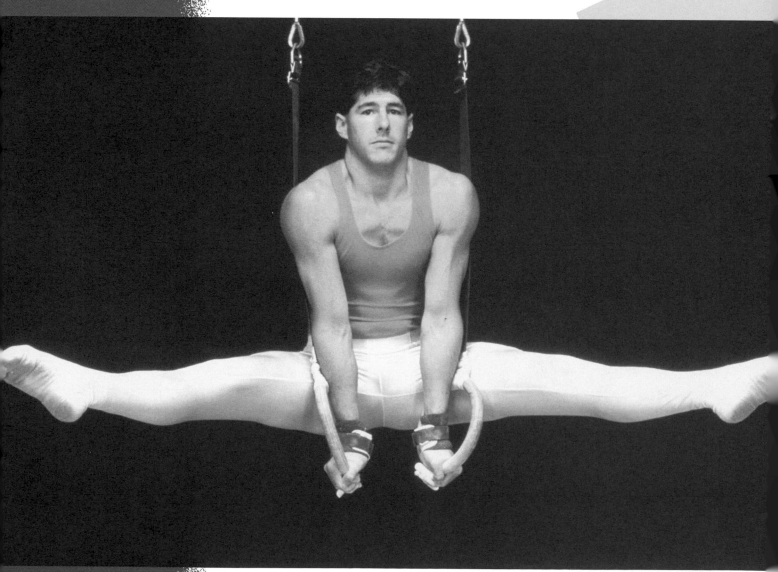

© Action Images/Brian Drake.

OBJECTIVES

After completing this chapter, you should be able to do the following:

1. Define tendinitis.
2. Discuss various etiologies of tendinitis.
3. Explain the inflammatory response of tendons.
4. Identify parameters governing the initial treatment for tendinitis.
5. Outline the progression of a tendinitis treatment program.

During her career, Misti Donns had seen many athletes with tendinitis. As much as she urged athletes to report early onsets of tendinitis, it seemed that they consistently waited until the problem became much more difficult to treat than it would have been if the athlete had been seen in the early stages of the condition.

Misti knew that tendinitis could not be treated like acute injuries, especially in the beginning. She enjoyed the challenge of treating cases of tendinitis because she had to be a detective to discover the cause and reduce the risk that the tendinitis would return later. As much as she enjoyed the challenge, she often became frustrated with the frequently slow progression of the treatment program. Of course, each patient responded differently to the treatment; but Misti realized that if the injury were treated early, improvements could occur much sooner than they would when the patient delayed reporting the injury, thinking it would go away on its own. If only there were some way she could impress on athletes the importance of early intervention.

No day in which you learn something is a complete loss.

–David Eddings, *King of the Murgos*

Although tendinitis can affect many body segments, it is worthwhile to discuss this condition in a separate chapter rather than including it in chapters on specific body segments. Looking at tendinitis separately makes sense because treatment of tendinitis differs from treatment of acute conditions, yet treatment of tendinitis in one area is similar to treatment of tendinitis in another area.

TERMINOLOGY

Tendinitis is the global, albeit inaccurate, term used to identify an inflammation in a tendon area.

There are many variations of tendinitis, and various terms are used to describe these conditions. These terms relate to the specific tissue involved. They can be confusing, so we will clarify them briefly here. **Tenosynovitis** is an inflammation of the synovial sheath that surrounds a tendon. **Paratendinitis** is an inflammation and thickening of the paratenon sheath of tendons that do not have synovial sheaths. **Tendinitis,** also spelled **tendonitis,** is the global term used to identify an inflammation of a tendon. **Tendinosis** involves microscopic tears of the tendon caused by repeated trauma. Whereas it is nearly impossible for the sport rehabilitation specialist to differentiate between a tenosynovitis and paratendinitis and because the symptoms and treatment are the same, the global term, tendinitis, is commonly used in referring to inflammations involving tendons or their sheaths. Although terms such as *tendinopathy* or *tendon stress syndrome* would be more accurate, the term tendinitis is the generally accepted, albeit incorrect, term used to describe inflammation of tendinous origin.

TENDON STRUCTURE

The basic structure of a tendon consists of collagen bundles containing fibroblasts and extracellular matrix. When a load is applied to a tendon it becomes stiffer and is subjected to stress-strain principles.

To develop an appreciation of tendinitis and its treatment, you must first understand the structure and function of the tendon. The specific structure varies somewhat from one tendon to another, but all tendons contain certain basic components. Normal tendon is composed of collagen bundles that contain fibroblasts and an extracellular matrix. The extracellular matrix primarily is composed of water, type I collagen, and ground substance. Type I collagen is a tendon's primary fiber component. Tendons are viscoelastic because of glycosaminoglycans, glycoproteins, and other substances in the ground substance that form a gel-like structure and support the extracellular matrix. Because they are viscoelastic, they take on all the properties of viscoelastic tissue discussed in chapter 5. The tendon's blood vessels and nerves are contained in the paratenon, the loose areolar tissue that surrounds the collagen bundles. Tendons that are subjected to greater than normal friction stresses, such as the Achilles and biceps tendons, are surrounded by synovial sheaths. If a sheath is present, it contains the primary blood supply for the tendon. The sheaths also normally contain a very small amount of fluid and serve to reduce friction in these high-stress areas.

In normal resting, a tendon has a crimped or wavy appearance, but as a load is applied to the tendon it becomes stiffer and is subject to the stress-strain principles discussed in chapter 5. A tendon's tensile strength is determined by how well it resists the stress applied to it. One estimate is that a tendon's tensile strength is about four times the maximal force produced by its muscle (Elliot 1965). Because tendon tensile strength is so much greater than muscle force generation, there must be factors other than tensile strength that enter into tendinitis injuries. Exactly what these additional factors are has yet to be determined.

ETIOLOGY

The fundamental cause of any form of tendinitis, including conditions resulting from repetitive stress and those resulting from acute trauma, is excessive stress on the tendon.

Although tendinitis may have several causes, the consequence is the same: excessive stress applied to the tendon. Excessive stress may take the form of cumulative trauma typically seen in overuse injuries, or may take the form of acute trauma such as a direct blow. Most cases of tendinitis are considered overuse injuries. In overuse injuries, cumulative trauma results from repetitive stresses that lead to a breakdown of otherwise normal tissue. In traumatic tendinitis, the tendon suffers a sudden severe injury and does not have sufficient time to recover before additional loads are applied to it, so breakdown occurs. In either cumulative stress injury or traumatic injury cases, normal tendon tissue breaks down; tendinitis is the result, and pain, swelling, and reduced functional ability are the clinical manifestations.

One of the most difficult problems for the sport rehabilitation specialist in dealing with overuse tendinitis is identifying where the tendon is in the healing process. This is not the case for traumatic tendinitis, because this condition results from a specific incident and the healing process is easy to identify. The injured athlete's symptoms and response to the first treatment may be the best means of identifying the healing stage for overuse tendinitis. The healing stage is important to pinpoint because this is what determines the treatment course, as outlined later in this chapter.

Tendinitis can occur in the upper and lower extremities. Rotator cuff tendinitis, bicipital tendinitis, and lateral and medial epicondylitis are common upper-extremity tendinitis conditions. Common lower-extremity tendinitis locations include the patella, posterior tibialis, peroneal, and Achilles tendons. Although most believe that tendinitis occurs because of chronic or overuse overload situations, the specific types of stress and the load magnitudes that lead to tendinitis are still mysteries.

Common etiology for tendinitis includes training errors; technique and execution errors; structural abnormalities; inappropriate equipment, playing conditions, and training surfaces; and muscle imbalances. Training errors include excessive increases in the progressive overload, excessive distances, and excessive increases in speed. Examples are increasing hill-running workouts in speed, distance, or incline; increasing the intensity of jump workouts; throwing too far, too hard, too fast, or for too many repetitions; and advancing the swimming distance too quickly or demanding speeds that are too great. Any type of training error for any sport can be the problem, but they all essentially increase the workload to a level greater than the tendon is able to tolerate. As a rule of thumb, an increased workload of 10% to 15% a week is usually safe and tolerable.

Technique and execution errors can place additional stress on a tendon. For example, if a tennis player hits a backhand late, extensor tendons on the lateral epicondyle incurs significant increases in stress.

Equipment and playing surfaces can alter forces placed on the body. For example, if the tennis player's racket grip is too big, the athlete must grip harder to hold onto the racket. This increases the stresses applied to the elbow where the tendons insert. If an athlete ties his or her shoes too tightly, the foot's extensor tendons incur increased pressure and tendinitis can develop. Playing basketball on a vinyl-covered concrete floor rather than a suspended wood floor can make a player susceptible to patellar tendinitis. The less force-absorbing the surface, the greater the stress the player's body incurs.

Structural abnormalities and muscle imbalances are intrinsic factors that place additional stresses on tendons. If an athlete excessively pronates when running, the medial Achilles and posterior tibialis tendons are placed on excessive stretch during the activity. If the rotator cuff is weak, the humerus does not glide into the inferior aspect of the glenoid during shoulder motion and becomes subject to impingement, especially during arm elevation activities.

Two additional factors that may lead to tendinitis are circulation and friction. Reduced circulation is a major detriment to a tendon's health. Two tendons particularly prone to tendinitis, the Achilles and the supraspinatus tendon, both have areas of reduced circulation that are frequent sites of tendinitis. Tendons that are compressed against bone or retinacular pulleys and tendons that are subject to high-friction forces are susceptible to tendinitis. For example, the biceps tendon's common site of inflammation is the point at which the transverse ligament holds the tendon in the bicipital groove.

Overload may include not only exaggerated tensile stresses, but also an accumulation of internal and external forces, producing stress during activity. These stresses cause the tendon to alter its behavior in an attempt to adapt to them. As with muscle, bone, and other structures, tendons respond to overload stresses by hypertrophying and remodeling. However, before their strength increases, they undergo a period of breakdown that leaves them weaker than normal. Although it is not known how long this process takes, one postulate is that if the tendon is overloaded again before it is permitted to remodel and adapt, breakdown can occur (Archambault, Wiley, and Bray 1995).

How much stress is enough to cause hypertrophy of the tendon, without overloading it to cause breakdown, becomes the question—a question that researchers have not yet answered. From a clinical standpoint, the best answer in the absence of definitive research conclusions must come from the observational skills of the sport rehabilitation specialist. Monitoring the patient's tendon responses to stress and adapting the therapeutic exercise program accordingly is the best method, at present, for determining appropriate load applications. Increase in pain, crepitus, or edema are clinical signs that overload has been excessive.

TENDON RESPONSE

Tendinitis involves changes within a tendon such as thickening of the tendon's sheath, areas of fibrosis and tissue thickening, and formation of nodules. Tendons break down when they incur stresses that are too great or when they are not given enough time to recover from a stress.

When a tendon becomes inflamed, a number of changes occur. The magnitude of these changes is governed by the extent of the inflammation. At the macroscopic level, the tendon's sheath is thickened. Additionally, areas of fibrosis and connective tissue thickening can often be palpated. Nodules can be palpated on superficial tendons, and adhesions can be present. At the histological level, chronic inflammatory cells, discussed in chapter 2, are prevalent, including myofibroblasts, fibroblasts, fibronectin, and fibrinogen. Additional changes include a reduction in vascularity, a fraying and splitting of collagen fibers, and the presence of type III collagen. As you will recall, type III collagen has less tensile strength than type I collagen. Its presence may lead to ruptures of inflamed tendons.

How a tendon responds to stresses depends on its circulation, its ability to withstand stresses, and the quantity of load applied. Healthy tendons that receive appropriate stress loads are able to increase strength through matrix adaptations. If loads are excessive and time for recovery is insufficient, the tendon eventually breaks down (figure 15.1) and symptoms occur. Rehabilitation intervention then becomes necessary for the tendon's recovery and ability to function normally.

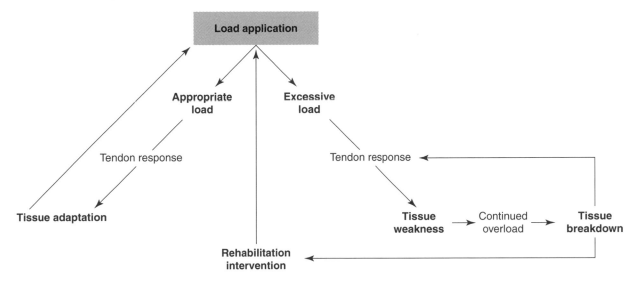

■ **Figure 15.1**   Load application and tendon response: When applied tendon loads are excessive without sufficient recovery time, tissue breakdown occurs. Healing tendons are maintained when load applications permit adequate tissue adaptation.

GENERAL TREATMENT

Guidelines for treatment that relate to all forms of tendinitis include two critical components: identifying the cause of the condition and modifying the causative factor. Selection of treatment depends on where in the healing process the tendon is.

Appropriate treatment of tendinitis conditions includes the identification and modification of those factors causing the patient's tendinitis. This aspect cannot be overemphasized. If the sport rehabilitation specialist does not correct the causative factor, the treatment will be in vain. The patient will be plagued with recurrent episodes of tendinitis and ultimately develop a chronic condition that will be frustrating for both the patient and the sport rehabilitation specialist.

To identify the cause, the sport rehabilitation specialist must take a thorough history, rely on the patient and/or coach for information about recent workouts and poor technique or personally observe the patient's execution, investigate equipment and playing surfaces, and evaluate for muscle imbalances and structural abnormalities. To prevent the tendinitis from recurring, each causative factor must be changed before the patient is allowed to return to full participation.

The initial treatment decision is the most difficult. The goal is to help the patient progress without aggravating the injury. Lacking knowledge of where in the healing process the tendon is makes accomplishing this goal challenging. Before therapeutic exercises can be instituted, the inflammatory process must be brought under control. The intensity of the symptoms can sometimes guide you in determining early treatments. Because pain is a highly subjective symptom, it can be difficult to accurately assess the intensity and stage of the inflammation. In these situations, it is better to err on the side of caution and do less treatment than to provide more treatment and increase the irritation. The accuracy of this trial-and-error approach to initial treatment depends on your knowledge of the patient's injury responses and tissue healing phases, skill in observation and history taking, and good judgment. If the tendon becomes more inflamed as a result of your treatment, you know that the tendinitis is now acutely inflamed, and you can gear future treatment accordingly. If the first treatment either improves the symptoms or has no effect, treatment can advance to the next level.

Although most chronic tendinitis is in the remodeling stage of healing, this is not always the case. As already noted, the symptoms serve as the primary guidelines for determining the intensity of the inflammation: The more intense and prolonged the symptoms, the more severe the inflammation. General guidelines based on work by Curwin and Stanish (1984) can help you ascertain the intensity of the inflammation and select an appropriate initial treatment (table 15.1). For example, if the patient has Achilles tendon pain while walking to class, you know that the inflammation is acute and that the patient will be able to tolerate little exercise. On the other hand, if the individual has Achilles pain only while running, the initial treatment can include therapeutic exercises.

Throughout the rehabilitation program it is important to continually monitor the tendon's response to treatment. Pain and swelling are key signs of inflammation that should be respected and regarded with care. Any increase in symptoms indicates an increase in the inflammation and is the result of recent activity. Thermal or electrical modalities and medication, as well as a reduction in activity can be used to relieve symptom exacerbations.

Therapeutic exercises are a critical aspect of tendinitis treatment, but they must be provided only when appropriate; otherwise they can aggravate the condition. When exercises are used, flexibility exercises are usually a chief component. Concentric and eccentric strengthening exercises stress the tendon and play a vital role in preparing the tendon to for normal functional activities.

Table 15.1   Tendinitis Classifications

Intensities	Level	Pain occurrence	Activity restriction
Mild	1	No Pain	No restriction
	2	Pain with extreme exertion that stops when activity stops	No restriction
Moderate	3	Pain with extreme exertion that lasts 1–2 h afterward	Can limit extreme exertion but has little effect on normal workouts
	4	Pain with moderate exertion that lasts 4–6 h afterward	Inability to perform at normal level or to perform some activities
Severe	5	Pain with any exertion that rapidly increases in itensity and lasts 8–24 h	Inability to perform any sport activity
	6	Pain during even daily activities	Inability to perform any sport activity and possible difficulty with some daily activities

Adapted from Curwin and Stanish 1984.

SPECIFIC TREATMENT

Components of specific treatment programs for tendinitis may include relief of pain and inflammation in addition to exercises in a progression that is consistent with the phases of the condition.

A tendinitis rehabilitation program follows a logical progression that is carefully designed for allowing the injured athlete to advance toward returning to full sport participation. Figure 15.2 depicts this rehabilitation progression for tendinitis. The progression consists of five phases that are determined by the tendon's healing stage and its response to the treatment parameters within each phase. Despite this outline of phases, each injured athlete's progression from one phase to another must be individually decided. At no time do you want an exacerbation of symptoms from one treatment session to the next. If this happens, it is essential that you return the patient to the previous level and allow the tendon time to adapt to that stress level before advancing the person to the next level.

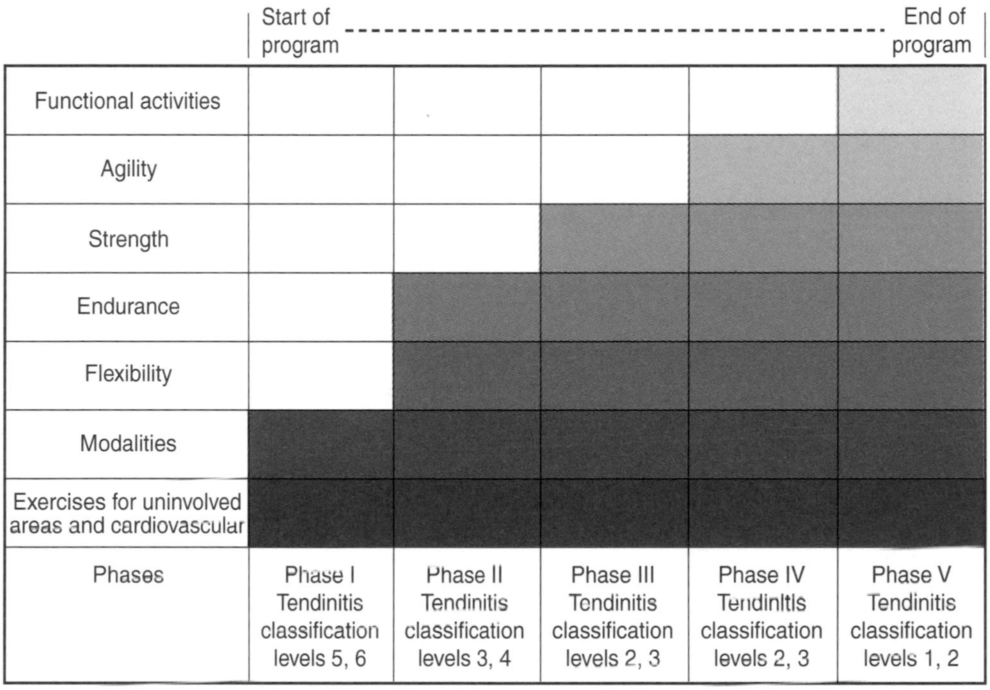

■ **Figure 15.2** Tendinitis treatment phases and rehabilitation: Emphasis in phase I is on reducing the inflammation. Phase II begins with flexibility exercises and low-resistance endurance exercises once the inflammation subsides. As the patient's injury improves, phase III includes the addition of strength exercises. Phase IV begins with agility activities and eventually progresses to phase V, where functional activities are added in preparation for return to full participation.

Adapted, by permission, from P.A. Houglum, 1986, "A clinical view of causes and cures for Achilles tendinitis in runners," *Topics in Acute Care Trauma Rehabilitation* 1 (2): 55–56. © 1986 by Aspen Publishers, Inc.

	Start of program				End of program
Functional activities					
Agility					
Strength					
Endurance					
Flexibility					
Modalities					
Exercises for uninvolved areas and cardiovascular					
Phases	Phase I Tendinitis classification levels 5, 6	Phase II Tendinitis classification levels 3, 4	Phase III Tendinitis classification levels 2, 3	Phase IV Tendinitis classification levels 2, 3	Phase V Tendinitis classification levels 1, 2

Early tendinitis rehabilitation is similar to early rehabilitation of other injuries. In addition to maintaining the injured athlete's cardiovascular conditioning level and the parameters of the uninvolved segments and extremities, the sport rehabilitation specialist uses techniques to relieve the pain and inflammation. The physician may have prescribed anti-inflammatory medication. Modalities that can be used to relieve the pain and inflammation include pulsed ultrasound, iontophoresis, phonophoresis, and electrical stimulation.

See Craig Denegar's (2000) text, *Therapeutic Modalities for Athletic Injuries*, for more specific information on modalities most appropriate for treatment of tendinitis.

Cross-friction massage, described in chapter 6, helps to release adhesions between newly formed collagen and adjacent structures. These adhesions can cause continued discomfort by preventing normal tissue mobility and irritating the local tissue when movement is attempted. The cross-friction massage can also exert tensile force on the tendon by causing a bowstring effect (Gross 1992).

As the tendon is able to tolerate additional stress, therapeutic exercises begin. The tendon should be at least in the proliferation phase. Exercises should certainly begin if the tendon is in the remodeling stage. In the inflammation phase, passive motion is useful because it does not stress the tissue but does assist in tissue organization. Loss of flexibility, a contributing factor to tendinitis, is seen in many cases. Flexibility exercises should almost always be a part of the program and should start in phase II.

Strengthening exercises can be stressful to a tendon. Low-load, high-repetition exercises can be useful for increasing muscle endurance and strength as discussed in chapter 7. Endurance activities put less stress on the tendon and still permit strength gains, but the patient's response to these activities should be carefully monitored. The patient begins strengthening with endurance exercises, but often he or she can advance relatively rapidly to exercises that emphasize strength. How quickly this occurs depends on the tendon's response to the activities.

Initial strength activities may include concentric activities. Eccentric exercises, however, are an important part of most therapeutic exercise programs for tendinitis. Curwin and Stanish (1984) advocate using three sets of 10 repetitions of eccentric exercise, beginning with a slow movement and progressing to a moderately fast and then to a fast motion as the tendon tolerates. Such a program for Achilles tendinitis, for example, starts with three sets of 10 heel raises at a slow speed on days 1 and 2, progresses to a moderate speed on days 3 and 4, and then progresses to a fast speed on days 5 and 6. This cycle is repeated when additional resistance is provided on day 7 (table 15.2). The patient performs stretching exercises before and after the series. If pain occurs during the first two sets, the stress is too much for the tendon, and the patient should return to the preceding level. Curwin and Stanish suggest that if pain occurs during the last set, the exercise is at an appropriate level for the tendon.

This progression is based on the force-velocity relationship of muscle, discussed in chapter 5; according to this principle, the faster the eccentric activity, the greater the force exerted. The tension on the tendon is increased when the speed of the eccentric movement is increased. This progression allows for a gradual buildup in overload and also increases strength output as the tendon's tolerance improves.

Table 15.2   Eccentric Exercise Progression

	Day	Speed of movement	Reps	Sets
	1	Slow	3	10
	2	Slow	3	10
Increase	3	Moderate	3	10
resistance	4	Moderate	3	10
	5	Fast	3	10
	6	Fast	3	10
	7			

Adapted from Curwin and Stanish 1984.

During the last half of phase III, in which strength is the primary emphasis and the tendon is tolerating eccentric and concentric exercises, the patient can progress to plyometric exercises. These should be low-level and low-impact exercises and should progress as the patient tolerates.

Within this period the patient transitions to phase IV, in which agility becomes the primary focus. Strength and flexibility exercises continue, but the activities become more strenuous as the patient is prepared for the final phase in which functional activities are the primary thrust. It bears repeating here that if symptoms return or become exaggerated during any progression, the patient should remain at the lower level for a couple of days more to allow the tendon additional time for adaptation to stress at that level.

EXAMPLES OF TENDINITIS CASES

The best way to demonstrate rehabilitation for tendinitis injuries is to provide examples. This section presents two examples, one for the lower extremity and one for the upper extremity. For one final example, you will be asked to outline an appropriate rehabilitation program.

LOWER-EXTREMITY CASE

A 20-year-old collegiate cross country runner, Sally, presented with complaints of right Achilles pain that had begun about three months earlier. She usually ran about 65 km (about 40 miles) a week on varying terrain. At first she had pain only when running hills, but at the time she came to the clinic she was experiencing pain even when walking across campus. She finally sought treatment because the intensity of the pain made it impossible to run.

Examination

On examination, Sally had a mildly antalgic gait. She had excessive pronation in weight bearing. She was unable to hop on the right leg because of pain. Although Sally said that she used stretching, her ankle dorsiflexion was 0° when the rearfoot was stabilized in subtalar neutral. Palpation revealed swelling along the Achilles tendon and a painful nodule about 8 cm (3 in.) above the tendon's distal insertion.

Treatment

Sally was instructed to stop running for the time being. She was advised to continue her cardiovascular conditioning either in a pool or by performing stationary cycling using only the left leg. She could continue any weight exercises with the upper extremities, left lower extremity, and trunk, but was instructed not to use the right leg for any exercise.

Sally was given crutches and instructed in partial weight bearing on the right. Right lower-extremity weight bearing was allowed only to the extent that the gait was pain free. Sally's first treatment included the use of phonophoresis, ice, and strapping to reduce her excessive pronation.

On the next day Sally returned, feeling better. The phonophoresis treatment was repeated. Cross-friction massage was used, first in nontender areas and then on the nodule and in other tender areas as Sally was able to tolerate. The strapping helped to reduce the pain, so Sally was measured for orthotics as a permanent correction for her excessive pronation. Ice was applied as a final treatment.

By her third visit Sally was able to walk around campus without pain, so the use of crutches was discontinued. She was instructed in proper stretching exercises for the gastrocnemius and soleus. She was also started on a progressive isotonic exercise program of three sets of 20 repetitions of bilateral heel raises, then unilateral heel raises, then heel raises with weights. She continued with the phonophoresis for one more week. She was taught how to self-administer cross-friction massage.

Exercises were then advanced to include trampoline jumping activities, rapid heel drops, lateral-movement exercises, and fast walking. Fast walking progressed to alternately walking and jogging, then jogging, then running on flat surfaces, and finally running hills.

UPPER-EXTREMITY CASE

Tom, a 24-year-old, right-handed baseball pitcher, was seen because of pain in the right shoulder. He reported that the pain was located over the deltoid tubercle and that it sometimes radiated down the lateral arm to the elbow. He was unable to sleep on his right side. The pain had started about two months before, in the beginning of the season, after Tom had pitched seven long innings in a game. He usually had pain during the last two innings that he pitched, especially with curve balls; the pain would last for about 2 or 3 h after he had finished pitching. He was pitching more during the current season than he had the year before. In the off-season, he had fallen while skiing, landing on his right shoulder, but did not think at the time that the shoulder was injured. It was just sore for a couple of days, and he did not seek any medical attention. During preseason, the flu had kept Tom out of most of the regular preseason conditioning program.

Examination

Active range of motion of the neck was normal. Shoulder range of motion was normal for a pitcher, but Tom had pain during the middle arc of shoulder elevation. Weakness was present, and Tom complained of pain with resisted manual muscle tests to external rotation and abduction in the scapular plane. He had shoulder tenderness when he put his hand behind his back and raised the hand upward along his back. There was tenderness to palpation of the greater tubercle. The findings were consistent with a tendinitis of the supraspinatus and infraspinatus. Tom's history indicated that the irritability stage of the tendon was moderate.

Treatment

Because the injury was in the irritability stage, Tom was able to begin exercises on the first treatment. The first treatment included concentric exercises consisting of manual resistance to the rotator cuff. Scapular rotator muscle exercises were also started. All exercises were performed in a pain-free range of motion. Ice application ended the treatment session. Home exercises included three sets of 20 repetitions with rubber bands for external rotation and abduction in a pain-free range of motion. Tom was told that he could also do scapular rotator exercises, such as push-ups, seated push-ups, and flys, as long as he could perform them pain free.

The rotator cuff exercises progressed with the shoulder at 90°. Agility and plyometric exercises with medicine balls and rubber tubing, as well as body weight-resisted exercises, were added.

A throwing progression similar to the one outlined in chapter 10 was given Tom. He began with tosses, progressed to throwing, and increased the speed and distance of the throws as he was able to tolerate.

A Challenging Case

Joe, a 19-year-old, right-handed tennis player, presents with complaints of right elbow pain. The pain is located over the outside of the elbow and sometimes radiates down the forearm. It began about four months ago, about three weeks after Joe had bought a new tennis racket and had started playing in two leagues. He stopped playing for a month until he was pain free, but when he went back to playing, the pain returned. He plays or practices tennis daily. He has noticed that the elbow especially bothers him on his tennis backhand, when he attempts to lift heavy objects, and when he shakes hands.

Examination

The right elbow and forearm have full range of motion in all planes. The neck and shoulder also have normal motion. There is pain to resisted wrist extension. Joe's grip strength on the right is 8 kg (17.6 lb) weaker than that on the left. Palpation of the lateral epicondyle reveals swelling over the epicondyle and tenderness to even light palpation. There is some tenderness to palpation extending into the proximal wrist extensor muscle bellies in the forearm.

Questions for Analysis

1. What will you include in your first treatment session?

2. What instructions will you give Joe about what he should and should not be doing at home?

3. How will you advance him in his program?

4. What exercises will you include?

SUMMARY

1. *Define tendinitis.*

   Tendinitis is an inflammation of a tendon, its paratenon, or its synovial sheath. Unless visualized in surgery, the precise structure involved is difficult to determine.

2. *Discuss various etiologies of tendinitis.*

   Tendinitis can occur as a traumatic or an overuse condition. The most common cause is excessive or repetitive stress: The tendon breaks down because cumulative trauma is applied without an opportunity for the tendon to recover before additional stress is applied. Abnormal stress resulting in tendon breakdown occurs most commonly because of training errors; technique and execution errors; inappropriate equipment, playing conditions, or training surfaces; structural abnormalities; or muscle imbalances.

3. *Explain the inflammatory response of tendons.*

   The inflammatory response in tendinitis reduces the tendon's tensile strength because the quantity of type I collagen normally present is reduced through damage, and type III collagen becomes a significant structure of the tendon. This makes the tendon susceptible to tears when tendinitis is present.

4. *Identify parameters governing the initial treatment for tendinitis.*

   Identifying the stage of the tendinitis is fundamental to deciding what should be included in the first treatment. The identification is based on the patient's history and complaints of pain and restriction of activity. The stage of the tendinitis determines the treatment; the more advanced the tendinitis, the more careful the sport rehabilitation specialist needs to be and the more conservative the course of treatment should be.

5. *Outline the progression of a tendinitis treatment program.*

Treatment for tendinitis is divided into five phases. In addition to correcting the cause and maintaining the conditioning status of unaffected segments, treatments should address restoration of flexibility, muscle endurance, strength, agility, and functional performance. These goals are accomplished by careful progression of the program, beginning with modalities if the tendon is very inflamed and progressing to cross-friction massage and exercises as tolerated. Observation by the sport rehabilitation specialist and reports by the patient regarding the tendon's response to treatment determine the rate of progression. If the tendon responds negatively to the treatment, the sport rehabilitation specialist should return the patient to the previous exercise stress level and resume modalities as indicated. To reduce the chance of recurrences, it is important that the sport rehabilitation specialist identify and correct the underlying precipitating factor.

CRITICAL THINKING QUESTIONS

1. A patient with Achilles tendinitis has advanced nicely over the past three weeks of treatment. He has responded well to all therapeutic exercises. Today, however, he returns for additional treatment, complaining that since yesterday's treatment he has experienced the same pain that he had at first. Yesterday you had increased the number of repetitions of the exercises he had been doing. What will your treatment today include? What will your criteria be for again attempting the program you tried yesterday?

2. A tennis player reports that she has tennis elbow for the second time this season. Last year she experienced the condition toward the end of the season, but with rest it went away. She wants to know what you will do for her, why this problem is recurring, and how it differs from a forearm strain she had two years ago. Explain how you will answer her questions.

3. A basketball player who has been unable to run for the past six weeks because of peroneal tendinitis has responded well to your rehabilitation program. He is now ready to start running. What will the first day's running program be, and how will you have him progress to normal running activities?

REFERENCES

Archambault, J.M., Wiley, J.P, and R.C. Bray. 1995. Exercise loading of tendons and the development of overuse injuries. *Sports Medicine* 20:77–89.

Curwin, S. and W.D. Stanish. 1984. *Tendinitis: Its etiology and treatment.* Lexington, MA: Heath.

Denegar, C. 2000. *Therapeutic modalities for athletic injuries.* Champaign, IL: Human Kinetics.

Elliot, D.H. 1965. Structure and function of mammalian tendon. *Biological Reviews* 40:392–421.

Gross, M.T. 1992. Chronic tendinitis: Pathomechanics of injury, factors affecting the healing response, and treatment. Journal of Orthopedic and Sport Physical Therapy 16:248–261.

PART FOUR

Specific Applications

Every exit is an entry somewhere else.

Tom Stoppard, British playwright, 1937

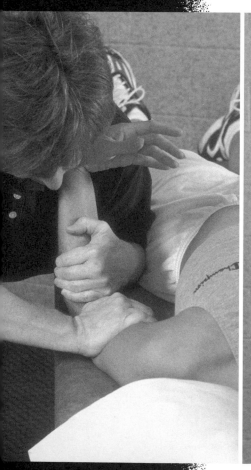

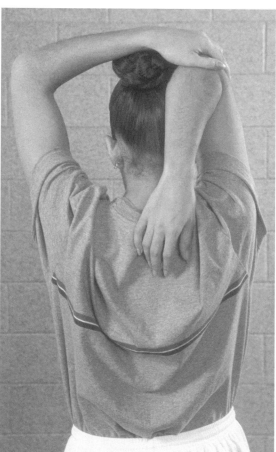

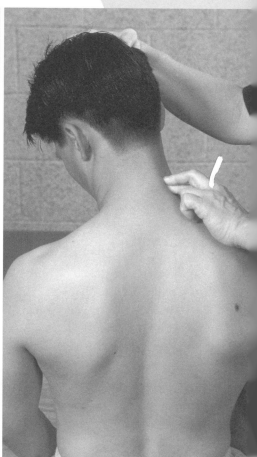

Parts I, II, and III have established the groundwork for this final part of the book. Having acquired the information from the earlier parts, you are now prepared to fully understand and appreciate the information presented in part IV. Part IV consists of therapeutic exercise programs for each body segment. The programs are not divided by sport, for an ankle sprain is an ankle sprain regardless of whether it occurs in basketball, volleyball, or track, and regardless of whether it is incurred by a teenager, college student, or professional individual who is physically active. The only point when a treatment program for an injury might deviate from one individual to another is in the final stages of therapeutic exercise, when the patient begins sport-specific functional exercises that will allow return to that sport.

Part IV is also not a cookbook for rehabilitation of injuries. A cookbook is not necessary, nor is it practical. Now that you have the information from parts I, II, and III, you have the tools to design your own rehabilitation programs. Because each patient must have an individualized program, a cookbook approach is irrelevant and useless. The information in part IV provides suggestions for exercises and treatment techniques; but for application, you will depend on the knowledge you have gained throughout this text to put those suggestions together in an appropriate and formidable program for each patient you work with.

By now it should be clear that the sport rehabilitation specialist is a detective, problem solver, innovator, and educator who follows laws of knowledge, skill application, logic, and common sense to achieve the final goal of returning a patient to full sport participation as efficiently and safely as possible. Detective work involves evaluation of the injury's status, assessment of the underlying causes of the injury to correct these causes and reduce the chance of reinjury, and continual reevaluation of the patient's response to the treatment so that the results are positive.

As a problem solver, the sport rehabilitation specialist must be able to adjust treatment programs, exercises, and progression sequences when a patient does not respond according to expectations. The program is always individualized, so the sport rehabilitation specialist must be alert to problems and must be able to adjust the program as needed for each patient.

As an innovator, the sport rehabilitation specialist attempts to achieve treatment goals and still make the program interesting and stimulating for the patient to help ensure compliance in the therapeutic exercise program. If equipment is limited, innovation becomes an even more important element, because making the program interesting using minimal materials presents an even greater challenge to the sport rehabilitation specialist's imagination. This situation of limited resources can make a therapeutic exercise program as interesting and challenging for you to design as it is for the patient to perform.

Throughout a therapeutic exercise program, the sport rehabilitation specialist is an educator. The patient is educated regarding the "dos and don'ts" following an injury—what activities are important to perform and what activities should be avoided to prevent further harm. The patient is educated about what to do to protect the injury and to promote an uneventful healing process. The patient is educated with regard to the injury, the rehabilitation program process, the rationale for specific exercises, and the importance of home exercises; each of these is vital to assuring the patient's compliance and the program's success. The sport rehabilitation specialist educates the patient throughout the program as the injury changes and the program evolves.

The sport rehabilitation specialist's knowledge, understanding, observation skills, evaluation skills, application skills, and ability to apply common sense and logic all contribute to the success of the rehabilitation process. Rehabilitation involves applying all these elements to provide a balanced program for the patient—one that provides appropriate stresses with the right degree of protection to advance the patient efficiently and effectively toward the goal of safe return to sport participation as soon as possible.

PROGRAM CONSIDERATIONS

The specific elements and the complexity of a rehabilitation program are determined by a variety of factors. These include the magnitude of the injury, the type of injury, the body segment involved, the patient's sport and position within the sport, the patient's response to the injury (physical, emotional, and psychological), and the patient's goals. All must be considered in the evaluation, design, and execution of the rehabilitation program.

EVALUATION

Before providing treatment in a rehabilitation program, the sport rehabilitation specialist must evaluate the injury to determine where in the healing process the injury is and how irritable it is. If the injury is very irritable, regardless of healing stage, the treatment must begin gently and include primarily modalities to calm the area. If the patient had reconstructive surgery three days ago, the initial treatments are not aggressive with respect to strengthening activities. If, on the other hand, the injury is not very irritable and is well into the healing process, the sport rehabilitation special-ist can be more aggressive in the first treatment. Whatever the initial treatment includes, careful observation for responses to the treatment is necessary, both during the first treatment session and before the next. The current treatment course is always determined by the injury's response to the previous treatment session.

MODALITIES

A total rehabilitation program includes the use of modalities to modulate pain and enhance the healing process. Modalities serve as preliminary adjuncts to the total program and should not be considered the primary means of returning the patient to full sport participation. Once pain modulation and healing are under way, therapeutic exercises become the primary emphasis in the rehabilitation process. Since this text includes information specific to therapeutic exercise, you should keep in mind as you read the following chapters that although a rehabilitation program may include pain-modulating modalities and efforts to manage and promote the healing process, these are not included in this text. *Therapeutic Modalities for Athletic Injuries* by Craig Denegar (2000) covers modalities used in athletic rehabilitation.

An injury does not have to become entirely pain free before exercises begin. In fact, most of the time it is not desirable to wait until the patient is completely pain free before starting exercises. Pain and swelling, however, are monitored throughout the rehabilitation process, especially in the first half of the therapeutic exercise program when the newly forming tissue is more susceptible to overstress from exercise than it will be later. Both pain and edema act as neural inhibitors, reducing the patient's rehabilitation output and ability to perform therapeutic exercises.

Remember the advice of Hippocrates: Do no harm. If you have any doubt about whether an exercise program may cause edema or increased pain later, it is advisable to apply ice following the exercise session to reduce the risk for these deleterious effects. As you obtain a more accurate impression of the patient's ability to tolerate the stresses applied during the therapeutic exercise program, and as the injury becomes more advanced in the remodeling phase, application of ice after a session becomes optional and relates more to the patient's preference or comfort level than to any physiological benefit.

MAINTENANCE OF CONDITIONING LEVEL

Throughout, this book has emphasized the importance of maintaining cardiovascular health and conditioning levels of noninjured body segments. Although this is a vital aspect of a total therapeutic exercise program, it is not addressed in the chapters in part IV; but you should always include exercises for these parameters in a rehabilitation program. The exercises discussed in this part of the book include only those relevant to the injured segment.

CHAPTER SEGMENTS

Each chapter in part IV includes specifics on various aspects of topics that have been covered in earlier chapters. The first portion of each chapter in part IV includes general considerations and specific techniques corresponding to concepts, theories, and applications presented in part II: soft-tissue and joint mobilization. The next portion deals with the progression of therapeutic techniques for achieving goals of normal range of motion, strength and muscle endurance, and coordination and agility. Once you are familiar with these elements, you will learn to apply them in the next section of the chapter, "Special Rehabilitation Applications." These sections address injuries that require special program considerations, precautions, or unique therapeutic exercise applications, followed by case studies. Specific answers are not given for the questions in these case studies because the studies are meant to stimulate discussion between students and instructor. There is no right answer for each question, because the answer is driven by the particulars of the case and is to some extent flexible, as dictated by the sport rehabilitation specialist's preferences and the equipment available. Of course, you must take into consideration specific precautions, contraindications, healing time line, and injury-unique information when creating a program for each case study.

SOFT-TISSUE MOBILIZATION

You may want to refer to earlier chapters that deal specifically with these techniques to review technique application. Soft-tissue mobilization techniques in the chapters to follow do not include the full range of soft-tissue techniques discussed in chapter 6. The primary techniques discussed are myofascial release and trigger point release. You should realize that these specific techniques or other soft-tissue mobilization techniques may or may not be indicated in individual situations; you must evaluate the patient's injury to decide whether they may be appropriate. The intent of the discussion of these techniques is to provide examples to help you appreciate the important role that soft-tissue mobilization can play in the total rehabilitation process.

The soft-tissue pain-referral patterns discussed in these chapters are based on the extensive work of Travell and Simons (1983, 1992). Other pain-referral patterns are based on common neurological patterns.

JOINT MOBILIZATION

As discussed in chapter 6, joint mobilization is a complex technique entailing either accessory movements or physiological movements. When using joint mobilization, the sport rehabilitation specialist should remember that the movement is produced not by the sport rehabilitation specialist's hands but by his or her body; this produces a better perception of the movement by the specialist and a more comfortable sensation for the patient. The hands are the vehicle through which the sport rehabilitation specialist's body produces the joint motion.

Joint mobilization is not used in all conditions. Positive results in mobilization should usually occur within four to five days (Maitland 1990). As discussed in chapter 6, joint mobilization is appropriate for treatment of pain using I and II grades of movement or treatment of joint stiffness using grade III or IV. These movements can be oscillatory motions or sustained. Please refer to chapter 6 for review of these techniques if necessary.

Most of the joint mobilization techniques presented in part IV are based on Maitland's work. Various scholars have developed a number of techniques, but probably the most widely used are those advanced by Maitland. At the back of this book is a listing of suggested readings that you can refer to for specific instruction in his techniques.

THERAPEUTIC EXERCISE PHASES

The therapeutic exercise phases differ to some extent from the rehabilitation phases outlined in chapter 2. The primary difference is that the therapeutic exercise program does not include very early aspects of rehabilitation. I recommend that you refer to

Therapeutic Modalities for Athletic Injuries (Denegar 2000) for information regarding the use of modalities in rehabilitation. Of course, the emphasis in the early stage of rehabilitation is to get the inflammation under control and protect the healing process, as dealt with in earlier chapters. Although the sport rehabilitation specialist must know what constitutes a total rehabilitation program and know how to administer such a program, only therapeutic exercises and manual techniques are addressed in the following chapters.

The therapeutic exercise aspect of a rehabilitation program can be divided into three phases: early, middle, and late. In administration of a program, the exercise progression is not so clearly defined; but the components of the progression are distinguished here to make the progression easier to comprehend and identify.

Early Phase

The early therapeutic exercise phase includes achieving gains in range of motion through joint and soft-tissue mobilization techniques, as well as range-of-motion exercises. Beginning-level strength and proprioception activities are also included at this time.

In the early phase, flexibility and range of motion are deficient. Weakness and loss of agility and coordination are also readily apparent when one compares the injured segment to the opposite side.

The intent of the early phase of therapeutic exercise is to achieve significant gains in range of motion and flexibility, to begin early strengthening activities, and to initiate low-level proprioception activities. Range-of-motion and flexibility gains come through the use of soft-tissue and joint mobilization techniques. Passive, active and assistive exercises can also be used to improve range of motion. Early strengthening exercises vary depending on the severity of the injury and include a range of activities, such as isometrics and concentric, concentric-eccentric, and/or eccentric exercises. Isometric exercises are often performed in either multiple angles, midrange, or in an anatomic position, depending on mobility and medical restrictions for motion. Strength exercises are usually performed in a straight plane, not progressing to diagonal or functional positions until the patient has achieved sufficient strength in straight-plane movement to control the extremity through a functional motion. It is not unusual for strength exercises to begin with high repetitions and low weights. This reduces stress on joints that may not be strong enough to tolerate the shear forces produced by heavy resistance. Proprioception exercises begin at a simple level and do not advance to more complex exercises until the patient demonstrates an ability to perform the lower-level activity well.

Middle Phase

By the time the patient progresses to the middle phase, range of motion is nearly or completely normal. Edema and pain have come under control. Strength and muscle endurance have improved but remain the greatest deficit. Because of weakness and incoordination, the patient is unable to perform high-level agility activities.

The middle phase includes primarily strength and muscle endurance exercises along with more advanced proprioception exercises. Flexibility exercises should continue in this phase to prevent a loss of motion with continued contraction that occurs because of the myofibril activity during the healing process. If flexibility is not yet normal, stretching exercises are a requirement during this phase. This is the time the patient begins more aggressive exercises, as discussed in chapter 1, including a progression of exercises that continue to work on range of motion and also advance strength, muscle endurance, and proprioception. Strength exercises here are in transi-tion. In the beginning of this phase, patients may perform the strength exercises primarily in a straight plane; but by the time a patient is nearing the next phase, many exercises include diagonal, functional patterns of movement. This is possible because the muscle strength has improved to a level that allows the patient to maintain extremity control while moving the segment.

Proprioception exercises are more complex in this phase. They may include multiple tasks, and the aim is to help prepare the patient for the stresses of functional activities in the next phase.

Late Phase

The middle phase readies the patient for the late phase, when power, strength, and coordination are jointly stressed in agility activities. By the time the patient reaches the final phase, flexibility, strength, and muscle endurance are all at near-normal levels; so the patient is ready for more advanced activities that further stress the injured area in preparation for return to sport activities. At this point the only real deficit lies in the patient's functional performance level. Flexibility and strength activities are now at a maintenance level, and the major emphasis is on fine-tuning the patient for a smooth transition and return to full sport participation. Although these chapters mention functional activities, they do not fully address sport-specific exercises because these are so numerous and so varied in their demands. You must remember, though, that functional activities are a vital part of the final phase and must always be part of a therapeutic exercise program. Functional activities should include a progression of sport-skill activities. These begin with less stress, speed, force, and distance and continue to increase these parameters as the patient's body adjusts to the stresses and the patient acquires better skill and ability to execute the specific activities appropriately.

EXERCISE CONTINUUM

The exercises for each phase can be placed on a rehabilitation continuum. On the continuum are all the parameters that have been discussed, as well as exercises corresponding to the phases as seen in the following figure. The diagram outlines the progression of a therapeutic exercise program according to parameter and divides those parameters according to the early, middle, and late phases of a program. The progression is a continuum in that exercises in a therapeutic exercise program flow from one level to the next. It is sometimes difficult to determine whether an exercise corresponds to the early or middle phase or to the middle or late phase, and a particular exercise can correspond to one phase with one injury and another phase with another injury. That is the essence of a continuum.

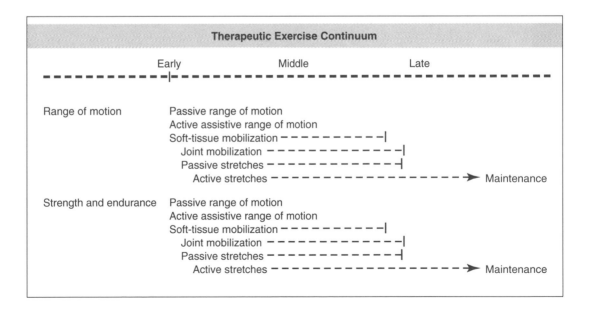

PUTTING IT ALL TOGETHER

The purpose of the phases and exercise continuum is less to delineate a specific program and progression for a patient than to give you a mental image that helps you identify how to advance a patient in a therapeutic exercise program. Understanding which phase an exercise corresponds to is not as important as recognizing the progression and level of difficulty of the exercise and identifying when the patient is able to move from one level to the next.

To make the rehabilitation program progression even less clear-cut and more confusing, a patient may be in the early phase with one parameter and in the middle phase with another parameter. For example, the patient may have good range of motion and grade 4/5 strength, indicating that he or she is in the middle phase of a therapeutic exercise program, but the balance ability of that patient may still be in the early phase. Each segment must be stressed to its capacity as long as this does not stress other segments inappropriately. As an example, a patient with a shoulder impingement and weakness of the scapular rotators should not be advanced to open chain exercises in the higher elevations of motion if such exercises will worsen the injury; if the scapular muscles lack sufficient strength, they will not be able to hold the scapula properly to prevent impingement. In that case, although coordination abilities of the patient may be able to advance, his or her strength remains deficient, so attempting to advance the coordination parameter before strength improves will aggravate the injury.

THERAPEUTIC EXERCISE INDIVIDUALIZATION

As has been mentioned throughout this book, it is important to design the patient's therapeutic exercise program for the individual patient. Even though two patients have ankle sprains, they will not necessarily progress at the same rate, so expectations of a specific time line of advancement are not appropriate. These patients may even have different exercises within their programs. The individual's injury and the body's response to the injury, the patient's abilities and goals, and the way the patient responds to both the program and the sport rehabilitation specialist all determine the exercises selected, the rate of progression, and the final outcome of the therapeutic exercise program. Expecting an individual to progress on the basis of any other guidelines leads to frustration for both the patient and the sport rehabilitation specialist.

The clinician should continually inspect the patient's activities; should evaluate before, during, and after treatment to see whether the treatment has had the desired effect; and should be ready to alter treatments if there are undesirable effects. It is essential to obtain information from the patient regarding posttreatment responses in order to further assess the effects of the treatment program. If increased pain, swelling, and other deleterious effects are recorded after treatment, the program has been too stressful on the injured part and needs to be revised to a less intense exercise level. Progress without regression should be the sport rehabilitation specialist's creed. In other words, the program should challenge the patient enough to improve all parameters without overstressing the injury to increase symptoms.

CHAPTER PROGRESSION

Part IV begins with the spine (**chapter 16**) and then moves to the upper extremities (**chapters 17–19**); the final chapters (**20–22**) include therapeutic exercise programs for the lower extremities. The material has been arranged this way because many upper- and lower-extremity problems can be related to the core, the spine. The spine is also an important consideration in rehabilitation of upper and lower extremities, because core strength is vital for both upper- and lower-segment stability and performance.

It would be nearly impossible to list all the exercises in a therapeutic exercise program. Those outlined in these chapters include the most commonly used activities, as well as some that are unique for each parameter. As always, the sport re-habilitation specialist's knowledge of injury healing, appreciation of the patient's abilities, the facilities and equipment available, and his or her own imagination are the only limiting factors of a therapeutic exercise program. A therapeutic exercise program can be fun and challenging for the patient as well as the sport rehabilitation specialist. The clinician can be imaginative in providing stimulating exercises for the patient so that both enjoy the rehabilitation process. So as you read through these next few chapters, see whether you can think of exercises in addition to those presented that would challenge and stimulate the patient in a therapeutic exercise program.

CHAPTER SIXTEEN

Spine and Sacroiliac

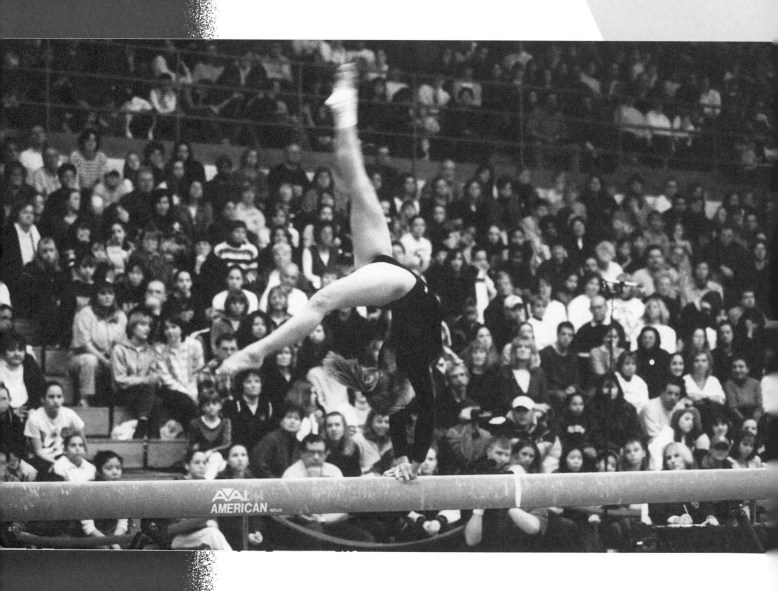

OBJECTIVES

After completing this chapter, you should be able to do the following:

1. Explain three flexibility exercises for the cervical spine and lumbar spine.

2. Explain three strengthening exercises for the cervical spine and lumbar spine.

3. Identify three progressive spinal stability exercises.

4. Identify three sacroiliac muscle energy release techniques and the indications for their use.

5. Outline a therapeutic exercise program for a cervical sprain.

6. List precautions for a therapeutic exercise program for disk lesions.

7. Discuss the difference in therapeutic exercise programs for a lumbar strain and a facet injury.

About half the patients Casey sees have back injuries. Mark, a high school athlete she is currently rehabilitating, is one of these. While practicing his high jump maneuver last week, he slipped during his approach and injured his back. Now that the muscle spasms are resolved, Casey is improving Mark's soft-tissue mobility with myofascial release (MFR) across the lumbar area. His sacroiliac became malaligned when he slipped, so Casey used muscle energy techniques and home exercises to correct the problem. Her initial evaluation revealed significant weakness of the trunk muscles, so she plans to develop Mark's abdominal and back strength. Casey is confident that this will not only protect Mark's back from further injury but may also improve his high jump.

It is our duty to remember at all times and anew that medicine is not only a science, but also the art of letting our own individuality interact with the individuality of the patient.

Albert Schweitzer, 1875–1965

This chapter begins the fun part of therapeutic exercise, applying the science that we have been discussing and letting our imaginations create therapeutic exercise programs. We will start the true blending of science and art in rehabilitation. We now have the opportunity to do what Schweitzer encourages us to do—apply our scientific knowledge in an artful manner to provide patients with a complete, stimulating, and challenging therapeutic exercise program that will allow those patients a safe and speedy return to sport participation.

The spine and sacroilium (SI) are composed of several different segments. Any segment can have separate injuries that do not affect the other spinal regions. They also can have injuries that affect or are affected by other regions. Since the spine and SI are interrelated, we are considering the spine and sacroilium together.

There are both similarities and unique characteristics among regions of the spine. For example, in the thoracic region, each vertebra is joined with a rib; the cervical spine has the atlas and brachial plexus; and the lumbar region has the lumbar plexus, larger vertebral bodies, and is connected to the sacrum. Examples of similarities are that all vertebrae have spinous and transverse processes and are separated by disks.

This chapter addresses general rehabilitation concepts for the spine. Some of the factors unique to the spine that influence a rehabilitation program are also introduced. Many texts are devoted to the spine, so this chapter by no means deals with all there is to know about the spine. The aim is to present key information that will enable you to treat most spine and spine-related injuries that you will encounter as a sport rehabilitation specialist.

Catastrophic injuries that include spinal cord injury resulting in paralysis are not among injuries seen for therapeutic exercise with the goal of returning the patient to sport participation, so they are not addressed here. Emergency treatment of these injuries is covered in *Assessment of Athletic Injuries* (Shultz et al. 2000), which readers should consult for information on this topic.

The spine is a complex structure that is often neglected in education programs because of its uniqueness in comparison to the upper and lower extremities. Rather than approach the spine as another segment that is subject to injury and in need of treatment, many approach the topic with apprehension because of ignorance and fear: ignorance because the spine seems to be a mystifying body segment that is far too complex to understand, and fear because its complexity gets in the way of appreciating its simplicity.

The spine is complex. So is the shoulder. So is the knee. There are many segments of the body that we still have much to learn about and understand, yet we do not hesitate to deal with injuries to these segments. The spine is like any other segment in that, regardless of its complexity, it is often injured in sport and needs to be addressed. This chapter deals with the most common injuries seen in the spine and outlines typical therapeutic exercise programs for them.

By the end of the chapter, you should view the spine not as a body segment to shy away from, but rather an area that you can approach with an appreciation of both its simplicity and its complexity.

GENERAL REHABILITATION CONSIDERATIONS

Treatment of spine injuries has changed greatly in the last few years. A therapeutic exercise program for the spine typically has many components, including instruction on posture and stability as well as exercises for flexibility, strength, and muscle endurance.

As recently as 10 years ago, conservative treatment of spine injuries, especially low back injuries, involved bed rest for extended periods of time. As medical professionals realized how detrimental immobilization and extended rest were, and noticed that those individuals who did not rest improved faster than those who did, the standard of care for spine injuries changed. Current treatment applications include minimal rest and progression into activity as quickly as is appropriate for the individual and the specific injury.

For many years, Williams flexion exercises were the accepted back-exercise regimen. Williams flexion exercises are a series of exercises that emphasize flexion and include activities such as the pelvic tilt, single and double knees-to-chest, and straight-leg raise. More recently, extension exercises became the exercises of choice because flexion exercises made many patients with disk injuries worse. Extension exercises, advanced by Robin McKenzie, a New Zealand physiotherapist, emphasize trunk extension aimed at relieving posterior pressure on disks. Many sport rehabilitation specialists today do not advocate a purist attitude of either flexion or extension exercises for spine patients. Rather, a program is individualized on the basis of the problems and needs of the patient.

A complete rehabilitation program for the spine typically involves modalities, therapeutic exercise, and manual techniques. Manual techniques include soft-tissue and joint mobilization. Spinal injuries respond well to Swiss ball, foam roller, and aquatic exercises. As you have learned, it is easy to incorporate these into a therapeutic exercise program.

It is important for spine injury programs to include cardiovascular exercises. The specific injury dictates the requirements for each program. The sport rehabilitation specialist must identify the patient's deficiencies before deciding on a precise therapeutic exercise program.

In addition to cardiovascular activities, a therapeutic exercise program for the spine should routinely include spinal stability instruction, posture correction, and body mechanics instruction. It should also include flexibility exercises, strengthening exercises, and muscle endurance activities. Hip tightness, especially in the external rotators, is often correlated with low back pain; so the program should include flexibility activities for those hip muscles that have been assessed as having restricted motion. The abdominals, obliques, and spine extension muscles are key muscle groups that provide support and stability to the spine, so strength exercises for these groups should also be included.

If one segment of the spine is hypomobile, it is common for an adjacent segment to be hypermobile. One must carefully assess each vertebra's mobility before applying joint mobilization. Random joint mobilization to any segment in the absence of an assessment of its mobility may increase, not decrease, the patient's symptoms. If you are ever in doubt whether to use joint mobilization, do not use it.

Although approaches to the various spinal segments have many similarities, and although the symptoms and treatment from one segment to an adjacent segment frequently overlap, this chapter deals with the segments separately to make it easier to identify and discuss treatment for each. You should keep in mind, however, that one segment and its injury are often intimately related to another spinal segment. For example, painful symptoms at T4 are often associated with cervical dysfunctions, and pain in the low back can be related to sacroiliac dysfunctions.

REHABILITATION TECHNIQUES

Rehabilitation techniques for the various segments of the spine include soft-tissue mobilization, joint mobilization, and exercises to improve parameters such as flexibility, postural and pelvic stability, strength, and agility.

Soft-tissue mobilization techniques are presented here before joint mobilization techniques; other types of exercises focusing on flexibility, stability, strength, and agility and coordination are presented in subsequent sections. Because there are so many types of soft-tissue mobilization techniques, only a couple are described. Keep in mind, however, that other soft-tissue mobilization techniques may be more appropriate than those presented here, depending on the individual and the specific injury.

SOFT-TISSUE MOBILIZATION

Although various techniques are available for soft-tissue mobilization as discussed in chapter 6, the techniques emphasized here are trigger point release and myofascial release. If the sport rehabilitation specialist observes pain-referral patterns identified with these muscles, he or she should use some of these techniques. Trigger points, referred pain, and release techniques presented here are based on the work by Trawell and Simons (1983).

Cervical Spine

The primary muscles of the cervical spine that often have soft-tissue restriction include the upper trapezius, levator scapulae, sternocleidomastoid, scalenes, spleni, and posterior cervical muscles. The following sections cover treatment of these muscles.

Upper Trapezius

This muscle commonly refers pain to the posterolateral neck, the mastoid process, the temple and posterior region of the head, occiput, and angle of the jaw (figure 16.1a). One or more of these areas may be a site of pain.

With the patient in supine, the sport rehabilitation specialist places the muscle on slight slack by having the patient move the ear toward the shoulder on the same side. The sport rehabilitation specialist can then either grasp the muscle at the juncture between the neck and shoulder portion of the muscle, or apply a caudal pressure directly over the area (figure 16.1b). If direct pressure is used, it is held until the muscle is felt to release and the patient's pain subsides. The pressure applied is uncomfortable but tolerable. An alternative treatment method is to use either the ice-and-stretch technique with the patient sitting, or deep massage with the patient supine while the sport rehabilitation specialist applies a mild stretch by rotating the head to the opposite side and flexing the neck (figure 16.1c). The direction of the ice strokes is upward from the acromion process toward the base of the skull.

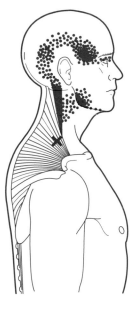

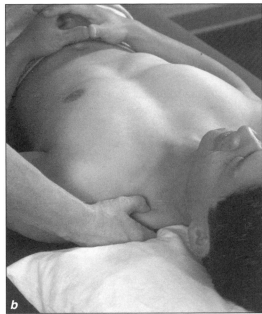

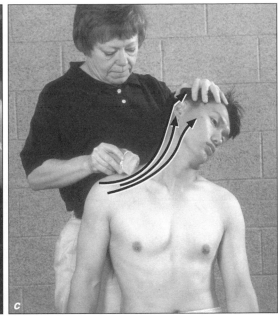

a

b

c

Figure 16.1 Upper trapezius: *(a)* pain pattern (x indicates trigger point), *(b)* myofascial release, *(c)* ice-and-stretch.
Pain pattern *(a)* adapted from Simons, Travell, and Simons 1999.

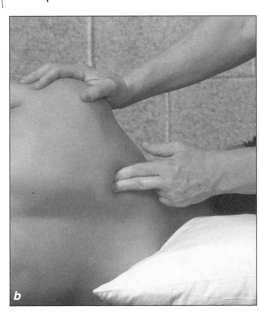

Levator Scapulae

The most common pain-referral pattern from the upper trapezius is at the angle between the neck and the shoulder with occasional referral along the vertebral border of the scapula or to the posterior shoulder (figure 16.2a). Trigger point release is performed as the patient is supine or side-lying with the sport rehabilitation specialist's fingers on the trigger points, indicated in figure 16.2b, either at the distal insertion of the levator scapulae on the vertebral angle of the scapula or at the angle of the neck. Ice-and-stretch is performed with the patient in sitting, the same-side arm anchored, and the head tilted forward and to the opposite side (figure 16.2c). A steady stretch is applied while the ice is stroked from the base of the skull downward along the path of the muscle.

a

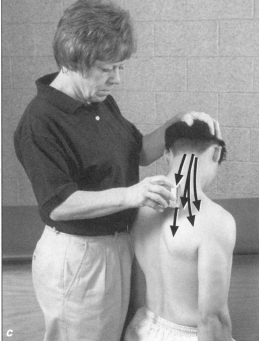

Figure 16.2
Levator scapulae myofascial release: *(a)* pain pattern (x indicates trigger point), *(b)* trigger point release, *(c)* ice-and-stretch.

b

c

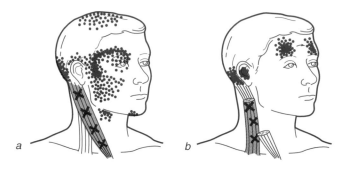

Sternocleidomastoid

Both the sternal and clavicular heads can refer pain into the face and head. The most common areas are in and behind the ear, around the eye, the forehead, cheek, teeth, tongue, pharynx, and the upper aspect of the sternum. There are multiple trigger points along this muscle as seen in figure 16.3, a and b. With the patient in supine and the head tilted to the same side, the sport rehabilitation specialist can either use a pincher grasp on the muscle at the trigger point or apply vertical pressure to it (figure 16.3c).

Ice-and-stretch is applied with the patient sitting, the same-side arm anchored, and the neck positioned in extension and rotation to the opposite side if the clavicular head is being treated (figure 16.3d). If the sternal head of the muscle is being treated, the neck is rotated to the same side and extended (figure 16.3e). The ice strokes are swept from the clavicle upward toward the head.

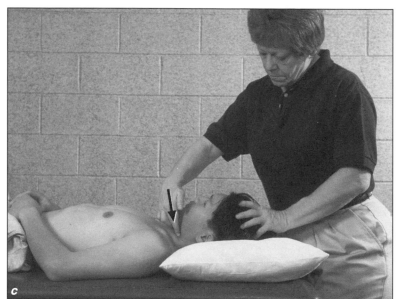

▌Figure 16.3
Sternocleidomastoid myofascial release: (a–b) trigger point pain-referral patterns (x = trigger point), (c) release of clavicular head, (d) ice-and-stretch of clavicular head, (e) ice-and-stretch of sternal head.

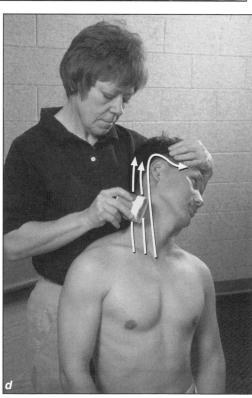

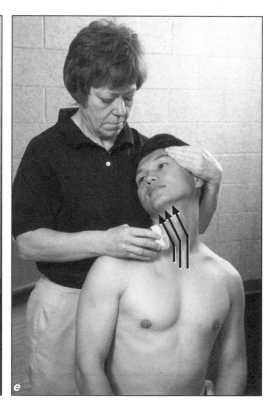

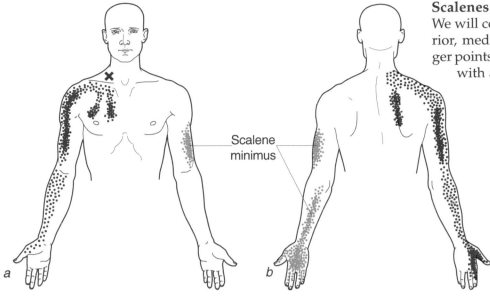

Scalene minimus

Scalenes

We will consider the scalene muscles—anterior, medius, and posterior—together. Trigger points of these muscles are seen in people with a forward-head posture. The pain-referral patterns for the scalenes include pain along the anterior chest, lateral shoulder and arm, vertebral border of the scapula, medial border of the forearm, and interscapular areas (figure 16.4, a and b). The trigger points for these muscles are located and treated with the patient in supine (figure 16.4c). The posterior sternocleidomastoid is first located cephalad to the clavicle. The scalenes lie just lateral to the sternocleidomastoid. The sport rehabilitation specialist identifies the external jugular vein and applies pressure to observe its expansion. This vein usually crosses over the anterior scalene. The anterior scalene's trigger point is just below the external jugular vein. The scalene medius is deep; it is found just lateral to the anterior scalene and just above the clavicle. The subclavian artery lies between the medius and anterior scalenes and can be palpated as it passes over the first rib behind the clavicle. The cervical transverse processes can be palpated when pressure is applied to the scalene medius. Trigger point treatment applied to these muscles often causes referral into the shoulder or arm. The sport rehabilitation specialist must take care to avoid applying pressure over the blood vessels in this area.

Ice-and-stretch is applied with the patient in sitting, the arm anchored (figure 16.4d). The neck is positioned in extension with the head rotated away from the side being treated. Ice stroking is applied from the cephalad insertion of the muscles downward and along the shoulder and arm.

■ **Figure 16.4** (*a*) Trigger point pain-referral pattern for scalene anterior and medius. (*b*) Trigger point pain-referral pattern for scalene posterior. (*c*) Scalenes myofascial release: with the two fingers of the left hand on either side of the anterior and medius scalenes, the right thumb is on the groove between these two muscles. (*d*) Ice-and-stretch for scalenes.

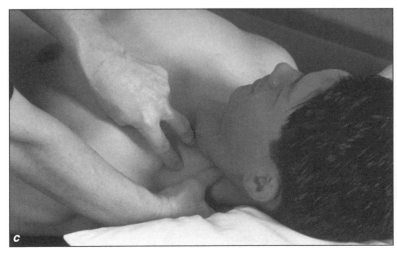

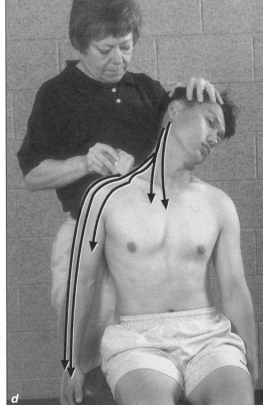

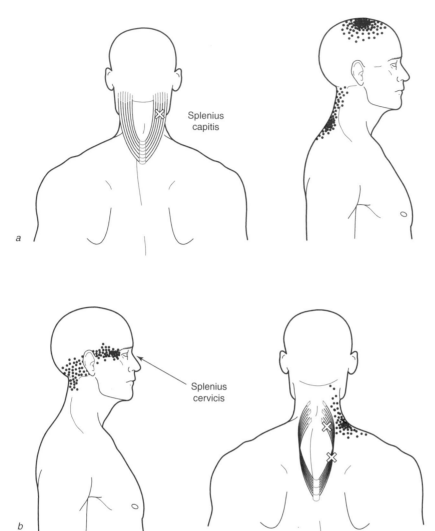

Spleni Muscles

As with the scalenes, we will look at treatment of the capitis and cervicis—the spleni group—together. These muscles also are frequent sites of trigger points in individuals with a forward-head posture. The spleni muscles refer pain to the top of the head, behind the eye, to the base of the neck, and along the side of the head (figure 16.5, a and b). Trigger point treatment is performed in supine or sitting. The splenius capitis trigger point is located just distal to its mastoid attachment (figure 16.5c).

The cervicis lies posterior to the lower cervical transverse processes and is located by laterally flexing the neck to the same side to relax the upper trapezius and levator scapula. The cervicis is palpated over the lower cervical transverse process. Its trigger point is located between the upper trapezius and sternocleidomastoid.

Ice-and-stretch is performed with the patient in sitting. The neck is rotated and laterally flexed to the opposite side, with the ice sweeps directed from the base of the neck upward and downward (figure 16.5d).

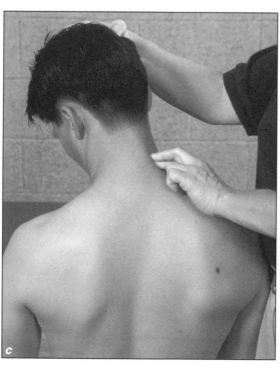
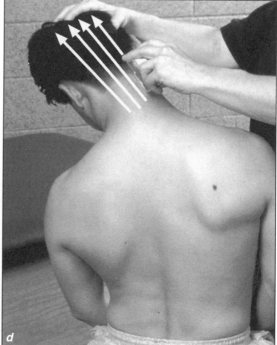

❚ **Figure 16.5**
Splenius myofascial release: (*a*) trigger point pain-referral pattern for splenius capitis, (*b*) upper and lower trigger point pain-referral patterns for splenius cervicis, (*c*) trigger point release, (*d*) ice-and-stretch.

Layer	Muscle	Fiber direction
1	Trapezius	
2	Splenii	
3	Semispinalis capitis	
	Semispinalis cervicis	
4	Multifidi	
	Rotatores	

a Adapted from Simons, Travell, and Simons 1999.

Posterior Cervical Muscles

There are two groups of muscles in the posterior cervical region, one superficial and the other deep. The more superficial group are referred to as posterior cervical muscles and include the semispinalis capitis, semispinalis cervicis, multifidi, and rotatores (figure 16.6a). Beneath the semispinalis muscles are several additional smaller muscles, termed the suboccipital muscles. These include the major and minor rectus capitis muscles and the superior and inferior oblique capitis muscles. The posterior cervical muscles commonly refer to the base of the neck and upward into the suboccipital area, down the neck to the vertebral border of the scapula, and in a horizontal band to the temple on the same side of the head (figure 16.6, b–f). The suboccipital muscles refer to the occiput, the eye, and the forehead. They often give the injured patient a sensation of pain inside the skull; sometimes the patient describes either a vague headache or a pain that is all over the head on one side.

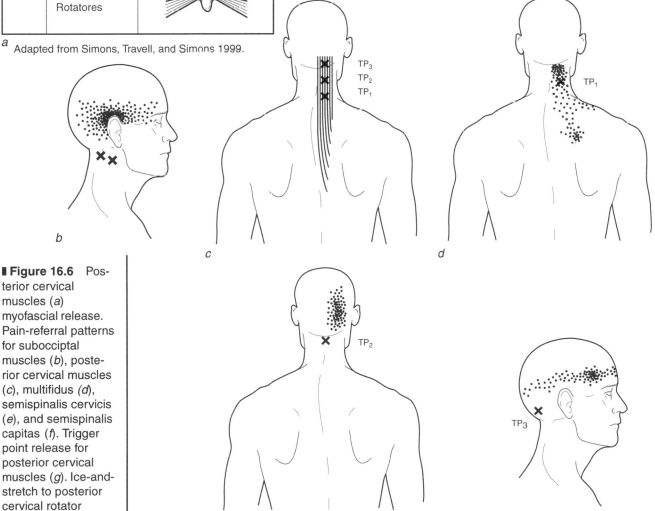

■ **Figure 16.6** Posterior cervical muscles (*a*) myofascial release. Pain-referral patterns for subocciptal muscles (*b*), posterior cervical muscles (*c*), multifidus (*d*), semispinalis cervicis (*e*), and semispinalis capitas (*f*). Trigger point release for posterior cervical muscles (*g*). Ice-and-stretch to posterior cervical rotator muscles (*h*).

(continued)

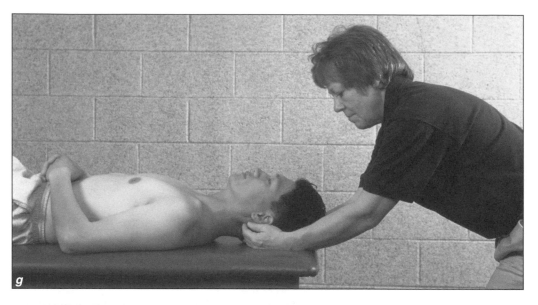

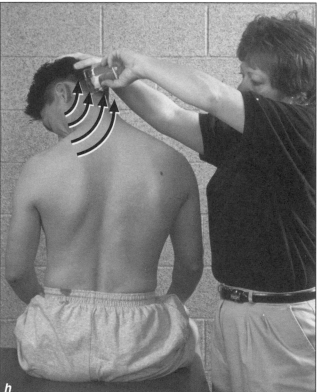

■ **Figure 16.6**
(continued)

For trigger point release, the patient is positioned in supine with the sport rehabilitation specialist at his or her head (figure 16.6g). The finger pads are applied over the trigger points.

Ice-and-stretch is applied in sitting. Head and neck position depends on the specific muscle being treated. The parallel semispinalis muscles can be treated bilaterally in a forward-head position. The rotator muscles that are angled from their distal to their proximal insertion are treated with the neck flexed forward and sideward and rotated to place the muscle on stretch (figure 16.6h). The ice is applied from the base of the neck upward toward the head.

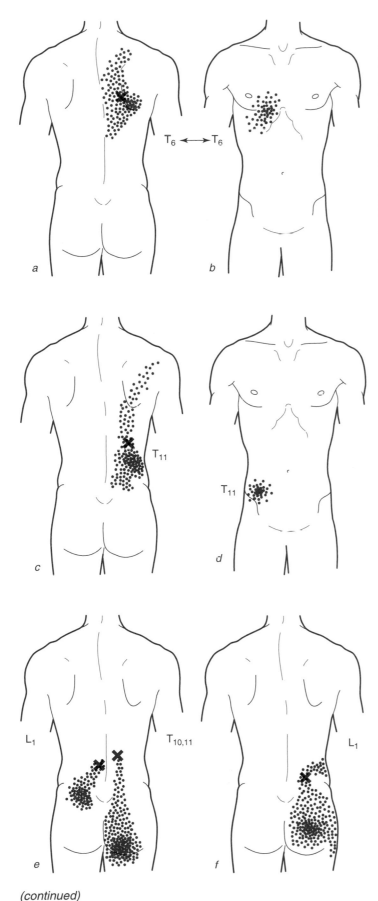

a

b

$T_6 \longleftrightarrow T_6$

c

d

T_{11}

T_{11}

e

f

L_1 $T_{10,11}$ L_1

(continued)

Thoracic and Lumbar Spine

Often the muscles treated with soft-tissue mobilization in the thoracic area are the shoulder and scapular muscles. Those are discussed in chapter 17. Some of the cervical muscles, as you have just seen, can refer into the scapular area; so if a patient describes pain around the scapula without any frank injury to the shoulder or thoracic region, you should evaluate the neck as a possible source of the pain. Likewise, some lumbar pain is referred from the gluteal and thigh muscles; this topic is discussed in chapters 21 and 22.

Because thoracic muscles commonly refer pain into the lumbar area, and because lumbar and thoracic muscles are extensions of the same muscles, the thoracic and lumbar muscles are discussed together. It is often very difficult to separate the two regions from each other. Treatment also often overlaps from one area to another, so it is logical to consider the two areas at the same time.

Muscles in the thoracic and lumbar regions that can refer pain into the thoracic, lumbar, and sacral areas include the thoracic and lumbar paraspinals, the quadratus lumborum, and the serratus posterior. The following sections cover their referral patterns and trigger point and ice-and-stretch treatments.

Paraspinals

This group of muscles includes deep and superficial paraspinal muscles. The superficial group, the iliocostals and longissimus muscles, are collectively referred to as the erector spinae. The deep muscles include the rotatores, semispinalis, and multifidi; among these, the multifidi group are the muscles that most commonly produce pain.

Midthoracic superficial paraspinals can refer pain into the scapula or anterior chest area (figure 16.7, a and b); the lower thoracic superficial paraspinals can refer pain upward into the scapula (figure 16.7c), anteriorly to the lower abdomen (figure 16.7d), or downward to the low back and buttock (figure 16.7, e and f).

∎ **Figure 16.7** Paraspinal pain-referral patterns (x indicates trigger point sites): *(a–f)* superficial paraspinals.

Thoracic multifidi refer pain to the spinous process near the trigger point (figure 16.7, g and h), while the lumbar multifidi can also refer pain into the abdomen (figure 16.7i). Multifidi at S1 can refer into the coccyx (figure 16.7h).

Treatment of the trigger points can be performed with the patient in side-lying or prone, if the neck can be comfortably positioned (figure 16.7j). To perform palpation the sport rehabilitation specialist applies trigger point treatment to the areas that reproduce pain. Ice-and-stretch is applied in a sitting position with the patient in a trunk flexion position (figure 16.7k). The ice is applied in a cephalad-to-caudal motion from the head to the sacrum. If the deep paraspinals are being treated, the stretch must involve rotation and flexion while the ice stroking is performed at an angle.

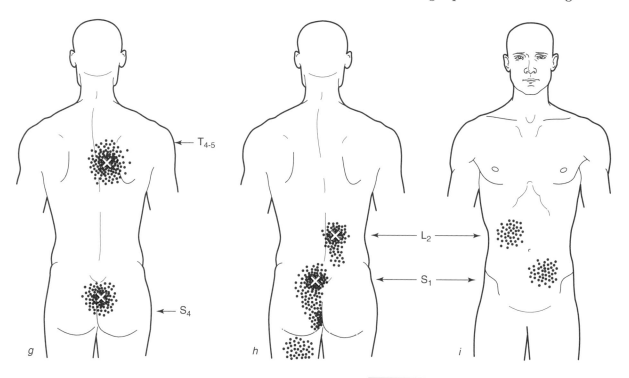

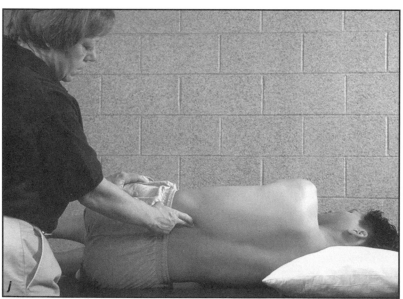

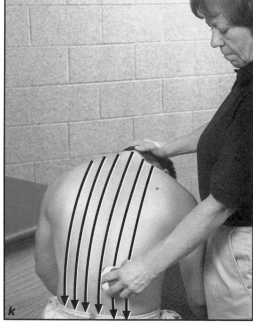

■ **Figure 16.7** *(continued) (g–i)* deep paraspinals, *(j)* myofascial release,*(k)* ice-and-stretch.

Quadratus Lumborum

The quadratus lumborum pain-referral pattern often gives the false sign of a disk syndrome and is neglected as a source of low back pain (Travell and Simons 1992). The pain, which can be intense, can accompany deep inhalation or make walking painful.

Typical quadratus lumborum pain can be either a deep ache or a sharp pain. The superficial fibers can refer pain along the iliac crest or greater trochanter or can wrap around to the outer groin. The deep fibers refer down to the sacroiliac joint or lower buttock (figure 16.8a).

For treatment, the patient should be positioned on the uninvolved side. If the area is not too tender, he or she can lie with the upper arm overhead to elevate the lower ribs, and the thigh and knee flexed with the knee on the table to lower the ilium (figure 16.8b). If the area is too tight or painful for the patient to lie in this position, the top knee should be placed on the bottom ankle or on a supportive pillow to reduce the stretch of the muscle. The superficial trigger points are located laterally, just cephalad to the iliac crest or distal of the 12th rib. The deep trigger points are located just lateral to the paraspinal muscles.

Ice-and-stretch treatment is applied with the patient in a position similar to that for trigger point release, but with the top leg forward of the bottom leg and distal thigh and leg positioned off the table to provide a stretch (figure 16.8c). The ice strokes are swept in a cephalad-to-caudad motion.

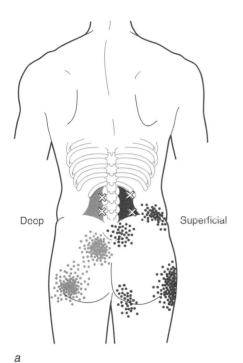

Deep   Superficial

a

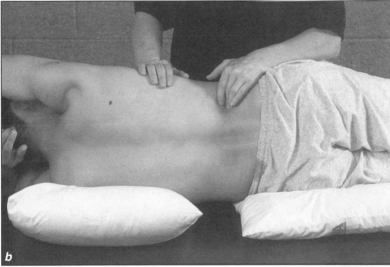

b

▮ Figure 16.8
Quadratus lumborum:
(a) pain-referral
pattern, *(b)* trigger
point release,
(c) ice-and-stretch.

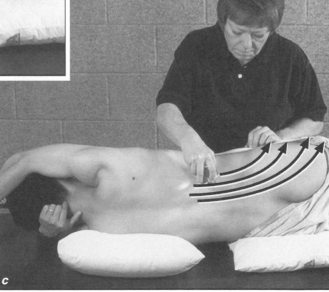

c

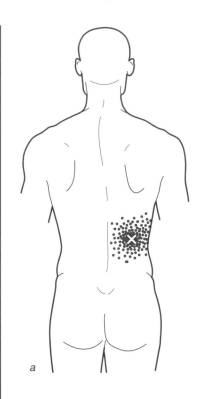

Serratus Posterior Inferior

This muscle causes an annoying ache in the posterior lower rib area in the site of its locale, from the posterior ninth rib medially to the L2 spinous process (figure 16.9a). Pain in this muscle usually remains localized and does not refer to other sites.

Trigger point treatment is performed with the patient in side-lying or prone. The trigger point is located in the lateral region of the muscle close to its rib insertion (figure 16.9b). Ice-and-stretch is performed with the patient in a sitting position. The trunk is flexed and rotated, and the ice is applied in upward and outward sweeps from the spine to the lateral trunk (figure 16.9c).

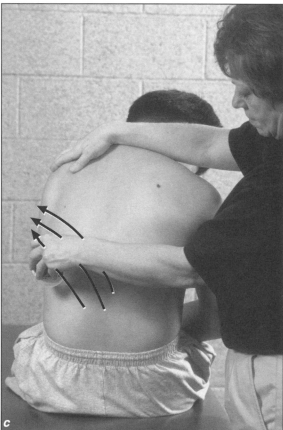

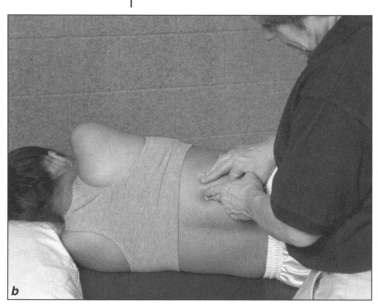

∎ **Figure 16.9**   Serratus posterior: *(a)* trigger point (x) with pain referral pattern, *(b)* trigger point release to right serratus posterior inferior, *(c)* ice-and-stretch to left serratus posterior inferior.

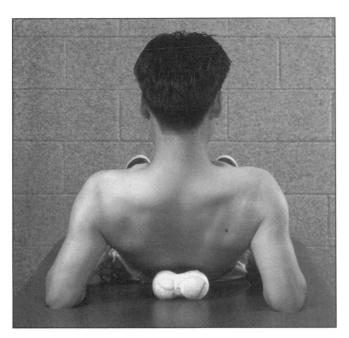

■ Figure 16.10 Tennis ball release.

Self Soft-Tissue Mobilization

This is a soft-tissue mobilization technique that you can instruct the patient in and that does not require assistance. It uses either one or two old tennis balls that have lost their compression. If two balls are used, they can be either taped together (figure 16.10) or placed together in a sock. The patient lies on the tennis balls, which are placed under a restricted soft-tissue area. The patient lies on the tennis balls until the tenderness is gone and he or she feels only the pressure of the tennis balls. The balls are then moved to another location of restriction and the technique is repeated. This technique can be performed in the thoracic and lumbar areas; it can also be used in other soft-tissue restricted areas of the body such as the hip and thigh.

JOINT MOBILIZATION

Obviously, the degree of movement in spinal joint mobilization accessory motion is very different from that in peripheral joints. Before you acquire the ability to determine normal movement, you will have evaluated many different vertebral movements on many different patients of varying ages and with various conditions. Normal accessory movement in the lumbar spine is different from that in the cervical spine, and joint accessory movement in a 19-year-old patient is different from that in a 40-year-old. You must recognize and consider these normal variations when assessing and treating a patient with joint mobilization.

It is necessary to outline some basic principles of application before discussing specific application techniques. When the cervical spine and head are in normal alignment, the lower cervical and lower lumbar spines are slightly extended. Because the best position for joint mobilization is an open-packed position, these areas of the spine should be placed in slight flexion to place the joints into a midposition before mobilization is performed. Rotating the head to the nonpainful side opens the vertebral foramen of C2 to C7. You can also open these by laterally tilting the patient's head away from the painful side. Mobilization techniques differ for the upper and lower cervical spine.

The sport rehabilitation specialist should use body weight and weight transfer as the force source, not the fingers, thumbs, or hands. Using the body as the source of force permits a finer sense of touch for joint movement; is more comfortable for the patient; imposes less stress on the fingers, thumbs, and hands; and conserves the sport rehabilitation specialist's energy.

Initial mobilization techniques should be gentle so that you can assess the patient's response to the technique. There should be no increase in symptoms as a result of the treatment. Assessment before, during, and after the application is necessary in order for you to decide the appropriate depth of treatment. The primary factors restricting the depth of mobilization application are muscle spasm and pain. Frequently, muscle spasm will not permit grades III or IV mobilization because of the increased pain that results from the pressure. When this occurs, gentle mobilization may be used. Mobilization that exacerbates distally referred pain should be modified to include a reduced amplitude or discontinued. Refer to chapter 6 for joint mobilization indications, precautions, and contraindications.

Although there are several mobilization techniques for use in the spine, only a couple for each area of the spine are discussed here. The primary techniques to be described include central posterior-anterior (PA) and unilateral PA mobilization. The symbols used to record these techniques are ↓ for central PA and ↓̣ or ↓̣ for right or left unilateral PAs, respectively. The symbols used to record rib mobilization are ̄↓ for right-rib and ↓ ̄ for left-rib mobilizations. In this section we will consider additional techniques for some specific sites. I recommend that you participate in continuing education courses to develop an understanding and appreciation of more complex maneuvers and to acquire application skills.

Cervical Spine

Description of these techniques will primarily emphasize hand placement. The specific grade to apply is determined by the patient's condition and the treatment goals. Refer to chapter 6 for a review of joint mobilization.

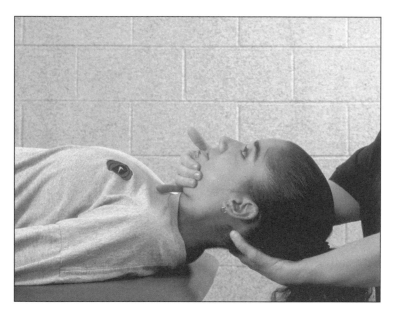

Longitudinal Movement

Longitudinal movement is a relaxing technique that can help you to gain the patient's confidence. It is often the technique used to initiate mobilization treatments. With the patient in supine, the head is grasped and supported with one of the sport rehabilitation specialist's hands behind the neck, and the fingers at the occiput. The other hand is placed under the chin (figure 16.11). The sport rehabilitation specialist leans back to produce a gentle longitudinal pull of the neck. The hand on the chin is for positioning only; no force is directed into the chin.

▌ **Figure 16.11**
Longitudinal cervical movement joint mobilization.

Central PAs

This technique can be used for midline or unilateral pain and spasm. The patient lies prone with his or her hands under the forehead and the chin slightly tucked. The sport rehabilitation specialist stands at the head and places the thumbs on the spine with the fingers relaxed, along the sides of the neck (figure 16.12). C1 and C3 are usually too difficult to palpate; but C2, C4, C5, C6, and C7 should be readily identified. The sport rehabilitation specialist applies PA pressure through movement of his or her trunk over the hands. The pressure should be gentle initially; adjustments are made according to the patient's response.

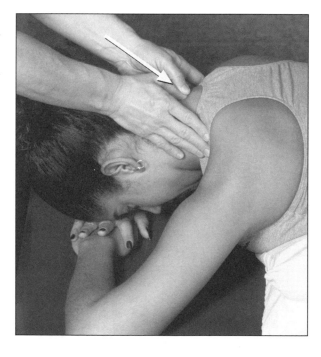

▌ **Figure 16.12**   PA central cervical mobilization.

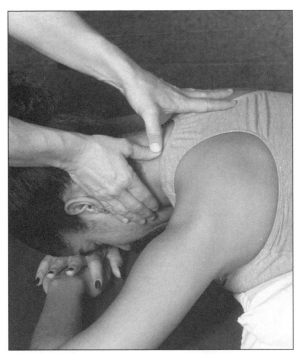

Figure 16.13 Unilateral cervical mobilization.

Unilateral PAs

The technique described here can be used for the lower cervical spine and for unilateral neck pain. The patient lies prone with the hands under the forehead and the chin slightly tucked. The sport rehabilitation specialist stands on the side that is to be treated. The thumbs are placed on the articular pillar and angled about 30° medially (figure 16.13). The pressure is applied in a PA direction with a constant medially directed pressure to maintain position on the articular pillar. The head may nod slightly, but there should be no rotation motion if the pressure is applied correctly.

Thoracic Spine

Look at the bony arrangement on a skeleton to see how the position and relative alignment of the spinous processes change from the cervical to the lumbar spine. The angle of the joint mobilization force must change to produce a force in the plane of the joint. This is a crucial point to keep in mind as you perform mobilization techniques along the spine.

Central PAs

This technique can be used for central or unilateral symptoms. The patient is in prone with the hands under the forehead and the chin slightly tucked. The specific thoracic segment being treated determines where the sport rehabilitation specialist stands. His or her position is at the head (figure 16.14a) if the upper segments are being treated and at the side (figure 16.14b) if the middle and lower segments are being treated. The thumbs are placed directly over the spinous process, with the fingertips spread across the back to act as a stabilizer for the thumbs. The pressure is applied at an angle perpendicular to the surface, so the position will change slightly as the hands move along the thoracic spine. The force is transmitted from the trunk through the arms to the thumbs. The fingers should remain relaxed.

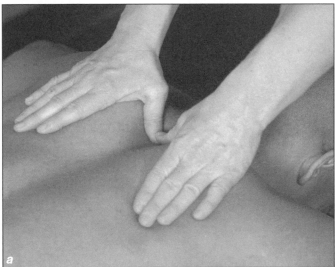

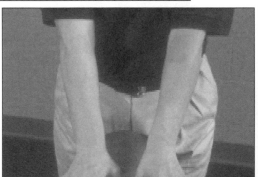
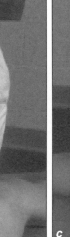
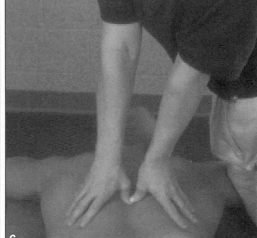

Figure 16.14 Central PA thoracic mobilization: *(a)* Thumbs are placed over the spinous process. One thumb can be used to reinforce the other thumb. *(b)* Upper thoracic mobilizations are most easily performed while standing at the patient's head. *(c)* Lower and middle thoracic mobilizations are performed while standing at the patient's side.

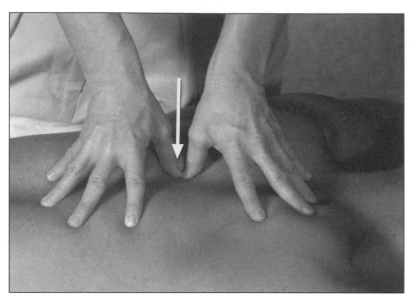

■ Figure 16.15   Unilateral PA thoracic mobilization.

Unilateral PAs

This technique can be used for unilateral symptoms. The patient lies prone with the head turned to the side being treated. The arms hang over the side of the table. The sport rehabilitation specialist stands on the side being treated and places his or her hands on the patient's back, with the thumb pads on the transverse process and the fingers buttressed over the back (figure 16.15). The sport rehabilitation specialist's shoulders and arms are directly over his or her hands; the force is directed at an angle perpendicular to the surface. Movement occurs as a result of trunk, not thumb, movement.

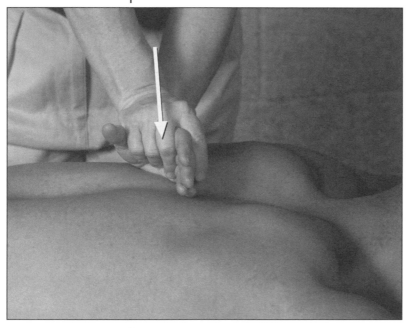

■ Figure 16.16
Unilateral costovertebral PA mobilization.

Unilateral Costovertebral PAs

This technique can be used for painful or restricted ribs. The patient lies prone with arms at his or her sides or hanging over the table. The sport rehabilitation specialist stands on the side being treated. The ulnar border of the sport rehabilitation specialist's hand is placed along the line of the patient's rib near the costovertebral joint, with the other hand placed on top of the second metacarpal and digit (figure 16.16). Placement of the ulnar border is approximately two finger-widths from the spinous process. The pressure is applied at an angle perpendicular to the joint surface from the trunk through the shoulders and into the hands.

Lumbar Spine and Sacroiliac

Like the cervical and thoracic areas, the lumbar spine can be treated with central and unilateral PA movements. In addition, rotation mobilizations can be performed as a gross technique affecting the lumbar spine as a whole rather than individual levels.

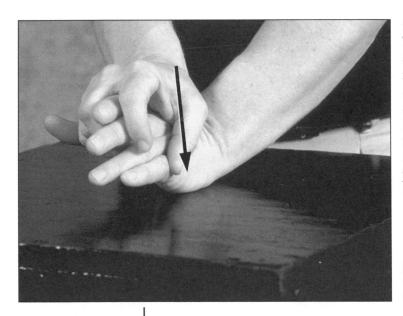

Central PA Mobilization

This technique can be used for hypomobility and central and unilateral pain and derangements. Lumbar spine PA movements can be applied using the pisiform area of the hand as the point of force application (figure 16.17). The patient lies prone and the sport rehabilitation specialist stands to the side. Pressure is applied perpendicularly to the joint surface through the shoulders from the trunk.

▌Figure 16.17   Central PA mobilization using the ulnar border of the left hand with reinforcement from the right hand.

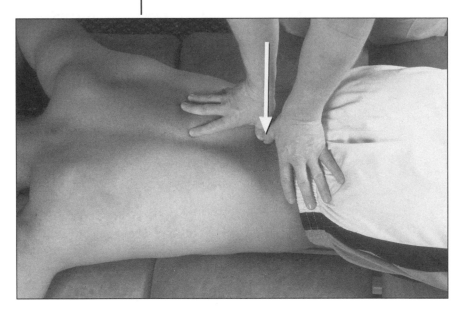

Unilateral PA Mobilization

This technique can be used for unilateral pain. The patient lies prone with the head turned to one side. The sport rehabilitation specialist stands on the side to be treated and places the thumbs lateral to the spinous process, at the level being treated, with the fingers spread across the back (figure 16.18). The sport rehabilitation specialist's shoulders are placed directly over his or her hands, and the pressure is applied directly perpendicular to the joint surface through the shoulders. The fingers remain relaxed; no pressure is applied through them.

▌Figure 16.18
Unilateral lumbar mobilization.

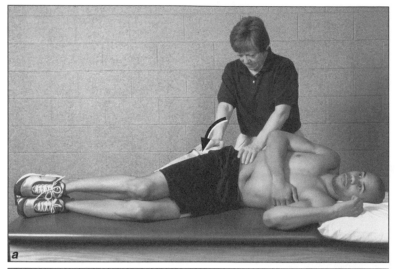

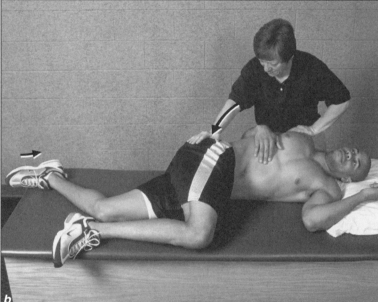

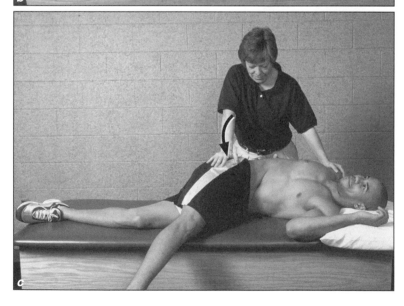

Rotation

This technique can be used in unilateral restriction of movement and unilateral back or leg pain. The patient lies on the unaffected side with a pillow under the head. The top shoulder is extended, and the elbow is flexed with the forearm resting on the side. The lower-extremity position depends on the grade of pressure being applied. For grades I and II, the hips and knees are flexed with the top leg slightly more flexed than the bottom leg. The lumbar vertebrae are positioned in midrange flexion-extension by the amount of hip flexion. The sport rehabilitation specialist places his or her hands on the pelvis and creates a gentle rocking motion of the pelvis (figure 16.19a).

In grade III, the shoulder is rotated slightly more posteriorly so that the chest faces the ceiling and the torso is in a three-quarter position. The bottom leg is more extended than in grades I and II; the top leg is flexed with the medial femoral condyle on the table or just off the edge, and the ankle is hooked around the bottom lower leg. The sport rehabilitation specialist places one hand on the patient's shoulder and the other on the pelvis with the fingers pointing forward. If the desired motion is more into extension, then the hand is placed over the iliac crest with the sport rehabilitation specialist standing near the shoulder (figure 16.19b); but if the desired motion is into flexion, the hand is placed over the greater trochanter with the sport rehabilitation specialist standing near the pelvis. The movement is caused by the hand at the pelvis, not the shoulder. Grade IV motion is produced with the top lower leg more extended and off the table. The sport rehabilitation specialist may need to kneel on the table behind the patient so that the force can be directed more easily from the shoulders to the hand on the pelvis. The sport rehabilitation specialist's knee behind the patient's back can also assist (figure 16.19c). Motion for each grade should be a rotatory motion of the pelvis, not posterior to anterior or inferior to superior.

∎ Figure 16.19 Unilateral lumbar mobilization: *(a)* grade I and II rotation, *(b)* grade III rotation, *(c)* grade IV rotation.

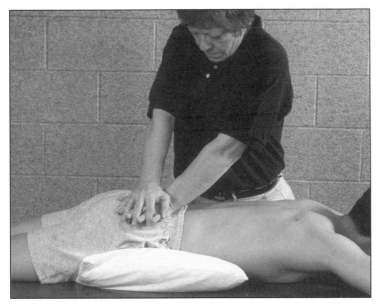

Figure 16.20 Sacroiliac posterior-anterior mobilization. Although the sport rehabilitation specialist is shown on the opposite side from the side being treated, this is only to allow better visualization of the technique.

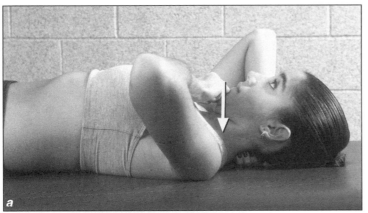

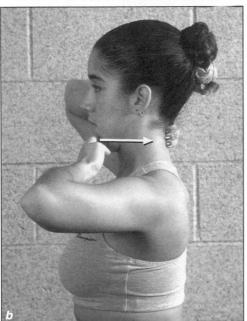

Figure 16.21 Axial extension in *(a)* supine and *(b)* sitting.

Sacroiliac Posterior-Anterior Pressures

These techniques can be applied centrally or unilaterally. The patient lies prone with the sport rehabilitation specialist standing on the side to be treated. The lateral aspect of one hand is reinforced with the other hand on top of it and is placed over the upper sacrum. Posterior-anterior pressure is applied at the S1 level and gradually continued distally to the distal end of the sacrum (figure 16.20). Because of the complexity of the SI joint, the PA pressure can be applied in a cephalic, caudal, medial, or lateral direction or in any combination of these.

FLEXIBILITY EXERCISES

Because the lower cervical spine is related to the upper thoracic spine and the lumbar spine is related to the lower thoracic spine, sacrum, and hips, some of the flexibility exercises for cervical and lumbar regions of the spine overlap into these other areas. Unless otherwise indicated, the stretch is held for about 20 s and repeated four to five times.

Cervical Spine

The description of each flexibility exercise in this section includes the correct manner of execution and common incorrect substitutions that should be avoided. These substitutions occur as the patient attempts to produce as much motion as possible. You should watch for these patterns carefully and correct them as they occur to prevent the patient from stretching ineffectively.

Axial Extension

This exercise helps the patient restore normal cervical alignment and correct posture. The patient lies supine on a firm surface, such as a tabletop or the floor. A pillow is not used. The patient places the fingertips of one hand on the cervical spinous processes and the other hand under the chin (figure 16.21a). The neck is then pushed into the fingertips as the patient pushes the tucked chin back with the front hand. As the patient finds this activity easier to perform, he or she can perform it in sitting. The patient places the index finger and thumb of one hand on the chin and the fingertips of the other hand along the upper cervical spine. With the chin tucked, the patient pushes the chin back with the chin hand and feels with the other hand as the cervical spine is pushed into that hand (figure 16.21b). In the common substitution for this exercise, the patient extends the cervical spine and presses the head backward rather than extending the cervical spine. If this occurs, have the patient move the chin downward first, then press the cervical spine into the fingertips.

Cervical Retraction

Also called the turtle exercise because of its motion, this exercise is used to stretch the posterior cervical muscles and improve posture. It can be performed in sitting or supine. The chin is tucked, and the head is pulled back while the chin stays at the same level (figure 16.22). The head does not tilt up or down during this activity. The common substitution for this exercise is cervical extension and lifting of the chin. Instruct the patient to keep the chin tucked if you observe the substitution.

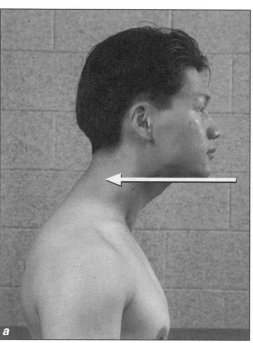
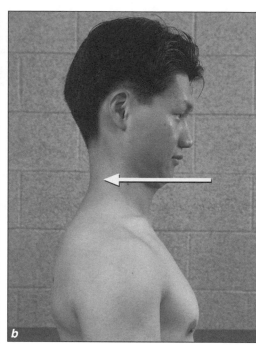

▌Figure 16.22
Cervical retraction: *(a)* forward, starting position; *(b)* retracted, end position.

Cervical Flexion

This exercise stretches the posterior cervical spinal muscles. With the chin tucked, the patient bends the head forward, attempting to touch the chin to the chest. Overpressure can provide additional stretch: The patient places his or her hands on top of the head and relaxes the shoulders. The weight of the arms will provide sufficient stretch, so instruct the patient not to pull the head but to let the arms relax and the elbows hang down (figure 16.23). The common substitution for this exercise is not to curl the neck but to use the lower cervical spine as a fulcrum while the upper cervical spine stays straight. If this occurs, instruct the patient to unwind the neck, beginning with the upper spine and moving downward.

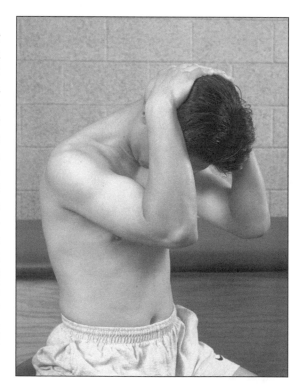

▌Figure 16.23
Cervical flexion.

Upper Trapezius Stretch

This stretch isolates the upper trapezius muscle. In sitting, the patient grasps the wrist of the side to be stretched and pulls it across the body. The head is tilted away from the shoulder (figure 16.24a). Leaning the head to the opposite side can increase the stretch. Common substitutions for this exercise are allowing the shoulder to shrug upward, rotating the neck, or bending the head forward, rather than directly sideways. If these substitutions occur, correct the patient by instructing him or her to stabilize the shoulder by sitting on the hand, and to keep the nose in a forward position. Sometimes it may be necessary to start the patient in a supine position so that rotation and forward bending are minimized.

An alternative stretch uses a stretch strap that is draped over one shoulder. The opposite foot's toes are used to anchor the strap to the floor (figure 16.24b). The patient aligns the strap from the anchoring toes to beneath the elevated heel and takes up the slack with the hands in front of the body. A towel or other pad is placed under the strap on the shoulder for comfort. The heel is then moved to the floor so that the strap becomes taut, applying pressure on the upper trapezius.

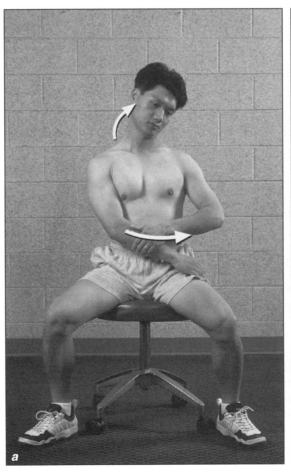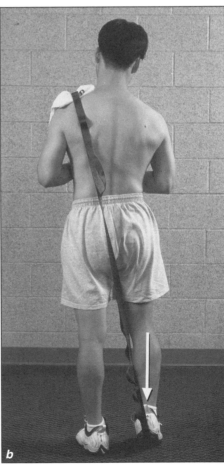

∎ **Figure 16.24** Upper trapezius stretch: (a) active stretch, (b) with stretch strap.

Scalene Stretch

Because the scalenes have three different parts, there are three positions to stretch them. These stretches can be performed in sitting or supine. The arm on the side being stretched is anchored under the hip in all positions, and the opposite hand is placed over the head and above the ear. For stretching the posterior, the face is turned to the opposite axilla (figure 16.25a). To stretch the medius, the face is kept looking forward while the head is tilted (figure 16.25b). To stretch the anterior, the face is turned to the side being stretched and the patient looks to the ceiling (figure 16.25c). The hand on top of the head applies a gentle stretch that produces a stretch sensation without discomfort or pain. The common substitution for this exercise is to move the shoulders during the stretch. If this occurs, have the patient perform the exercises in supine.

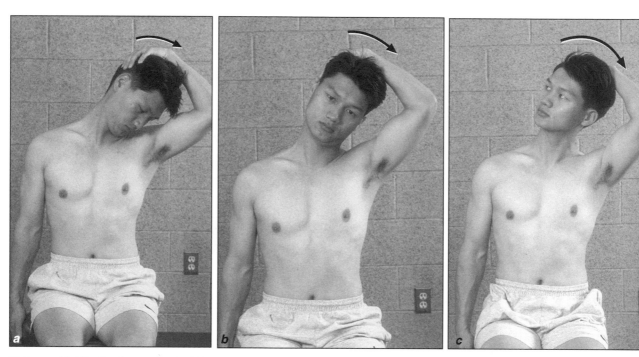

■ **Figure 16.25**   Scalene stretch: *(a)* posterior, *(b)* medius, *(c)* anterior.

For additional information about physiotherapy, see **www.physio-net.com/aboutphysio/**.

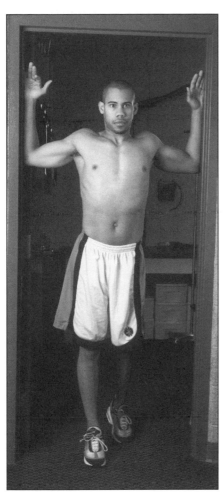

■ Figure 16.26
Stretch to middle
pectoralis.

Pectoral Stretch

This exercise stretches the pectoral muscles, a common source of poor cervical posture. The patient stands in a doorway with the forearms on the door frame and elbows at shoulder level. With one foot in front of the other, the patient attempts to push through the doorway (figure 16.26). This exercise can also be performed in a corner, although empty corners are often difficult to find. The common substitution for this exercise is rotating the body toward the tight shoulder, especially if patients are small and the door frame is too wide. If this occurs, have the patient keep both arms at the same level on the door frame. Using a corner instead of a door frame also helps improve execution of the exercise.

Sternal Raise

This exercise for the cervical and upper thoracic spine assists in improving posture. The patient elevates the sternum while moving the scapulae downward toward the back pockets. A common substitution for this exercise is to hyperextend the lumbar spine rather than elevate the sternum. You can limit the substitution if you instruct the patient to simultaneously contract the abdominals to stabilize the lumbar spine.

Thoracolumbar Spine

Because the ribs restrict mobility of the thoracic spine, thoracic motion is possible but limited. Abnormally limited motion in the thoracic ribs or spine can reduce shoulder motion and lung inhalation.

For links to a wide range of sports medicine resources, see *The Physician and Sportsmedicine* Web site at **www.physsportsmed.com/links.htm**.

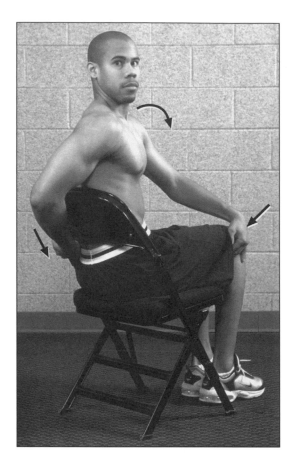

Spinal Twist

This exercise stretches the middle and low back and buttocks. It can be performed sitting on the ground or in a chair. On the ground, the patient crosses one leg over the other outstretched leg so that the crossing foot is placed on the outside of the outstretched leg. The elbow on the outstretched-leg side is placed on the outside of the bent knee, and the other arm is placed behind the body with the elbow straight. The patient then twists the body around toward the outstretched arm. If performing this exercise in a chair, the patient uses a straight-backed chair without arms. The feet are firmly planted on the floor, and the trunk is rotated toward the back of the chair. With one hand placed on the chair back, the other hand is placed on the outside of the knee as shown in figure 16.27. The patient uses the hands to pull around and provide the stretch. The thighs should not move but should remain in place during the stretch. A common substitution for this exercise is to allow the hips to rotate with the stretch. Instruct the patient to apply a hand on the outside of the thigh during the chair-twist stretch. To correct substitution in the stretch when it is performed on the floor, the patient should use the hand on the thigh to apply additional stabilizing force.

▌**Figure 16.27** Spinal twist stretch.

Quadratus Lumborum Stretch

This exercise stretches the quadratus lumborum and latissimus dorsi. The patient sits on the floor. One thigh is parallel to the wall and flexed at the knee so that the sole of the foot of that leg is placed on the inner thigh of the opposite leg, which is extended out to the side (figure 16.28). The arm farther from the wall is in front of the

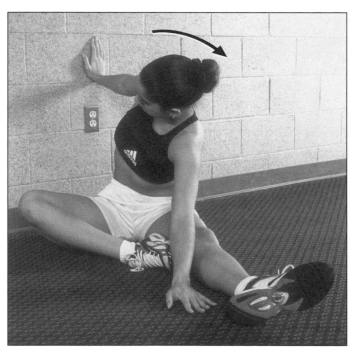

same-side leg and the hand nearest the wall is placed on the wall to push the trunk away from the wall. In an alternative position that offers more stretch, the patient places the wall arm over the head in external rotation and full abduction and leans toward the opposite side. The patient should maintain pelvic neutral during the stretch. A common substitution for this stretch is to move out of pelvic neutral and flex the trunk. Instruct the individual to maintain pelvic neutral and lean only as far as possible while in pelvic neutral.

▌**Figure 16.28**
Quadratus lumborum stretch.

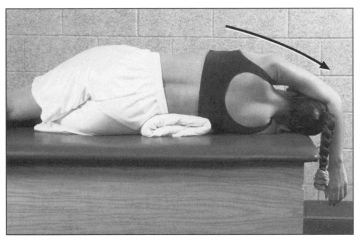

■ Figure 16.29 Prolonged side-bending stretch.

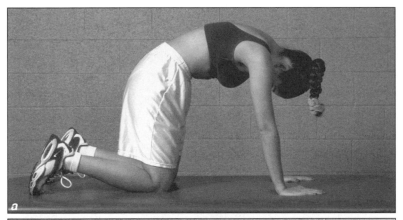

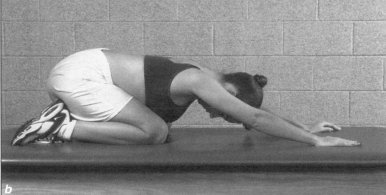

■ Figure 16.30
Lumbar rock stretch:
(a) start position, *(b)*
end position for
lumbar flexion portion
of the lumbar rock,
(c) end position for
lumbar extension
portion of the lumbar
rock.

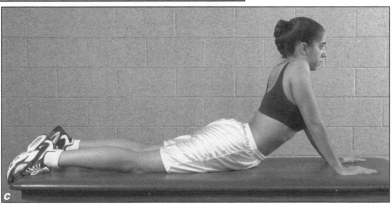

Prolonged Side-Bending

This exercise stretches out the trunk area. It can also be used to open up a facet joint. Depending on the position, it can be used to stretch out the middle or lower thoracic area or the lumbar area. The patient is in sidelying with the tight region on the top and a rolled towel or pillow supporting the portion of the trunk that is underneath the tight region. The top arm is placed overhead, and the top leg is straight in extension (figure 16.29). The degree of stretch can be altered by increasing or decreasing the size of the rolled towel or pillow. Trunk flexion is the common substitution for this exercise. The patient must remain in a straight-aligned position of the trunk relative to the pelvis to attain maximum results.

Lumbar Rock

This exercise stretches the low back and hips. The patient is positioned on hands and knees with elbows straight, hands shoulder-width apart, knees under the hips, and hands under the shoulders. The back is arched, and the hips are pushed back toward the ankles as the shoulders go down toward the floor (figure 16.30, a and b). Without moving the hands or knees, the patient then moves forward to the starting position and continues forward until he or she is in a press-up position (figure 16.30c). A common substitution is to move the hands rather than keeping them stationary. If you observe this, remind the patient to maintain hand positions.

Bent-Over Stretch

This exercise stretches the lumbar and thoracic spine. The patient sits in a chair with feet flat on the floor and apart. Starting from the neck, the patient slowly flexes forward and continues to bend the spine as the body flexes forward. The patient can wrap the hands around the ankles from inside the legs to outside the ankles and pull in order to give an extra stretch. When returning to the starting position, the patient places the hands on the knees and pushes with the arms to move upright rather than using the trunk muscles. Bending from the hips is the most common substitution for this exercise. Instruct the patient to roll and attempt to feel each segment moving as he or she curls through to the end position.

Knees-to-Chest

This exercise stretches the low back and hips. The patient lies supine with the knees flexed. For a single knee-to-chest exercise, the patient first tightens the abdominals to stabilize the pelvis, then lifts one knee to the chest. The knee is held to the chest passively by the arms. In the more aggressive double knee-to-chest stretch, the patient stabilizes the pelvis by tightening the abdominals, then raises one knee to the chest. While keeping the knee up, the patient raises the other knee to the chest and pulls both knees to the chest with the arms. In a double knee-to-chest stretch, one leg at a time is raised and lowered to prevent the back from arching.

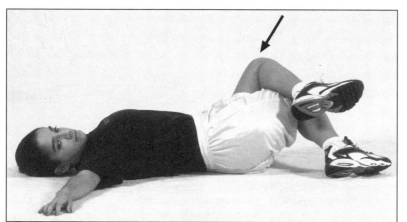

■ **Figure 16.31** Lateral trunk stretch.

Lateral Trunk Stretch

This exercise stretches the lateral lumbar area. The patient is in supine with the knees flexed, feet flat on the floor, and arms outstretched. One knee is crossed over the other, and the top leg pulls the bottom leg toward the top-leg side while both shoulders remain in contact with the floor (figure 16.31). A common substitution is to allow the shoulders to come off the floor so that less stretch is applied. Remind the patient of the importance of shoulder stabilization if you observe this error.

Thomas Hip Flexor Stretch

This exercise stretches the hip flexors. The patient sits on a table so that the thigh is halfway off the table. The patient lies supine with both knees to the chest. One leg is grasped behind the knee, and the leg being stretched is lowered to the table. The thigh of the leg being stretched (the lowered leg) should be kept in proper alignment with the body's midline, without hip rotation or abduction and with knee flexion to 90° (figure 16.32). If the patient has normal flexibility, the thigh should rest comfortably on the table with the back in full contact with the table. A common substitution for this exercise is hyperextension of the lumbar spine. If you observe a lift of the lumbar spine, have the patient bring the opposite leg up closer to the chest.

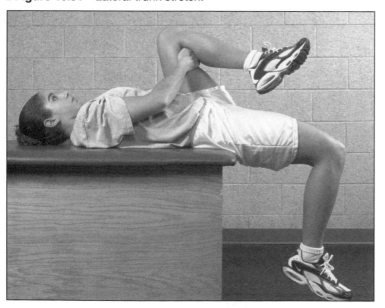

■ **Figure 16.32** Thomas hip flexor stretch.

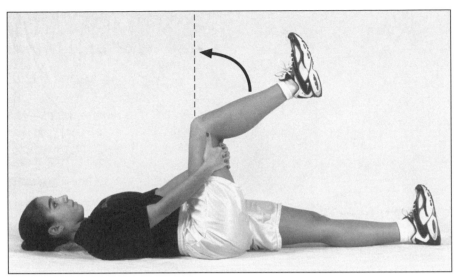

■ Figure 16.33
Hamstring stretch.

Straight-Leg Raise

This exercise stretches the hamstrings. Hamstring tightness can contribute to low back inflexibility. Although a variety of methods are available to stretch the hamstrings, this exercise places minimal stress on the spine. In supine the patient places the hands behind the thigh of one leg while the other leg remains extended. The patient then straightens the knee of the leg that the hands are on until he or she feels a stretch in the thigh or behind the knee (figure 16.33). The common substitution for this exercise is to flex the opposite hip to relieve the stretch. The patient should keep the other leg in a fully extended position throughout the exercise.

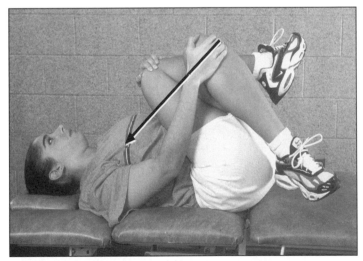

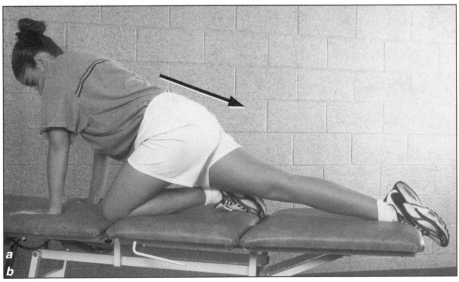

Piriformis Stretch

This exercise stretches the external hip rotators, a common source of low back pain. The patient lies supine with the knees flexed and feet flat on the floor. The knee of the involved leg is crossed on top of the other, and both knees are brought to the chest. The patient grasps the lower knee and pulls both knees toward the chest (figure 16.34a). A common substitution is to provide less rotation of the stretched hip. The knees should be adequately crossed to aim the knee toward the opposite shoulder when the knees are brought to the chest.

In an alternative piriformis stretch, the patient is on hands and knees with the uninvolved leg crossed over the involved leg and behind the involved hip. The patient moves the hips backward, keeping the uninvolved leg straight and bending the knee of the involved leg (figure 16.34b). A common substitution is moving the hips toward the extended leg rather than keeping the weight equally distributed over both hips. If you observe this substitution instruct the patient not to rotate, but to move straight back.

■ Figure 16.34 Piriformis stretch: *(a)* supine, *(b)* quadruped.

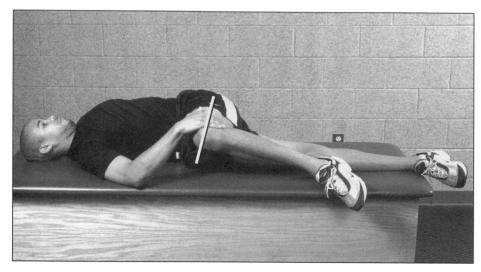

■ **Figure 16.35**   Iliotibial band stretch.

Iliotibial Band Stretch

This exercise stretches the lateral thigh. Tightness in this area can influence the low back. The patient lies supine with the knees straight. One leg is crossed over the other so that the foot of the crossed-over leg lies on the outside of the opposite knee. The hand on the opposite side grasps the crossed-over knee and pulls it toward the floor (figure 16.35). The common substitution for this exercise is to lift the ipsilateral shoulder off the floor. Instruct the patient in proper stabilization of the trunk for this exercise.

Lateral Shift

This exercise is used to correct a lateral shift. The patient stands next to the wall, with the side that has the lumbar lateral shift away from the wall. Keeping the shoulders level, the patient shifts the pelvis laterally to the wall (figure 16.36a). To perform this stretch passively, the sport rehabilitation specialist stands facing toward the side with the shift. The sport rehabilitation specialist then grasps around the patient's waist and clasps his or her hands together on the opposite hip (figure 16.36b). The sport rehabilitation specialist applies pressure with the shoulder into the patient's waist while pulling the pelvis toward him- or herself. The common substitution for this exercise is a tilting of the shoulders away from the wall, or a leaning of the hips into the wall, or both. If this occurs, either have the patient

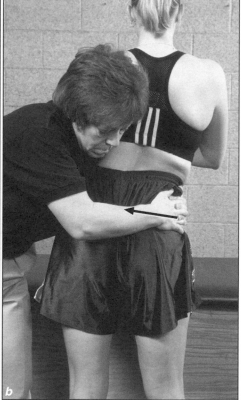

■ **Figure 16.36**
Lateral shift:
(a) independent,
(b) assisted.

perform the exercise in front of a mirror or place your hands above the shoulders, but not touching them, and instruct the patient to perform the exercise without letting the shoulders touch your hands.

Standing Extension
This exercise increases trunk extension and relieves tension after prolonged sitting or forward bending. The patient is in standing and places the hands in the small of the back. The patient then leans backward, leading with the head and keeping the knees and hips extended. A common substitution is extending the hips and bending the knees, leaning back from the knees. If this occurs, have the patient perform the exercise with his or her back against a countertop to stop the hips from moving backward.

POSTURE AND PELVIC STABILIZATION EXERCISES

Any patient who has a spinal injury should be assessed for posture. Posture plays a vital role in both recovery from and prevention of injuries. If a patient has poor posture and nothing is done to correct it, the poor posture will continue to exacerbate the injury and make recovery difficult. Instruction in techniques to maintain proper posture and in use of proper body mechanics should also be a part of the rehabilitation program. Refer to the discussion of posture in chapter 11 as necessary.

A progression of exercises designed to assist the patient in spine stabilization includes exercises in the supine and quadruped positions. The intent is to strengthen the lower back and abdominal muscles and provide spinal stability during arm and leg motion. These exercises constitute the initial step toward movement without stress to the spine and should be a part of the rehabilitation program if a patient has difficulty grasping the spinal alignment concept and maintaining good spinal alignment during activities.

The supine exercises are often referred to as "bug exercises" or "dead-bug exercises," presumably because of the position they are performed in and the arm and leg movement that occurs. The supine and quadruped exercises are outlined here progressively, from the easiest to the more difficult. Once the patient masters one exercise, he or she can progress to the next one. These may seem to be simple exercises, but if you try them, you quickly realize that they may not be as simple to perform as they look.

Not all patients with back injuries need to perform these exercises; but for those who do, the sport rehabilitation specialist should assess their ability to maintain pelvic stability throughout the exercises. Any difficulty the patient has with any of these exercises indicates that pelvic stabilization is limited, and that the patient should do the exercise until he or she is able to perform it correctly.

Spinal stabilization work moves from these basic exercises to more functional activities. It is important that the patient maintains good trunk stability during all activities. This protects the spine and also allows the patient to perform athletic activities more skillfully and with greater force, because with good pelvic stability the lower-extremity forces can be more readily transmitted to the upper extremities. Activities in the final phase of pelvic stabilization include performance of skill drills while in pelvic neutral. From skill drills the patient advances to functional sport movement.

It is important to remember that spinal stability must be maintained throughout each of these exercises. The hips should not roll; the lumbar spine should not flex or extend; and there should not be an anterior or posterior pelvic tilt. If the patient is unable to maintain stability during any exercise, it may be necessary to return to exercises at the previous level of difficulty before advancing. The abdominal and buttock muscles should be tensed in each of these exercises to provide the stabilization necessary for correct performance. You should instruct or remind the patient regarding this until he or she can perform the exercise without verbal cueing. Before using any of these exercises, you should instruct the patient in how to find and maintain a pelvic neutral position. Once the patient can find pelvic neutral, the exercises can begin.

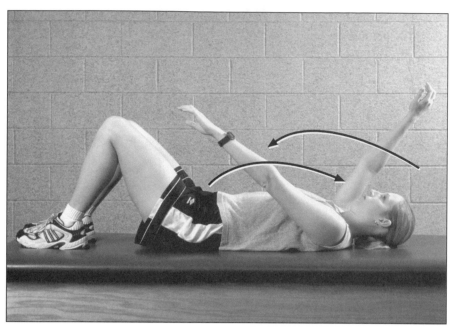

I Figure 16.37 Spine stabilization with arms.

Supine Stabilization With Arm Movement

This exercise provides arm resistance to pelvic stabilization. The patient lies supine with the knees bent. The abdominals are contracted to maintain a neutral spine position. One arm is raised overhead, and then the other, in an alternating fashion (figure 16.37). The trunk is stabilized, with no movement occurring in the spine or pelvis while the arms are moving. The patient must maintain pelvic neutral and breathe while performing the movement.

Supine Stabilization With Leg Movement

This exercise strengthens the lower abdominals and provides increased resistance to pelvic stabilization. The patient lies supine with the legs bent. While in a neutral spine position, the patient raises one knee up toward the chest and then extends the leg from the knee without moving the hips as the abdominals are contracted more tightly to maintain pelvic neutral (figure 16.38). The hips should not rise up or rotate, and the back should not arch. The motion should be smooth. The patient returns the leg to the starting position and repeats the movement with the opposite leg.

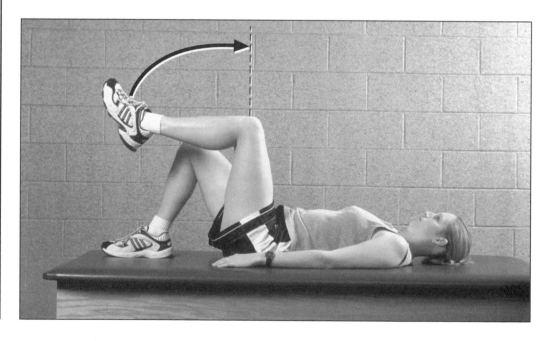

I Figure 16.38 Spine stabilization with legs.

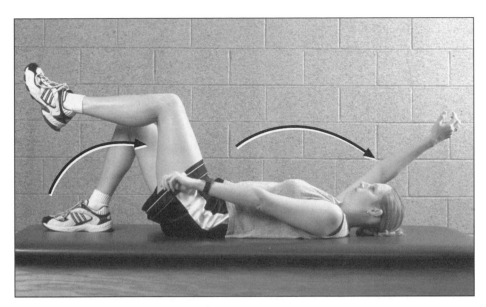

▌Figure 16.39 Spine stabilization with arm and leg movement.

Supine Stabilization With Arm and Leg Movement

This exercise is designed to strengthen the abdominals and stabilize the spine while the arms and legs move independently of the spine. The patient lies supine with the knees bent and the spine in a neutral position. One arm and the opposite leg are raised simultaneously and then lowered while pelvic neutral is maintained (figure 16.39). The movement is repeated with the contralateral arm and leg. The movement should be smooth, and no trunk motion should occur. The pelvis is maintained in neutral throughout. The back should not roll from one side to another and should not arch off the floor.

Supine Stabilization With Arms and Unsupported Legs

This is a more severe exercise for strengthening the abdominals and maintaining pelvic neutral during independent arm and leg movement. The patient lies supine with the knees bent and the spine in pelvic neutral. The neck and shoulders should remain relaxed throughout the exercise. The abdominal muscles remain tightened as the patient lifts the arms and legs off the floor. The patient gradually straightens the leg while raising the arm on the same side (figure 16.40). The back should not lift off the floor, and the hips should not roll.

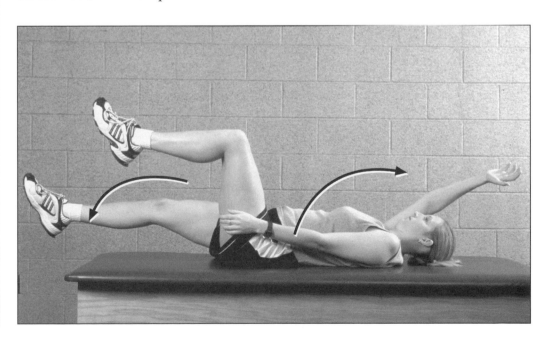

▌Figure 16.40 Spine stabilization with arms and unsupported legs.

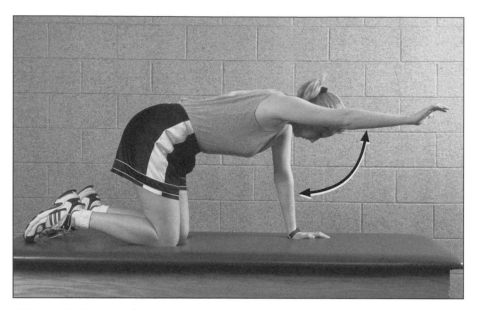

■ Figure 16.41
Quadruped arm raise.

Quadruped Arm Raise

This exercise is for spinal stabilization. The patient is in a quadruped position, and the abdominal muscles are tightened to stabilize the pelvis. One arm is raised and lowered, and the movement is then repeated on the opposite side (figure 16.41). The hips and back should not move throughout the exercise. A good feedback technique to help the patient detect hip motion during these exercises is to place a 0.9- to 1.2- m (3- to 4-ft) stick or dowel across the low back. The dowel should be balanced on the back. If the patient sees the stick drop on one side during the exercise, he or she knows that the hips have rotated and that pelvic neutral has not been maintained.

Quadruped Leg Raise

The purpose of this exercise is to enhance pelvic stabilization. The patient is in a quadruped position with the abdominals tightened to stabilize the lower spine and pelvis. The patient raises one leg, rather than an arm, and extends it backward by tightening the buttocks and hamstrings. No movement of the pelvis, trunk, or back occurs throughout the motion. The extremity motion should be smooth and steady.

Quadruped Arm and Leg Raise

This exercise enhances stabilization and strengthens the spinal extensors. With the patient in a quadruped position and the abdominals tightened to stabilize the spine in neutral, the patient lifts one arm and the opposite leg and then repeats the motion with the other arm and leg (figure 16.42). The shoulders, hips, and back should not move throughout the exercise. The hip should not drop or lift, and the back should not roll.

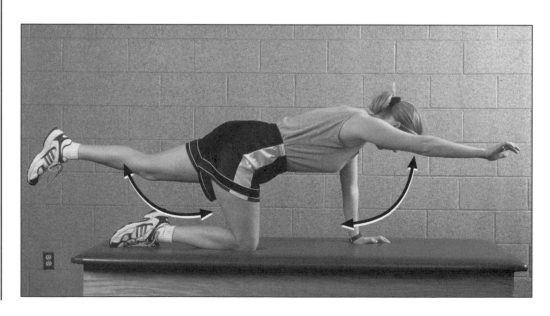

■ Figure 16.42
Quadruped arm and leg raise.

STRENGTHENING EXERCISES

These exercises are used in the strength and muscle endurance component of the therapeutic exercise program. We begin with the mildest and proceed to more challenging exercises, first for the neck and then for the lower back. Keep in mind that other exercises you can use for strengthening include the aquatic exercises discussed in chapter 13 and the Swiss ball and foam roller exercises discussed in chapter 14.

Cervical Exercises

Distinct advantages of isometric exercises are that they can be initiated early in the therapeutic exercise program and that the patient can perform them independently throughout the day.

Cervical Isometrics

Each isometric exercise is held for 10 s. These exercises are performed in either an anatomical or a midrange position. In the forward flexion exercise, the patient places the palms of the hands on the forehead and attempts to touch the chin to the chest while providing resistance to the motion with the hands on the forehead (figure 16.43a). In the extension exercise, the patient places both hands behind the back of his or her head while attempting to tilt the head backward, resisting the motion with the hands (figure 16.43b). To perform lateral flexion, the patient places one hand near the ear, resisting the motion of bringing the ear to the shoulder on the same side (figure 16.43c). The exercise is repeated on the opposite side. In isometric rotation, the patient places one hand on the side of the face and resists the movement of rotating to look over the same-side shoulder (figure 16.43d). The exercise is repeated on the opposite side. A common substitution for each of these exercises is to perform them out of cervical alignment. Each exercise should be performed with the head and neck in correct postural alignment. If the patient has difficulty identifying correct postural alignment, he or she should perform the exercises in front of a mirror until the concept is clear.

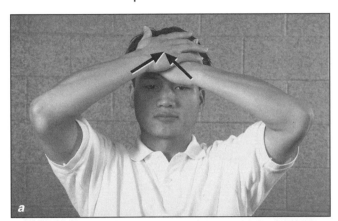

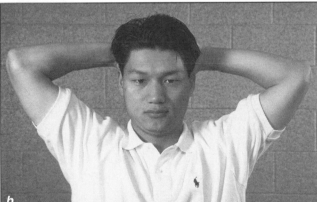

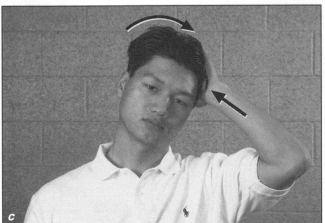

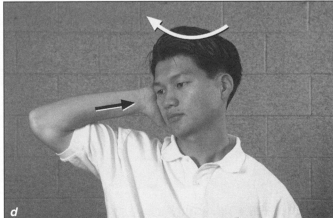

∎ **Figure 16.43** Cervical isometric exercise: *(a)* flexion, *(b)* extension, *(c)* lateral flexion, *(d)* rotation.

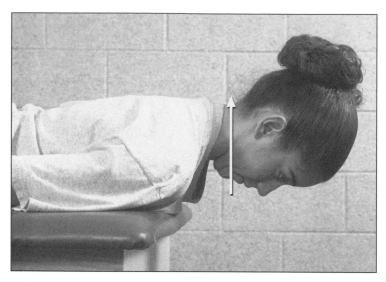

Figure 16.44   Prone cervical retraction.

Prone Neck Retraction

This exercise strengthens the posterior cervical muscles and encourages correct cervical spine alignment. The patient lies prone with his or her head and neck off the table. Keeping the chin tucked, the patient lifts the back of the head toward the ceiling (figure 16.44). The shoulder blades can also be squeezed together. At the top of the movement, the position is held for 5 to 10 s. This exercise is often incorrectly performed with the neck in extension and the head tilted upward. Instructing the patient to keep the chin tucked and describing the activity as, "like opening and closing a drawer," may give the patient a visual image that will help.

Side-Lying Head Lifts

This exercise strengthens the lateral neck muscles. The patient is in side-lying with the head hanging down to the table or off the table. The individual then lifts the head toward the top shoulder, going through a full arc of motion. An incorrect performance often seen is with the neck in a forward-head position. Correct posture should be maintained throughout the exercise.

Resisted Cervical Exercises

These are more aggressive exercises for strengthening the cervical muscles. They can be performed with rubber tubing, pulleys, or machines applied to the head. It is important to be careful using the machine exercises, because if applied inappropriately, they can place too much stress on the cervical spine and increase the risk of injury. Proper cervical alignment must be maintained throughout the exercises with movement occurring at each segment—the lower cervical spine should not be used as a fulcrum.

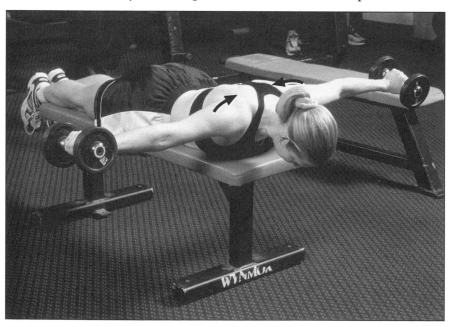

Figure 16.45   Prone flys.

Upper Back Exercises

Many upper back exercises are also shoulder exercises, because many of the shoulder muscles are located in the upper back region.

Prone Flys

This exercise strengthens rhomboids, middle trapezius, and cervical and thoracic spine extensors. The patient lies prone on a bench with the arms hanging down to the floor. The patient lifts dumbbells toward the ceiling while squeezing the scapulae together (figure 16.45). People often perform this exercise incorrectly by raising the arms but not squeezing the scapulae together. The patient should be instructed to go through the full scapular retraction motion.

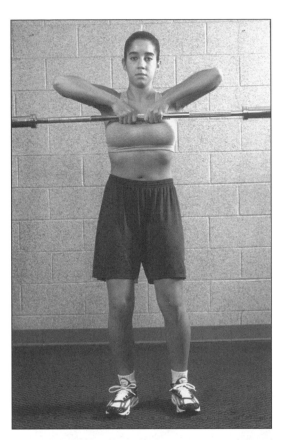

■ **Figure 16.46**
Upright row.

Upright Row

This exercise strengthens the upper back, trapezius, and deltoids. The patient uses pulleys, weights, or rubber tubing with hands close together while standing erect. With the abdominals tightened to maintain a pelvic neutral position, the patient lifts the device upward toward the chin, keeping the elbows higher than the wrists (figure 16.46). Keeping the elbows down rather than up provides less resistance for the deltoids and rotator cuff.

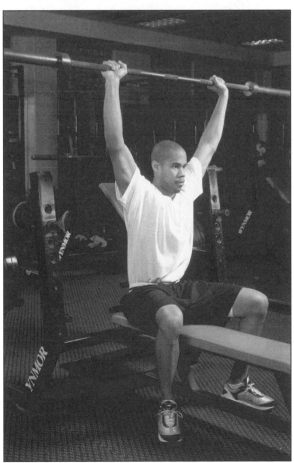

■ **Figure 16.47**
Upright press.

Upright Press

This exercise strengthens the deltoids and trunk stabilizers. It is also called a seated press or a military press. The patient can be standing or seated. The weight is grasped in the hands; with the elbows bent, the weights start at shoulder level. The abdominals are tightened to maintain trunk stability and prevent the back from arching as the patient lifts the weight straight up and overhead (figure 16.47). The patient should also be instructed not to shrug the shoulders, a common error in execution of this exercise.

Bouhler Exercises

These exercises strengthen the middle back muscles and lower trapezius. The patient stands with back to the wall, arms overhead with elbows next to the ears, and elbows straight. In the first exercise the patient pushes the thumbs to the wall, holds the position for 5 s, relaxes, and then repeats (figure 16.48a). In the second exercise, the patient, positioned with the thumbs facing each other, repeats the movement of the arms to the wall (figure 16.48b). In the third exercise, the arms are positioned at a 45° angle from the horizontal and then pushed to the wall, with the elbows straight and the scapulae retracted together (figure 16.48c). In each position the patient must tighten the abdominals to stabilize the trunk and prevent the back from arching. A progression of these exercises is to position the patient in prone to perform the exercises (figure 16.48d) or to add weights while in prone. Common errors in execution include arching the back and standing too far from the wall. Good lumbar stability helps to ensure correct execution.

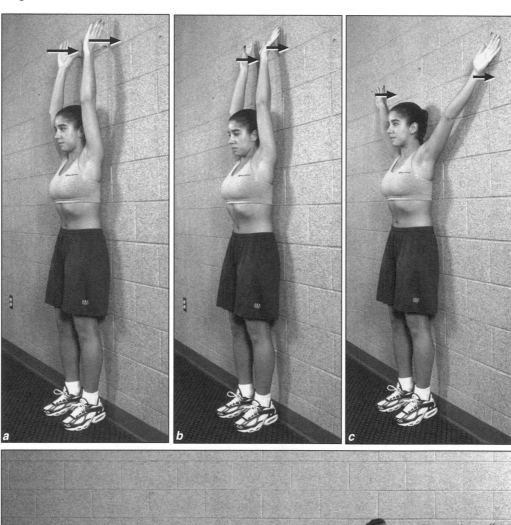

❚ **Figure 16.48**
Bouhler exercises:
(a) thumbs to wall,
(b) thumbs facing
each other, *(c)* 45°
angle, *(d)* prone.

Lower Back, Abdominal, and Pelvic Exercises

You may recall the abdominal and trunk exercises using the Swiss ball and foam roller (chapter 14) and the medicine ball (chapter 9). It is easy to incorporate these exercises into a progressive strengthening exercise program for the abdominals and lower back. You must be able to judge the degree of difficulty of each of these exercises and incorporate them at an appropriate time in the strengthening program.

Posterior Pelvic Tilt

This exercise strengthens the abdominals and gluteals and encourages the patient to maintain a pelvic neutral. It can also increase pelvic mobility. The patient lies supine with the legs straight, or with legs flexed and feet flat on the floor, and arms relaxed at the sides. The patient tightens the abdominals, tightens the buttocks, and pushes the back to the floor. The pelvis should roll posteriorly (figure 16.49). Once the patient is able to perform this exercise in supine, he or she can also perform it in sitting and standing. Common errors include using the legs to move the pelvis rather than the abdominal and back muscles, arching the back rather than performing a pelvic tilt, and pushing the abdomen outward rather than tensing the abdominal muscles.

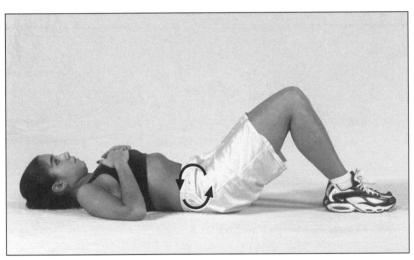

❚ Figure 16.49   Posterior pelvic tilt.

Trunk Curl

This exercise strengthens the upper rectus abdominis and obliques. The patient lies supine with knees straight and hands on top of the head. The chin is tucked to the chest and the upper trunk is slowly curled toward a sitting position (figure 16.50). The end position is not a full sitting position. The abdominal muscles should be tensed so that the umbilicus moves toward the spine. A curl should occur throughout the movement. Holding the top of the position for several seconds or holding weights in the hands makes the exercise more difficult. The feet are not anchored in this exercise because this would permit the hip flexors to perform the exercise instead of the abdominals. Hips and knees should be straight to prevent hip flexor activity during the curl. The patient should curl the upper spine rather than lift the trunk from the hips.

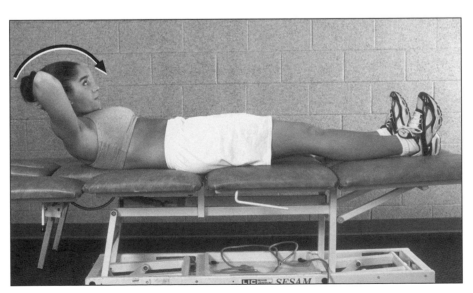

❚ Figure 16.50   Supine trunk curl.

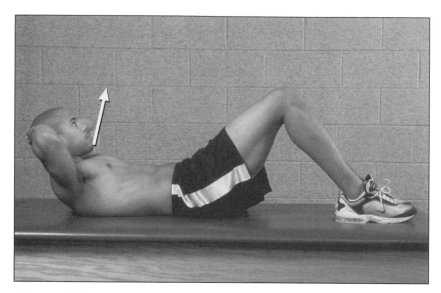

Figure 16.51
Abdominal crunch.

Crunch

This exercise strengthens the upper abdominal muscles. The patient lies supine with the knees bent, feet flat on the floor, and hands behind the neck. The abdominals are tightened, and the head and shoulders are lifted upward toward the ceiling. There is no curling movement. The position is held for 10 to 20 s at the top of the motion (figure 16.51). The exercise becomes more difficult if the patient has the legs in an unsupported position with the feet off the floor. This exercise can serve as a progression toward abdominal crunch exercises combined with medicine-ball tosses as introduced in chapter 9. The patient is performing this exercise incorrectly if he or she moves toward the knees rather than toward the ceiling. The elbows should remain back with the scapulae retracted as the patient lifts the upper trunk upward.

Oblique Abdominal Curl

This exercise strengthens the oblique muscles. The patient lies supine with knees bent and feet flat on the floor. The patient rotates the hips to one side so that he or she is lying on the back while on one hip and the other hip is facing the ceiling (figure 16.52). With hands on shoulders, or in the more difficult position, behind the head, the patient curls toward the top hip, attempting to lift upward and forward as much as possible. So that the obliques, not the hip muscles, perform the exercise, the feet are not anchored. A common error is beginning the rotation at the end of the motion rather than beginning the rotation at the onset and continuing through the range of motion. An alternative method is for the patient to lie supine and rotate one elbow toward the opposite knee while performing a crunch. Difficulties with this method are that hip rotation can be easily substituted, the rotation can begin too early or too late in the motion before the patient lifts the shoulders upward, or the rotation can be performed with too much momentum.

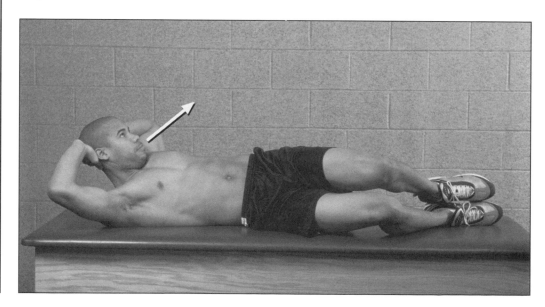

Figure 16.52
Oblique abdominal curl.

Supine Leg Exercises

These exercises strengthen the lower abdominal muscles and facilitate maintenance of pelvic neutral. The patient lies supine with the knees bent and feet flat on the floor. The arms should be across the stomach, but if the patient has difficulty with the exercise, initial performance may be with arms at the sides; however, this position should be changed to the correct arm position before the exercise is advanced. The spine is kept in neutral throughout the exercise with tension in the abdominals. One leg is raised with the knee extended, foot pointing toward the ceiling. The leg is slowly lowered to the floor (figure 16.53a). The back should not arch or roll, and the abdominals should not push upward during the movement. As patient gradually lowers the leg, he or she must progressively tighten the abdominals to maintain a pelvic neutral position. The patient can progress in this exercise by performing leg thrusts. With the spine in a neutral position and the abdominals tightened, the patient has both knees and hips flexed and the feet off the floor. One leg is thrust outward into extension and returned to the starting position. The other leg then performs the same exercise (figure 16.53b). In the more advanced version of this exercise, the patient alternately moves one leg out into extension while bringing the other leg toward the starting position so that both legs are moving simultaneously.

In the next progression of this exercise, the patient is in supine with both legs raised toward the ceiling and knees straight. As with the other exercises, the abdominals must control and keep the spine in a neutral position. The patient slowly lowers the legs to the floor without letting the low back arch (figure 16.53c).

A final progression includes the V-sit-up (figure 16.53d). It is important that the patient maintain pelvic neutral and have control of the low back—that there is no arching of the back. If the patient is unable to maintain a pelvic

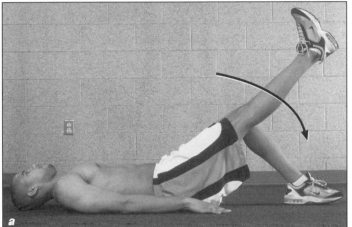

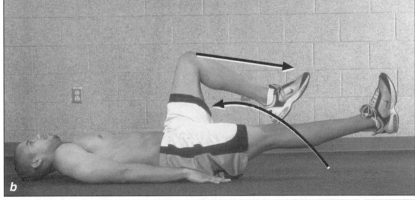

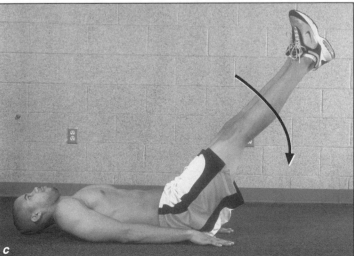

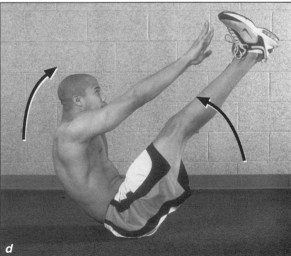

Figure 16.53 Supine leg exercises: *(a)* leg lowering, single; *(b)* leg thrusts; *(c)* leg lowering, bilateral; *(d)* V-sit-up.

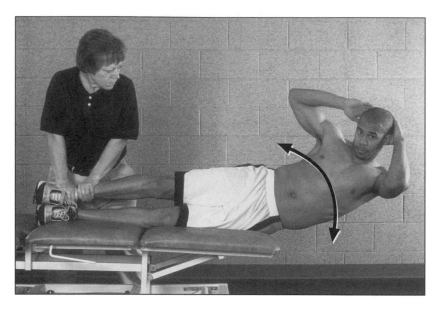

neutral position and arches the low back, the person should return to the preceding exercise level until he or she achieves greater strength and control.

Side-Lying Sit-Up

This exercise strengthens the quadratus lumborum and the obliques. The patient is in side-lying with the feet anchored. The hands are placed across the chest or in the more difficult position behind the head. The patient curls sideways toward the top hip as much as possible, attempting to curl rather than just lift from the hips (figure 16.54).

∎ **Figure 16.54**   Side-lying sit-up.

Bridging

This exercise strengthens the abdominals and back extensors and emphasizes trunk stabilization. The patient lies supine with the knees bent and feet flat on the floor. The abdominals are tightened to keep the spine in neutral. The gluteals are tightened to lift the hips off the floor until the thighs and trunk form a straight line (figure 16.55a). This position is held for 15 to 60 s.

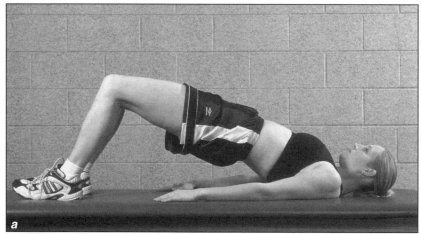

The next progression of this exercise is to perform the bridge and then lift each leg to march in place while maintaining the bridge in pelvic neutral. The patient must use the abdominals and buttocks while performing this exercise to maintain a straight line from the trunk to the supporting thigh.

A more advanced version of this exercise has the patient in the same bridging position, keeping abdominal, buttock, and lower back muscles in good tension to maintain the position. The patient first brings one knee into full extension without moving the hips, then lowers it, and then performs the motion with the other leg (figure 16.55b). The hips should not drop or roll throughout the exercise. A stick placed across the hips and parallel to the floor will easily inform the patient of any change in pelvis position during the activity. If the stick either falls off or dips on one side, pelvic stability has not been maintained.

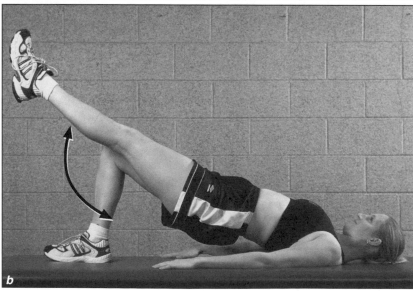

∎ **Figure 16.55**   Bridging progression: *(a)* bridging, *(b)* leg lift.

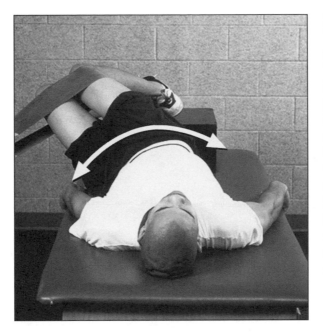

Lateral Trunk Rotation

This exercise strengthens the obliques and quadratus lumborum. The patient lies supine with knees bent. Rubber tubing or a pulley system is secured around both knees. The feet can be up on a stool or flat on the floor. The patient lets the pulley or tubing pull the knees downward to the side and then brings the knees upright by tilting the pelvis to flatten the back onto the floor, initiating the movement from the abdominals and back muscles rather than from the knees (figure 16.56).

■ Figure 16.56
Lateral trunk rotation: start position—hips and knees flexed with knees together.

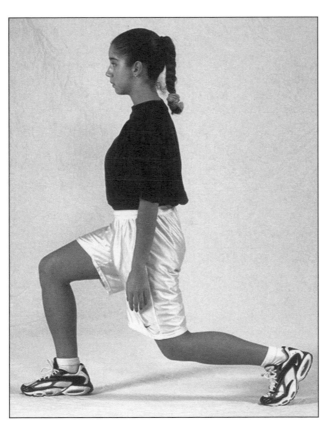

Lunges

This exercise strengthens the abdominal, leg, and gluteal muscles. It also facilitates correct trunk stability during lower-extremity activities. The patient begins in a standing position with the spine in neutral. Keeping the abdominals tightened and the back straight, the patient moves to a lunge position, going down smoothly, and then returns to a standing position (figure 16.57).

In the reverse lunge, the patient starts in the same position with the spine in neutral and the abdominals tightened. He or she steps backward and lowers the trunk in one smooth motion, keeping an upright position. The trunk should not tilt or rotate during either a forward or reverse lunge exercise. People often perform these exercises incorrectly with trunk rotation or flexion. The hips and shoulders should remain in the same plane throughout the exercise.

■ Figure 16.57
Lunge.

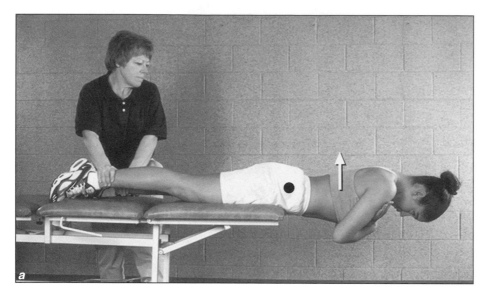

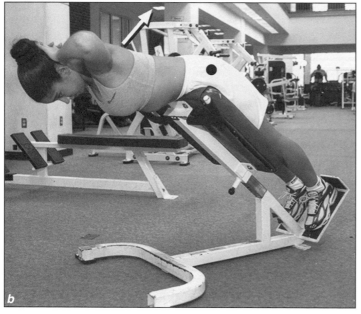

Prone Trunk Extension

This exercise strengthens the lower back extensors and buttock muscles. The patient lies prone over the seat of a chair, a table, a Roman chair, or a Swiss ball. The feet are anchored either by another person (figure 16.58a) or by equipment (figure 16.58b). The easiest position is with the hands placed behind the back or at the side; the exercise is more difficult with the hands placed farther away from the body's center of gravity to increase the lever-arm length for additional resistance. Weights can be placed in the hands with the arms overhead for the most difficult position. The patient begins in a slightly downward position, flexed approximately 30° at the hips. The buttocks are then tightened to lift the patient upward without curling backward. The lift is a straight lift and not a backward roll; and the patient should not start in a full trunk flexion position, because this can put unwanted stress on the intervertebral disks.

Once the patient has mastered the straight-plane extension exercises on the Roman chair, a progression can include trunk rotation during trunk extension exercises. The patient can perform this exercise similarly to a rotational abdominal curl but in reverse motion, or the exercise becomes more difficult if the patient uses a medicine ball, rotating with the ball in the hands while going into extension. Patients cannot perform this exercise until they have good strength in the abdominals and trunk extensors; they must also be able to perform side sit-ups and trunk rotations in standing with a medicine ball without difficulty or pain.

❚ **Figure 16.58**
Prone trunk extension: *(a)* with assist on a table, *(b)* independently on Roman chair. Movement comes from the hip with the contraction of the gluteus maximus. The back should remain straight throughout the exercise, regardless of position of equipment on which it is performed. Dot indicates point from which movement occurs.

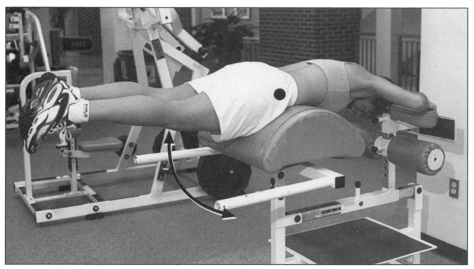

Prone Leg Lift

This exercise strengthens the lower back extensors, abdominals, and buttocks. With the patient in a position that is the reverse of the position for the prone trunk lift, the trunk is supported on the table or a Roman chair, and the legs hang downward to the floor. The buttocks are squeezed to lift the legs until they are parallel with the floor. The pelvis must be positioned on the support structure, and the bend occurs at the hips, not at the back (figure 16.59).

■ **Figure 16.59**
Prone leg lift. Dot indicates point from which movement occurs.

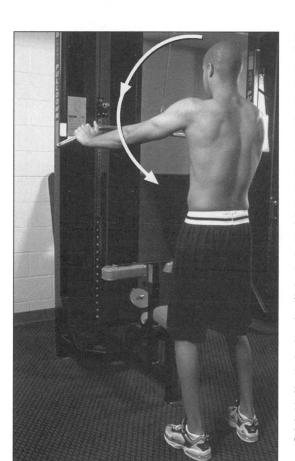

■ **Figure 16.60**
Latissimus pull-down.

Latissimus Pull-Down

This exercise is used to strengthen the latissimus dorsi. The latissimus dorsi is important in providing stabilization to the thoracolumbar spine because the muscle originates from the lower thoracic spinous processes, lumbar fascia, and iliac crest and has interdigitations with the external oblique muscles. The exercise uses an overhead pulley bar, with the patient's hands positioned shoulder-width or slightly farther apart and the elbows extended. The abdominals remain taut throughout the exercise to provide pelvic stability. The patient brings the bar downward toward the thighs while keeping the elbows fairly straight (figure 16.60). Common errors are to flex the elbows too much, shrug the shoulders, or flex the lumbar spine. You should instruct the patient in proper technique before he or she performs the exercise and correct the execution as needed.

AGILITY AND COORDINATION EXERCISES

Once patients have mastered the strengthening exercises, they should be ready for the trunk rotation and plyometric exercises that involve higher forces, quicker movements, and functional multiplanar motions. Pelvic stability should always be maintained throughout execution of any of these exercises.

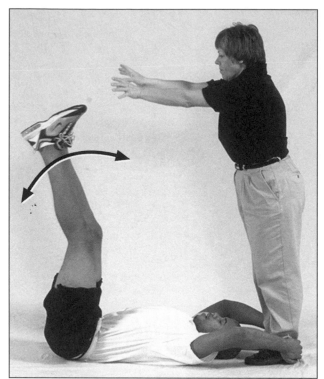

Resisted Leg Lifts

This exercise is performed with the patient supine on the floor and the sport rehabilitation specialist standing at the patient's head. The patient's legs are straight, and the hips are flexed to approximately 90°. The patient attempts to lift the legs upward as the sport rehabilitation specialist attempts to push them back down (figure 16.61). This exercise is performed quickly but with control. It is important that the patient maintain pelvic neutral and that the back not arch throughout the exercise.

■ **Figure 16.61**
Resisted leg lifts.

Medicine-Ball Exercises

Many of these medicine-ball exercises are listed in chapter 9. As a reminder, figure 16.62 depicts some of them. These exercises include activities such as ball passing low or high, trunk rotations, and abdominal curls with ball catching.

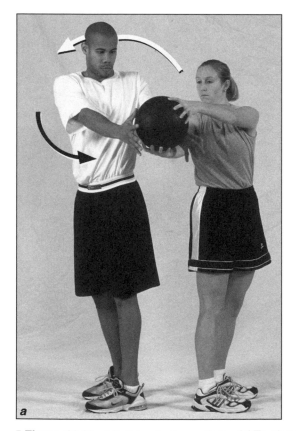

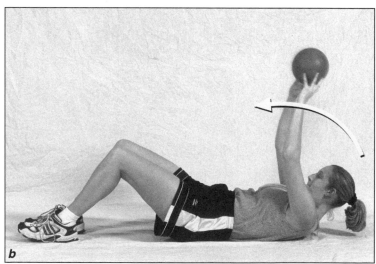

■ **Figure 16.62** Medicine-ball exercises: *(a)* Trunk rotations. *(b)* Medicine-ball toss on floor can be performed in straight plane to body or rotationally to facilitate oblique activity.

Many other exercises can be used to increase agility and resistance. A couple of additional exercises are ball tossing on the Roman chair to increase trunk extension activity and adding rotation with the medicine ball to the Roman chair exercise.

SPECIAL REHABILITATION APPLICATIONS

Specific types of back injuries call for particular kinds of exercises. Back problems that the sport rehabilitation specialist often encounters include sprains and strains; spondylosis, spondylolysis, and spondylolisthesis; disk lesions; facet injuries; sacroiliac joint injuries; and thoracic outlet syndrome.

Before we look at specific injuries and the corresponding programs, let's use our artillery of exercises and progressions to put together a generic outline of a spinal rehabilitation program. We should keep in mind that modalities may be required initially to provide pain modulation and control inflammation. Soft-tissue mobilization and joint mobilization, if appropriate, are also part of the program. Flexibility exercises to improve range of motion of deficient areas are usually incorporated in the early days of the program, with instructions to perform the exercises frequently throughout the day. Instruction in pelvic neutral, pelvic stabilization exercises, and body mechanics is also part of the early portion of the program. Once the patient has grasped the concept of pelvic neutral and is able to maintain it in simple dead-bug exercises, he or she can progress to pool exercises and trunk-strengthening exercises. Early trunk-strengthening exercises include abdominal crunches and curls, oblique exercises, and bridging exercises. The latissimus pull-down is included as part of the strengthening exercises. As the patient is able to maintain a proper pelvic-neutral position, he or she performs lower extremity-strengthening exercises. Swiss ball exercises such as crunches, bridges, leg lifts, side sit-ups, and progressions of strengthening exercises for the abdomen and trunk can begin in the middle phase of the program once the patient demonstrates good pelvic stability during arm and leg movements.

More aggressive strengthening exercises for the trunk begin when the patient is able to demonstrate good pelvic control and strength with the Swiss ball and weight exercises. Examples of these more aggressive exercises include trunk and leg extension exercises on the Roman chair and abdominal crunches and standing trunk rotations using the medicine ball.

The final aspect of the program includes incorporation of drills that mimic sport-specific activities. The patient should be able to maintain good spinal stability and alignment throughout the activities. When the individual is pain free, has good strength and flexibility, and is able to perform functional activities without difficulty, return to full sport participation is indicated.

The spine is subject to a few unique injuries that require special consideration in an injury-specific therapeutic exercise program. The following sections present these injuries and therapeutic exercise programs to address them.

SPRAINS AND STRAINS

Sprains and strains are among the most common back injuries. If they are not appropriately evaluated and treated, sprains and strains become frustrating and aggravating injuries because they can linger and cause lasting disability.

Program Considerations

The resulting pain and muscle spasm from acute sprains and strains must first be resolved with modalities and mild stretching exercises. Sometimes these conditions respond to grade I and II mobilization, but the response may depend on the severity of the pain and spasm and on the effectiveness of the modalities in relieving these problems.

Acute conditions require primarily modalities in the initial treatment phase along with limited activity and stretching exercises. As spasm and pain are reduced, soft-tissue mobilization is indicated if restriction is noted with palpation. Joint mobilization may be useful if the restriction is the result of joint hypomobilization.

As with all spinal injuries, posture and body mechanics should be assessed and corrected as needed. Spasm will persist if the muscles are required to work more than they should because poor posture or body mechanics is present.

A progression of strengthening exercises should begin once the pain and spasm are under control. The muscles requiring the greatest emphasis are the abdominals, especially the obliques, the trunk extensors, and the gluteals.

Case Study

A javelin thrower injured his back last week in practice when he attempted to throw the javelin and felt a sudden pain in the right low back area. He comes to you stating that he applied ice to the injury when it occurred. The pain is now better than it was last week, but he still has pain when he rotates his trunk to the left and to the right. He has pain when he gets up from a chair and when he gets out of bed in the morning. His pain is worse at the end of the day. He has been taking it easy for a couple of days but is still unable to practice because of the pain. His pain is located on the right side of his low back area. He has no radiation of symptoms into the lower extremities, but he does get pain in the right buttock. When you examine him you find that he is unable to forward bend because of pain; side-bending to the left is too painful to perform, but side-bending to the right is better. Trunk rotation is more painful to the left than to the right. His spine has a lateral shift to the right in the lumbar region. Palpation reveals muscle spasm with tenderness in the right paraspinals and quadratus lumborum muscles. Pressure over the multifidi reproduces his buttock pain.

Questions for Analysis

1. What is your first treatment?

2. What is your treatment progression and what guidelines will you use to advance this patient from one level to the next?

3. What are some examples of specific exercises, including functional activities you should use before the patient's return to full participation?

SPONDYLOSIS, SPONDYLOLYSIS, AND SPONDYLOLISTHESIS

Before presentation of the case study is a brief outline of considerations to keep in mind in a therapeutic exercise program for spondylosis, spondylolysis, and spondylolisthesis.

Program Considerations

Although these three conditions differ from one other, they all most often involve the lower lumbar spine and become irritated with extension movement. Patients with any of these conditions should be taught to maintain a posterior pelvic tilt and should attempt to avoid hyperextension movements as much as possible. It is vital that these patients establish and maintain pelvic stability and strengthen the abdominals. In spondylolisthesis, the most severe of the three conditions, there can be a forward displacement of the vertebrae.

Case Study

A gymnast has seen an orthopedic physician because of persistent complaints of low back pain that did not resolve after two weeks of modality treatments and reduced activity. The physician's diagnosis is a spondylolysis. The patient needs a rehabilitation program before she can return to competition.

Questions for Analysis

1. What exercises would you have this patient avoid?

2. What progression of exercises and activities should her therapeutic exercise program include to return her to full participation?

DISK LESIONS AND SCIATICA

Disk lesions can be unnerving conditions for both a patient and the sport rehabilitation specialist. You should be familiar with the factors identified here and consider them before establishing care.

Program Considerations

A protruding or herniated disk can be a serious problem and most often cause radiculopathy down one or both extremities, depending on the location of the protrusion. The mere presence of pain or symptoms down the leg does not mean that there is a disk herniation, but you should consider this a possibility until it has been ruled out. Other conditions such as facet injuries, muscle spasm, and myofascial restriction can also cause pain down the leg.

Patients who have been diagnosed with disk lesions should avoid those positions and motions that aggravate or produce the sciatica symptoms. These motions most commonly are forward bending and bending or twisting in the direction that further compresses the disk protrusion.

Patients who have disk lesions must learn to find and maintain pelvic neutral and must strengthen the abdominals, obliques, back extensors, and gluteal muscle groups. They should learn correct body mechanics and posture and should eventually progress to sport-activity execution while in a neutral spine position.

Although not all authorities agree on its importance, some advocate the centralization of pain for disk lesions. What this means is that if the treatment is appropriate, the patient will experience a gradual and progressive retreat of the sciatic pain until the only pain remaining is the original back pain. It is the goal of treatment to also relieve this central pain. Most often, the use of extension exercises, flexibility and strengthening activities, and pelvic-neutral exercises will accomplish this goal. Exercises progress at the patient's own rate. Progression depends on the treatment results and the patient's feedback regarding the pain. If the pain is receding, the progression of exercises can continue; but if the sciatic pain worsens, you must reevaluate the most recently performed exercises and activities, first for possible incorrect execution and secondly for appropriateness. It may be too soon for the patient to tolerate the severity of the exercise. Use of the wrong exercises or failure to correct body mechanics and posture may aggravate the disk lesion. It is vital that the sport rehabilitation specialist have a good understanding of the correct exercises and of the stresses that are applied with each exercise.

Those patients who have undergone microdiscectomies follow a course of treatment similar to that for patients who have disk pathology but have not had surgical correction. In a typical time line, treatment begins about one week postoperatively and follows a progression, including pain modulation, pelvic stabilization, and flexibility and strength exercises of increasing difficulty as already outlined. If postsurgical muscle tightness and soft-tissue restriction are present, they are treated with soft-tissue release and modalities.

Case Study

A football lineman injured his back in a game four weeks ago. He was referred to an orthopedic surgeon because of continued low back and right lower-extremity pain. Magnetic resonance imaging (MRI) revealed that he has a disk bulge of 3 mm at L4-5. The physician indicates that this patient is not a surgical candidate because the problem may be resolved with rehabilitation, corticosteroid injections, or Medrol dose pack. The patient has had two of the three injections and reports significant relief of his back and leg pain. He is now coming to you for a rehabilitation program. He moves pretty well when he enters the examination room. He does not appear to hesitate to walk or get up from a chair. When he moves around the room, however, you notice that he has very poor body mechanics, bending from the back to sit down and bending and twisting sideways to retrieve his backpack. His examination reveals a straight-leg raise to 50° on the right and 55° on the left, and his internal hip rotation is 20° bilaterally. In a forward bend, he is able to touch his fingers to his knees; in a side-bend he can touch 10 cm above his knee; and in backward bending he has good motion. Forward bending produces some discomfort. You notice that when he bends, most of the motion comes from the thoracic spine, with the lumbar spine remaining essentially flat. The neurological examination reveals no deficiencies in sensory, motor, or reflex innervation. The patient's gluteal muscles and abdominals each test at 4/5 strength. He is unable to perform a side sit-up on the right side. The paraspinals, quadratus lumborum, and hip external rotators are all tender to palpation, especially on the right; and you are able to palpate restriction of soft-tissue mobility in those tender areas. There is some restriction of joint mobility to PA tests in the lower lumbar spine.

Questions for Analysis

1. What precautions would you observe in treating this patient?
2. What would your initial treatment program include?
3. What techniques would you include in your first three treatment sessions?
4. What progression of exercises would you select for this patient, and what criteria would you use for progression from one level to the next in the program?

FACET INJURIES

Facet injuries can be frustrating to treat, especially if you do not consider the factors listed here. Facet injuries can also be difficult to identify. The sport rehabilitation specialist must use his or her deductive tools if there is a possibility of facet injury.

Program Considerations

Although facet injuries may result from either an impingement or a sprain of the facet, symptoms will be similar for any facet joint syndrome, regardless of the cause. The patient usually presents with posture that is locked in a side-bending and rotated position. In the cervical area, the side-bending and rotation are to the same side as the injury. In the thoracic and lumbar spine, rotation and side-bending can be restricted in the same or the opposite direction. If the patient attempts to move out of the locked position, he or she will experience pain and have a reduced range of motion. For example, if the patient is locked in a cervical side-bend and rotation to the right, the right facet is impinged, and the patient has pain and reduced motion when side-bending to the left and rotating the head to the left. In the lumbar spine, if the patient is locked in side-bending to the right and rotation to the left, pain and reduced motion can occur in side-bending to the left and rotation to the right. Radiating facet pain can mimic dermatomal distribution into the lower extremity. Palpation of the specific spinous process causes tenderness. There may also be reflex muscle spasm in the region.

Facet impingement occurs when the facet joint capsule and synovium are impinged between the joint surfaces. It results from sudden extension, side-bending, or rotation movements or a combination of these movements, but the causative injury may seem minor. The patient reports pain with motion and relief with rest. Treatment for cervical facet impingement includes manual traction, joint mobilization, and treatment for relief of muscle spasm, if present. Gentle rotation and side-bending in the pain-free range of motion are followed by gradual progression of motion into the painful range with simultaneous application of manual traction. Extension is initially avoided because it is an aggravating position. Traction is more difficult to apply and usually less effective in the lumbar spine, but gentle motion and mobilization techniques are used in this region as well.

Facet sprains are different from facet impingements in that the trauma is usually more profound; tissue injury is thus greater, and a more conservative treatment approach is warranted. Because of the more severe forces, soft tissue around the joint may also have been injured, and swelling and muscle spasm are commonly associated with facet sprains. A cervical collar may be necessary to prevent the patient from assuming a forward-head posture and causing complications of poor posture and stiffness. The patients tend to want to maintain a forward-head position because extension is painful. Gentle range of motion in pain-free movements and joint mobilization are performed following modalities to relieve muscle spasm, pain, and edema.

Case Study

A diver landed poorly in a dive during practice four days ago. She has had a stiff neck since that time. This morning she awoke and could not turn her head to the left. She presents to you with her head laterally flexed about 20° to the right and is unable to look straight ahead. Her head is rotated to the right about 15°. It is painful for her to attempt to place her head in an upright and straight position, but she has no difficulty turning her head all the way to the right and looking over her right shoulder. She also reports some tingling along the right lateral upper arm and into the lateral forearm. Your palpation reveals tenderness over the C5 and C6 spinous processes, and there is some tightness in the muscles in the same area.

Questions for Analysis

1. What do you believe her problem is?
2. Outline your treatment program, sequencing your treatment in a logical progression.

SACROILIAC JOINT

Although the impact of the SI joint on low back pain is controversial, most clinicians agree that the SI is a complex structure. Those who believe that the SI is important in low back pain argue that it can refer pain into the back, and that the back can refer pain into the SI. The SI and hip can also refer pain to each other. An examination of the SI should be part of the evaluation of any patient who complains of back or hip pain.

Patients who have excessive lumbar lordosis with an exaggerated sacral forward tilt can place excessive stress on the SI joint and cause pain in the area. Patients who have a leg-length discrepancy, who fall on the side or buttocks, who misstep off a curb while running, who run while twisting, or who bend and twist can damage the SI joints. The patients most susceptible to SI injuries because of the stress of their sports are soccer, basketball, and football players; gymnasts; wrestlers; and track and field athletes.

Some SI joint injuries result from classic types of injuries. Up-slips, inflares or outflares, and pubic subluxations can occur when there is a sudden, sharp jolt to the leg as a person steps off a curb or steps down and does not realize that there is another step. Landing on the buttock can lead to sacral flexion, pubic subluxations, and up-slip injuries. Trunk rotation and bending activities can cause sacroiliac dysfunctions. Knowing the history will help to identify the problem. Treatment is directed toward relieving and correcting the SI joint alignment, stabilizing the joints, and correcting posture or faulty techniques. The techniques used to correct alignment are referred to as muscle energy techniques. The specifics of theory and application for these are presented in chapter 6. The muscle energy techniques discussed here are treatments for specific SI dysfunctions.

Muscle Energy Techniques

Muscle energy techniques are a form of manual therapy that lend themselves well to the sacroiliac region. Listed here are a few muscle energy techniques. Remember, only two ounces of resistance is necessary for muscle energy techniques.

Anterior Iliac Subluxation: Up-Slip

This treatment is for an iliosacral lesion—an up-slip of the ilium whereby the ilium on the right is higher than the one on the left. This injury can occur when someone falls on the buttock or steps down off a curb. It is also seen in sports such as basketball and hockey. Although it always occurs on the right, the pain is sometimes on the left. Pain can also be located in the low back or coccyx or can mimic nerve root pain. The right leg appears shorter than the left leg, and the right iliac crest is higher. When palpated, the right sacrotuberous ligament feels slack compared to that on the left side.

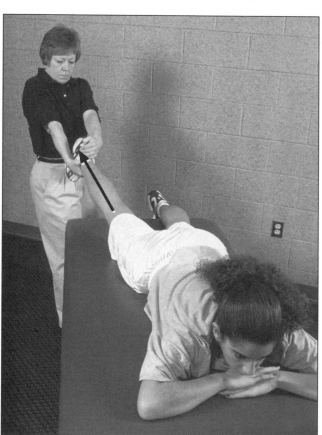

The muscle energy treatment is to have the patient lie prone with the right leg in 30° of abduction and extension. The sport rehabilitation specialist grasps the tibia and fibula above the ankle to maintain the leg position and takes up the slack of the leg. The patient takes in a deep breath and blows it out as the sport rehabilitation specialist takes up the slack of the leg again (figure 16.63). This is repeated three or four times, and on the last repetition the sport rehabilitation specialist has the patient cough twice and simultaneously provides a quick pull on the leg in the long axis of the leg.

∎ **Figure 16.63**   Anterior iliac subluxation: up-slip treatment.

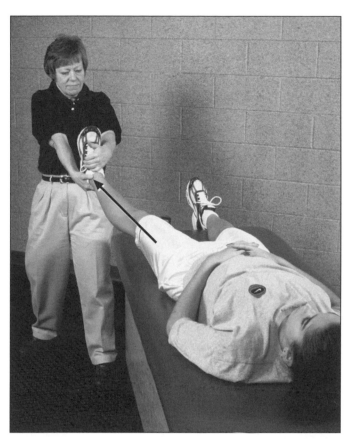

Posterior Iliac Subluxation: Up-Slip

This treatment is for an iliosacral lesion. This up-slip always occurs on the left. It commonly occurs with other spinal problems and should be investigated if the pain does not respond to treatment. The left leg is the short leg this time, and the left sacro-tuberous ligament is slack when palpated. The left iliac crest appears higher than the right.

Treatment is performed with the patient in supine and the left leg held by the sport rehabilitation specialist, proximal to the ankle in 30° of abduction and flexion (figure 16.64). The slack is taken out of the leg, and the patient is instructed to take a deep breath in and then let it out as the sport rehabilitation specialist takes out additional slack. After the final repetition, the patient is asked to cough, and simultaneously with the cough the sport rehabilitation specialist provides a quick longitudinal pull on the leg.

I Figure 16.64   Posterior iliac subluxation: up-slip muscle energy treatment.

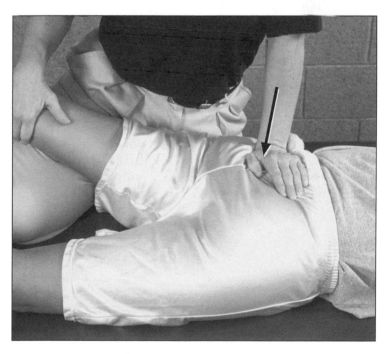

Sacral Flexion

This treatment is for a sacroiliac lesion that can occur with a bending-and-twisting activity. Push-pull activities can also cause a sacral flexion injury. This injury is more commonly seen on the left than on the right, but it can occur on either side. The pain may sometimes be on the side opposite the injury. If the injury is on the left side, the left sulcus will appear deeper (more anterior) than the right, and the left inferior lateral angle of the sacrum (ILA) is palpated more posteriorly.

Treatment is to have the patient lie prone with the leg in 30° abduction and internally rotated. The patient's thigh is stabilized on the thigh of the sport rehabilitation specialist, whose hand applies pressure to the left ILA (if the injury is on the left) (figure 16.65). The patient takes a deep breath in and holds it, then breathes out while the sport rehabilitation specialist continues to exert constant pres-

I Figure 16.65
Sacral flexion muscle energy treatment.

sure over the ILA. The pressure is maintained as the patient breathes in again. This technique is performed three times. Sometimes a click can be palpated or heard on the maneuver.

In an exercise that can accompany this treatment, the patient lies with both knees to the chest. This facilitates sacral extension because the sacrum moves in the opposite direction of the lumbar spine. As the lumbar spine moves into flexion, the sacrum should extend; and as the spine extends, the sacrum flexes.

Forward Torsion

A sacroiliac lesion of a forward torsion occurs primarily on the left and is more common than a backward torsion. Simultaneous bending and twisting is the most common mechanism for this injury. The pain may be present in the back, buttock, or leg, and it may occur on the opposite side. Because this is a torsion injury, one side of the sacrum is twisted, or torqued, on the other. For example, if the torsion is on the left, the left ILA is more posterior than the right; but the right sulcus lies deeper than the left. The left piriformis is tight.

Treatment is delivered with the patient lying on the side of the injury, usually the left, with the knees and hips flexed to 90°. The patient then pushes up with his or her top hand to lift the trunk off the table and places the bottom arm behind the back.

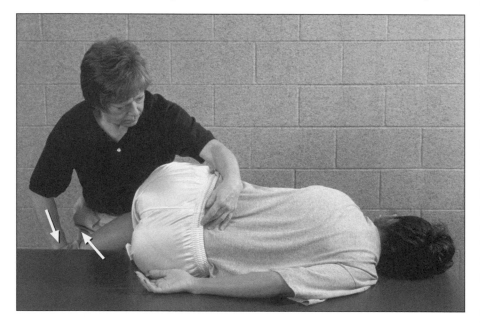

▌Figure 16.66 Forward torsion muscle energy treatment.

The patient then lies back down with the top arm hanging over the table toward the floor. The sport rehabilitation specialist places a hand in the L5–S1 joint space to monitor and maintain the spine in neutral (figure 16.66). The patient's thighs are supported on the table to the knee, and the lower legs are off the table. The sport rehabilitation specialist provides light resistance as the patient produces an isometric lift of the feet toward the ceiling. The muscles relax, and the feet drop to the floor to stretch the area.

The exercise that helps correct a forward torsion is similar to the treatment. The patient takes a side-lying position; the bottom arm is behind the trunk and the top arm hangs to the floor while the knees and hips are flexed to 90° with the lower legs over the edge of the bed or table. This position is held for 5 to 10 min. This exercise is performed until the area is stable.

Backward Torsion

This treatment is for a sacroiliac impairment that has classic signs. The patient is unable to stand upright because extension is too painful. He or she may waddle like a duck and is unable to walk normally. Pain may be in the low back or buttock or may mimic nerve root pain. Treatment for this injury has the patient standing facing a table and leaning onto it with the anterior superior iliac spine (ASIS) on the edge of the table. The trunk is supported on top of the table. The sport rehabilitation specialist applies firm pressure on the sacrum, with the heel of the hand at the base and the fingers pointing toward the sacral apex (figure 16.67a). The pressure should be downward and firm throughout the motion. The patient then walks with the hands on the table to a standing position (figure 16.67b). The movement may be uncomfortable, but the patient should be encouraged to continue to the end of the motion.

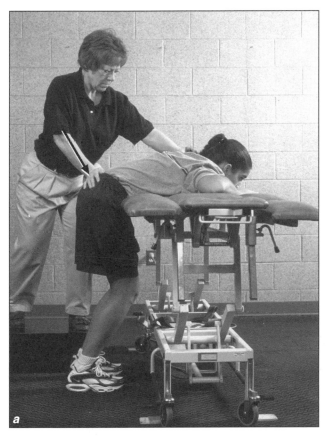 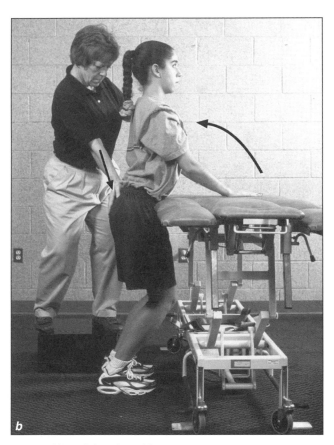

▌Figure 16.67 Backward torsion muscle energy treatment: *(a)* start position, *(b)* end position.

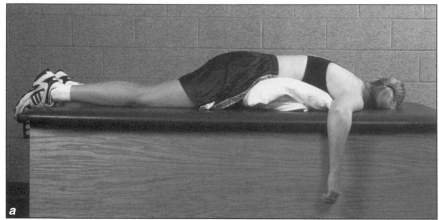

The exercises that the patient should do to promote correction of the backward torsion are press-ups or standing trunk extensions. If standing extensions are too painful, start with press-ups. If press-ups are too uncomfortable, the patient can begin by lying prone on a pillow (figure 16.68a), progressing to lying prone without a pillow (figure 16.68b), and then progressing to lying prone on elbows (figure 16.68c) before advancing to a press-up (figure 16.68d).

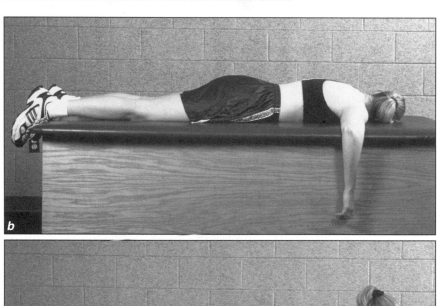

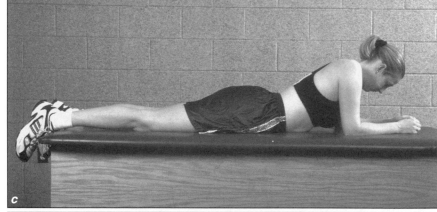

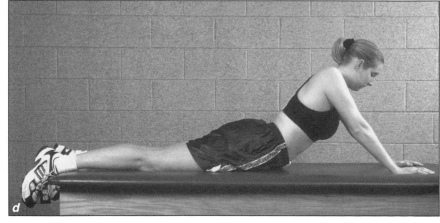

▋ Figure 16.68 Extension progression: *(a)* prone with pillows, *(b)* prone without pillows, *(c)* prone on elbows, *(d)* press-ups.

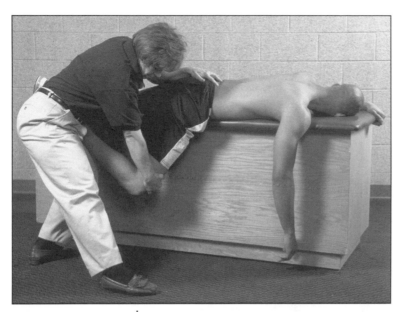

■ Figure 16.69 Anterior iliac rotation muscle energy treatment.

Anterior Iliac Rotation

The dysfunction known as anterior iliac rotation usually occurs with other lesions. It is an iliosacral lesion and is also called an anterior innominate lesion. It usually occurs on the right, and the patient can complain of cervical or lumbar symptoms. The iliac crest may be low on the same side as the injury, whereas the posterior superior iliac spine (PSIS) is high and the ASIS is low.

For treatment of this injury, the patient lies prone on the table with the leg of the involved side positioned over the side of the table and the foot on the floor. The sport rehabilitation specialist places his or her thumb in the sacral sulcus to monitor the SI joint. For control of the leg, the foot is placed on the sport rehabilitation specialist's thigh and the knee is grasped (figure 16.69). The patient's 3 to 10 s isometric contraction toward extension is resisted. The patient is instructed to relax, and the leg is moved into flexion until its barrier is felt. This exercise is repeated three to five times.

The exercises used to facilitate correction are a pelvic tilt and both knees to chest.

Posterior Iliac Rotation

This iliosacral lesion is also called a posterior innominate lesion. It commonly occurs on the left side and is seen following a fall or sudden hamstring contraction. The patient may use an antalgic gait and walk with reduced hip extension movement. Patients with this injury usually complain of a lot of pain that can be located in the buttock or knee. The ilium is posteriorly rotated, and the ASIS, PSIS, and iliac crest can appear high. There may also be a short-leg appearance on the same side.

For treatment, the patient is placed in a prone position. The sport rehabilitation specialist places one hand on the ilium to monitor stability of the joint and the other on the anterior thigh proximal to the knee. The hip is extended while the pelvis maintains neutral until the barrier is felt (figure 16.70). The barrier occurs when the monitor hand feels ilium movement as the leg is extended. The patient is instructed to attempt to push the thigh to the table isometrically for 3 to 10 s. The patient then relaxes, and the thigh is passively moved into extension to its next barrier. The procedure is repeated three to five times.

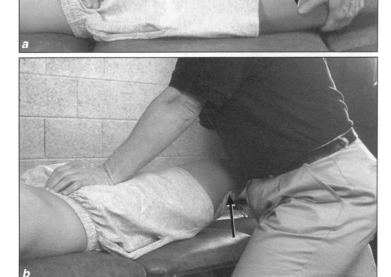

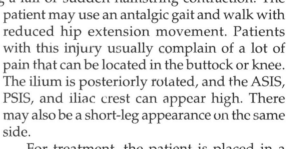

■ Figure 16.70 Posterior iliac rotation muscle energy treatment: *(a)* Start position—patient is prone; sport rehabilitation specialist's monitor hand is on the ilium and the movement hand is under the patient's knee. *(b)* Once relaxed after isometric hip flexion, the thigh is passively moved into extension to the barrier.

Exercises that accompany this technique include press-ups and hip-flexor stretches.

Pubic Subluxation

This is an iliosacral lesion that occurs in soccer players. It occurs also during pregnancy or delivery of a child. These lesions are commonly found in combination with other SI lesions, especially up-slips, or low back injuries. The patient may complain of only low back pain or may have groin or buttock pain. Pushing down on the left or right pubic bones produces pain (spring test). If it is a superior lesion, the leg will appear shorter, but if it is an inferior lesion, the leg will appear longer.

Treatment depends on whether the pubis is superior or inferior and involves a contract-relax-stretch technique. For a superior subluxation, the patient lies supine with the leg over the edge of the table. The sport rehabilitation specialist supports the hanging leg under the patient's thigh and stabilizes the ASIS on the opposite side (figure 16.71). The patient performs isometric hip flexion for 5 to 10 s against the sport rehabilitation specialist. The leg is relaxed and the hip is passively stretched into extension.

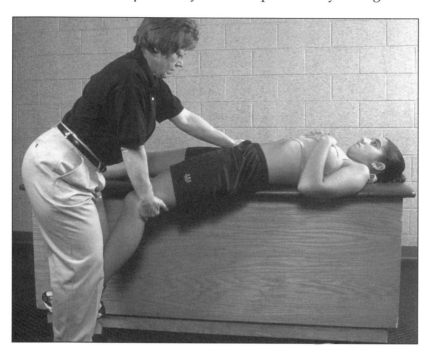

▌Figure 16.71   Superior pubic subluxation muscle energy treatment.

For an inferior subluxation, the patient lies with the hip in flexion while the sport rehabilitation specialist places a hand under the ischial tuberosity to monitor its stability. The patient performs isometric hip extension against the sport rehabilitation specialist's hand on the proximal lower leg (figure 16.72). A stretch into hip flexion is performed after the patient has relaxed the muscles.

▌Figure 16.72   Inferior pubic subluxation muscle energy treatment.

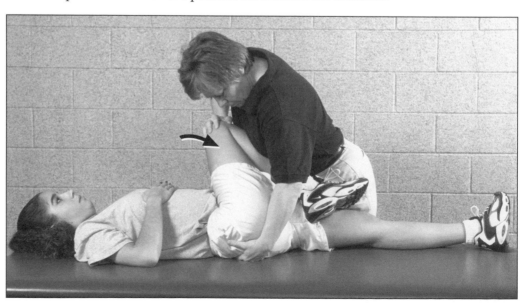

Occasionally, a treatment technique specific to superior subluxations or one specific to inferior subluxations can be successful for either problem. The patient is supine with the hips and knees flexed and the feet on the table. The patient performs a series of isometric abduction exercises of both legs simultaneously as the sport rehabilitation specialist resists the movement (figure 16.73a). This is followed by a series of isometric adduction exercises with the sport rehabilitation specialist's forearm placed between the patient's knees during the isometric exercise (figure 16.73b). Sometimes a pop of the pubic bones may be heard.

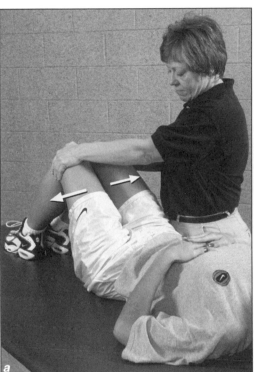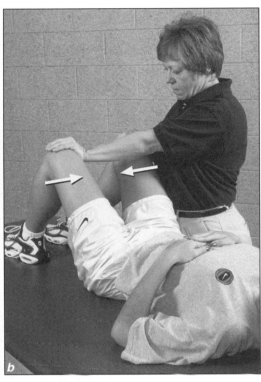

Figure 16.73 Inferior or superior pubic subluxation muscle energy treatment: *(a)* isometric abduction, *(b)* isometric adduction.

Exercises the patient should perform for superior subluxation include a Thomas stretch. The inferior subluxation exercise is a single-knee-to-chest stretch.

Inflares and Outflares

Inflares and outflares are also referred to as innominate internal and external rotations, respectively. These iliosacral conditions often produce groin pain. Leg and hip pain may or may not be present as well. This occurs in soccer players and can result from a direct blow on the ilium. In an inflare, the distance from the ASIS to the umbilicus is shorter on the affected side. In an outflare, the distance is greater on the affected side than on the opposite side.

Treatment for an inflare is to have the patient lie supine with the leg on the involved side flexed and the foot flat on the table. The sport rehabilitation specialist's hand is on the medial malleolus, with the forearm against the lower leg. The patient's knee rests against the sport rehabilitation specialist's hip. The sport rehabilitation specialist's other hand is used to stabilize the opposite ASIS. The patient performs an isometric hip adduction exercise for 5 to 10 s. When the muscle relaxes, the patient's leg is passively moved into hip abduction. When the exercise series is complete, the patient's leg is passively moved into extension.

The exercise for an inflare is performed with the patient lying supine, the leg flexed at the hip and knee, and the foot on the table. The knee is dropped out to the side to move the hip into abduction.

An outflare is treated with the patient in supine and the knee of the affected side brought toward the opposite shoulder. The sport rehabilitation specialist places his or her hand on the sulcus of the involved side. The hip is internally rotated. While maintained in this position, the patient performs a series of isometric exercises in hip flexion, adduction, and internal rotation (figure 16.74). The leg is returned passively to full extension when the series is complete.

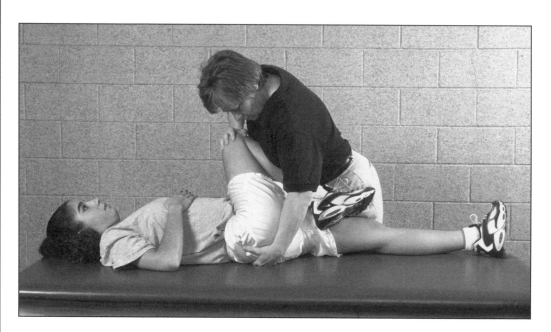

▌Figure 16.74
Outflare muscle
energy treatment.

To perform the exercise for this dysfunction, the patient moves the knee to the opposite shoulder and produces a series of hold-relax techniques.

Program Considerations

When the SI is being treated, the low back and hip areas should also be addressed to eliminate other sites of injury or referral. Muscle energy techniques are used in combination with flexibility and strengthening exercises. The cause, if it was not a traumatic injury, should also be corrected to prevent a recurrence.

If the SI joint is the source of pain, muscle energy techniques are usually very effective in relieving or reducing the pain. Provided that the problem has not been long-standing, the patient experiences significant resolution within a few treatments, in many cases.

Case Study

In last week's game, a basketball player was going in for a layup when she collided with an opponent whose knee hit her on the front of the left hip. She had an initial bruise over the anterior ilium but since then has noticed persistent left groin pain. She also has pain that goes into the left leg. Examination shows that she has normal lumbar range of motion. There is no spasm or pain in the low back area. In supine, the distance from the umbilicus to the ASIS is 0.5 cm ($\frac{1}{5}$ in.) longer on the left than on the right.

Questions for Analysis

1. What do you suspect this patient has, and what is your treatment program?

2. What exercises would you include in her home program?

THORACIC OUTLET SYNDROME

Thoracic outlet syndrome (TOS) can be classified as a cervical injury or a shoulder injury. The classification depends on your orientation. Because the syndrome can be caused by structures in the neck region, some feel it is related to the cervical spine. Many of the structures contributing to it, however, are shoulder based; and certainly many of the exercises used to correct the problem are shoulder exercises. It would be logical to include TOS in a discussion of either cervical or shoulder injuries. The syndrome is discussed here, but you should keep in mind that assessment of shoulder injuries and development of shoulder rehabilitation programs should also include consideration of possible TOS manifestations, particularly if the patient does not respond as expected to a shoulder rehabilitation program.

Program Considerations

Although the diagnosis of TOS can be difficult and the signs and symptoms complex, the treatment program is simple. Symptom control is the first goal; this should include the use of modalities as needed and instruction in positions that relieve the tension or compression on the brachial plexus. The position that best relieves TOS in the supine position for sleeping is with the scapula in protraction and elevation and the shoulder in internal rotation and adduction. Pillows should be used to support and position the shoulder and scapula as seen in figure 16.75. In severe cases, it may be necessary for the patient to wear a sling during the day. In less severe cases, the patient can obtain relief during the day by placing his or her hand in a front pant pocket or in the waistband when standing and by supporting the arm when sitting.

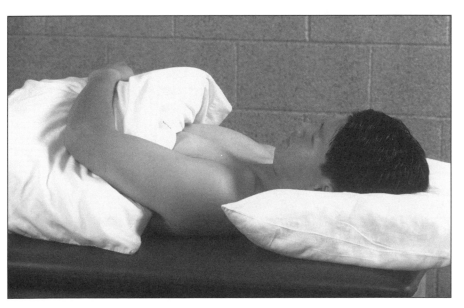

∎ **Figure 16.75** Resting position for TOS.

Soft-tissue mobilization of the cervical spine and scapular muscles—especially the upper trapezius, scalenes, pectoralis minor, and occasionally the cervical paraspinal muscles—is often effective in relieving pain and tenderness if the muscle tension in these muscles is contributing to the symptoms.

Improving joint mobility of the first rib may also help to relieve symptoms if the rib is restricted and impinging on the brachial plexus. If the sport rehabilitation specialist is comfortable with spine mobilization techniques, he or she should perform cervical spine and thoracic spine mobilization if areas of restriction are present.

Once the inflammation has subsided, flexibility and strengthening exercises should begin. The brachial plexus is stretched using the upper-limb tension tests (ULTT) described in chapter 6. These are reviewed in figure 16.76. These stretches are performed to the point of pain, not beyond, because pushing into the pain may reinflame the nerve.

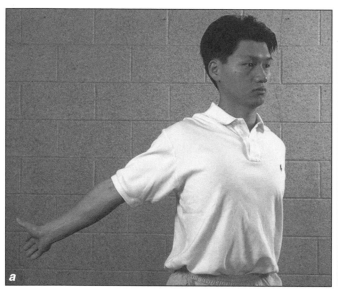
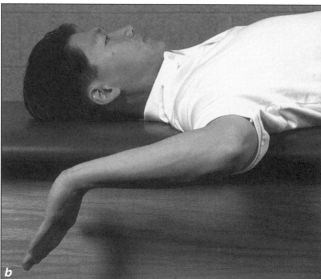
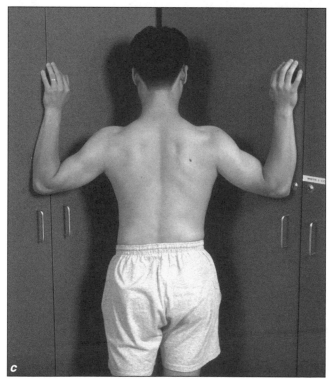

■ **Figure 16.76**
Brachial plexus stretches for TOS: *(a)* ULTT with elbow extended, *(b)* ULTT with elbow flexed, *(c)* ULTT with elbow flexed into a corner.

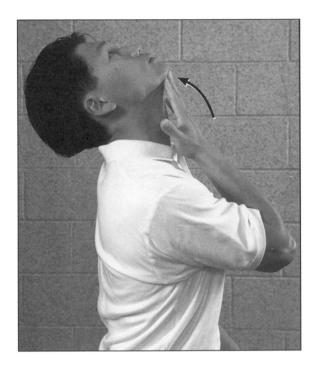

▌Figure 16.77
Cervical extension
with overpressure.

Flexibility exercises for the cervical and thoracic spine should also be included. Axial extension and cervical retraction exercises (figures 16.21 and 16.22) are simple beginning exercises. Additional flexibility exercises include cervical extension, lateral flexion, and forward flexion exercises. Cervical extension is performed with the neck maintained in a slightly retracted position as the patient extends the neck beginning from the upper spine and moving through the lower spine. If tolerated, overpressure with the hand on the chin can be added (figure 16.77). Lateral flexion is essentially an upper trapezius stretch as seen in figure 16.24. The patient may find it more comfortable to perform the lateral flexion exercise in supine, but it is also effective when performed either in sitting or supine.

Because thoracic mobility can influence cervical range of motion, flexion and extension flexibility exercises of the thoracic spine should also be part of a program for TOS. These are performed in sitting with the hands clasped behind the neck. A rolled towel can be placed around the neck at the restricted level and pulled downward from the front with the hands as the neck is extended. For extension, the elbows are raised toward the ceiling and the patient looks upward (figure 16.78). For flexion, the patient lowers the elbows toward the chest with hands clasped together at the base of the neck. The movement should come from the thoracic spine without pressure on the neck from the hands.

Because brachial plexus mobility can be restricted by shoulder positioning and associated scapulothoracic and glenohumeral soft-tissue tightness, shoulder flexibility exercises should also be included in a TOS program if there are deficiencies in the shoulder motions of external rotation, internal rotation, or flexion or scapulothoracic motions of retraction, rotation, and elevation. Stretches for these muscles are presented in chapter 17.

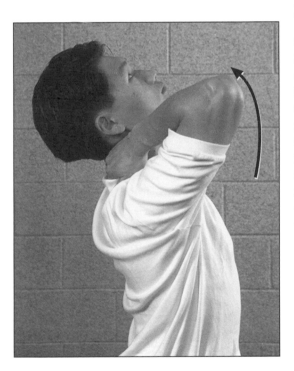

▌Figure 16.78
Thoracic extension
with overpressure.

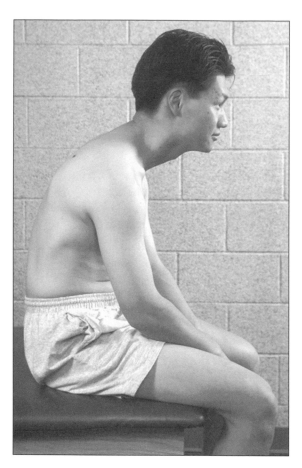

Figure 16.79 Poor posture associated with TOS.

Correction for posture and body mechanics is vital to correcting and preventing recurrence of TOS. A typical posture held by persons with TOS is a forward-head, round-shoulder posture as seen in figure 16.79. The patient should be made aware of his or her current posture and receive instruction in how to correct it. It may be difficult for the patient to assume normal posture initially because of pain, habit, reduced flexibility of muscles, and weakness of opposing muscles; however, it is important for the individual to gain posture awareness and begin posture correction early in the program.

Strength exercises are designed to restore correct muscle balance of the neck and upper back so that normal movement of the brachial plexus and related soft tissue can occur and stress is reduced. The sport rehabilitation specialist should assess balance of respiratory muscles by determining how the patient breathes. It is common for patients with TOS to breathe using primarily upper respiratory muscles, the sternocleidomastoid and scalenes. These patients should be taught how to do diaphragmatic breathing or belly breathing in addition to using a combination of upper and lower respiratory muscles.

Other strengthening and muscle balance activities include exercises for the rotator cuff, especially external rotators, rhomboids, and middle trapezius for scapular retraction, and cervical and thoracic extensors. These are commonly the weakest muscle groups in patients with TOS and should be strengthened to create a balance with their opposing muscles.

Case Study

A 20-year-old wrestler reports that for the past week he has had trouble sleeping at night. He awakens with severe numbness and tingling in the right hand and a feeling of pressure in the forearm. The problem has been getting progressively worse since it started. He has some pain if he carries a lot of books between classes, but feels all right when he is sitting in class. He does not recall having incurred a specific injury. He has been wrestling for eight years and lifts weights during the preseason. His shoulder weight program includes bench press, military press, push-ups, flys, and biceps curls. Your examination confirms the doctor's diagnosis of TOS; although the Adson maneuver is negative, you can reproduce his hand's tingling symptom when you perform a hyperextension maneuver. His posture is one of forward-head and round-shoulder alignment. He has limited shoulder range of motion in elevation and external rotation, and he is unable to move his elbow behind his shoulder in horizontal extension without discomfort in the chest. He has well-pronounced pectoralis and anterior deltoid muscles, but his rhomboids appear diminished and his rotator cuff muscles are weak.

Questions for Analysis

1. What instructions on posture will you give this patient?

2. What flexibility exercises will you give him, and what guidelines will you use in determining when to begin them?

3. What are his strength deficiencies and muscle imbalances, and what exercises will you use to restore muscle balance?

SUMMARY

1. *Explain three flexibility exercises for the cervical spine and lumbar spine.*

   Cervical flexion: Bring the chin down to the chest, attempting to move one cervical level at a time. Rotational stretch: While sitting in a chair, reach behind to grasp the back of the chair with the near hand, and use the opposite hand to keep the legs stable. Both knees to chest: In a supine position, bring one leg to the chest, then the other leg; return to the starting position by reversing the procedure.

2. *Explain three strengthening exercises for the cervical spine and lumbar spine.*

   Isometrics: In a proper posture, place the right hand along the right side of the head; push the head against the hand while not allowing any movement. Prone leg lift: Lying prone in a neutral spine position, squeeze the buttocks and lift the legs upward. Abdominal crunch: in a hook-lying supine position with hands behind the head, lift the chest and head toward the ceiling.

3. *Identify three progressive spinal stability exercises.*

   Dead-bug, quadruped, and abdominal exercises.

4. *Identify three sacroiliac muscle energy release techniques and the indications for their use.*

   Up-slip: Up-slip is always on the left and often accompanies other spinal problems. A leg pull is performed with the patient in supine and the leg positioned in 30° abduction and flexion. Forward torsion: This occurs primarily on the left and occurs with twisting and bending motions. With the patient lying on the involved side, the legs are off the table, where resistance is provided to leg movement toward the ceiling. Posterior iliac rotation: This occurs primarily on the left side as a result of a fall or sudden hamstring contraction. With the patient prone, the hip is passively extended; the isometric force occurs in hip flexion.

5. *Outline a therapeutic exercise program for a cervical sprain.*

   The program should begin with modalities for pain and spasm, soft-tissue mobilization, and joint mobilization if there is soft-tissue or joint restriction. Range-of-motion exercises begin with active motion within a pain-free range of motion. Overpressure can occur as the tissue continues to heal. Isometric exercises can be initiated after pain and spasm are relieved. Other exercises can include strengthening exercises such as machine resistance and manual resistance through a full range of motion. Strengthening exercises should address the abdominals, trunk extensors, and gluteals for a foundation for the cervical spine. Agility and coordination exercises with medicine balls for the upper extremity and abdominals are included once strength and endurance are good. Functional exercises are the final phase of the program and depend on the patient's specific sport.

6. *List precautions for a therapeutic exercise program for disk lesions.*

   Avoid positions that aggravate the sciatica; rule out other causes of sciatica; strengthen abdominals, gluteals, and back extensors; have the patient maintain a pelvic neutral position during activities; exercises should progress at the patient's own pace; and the sport rehabilitation specialist should have a good understanding of the exercises and the stresses that are imposed by each exercise.

7. *Discuss the difference in therapeutic exercise programs for a lumbar strain and a facet injury.*

Facet injury treatment includes gentle rotation and side-bending in a pain-free range of motion, as well as avoiding extension activities (pain will occur in rotation to one side and side-bending to the opposite side). Extension exercises do not have to be avoided in lumbar strains; rotation and side-bending are painful in the same direction and should occur in pain-free motions.

CRITICAL THINKING QUESTIONS

1. Referring to the scenario presented at the beginning of this chapter, identify a myofascial release technique Casey probably used on Mark. Why did you select the technique you did?

2. What exercises would you give Mark to strengthen his trunk muscles? What progression would you include for each exercise, and what are your criteria for progression?

3. With reference to the example of the gymnast with spondylolysis mentioned in the chapter, extension exercises should be avoided. How can you strengthen her back muscles without aggravating her injury? Will your attempts to strengthen her abdominals irritate the spondylolysis? Why or why not?

4. A football lineman who has been diagnosed with a disk herniation is attempting conservative rehabilitation to avoid surgery. What will your program of therapeutic exercises include? What will you avoid in the exercises? Does body mechanics impact his injury, and if so, how?

REFERENCES

Shultz, S.J., Houglum, P.A., and D.H. Perrin. 2000. *Assessment of athletic injuries*. Champaign, IL: Human Kinetics.

Travell, J.G., and D.G. Simons. 1983. *Myofascial pain and dysfunction. The trigger point manual.* Vol. 1. Baltimore: Williams and Wilkins.

Travell, J.G., and D.G. Simons. 1992. *Myofascial pain and dysfunction. The trigger point manual.* Vol. 2. Baltimore: Williams and Wilkins.

SUGGESTED READING

Cibulka, M.T. 1992. The treatment of the sacroiliac joint component to low back pain: A case report. *Physical Therapy* 72:917–922.

Corrigan, B., and G.D. Maitland. 1989. *Practical orthopaedic medicine.* Boston: Butterworths.

Erhard, R.E., Delitto, A., and M.T. Cibulka. 1994. Relative effectiveness of an extension program and a combined program of manipulation and flexion and extension exercises in patients with acute low back syndrome. *Physical Therapy* 74:1093–1100.

Foster, D.N., and M.N. Fulton. 1991. Back pain and the exercise prescription. *Clinics in Sports Medicine* 10:197–209.

Hodges, P.W., and C.A. Richardson. 1997. Contraction of the abdominal muscles associated with movement of the lower limb. *Physical Therapy* 77:132–144.

Hopkins, T.J., and A.A. White. 1993. Rehabilitation of athletes following spine injury. *Clinics in Sports Medicine* 12:603–618.

Johannsen, F., Remvig, L., Kryger, P., Beck, P., Warming, S., Lybeck, K., Dreyer, V., and L.H. Larsen. 1995. Exercises for chronic low back pain: A clinical trial. *Journal of Orthopaedic and Sports Physical Therapy* 22:52–59.

Kuzmich, D. 1994. The levator scapulae: Making the con-NECK-tion. *Journal of Manual and Manipulative Therapy* 2:43–54.

Lee, H.W.M. 1994. Progressive muscle synergy and synchronization in movement patterns: An approach to the treatment of dynamic lumbar instability. *Journal of Manual and Manipulative Therapy* 2:133–142.

Maitland, G.D. 1990. *Vertebral manipulation.* Boston: Butterworth-Heinemann.

Oliver, J. 1994. *Back care. An illustrated guide.* Boston: Butterworth-Heinemann.

Saudek, C.E., and K.A. Palmer. 1987. Back pain revisited. *Journal of Orthopaedic and Sports Physical Therapy* 8:556–566.

Smith, K.F. 1979. The thoracic outlet syndrome: A protocol of treatment. *Journal of Orthopaedic and Sports Physical Therapy* 1:89–99.

Tan, J.C., and M. Nordin. 1992. Role of physical therapy in the treatment of cervical disk disease. *Orthopedic Clinics of North America* 23:435–449.

Walker, J.M. 1992. The sacroiliac joint: A critical review. *Physical Therapy* 72:903–916.

Watkins, R.G. 1996. *The spine in sports.* St. Louis: Mosby.

CHAPTER SEVENTEEN

Shoulder and Arm

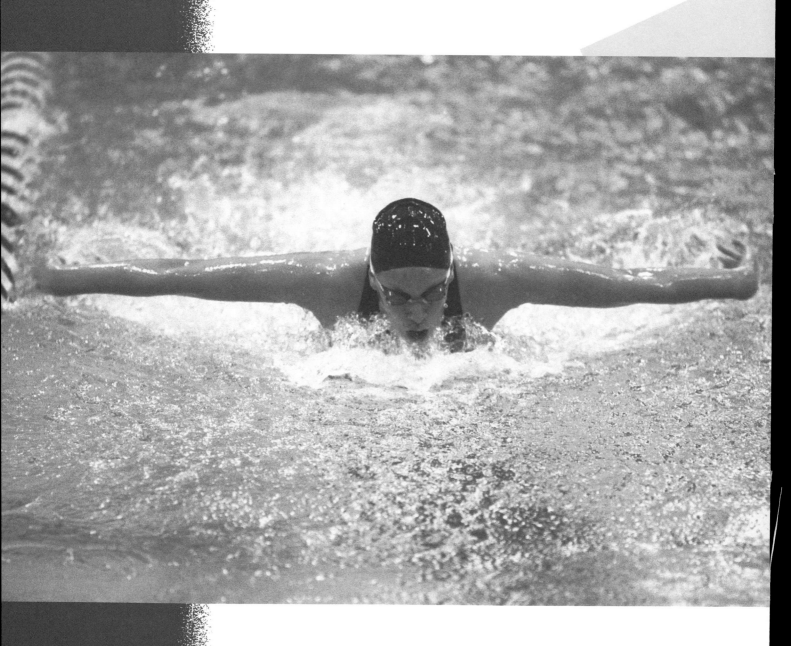

OBJECTIVES

After completing this chapter, you should be able to do the following:

1. Explain how knowledge of the mechanics of sport performance impacts the establishment of a therapeutic exercise program.

2. Discuss the importance of stability in shoulder rehabilitation.

3. Explain the role of scapular stabilization in shoulder function.

4. Describe two soft-tissue mobilization techniques for the shoulder.

5. List three joint mobilizations for the shoulder.

6. Identify three strengthening exercises for the scapula and three for the glenohumeral muscles.

7. Discuss the general progression of strengthening exercises for the shoulder.

8. List precautions for a therapeutic exercise program following a rotator cuff repair.

9. Outline key factors for a program for a biceps rupture.

Mac Deane, certified athletic trainer for the local baseball farm team, sees several shoulder injuries each season. He is very familiar with the shoulder rehabilitation process, having successfully treated many players over the years.

His latest patient, Jason, is one of the more promising pitchers Mac has seen in recent years. Jason began having shoulder pain as a result of scapular muscle weakness and fatigue. Although he didn't have any capsular tightness in the shoulder that would have necessitated joint mobilization techniques, he did have the external rotator tightness that pitchers often acquire. Mac has provided Jason with a good rehabilitation program that has resolved the shoulder's motion and strength deficits, and Jason is about to begin a plyometric exercise program before beginning throwing activities.

Mac likes to make the rehabilitation program interesting for the baseball players. On different days he provides different exercises that can produce the same result. He uses rubber bands, manual resistance, and medicine balls instead of machine weights or dumbbells, because he feels that the patients find these more interesting and fun than weights.

Happy the man who finds wisdom, the man who gains understanding! For the profit is better than profit in silver, and better than gold is the revenue.

Proverbs 3:13–14

The purpose of the shoulder is to position the hand for function. The shoulder provides the impetus for propelling objects from the hand; it also places the hand in a position that enables you to catch or propel an object or to make contact with an object or surface. For these activities to occur, the entire shoulder complex, including its related joints and muscles, must operate with precise timing, intensity, positioning and speed of movement.

The shoulder has more mobility than any other joint in the body. Differentiated into one-degree increments, there are approximately 16 000 different possible shoulder positions (Perry 1978). The shoulder is designed for large ranges of motion, making thousands of hand placements possible. People who participate in overhead sports, such as baseball; softball; golf; football; swimming; volleyball; racket sports; and field events including javelin, discus, and shot put, utilize the shoulder's expansive mobility repetitively throughout each day of practice and participation. Overhead sports entail the use of tremendous forces to produce great upper-extremity velocity. During the acceleration phase of pitching, for example, arm movement at a velocity of around 7500°/s has been recorded (Pappas, Zawacki, and Sullivan 1985). Rotational velocity in a tennis serve is 1500°/s, and hand speed at ball impact has been clocked at 75.6 kph (47 mph) (Kibler 1995). These velocities are generated from the shoulder starting essentially at rest in the cocking phase of a movement, accelerating to these top speeds and then suddenly decelerating in the follow-through, all in the space of less than 180° of rotation and milliseconds of time. For the shoulder to withstand these repeated stresses, the joints and muscles must all work as a highly synchronous, well-balanced unit. If a joint fails to move correctly or the muscles are imbalanced, an injury is sure to occur.

The risk of injury makes it vital for the sport rehabilitation specialist to understand the mechanics of normal shoulder motion and to have the knowledge, wisdom, and good judgment for appropriate rehabilitation progression. Before presenting specific therapeutic exercises for the shoulder, this chapter introduces the mechanics of overhead activities and basic considerations that are unique to the shoulder. As a sport rehabilitation specialist you must be aware of these elements to design an appropriate rehabilitation program for an injured shoulder.

MECHANICS OF OVERHEAD SPORT ACTIVITIES

Overhead motions, such as those that athletes perform in baseball, tennis, swimming, and golf, place particular types of stresses on the shoulder.

All overhead activities impart stress to the shoulder and other upper-extremity segments. An appreciation of these stresses and of the biomechanics in overhead sports can help you develop suitable rehabilitation programs.

The muscles to be discussed in relation to each motion include only those that have been investigated by researchers. Even though the research on shoulder biomechanics and muscle activity is extensive, we still have much to learn before we will have a complete picture of the shoulder in overhead sports. Meanwhile, you need to realize the importance of your own observations, your knowledge of shoulder function, and your knowledge of the muscles that produce those functions. Even though research may not have yielded all the answers you need, your clinical skills, knowledge, and observations will help you identify and correct a patient's deficiencies to permit a safe return to full sport participation.

PITCHING

Pitching has been investigated more thoroughly than any other overhead sport activity, with the shoulder most often the primary focus. It is recognized that the baseball pitcher uses the entire body in the pitching motion, beginning with the lower extremities and advancing to the trunk, shoulder, elbow, wrist, and hand. An alteration in any segment of this chain can affect the result. Consistent accuracy through repetition of coordinated high-velocity activity is the key to successful pitching. It is also the source of injury.

Pitching is a smooth, continuous motion that occurs during a relatively brief period of time. It can be divided into four segments—windup, cocking, acceleration, and follow-through (figure 17.1).

Windup

Windup, the setting phase of the pitching motion, occurs when the individual positions the body such that the glove (non-throwing) side is facing the target. In the beginning of windup, the two hands are together and near the chest. As the movement begins, the athlete takes a step toward the target with the foot opposite the throwing arm. This phase is a minimally demanding portion of the pitching motion. Speed, energy expenditure, and forces generated are all at low levels.

■ Figure 17.1
Throwing motion: *(a)* windup, *(b)* late cocking, *(c)* acceleration, *(d)* follow-through.

Reprinted from Jobe and Ling 1988.

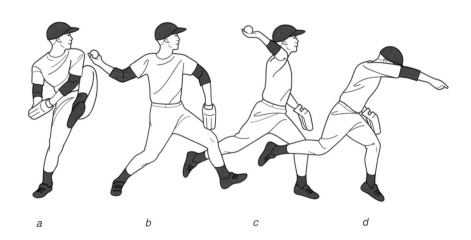

a   b   c   d

Cocking

Cocking begins when the hands separate and ends when maximum external rotation and abduction of the shoulder have been achieved. Cocking is divided into early cocking and late cocking according to the contact of the forward foot on the ground. In early cocking, the scapula is retracted and the humerus is abducted, externally rotated, and horizontally extended. The elbow is flexed, and the forward leg advances toward the target almost directly in front of the back leg. At the time of foot contact, both arms are elevated about 90° and in line with each other along the plane of the shoulders. Anterior stress on the glenohumeral joint is predominant at this time, with the body in front of the arm. The deltoid is strongly active during early cocking. When maximum shoulder external rotation and abduction to 90° occur, the static stabilizers of the shoulder, the glenohumeral capsule and ligaments, serve to limit further motion. Active stabilizers, including the forward flexors, external rotators, the subscapularis, pectoralis major, and latissimus dorsi, act as additional restraints to control motion. Scapular stabilizers such as the pectoralis minor and serratus anterior are also active in late cocking. Reciprocal inhibition of the other rotator cuff muscles, the teres minor, supraspinatus, and infraspinatus, is also taking place as these muscles attempt to resist the superior subluxating forces that occur when the trunk is in a forward lean and the shoulder is maximally externally rotated. The supraspinatus and infraspinatus are particularly active in late cocking. By the end of this phase, the shoulder internal rotators are on maximum stretch, the body is "wound" optimally for the elastic energy transfer, and the legs and trunk begin their acceleration for energy release.

Acceleration

Acceleration starts with maximum shoulder external rotation and abduction and ends when the ball leaves the fingers. The movements in this phase include scapular protraction, humeral horizontal flexion and internal rotation, and elbow extension. At ball release, the shoulder is still in about 90° abduction. This helps to reduce impingement during acceleration. During this phase the speed of the arm has increased significantly in a relatively brief period of time, beginning from almost 0°/s at the end of cocking to 7500°/s by the end of acceleration (Pappas, Zawacki, and Sullivan 1985). The serratus anterior and pectoralis major are strongly active during this phase as the arm moves forward and the scapula protracts. The subscapularis and latissimus dorsi are contracting concentrically as the arm is moved into internal rotation during acceleration.

Follow-Through

Follow-through occurs from the point of ball release to the completion of the motion. It is divided into early and late follow-through according to the point of maximal shoulder internal rotation. Early follow-through is completed rapidly, in less than 0.1 s (Moynes et al. 1986). Trunk rotation and scapular motions occur and are diminished to a varying extent from one style to another, depending on the individual thrower. The deltoid is strongly active during early follow-through. The rotator cuff, especially the external rotators, must decelerate the arm after ball release and also work against the momentum distraction forces occurring at the shoulder. The biceps is also working eccentrically to reduce distraction forces at the elbow. It is during the follow-through that injuries to the posterior shoulder occur. The energy that has been developed to accelerate the ball must now be dissipated by the body. This is one reason it is important for the body to continue to move after the ball is released. An abrupt stop in arm motion will prevent this energy dissipation and cause these tremendous forces to be absorbed primarily by the shoulder. Flexing the trunk, extending the supporting knee, and allowing the arm to continue along its path of movement across the body and to the opposite leg all assist in dissipating this energy and reducing distraction forces on the shoulder.

TENNIS

The repetitive motions and forces applied to the shoulder in tennis are a frequent cause of tennis injuries. Overhead serves and hits require more muscle activity of the shoulder than other motions and are the leading cause of shoulder injuries in this sport. The three main activities in tennis are the serve, the forehand ground stroke, and the backhand ground stroke. Each deserves a brief discussion because the sport rehabilitation specialist must understand the motions involved and the demands placed on the shoulder to effectively and safely advance the patient in a functional therapeutic exercise program.

Serve

The serve is divided into four phases–windup, cocking, acceleration, and follow-through (figure 17.2).

Windup
Windup, the setting phase of the serve, takes place when the athlete prepares for the motion. The serve stance is taken in preparation for the ball toss. The body is perpendicular to the service line, with the weight on the back leg and the front leg facing the target. The shoulder muscles are relatively quiet. The shoulder is in slight abduction, extension, and external rotation. The trunk is slightly laterally flexed and rotated, and the legs are rotated.

Cocking
Cocking begins with ball release from the opposite arm and continues to the point at which the racket shoulder is at maximum external rotation. The scapula is upwardly rotated and adducted, the shoulder is abducted and externally rotated, and the elbow is flexed. The supraspinatus, infraspinatus, and subscapularis muscles are very active, stabilizing the humerus in the glenoid and positioning the shoulder. The subscapularis also works to decelerate external rotation in preparation for acceleration.

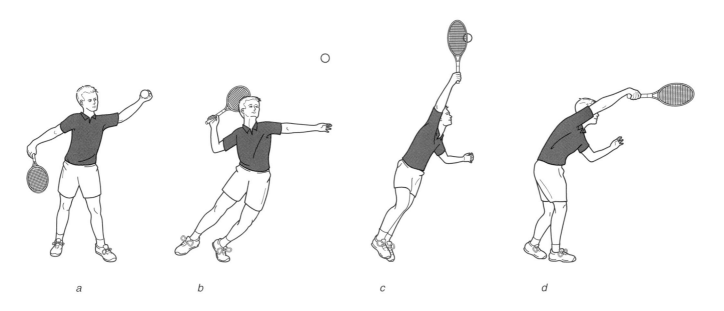

a   *b*   *c*   *d*

▌Figure 17.2   Tennis serve: *(a)* windup, *(b)* cocking, *(c)* acceleration, *(d)* follow-through.

The serratus anterior is active to stabilize the scapula on the thoracic wall, rotating the scapula into the correct position to serve as a platform from which the glenohumeral joint moves (Ryu et al. 1988). The posterior deltoid and trunk lean are responsible for shoulder abduction. Biceps activity is moderately high during this phase so that the racket is held in the correct position with the elbow flexed overhead.

Acceleration

Acceleration begins with internal rotation movement of the shoulder and ends with ball contact. Glenohumeral internal rotation is rapid and forceful, occurring with shoulder adduction, elbow extension, and trunk flexion. It is the quickest and briefest phase of the serve. The subscapularis is very active to produce internal rotation. The pectoralis major and latissimus dorsi work to adduct the arm. Scapular stabilizers, performing a critical function, are active as they continue to maintain good scapular positioning and stabilization on the thoracic wall. The biceps is eccentrically controlling elbow extension and pronation.

Follow-Through

The last phase of the serve, follow-through, occurs from ball impact to the end of the motion. As with pitching, the rapid change from acceleration to deceleration places tremendous forces on the shoulder and causes the scapular and glenohumeral muscles to work at moderate to high levels primarily to decelerate and protect the shoulder. Most of these muscles work intensely in the early part of follow-through, their activity declining as the motion continues. The latissimus dorsi and pectoralis major decelerate forward shoulder motion; the rotator cuff muscles work eccentrically to provide deceleration of the forward momentum and distraction pull on the humerus in the glenoid; the serratus anterior (the most thoroughly investigated scapular rotator) is active eccentrically; and the biceps continues its eccentric control of the elbow.

Forehand Ground Stroke

The forehand ground stroke is divided into three phases—racket preparation, acceleration, and follow-through (figure 17.3).

Racket Preparation

The racket preparation phase begins with the shoulder turn and ends with the initiation of weight transfer onto the front foot. The trunk and hips are rotated away from the front foot. The arm is positioned into abduction and external rotation, and the weight is on the back foot. The shoulder positioning is primarily the result of hip and trunk rotation; little muscle activity occurs in the shoulder.

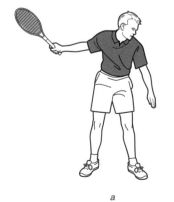 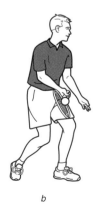 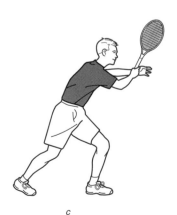

▌Figure 17.3 Forehand ground stroke: *(a)* racket preparation, *(b)* acceleration, *(c)* follow-through.

a   b   c

Acceleration

This phase begins with weight transfer onto the front foot and ends at ball impact. During this phase the body and racket are moved forward, and the hips and trunk begin to rotate. A rapid internal rotation of the shoulder and adduction occur. Internal rotation results from strong contraction of the subscapularis, and adduction occurs because of activity of the pectoralis major. The serratus anterior also works actively to continue protraction and scapular stabilization. The biceps works to keep the elbow slightly flexed.

Follow-Through

Follow-through occurs from ball contact to the end of the motion. The serratus anterior, biceps, infraspinatus, and supraspinatus are highly active as during other follow-through motions.

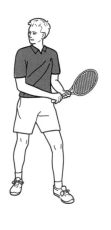
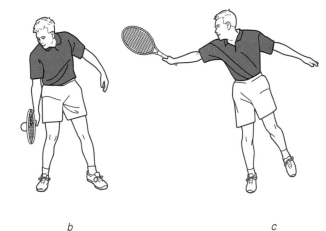

a　　　　　　　　　　b　　　　　　　　　　c

■ **Figure 17.4** Backhand ground stroke: *(a)* racket preparation, *(b)* acceleration, *(c)* follow-through.

Backhand Ground Stroke

The backhand ground stroke is similar to the forehand ground stroke in having three phases: racket preparation, acceleration, and deceleration (figure 17.4).

Racket Preparation

This phase begins with shoulder turn to place the racket shoulder to the net and ends with weight-transfer initiation to the front foot. The trunk and hips are rotated with the weight primarily on the back foot, the shoulder is in internal rotation and adduction, and the elbow is flexed. As with other preparatory phases, shoulder muscle activity is relatively quiet.

Acceleration

Acceleration begins with weight transfer to the front foot and ends with ball contact. The hips and trunk begin rotation; and as the weight is transferred, the scapula retracts, the shoulder abducts and externally rotates, and the elbow extends. This movement occurs with strong, forceful shoulder external rotation caused by the rotator cuff) supraspinatus, infraspinatus, and teres minor). The middle deltoid is also active as the shoulder is abducted. The serratus anterior, acting as a scapular stabilizer, and the biceps, working as an elbow decelerator, are also active during this phase.

Follow-Through

Follow-through takes place from ball contact to the end of the stroke. The most active muscles during this phase are the middle deltoid, biceps, supraspinatus, and infraspinatus.

SWIMMING

Shoulder pain is common in swimmers. The shoulder provides the propulsive force to permit use of the hand as a paddle for moving the body through the water (Perry 1983). The legs provide less propulsion than the arms in swimming, and they are important for smoothing out the stroke and making it more efficient. The legs also provide a base for body roll during the stroke, so therapeutic exercise programs for injured swimmers should include lower-extremity exercises.

Each of four primary swimming strokes—the freestyle, the backstroke, the breaststroke, and the butterfly—has unique characteristics, but they all have two phases of motion, pull-through and recovery (figure 17.5a). With the exceptions of the backstroke and the recovery phase in the breaststroke, which are performed out of the water, all are performed in a prone position. Because most shoulder injuries in swimming occur with the freestyle stroke, this is the stroke we will consider here.

Pull-Through

The pull-through phase is the propulsive phase of the freestyle stroke and is similar to the acceleration phase in throwing. In contrast to the acceleration phase in throwing, though, pull-through is the longest phase in swimming. This requires sustained activity of the muscles producing the movement. Pull-through occurs during 65% to 70% of the freestyle stroke (Nuber et al. 1986). The shoulder begins in external rotation and abduction at hand entry into the water and ends internally rotated and adducted just before leaving the water. The elbow moves from flexion to extension. The body rolls to a maximum of 40° to 60° from horizontal, and the shoulder is at 90° abduction and neutral rotation during the middle of the pull phase (Richardson,

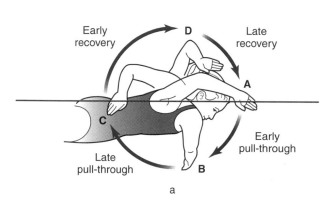

Jobe, and Collins 1980). In the early portion of pull-through, the arm reaches forward underwater with the hand lateral to the head, but medial to the shoulder, and becomes positioned for the pulling aspect of the phase. The fingers enter the water first. Pulling begins after the arm is positioned in the water and continues until the hand is near the thigh, before the hand exits the water. During the most propulsive portion of the pull-through phase, the arm moves in an S-shaped curve: The hand moves across the chest as the shoulder adducts, then moves laterally as it passes by the pelvis. Before lifting the hand out of the water, the shoulder internally rotates to turn the palm to reduce drag (figure 17.5b). During hand entry and early pull-through when the hand crosses the body, the shoulder is in adduction, flexion, and internal rotation; this position can produce mechanical impingement on the biceps tendon and the supraspinatus tendon.

Muscles active during the early pull-through phase include the upper trapezius to upwardly rotate the scapula, the rhomboids to retract the scapula, and the supraspinatus and anterior and middle deltoids to work as a force couple to stabilize the humerus. During later pull-through, the pectoralis major and latissimus dorsi act as the propulsive muscles; the deltoids lift and place the arm in preparation for hand exit from the water; the serratus anterior stabilizes the scapula and the teres minor and the subscapularis stabilize the humerus, as well as performing their movement activities. The serratus anterior and rhomboids downwardly rotate the scapula as the shoulder moves into extension. The teres minor assists with shoulder extension, and the subscapularis internally rotates the humerus. (Pink et al. 1991).

Recovery

The recovery phase begins when the arm leaves the water and continues until hand entry. This phase, used as a preparation for the pull phase, is equivalent to the cocking phase in pitching. During recovery, the shoulder abducts and is in internal rotation but moving into external rotation as the elbow is lifted and the body rolls to the opposite side, as during early pull-through (Richardson, Jobe, and Collins 1980). It is during this time that impingement can occur. This is especially true if weakness prevents the swimmer from lifting the elbow out of the water first or if weak rotator

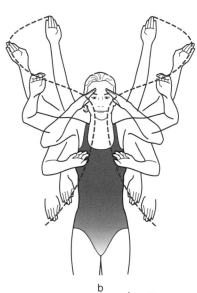

I Figure 17.5 Swim stroke: *(a)* swimming phases, *(b)* S-curve of pull-through.

Adapted from Pink et al. 1991.

cuff and biceps muscles prevent adequate humeral head depression. By mid-recovery, the shoulder is abducted to 90° and in external rotation. The body roll reaches its maximum of 40° to 60° as the athlete breathes. By the time the hand enters the water, the shoulder is maximally externally rotated and abducted, and the body roll is back to a neutral position.

Early recovery is initiated by the muscles abducting and rotating the humerus and rotating the scapula, the supraspinatus and middle deltoid. As recovery progresses, the rhomboids retract the scapula; and the subscapularis internally rotates the shoulder from a maximally externally rotated position at middle recovery and assists the infraspinatus in depression of the humerus in the glenoid before hand entry.

The subscapularis and the serratus anterior work consistently throughout the entire swimming stroke. The range of activity varies according to the arm position and the activity occurring, but the sustained activity of these muscles is significant and should be taken into account in the design of a therapeutic exercise program. Therapeutic exercise programs for these two muscles must include both high-endurance and strength exercises to provide proper shoulder positioning during swimming and to prevent fatigue.

GOLF SWING

There are four phases of the golf swing: take-away, forward swing, acceleration, and follow-through (figure 17.6). Research on the golf swing has been limited. The information presented here is based primarily on the work of Jobe, Moynes, and Antonelli (1985). These investigators looked only at the supraspinatus, subscapularis, infraspinatus, latissimus dorsi, pectoralis major, anterior deltoid, middle deltoid, and posterior deltoid.

The shoulders do not elevate in golf as they do in other overhead sports. For this reason, the deltoids do not play as important a role in golf as they do in throwing, tennis, and swimming. The major muscles in golf, according to the investigation by Jobe, Moynes, and Antonelli, include the rotator cuff, especially the subscapularis, the latissimus dorsi, and the pectoralis major. Keep in mind that the researchers did not investigate all the muscles surrounding the shoulder complex. Other muscles may play an important role in the golf swing and in injury etiology and treatment.

Take-Away

This phase begins when the golfer addresses the ball, and it ends at the top of the backswing. The body is positioned with the front leg and arm facing the direction the ball is to be hit. During take-away, the front shoulder has low-level activity except in the subscapularis. The primary activity of the back shoulder is in the supraspinatus.

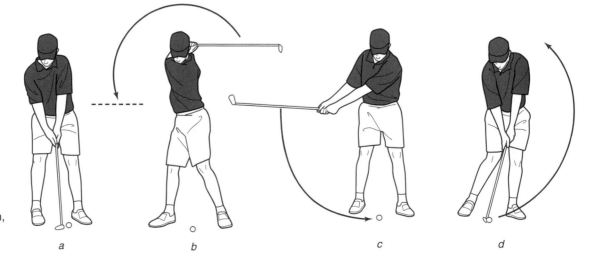

■ **Figure 17.6** Golf swing: *(a)* take-away, *(b)* forward swing, *(c)* acceleration, *(d)* follow-through.

a   b   c   d

Forward Swing

This phase begins at the end of backswing and continues until the club becomes horizontal. The front arm has moderate activity of the subscapularis and latissimus dorsi, whereas the back arm has more activity of the other rotator cuff muscles—the infraspinatus and subscapularis—and less of the supraspinatus. The pectoralis major and latissimus dorsi of the back arm also increase their activity.

Acceleration

Acceleration occurs from the time the club becomes horizontal to the time of ball contact. The front and back arm muscles that are highly active at this time are the same; these include the pectoralis major, latissimus dorsi, and subscapularis.

Follow-Through

Follow-through begins with ball contact and continues to the end of the stroke. The front shoulder's subscapularis continues at high activity levels, but the activity of the pectoralis major and latissimus dorsi subsides. The infraspinatus produces increased activity during this phase. In the back arm, the subscapularis, pectoralis major, and latissimus dorsi continue high activity output.

GENERAL REHABILITATION CONSIDERATIONS

To function normally, the shoulder must have stability, scapular muscle strength, and balance within force couples. Other elements affecting shoulder function include the relationship between the shoulder and other body segments, as well as posture.

The shoulder is a unique area that is composed of several joints: the sternoclavicular, acromioclavicular, scapulothoracic, and glenohumeral joints. Not only must these joints possess appropriate mobility and provide stability, but the muscles that surround and control these joints must all work synchronously to provide normal shoulder function and timing of movement.

STABILITY

Fundamental to normal joint function is stability. When an injury occurs, normal joint stability is compromised, and full recovery is threatened unless the stability is restored. Joint stability is provided by static and dynamic factors. Static stability is provided by the inert structures. In the shoulder, these inert structures include the joint capsule, ligaments, and glenoid labrum. Dynamic stability is the responsibility of the nerves and muscles, including appropriate input from the afferent receptors to the central nervous system to provide timely support through balanced muscle activity as discussed in chapter 8. When the joint's ligaments are injured, the afferent receptors located in those ligaments are unable to provide adequate sensory input. This leads to insufficient neural input and, in turn, inappropriate muscle responses. The end result is a deficiency in static stability because of the injury itself, and a secondary dynamic instability caused by the damage to the afferent receptors. These conditions set up a continuous injury cycle in which continued dynamic and static instability causes functional instability. The cycle continues and leads to progressive injury (figure 17.7).

If muscles surrounding the shoulder are imbalanced, dynamic instability results. If the agonist and antagonist groups are not balanced, there is loss of proprioceptive and kinesthetic control. Dynamic instability results. Muscle imbalance, if not corrected, can be the primary cause of shoulder injury.

The sport rehabilitation specialist is able to break this cycle by providing a rehabilitation program for restoring dynamic stability. Rehabilitation programs include re-education of the neuromuscular system and exercises to restore balance between agonists and antagonists. Sometimes, this is enough to restore the patient to full sport participation. When the static instability is too great,

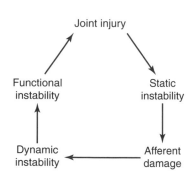

■ **Figure 17.7** Joint instability cycle.

surgical intervention is necessary. Rehabilitation of dynamic stabilizers is just as important after surgical correction of static instability as it is in cases without surgical intercession.

SCAPULAR MUSCLES

Fundamental to all shoulder rehabilitation is rehabilitation of the scapular stabilizers. These are the muscles that control scapular motion. Their strength and control are crucial to the shoulder because the scapula serves as a platform for the shoulder to move from. The difference for the shoulder between a stable and an unstable scapula is similar to the difference between running on firm ground and running on a suspended wood-and-rope footbridge. The ground provides the runner with a stable base from which to move the body forward smoothly and efficiently. Running on an unstable footbridge places high energy demands on the individual's leg muscles, causes incoordination and inefficiency of movement, and increases risk of injury. So, too, a shoulder that has an unstable scapula moves inefficiently and is at risk for injury. With an unstable scapula, the glenohumeral joint tends to migrate superiorly. This leads to impingement and biceps or rotator cuff tendinitis. It is imperative, then, that any therapeutic exercise program for the shoulder include exercises for the scapular stabilizing muscles.

Fatigue of scapular muscles can also affect shoulder motion and performance. The scapular muscles' role as a stabilizer is disrupted when the muscles are fatigued. This disruption occurs as a result of changes in normal scapulohumeral rhythm with fatigue of the scapular muscles, as shown by McQuade, Dawson, and Smidt (1998). The results of their study point to the importance of endurance activities in a therapeutic exercise program.

Because scapular muscle strength is so important to the function and stability of the shoulder, exercises for these muscles should begin early in the rehabilitation program, even after surgical repair. You can start strengthening exercises for these muscles without stressing the glenohumeral joint by using manual resistance in all scapular motions. In many cases, the upper trapezius and levator scapulae muscles are not weak, but the other scapular muscles are and, therefore, need re-education and rehabilitation. Scapular depression, protraction, retraction, and upward and downward rotation are all motions that can and should be manually resisted early in the rehabilitation process.

If the upper trapezius and levator scapulae are weak, of course, strengthening of these muscles is in order. Often, however, these muscles compensate for weak shoulder muscles and are used incorrectly. If the rotator cuff is weak, the upper trapezius may work with the deltoid to elevate the shoulder, enhancing muscle imbalances, encouraging incorrect mechanics, and aggravating the shoulder injury. Two techniques that can be used to control and retrain the upper trapezius are biofeedback and taping. Biofeedback can be used to either facilitate rotator cuff activity or reduce upper trapezius activity during shoulder elevation exercises (figure 17.8). The specific application depends on the electrode placement, machine settings, and motions desired.

Scapular taping can be useful in cases of secondary impingement in which faulty positioning of the scapula during overhead movements causes impingement of the rotator cuff tendons. The taping must be accompanied by retraining exercises to re-educate the scapular muscles so that they position the scapula correctly during shoulder motions. The taping technique was introduced by Jenny McConnell, an Australian manipulative physiotherapist. Limited research has demonstrated that tape application inhibits upper trapezius and facilitates middle and lower trapezius activation (Morin, Tiberio, and Austin 1997). This can improve scapular stability by facilitating muscle balance during motion to permit arm movement without impingement pain;

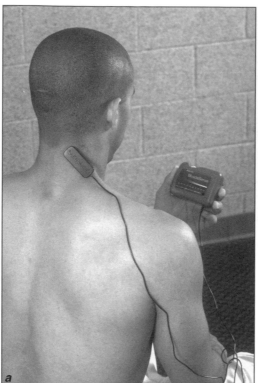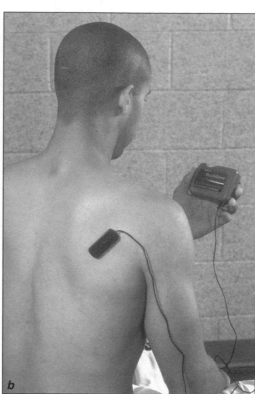

Figure 17.8 Biofeedback: electrode placement for upper trapezius inhibition to decrease activity *(a)*, and for infraspinatus facilitation to increase activity *(b)*.

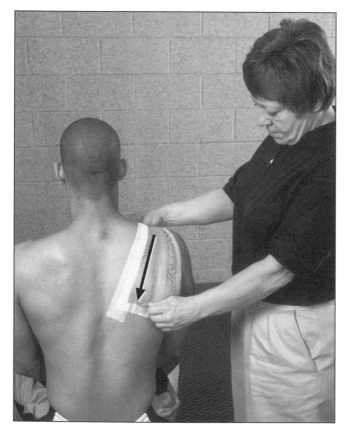

Figure 17.9 Scapular taping support.

it can also enhance muscle re-education for normal scapular alignment and positioning (Host 1995). Two types of tape are used together: a protective stretch tape called Cover-roll stretch, and a support tape, Leukotape P (both distributed by Beiersdorf, Inc., Norwalk, CT). Two to three strips of the protective stretch tape are applied to the skin over the shoulder from the clavicle anteriorly and across the upper trapezius to below the scapula toward the lower thoracic spinous processes posteriorly. With the patient in a proper posture position, the support tape is applied in several strips from the middle aspect of the upper trapezius muscle belly, in a direction downward and medially to the inferior angle of the scapula (figure 17.9). When applying the tape, the sport rehabilitation specialist should support the shoulder under the axilla so that the upper trapezius can stay relaxed. The tape should be snug but still loose enough to permit scapular motion during shoulder elevation.

FORCE COUPLES

Force couples—two equal forces acting in opposite but parallel directions—produce rotatory motion. The shoulder has several force couples that function during arm movement. It is important that the muscles within each of these force couples are balanced to provide optimal function. In the glenohumeral joint, the infraspinatus and teres minor form a force couple with the subscapularis, and the rotator cuff forms a force couple with the deltoid. Scapular force couples include the upper and lower trapezius and serratus anterior, which work together to upwardly rotate the scapula, and the pectoralis minor, levator scapulae, and rhomboids working together to downwardly rotate the scapula. The muscles within each force couple must work cooperatively in timing and level of intensity to produce the desired activity. For example, if the deltoid overpowers the rotator cuff, the glenohumeral joint becomes unstable during elevation. If the scapular upward rotators are stronger than the downward rotators, or if one upward rotator overpowers another upward rotator, the scapula is not positioned correctly during arm elevation, and impingement of the rotator cuff occurs.

RELATIONSHIP BETWEEN TRUNK/HIP AND SHOULDER

Just as scapulothoracic stability and strength are important for glenohumeral function, trunk and lower-extremity stability and strength are important for scapular function. The trunk must have the strength to maintain a stable base for the functioning of the scapula. The legs and trunk provide 51% to 55% of the total kinetic energy and total force for overhead activities (Kibler 1995). The shoulder contributes 13% to the total energy production and 21% of the total force. For this reason, exercises for hip rotators, extensors, and abductors, as well as for abdominals, obliques, and trunk extensors, should all be included in a shoulder rehabilitation program.

The forces generated from the legs, hips, trunk, shoulder, and arm are delivered

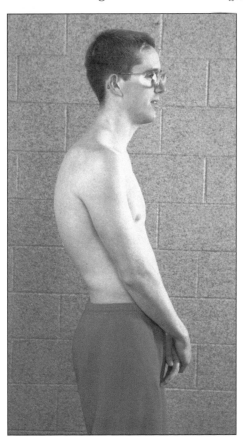

through summation via the body's kinetic chain and are ultimately delivered to the hand and transferred to the object within the hand. These forces must be regulated, directed, and applied in a specific sequence if the body is to work efficiently and effectively. This requires a balance of muscle strength throughout all the delivery systems involved.

POSTURE

Any patient with a shoulder injury should have a posture evaluation. Correct posture is crucial to shoulder balance and function. If a patient has a forward-head posture with a thoracic kyphosis, the shoulders are drawn forward and internally rotated (figure 17.10). This causes a protraction of the scapula and internal rotation of the humerus. It prevents full elevation of the shoulder and leads to subacromial impingement that will cause rotator cuff tendinitis. A forward-head posture also causes a muscle imbalance, shortening the anterior muscles and lengthening and weakness of the posterior muscles. Posture must be corrected if the rehabilitation program is to be successful.

▌ **Figure 17.10**
Forward-head, kyphotic posture.

CERVICAL INFLUENCE

There is an intimate relationship between the cervical spine and shoulder. Patients who complain of shoulder pain without a frank shoulder injury should be evaluated for cervical involvement. Cervical disk pathology can refer pain along the medial border of the scapula, into the shoulder joint, or down the arm. If shoulder symptoms increase with movement, palpation, or joint mobilization of the spine, the cervical spine may be the source of shoulder pain. It is sometimes difficult to determine whether the cervical spine or the shoulder is the primary source of pain. A quick quadrant test can rule out the possibility of cervical involvement. If the test is negative, the neck may not be the source of pain; however, if the patient does not respond to treatment, reassessment of the cervical spine is in order. Reproducing the patient's pain is a key component of the rehabilitation assessment for determining the origin of the patient's complaints.

THORACIC INFLUENCE

Shoulders lacking full range of motion may have joint mobility restriction in the ribs and thoracic spine. If a patient lacks full elevation of the glenohumeral joint and the shoulder complex has been mobilized with good results, the thoracic spine and costothoracic joints should be assessed for hypomobility. Restricted costothoracic and thoracic spine mobility can restrict the shoulder's movement by limiting the expansion of the trunk that is necessary for full shoulder motion. This is particularly true if the patient has habitually poor posture. Application of posterior-anterior movements of the thoracic spine or rib mobilization techniques, or both, should restore normal shoulder mobility if thoracic hypermobility is a factor in a patient's having difficulty achieving the last few degrees of glenohumeral motion.

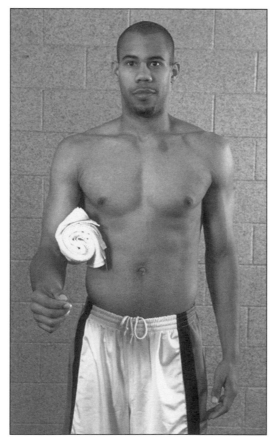

▌Figure 17.11
Using a rolled towel under the arm helps to position the shoulder in the scapular plane during internal rotation/external rotation exercises.

SCAPULAR PLANE

It is important to exercise the rotator cuff in the scapular plane. This is a position about 30° forward of the coronal plane. In this position, the arm is in line with the scapula as it lies on the ribs. It is a functional position for the rotator cuff. Often, exercises for the rotator cuff performed in the coronal plane are too uncomfortable for the rotator cuff and encourage impingement of its tendons. Placing the arm in a scapular plane reduces this possibility and is generally more comfortable for the patient.

When internal and external rotation exercises are performed, a roll should be placed between the arm and the ribs (figure 17.11). This positions the arm in a scapular plane. This position also reduces the tension on the supraspinatus tendon, lessening irritation to the tendon (Kelley 1995). In addition, this position may improve the subscapularis alignment to more effectively depress the humeral head.

PLANE EXERCISE PROGRESSION

Strength exercises may begin as isometrics and progress to concentric and eccentric exercises. When agonists are weak and are imbalanced with their antagonists, the exercises should be initially performed in straight-plane motions. As strength improves and control of motion becomes possible, the exercises progress to diagonal, multiplane, functional motions. Patients should not perform diagonal motions until they have adequate muscular strength, because the complexity of the shoulder's motions requires good control. Good straight-plane strength permits the patient to perform functional activities without aggravating the shoulder or using stronger muscles to produce the motion instead of strengthening the weaker muscles.

Exercises are usually kept to less than 60° elevation in the initial strengthening stages because little scapular motion occurs in the first 60° of glenohumeral motion, so scapular muscles exercised below 60° work primarily as stabilizers, not scapular movers. Elevation higher than 90° is an unstable position for the glenohumeral joint, and shoulder strength in the early stages is not adequate to keep the shoulder stabilized. The scapular muscles are also not strong enough in their shortened range to provide the scapular stabilization necessary for glenohumeral motion above 60° elevation. Once scapulothoracic and glenohumeral muscles have adequate strength to control shoulder motion and provide the stabilization necessary for activity to 90°, progression of exercises to the fully elevated ranges is appropriate after strength at 90° is achieved.

REHABILITATION TECHNIQUES

Two rehabilitation techniques for the shoulder are soft-tissue mobilization and joint mobilization. Trigger point release and ice-and-stretch are soft-tissue mobilization techniques used to improve parameters in the rotator cuff muscles, the scapular muscles, and the large glenohumeral muscles. The sport rehabilitation specialist uses joint mobilization techniques to improve mobility in the gleno-humeral joint, the scapulothoracic joint, and the clavicular joints.

SOFT-TISSUE MOBILIZATION

Because of the intimate relationship between the cervical spine and the shoulder, some of the muscles discussed in the preceding chapter are also relevant here. Refer to chapter 6 for details on soft-tissue mobilization theory, physiology, and application. Trigger point release and ice-and-stretch techniques are the primary treatment approaches discussed here. These techniques and the pain referral patterns described here are based on the work of Travell and Simons (1983).

Rotator Cuff Muscles

Each rotator cuff muscle has distinct pain-referral patterns. The sport rehabilitation specialist should be aware of these differences to make an accurate differential diagnosis and correctly treat the patient's injury.

Supraspinatus

The muscle and the tendon have trigger points and can refer pain into the arm. The referred pain pattern is a deep ache that occurs around the shoulder in the middle deltoid area down to the deltoid insertion (figure 17.12, a and b). The pain can also be referred to the elbow's lateral epicondyle.

Trigger point treatment can be performed with the patient in side-lying on the opposite side or sitting. The medial trigger point is often the most sensitive site. With the patient's arm in a relaxed position, sustained pressure is applied over the muscle just above the clavicular spine, 2 to 3 cm (0.8–1.2 in.) lateral to the vertebral border (figure 17.12c). The rehabilitation specialist should palpate an expansion, tightening, or nodule within the soft tissue over the trigger point site.

Ice-and-stretch is applied with the patient in sitting and the forearm behind the waist. Ice strokes are swept from the proximal supraspinatus insertion, across the muscle and acromion, over the deltoid, and down the arm to the elbow (figure 17.12d). The sport rehabilitation specialist applies the stretch by raising the patient's hand behind the back upward toward the opposite scapula.

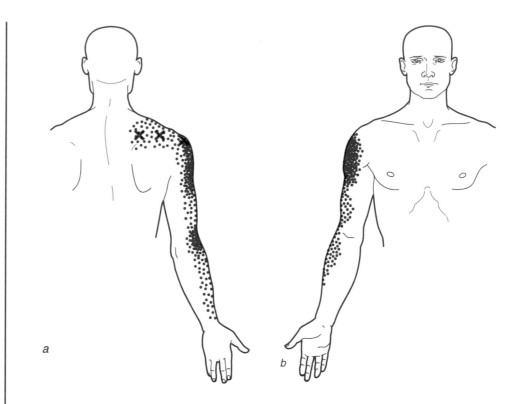

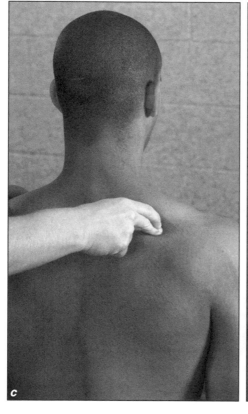

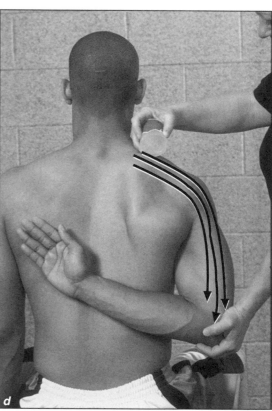

▌ Figure 17.12
Supraspinatus: *(a–b)* pain-referral pattern, *(c)* trigger point release, *(d)* ice-and-stretch.

Subscapularis

The subscapularis refers pain to the posterior shoulder and around the wrist. It can also refer pain into the scapula and down the posterior arm to the elbow (figure 17.13, a–b).

Trigger point release is performed with the patient in supine and the arm abducted comfortably away from the body to about 60° to 90°. The sport rehabilitation specialist supports the patient's arm while applying traction to keep the scapula away from the ribs, then moves his or her fingers past the teres major and latissimus dorsi and palpates the anterior surface of the scapula. A sustained pressure in a cephalic direction toward the spine is applied once the trigger point has been located (figure 17.13c).

Ice-and-stretch is applied with the patient supine and the arm in partial abduction and external rotation. Ice sweeps start at the side and move over the axilla and along the posterior arm. As the sweeps are repeated, the arm is moved into more abduction and external rotation until it is positioned overhead in full abduction and external rotation (figure 17.13, d–e).

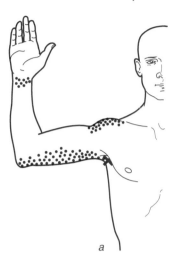
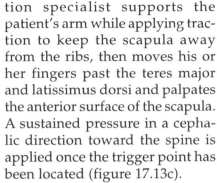

a *b*

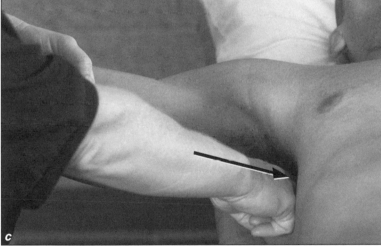

c

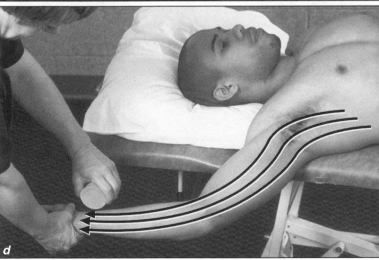

d

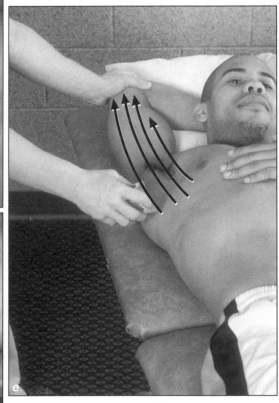

e

∎ **Figure 17.13** Subscapularis: *(a–b)* pain-referral pattern, *(c)* trigger point release, *(d)* ice-and-stretch in moderate stretch position, *(e)* ice-and-stretch in stretch position.

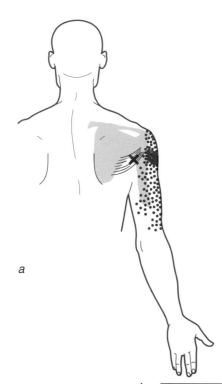

a

Teres Minor

The teres minor muscle refers pain to the posterior deltoid, proximal to the deltoid attachment and about 5 cm (2.0 in.) in diameter (figure 17.14a). The pain is frequently described as deep and sharp. The spillover area of pain referral is the posterior upper arm.

Trigger point release is performed with the patient in side-lying on the opposite side with the arm comfortably supported. The trigger point is located in the teres minor muscle belly along the lateral scapular border between the teres major inferiorly and the infraspinatus superiorly (figure 17.14b).

Ice-and-stretch is applied with the patient in side-lying on the opposite side. The ice sweeps begin low on the side and move along the lateral border of the scapula over the teres minor and along the posterior arm. As the ice is applied, the arm is moved overhead and internally rotated (figure 17.14c).

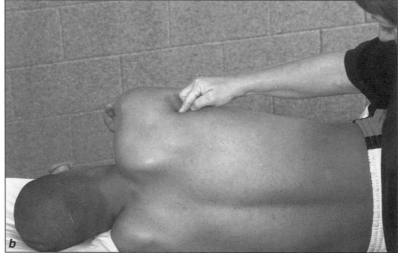

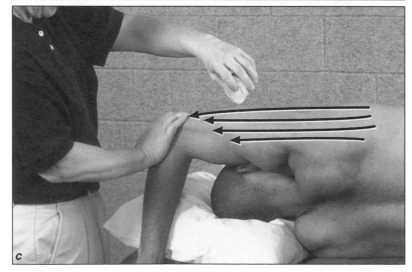

▌Figure 17.14
Teres minor: *(a)* pain-referral pattern, *(b)* trigger point release, *(c)* ice-and-stretch.

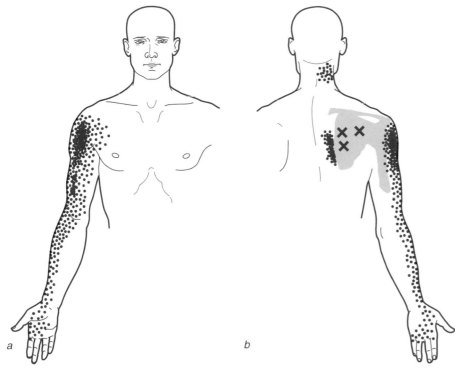

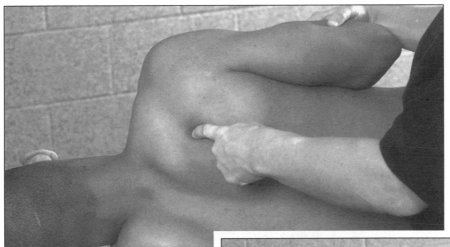

Infraspinatus

The infraspinatus refers pain most often to the anterior shoulder, to the anterior arm, to the wrist, and to the radial fingers (figure 17.15, a–b). On occasion, vertebral border scapular pain or pain at the base of the skull can also occur.

The most commonly irritated trigger points are in the superior aspect of the muscle inferior to the scapula spine. Trigger point release is performed by application of sustained pressure over the muscle with the patient in sitting or side-lying on the opposite side. The trigger point sites are easily located as tender bands within the muscle (figure 17.15c). Ice-and-stretch is applied with the patient in side-lying on the opposite side or sitting. The muscle can be progressively stretched by moving the arm either behind the back with the shoulder in internal rotation, or horizontally in front and across the body with internal rotation. The ice is applied from the vertebral border upward to the shoulder and then either up to the head or down the arm (figure 17.15d).

▌Figure 17.15   Infraspinatus: pain-referral patterns *(a)* anterior and *(b)* posterior; *(c)* trigger point release; *(d)* ice and stretch.

Scapular Muscles

Although the scapular muscles refer pain primarily to the upper back, they can also refer pain to the chest and upper extremity. As with the rotator cuff muscles, the scapular muscles have pain-referral patterns that are unique for each muscle.

Upper Trapezius and Levator Scapulae

Trigger points and treatment of these muscles are described in chapter 16. Refer to figures 16.1 and 16.2 for details.

Serratus Anterior

This muscle refers pain laterally to the midchest area or to the inferior angle of the scapula (figure 17.16, a–b). Spillover referral pain can also be experienced as abnormal breast sensitivity, pain down the anteromedial forearm to the palm and ulnar digits, or pectoralis major pain. Trigger point release is performed with the patient in supine and the arm positioned slightly behind the trunk. Sustained pressure is applied over the level of the fifth or sixth rib just anterior to the midaxillary line at the nipple level (figure 17.16c).

Ice-and-stretch is performed with the patient in side-lying. Ice stroking is applied from the trigger point outward anteriorly and posteriorly over the muscle (figure 17.16d). The progressive stretch is applied with backward and downward pressure on the arm. An additional stretch can be applied to the muscle if the patient takes a deep breath and holds it during the stretch.

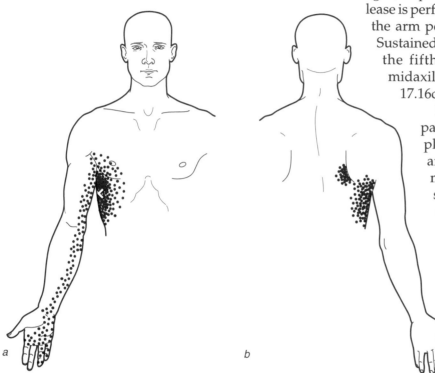

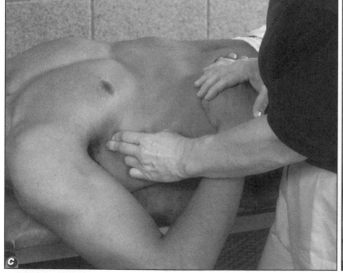

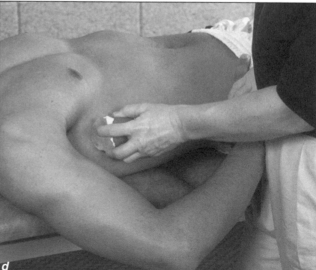

∎ **Figure 17.16**   Serratus anterior: *(a–b)* trigger points and referral points, *(c)* trigger point release, *(d)* ice-and-stretch.

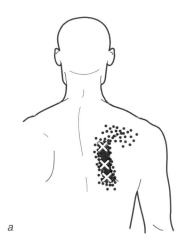

a

Rhomboids

These muscles have pain-referral patterns similar to those of the levator scapulae except that there is no neck component. The pain-referral pattern is along the vertebral border of the scapula, with some pain possible into the supraspinatus area (figure 17.17a).

Trigger point release is performed with the patient in prone or sitting. The area of restriction is often palpated as tender bands in the muscle along the vertebral border. Sustained pressure over this area should be maintained until the pain subsides (figure 17.17b).

Ice-and-stretch is applied with the muscle on stretch. The patient is in a relaxed sitting position with the thoracic spine flexed and the arms hanging forward or across the chest to protract the scapula. Ice sweeps are made in parallel strokes across the back in the direction of the muscle fibers from the vertebral border and upward to the shoulder (figure 17.17c).

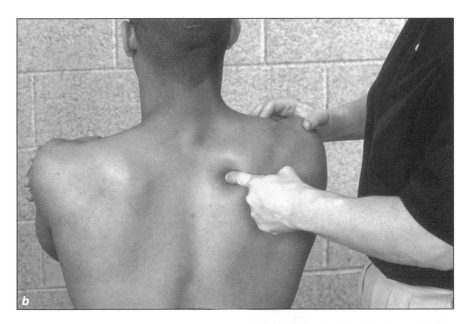

b

▌Figure 17.17
Rhomboids: *(a)* pain-referral patterns, *(b)* trigger point release, *(c)* ice-and-stretch.

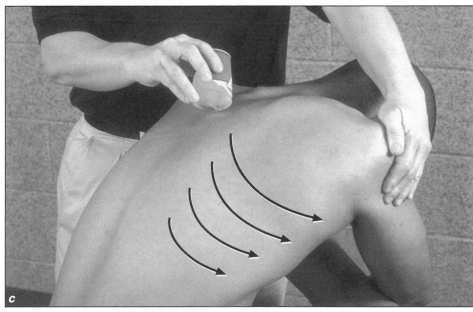

c

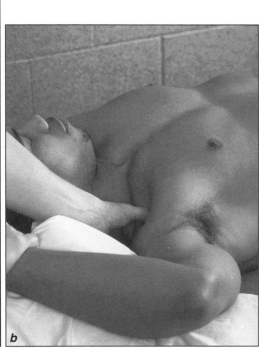

Pectoralis Minor

This muscle refers pain over the anterior deltoid with some spillover into the subclavicular area, pectoral area, and ulnar aspect of the arm, forearm, palmar hand, and fingers (figure 17.18a).

Release of the active trigger point can be performed with the patient supine. The forearm should be supported on the abdomen to keep the pectoralis major lax. The sport rehabilitation specialist counts the ribs down from the concave aspect of the clavicle to the third and fourth ribs. The cephalic trigger point or taut band in the pectoralis minor should be palpated in this region (figure 17.18b). The more distal trigger point is located one rib down and slightly medial to the cephalic trigger point.

Ice-and-stretch is performed with the patient seated. The arm is abducted, and the shoulder is pulled posteriorly in horizontal extension and external rotation to elevate and retract the scapula to put the pectoralis minor on stretch. Ice sweeps are made from the anterior chest region upward to the anterior shoulder, along the medial upper arm and forearm to the ulnar fingers (figure 17.18c).

■ **Figure 17.18**
Pectoralis minor: *(a)* pain referral and trigger points, *(b)* trigger point release, *(c)* ice-and-stretch.

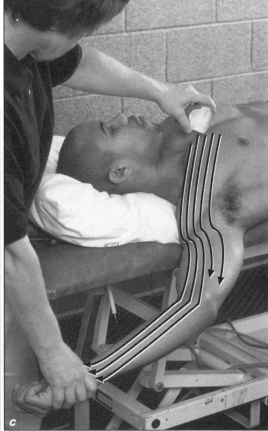

Large Glenohumeral Muscles

Some of the large glenohumeral muscle pain-referral patterns can closely resemble those of other shoulder muscles, including the rotator cuff and scapular rotators. Careful observation and testing are necessary in order to focus in on the proper muscle to treat.

Latissimus Dorsi

A constant aching in the inferior angle of the scapula and midthoracic area is typical of a pain referral with this muscle. Spillover pain referral can also occur in the posterior shoulder, down the medial arm and medial forearm, and to the hand and ulnar fingers (figure 17.19a–c).

Release of this trigger point can be performed with the patient supine and the arm abducted to about 60° to 90°. The sport rehabilitation specialist can palpate myofascial bands by grasping the muscle a couple of centimeters below the top of the arch of the posterior axillary fold at the midscapular level (figure 17.19d).

Ice-and-stretch is performed with the patient in supine or side-lying on the opposite side. Ice sweeps are performed in parallel strokes, from the distal insertion of the muscle upward over the axilla and along the arm and ulnar aspect of the forearm to the hand (figure 17.19e). The muscle is stretched upward so that the arm is eventually placed behind the ear.

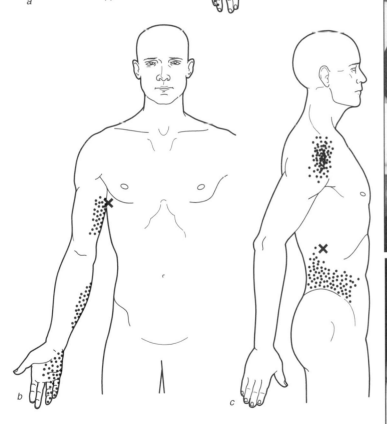

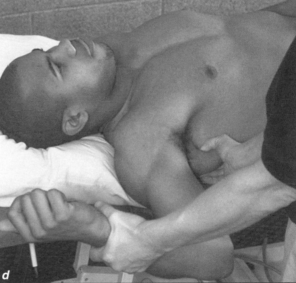

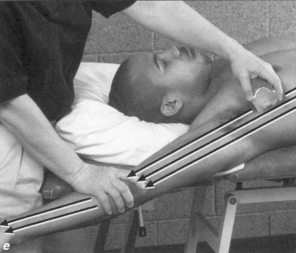

▮ Figure 17.19 Latissimus dorsi: *(a–c)* trigger point and pain referral, *(d)* trigger point release, *(e)* ice-and-stretch.

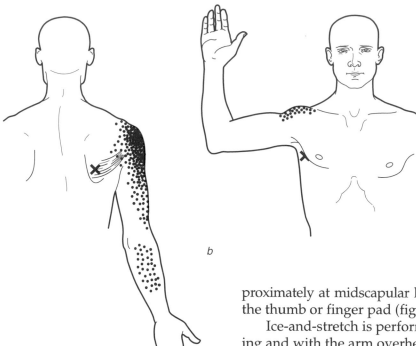

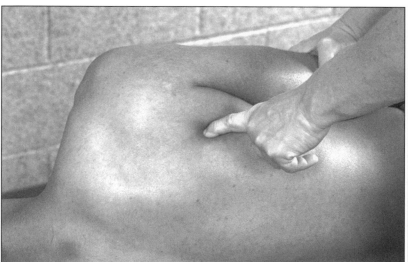

Teres Major

The teres major refers pain over the posterior deltoid, over the triceps long head, and occasionally into the posterior forearm (figure 17.20, a–b).

Trigger point release is performed with the patient in supine and the arm abducted to 90°. The groove between the lateral lower edge of the scapula and the axillary fold is palpated; the muscle is grasped by the thumb and index finger, whose web space surrounds the latissimus dorsi. A tender, taut band can usually be palpated. When the patient is in sitting or side-lying, the muscle is located near the scapula's lateral border approximately at midscapular level and released with pressure using the thumb or finger pad (figure 17.20c).

Ice-and-stretch is performed with the patient supine or side-lying and with the arm overhead in shoulder abduction and external rotation and elbow flexion. Ice strokes are swept from the lateral inferior border of the scapula along the triceps as the arm is moved into internal rotation (figure 17.20d).

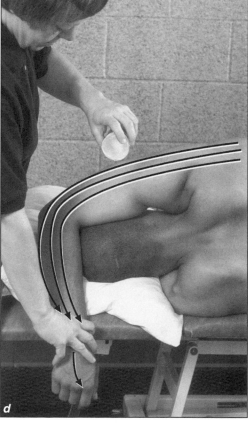

■ **Figure 17.20** Teres major: *(a, b)* pain referral patterns and trigger points, *(c)* trigger point release, *(d)* ice-and-stretch.

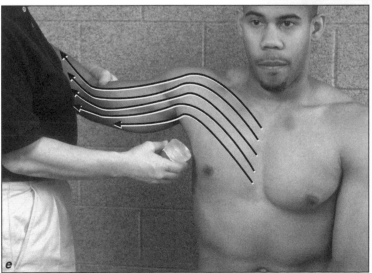

Pectoralis Major

This muscle refers pain to the anterior chest, anterior deltoid, medial epicondyle, sternum, and breast. Overspill referral pain can also occur in the medial arm and ulnar digits (figure 17.21, a–c).

Myofascial release of the pectoralis major can be performed with the arm in 90° abduction. Consistent upward pressure is applied to the muscle between the fifth and sixth ribs (figure 17.21d). Other areas of localized tenderness can be treated in the trigger point regions of the muscle.

Ice-and-stretch is applied with the patient either supine or sitting. The various heads of the pectoralis major are stretched in different positions. The clavicular portion is stretched with the patient in sitting, with the shoulder in 90° of abduction and horizontally extended (figure 17.21e). The sternocostal portion is stretched in sitting or supine, with the shoulder in abduction and external rotation moving into full flexion. If the application is performed with the patient supine, care must be taken to keep the scapula unimpeded during the treatment. Ice strokes are swept from the sternum to the shoulder, along the medial arm, to the ulnar aspect of the hand as the stretch is applied. Traction should be applied to the arm throughout the treatment.

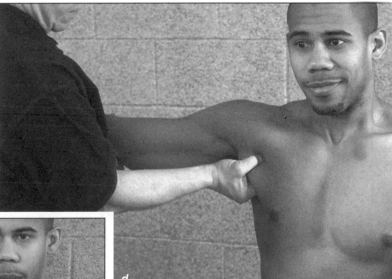

∎ Figure 17.21 Pectoralis major: *(a–c)* pain patterns and trigger points, *(d)* trigger point release, *(e)* ice-and-stretch, clavicular portion.

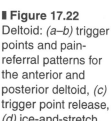

Deltoid

The anterior and posterior deltoid portions can refer pain over the anterior, posterior, and middle deltoid locations with some spillover into adjacent areas of the arm (figure 17.22, a–b). The taut bands and trigger points can be treated with the arm in 30° to 90° of abduction. Pressure is then applied to the trigger point areas (figure 17.22c).

Ice-and-stretch is applied with the patient in sitting. The arm is positioned in horizontal flexion and internal rotation to stretch the posterior deltoid, and in horizontal extension and external rotation to stretch the anterior deltoid (figure 17.22d). As the muscle is being stretched, the ice strokes are swept from the origin of the specific muscle portion, and over the shoulder and arm. For the posterior deltoid ice strokes, move from posterior to anterior; reverse the direction for the anterior deltoid.

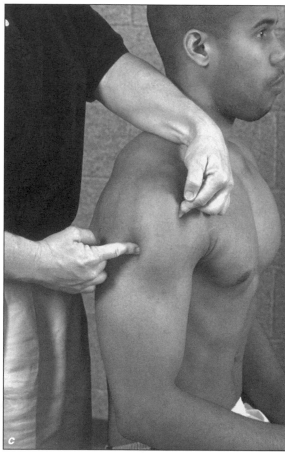

■ Figure 17.22
Deltoid: *(a–b)* trigger points and pain-referral patterns for the anterior and posterior deltoid, *(c)* trigger point release, *(d)* ice-and-stretch.

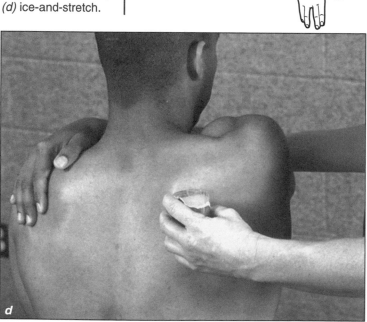

Supraspinatus Friction Massage

This massage technique is used to treat supraspinatus tendinitis. The patient is in sitting with his or her hand behind the back to expose the supraspinatus tendon. The sport rehabilitation specialist's index finger is reinforced by the middle finger and placed on top of the tendon about two finger-widths inferior to the acromion. Cross-friction pressure is applied to the tendon for 1 to 2 min or until the tenderness subsides (figure 17.23).

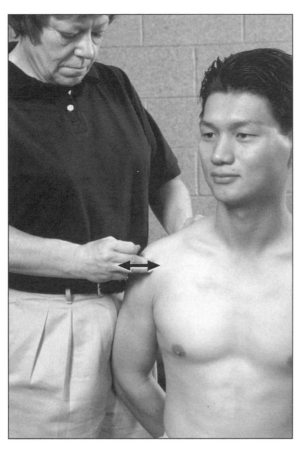

∎ **Figure 17.23**
Cross-friction massage to supraspinatus tendon.

Arm Pull

This technique is a general myofascial stretching technique for stretching or mobilizing soft tissue. With the patient in supine, a longitudinal traction is applied to the patient's arm, with the sport rehabilitation specialist grasping the patient's hand. While traction is applied, the arm is in external rotation, and a gradual, passive movement of the arm into abduction occurs (figure 17.24). When the sport rehabilitation specialist feels a barrier to motion, the position is held until a release is felt. This procedure is repeated with the arm in horizontal adduction. The scapula is protracted, and the patient rolls to the side. A final arm-pull technique is performed with the patient supine. As traction is applied to the arm, the arm is internally rotated and adducted.

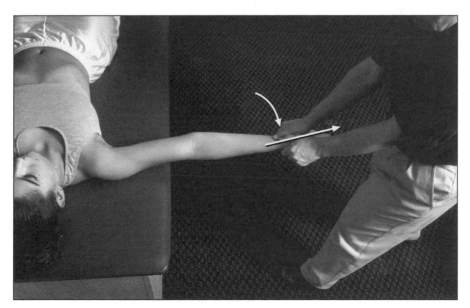

∎ **Figure 17.24** Arm pull.

JOINT MOBILIZATION

Joint mobilization can be performed on all joints of the shoulder complex. Findings from the initial assessment will determine the specific joints requiring mobilization treatment. Shoulder joint mobility is also influenced by the mobility of the ribs and thoracic spine. If a shoulder lacks full range of motion and appears to have good mobility in its joints, assessment of rib and thoracic spine mobility may demonstrate restriction of these joints. If this proves to be the case, mobilization techniques discussed in chapter 16 for these areas may be helpful in restoring full shoulder motion.

Capsular restriction of the glenohumeral joint follows a capsular pattern: more restricted motion in external rotation than in abduction, more restricted motion in abduction than in flexion, and more restricted motion in flexion than in internal rotation. For example, if a patient's shoulder has 100° flexion, 90° abduction, and full external rotation, the joint capsule is not the primary structure limiting full motion. However, if the joint measures 100° flexion, 90° abduction, and 60° external rotation, the joint capsule is probably restricting full motion. If a patient's shoulder presents with this loss-of-motion profile, the capsule is restricted, and joint mobilization is needed to restore glenohumeral motion. If a shoulder does not demonstrate this capsular pattern, loss of motion is not limited primarily by the capsule.

Initial glenohumeral mobilizations should be applied with the joint in a loose-packed position—55° flexion and 20° to 30° horizontal abduction. As additional mobility is achieved but full mobility is still lacking, the joint may need to be mobilized out of the loose-packed position. The extreme close-packed position for the glenohumeral joint is full abduction with full external rotation. Mobilization of the loose-packed position is not used, however, until later in the rehabilitation process when full elevation is lacking because of glenohumeral joint restriction.

While applying joint mobilization, the sport rehabilitation specialist should always use good body mechanics. The hand applying the force should be positioned as close to the joint as possible to act as a fulcrum. The mobilization force should be directed from the legs, not the arms.

The sport rehabilitation specialist needs to remember the principles of glide, roll, and spin so that the force application is proper for the desired movement. The humerus is a convex surface moving on a concave surface, so the convex-concave rule applies. The joint mobilization techniques presented here are the most commonly used techniques. As with any joint mobilization procedure, it is important for the sport rehabilitation specialist to visualize the joint surfaces and apply the mobilization force parallel to the surface. As the arm is moved into different positions, the angle of the glenoid changes; you must take this into account as you determine the angle of force application.

Precautions and contraindications should be respected. The time line for tissue healing and the status and strength of new tissue must be considered when one is deciding whether to apply joint mobilization or how much force to use. Joint mobilization applied to hypermobile joints can increase instability and cause further damage, and is contraindicated. Improper technique, incorrect force application, excessive force, and inappropriate timing of application can all result in unnecessary injury or damage to the joint's structures.

Glenohumeral Joint

During most mobilization techniques for the glenohumeral joint, a sustained joint distraction force is applied in addition to the mobilization force. The techniques are usually named according to the direction of the mobilization force.

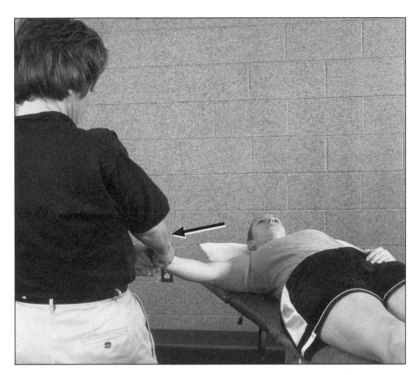

Distraction With Oscillation

This type of mobilization, a relaxation technique, is a good way to begin and end mobilization treatment; it relaxes the joint before and after treatment. The patient lies supine, and the sport rehabilitation specialist grasps the patient's distal forearm and wrist with two hands. The shoulder should be in the loose-packed position, about 55° of flexion and 30° of horizontal abduction. The sport rehabilitation specialist applies mild distraction to the glenohumeral joint while performing oscillations (figure 17.25).

▌**Figure 17.25** Joint mobilization: distraction with oscillation.

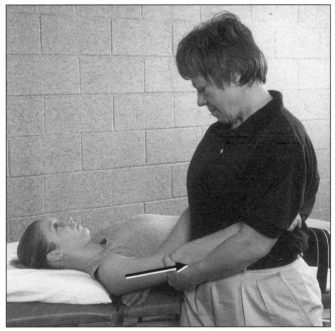

▌**Figure 17.26** Joint mobilization: longitudinal distraction.

Longitudinal Distraction

The loose-packed position, the most comfortable position for the glenohumeral joint, is the position used for longitudinal distraction. This is a good beginning technique for improving inferior capsule mobility. The patient is supine with the involved shoulder as close to the edge of the table as possible. For a right shoulder, the sport rehabilitation specialist places his or her right hand in the axilla to stabilize the glenoid. The left hand grasps just above the elbow joint and applies a distraction force to the humerus (figure 17.26). Although a prolonged force is more effective, an oscillation can also be used.

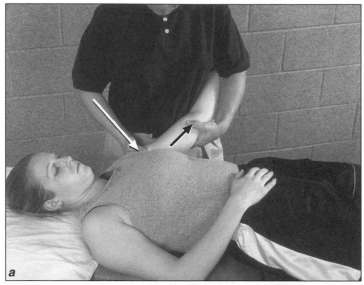

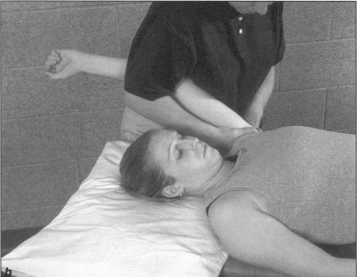

Inferior Glide

This technique is used to improve inferior capsular mobility by stretching the inferior capsular pouch. The patient lies supine with the involved shoulder as close to the edge of the table as possible. A stabilization strap can be placed around the chest to stabilize the scapula. The sport rehabilitation specialist places the stabilizing hand on the proximal humerus and places the mobilizing hand on superior aspect of the humerus as close as possible to the acromion. The mobilizing hand web space should be over the superior humeral head. The stabilizing hand maintains the shoulder in a loose-packed position with some distraction as the mobilizing hand applies a glide force in a caudal direction parallel to the joint's surface (figure 17.27a). The arm can be abducted to a maximum of 60°, but initial glides should be performed in a loose-packed position. Once approximately 120° of flexion has been attained, an inferior glide can be performed with the arm in an elevated position. As the shoulder's position changes, the glenoid joint surface changes; the mobilization force is directed more inferiorly and downward in this position (figure 17.27b).

∎ **Figure 17.27**   Joint mobilization—inferior glide: *(a)* initial position, *(b)* advanced position.

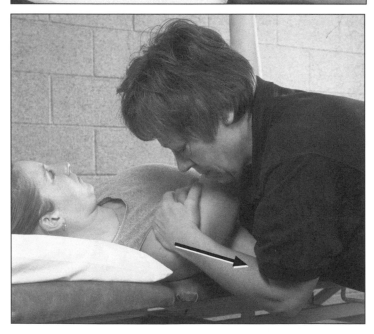

This technique is useful for improving inferior capsule mobility. The patient lies supine with the involved shoulder flexed to 90°. The sport rehabilitation specialist's hands grasp the humerus as close as possible to the shoulder joint. The patient's upper arm rests on the sport rehabilitation specialist's shoulder. An inferior force is applied by the sport rehabilitation specialist's hands (figure 17.28). A prolonged or oscillation technique can be used.

∎ **Figure 17.28**   Joint mobilization: caudal glide.

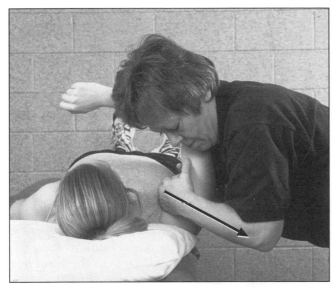

■ **Figure 17.29** Joint mobilization: lateral glide.

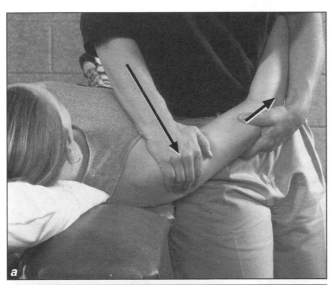

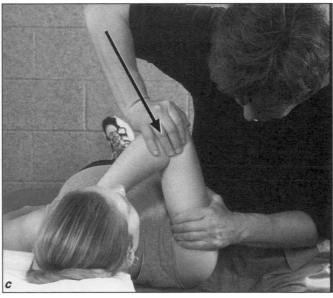

■ **Figure 17.30** Joint mobilization: *(a)* posterior glide, *(b)* posterior glide with internal rotation, *(c)* posterior glide with flexion.

Lateral Glide

This technique is used to increase all motions of the glenohumeral joint. The patient lies supine with the involved shoulder as close to the edge of the table as possible. A strap can be used to stabilize the scapula. The sport rehabilitation specialist faces the patient at shoulder level and grasps the patient's humerus as proximally as possible with the patient's shoulder flexed to 90° and the patient's upper arm resting on the sport rehabilitation specialist's shoulder. A lateral force is applied to the humerus (figure 17.29).

Posterior Glide

This technique is used to improve flexion and internal rotation motions by improving posterior capsule mobility. The patient lies supine with the shoulder as close to the edge of the table as possible. A towel roll or wedge is placed under the scapula for stabilization. The sport rehabilitation specialist abducts the patient's arm; standing between the patient's arm and trunk, the sport rehabilitation specialist places the stabilizing hand at the elbow and the mobilizing hand just distal to the acromion, as close to the humeral head as possible. A downward and slightly lateral force is applied by the mobilizing hand, and slight traction of the patient's glenohumeral joint is applied by the stabilizing hand at the patient's elbow (figure 17.30a). An alternative technique is performed with the patient's shoulder in internal rotation to gain additional motion in that direction (figure 17.30b). An advanced flexion technique can be performed with the patient's shoulder flexed to 90° and adducted with the elbow flexed. In this position the sport rehabilitation specialist stabilizes the arm with a hand on the proximal humerus. A downward mobilization force is applied with the other hand on the patient's elbow and the sport rehabilitation specialist's forearm in line with the patient's arm (figure 17.30c).

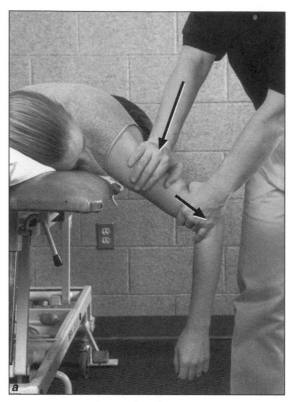

Anterior Glide

This technique is used to increase anterior capsule mobility for improving extension and external rotation. The patient lies prone with a towel or wedge support under the anterior clavicle and coracoid process to stabilize the shoulder. The glenohumeral joint is off the edge of the table, and the arm is abducted in the scapular plane. The sport rehabilitation specialist stands between the patient's arm and side, facing the shoulder, and places the stabilizing hand on the distal humerus and the mobilization hand on the posterior aspect of the humeral head just distal to the acromion. As a distraction force is applied by the stabilizing hand, an anterior and slightly medial mobilization force is applied by the proximal hand (figure 17.31a). As additional motion is achieved but restriction in the anterior-inferior capsule remains, an alternative position for mobilization is with the arm in elevation (figure 17.31b). An alternative technique can be used to increase external rotation by positioning the arm in additional external rotation during the mobilization. With another technique, one that is less comfortable for the sport rehabilitation specialist, the patient is supine and a force from the posterior aspect of the shoulder is applied (figure 17.31c).

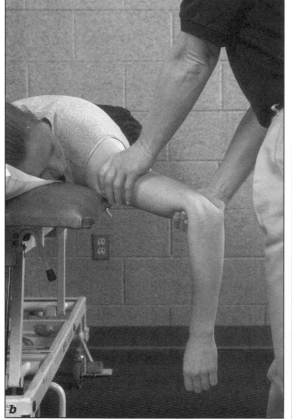

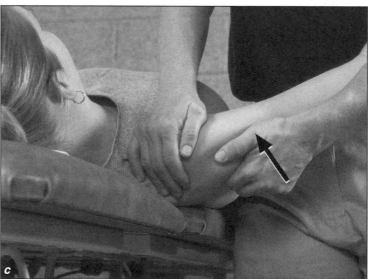

❚ Figure 17.31 Joint mobilization—anterior glide: *(a)* initial position, *(b)* alternative position, *(c)* supine position.

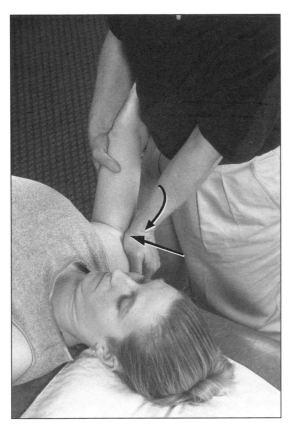

Figure 17.32 Joint mobilization: external rotation.

External Rotation

This technique is used to improve external rotation motion. The patient lies supine with the arm abducted in the scapular plane. The sport rehabilitation specialist places the distal hand over the distal humerus and the heel of the proximal hand over the humeral head. As the distal hand stabilizes the arm in external rotation, the proximal hand applies a simultaneous external rotation and inferior glide force (figure 17.32).

Scapulothoracic Joint

These mobilization techniques for the scapulothoracic joint are possible only if the patient remains relaxed. If a patient is not relaxed, the sport rehabilitation specialist will be unable to position his or her hands between the scapula and ribs to apply the techniques.

Scapular Distraction

This technique is used to improve subscapularis mobility. The patient is in side-lying with the involved arm on top. The sport rehabilitation specialist positions his or her lower hand between the patient's arm and rib cage and grasps the inferior angle of the scapula. The upper hand grasps the scapula's upper vertebral border. For personal comfort and professional consideration, a pillow should be placed between the patient and the sport rehabilitation specialist. As the shoulder is stabilized by the sport rehabilitation specialist's abdomen against the anterior shoulder, both hands apply a force to tilt the vertebral border of the scapula up and away from the ribs (figure 17.33a). An alternative position is with the patient prone. The arm is extended alongside the body, supported on the table. The sport rehabilitation specialist stands beside the patient, facing the patient's head, and places one hand on the anterior humeral head and the other under the inferior angle of the scapula. Simultaneously the hands are moved toward each other, the hand under the humerus lifting upward and medially, and the hand under the scapula moving laterally under the scapula (figure 17.33b).

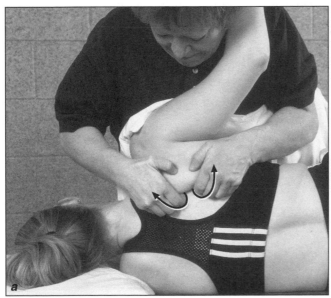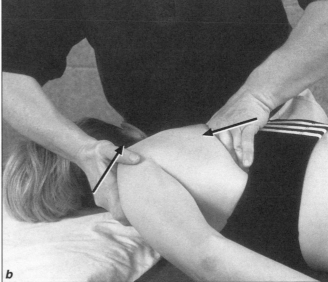

Figure 17.33 Joint mobilization—scapular distraction: *(a)* in side-lying, *(b)* alternative technique in prone.

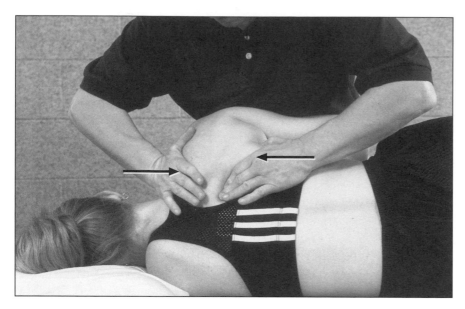

Scapular Inferior Glide

This technique is used to improve downward mobility of the scapula. The patient is in side-lying, and the sport rehabilitation specialist faces the patient. The sport rehabilitation specialist's cephalad hand is placed over the superior scapula, and the caudad hand is positioned with the web space cradling the inferior angle of the scapula. As the superior hand pushes the scapula in a caudal direction, the inferior hand moves under the inferior angle of the scapula (figure 17.34).

∎ Figure 17.34   Joint mobilization: scapular inferior glide.

Clavicular Joints

Because clavicular motion contributes 60° to glenohumeral motion, it is important for clavicular joint mobility to be intact. After shoulder immobilization, these joints may become restricted and should be mobilized if hypomobility is present.

Four mobilization techniques are used at the sternoclavicular and acromioclavicular (AC) joints: inferior, superior, anterior, and posterior glides. The force is applied with the thumb pad of one hand, reinforced with the other thumb.

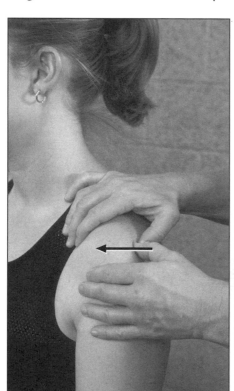

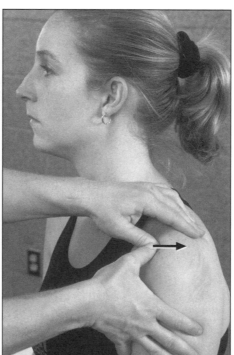

Acromioclavicular Glides

These techniques are performed with the patient supine and the arm supported on the table, or with the patient sitting. When the patient is supine, the sport rehabilitation specialist stands at the waist for superior glides, at the head for inferior glides, and at the side for posterior glides. To perform anterior glides with the patient sitting, the sport rehabilitation specialist is behind the patient (figure 17.35a) and in front of the patient for posterior glides (figure 17.35b). With each technique, the sport rehabilitation specialist applies a force on the end of the the lateral clavicle, parallel to the joint-surface plane.

∎ Figure 17.35   Joint mobilization—AC glides: *(a)* anterior glide, *(b)* posterior glide.

Sternoclavicular Glides

For these techniques, the patient is supine, and his or her arm is supported on the table. The sport rehabilitation specialist stands at the patient's waist for superior glides, at the head for inferior glides (figure 17.36a), and at the side for posterior glides. The force is applied parallel to the joint surface on the medial end of the clavicle.

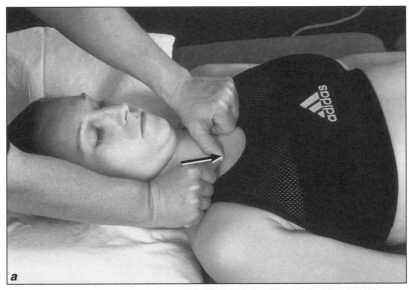

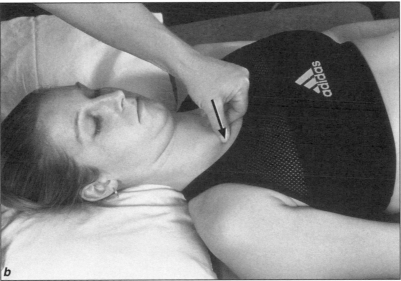

❚ **Figure 17.36** Joint mobilization—sterno-clavicular glides: *(a)* inferior glide, *(b)* posterior glide.

FLEXIBILITY EXERCISES

Flexibility exercises for the shoulder include pendulum exercises, active and assistive stretches, wand exercises using the uninvolved extremity, and pulley exercises.

As with other flexibility exercises, the stretch force should be such that the patient feels a stretch sensation without pain. Pain indicates that the stretch force is too aggressive and should be reduced. Stretches can be either short term or prolonged. Recent injuries with newly formed scar tissue can be effectively treated with short-term stretches. Injuries that occurred several months before treatment and that contain scar tissue that is more mature will benefit from prolonged stretches.

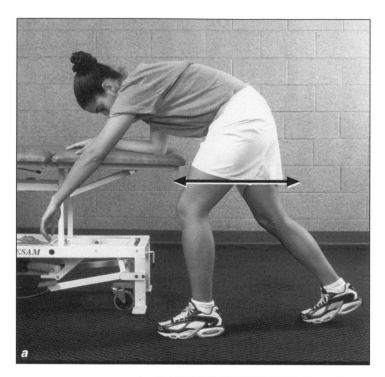

▌Figure 17.37
Codman's exercises:
(a) flexion-extension,
(b) horizontal flexion-extension. Passive
motion of the shoulder
occurs because of
weight transfer back
and forth between the
left leg and the right
leg while the arm
remains relaxed.

PENDULUM EXERCISES

These exercises can be performed after other exercises in the early rehabilitation phase to distract the glenohumeral joint, relax the muscles around the shoulder, and provide pain modulation. They are also called Codman's exercises. The patient lies prone or stands with the arm hanging freely over the edge of the table. A cuff can be applied to the wrist. If a weight is used, it is important for muscle relaxation that the patient not hold on to the weight with the hand; it should be passively secured to the wrist.

Codman's exercises are performed with the patient bent over at the waist and supported by the uninvolved arm on a table. Arm movement is initiated from the hips, not the arm. The arm should remain relaxed throughout the motions. Passive flexion-extension motion of the shoulder occurs with the patient's legs in a forward-backward straddle position. Body weight is transferred from the front to the back leg to provide momentum for arm movement (figure 17.37a). Horizontal flexion-extension movement occurs with the patient standing in a side-to-side straddle position, and body weight is transferred from the left leg to the right leg to produce sideward arm motion (figure 17.37b). Circular motion of the shoulder is produced by the hips as the patient moves in a circular direction with the body while the arm hangs passively, swinging with momentum produced from the hips. Circular motion can occur in a clockwise or counterclockwise direction.

ACTIVE STRETCHES

Selection of these stretches is based on areas of the capsule that are tight. These exercises are often used in conjunction with joint mobilization.

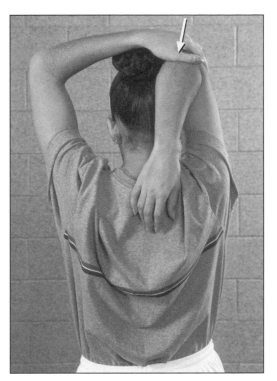

■ Figure 17.38
Flexibility exercise: inferior capsule stretch.

Inferior Capsule Stretch

This exercise increases inferior capsular mobility to improve shoulder elevation. The patient positions the arm overhead with the elbow flexed and the forearm behind the head. The uninvolved hand, placed on the elbow, pulls the elbow behind the head (figure 17.38). A common error with this exercise is lateral trunk lean away from the shoulder being stretched. If this occurs, the patient should perform the exercise in front of a mirror to monitor and correct trunk position.

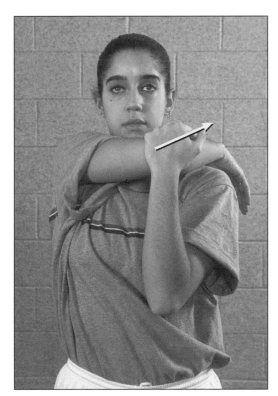

■ Figure 17.39
Flexibility exercise: posterior capsule stretch.

Posterior Capsule Stretch

This stretch, used to gain internal rotation and horizontal flexion, is for the posterior rotator cuff. The patient positions the involved arm at shoulder level and grasps the elbow with the opposite hand. The patient pulls the arm across the body, attempting to place the involved hand behind the opposite shoulder and the elbow close to the chin (figure 17.39). A common error is to rotate the trunk rather than pull the arm across the body. The patient may also tend to lower the elbow below shoulder level. The sport rehabilitation specialist uses verbal cueing to correct for proper execution. If necessary, the patient can also stand in front of a mirror to receive visual feedback.

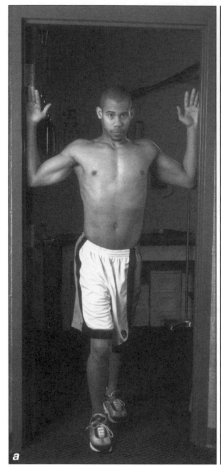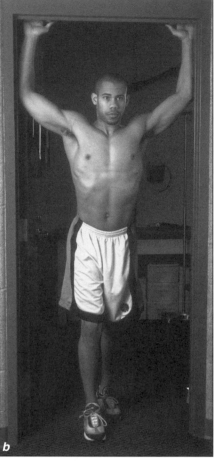

■ **Figure 17.40**   Flexibility exercise: anterior capsule stretch: *(a)* upper, *(b)* lower.

Anterior Capsule Stretch

This stretch is used to gain horizontal extension and external rotation. It stretches the anterior capsule and pectoralis major. The patient stands in a doorway with the elbows and forearms on the door jamb. To stretch upper pectoralis fibers, the elbows are positioned below the shoulders (figure 17.40a). To stretch middle fibers, the elbows are positioned at shoulder level. To stretch lower fibers, the elbows are positioned above the shoulders (figure 17.40b). With one foot placed in front of the other, the patient pushes from the back foot to lean through the doorway and feel a stretch in the anterior chest area. Common substitutions include arching the back, moving the elbows off the door jamb, and keeping the involved shoulder behind the uninvolved shoulder so that the trunk is at an angle to the doorway. Verbal cueing for proper technique should be used to correct these substitutions.

Superior Capsule Stretch

This exercise increases superior capsule mobility. The patient places a rolled towel under the arm and positions the elbow next to his or her side. With the uninvolved hand, the patient pulls the elbow toward the side (figure 17.41). A common error is to use a roll that is not large enough to provide adequate stretch. Applying the stretch force too high on the arm delivers less stretch force.

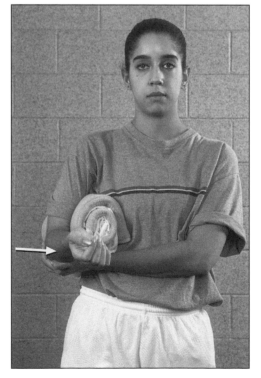

■ **Figure 17.41**
Flexibility exercise:
superior capsule
stretch.

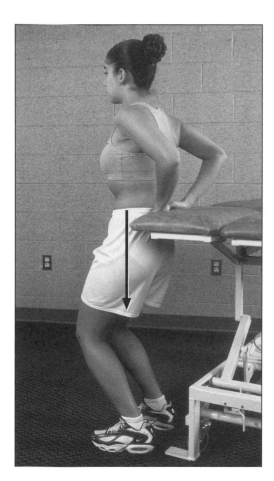

■ Figure 17.42
Flexibility exercise:
internal rotation
stretch.

Internal Rotation Stretch

This exercise increases internal rotation and stretches the posterior capsule. The patient stands with his or her hands behind the back and on a countertop. The feet are shoulder-width apart. The patient squats down while maintaining a grasp on the countertop (figure 17.42). The hands may start in a shoulder-width grip, but the patient should move the hands closer together as possible until one hand is on top of the other. The most common substitutions are bending over at the waist, looking down at the floor, and flexing the wrist. The wrist should remain straight, and the patient should maintain an erect position. Giving the patient a verbal cue to keep the head up or to look at the ceiling will help correct the posture.

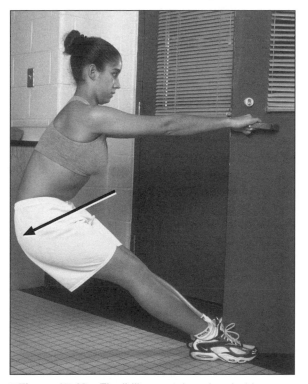

■ Figure 17.43   Flexibility exercise: rhomboid stretch.

Rhomboid Stretch

This exercise stretches the rhomboids and posterior capsule. The patient stands facing the edge of a door, with the feet placed on either side of the door and the hands on the doorknobs. With the legs straight, the patient leans the hips backward. The arms should remain straight and relaxed as the body moves backward (figure 17.43). A common error is not allowing the body weight to stretch the shoulders. If this error occurs, instruct the patient to relax the arms and let the hips move backward and downward.

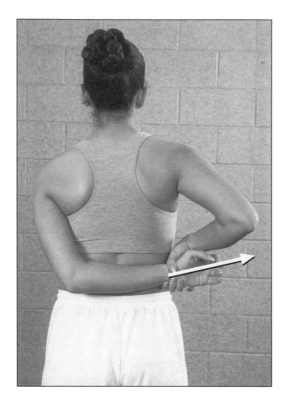

Supraspinatus Stretch

This stretch increases supraspinatus flexibility and superior capsular mobility. The patient positions the involved arm behind the body with the elbow flexed and grasps a chair back with the hand. The patient then leans away from the hand. An alternative technique is to grasp the hand behind the back with the opposite hand and pull the involved arm toward the uninvolved side (figure 17.44). A common substitution is twisting the body. Bending the trunk rather than leaning is also a substitution.

ASSISTIVE STRETCHES

These stretches require the assistance of the sport rehabilitation specialist. They can be combined with contract-relax-stretch techniques to give the stretch a neuromuscular facilitation component. Improper technique and substitutions should be corrected so that the intended structures are appropriately stretched.

Supraspinatus Stretch

This exercise increases supraspinatus motion and superior capsular mobility. The patient's arm is placed behind the low back with the elbow flexed similarly to as shown in figure 17.44. The sport rehabilitation specialist pulls the arm across the body and maintains internal rotation of the shoulder. The trunk should not be permitted to laterally flex toward the shoulder that is being stretched. To prevent this movement, you can place a hand on the opposite shoulder to stabilize the trunk.

Infraspinatus Stretch

This stretch increases infraspinatus flexibility and posterior capsular mobility. The patient's arm is positioned in internal rotation and in front of the body. The sport rehabilitation specialist grasps the elbow and pulls the arm across the body while maintaining internal rotation (figure 17.45). To prevent trunk rotation and lean, place a stabilizing hand on the patient's opposite shoulder.

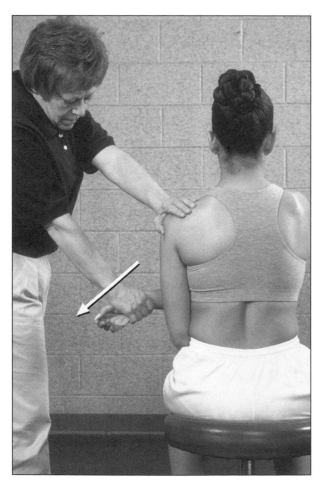

▮ Figure 17.45   Assistive infraspinatus stretch.

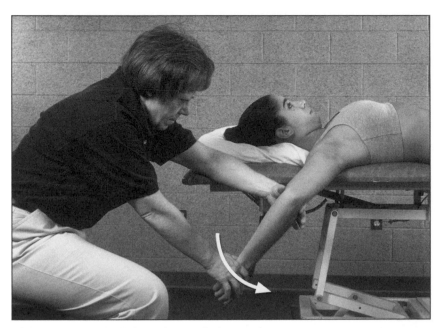

■ **Figure 17.46**   Assistive subscapularis stretch.

Subscapularis Stretch

This stretch increases subscapularis flexibility and improves inferior capsular mobility. The patient lies supine, and the sport rehabilitation specialist moves the arm into abduction and external rotation (figure 17.46). A stretch force is applied into external rotation. The back and chest should remain flat on the table. Care must be taken to avoid excessive elbow stress.

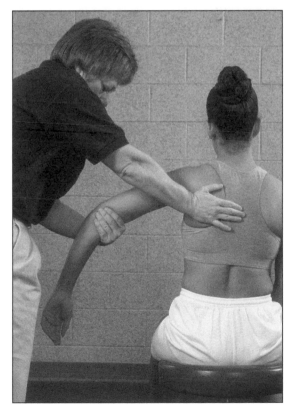

■ **Figure 17.47**
Assistive teres minor stretch.

Teres Minor Stretch

This stretch increases teres minor flexibility and stretches the inferior capsule. The patient is sitting with the arm elevated overhead and next to the ear. The arm is internally rotated (figure 17.47). The scapula should be stabilized to isolate teres minor movement.

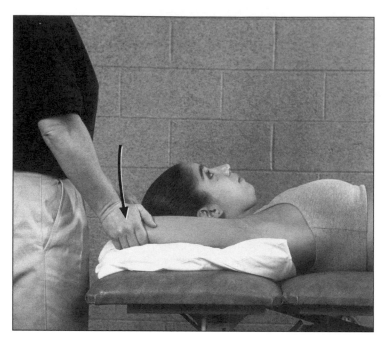

Figure 17.48 Assistive teres major stretch.

Teres Major Stretch

The teres major is stretched with the patient supine and the arm overhead in flexion and external rotation. The stretch force is applied into flexion and external rotation (figure 17.48). The thorax should not rise up from the table.

Latissimus Dorsi Stretch

This stretch increases latissimus dorsi flexibility. The patient lies prone with the arm overhead. The sport rehabilitation specialist grasps the forearm and then distracts and externally rotates the shoulder as the arm is lifted toward the ceiling (figure 17.49). The trunk should not rotate, and the elbow should remain extended.

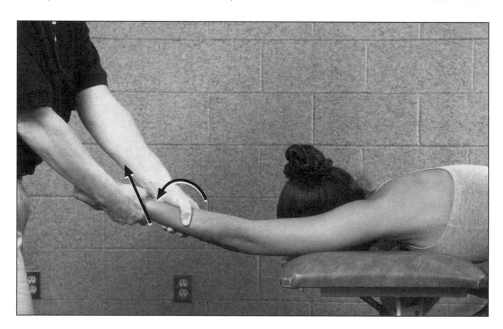

Figure 17.49
Assistive latissimus dorsi stretch.

WAND EXERCISES

These exercises, performed with a wand, use the uninvolved contralateral arm to provide the stretch force. Commercial wands and T-bars can be used; but a 2.5-cm (1-in.) diameter dowel, broom handle, cane, and other such items are readily available, inexpensive, and easy to use.

The patient uses the uninvolved arm to guide the wand in the desired direction to provide the stretch force needed to increase motion. He or she holds the end position 5 to 10 s and repeats each motion several times. The advantage of these exercises is that the patient can perform them independently several times throughout the day.

Wand Flexion

This wand exercise increases flexion motion. The patient can perform this exercise in sitting, standing, or supine; but because strength may be a factor in the sitting and standing positions, supine is the recommended position. The patient grasps the wand in each hand, with the hands shoulder-width apart. He or she moves the arms overhead, keeping the elbows straight throughout the exercise (figure 17.50). Substitutions include arching the back, bending the elbows, and hyperextending the wrists.

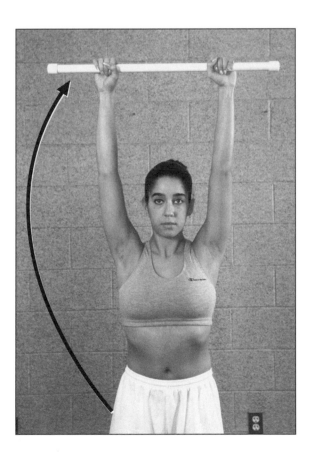

❚ **Figure 17.50**
Wand flexion.

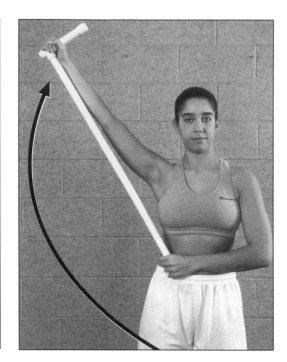

Figure 17.51 Wand abduction.

Wand Abduction

This exercise increases shoulder abduction. The patient can stand or lie supine. He or she grasps the end of the wand with the involved hand and places the uninvolved hand toward the other end of the wand. The uninvolved arm pushes the involved arm upward into abduction (figure 17.51). Substitutions include leaning sideways, moving the shoulder into the flexion plane, and bending the elbow.

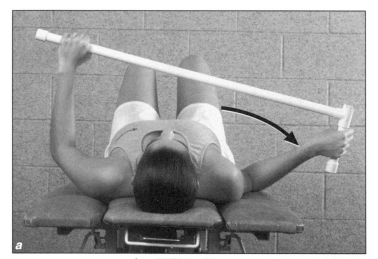

Wand External Rotation

This exercise increases external rotation. The patient lies supine with the involved hand on one end of the wand and the uninvolved hand toward the other end. The involved elbow is kept next to the side in 90° of flexion throughout the exercise. With the wand, the patient pushes the involved hand away from the body to externally rotate the shoulder (figure 17.52a). Common substitutions here include extending the elbow as the wand is pushed laterally, and abducting the shoulder. A more advanced external rotation exercise can be performed with the hands shoulder-width apart on the wand. The patient raises the wand overhead and then bends the elbows to attempt to place the wand behind the neck (figure 17.52b). Neck flexion, trunk flexion or rotation, elbow extension, and wrist hyperextension are common errors with this exercise.

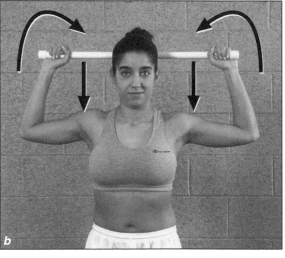

Figure 17.52 Wand external rotation: (a) supine, (b) advanced.

Internal Rotation

This exercise increases shoulder internal rotation. The patient stands with the wand behind the waist, hands placed shoulder-width apart. The bar is raised along the back as high as possible (figure 17.53a). Common substitutions include excessive wrist flexion and trunk lean. An alternative stretch is with the wand placed vertically behind the back. The involved hand is at the waist, and the uninvolved hand is at the top of the wand. The wand is pulled upward with the top hand (figure 17.53b). Trunk flexion is a common substitution with this alternative stretch.

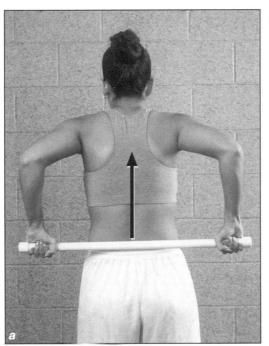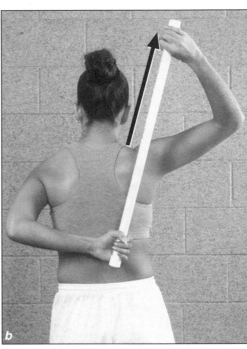

▌Figure 17.53 Wand Internal rotation: *(a)* initial position, *(b)* alternative position.

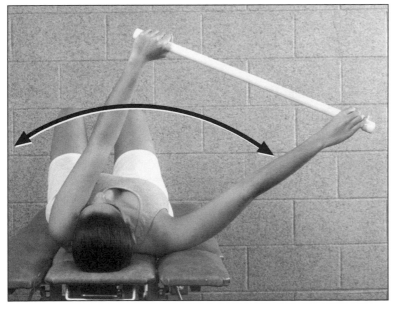

Horizontal Flexion-Extension

This exercise increases horizontal movements. The patient lies supine with the hands overhead, shoulder-width apart on the wand, and the elbows straight. The uninvolved arm pushes the involved arm away from the body as far as possible, then pulls the arm across the body as far as possible (figure 17.54). Throughout the exercise the hands remain at shoulder level and the elbows remain straight. Common errors include elbow flexion, trunk rotation, moving the arms into extension, and shoulder rotation.

▌Figure 17.54 Wand horizontal flexion-extension.

PULLEY EXERCISES

These exercises can be performed with a pulley, rope, or stretch strap. They are easy to incorporate into a home exercise program that the patient can perform independently. The patient must be careful to avoid driving the humeral head into the glenoid socket, especially when using the pulleys for frozen-shoulder exercises. The patient should be instructed to maintain the scapula in a depressed position during the motion.

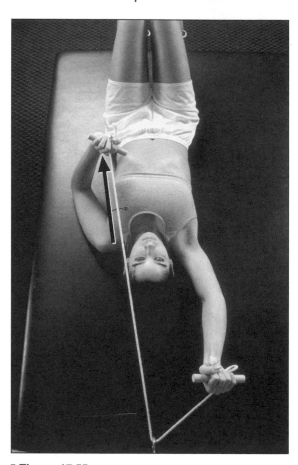

■ **Figure 17.55**
Pulley: shoulder flexion.

Shoulder Flexion

For this exercise, an overhead rope and pulley or a stretch strap and hook are attached in a doorway or on a wall. The patient sits with his or her back to the door or wall. The hands are positioned with the thumbs facing upward. The uninvolved arm pulls the rope or strap down to elevate the involved arm into flexion as high as possible. The involved arm is lowered and the motion is repeated several times. One alternative stretch uses a stretch strap placed over the top of a door. The patient reaches up as high as possible on the strap, then bends the knees to lower the body and apply the stretch force to the shoulder. Another alternative position is with the patient supine and the pulley attached to the wall or doorjamb (figure 17.55).

Shoulder Abduction

This exercise is similar to the shoulder flexion exercise except that the arm is raised in abduction from the side of the body.

STRENGTHENING EXERCISES

Exercises for strengthening the shoulder begin with isometric activities and straight-plane isotonic exercises, then progress to multiplane and diagonal exercises.

These exercises incorporate a broad spectrum of degrees of difficulty and of stresses applied to the shoulder. They are presented here from easiest to more advanced exercises, beginning with early-phase isometric exercises and progressing to later-phase plyometric exercises. As the exercises become more difficult, they advance from straight-plane to diagonal exercises. We will consider the diagonal exercises, which combine movement planes to stress muscles for all the shoulder joints, in terms of their function and goals within a therapeutic exercise program. The sport rehabilitation specialist should note and correct substitution patterns to achieve optimal strengthening of intended muscles and facilitate appropriate muscle firing patterns.

ISOMETRICS

Isometrics begin early in a rehabilitation program when the patient is limited in shoulder mobility and strength. They are used to minimize atrophy during times when use of the shoulder is limited. They are performed in a pain-free position and may be performed at multiple angles of a motion, if motion is permitted. If motion is limited, the exercises are performed in non-aggravating, acceptable positions. Each isometric contraction is gradually increased to a maximum, held at a maximum, and then decreased gradually until the muscle is relaxed. The patient must be instructed to avoid sudden maximal contractions to avoid injury or undue strain of the muscle. The patient should maximally contract only if no pain is produced. If pain occurs, effort should be limited to a submaximal contraction until the greater force is non-irritating. Each isometric is held for 5 to 10 s and repeated 10 times. These exercises are performed frequently throughout the day.

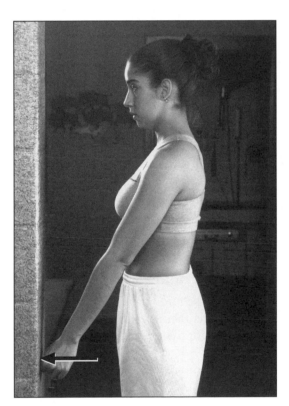

■ **Figure 17.56**
Isometric flexion.

Shoulder Flexion

This exercise strengthens the shoulder flexors. The patient stands facing a doorway, with the involved arm slightly forward and the hand on the door frame. The patient attempts to move the arm forward while pushing the hand against the door frame (figure 17.56).

Shoulder Abduction

This exercise strengthens the shoulder abductors. The patient stands with the involved side facing a wall or doorway. The arm is positioned in slight abduction with the dorsum of the hand against the wall. The patient keeps the elbow extended and pushes the arm against the wall, attempting to move the arm into abduction.

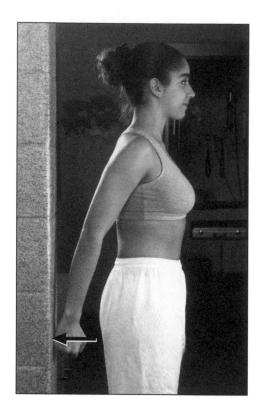

Shoulder Extension

This exercise strengthens the shoulder extensors. The patient stands with back to the wall and positions the arm slightly behind the body, with the hand against the wall. The patient pushes the hand backward to the wall, keeping the elbow extended (figure 17.57).

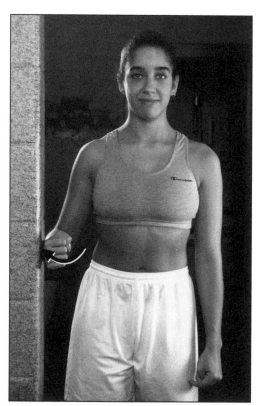

▌ Figure 17.58   Isometric shoulder external rotation.

Shoulder Internal Rotation

This exercise strengthens the internal rotators. The patient stands facing a doorway with the elbow flexed to 90° and the anterior distal forearm placed against the surface of the door frame. With the elbow at his or her side, the patient attempts to roll the forearm inward toward the abdomen.

Shoulder External Rotation

This exercise strengthens the shoulder external rotators. The patient stands facing a doorway with the elbow flexed to 90° and the posterior distal surface of the forearm against the door frame. The elbow is kept in to the side as the patient attempts to roll the forearm outward (figure 17.58).

ISOLATED-PLANE ISOTONIC EXERCISES

As mentioned previously, initial strengthening exercises should include primarily straight-plane activities. Once strength is sufficient to control the joint during motion, multiplane and diagonal exercises can begin. Here we look first at straight-plane exercises and then move to multiplane exercises. Keep in mind that although this section includes many of the commonly used exercises, the listing here is far from exhaustive.

Although shoulder motion includes muscle function of scapulothoracic and glenohumeral muscles, patients can and should perform isolated exercises of the muscles for each joint until the muscles have sufficient strength to control the joints during functional motions. To make it easier to identify specific exercise functions, the straight-plane exercises for the scapulothoracic and glenohumeral muscle groups are presented separately. Most are considered relative to the specific motion and muscles they address and are presented from easiest to more difficult.

Scapulothoracic Exercises

If the patient has pain with the shoulder in elevated positions, it is best to provide manual resistance with the shoulder in the lower planes of motion. An advantage of manual resistance is that it can be offered in any position. As the patient's strength increases, resistance can be offered in planes of motion that are more elevated.

Manual Resistance to Scapula

Patients can do this exercise early in the rehabilitation program for glenohumeral injuries, because it does not stress the glenohumeral joint and assists in minimizing atrophy of scapular rotators. The patient is side-lying with his or her hand on the table to isolate the scapular muscles (figure 17.59a). If glenohumeral joint adduction is uncomfortable, the hand need not be placed on the table, and the sport rehabilitation specialist can support the arm between his or her side and arm (figure 17.59b). The sport rehabilitation specialist faces the patient and places his or her hands on the medial scapular border to resist the combined movements of retraction and depression of the scapula; he or she places the other hand on the anterior shoulder to resist protraction and elevation of the scapula in the opposite direction. Manual resistance can also be offered to isolated scapular movements if there is weakness in specific muscles.

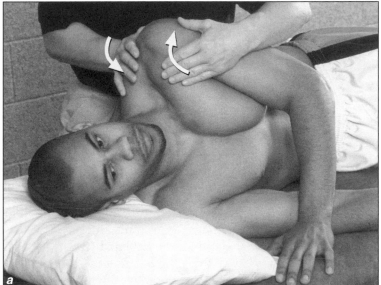
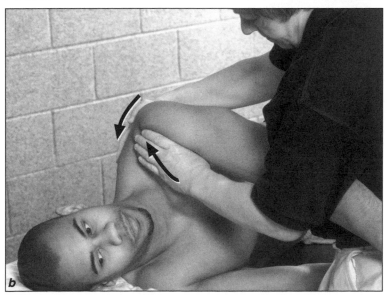

■ **Figure 17.59** Manual resistance to scapula: (a) with hand on table, (b) with arm supported in non-weight-bearing position.

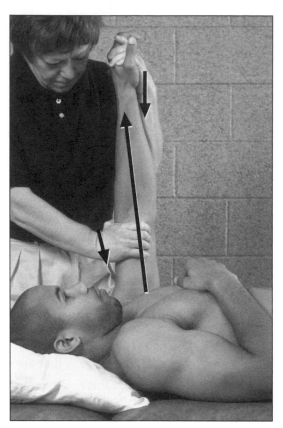

Figure 17.60
Serratus anterior.

Scapular Protraction

The serratus anterior is the primary muscle providing this motion. The patient lies supine with the arm flexed to about 110° to 120° and the elbow extended. The hand is pushed toward the ceiling, with the movement coming from the scapula as it moves forward around the ribs. This motion can be resisted manually, with a dumbbell in the hand, or on a bench-press machine with the bar lifted into position by the sport rehabilitation specialist (figure 17.60).

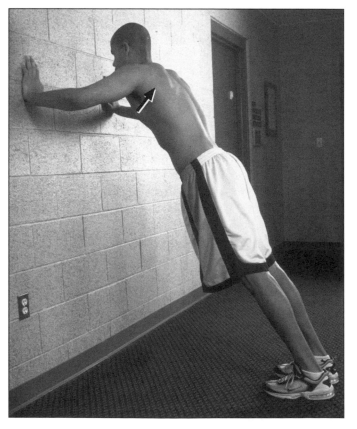

The serratus anterior can also be strengthened using a push-up plus. The patient performs a push-up with the emphasis on the additional push at the end to facilitate the serratus anterior; once the elbows are extended, the patient attempts to push the body away from the hands an additional distance by moving the scapulae forward around the rib cage. The lowest-level resistance for this exercise is with a wall push-up (figure 17.61); progression is to an incline push-up, then to a modified position on hands and knees, then to a regular push-up position, and finally to a decline push-up position with the feet higher than the hands. With the feet higher than the hands, the serratus anterior and the upper trapezius are particularly facilitated (Lear and Gross 1998). Patients with anterior instability or who have had recent shoulder surgery should avoid lowering the body so that the shoulders move in front of the plane of the elbows during push-ups so undue stress on the anterior shoulder is prevented.

Figure 17.61 Push-up plus.

The serratus anterior can also be strengthened using rubber tubing or pulleys. The tubing or pulleys are anchored just below shoulder level, and the patient stands or sits with his or her back to the anchor. With the elbow flexed, the patient pushes the band forward and slightly upward, reaching as far as possible with the elbow extended and the scapula punched forward (figure 17.62). A substitution to avoid in this exercise is using the trunk to rotate the arm forward rather than using the serratus anterior to punch the scapula forward.

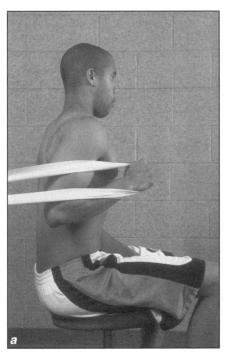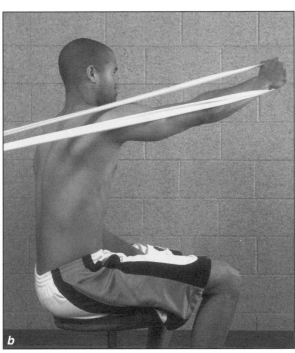

Figure 17.62
Serratus anterior with rubber tubing: *(a)* start position, *(b)* end position.

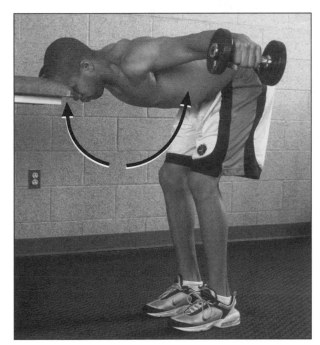

Figure 17.63
Reverse flys.

An alternative exercise using rubber tubing can be performed with the patient supine and the tubing under the shoulder and back area. The patient grasps the ends of the tubing and starts with the elbows extended and the shoulders flexed to 90° so that the hands are toward the ceiling and the tubing is taut. The patient punches the hands toward the ceiling, rolling the scapulae around the ribs.

Scapular Retraction
Scapular retraction is produced by the rhomboids and middle trapezius. An early-phase exercise for strengthening these muscles is a scapular squeeze. The patient keeps his or her elbows at the sides and squeezes the shoulder blades together, holding for 5 to 10 s. This exercise can be performed frequently throughout the day.

Prone flys and rows strengthen these muscles. Prone flys, also called reverse flys, can be performed with the patient prone and the arm hanging over the table. An alternative position is shown in figure 17.63, with the patient flexed at the hips and the head supported on the table so that the back is straight. The patient lifts a weight in horizontal extension as the scapulae are squeezed together. The elbows remain extended but not locked throughout the movement. Although the patient need perform the exercise with only the involved extremity, a greater facilitation of the muscles occurs if both arms perform the exercise simultaneously. A substitution seen in this exercise is shoulder horizontal extension without scapular retraction.

A row exercise can be performed in prone or sitting. In prone, the patient stands bent over at the waist or lies prone with the arm over the edge of the table. The patient lifts the weight toward the ceiling as high as possible; the elbow bends as the weight moves close to the shoulder.

If performing the row in sitting, the patient faces rubber tubing or pulleys that are anchored to a door at or below shoulder level. The patient leans forward from the hip, keeping the back straight, with the scapulae in a protracted position and then moves to an erect position and simultaneously pulls to retract the scapulae, squeezing them together and keeping the elbows at the sides (figure 17.64). A substitution in this exercise is moving the pulley or tubing primarily with the trunk, hips, or shoulder extensors and not retracting the scapulae.

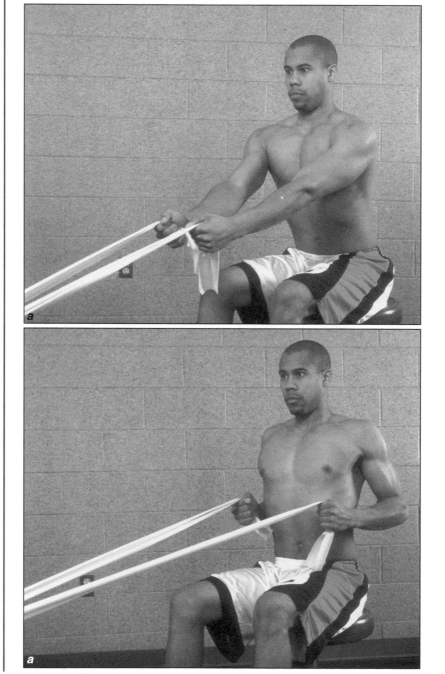

▌Figure 17.64 Row, seated: *(a)* start position, *(b)* end position.

Scapular Depression

This motion is performed by the lower trapezius and pectoralis minor. The patient performs the seated push-up or press-up while seated in a chair with the hands on the chair seat. The patient pushes down to lift the hips off the chair (figure 17.65a). These muscles can also be strengthened with the use of a pulley or rubber tubing. The pulley or tubing is positioned high overhead, and the patient grasps the handle with the elbow straight and the shoulder in flexion (figure 17.65b). Keeping the shoulder and elbow in the same position throughout the exercise, the patient pulls the scapula downward toward the back pants pocket. A latissimus pull-down bar using both hands, the involved arm positioned at the end of the bar and the uninvolved arm positioned closer to the middle of the bar, can also be used for this exercise. Substitutions most common in this exercise are shoulder extension and elbow flexion. You must take care to have the patient maintain the same shoulder and elbow position throughout the exercise.

An alternative for this exercise can be performed with the resistance device anchored to the shoulder; in this position the shoulder is not placed in an elevated position (figure 17.65c). This exercise isolates the depressors and does not put stress on the glenohumeral joint.

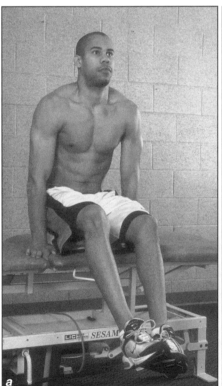
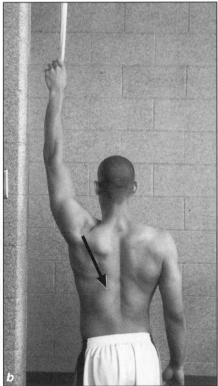
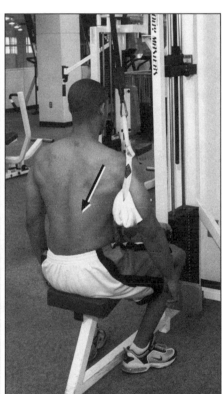

■ **Figure 17.65**   Scapular depressors: *(a)* seated press-up, *(b)* overhead depression, *(c)* alternative scapular depressor exercise position.

Bouhler Exercises

These three exercises strengthen the lower trapezius as it functions in upward rotation of the scapula. The patient stands with the back and heels near a wall. With the abdominals tightened to prevent the back from arching, the patient raises the arms overhead with the elbows straight and close to the ears. In the first exercise, the thumbs face the wall and are pushed to the wall (figure 17.66a). In the second exercise, the arms are in the same position as in the first exercise, but the thumbs face each other as the arms are moved to the wall (figure 17.66b). In the last exercise, the arms are positioned at a 45° angle from the body and are moved to the wall as the shoulder blades are squeezed together (figure 17.66c). In each exercise the patient holds the position for 5 to 10 s and repeats the exercise several times. To perform these exercises at a more advanced level, the patient is prone, either on a table or on a Swiss ball. Weights can be added to the hands for additional resistance (figure 17.66d). Substitutions for this exercise include arching the back, bending the elbows, abducting the arms, and standing away from the wall.

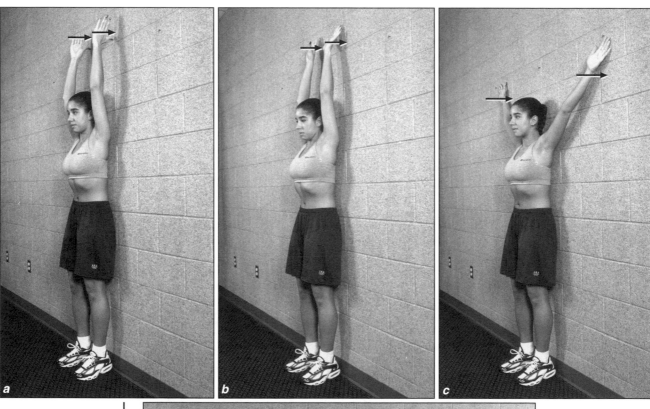

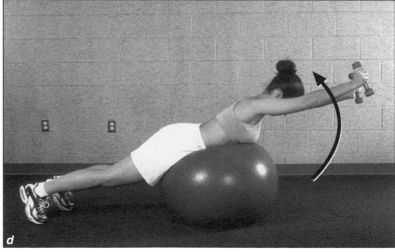

▌Figure 17.66
Bouhler exercises: *(a)* thumbs to the wall, *(b)* thumbs facing each other, *(c)* arms at 45° angle, *(d)* progression in an antigravity position with weights.

Scapular Elevation

This motion is performed by the upper trapezius and levator scapulae. These muscles are normally not weak and often overpower their synergists and their antagonists, resulting in a muscle imbalance. They are often used incorrectly during shoulder elevation as substitution for weak rotator cuff muscles, contributing to faulty mechanics, muscle imbalance, and prolonged injury recovery. In patients who have weakness of these muscles, initial strengthening can include shoulder shrugs and manual resistance to shrugs. A more advanced exercise uses weight during shrugs. Once the patient is able to elevate the shoulder without pain, he or she can perform additional exercises such as an upright row; however, to reduce the risk of rotator cuff impingement, the patient should not elevate the elbows higher than the shoulders. An advanced exercise that can be used in the later stages of strengthening is the upright press with dumbbells or machines, also known as the overhead press or military press. Impingement can be a problem with this exercise, so the sport rehabilitation specialist must use caution in determining whether to include this exercise.

Scapular Rotation

Upward rotation is performed by the serratus anterior and trapezius muscles. Downward rotation is performed by the levator scapulae, rhomboids, and pectoralis minor. Full range-of-motion exercise for scapular rotation also includes glenohumeral motion, so it is important for the sport rehabilitation specialist to be sure that glenohumeral joint stability is adequate before including these full-motion scapular activities in the rehabilitation program.

An upward scapular rotation exercise uses full shoulder elevation in either flexion or abduction. These exercises are performed with the elbow straight and the thumb facing upward to reduce rotator cuff impingement. The arm is elevated until the hand is overhead (figure 17.67).

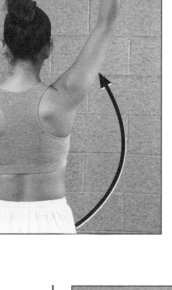

∎ Figure 17.67 Scapular upward rotation.

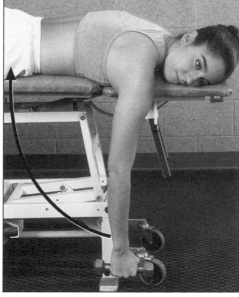

∎ Figure 17.68
Scapular downward
rotation.

Downward scapular rotation occurs during shoulder extension. In a prone position with the arm over the edge of the table, the patient lifts the hand toward the hip, keeping the elbow straight (figure 17.68).

Latissimus pull-downs are an advanced exercise for downward rotation. The hands are shoulder-width apart on the lat bar, and the elbows are kept straight throughout the exercise. Keeping the scapulae set, the patient brings the arms down to the front of the thighs.

In performing each of these exercises, the patient must maintain scapular control and correct glenohumeral positioning. The most frequent substitution in these exercises is shrugging the scapula and initiating the movement with the upper trapezius rather than allowing all scapular rotators to work correctly.

Glenohumeral Exercises

Glenohumeral exercises performed in the lower levels of shoulder elevation empha-size the glenohumeral muscles. Once the shoulder is elevated, scapular muscles are also stressed with the exercise to maintain the shoulder position. Early strengthening of the shoulder may nec-essarily start in the lower levels of elevation until suffi-cient scapular muscle strength is present for stabilizing the shoulder in its correct position. Shoulder exercises should be divided into three levels: below 60°, 60° to 100°, and above 100°. Because scapular stabilization is a prerequisite to good shoulder motion, scapular muscle strength in the low and middle ranges of shoulder mo-tion should be achieved before advancing to middle and higher ranges of motion. As shoulder elevation increases, scapular muscles must work harder to provide both scapular stabilization and scapular motion.

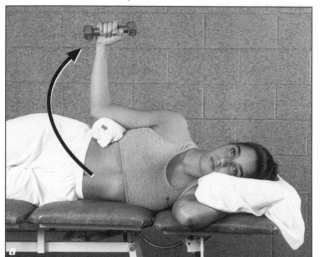

External Rotation

This motion is performed by the infraspinatus, teres minor, and posterior deltoid. The exercises should be performed in the scapular plane. In side-lying on the uninvolved side with a towel roll placed under the arm, the patient positions the elbow at 90° and lifts the weight upward toward the ceiling (figure 17.69a). Sub-stitutions to watch and correct for include shoulder ex-tension, shoulder abduction, elbow extension, wrist extension, and rolling the trunk backward. Stabiliza-tion is important if the patient is to achieve the desired gains from the exercise. This exercise can also be per-formed in prone (figure 17.69b), or in standing with rubber tubing or pulleys with the elbow at the side (fig-ure 17.69c). Once scapular stability is achieved, this ex-ercise can be performed with the arm abducted to 90°.

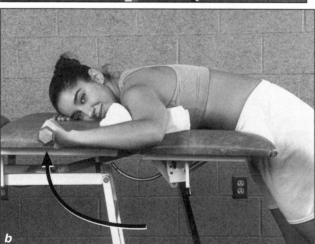

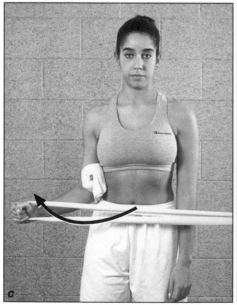

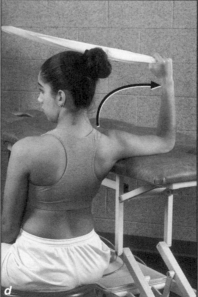

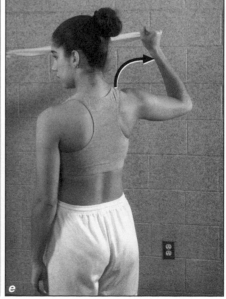

▌Figure 17.69   External rotation: *(a)* side-lying, *(b)* prone, *(c)* standing, *(d)* in 90° of abduction with support, *(e)* without support.

Initially, it may be necessary to support the elbow (figure 17.69d); but as strength improves, elbow support becomes unnecessary (figure 17.69e). In the elevated position, the elbow should remain elevated, and the shoulder should be maintained at 90° abduction without horizontal adduction or abduction.

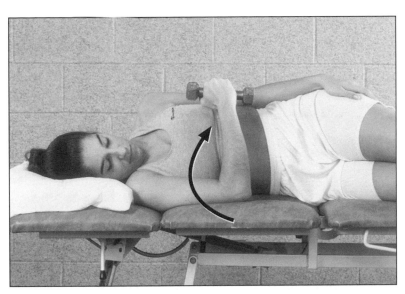

■ Figure 17.70   Internal rotation.

Internal Rotation

The subscapularis is the primary muscle responsible for internal rotation. It receives assistance from other muscles including the teres major, latissimus dorsi, anterior deltoid, and pectoralis major.

The patient can be side-lying on the involved side or supine. The elbow is flexed to 90°. If the patient is supine, the arm is abducted slightly. If the patient is side-lying, the elbow is next to the side. The elbow position is maintained as the hand is moved toward the abdomen (figure 17.70).

This exercise can also be performed in standing using rubber tubing or pulleys and following the progression discussed for external rotation. A towel roll is placed between the trunk and arm, with the forearm kept parallel to the floor similar to the position shown in figure 17.69c. From a starting position away from the body, the patient moves the forearm toward the abdomen. Common substitution patterns are rotation of the trunk, horizontal flexion of the shoulder, forward motion of the elbow, and elbow motion.

Once the scapular muscles are able to stabilize the scapula, the motion is performed with the arm abducted to 90°. Initially, the elbow can be supported, but progression should be toward the more aggressive position for the exercise without elbow support.

Abduction

This motion is produced by force-couple activity of the deltoid with the supraspinatus. The other rotator cuff muscles also play an important role during shoulder abduction and flexion as they co-contract during abduction to depress the humeral head into the glenoid. Thus, the rotator cuff and deltoid collectively stabilize the glenohumeral joint during elevation activities. It is important that the scapular stabilizers also work to position the scapula during abduction. In the early strengthening stages it may be necessary to remind the patient to fix the scapula or set the scapula before moving the humerus so that proper sequencing of shoulder motion occurs.

Abduction can be performed in the coronal plane, but the recommendation is to perform this exercise in the scapular plane, approximately 30° forward of the frontal plane. This position maximally facilitates the rotator cuff muscles. This position of the humerus in the plane of the scapula is called **scaption**.

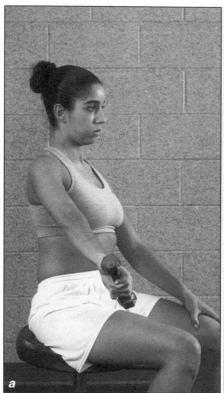 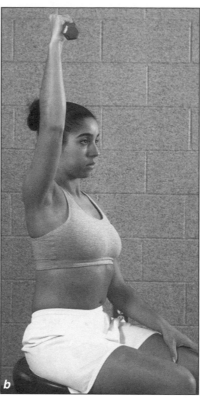

▌ Figure 17.71
Shoulder abduction in scapular plane (scaption): *(a)* thumbs down with internal rotation, *(b)* thumbs up with external rotation.

Abduction can be performed in side-lying with the elbow extended and the arm resting along the length of the trunk and thigh. The scapula is set and the arm is lifted into scaption. Two alternative positions are both performed in sitting. The patient sets the scapula and raises the arm with the elbow straight in a scapular plane. In one exercise, the thumb is pointed toward the floor so that the arm is in internal rotation (figure 17.71a). Although this position facilitates the greatest response from the supraspinatus, it may also aggravate the supraspinatus tendon by impinging it. If this occurs, the patient should limit elevation to within a pain-free range of motion. The second position is performed with the thumb pointed toward the ceiling (figure 17.71b). This position facilitates the scapular stabilizers. You should correct substitutions for these exercises, which include trunk lateral flexion, shoulder shrugging, moving the arm more into flexion and out of the scapular plane, and flexing the elbow.

Horizontal Abduction (Extension)

Horizontal abduction or extension, performed in the prone position with the arm in external rotation, demands output from the teres minor and infraspinatus muscles. This exercise also strengthens the posterior deltoid and scapular stabilizers. The patient lies prone with the arm over the edge of the table. The arm is elevated into horizontal extension (abduction) with the arm in external rotation. Common substitutions are rolling the trunk rather than lifting the arm, moving out of the plane of motion and placing the hand closer to the hip, and bending the elbow.

Key Shoulder Exercises

For several years many sport rehabilitation specialists advocated specific exercises to strengthen the shoulder, but few offered concrete evidence that their exercises were beneficial. Although the results are arguably inconclusive, the findings presented by Bradley and Tibone (1991) shed some light on what many consider significant exercises that should be part of a general shoulder rehabilitation program (table 17.1). The authors defined a significant exercise as one that produced substantial effort in more than one muscle investigated. In their research, the four scapular rotator exercises that met this criterion were scaption with thumbs up, rowing, push-up plus, and the seated press-up. The glenohumeral exercises that met this criterion were scaption with internal rotation, horizontal abduction with external rotation, and the seated press-up. Other exercises beneficial to at least one muscle included internal rotation, external rotation, coronal plane abduction, flys (horizontal adduction), a regular push-up without the plus, a push-up with the hands apart, bench press, military press, and shoulder extension in prone.

Table 17.1 Shoulder Rehabilitation Exercises	
Exercises	**Muscles Significantly Activated**
Scaption with thumbs up	Scapular stabilizers
Rowing	Rhomboids, trapezius
Push-up plus	Serratus anterior, pectoralis minor
Seated press-up	Scapular rotators, pectoralis major, lattisimus dorsi
Scaption with thumbs down	Subscapularis, anterior deltoid, posterior deltoid, supraspinatus
Horizontal abduction in external rotation	Infraspinatus, teres minor, posterior deltoid

Based on Bradley and Tibone 1991.

STABILIZATION EXERCISES

Several kinds of stabilization exercises help to restore the scapular stability crucial to shoulder motion. Advanced open chain exercises for shoulder stability include isokinetic exercises and open chain elastic-band exercises.

The importance of stability during shoulder motion cannot be overstated. Trunk stabilization must provide a firm base for the scapula to operate from. Scapular stabilization must provide a firm foundation for shoulder movement. Rotator cuff stabilization allows the humerus smooth, synchronous glenohumeral motion for functional upper-extremity activity.

Trunk stabilization exercises are discussed in chapter 16. A few will be mentioned later in this chapter, but only as they relate to shoulder exercises. Refer to chapter 16 for specific trunk stabilization exercises.

Shoulder stabilization exercises are important in that they aid strength development and also facilitate neuromuscular re-education of the shoulder. They stimulate the afferent receptors to provide appropriate feedback into the central nervous system, to re-educate and reactivate the proprioceptive pathways that will eventually lead to proper functional performance.

Although some of these exercises are open kinetic chain activities, many are closed kinetic chain activities. One can argue that because most people involved in physical activity do not perform closed kinetic chain activities, use of closed kinetic chain exercises for the upper extremities is not germane in a rehabilitation program. Closed kinetic chain exercises are useful for the upper extremity for a couple of reasons. In a close-packed position, the shoulder has more stability through increased joint congruity; less stress is applied to the ligaments, and joint proprioceptors are stimulated. Closed kinetic chain exercise also facilitates co-contraction of muscles around the shoulder. This co-contraction during closed kinetic chain exercises permits stabilization activities to be initiated with less shear force applied to the static structures and also facilitates dynamic stabilization of the joints (Lephart and Henry 1996).

It is not necessary that every exercise mimic functional motions. In fact, in the early and middle stages of rehabilitation, it is important to improve muscle strength before functional movements can be safely executed. Neither straight-plane exercises nor pure closed kinetic chain exercises are functional; they do not mimic the shoulder's functional movements. They are crucial in a therapeutic exercise program, though, in that they facilitate, develop, and improve specific muscle activity that permits functional shoulder movement.

SCAPULAR STABILIZATION

Because scapular stability is vital to functional shoulder motions, scapular stabilization exercises should begin early in the rehabilitation program. A variety of scapular stabilization exercises are outlined here. The progression begins with isometric stabilization exercises and advances to stabilization during arm movement, first in simple planes and then in diagonal planes. The progression also begins with movements in the lower shoulder positions (30°–60° elevation) where the scapula has relatively little motion and advances to middle-range positions of shoulder elevation (60°–100°) where the scapular muscles must work to stabilize and move the scapula simultaneously. In the final phases of stabilization, movements include both high (over 100° elevation) and low joint positions, use increased resistance, and are performed with greater speeds. These activities then become more functionally based.

Swiss Ball Stabilization

Various exercises using Swiss balls can facilitate scapular stabilization. In a basic exercise that can begin early in the rehabilitation program, the ball is placed on a table or on the floor, and the patient bears weight through the shoulder as he or she moves the ball from side to side, forward and back, and in circles. The patient can also lie prone on the Swiss ball with the feet off the floor and the body anchored with the hands on the floor, shoulder-width apart. The patient then moves the body forward and back and from side to side on the ball while maintaining weight bearing through the arms (figure 17.72a).

A more advanced weight-bearing exercise with the Swiss ball has the patient's lower body on a table and the hands placed on the ball while the upper body is over the edge of the table. The patient moves the ball out and away from the body as far as possible, then moves the ball closer (figure 17.72b).

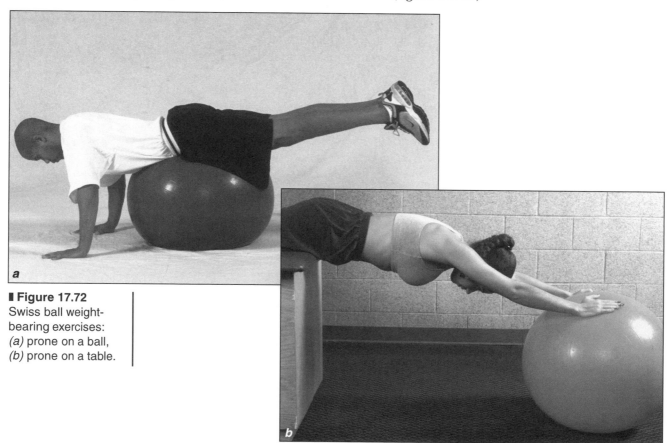

▌ Figure 17.72
Swiss ball weight-bearing exercises:
(a) prone on a ball,
(b) prone on a table.

Distal Movement Stabilization

These activities involve movement of the distal extremity, requiring movement control and strength as well as stabilization of the shoulder. You must be careful to have the patient maintain correct scapular position throughout each of these exercises. Verbal cueing may be necessary as a reminder to maintain proper scapular positioning. In one activity the patient lies prone on a roller stool with feet off the floor and hands on the floor. The patient then moves across the floor using only the arms (figure 17.73a). Another distal movement activity is performed with a weighted ball in the hand. The patient stands with the arm outstretched at from 60° to 110° elevation in the scapular plane. In this position the patient spells out the alphabet with the ball (figure 17.73b). Heavier balls provide additional resistance.

The Body Blade (Hymanson, Inc., Los Angeles, CA), B.O.I.N.G. (exclusively distributed by OPTP, Minneapolis, MN), and other commercially available rhythmic-wand equipment are useful in rhythmic stabilization exercises. They can be used in different positions, beginning in the scapular plane at 30° elevation (figure 17.73c) and advancing to overhead positions.

Upper-body ergometers are another means of offering distal movement and proximal stabilization. These machines also provide cardiovascular exercise.

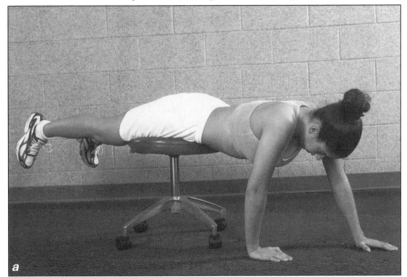

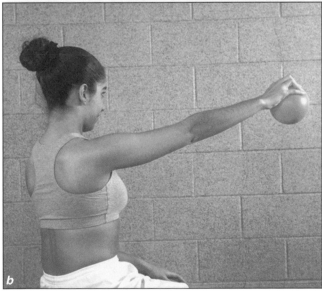

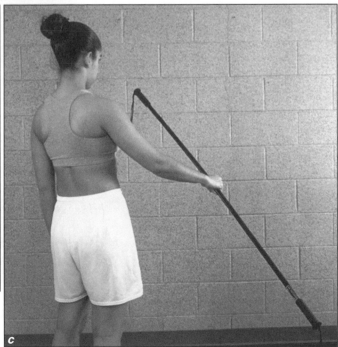

■ **Figure 17.73** Distal movement stabilization exercises: *(a)* walk while prone on roller stool, *(b)* alphabet with distal weight, *(c)* rhythmic wand.

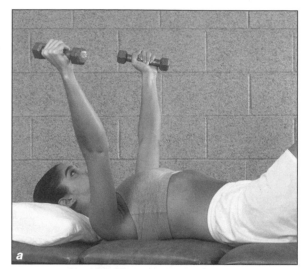

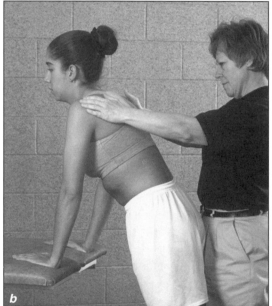

Rhythmic Stabilization

These exercises assist in re-educating the proprioceptors and improve kinesthetic awareness. In the first exercise, the patient lies supine and places the arm in a scapular plane at approximately 100° elevation (figure 17.74a). The patient can hold a weight in this position, maintaining the angle with eyes closed, or the sport rehabilitation specialist can offer manual resistance in different directions while the patient provides an isometric resistance to the movements. You can repeat the exercise in different positions, each time requiring the patient to position and maintain the arm at the desired angle with the eyes closed.

Another rhythmic stabilization exercise can be performed with the patient in standing and bearing weight on the arms on a tabletop. The sport rehabilitation specialist offers resistance to the patient as the patient shifts weight from one arm to the other (figure 17.74b).

Additional weight-bearing exercises are performed with the patient in a quadruped position. The shoulders should be directly over the hands, and the hips should be forward of the knees so that the weight is primarily borne on the upper extremities. If the patient is unable to hold this position, the hips may be positioned directly over the knees to equalize weight distribution between the upper and lower extremities. The simplest exercise is to have the patient shift weight from the left to the right arm. You can offer manual resistance as the patient attempts to stabilize in the quadruped position (figure 17.74c). Once the patient can do this without difficulty, he or she balances in a tripod position with the uninvolved arm off the table (figure 17.74d). From this exercise the patient can advance to a biped position and have the involved arm and the opposite leg bear the weight (figure 17.74e). Once again, the patient's hips should be ahead

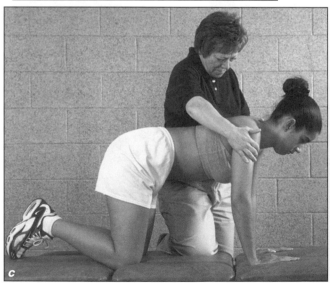

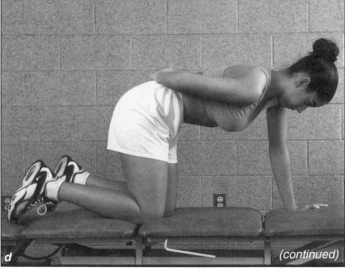

(continued)

■ **Figure 17.74** Rhythmic stabilization: *(a)* open-kinetic chain, *(b)* weight bearing in standing, *(c)* quadruped weight bearing, *(d)* tripod weight bearing, *(e)* bipod weight bearing *(f)* with rubber-tubing resistance to involved extremity, *(g)* with PNF manual resistance to uninvolved extremity, *(h)* unilateral weight bearing

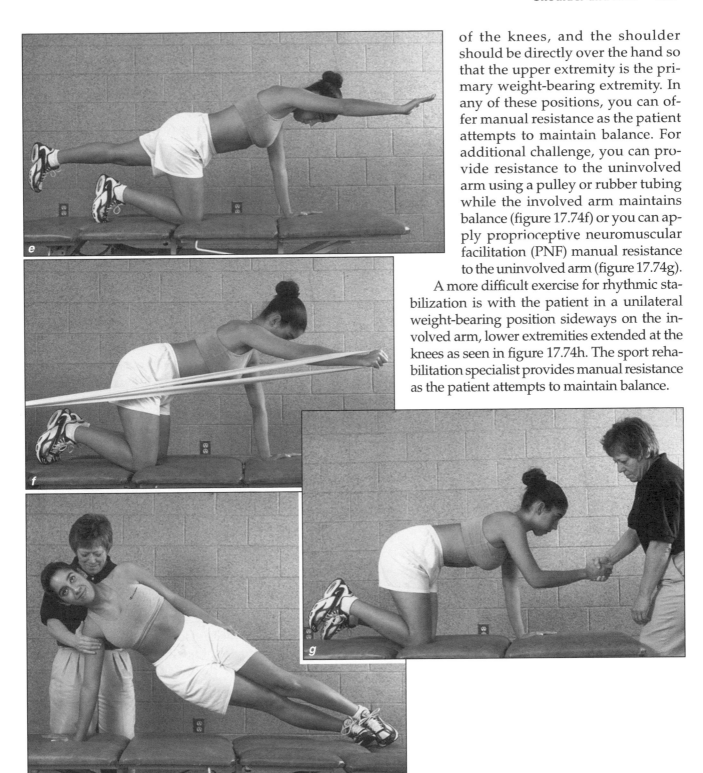

of the knees, and the shoulder should be directly over the hand so that the upper extremity is the primary weight-bearing extremity. In any of these positions, you can offer manual resistance as the patient attempts to maintain balance. For additional challenge, you can provide resistance to the uninvolved arm using a pulley or rubber tubing while the involved arm maintains balance (figure 17.74f) or you can apply proprioceptive neuromuscular facilitation (PNF) manual resistance to the uninvolved arm (figure 17.74g).

A more difficult exercise for rhythmic stabilization is with the patient in a unilateral weight-bearing position sideways on the involved arm, lower extremities extended at the knees as seen in figure 17.74h. The sport rehabilitation specialist provides manual resistance as the patient attempts to maintain balance.

■ **Figure 17.74**   *(continued)*

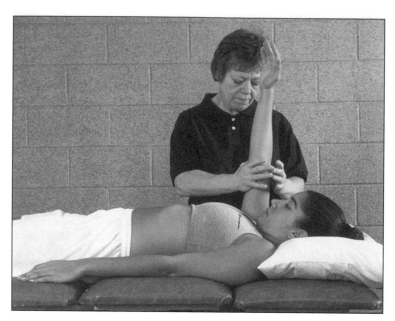

Figure 17.75   Proprioceptive neuromuscular facilitation: rhythmic stabilization.

Proprioceptive Neuromuscular Facilitation

Proprioceptive neuromuscular facilitation is useful in shoulder rehabilitation. There are a number of advantages to using PNF. There is no cost, because this form of exercise uses the sport rehabilitation specialist's manual resistance; PNF is appropriate throughout most of the program. In the early rehabilitation stages, PNF can enhance neuromuscular control, and at later stages it can improve strength and coordination of muscle firing. Techniques include iso-metrics, concentrics, eccentrics, and rhythmic stabilization. Proprioceptive neuromuscular facilitation incorporates functional positions because it uses multiplane motions.

In the early rehabilitation stages, PNF is commonly used for rhythmic stabilization (figure 17.75). This assists in re-educating synchronous muscle firing and providing joint stability. Moving through functional patterns can stimulate neuromuscular control for stability and synchronous patterns of movement. The sport rehabilitation specialist provides isometric resistance at points in the range of motion that are weak.

In later rehabilitation stages, PNF can increase coordination through use of eccentric resistance in functional planes and through use of combinations of eccentric with concentric and isometric resistance as the arm moves through its motion patterns. In this activity the patient attempts to move the arm through either a D1 or D2 flexion-extension pattern at a constant rate of speed as the sport rehabilitation specialist provides various types of resistance—eccentric, concentric, and isometric.

ADVANCED OPEN CHAIN EXERCISES

These exercises can incorporate various types of equipment. They are performed unsupported, first in straight-plane and then in diagonal positions. The unsupported position is the primary distinction between these and earlier exercises.

Isokinetic Exercises

Many rehabilitation facilities have isokinetic machines. These machines can be useful for monitoring and advancing shoulder strength. Early exercises are performed in straight-plane motions, isolating specific muscles to perform the desired activity. As the patient's strength improves, diagonal patterns are used and the patient performs a more normal movement pattern using a summation of trunk and hip forces to produce normal shoulder motion (figure 17.76).

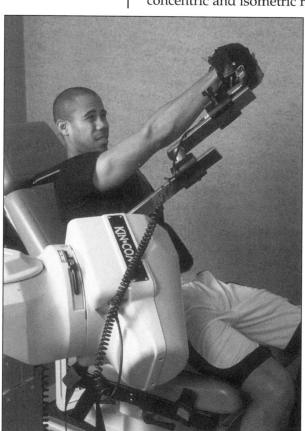

Figure 17.76   Isokinetic exercises for the shoulder.

Open Chain Elastic-Band Exercises

Once the patient achieves appropriate strength levels for shoulder stabilization during arm movement, elastic band or rubber tubing activities in an open kinetic chain can provide additional resistance and challenge. The challenge is to maintain stability during resisted arm movement. This is the next step once closed kinetic chain stabilization has been achieved. The patient is now required to execute resistive exercises without the feedback of the sport rehabilitation specialist in PNF and without the feedback of joint compression that closed kinetic chain activities provide. These exercises include a combination of concentric and eccentric resistance. The need for dynamic stabilization during these exercises more closely resembles functional activity demands; and these exercises are designed to prepare the shoulder for the next level of resistive exercises, plyometrics.

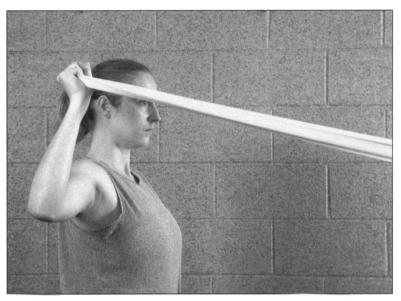

▮ Figure 17.77 Straight-plane external elastic-band exercises.

Straight-Plane Exercises

By now the patient should be able to maintain joint stability with the arm in at least 45° of elevation. Straight-plane exercises include internal and external rotation with the elbow at shoulder level and in the scapular plane. As control is achieved, the arm is elevated to 90° (figure 17.77). You must correct errors in execution. Common errors include dropping the elbow, horizontally extending the arm during external rotation and horizontally flexing it during internal rotation, and flexing the elbow during external rotation and extending it during internal rotation.

For shoulder-related fact sheets and patient information brochures and booklets, see the American Academy of Orthopaedic Surgeons Web site at: **http://orthoinfo.aaos.org/ category.cfm?topcategory=Shoulder**.

Diagonal-Plane Exercises

These exercises are performed once the patient demonstrates proper stabilization and control in the straight-plane exercises. Proprioceptive neuromuscular facilitation movements in D1 and D2 flexion and extension patterns are used (figure 17.78). It is important for the patient to execute the motion correctly and to maintain appropriate joint stability throughout the motion.

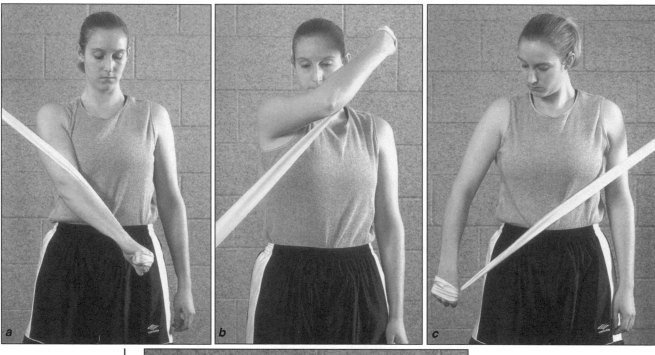

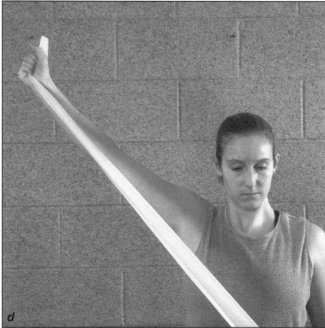

■ **Figure 17.78**   Diagonal-plane exercises: *(a)* D2 extension, *(b)* D1 flexion, *(c)* D1 extension, *(d)* D2 flexion.

PLYOMETRIC EXERCISES

Patients who have achieved strength and stability of the shoulder can go on to perform plyometric exercises on unstable surfaces, plyometric push-ups, weight-bearing activities, and medicine-ball exercises.

Once the patient has achieved strength, and static and simple dynamic stabilization control, he or she progresses to plyometric exercises before performing functional activities. Plyometrics are the most demanding in the series outlined because they require maximum strength, optimal joint stabilization during high-level dynamic activities, and agility and coordination throughout the activity.

UNSTABLE SURFACES

Exercises on unstable surfaces provide dynamic stabilization stress to the shoulder. Muscles must provide dynamic shoulder stability while simultaneously maintaining balance on a moving surface. A slide board can be used to stress joint stabilization during flexion-extension and horizontal abduction-adduction movements. In the progression, the patient is first on hands and knees and then on hands and feet. It is important that the weight be forward on the hands with the knees ahead of the hips. As the progression continues, the patient's feet are raised on a bench or stool, and finally the patient is positioned on a Swiss ball.

A Fitter (Fitter International, Calgary, AB, Canada) or simple device, such as a slide board or balance board, can be used to provide an unstable surface. The patient begins on hands and knees with the hands on the apparatus and moves the hands from side to side and forward and backward. Circular patterns can be used on the slide board (figure 17.79a). The board can also be balanced or can be moved from side to side while the ends of the board are kept off the floor. Progression for this exercise includes advancing to a hands-and-feet position and finally to placing the legs on a Swiss ball (figure 17.79b).

If available, more elaborate devices such as a computerized balance system or other commercially available balance system can be useful in providing an unstable base for dynamic stabilization exercises (figure 17.79c).

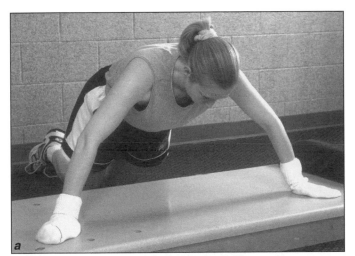

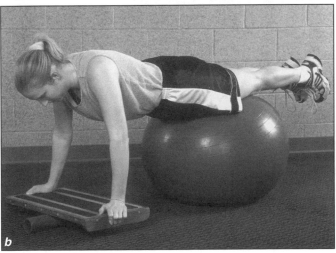

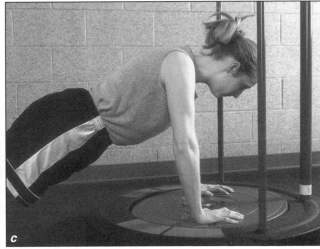

■ Figure 17.79 Unstable surface exercises: *(a)* Slide board while on knees, *(b)* balance board, *(c)* commercially available balance system.

PLYOMETRIC PUSH-UPS

The progression of plyometric push-ups begins with a wall push-up. The patient pushes him- or herself away from the wall with enough force to remove the hands from the wall. When the patient's hands come off the wall, the sport rehabilitation specialist pushes the patient back toward the wall and the patient stops his or her movement toward the wall by "catching" him- or herself with both hands on the wall. The impact force is absorbed by bending the elbows as the body returns to the starting position. This exercise progresses to an incline push-up. The patient pushes off the incline support, such as a tabletop or counter, to lose hand contact and is pushed back to the starting position by the sport rehabilitation specialist, as with the wall push-ups.

An additional progression involves having the patient perform a regular or modified push-up, first with the uninvolved hand on a medicine ball and the involved hand on the floor, then with both hands on the ball (figure 17.80, a and b).

Push-ups can also be performed on a trampoline. With the patient in a regular push-up position and the hands on the trampoline, the individual "jumps" the hands off the trampoline and lands them out to the side, and then "jumps" them back to the center on the next push-up movement.

The most difficult plyometric push-up is performed with boxes. Two boxes of the same height are placed on either side of the patient. The recommended starting height is 10 to 15 cm (3–6 in.). The patient begins with the hands on the floor and pushes up and away from the floor to position each hand on the box adjacent to each arm. The patient then drops the hands to the floor and repeats the push-up to the boxes (figure 17.80c).

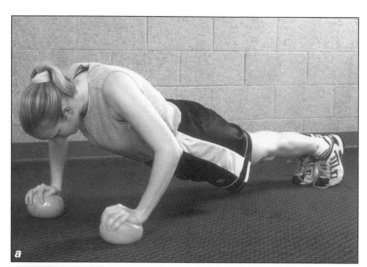
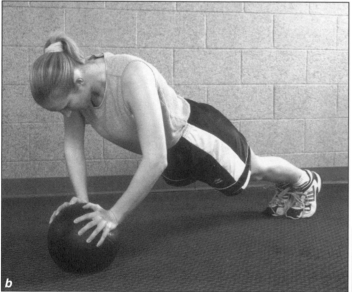
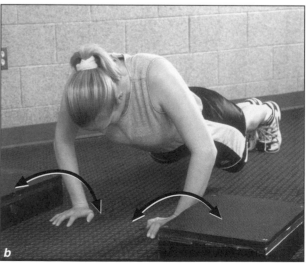

Figure 17.80 Plyometric push-up variations: *(a)* push-up with hands on small medicine balls, *(b)* push-up with both hands on one large medicine ball, *(c)* box jump.

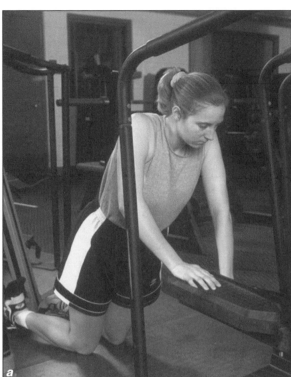

■ **Figure 17.81** Resisted movement in weight bearing: *(a)* on stair machine on knees, *(b)* on treadmill on toes.

RESISTED MOVEMENT IN WEIGHT BEARING

These exercises require good strength, control, and endurance. A stair machine, a step machine, or a treadmill can be used. The patient begins with hands on the machine and knees on the floor (figure 17.81). The patient "walks" the hands as the treadmill's belt or stair machine's steps move. The speed of the machine depends on the patient's abilities. The recommendation is to use a manual setting initially, but a random setting may be appropriate as the patient progresses. Bouts of 30 s to 1 min provide the patient ample challenge, initially. As the patient improves, speed, time, and resistance may be increased. The use of gloves will protect the patient's hands.

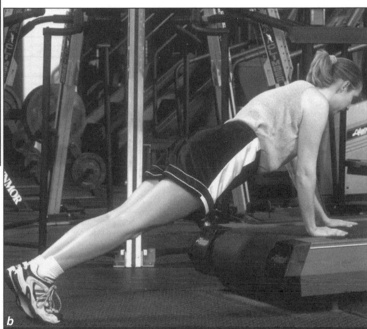

MEDICINE-BALL EXERCISES

These exercises begin with a lightweight ball—approximately .9 kg (2 lb)—and can increase as the patient is able to maintain control and still execute the exercise correctly.

Rotation Progression

A beginning exercise is performed with the patient in supine and the shoulder at 90° abduction and externally rotated, supported on the table. The forearm should be supported on the table to prevent excessive external rotation during the initial phases of this progression. The medicine ball is dropped from the level of the sport rehabilitation specialist's shoulder to the patient's hand. Initially, the patient only catches the ball, but the patient should quickly advance to catching and tossing the ball back (figure 17.82a). When the individual can perform this exercise without pain and through good motion, the sport rehabilitation specialist stands away from the patient toward the patient's feet and tosses the ball to the patient. The patient catches the ball and returns the toss, keeping the shoulder at 90° abduction and allowing it to externally rotate as the ball is caught. The arm should move into internal rotation when the ball is thrown back to the sport rehabilitation specialist. If this is not difficult, the patient performs the exercise with the forearm unsupported and then with the upper arm off the table as well. When the patient demonstrates good control,

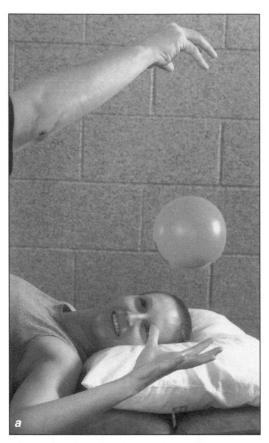

ease in allowing external rotation in the catch, and smooth internal rotation during the throw, he or she performs the exercise in a standing or kneeling position (figure 17.82b). The patient must maintain an elevated elbow at 90° of shoulder abduction and elbow flexion at 90°. This exercise is also performed with the patient's back to the sport rehabilitation specialist (figure 17.82c). The patient tosses the ball backward as the arm is moved into external rotation. The arm is maintained at 90° abduction throughout the exercise.

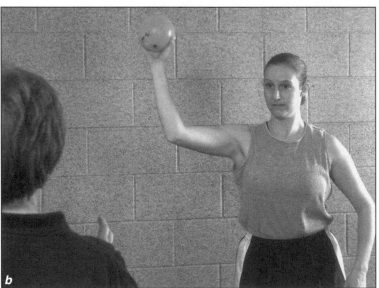

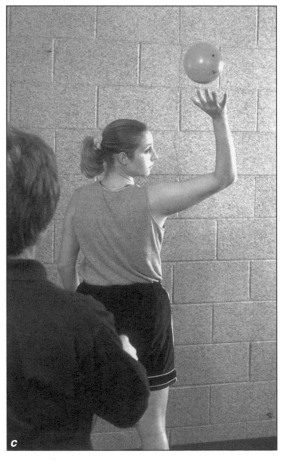

❚ **Figure 17.82** Medicine-ball progression: *(a)* drop-and-catch, *b)* standing forward toss, *(c)* backward toss.

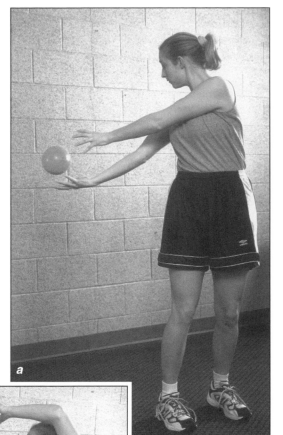

Rotational Tosses

Additional medicine-ball exercises include rotational tosses. The patient should perform these initially with the hands at hip level, as scapular muscles are less stressed in this position than they are with the arms more elevated. The trunk is rotated from one side as the ball is thrown and continues to rotate during a full follow-through position. This exercise is performed to both sides and facing the wall or the sport rehabilitation specialist and with the back to the wall or sport rehabilitation specialist (figure 17.83a). This activity is important in facilitating a functional motion, and it also assists in trunk strengthening.

In this exercise's progression, the arms are kept at a low level at first and then placed in the more stressful elevated position, at shoulder level. In the final position, the patient tosses the ball overhead (figure 17.83b). The overhead exercises can be performed in a standing or kneeling position or in the more difficult supine position (figure 17.83c). The supine position adds more resistance to the abdominals.

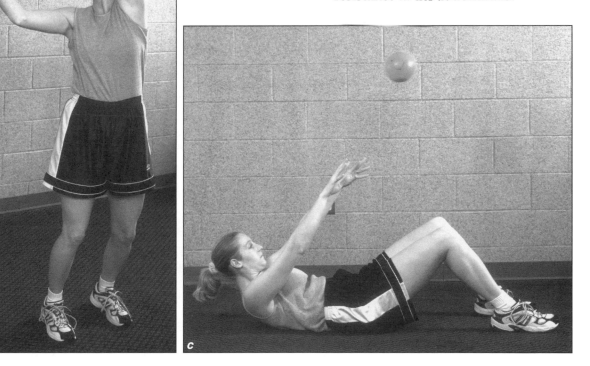

■ **Figure 17.83**   Rotational medicine-ball tosses: *(a)* backward toss with arms at low level; *(b)* backward overhead toss, standing; *(c)* overhead toss, supine.

FUNCTIONAL ACTIVITIES

Functional exercises for patients with shoulder injuries progress gradually in time, resistance, and/or distance. For overhead activities, the progression is from lower to higher movements.

At this point, the specifics of the program are dictated by the patient's sport. If a patient participates in a throwing sport, during the plyometric exercise phase he or she can begin throwing a foam rubber ball or knotted sock toward a mirror, watching for form and motion pattern (figure 17.84). A tennis player can begin forehand and backhand strokes in the same manner in front of a mirror. This helps to promote proprioception and correct technique through the additional afferent feedback that comes from the visual system.

Chapter 10 covers progressive functional programs, outlining specific sequences of exercises as a guide for setting a patient on a course of functional return to full activity participation. The most important point to remember is that the program must present a gradual progression of time, resistance, and/or distance. If one element is increased, another may be decreased to allow the body to adjust to new stresses. For example, if a pitcher increases throwing speed from 50% to 75% of his or her normal speed, a reduction in throwing distance or a reduction in repetitions may be necessary. An increase in the program is usually added only every third day of activity. This allows the body the time it needs for adjustment to new levels of stress before application of additional levels. For example, if a golfer is now able to perform a full swing with the long irons, it will be three days before he or she advances to using the woods.

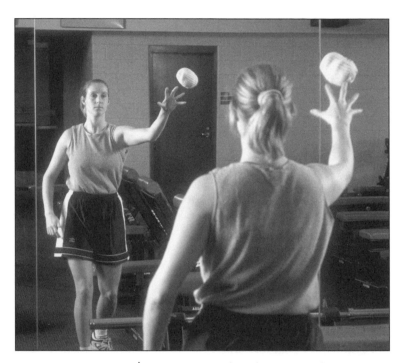

Figure 17.84   Mirror feedback.

In overhead events, the patient progresses through a program of low- and medium-height movements and attempts high movements last. For example, a tennis player begins functional activities with forehand and backhand ground strokes. It is not until the individual accomplishes full-distance and full-force hits with these strokes that he or she progresses to overhead strokes. Because serves are the most strenuous activity, they are the last stroke the patient attempts. Partial force is used in the initial stages of serve activities, with progression to normal serves.

SPECIAL REHABILITATION APPLICATIONS

Among the types of shoulder injuries that raise special concerns and call for particular exercise approaches are instability, impingement, traumatic rotator cuff conditions, glenoid labral tears, adhesive capsulitis, acromioclavicular sprains, and biceps tendon injuries.

The combination and progression of exercises used in each rehabilitation program are determined individually according to the patient and the injury. Some injuries dictate special concerns for the sport rehabilitation specialist. Some of these injuries and the concerns unique to them are addressed here.

SHOULDER INSTABILITY

The shoulder has two systems of stability, the **static restraints** and the **dynamic restraints.** The static restraints include the ligaments, capsule, and glenoid labrum. The dynamic restraints are the neuromuscular components. If the static restraint is damaged by joint sprains, subluxations, or dislocations, the neural input from the proprioceptors located within the static structures is compromised. Damage to static restraints also causes a deficiency in muscle function. Instability is the result. A secondary problem that can result from instability is rotator cuff tendinitis that can lead to rotator cuff tears with repetitive impingement and breakdown. If instability is not corrected either by surgery to reinforce static structures, or by rehabilitation to restore dynamic structures, or both, reinjury is perpetuated with continued activity until the joint becomes so unstable that it may sublux or dislocate with relatively little stress.

Before you design a therapeutic exercise program for a patient with shoulder instability, you must consider several factors. The most common instability is anterior instability, which occurs when anterior structures become damaged. Inferior instability is the result of injury and laxity of the inferior capsule and support structures. Posterior instability, which is less common, occurs with damage to the posterior joint structures.

Two acronyms, AMBRI and TUBS, indicate the difference between nontraumatic and traumatic shoulder instability and present guidelines for treatment. The acronym **AMBRI** stands for "**A**traumatic, **M**ultidirectional, **B**ilateral, **R**ehabilitation effective, **I**nferior capsular shift required." Patients with this condition usually have bilateral shoulder laxity, as well as hypermobility in most joints. The instability is multidirectional but usually responds well to the conservative treatment of rehabilitation. If surgery is necessary, an inferior capsular shift is usually the procedure of choice.

Shoulders with **TUBS** (**T**raumatic, **U**nilateral, **B**ankart lesion, **S**urgery required) are shoulders that have incurred a traumatic injury. A **Bankart lesion**, or tear of the anterior capsulolabral complex, is present and surgery is required to relieve the problem.

Patients in overhead-throwing sports commonly develop anterior instability because the throwing motion places repetitive stresses on the anterior joint structures. Often accompanying and encouraging this problem is a concomitant posterior capsule and rotator cuff tightness of the internal rotators. In these patients, the rehabilitation program for instability should include stretching of these structures.

The rehabilitation processes for surgically corrected anterior instability and nonrepaired instability are similar. The greatest differences may be their time lines, but the exercise sequence is essentially the same. A nonrepaired shoulder may require longer immobilization time and, thus, a delay in the total rehabilitation process. The arm is immobilized in a sling for approximately three to four weeks for the surgically repaired shoulder, but the time in a sling can be longer for the nonrepaired shoulder. Older patients are the exception. Generally, patients over 40 are started on early postoperative exercise intervention because a frozen shoulder is a common complication if motion is not initiated soon after any shoulder surgical procedure. The time required for a complete rehabilitation program varies from younger to older patients and from one sport to another. Patients in overhead sports such as baseball or volleyball may require a longer rehabilitation process than those whose shoulder demands are minimal, such as soccer players. An average program may take anywhere from 15 to 26 weeks.

After the first week following surgery or injury, the shoulder is taken out of the sling to permit active assistive range of motion in straight-plane flexion. Gentle, passive motion to no more than 0° external rotation with the elbow at the side can also begin. Abduction to 30° is also permitted. Isometrics in non-stress positions are initiated after the first week. Care must be taken to avoid external rotation greater than 20° to 30° and abduction greater than 30° to 40°. The anterior shoulder joint should be minimally stressed during the first three weeks. Manual resistance to scapular stabilizers, avoiding stress to the glenohumeral joint, should begin at this time. The most stressful position for the anterior joint is external rotation with abduction; this position should be avoided for the first several weeks.

By the sixth week, passive shoulder flexion range of motion should be normal, and passive external rotation should be approximately 50° to 60° with the elbow at the side. By the 8th to 10th week, full passive range of motion should be present in all motions except external rotation, which should be at approximately 75°. Between weeks 10 and 12, full passive motion should be possible in all movements.

After the third week, gentle, active resistive isotonic exercises for internal rotation, external rotation to about 20° to 30° with the elbow near the side, and abduction to 20° can begin in a scapular plane. Scapular exercises should advance as tolerated without the imposition of additional stress on the glenohumeral joint.

By the end of the third or fourth week, the shoulder sling is removed. This can be an apprehensive time for the patient. The lack of support can also be initially fatiguing for the shoulder. The patient should be encouraged to support the arm throughout the day by placing it on top of a table or desk while sitting, and by putting the hand in a pocket when standing to permit some muscle rest.

By the 6th to 10th week, the rotator cuff exercises can go through increased ranges of motion as long as the anterior joint is not stressed. The program should continue with low weights and high repetitions. The elbow is kept near the side, but external rotation can progress to approximately 45°. Mild isokinetic exercises with the shoulder stabilized can begin during this time.

When the patient has full external rotation, eccentric exercises can begin. These start with the arm in the low position, less than 60°, and progress to the higher positions as tolerated. Once strength and control of the joints during motion are achieved, overhead activities, plyometrics, and finally functional activities can be added to the therapeutic exercise program.

Throughout the program, the sport rehabilitation specialist must receive feedback from the patient about the shoulder's response to activity. Pain should not be present with any activities. Scapular stability must be present before the patient advances to activities that place the arm above shoulder level. If this precept is not respected, rotator cuff tendinitis may occur and delay the patient's return to sport participation.

In posterior instability, positions to avoid initially are those that put stress on the posterior capsule. Excessive internal rotation, abduction, and horizontal adduction should be performed carefully after the first three to four weeks. Weight-bearing activities in a quadruped position should be avoided initially. These can put undue additional stress on the posterior capsule and cause additional damage. Other exercises that should be modified or avoided because of the posterior capsule stress they impose include chest flys, bench press, and push-ups. These activities should be added to the program carefully and not until the later stages of therapeutic exercise. In the early and middle phases, exercises should be performed with the shoulder in some external rotation and abduction. Scapular stabilization exercises should be performed in a supine position with glenohumeral external rotation and should advance to a sitting position, in which joint stability is more difficult to maintain than it is in supine. Seated, weight-bearing exercises that do not stress the posterior capsule can start earlier than quadruped weight-bearing exercises. Internal rotation exercises are performed from full external rotation to neutral in the early phases. Horizontal adduction exercises are avoided early in the program. When added later, they begin with horizontal adduction limitations to approximately 45° forward of the frontal plane. Gradually, full horizontal adduction is instituted in the later stages. Quadruped weight-bearing exercises for the shoulder begin in the later phase of rehabilitation after the patient has achieved stabilization and adequate strength and after adequate tissue-healing time has passed. When the bench press is initiated in the later phases, it should be performed with a wide grip so that the arms are in abduction and horizontal extension.

Initial positions to avoid with inferior instability injuries include placing the arm overhead and allowing it to hang at the side unsupported. The upright press and shrugs are exercises that the patient should avoid because of the stress they place on the inferior capsule.

Case Study

A 16-year-old basketball player was seen by the physician after experiencing a right shoulder subluxation. The injury occurred as he was going under the basket for a layup and his arm was caught and pulled into horizontal extension with external rotation. He has no history of prior injury. The physician has placed the arm in a sling and instructed you to begin a rehabilitation program for this patient. It has been one week since the injury. The patient reports some difficulty sleeping at night; he cannot get comfortable as a result of the pain. He reports that he wears the sling all the time except for showers, as the physician has instructed. On examination, you find some discoloration in the upper arm, but the swelling of last week is gone. There is some muscle spasm and tenderness to palpation of the infraspinatus, supraspinatus, teres minor, rhomboids, upper trapezius, and levator scapula. You notice that atrophy of the supraspinatus is already evident after one week. Range of motion of the shoulder is 40° flexion, 20° abduction, and −10° external rotation.

Questions for Analysis

1. What will be your initial treatment?

2. Outline the exercises you will use for this patient during the first week of treatment.

3. What precautions must you take with his treatments?

4. Give a general outline of progression for his rehabilitation program, specifying what guidelines you will use to move from one stage to the next.

SHOULDER IMPINGEMENT

Shoulder impingement is associated with unique factors that you must consider in developing and executing a therapeutic exercise program. These are discussed as program considerations before the case study is presented.

Program Considerations

The subacromial space is not a large area—a little wider than a pencil. Because the space is not large to begin with, even a slight alteration in its normal structure can have significant consequences, especially to a patient who places great stresses on the joint.

There are two types of impingement, primary and secondary. Primary impingement is the result of structures present within the subacromial space that narrow the normal size of the space to compromise the soft-tissue structures within it—the rotator cuff tendons (supraspinatus and infraspinatus), biceps tendon, and subacromial bursa. Among these structural factors are a congenital anomaly of the acromion structure, an osteophyte on the distal acromion, a narrower-than-normal subacromial space, and a larger-than-normal tendon. All these structural variations narrow an already small space and cause the soft-tissue structures to become impinged. Most often the cause of primary impingement is either a congenital anomaly in the distal acromion configuration or a bony spur.

Acquired or secondary impingement reduces the subacromial space and occurs because of alterations in the shoulder's function that lead to instability. These factors can include capsular laxity or tightness, postural deviations, rotator cuff weakness, and scapular rotator muscle imbalances. Cervical radiculopathy can also result in impingement if muscle weakness occurs and causes muscle imbalances during shoulder motion. If the capsule is loose, the humerus moves forward during follow-through of throwing motions. If the posterior capsule is tight, it tends to push the humerus upward into the anterior joint during shoulder motions, narrowing the subacromial space. Normal function of the rotator cuff is to depress the humeral head during shoulder elevation motions to provide for adequate subacromial space; but if the rotator cuff is weak, the humeral head will ride higher in the glenoid and cause impingement. When the scapular rotator muscles are imbalanced, the upper trapezius and levator scapulae usually overpower the weaker lower trapezius. This causes poor scapulohumeral rhythm and narrows the subacromial space under the coracoacromial arch during shoulder motion because scapular elevation and upward rotation will not occur with shoulder elevation (Kamkar, Irrgang, and Whitney 1993). Poor posture causes the shoulders to round forward so that the greater tubercle is more directly under the acromial arch to cause impingement earlier in the range of motion. Each of these secondary problems can result in subacromial impingement. Uncorrected secondary impingement leads to a gradual, progressive shredding of the rotator cuff tendon and ultimately results in rotator cuff tears. Secondary impingement and rotator cuff tears are more common in athletes over the age of 30 than in those who are younger.

Secondary and primary impingement both result in inflammation of the soft-tissue structures in the subacromial space. This inflammation most commonly includes the supraspinatus tendon. The infraspinatus tendon can sometimes be affected as well. The subacromial bursa and biceps tendon can also be involved. Impingement, then, causes tendinitis or bursitis. Inflammation of the rotator cuff tendons weakens the tendon and can lead to tendon rupture if the condition is poorly managed or untreated.

Secondary impingement can be resolved through conservative efforts if the cause of the impingement is corrected. The cause must be determined before treatment can be successful. Secondary factors of muscle imbalance and asynchronous shoulder motion are commonly seen in primary impingement, leading to pain and rotator cuff tendinitis. Primary impingement is surgically corrected, but both primary and secondary problems should be treated with rehabilitation. The most common surgical correction is either removal of the osteophyte (if present) or an anterior acromioplasty.

Rehabilitation emphasizes control of the inflammation, correction of the secondary cause, and restoration of normal shoulder function. Initially, the focus is on pain and inflammation control and achievement of full range of motion. Placing the shoulder in a loose-packed position with the arm slightly abducted and flexed helps to provide optimal circulation to the tendons. Gentle grade II mobilizations can be helpful in relieving pain. If inferior capsule tightness is present, inferior glenohumeral glide mobilizations should be used to increase capsule mobility, permitting the rotator cuff to position the humerus caudally during arm elevation. The sport rehabilitation specialist can massage the supraspinatus tendon by placing the patient's hand behind the hip to expose the anterior humerus and providing deep cross-friction to the tender area until the pain subsides (figure 17.23). Scapular stabilization strengthening exercises can take place, without stress applied to the rotator cuff tendons, and should be a part of the early program. Early on, the program should incorporate neuromuscular re-education for proprioception and improved kinesthetic awareness of the scapular rotators for correct scapular positioning during arm movement. Rotator cuff exercises in a pain-free range of motion are important at this time as well. Most rotator cuff exercises should be performed in the lower positions (below 60°), and the scapula should be in a set position. Resistive exercises should begin with high repetitions and lower weights.

Progression of exercises is based on the patient's pain and strength. Exercises that produce pain should be avoided. In the early stages, these exercises include activities that place the arm above 60° to 90° or behind the back, as well as diagonal-plane motions. As the tendon's inflammation subsides and the patient achieves scapular stabilization strength, he or she can begin to use higher shoulder positions and more stressful exercises. Finally, the plyometric and functional exercises are incorporated into the program before the patient returns to full activity.

Case Study

A 40-year-old, competitive tennis player reports to you that she has had shoulder pain since the first half of the tennis season. She is now unable to serve without pain. She has pain in the beginning of her warm-ups but before a match begins, the pain goes away. About 2 h after a match, her pain is significant. She has pain in the deltoid insertion area. The doctor has ruled out primary impingement but feels that a course of rehabilitation is necessary before the patient returns to tennis. On examination this patient has full range of motion except that she is lacking about 10° in elevation. Pain occurs in the end ranges of movement and above 90° of elevation. She has a forward-head, round-shouldered posture. Her glenohumeral rotators and abductors are weak and painful. She has weakness in the lower trapezius and rhomboids.

Questions for Analysis

1. What is the cause of her secondary impingement?
2. What will you do to relieve the causes?
3. What will your first treatment include?
4. How will you help the patient progress in her rehabilitation program?
5. What guidelines will you use for her progression?
6. What functional program will you use to prepare her for her return to tennis?

TRAUMATIC ROTATOR CUFF CONDITIONS

Traumatic rotator cuff injuries are different from degenerative tears that occur in older patients. You must take into account several unique factors associated with traumatic rotator cuff injuries before developing a therapeutic exercise program for a patient with this type of injury.

Program Considerations

Traumatic rotator cuff conditions can include acute rotator cuff strain, a partial tear, a complete tear, and postsurgical conditions. Although rotator cuff tears are more commonly seen in athletes who are older, patients now begin sport participation at an earlier age and at a greater intensity level than earlier generations did, so rotator cuff tears are increasingly seen in younger patients as well. A sudden traumatic event such as a shoulder dislocation or a fall on the outstretched, externally rotated arm can cause rotator cuff tears at almost any age, and may occur in a healthy rotator cuff or in one that has minor asymptomatic changes. Rotator cuff tears can also occur in rotator cuffs that have undergone repetitive stresses over time. These conditions are associated especially with overhead athletic activities in which the musculotendinous unit has encountered chronic stress and fiber damage. An open repair is necessary for most rotator cuff tears in patients who wish to remain active. Following surgical repair, the starting point, duration, and progression of the rehabilitation process depends on the size of the tear, the extent of the surgical repair, the state of integrity of the deltoid (whether it was split or preserved in surgery), and the age of the patient. A sling or abduction brace may be used immediately postoperatively and continued for about six weeks. After 7 to 10 days of immobilization, mild passive and active assistive range-of-motion exercises may be possible, but this depends on the surgeon's preference. Early exercises can include passive and active assistive elevation and external rotation, extension, and internal rotation. Pendulum exercises are also appropriate. Joint mobilization for pain relief (grades I and II) can be used. Active external and internal rotation can be performed with the elbow at the side and extended. Manual resistance to scapular rotators in side-lying and with the arm at the side can be useful. Distal joint movements such as elbow and wrist flexion and extension and ball squeezes should be performed to minimize atrophy of the muscles in these areas. At the end of the first three weeks, rubber tubing or manual-resistance internal and external rotation with the elbow at the side, and rhythmic stabilization with the arm at 100° to 120° flexion, can begin.

The time to start active exercises depends on the size of the tear and the type of repair, but an average time point is approximately six to eight weeks after the surgery. At this time, joint mobilization for increased mobility can begin. Active range of motion can be performed in the scapular plane and can be accompanied by isometric exercises in different arm positions as long as the motion is pain free. Resistive exercises such as those done with rubber tubing should continue for the rotator cuff if the arm is kept at the side. If scapular stabilization is adequate, gentle guided internal and external rotation with the arm at 90° abduction can begin. Biceps and triceps exercises can be performed against resistance. Antigravity shoulder extension, supine flys, and prone flys to no more than a horizontal neutral position, as well as weight-bearing scapular stabilization exercises, are suitable at this time. Exercises are kept in a straight plane.

At 10 to 12 weeks, the patient should have nearly full range of motion. More vigorous stretching exercises, such as overhead hangs, are permissible if full motion is not present. Exercises should remain in a pain-free range. Side-lying exercises for the external and internal rotators can begin; these should initially use low resistance and high repetitions. Isokinetic exercises in the scapular plane are also appropriate. Proprioceptive neuromuscular facilitation patterns of resistance can be used.

After 12 weeks, the scapular stabilizers should have adequate strength to control the scapula in planes higher than 60° elevation. The shoulder should be able to tolerate an aggressive strengthening program. Resisted diagonal movements can begin in the lower levels, progress to shoulder level, and then progress to above shoulder levels. Plyometrics such as medicine-ball exercises can be started.

At 15 to 18 weeks, resisted rotation exercises with the arm at 90° abduction can be performed, as can aggressive resistive exercises for all shoulder muscle groups. Toward the end of this time, a progression of functional activities can begin—when the patient has full pain-free motion, normal strength of all shoulder muscles, and normal scapulohumeral synchronized motion. By 21 to 26 weeks the patient should be able to return to full sport participation.

The difference in rehabilitation for a conservatively managed and postoperative rotator cuff injury lies primarily in the initial treatment and the progression. In conservative treatment, the inflammation following injury must be initially treated with modalities and activity modification. Isometric exercises can begin earlier for conservatively treated injuries, and active motion can be initiated early as long as the shoulder remains pain free and scapular strength is sufficient to maintain proper scapular stabilization during shoulder motion. Early shoulder internal and external rotation motions are performed with the elbow near the side in a scapular plane. Shoulder elevation can occur to 90° as long as the shoulder is pain free and scapular stabilization is maintained. Resistance exercises begin with high repetitions and low resistance and progress to higher resistance with increased scapular and glenohumeral control.

Case Study

An 18-year-old baseball pitcher with shoulder instability underwent a glenohumeral capsular shift reconstruction one week ago. The surgeon wants you to begin the rehabilitation process today. The patient's shoulder is in a bolster, with the arm supported in partial abduction and internal rotation. Examination reveals a nicely healing surgical scar over the anterior-inferior aspect of the shoulder. Passive range of motion measures 80° flexion, 80° abduction, and −10° external rotation. There is tenderness over the supraspinatus muscle belly, and the upper trapezius and levator scapula muscles are tense and tender to palpation.

Questions for Analysis

1. What will your treatment session today include?

2. Give this patient an outline of your rehabilitation program with an estimate of how long it will be before he begins a pitching program.

3. Outline his pitching progression program.

ARTHROSCOPIC DECOMPRESSION

The advancement of arthroscopic procedures to improve subacromial arch space has permitted a relatively rapid recovery following surgery to relieve subacromial impingement.

Program Considerations

Debridement of rotator cuff tendons and decompression of the subacromial space via an **arthroscopy** permits early rehabilitation because there has been no disruption of the deltoid and the surgical insult is less than in open surgical repairs and techniques. A decompression is used to relieve primary impingement, and a debridement is used to relieve chronic tendinitis or synovitis.

Rehabilitation following arthroscopic decompression can begin immediately after surgery. The first week or two involves primarily pain and swelling modulation and range-of-motion exercises. Early motion exercises can include Codman's exercises and active assistive range-of-motion exercises with a wand, pulley, or the sport rehabilitation specialist. Internal and external rotation motion exercises start with the elbow near the side and progress to 45° and then 90° of abduction. Motion activities can also include capsular stretches and joint mobilization. Submaximal isometric exercises can be initiated in the first two weeks postoperatively. Scapular stabilization exercises and biceps and triceps exercises are important in the early program as well. Early neuromuscular control exercises such as proprioception drills for glenohumeral positioning with eyes closed can be started early.

Once pain is under control and near-full motion is possible, straight-plane resistive exercises can be initiated, first below 60° in the scapular plane. As scapular stabilization improves, external and internal rotation can be performed at 90° of abduction. Isokinetics in the scapular plane can begin. Full range of motion and good capsular mobility should be present before the patient moves to the next step of the progression. Once scapular stabilization and straight-plane strength are good, diagonal-plane exercises using pulleys or rubber tubing can begin. These are followed by first low-level, then higher-level, and finally overhead medicine-ball activities. Plyometrics are followed by functional exercises before the patient finally returns to full sport participation. The entire rehabilitation process may average three to five months.

Case Study

A 19-year-old volleyball player underwent an arthroscopic decompression of her right-dominant shoulder after an eight-week course of rehabilitation did not alleviate her shoulder pain. The surgery was two days ago. The surgeon wants her to begin a rehabilitation program today. On examination she reports normal postoperative shoulder pain, but no more rotator cuff pain. There is minimal ecchymosis around the shoulder. The surgical portal sites are covered with adhesive suture strips. There is some spasm in the rotator cuff muscles and upper trapezius. Range of motion of the shoulder is 150° flexion, 100° abduction, 80° external rotation, and 90° internal rotation. Her strength has diminished from preoperative levels and is now 3/5 in the rotator cuff muscles, 3–/5 in shoulder abduction, 3/5 in shoulder flexion, and 4–/5 in the scapular rotators. The patient tends to shrug her shoulder when she elevates the arm.

Questions for Analysis

1. What will you include in your treatment today?

2. What instructions will you give the patient today?

3. What will the next three treatment sessions include?

4. Explain what you will use as guidelines to determine when she is ready to progress from straight-plane to diagonal-plane exercises, from diagonal plane to plyometrics, and from plyometrics to functional exercises.

5. List four exercises for each exercise level and indicate your justification for their inclusion.

6. Describe the functional program you will use before the patient's return to volleyball.

GLENOID LABRAL TEARS

Glenoid labral tears are difficult to identify. Nevertheless, when they are diagnosed, and whether an anterior or posterior tear is present, special considerations are warranted in the development of a therapeutic exercise program. We look at these considerations first and then at a case study.

Program Considerations

Glenoid labrum tears are primarily the bane of throwing athletes. The large compression and shear forces generated during deceleration in throwing are mainly responsible for causing degenerative tears, abrupt tears, or detachments of the glenoid labrum. The labrum frequently tears superiorly either on the posterior or anterior glenoid in throwers. This type of lesion is referred to as a **SLAP** lesion—**S**uperior **L**abrum tear **A**nterior and **P**osterior in location. The anterior-superior lesion occurs because of the tremendous throwing deceleration forces applied in this area where the long head of the biceps tendon attaches to the labrum. The posterior-superior lesions are thought to occur because of glenohumeral joint instability. If a glenoid labrum tear is present, instability is frequently an accompanying problem and should be assessed and treated as part of the total rehabilitation process.

Whether or not instability is present, the usual treatment choice is to try conservative rehabilitation first. If this is unsuccessful, excision of the torn segment may be necessary. If instability is present, open reduction to remove the avulsed segment and stabilize the joint may be necessary. A variety of surgical repairs are used for this problem, including a Bankart repair and capsulolabral reconstruction.

If the patient undergoes an arthroscopic excision, the rehabilitation process follows the program used for arthroscopic debridement discussed earlier. If an open repair is necessary, the rehabilitation program must be delayed because of the required additional immobilization; the rehabilitation program proceeds more slowly and cautiously because of the risk of damaging the surgical repair if the rehabilitation is too aggressive. In these cases, the process will more closely follow the time line outlined for the rotator cuff repair program as discussed previously.

Case Study

A 17-year-old lacrosse player injured his right-dominant shoulder when another player ran into him while his arm was abducted. He suffered a torn glenoid and was in rehabilitation for three weeks following the injury. Two weeks ago the shoulder subluxed when he slipped on the ice and fell on an outstretched arm. He underwent an open debridement and anterior capsular reconstruction last week and is now ready for rehabilitation. The arm is in an abduction bolster harness, but the surgeon wants it removed during therapeutic exercises. Shoulder motion is 60° flexion, 60° abduction, and −10° external rotation. Rotator cuff strength in the middle of available range is 3+/5. The surgical scar is well healed, but there is ecchymosis surrounding the anterior shoulder area and into the upper arm. The upper trapezius and pectoralis major muscles are tender to palpation and in spasm.

Questions for Analysis

1. What will be your first treatment?

2. What will be included in your first two weeks of treatment?

3. When will you begin passive range of motion?

4. When will you begin resistive exercises, and what will they first include?

5. What precautions must you be aware of in this case?

ADHESIVE CAPSULITIS

Adhesive capsulitis is more commonly seen in older patients than in younger patients but can also occur in younger age groups. Understanding the condition is essential to designing a therapeutic exercise program. Elements unique to this injury are discussed and a case study is then presented.

Program Considerations

Adhesive capsulitis is commonly referred to as a frozen shoulder. The generic term for adhesions in the capsule is arthrofibrosis. An idiopathic frozen shoulder occurs spontaneously with no known trauma or aggravating incident. Idiopathic frozen shoulder occurs predominantly in middle-aged patients—usually over 40, usually female—and typically in the nondominant shoulder. Although adhesive capsulitis is a malady of older patients, the shoulder can become restricted in its motion in younger patients because of a variety of predisposing factors. These factors can include surgery that changes the biomechanics of the shoulder; prolonged immobilization of the shoulder; scar-tissue adhesions in the capsule or ligaments surrounding the shoulder; and prolonged inflammation of the tendons, bursa, and other soft tissue around the shoulder. This condition is termed traumatic or secondary adhesive capsulitis when there is a sudden onset of injury or of immobilization resulting in loss of motion.

Immobilization causes adhesions in the intermuscular connective tissue that can reduce muscular tissue mobility. Reduced muscle tissue mobility decreases the number of sarcomeres present in the muscle (Akeson et al. 1973). The additional changes that occur with immobilization in muscle, joints, and supportive tissue were discussed in chapter 2. When the joint capsule is affected, loss of motion is most notable in external rotation, abduction, and flexion of the shoulder. A capsular pattern of motion loss becomes apparent, with external rotation more limited than abduction, abduction more limited than flexion, and flexion more limited than internal rotation (Cyriax 1975).

When adhesive capsulitis is in stage I, shoulder pain, pain at end ranges of movement, difficulty sleeping on the shoulder, and progressive loss of motion are hallmark signs. It is during this time that the capsular scar tissue is forming and maturing. External rotation will demonstrate loss of available motion, but other movements may or may not show evidence of lost motion. The most effective treatment at this time is active range-of-motion exercise. Joint mobilization should not be painful and should be oriented more toward pain relief than mobility gains. Stronger mobilization grades only aggravate the capsule and may promote an inflammatory response or cause a reactive muscle spasm that will increase pain. Active range-of-motion exercises maintain muscle length. Attempts at stretching the capsule at this time cause pain but little change in mobility.

In stage II, adhesive capsulitis has become mature, the glenohumeral joint has lost its normal mobility, and the shoulder is very stiff. Pain is present at the end of available motion. The patient may complain of pain in the elbow and is unable to lie on the shoulder. At this time more aggressive joint mobilization can be used as long as an inflammatory response is not created. Continued active stretches should also be used. Strengthening exercises in the available ranges should be a part of the program. Ultrasound before joint mobilization may permit more optimal results from the mobilization.

In the third stage, the patient's pain is evident before the end of capsular restriction is reached. The primary area of pain is distal on the arm, not in the shoulder. Pain is present at rest as well as during activity. Passive range-of-motion assessment demonstrates a hard leathery end-feel in a limited capsular pattern. Scapulohumeral rhythm is lost because glenohumeral capsular restrictions prevent normal motion between the scapulothoracic and glenohumeral joints. Because glenohumeral rhythm is lost, attempts at arm elevation include shoulder shrugging, and the scapula moves at the same time and rate as the humerus. Grades III and IV joint mobilizations can be used at this time. Continued range-of-motion exercises and active stretches are used throughout the day to promote mobility gains. Self-mobilization techniques are taught to the patient. Strength exercises for the scapular rotators, rotator cuff, and large glenohumeral muscles (deltoid, pectoralis major, teres major, and latissimus) should be provided in a progressive program.

If the patient is not seen until the third stage, treatment for 3 to 6 months may be necessary to resolve the condition. Without treatment, the adhesive capsulitis takes longer to resolve, perhaps between 18 and 24 months.

Case Study

A 45-year-old golfer had noticed a gradual loss of motion in his left nondominant shoulder over the past several months. He went to the physician when he was unable to retrieve his wallet out of his back pocket and was diagnosed with a frozen shoulder. He is unable to lie on the left side and has pain with sudden movements and when just sitting. He is concerned about getting his shoulder ready for golf season, which begins in three months. On examination, you find that he has 120° of flexion, 80° of abduction, 35° of external rotation, and 60° of internal rotation and that he is able to reach across in horizontal adduction to get his elbow even with his left ear. He has pain about 10° to 15° before the end range of all motions, and you observe a stiff end-feel at the end of each movement. Joint mobilization assessment indicates tightness throughout the capsule, especially the inferior and posterior capsule. Palpation reveals tenderness in all the rotator cuff muscles and some tension in the pectoralis major, upper trapezius, and levator scapulae. The patient's posture is good, but when he moves the arm there is no scapulohumeral rhythm, and he shrugs the shoulder toward his ear during flexion motions.

Questions for Analysis

1. What stage of adhesive capsulitis is he in?

2. What will be your first treatment for him?

3. What home exercises will you give him on the first day?

4. Outline a progressive program for him including modalities, exercises, mobilization techniques, and functional progression for returning to golf.

ELECTROTHERMALLY ASSISTED CAPSULAR SHIFT

Electrothermally assisted capsular shift is a procedure for which long-term results have not been defined because of its newness to medicine. There remain many unanswered questions regarding the proper rehabilitation course. There is little research on postoperative treatment procedures. One study indicated that early range of motion and a slow but progressive strengthening program produce successful results over a 12-week therapeutic exercise treatment course (Ellenbecker and Mattalino 1999). This section presents the information currently available about the procedure and the postoperative course.

Program Considerations

The electrothermally assisted capsular shift procedure is a relatively new arthroscopic technique used to address glenohumeral instability. The long-term effects of the procedure are still being investigated and are at this point unknown because the technique has been used only since the late 1990s. The arthroscopic technique incorporates the use of a thermally assisted coagulator probe that is set at or above 65° F and is swept along the capsule between the glenoid and the humeral head (Hayashi et al. 1997). The capsule immediately shrinks like a plastic shrink-wrap, reducing the joint's laxity.

It is thought that the heat causes the collagen to denature and fuse when the fibroblasts invade the area. The fibroblasts are thought to use the denatured collagen as a scaffold in the new collagen matrix formation during the inflammatory healing phase (Hayashi et al. 1996). It is during this time that immobilization of the shoulder must occur so that the collagen matrix formation will result in appropriate capsular tightening.

The shoulder is kept immobilized for 7 to 14 days, although wrist and elbow motions are permitted. Active abduction is initiated about 10 to 14 days postoperatively. External rotation is permitted to 45° with the elbow at the side and at 90° abduction after about two weeks. Forward flexion is kept to 90°, and extension is limited to 20° hyperextension.

Strengthening exercises can be performed as long as the patient stays within the range-of-motion restrictions. Resistance consists of high repetitions with low resistance. Scapular stabilization exercises can be performed without placing undue stress on the glenohumeral joint. Resisted elbow and wrist motions should also be a part of the program.

At four to eight weeks, all motions should be within normal limits except external rotation, which is limited to 15° less than that on the contralateral side. Strength exercises continue as with other programs. Strenuous overhead activities should be avoided at this time, but controlled diagonal movements can be initiated.

After week 12, the patient should be able to tolerate plyometric exercises. The progression is the usual one previously discussed, starting with low-level movements and progressing to overhead movements once control is achieved at the lower elevation levels. The final step consists of functional activities and drills before return to full sport participation.

Case Study

A 21-year-old swimmer underwent an electrothermal capsular shift 10 days ago for anterior instability. The physician reports that the patient had no other joint damage and that no other surgical procedure was necessary. She is now to begin rehabilitation. She has some mild postoperative pain, but nothing unusual. She is to wear a sling for another four weeks but is permitted to remove the sling for rehabilitation. Her shoulder range of motion is 40° flexion, 30° abduction, and −5° external rotation. The rotator cuff and scapular rotators are grossly 4−/5 in strength, but there is more weakness in the scapular rotators than in the rotator cuff.

Questions for Analysis

1. What will be your first day's treatment?

2. What precautions will you provide this patient?

3. Outline your treatment progression for her.

4. What will you include in your functional program before her return to full sport participation?

ACROMIOCLAVICULAR SPRAIN

Although first-degree sprains are not usually difficult to manage, the treatment approach to more severe AC sprains is more complex. Considerations for the various degrees of AC sprains are presented, followed by a case study.

Program Considerations

Most sprains, regardless of severity, are not surgically repaired and are treated conservatively. The speed with which conservative care is advanced depends on the severity of the injury. In mild sprains, the shoulder may be immobilized in a sling for a few days to relieve the traction discomfort caused by the weight of the arm pulling on the AC joint. Modalities are used to relieve pain, swelling, and muscle spasm. Active and active assistive range of motion are initiated on day 1 or 2 following the injury. Isometrics to tolerance can also begin immediately. Once full motion is restored, a progression of strengthening exercises is used until the patient has full function without pain and is able to return to full sport participation.

In type II and III sprains, the AC ligament is torn. In type II sprains the coracoclavicular ligament is intact, but in type III sprains it is not. Some deformity is present in both type II and type III sprains. Attempts at immobilization are made, but they are often unsuccessful because of the discomfort and restriction of the immobilizing device and the difficulty in stabilizing the AC joint. The benefits of surgical repair for type III sprains are disputable. Most often the treatment option selected is nonsurgical: a sling is used to relieve the distraction force of the weight of the arm on the AC joint. Some deformity usually persists, but this is a cosmetic issue and does not interfere with activity and shoulder function. The more severe injuries (types IV, V, and VI) are often surgically repaired, because significant damage to both static and dynamic structures around the joint has occurred.

In the type II and III injuries, the shoulder may be immobilized for one to three weeks. Active assistive range of motion of the glenohumeral joint may begin early. Strengthening exercises (below 60°) follow a normal progression from stabilization, straight-plane, and low-level exercises to higher-level exercises and diagonal movements. Plyometric exercises are followed by functional exercises. Normal progression to heavy lifting occurs at about 8 to 12 weeks postinjury, and the patient returns to sport participation after having performed functional exercises correctly.

Case Study

A 17-year-old wrestler incurred a type II sprain of his right AC joint in last week's match. He is to begin rehabilitation today. The shoulder has been in a sling for the past week. The patient is able to take the arm out of the sling for brief periods of time, but he reports that keeping the sling off for longer than 4 h causes an ache in the top of the shoulder. The muscles also feel tired. Examination reveals 150° of shoulder flexion, 120° of shoulder abduction, 60° of external rotation, and 75° of internal rotation. Strength tests reveal grades of 4–/5 in the pectoralis major and rotator cuff; 3+/5 in the rhomboids, lower trapezius, and serratus anterior; and 4/5 in the deltoid and latissimus dorsi. You can palpate trigger points in the upper trapezius, pectoralis major, and supraspinatus muscles.

Questions for Analysis

1. What will your first treatment session include?
2. What are your goals for the first treatment session?
3. What instructions will you give the patient before he leaves today?
4. Outline the rehabilitation course, including a time line you anticipate for program changes and four examples of each type of exercise.
5. What will your functional exercise program include before return to sport participation?

BICEPS TENDON INJURIES

Although it might seem appropriate to deal with the biceps tendon in the chapter on the elbow, the biceps tendon plays an important role in shoulder stabilization. For this reason, injuries to the biceps tendon are discussed here.

Program Considerations

The most common injury seen in the biceps tendon is tendinitis. Tears, subluxations, and dislocations can also occur. Bicipital tendinitis occurs primarily in the long head and is usually secondary to shoulder instability, impingement, rotator cuff pathology, or other inflammations of the shoulder. The patient reports tenderness in the bicipital groove. Cervical pathology can refer into the biceps area and must be ruled out if no frank injury has occurred to cause the pain.

Biceps tendon ruptures are often associated with rotator cuff pathology, and most occur in middle-aged athletes. A sudden muscle contraction while the muscle is on stretch is a common mechanism of injury. Complete ruptures may display a "Popeye" muscle, but partial ruptures are not as obvious. Pain, spasm, and swelling are immediate signs. If the long head of the biceps is ruptured in a young patient, surgery may be indicated. The same injury in an older patient may or may not require surgery. Because the long head of the biceps provides glenohumeral stability, its surgical repair can be important in the younger and more active population.

Rehabilitation treatment must include an assessment of the rotator cuff, because pathology in this location is often related to biceps pathology. Control of pain, swelling, and inflammation is an initial goal of treatment. Use of modalities, anti-inflammatories, and rest initially may be beneficial. Rest is usually accompanied by active assistive range-of-motion exercises. Therapeutic exercises progress as tolerated to include a strengthening sequence similar to that listed for conditions discussed earlier. It should also obviously include supination and elbow flexion exercises.

Case Study

Three days ago a 21-year-old gymnast experienced a ruptured biceps injury while practicing on the rings. He is now ready to begin a rehabilitation program. There is ecchymosis in the distal arm and into the forearm. The area has swelling, and the biceps muscle feels tight from spasm. Elbow motion is −15° extension and 120° flexion. The patient has full passive supination but actively supinates 45°. Elbow flexion is 3+/5 and painful. The patient admits to having had shoulder pain last season that kept him out of competition for one month. This season the pain has been present but tolerable. He indicates that he has never injured his neck but that sometimes it feels stiff.

Questions for Analysis

1. What will your first treatment include, and what are your goals for the first treatment?

2. What other areas should you investigate before deciding on your course of treatment?

3. When do you expect to achieve full range of motion in the elbow?

4. When will you begin strengthening exercises, and what will your first week of exercises include?

SUMMARY

1. *Explain how knowledge of the mechanics of sport performance impacts the establishment of a therapeutic exercise program.*

   The shoulder is a complex structure composed of several joints and many muscles that must work synchronously to produce injury-free motion. When activity is not synchronous or when trauma occurs, the result is an injury that can affect the entire shoulder function. During specific motions such as pitching, swinging a golf club, swimming, or performing hits and serves in tennis, the shoulder and its joints and muscles must work in a specifically timed and synchronous manner to produce the desired effect with minimal risk of injury. The sport rehabilitation specialist must have an awareness and appreciation of these activities to properly rehabilitate the patient for return to full sport participation.

2. *Discuss the importance of stability in shoulder rehabilitation.*

   Stability of the glenohumeral and scapulothoracic joints is crucial to performance and to reduced injury risk for the shoulder. Studies have demonstrated the significance of good stabilization of these joints and the importance of good therapeutic exercise programs to permit restoration of stability of these areas.

3. *Explain the role of scapular stabilization in shoulder function.*

   Basic to shoulder function is scapular stabilization during shoulder activities. Scapular muscles serve as the foundation from which the shoulder moves; so when scapular muscles do not function properly, either because of weakness, loss of motion, or reduced endurance, the shoulder is at great risk of injury.

4. *Describe two soft-tissue mobilization techniques for the shoulder.*

   Cross-friction massage to the biceps tendon and anterior rotator cuff muscles is commonly performed with tendinitis injuries. Trigger point releases to rotator cuff muscles, such as the supraspinatus in the supraspinatus fossa or the teres minor at the lateral border of the scapula, are commonly performed to relieve pain and improve motion.

5. *List three joint mobilizations for the shoulder.*

   Shoulder joint mobilization techniques should include techniques for the specifically restricted joints. If the AC joint is restricted, posterior-anterior, superior, and inferior glides can be used. If the scapula is restricted, scapular distraction is appropriate. If the glenohumeral joint is restricted, an arm pull is a gross technique, and an inferior glide is a more specific technique for improving joint mobility.

6. *Identify three strengthening exercises for the scapulae and three for the glenohumeral muscles.*

   Scapular muscle-strengthening exercises can include maneuvers such as push-up-plus exercises, prone flys, and Bouhler exercises. Glenohumeral muscle strengthening exercises can include internal and external rotation exercises starting with isometric exercises and moving to rubber tubing and free-weight exercises, as well as abduction in the scapular plane.

7. *Discuss the general progression of strengthening exercises for the shoulder.*

   The specific progression depends on the specific injury and its severity. A general progression of strengthening exercises begins with scapular stabilization exercises and isometric rotator cuff exercises. Manual resistance to the scapular muscles can begin early in the program. From there the exercises include active resistive exercises in the lower third of shoulder motion until the scapular muscles are strong enough to provide scapular control in the middle ranges of motion and finally in motion over 100°, so overhead exercises can be performed without loss of control of scapular and glenohumeral positioning. Eccentric exercises for the rotator cuff using rubber tubing, medicine balls, and even manual resistance begin in straight planes and progress to diagonal planes. Exercises in both weight bearing and non-weight bearing are used for stabilization and strengthening. Plyometric activities begin slowly and progress as the patient gains proficiency. Functional exercises using sport equipment such as a tennis racket or golf club then begin, at first in low ranges of motion with reduced force until control and proficiency have been demonstrated. Exercises next progress to greater ranges of motion and begin to mimic the actual activity. Functional overhead activities are the last item to be added to the program. In addition to the shoulder, the biceps, triceps, and abdominal muscles must also be included in the program.

8. *List precautions for a therapeutic exercise program following a rotator cuff repair.*

   Care must be taken to allow tissue healing before exercises begin. Range of motion usually begins at 7 to 10 days. If immobilization continues for an extended period of time, there can be complications such as adhesive capsulitis, especially in older patients. Range-of-motion exercises begin with activities such as Codman's and must progress on the basis of the status of the healing tissues. Strength exercises begin slowly with high endurance and low resistance, progressing as the patient gains control and strength. Scapular exercises can be initiated early, but rotator cuff exercises begin with submaximal isometrics. Range-of-motion gains in external rotation occur slowly and cautiously.

9. *Outline key factors for a program for a biceps rupture.*

   Active range of motion for shoulder, elbow, and forearm is followed by strengthening exercises for motions including elbow flexion, supination, and shoulder flexion and extension. Progression of exercises follows a pattern similar to that for other shoulder programs, according to considerations regarding pain, control, and tissue healing.

CRITICAL THINKING QUESTIONS

1. If you were Mac in the opening scenario for this chapter, what techniques would you have used to relieve Jason's posterior shoulder tightness and the scapular muscle weakness? What plyometric progression would you have used to advance him to functional activities? What criteria would you have used to begin his functional activities, and what would your throwing progression have been?

2. If an injured wrestler who experienced a shoulder dislocation two weeks ago comes to you to begin rehabilitation, what must be your greatest precaution with him? How much elevation can you safely place the shoulder in? What is your reasoning for this amount of motion? What exercises should you be able to do with him at two weeks postinjury?

3. If the rehabilitation process and the results for electrothermally assisted capsular shift procedures have not yet been fully documented, what guidelines can you use when a patient comes to you after this procedure has been performed on his or her shoulder? Based on your knowledge of healing and the shoulder, what precautions should be taken, and what exercises can you perform in the first three to six weeks postoperatively?

4. Recall the case of the 40-year-old tennis player presented in the section on impingement in this chapter. Have you figured out the cause of her problem? If posture is a primary contributing factor, what instructions will you give her to relieve the cause? What exercises will reinforce your efforts to change her posture? If her posture has been incorrect for some time, what soft-tissue changes would you expect will need to be treated?

5. If you have a patient whose diagnosis has been narrowed down to a rotator cuff tendinitis, shoulder instability, shoulder impingement, capsulitis, and cervical radiculopathy, how will you determine which diagnosis is correct? What tests will you use to differentiate between these diagnoses? Would the rehabilitation program change with different diagnoses? Why or why not?

REFERENCES

Akeson, W.H., Woo, S.L-Y., Amiel, D., Coutts, R.D., and D. Daniel. 1973. The connective tissue response to immobility: Biochemical changes in periarticular connective tissue of the immobilized rabbit knee. *Clinical Orthopedics* 93:356–365.

Bradley, J.P., and J.E. Tibone. 1991. Electromyographic analysis of muscle action about the shoulder. *Clinics in Sports Medicine* 10:789–805.

Cyriax, J.H. 1975. *Textbook of orthopaedic medicine. Vol. 1. Diagnosis of soft tissue lesions.* 6th ed. Baltimore: Williams & Wilkins.

Ellenbecker, T.S., and A.J. Mattalino. 1999. Glenohumeral joint range of motion and rotator cuff strength following arthoscopic anterior stabilization with thermal capsulorrhaphy. *Journal of Orthopaedic and Sports Physical Therapy* 29:160–167.

Hayashi, K., Thabit, G. III, Bogdanske, J.J., Mascio, L.N., and M.D. Markel. 1996. The effect of nonablative laser energy on the ultrastructure of joint capsular collagen. *Arthroscopy: The Journal of Arthroscopic and Related Surgery* 12:474–481.

Hayashi, K., Thabit, G. III, Massa, K.L., Bogdanske, J.J., Cooley, A.J., Orwin, J.F., and M.D. Markel. 1997. The effect of thermal heating on the length and histologic properties of the glenohumeral joint capsule. *American Journal of Sports Medicine* 25:107–112.

Host, H.H. 1995. Scapular taping in the treatment of anterior shoulder impingement. *Physical Therapy* 75:803–812.

Jobe, F.W., Moynes, D.R., and D.J. Antonelli. 1985. Rotator cuff function during the golf swing. *American Journal of Sports Medicine* 14:388–392.

Kamkar, A., Irrgang, J.J., and S.L. Whitney. 1993. Nonoperative management of secondary impingement syndrome. *Journal of Orthopaedic and Sports Physical Therapy* 17:212–224.

Kelley, M.J. 1995. Anatomic and biomechanical rationale for rehabilitation of the athlete's shoulder. *Journal of Sports Rehabilitation* 4:122–154.

Kibler, W.B. 1995. Biomechanical analysis of the shoulder during tennis activities. *Clinics in Sports Medicine* 14:79–85.

Lear, L.J., and M.T. Gross. 1998. An electromyographical analysis of the scapular stabilizing synergists during a push-up progression. *Journal of Orthopaedic and Sports Physical Therapy* 28:146–157.

Lephart, S.M., and T.J. Henry. 1996. The physiological basis for open and closed kinetic chain rehabilitation for the upper extremity. *Journal of Sport Rehabilitation* 5:71–87.

McQuade, K.J., Dawson, J., and G.L. Smidt. 1998. Scapulothoracic muscle fatigue associated with alterations in scapulohumeral rhythm kinematics during maximum resistive shoulder elevation. *Journal of Orthopaedics and Sports Medicine* 28:74–80.

Morin, G.E., Tiberio, D., and G. Austin. 1997. The effect of upper trapezius taping on electromyographic activity in the upper and middle trapezius region. *Journal of Sports Rehabilitation* 6:309–318.

Moynes, D.R., Perry, J., Antonelli, D.J., and F.W. Jobe. 1986. Electromyography and motion analysis of the upper extremity in sports. *Journal of the American Physical Therapy Association* 66:1905–1911.

Nuber, G.W., Jobe, F.W., Perry, J., Moynes, D.R., and D. Antonelli. 1986. Fine wire electromyography analysis of muscles of the shoulder during swimming. *American Journal of Sports Medicine* 14:7–11.

Pappas, A.M., Zawacki, R.M., and T.J. Sullivan. 1985. Biomechanics of baseball pitching, a preliminary report. *American Journal of Sports Medicine* 13:216–222.

Perry, J. 1978. Normal upper extremity kinesiology. *Physical Therapy* 58:265–278.

Perry, J. 1983. Anatomy and biomechanics of the shoulder in throwing, swimming, gymnastics, and tennis. *Clinics in Sports Medicine* 2:247–270.

Pink, M., Perry, J., Browne, A., Scovazzo, M.L., and J. Kerrigan. 1991. The normal shoulder during freestyle swimming. *American Journal of Sports Medicine* 19:569–576.

Richardson, A.B., Jobe, F.W., and H.R. Collins. 1980. The shoulder in competitive swimming. *American Journal of Sports Medicine* 8:159–164.

Ryu, R.K.N., McCormick, J., Jobe, F.W., Moynes, D.R., and D.J. Antonelli. 1988. An electromyographic analysis of shoulder function in tennis players. *American Journal of Sports Medicine* 16:481–485.

Travell, J.G., and D.G. Simons. 1983. *Myofascial pain and dysfunction. The trigger point manual.* Vol. 1. Baltimore: Williams & Wilkins.

SUGGESTED READING

Allegrucci, M., Whitney, S.L., and J.J. Irrgang. 1994. Clinical implications of secondary impingement of the shoulder in freestyle swimmers. *Journal of Orthopaedic and Sports Physical Therapy* 20:312–318.

Andrews, J.R., and K.E. Wilk. 1994. *The athlete's shoulder.* New York: Churchill Livingstone.

Bonci, C.M., Sloane, B., and K. Middleton. 1992. Nonsurgical/surgical rehabilitation of the unstable shoulder. *Journal of Sport Rehabilitation* 1:146–171.

Braatz, J.H., and P.P. Gogia. 1987. The mechanics of pitching. *Journal of Orthopaedic and Sports Physical Therapy* 9:56–69.

Brewster, C., and D.R. Moynes Schwab. 1993. Rehabilitation of the shoulder following rotator cuff injury or surgery. *Journal of Orthopaedic and Sports Physical Therapy* 18:422–426.

Culham, E., and M. Peat. 1993. Functional anatomy of the shoulder complex. *Journal of Orthopaedic and Sports Physical Therapy* 18:342–350.

Davies, G.J., and S. Dickoff-Hoffman. 1993. Neuromuscular testing and rehabilitation of the shoulder complex. *Journal of Orthopaedic and Sports Physical Therapy* 18:449–458.

Dillman, C.J., Fleisig, G.S., and J.R. Andrews. 1993. Biomechanics of pitching with emphasis upon shoulder kinematics. *Journal of Orthopaedic and Sports Physical Therapy* 18:402–408.

Grubbs, N. 1993. Frozen shoulder syndrome: A review of literature. *Journal of Orthopaedic and Sports Physical Therapy* 18:479–487.

Jobe, F.W., and J.P. Bradley. 1989. The diagnosis and nonoperative treatment of shoulder injuries in athletes. *Clinics in Sports Medicine* 8:419–438.

Jobe, F.W., Moynes, D.R., and C.E. Brewster. 1987. Rehabilitation of shoulder joint instabilities. *Orthopedic Clinics of North America* 18:473–482.

Litchfield, R., Hawkins, R., Dillman, C.J., Atkins, J., and G. Hagerman. 1993. Rehabilitation for the overhead athlete. *Journal of Orthopaedic and Sports Physical Therapy* 18:433–442.

McQuade, K.J., and G.L. Smidt. 1998. Dynamic scapulohumeral rhythm: The effects of external resistance during elevation of the arm in the scapular plane. *Journal of Orthopaedic and Sports Physical Therapy* 27:125–133.

Meister, K., and J.R. Andrews. 1993. Classification and treatment of rotator cuff injuries in the overhand athlete. *Journal of Orthopaedic and Sports Physical Therapy* 18:413–421.

Moynes, D.R. 1983. Prevention of injury to the shoulder through exercises and therapy. *Clinics in Sports Medicine* 2:413–422.

Pappas, A.M., Zawacki, R.M., and C.F. McCarthy. 1985. Rehabilitation of the pitching shoulder. *American Journal of Sports Medicine* 13:223–235.

Payne, R.M., and M. Voight. 1993. The role of the scapula. *Journal of Orthopaedic and Sports Physical Therapy* 18:386–391.

Pezzullo, D.J., Karas, S., and J.J. Irrgang. 1995. Functional plyometric exercises for the throwing athlete. *Journal of Athletic Training* 30:22–26.

Plancher, K.D., Litchfield, R., and R.J. Hawkins. 1995. Rehabilitation of the shoulder in tennis players. *Clinics in Sports Medicine* 14:111–137.

Stone, J.A., Lueken, J.S., Partin, N.B., Timm, K.E., and E.J. Ryan. 1993. Closed kinetic chain rehabilitation for the glenohumeral joint. *Journal of Athletic Training* 28:34–37.

Wilk, K.E., and C. Arrigo. 1993. Current concepts in the rehabilitation of the athletic shoulder. *Journal of Orthopaedic and Sports Physical Therapy* 18:365–378.

Wilk, K.E., Voight, M.L., Keirns, M.A., Gambetta, V., Andrews, J.R., and C.J. Dillman. 1993. Stretch shortening drills for the upper extremities: Theory and clinical application. *Journal of Orthopaedic and Sports Physical Therapy* 17:225–239.

Zmierski, T., Kegerreis, S., and J. Scarpaci. 1995. Scapular muscle strengthening. *Journal of Sport Rehabilitation* 4:244–252.

CHAPTER EIGHTEEN

Elbow and Forearm

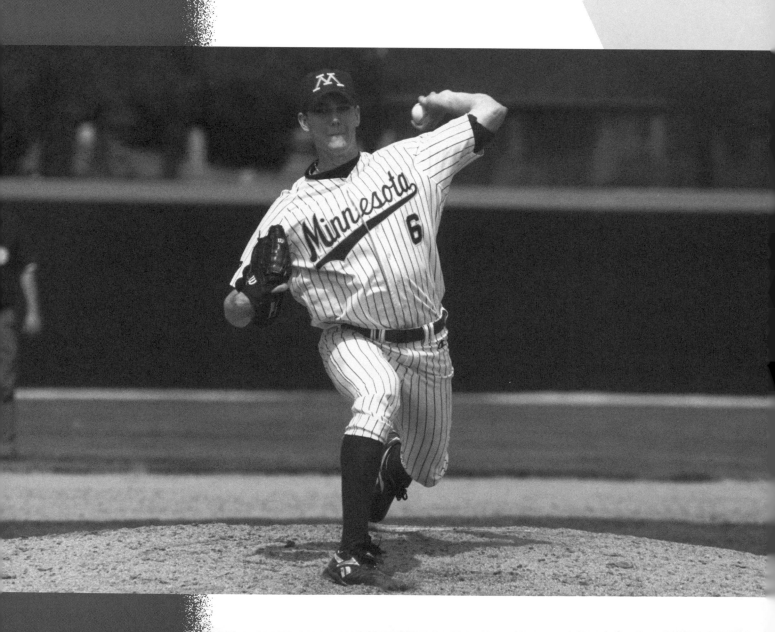

OBJECTIVES

After completing this chapter, you should be able to do the following:

1. Discuss why you should avoid overstretching the elbow, especially during the inflammation phase of healing.

2. Describe the convex-concave rules for the various elbow joints.

3. Identify the loose-packed positions for the elbow joints.

4. Identify three soft-tissue mobilization techniques for the elbow.

5. List three joint mobilizations for the elbow.

6. Explain three strengthening exercises for the elbow, and their purpose.

7. Discuss the general progression of strengthening exercises for the elbow.

8. Outline a therapeutic exercise program for epicondylitis.

9. Indicate precautions to consider in a Little League elbow therapeutic exercise program.

10. List precautions, following an ulnar nerve transposition, for a therapeutic exercise program.

11. Explain the differences in rehabilitation programs for an arthroscopic debridement and a medial collateral reconstruction.

Rita Jolley has worked as the certified athletic trainer in the local high school for the past 10 years. Occasionally a parent brings a preteen athlete to her, knowing that she has worked successfully with the child's older sibling. She normally provides an evaluation of the youngster's injury and makes recommendations to the parents for first-aid treatment or referral to the family physician.

Today she is visited by a parent who is familiar to Rita because he has had two teenagers pass through Rita's athletic training room during their high school careers. Mr. Skully reports that his youngest son, 10-year-old Pat, developed medial elbow pain while pitching in a Little League baseball game last week. Although it had been bothering him for a couple of weeks before last week's game, Pat hadn't complained about it until the pain had become too intense.

From her past experience, Rita suspected Little League elbow. But she knew she should not assume anything and should perform an evaluation with an open mind before she came to any conclusions.

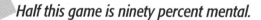

Half this game is ninety percent mental.

Danny Ozark, Philadelphia Phillies manager

Like the spine and the shoulder, the elbow has special and distinct characteristics that must be considered in developing rehabilitation programs for elbow injuries. As the joint between two long lever arms, the elbow can experience large force applications from its proximal and distal arms. Open chain activities apply large velocities with sudden acceleration and deceleration forces from the proximal arm of the joint, while closed chain activities apply compressive stresses and torsional forces from the distal arm. The elbow muscles must work synchronously with adjacent structures, and the joint and muscles must have the flexibility necessary to withstand these forces.

Because the elbow lies between the shoulder and wrist, some muscles that traverse the elbow also affect the shoulder or wrist. It is difficult to separate these and thus was difficult to decide which chapter some of the techniques and exercises should be delegated to. It may seem that some of the techniques and exercises presented in this chapter would be better suited to the shoulder chapter or the wrist chapter. That may be the case, but how best to classify the exercise depends on the injury. For example, if a patient has a tennis-elbow injury, exercises and techniques for wrist extensor muscles are appropriately discussed in the context of the elbow. However, if a patient has a wrist sprain, those same techniques and exercises for wrist extensor muscles are best addressed in a discussion of wrist injuries. For this reason, some of the techniques and exercises you read about in this chapter are also referred to in the next chapter on the wrist and hand.

This chapter outlines basic considerations for elbow rehabilitation and then presents soft-tissue and joint mobilization techniques, flexibility and strength exercises, and plyometric and functional considerations. Distinctive considerations for some of the more commonly seen elbow injuries are discussed, and case studies for these injuries are presented so that you can problem solve and devise your own rehabilitation program.

GENERAL REHABILITATION CONSIDERATIONS

The design and execution of a therapeutic exercise program for the elbow must take into account the types of joint stresses incurred by the elbow, its unique structure, the mobility of its joints, and the amount of force application that is appropriate.

The elbow is unique in several ways, and the sport rehabilitation specialist needs to understand its distinctive characteristics to properly design and execute a therapeutic exercise program. The following sections focus on these characteristics.

JOINT STRESSES

As mentioned in chapter 17, overhead motions are actually a total body movement that includes a summation of forces and properly timed execution of movement, started in the lower extremities and trunk and transferred to the shoulder, elbow, and hand. As the summation of forces accelerates the arm in throwing sports, the elbow and forearm velocity must occur at high rates to successfully propel the hand or object at the desired speed. Researchers have reported different angular velocities for different sports. Baseball pitching produces the highest velocity at 2300°/s (Feltner and Dapena 1986). Javelin athletes experience an angular velocity of 1900°/s (Mero et al. 1994); the tennis serve has been recorded at 982°/s (Kibler 1995); and in fast-pitch softball, 680°/s velocities have been recorded (Ellenbecker and Mattalino 1997).

Most of these overhead motions place additional valgus or varus stress on the joint. The greatest speeds and force applications occur during acceleration and deceleration phases of movement. High demands are placed on the biceps, brachioradialis, and brachialis during deceleration to slow down forearm motion and prevent overextension and injury to the elbow. During acceleration the elbow experiences compressive forces laterally and distraction forces medially. The medial stresses can result in injuries such as neuritis, tendinitis, and medial joint sprains and muscle sprains. The lateral stresses can cause osteochondritis dissecans in young athletes, and bony osteophytes, articular damage, and degeneration in older athletes. It is common for athletes with an extended throwing career to develop flexion contractures because of articular and muscular changes. Proper mechanics, timing, and balanced joint and muscle function are crucial in the prevention of elbow injuries. If biomechanics are altered because of these deficiencies, the stresses are magnified. In pitching, the forces applied are a valgus distraction stress medially with a lateral compressive force. Tennis produces stress over the lateral epicondyle during the backhand stroke and medial epicondyle stresses during overhead serves and late-hit forehand strokes. Gymnastics, an upper-extremity weight-bearing sport, places excessive lateral stress on the joint because of the elbow's normal valgus position. Golfers with incorrect mechanics can place excessive medial force on the trailing elbow or excessive lateral force on the leading elbow. Pitchers with inflexibility of hips, trunk, or shoulder open up too soon and increase the elbow's medial joint stress. If tightness, weakness, or fatigue causes the elbow to drop, increased medial joint stresses are placed on the elbow during the cocking phase in pitching. In tennis, increased lateral stress is placed on the elbow when the player leads with the elbow on the backhand, and increased medial stress is applied on the forehand stroke when the ball is hit late.

It is important for the sport rehabilitation specialist to understand these concepts because the rehabilitation program should include an assessment of the patient's skill execution. Incorrect techniques may be the underlying cause of the problem, and the program must include correction of those techniques to prevent recurrence of the injury.

UNIQUE STRUCTURE

The elbow has unique anatomical characteristics that can be advantageous or disadvantageous. The joint has a high degree of congruency within the ulnohumeral joint. That makes it stable. One of the more distinctive characteristics is that a muscle, not it's tendon, traverses the joint. The brachialis muscle not only traverses the joint, but it also inserts onto the elbow's anterior superior capsule. This can cause problems when elbow immobilization is required following injury. Scarring and limitation of motion can easily occur in this area. Immobilization should be used cautiously, and extended immobilization should be avoided. More than two weeks of immobilization can cause severe restrictions of the elbow's joint mobility. Complicating this reality that adhesions occur relatively easily in the elbow is the fact that the joint's anterior capsule is relatively thin and can easily incur damage with aggressive stretching, resulting in additional scarring. For this reason, it is important that aggressive, high-intensity stretching at the elbow be avoided. This is particularly crucial during the inflammation phase when the area is weaker and more easily aggravated than will be the case later. Soft-tissue tearing, scarring, and loss of joint motion can occur with passive overstretching. Early stretching techniques should include primarily active stretches. Passive range-of-motion exercises are permissible, but they should be pain free and should be performed in controlled and monitored situations.

JOINT MOBILITY

The elbow has three joints that should be assessed for joint mobility: the ulnohumeral, humeroradial, and radioulnar joints. Each joint has different **loose-packed** and **close-packed positions** that you should recall when performing mobilization techniques. The ulnohumeral joint's loose-packed position is at 70° elbow flexion with 10° supination, and its close-packed position is in full extension. The humeroradial joint's loose-packed position is at full extension and full supination, and its close-packed position is at midflexion with midpronation. The radioulnar joint's loose-packed position is at 70° elbow flexion with 35° supination, and its close-packed position is at full pronation or full supination. Joint mobilization should be performed initially in the loose-packed position, where there is the greatest mobility and the least stress is applied to the joint. In later stages, it may be necessary to move the joint toward the close-packed position to perform mobilizations. The close-packed position can also be used as an exercise position for unstable joints to provide increased stability during resistance activities.

Because the ulnohumeral and radiohumeral joints have the concave ulna and concave radius moving on the convex humerus, the **concave-convex rule** applies for mobilization techniques to these joints. The mobilization force application should be in the same direction as the restricted movement. Joint distraction applied in a loose-packed position will stretch the anterior and posterior capsule. If the elbow is placed in flexion, and distraction is applied, the posterior capsule is stretched to increase elbow flexion; but if distraction is applied with the joint in extension, the anterior capsule is stretched to increase elbow extension.

The radius and ulna are connected by two joints, the proximal radioulnar joint at the elbow and the distal radioulnar joint at the wrist. Both joints must have normal movement to produce full supination and pronation. The proximal joint at the elbow is formed by the convex radial head in the concave ulnar notch. This joint abides by the convex-concave mobilization rule. The mobilization force application is in the opposite direction of restricted movement. To improve supination, the force is applied anterior to posterior; to improve pronation, the force is applied posterior to anterior.

FORCE APPLICATIONS

Depending on the specific injury, the sport rehabilitation specialist may need to take special precautions with some strength exercises. Stresses applied to the elbow during strengthening can be excessive, depending on the arm position and the weight lifted. Lifting weights with the elbow extended places more stress on the anterior elbow, while lifting weights with the elbow flexed places more stress on the posterior elbow. Because of lever-arm lengths, a resultant force of up to three times body weight occurs when the elbow is flexed 30° (Ellenbecker and Mattalino 1997). Lighter weights or cuffs attached to the mid-forearm reduce these stresses.

An exercise such as a push-up delivers stress to the elbow, but the arm position determines the degree of stress. In a normal push-up position, the greatest compression force at the elbow is 45% of body weight, but the compression force is decreased if the hands are moved farther apart. In the superior position the compression force is decreased in the elbow, but the valgus torque is increased by 54% (Donkers et al. 1993).

Low-resistance, high-repetition strength exercises are commonly used in the early phases of elbow rehabilitation to reduce excessive stresses such as these on the joint. Once healing of tissue has occurred and neuromuscular control and strength gains are such that good joint control is possible, increased weights can be used.

SOFT-TISSUE MOBILIZATION

A therapeutic exercise program for the elbow includes trigger point release, ice-and-stretch, and cross-friction massage for the elbow movers and the wrist and finger movers, as well as cross-friction massage for elbow tendinitis.

The techniques addressed here are primarily trigger point release, ice-and-stretch, and cross-friction massage techniques. The trigger point referral patterns, trigger point release, and ice-and-stretch procedures described here are based on the work of Travell and Simons (1983). The muscles mentioned here are also muscles that are addressed in chapter 19 on the wrist and hand, because most of the muscles originating at the elbow function at the wrist and hand.

It is important to note the locations of the patient's pain. Pain assessment necessitates investigation and elimination or confirmation of trigger points, neurological pathology, or localized injury as the source of the pain. If pain is not neurologically based, trigger points may often be the source, especially in situations in which the site of injury is different from the location of pain.

ELBOW MOVERS

Along with pure elbow muscles, elbow movers also include muscles that cross the shoulder, biceps, and triceps but whose primary function is at the elbow.

Biceps Brachii

This muscle refers pain to the anterior deltoid and antecubital space, as well as into the suprascapular and distal biceps regions (figure 18.1, a and b). Trigger point release is performed with the patient supine or seated and the elbow slightly flexed and supinated. The trigger points on the distal one third of the muscle are palpated first superficially, then more deeply for tender areas or taut bands. A strumming of the taut band, a deep pressure over the trigger point, or a pincher grasp on the muscle can be used (figure 18.1c).

Ice-and-stretch is performed with the patient sitting. The shoulder is abducted to 90°, externally rotated, and horizontally abducted. The elbow is extended and the forearm pronated to put the biceps on stretch as ice sweeps are made from distal to the elbow proximally along the upper arm and to the shoulder (figure 18.1d).

Brachialis

The brachialis refers pain to the anterior carpometacarpal thumb joint and thumb's dorsal web space (figure 18.2a). It can also refer to the anterior arm and antecubital space (figure 18.2b). Trigger point release is performed with the patient supine or sitting and the elbow flexed about 45°. The biceps muscle is pushed medially to gain access to the brachialis (figure 18.2c). The distal trigger points most commonly refer to the thumb or antecubital space, and the more proximal points refer to the arm.

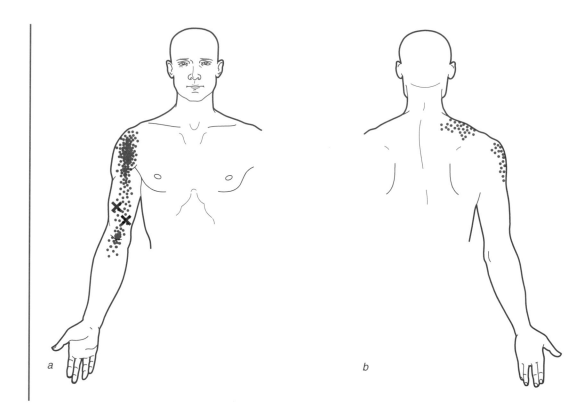

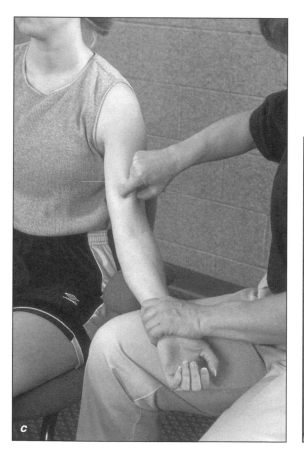

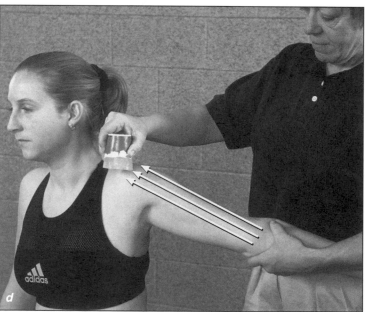

▌Figure 18.1 Biceps brachii pain referral patterns *(a–b)*, trigger point release *(c)*, and ice-and-stretch *(d)*.

Ice-and-stretch is performed with the muscle on stretch and the patient in sitting or supine. The elbow is extended with support behind it as ice is stroked in the direction of pain referral from the elbow, either proximally along the arm or distally along the forearm to the thumb (figure 18.2d).

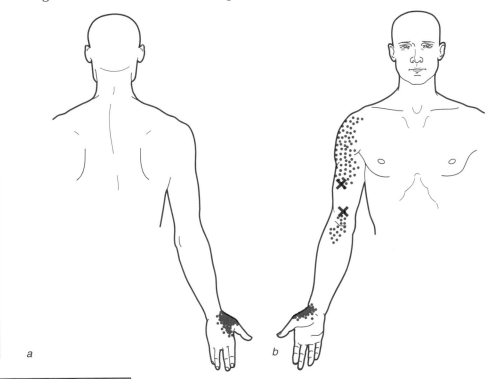

a   b

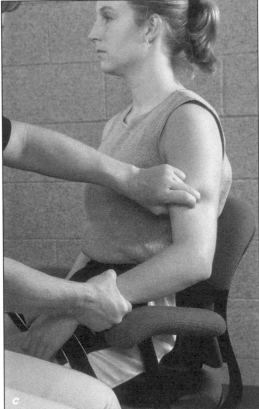

c

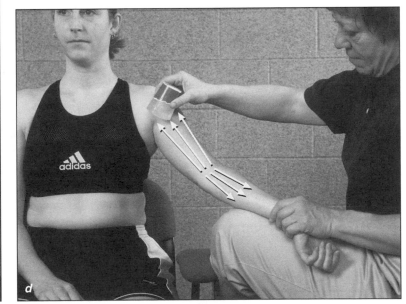

d

Figure 18.2 Brachialis pain referral patterns *(a–b)*, trigger point release *(c)*, and ice-and-stretch *(d)*.

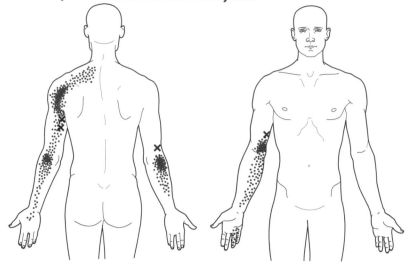
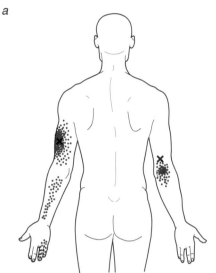
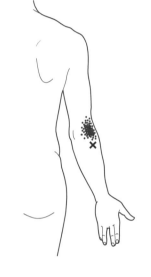

a

b

c

d

Triceps Brachii and Anconeus

The three heads of this muscle refer pain along the posterior arm to the shoulder and sometimes into the upper trapezius. They can refer pain into the lateral epicondyle, medial epicondyle, and olecranon process; along the lateral or posterior forearm; and to the fourth and fifth digits (figure 18.3, a–c). The anconeus muscle refers pain locally to the lateral epicondyle (figure 18.3d).

Trigger point release is performed with the muscle relaxed, the elbow in slight flexion, and the patient in supine. The taut band can be treated with a pincher grasp, or deep pressure over the trigger point sites can be used (figure 18.3e).

Ice-and-stretch is performed with the patient supine or sitting. The triceps is placed on stretch with the shoulder and elbow flexed as the ice is applied from the scapula along the posterior arm and forearm (figure 18.3f).

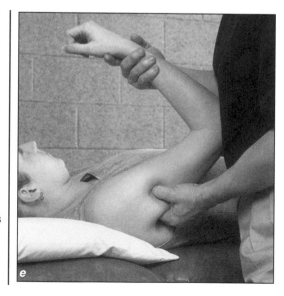
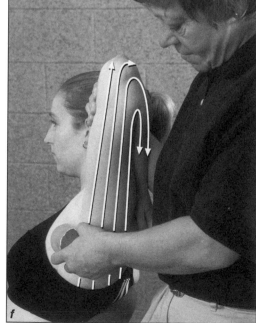

■ **Figure 18.3**
Triceps and anconeus pain referral patterns *(a–d)*, trigger point release *(e)*, and ice-and-stretch *(f)*.

Supinator

The most common site of pain referral for this muscle is locally around the lateral epicondyle and lateral elbow region (figure 18.4a). The supinator can also refer to the dorsal thumb web space (figure 18.4b). A supinator trigger point is commonly seen with tennis elbow. Trigger point release is performed with the elbow slightly flexed and fully supinated. Deep pressure is applied between the biceps tendon and brachioradialis muscle (figure 18.4c).

Ice-and-stretch is applied with the patient relaxed in supine or sitting. With the elbow in extension and the forearm in pronation, ice strokes are swept from the elbow in the direction of referred pain, either superiorly along the lateral arm or inferiorly along the radial aspect of the forearm to the thumb (figure 18.4d).

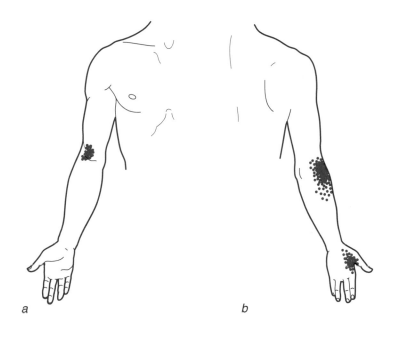

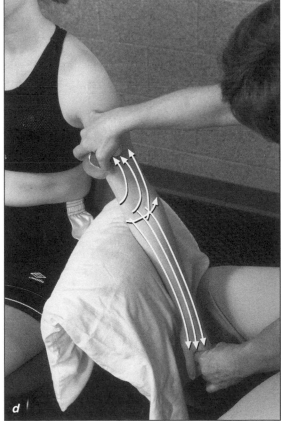

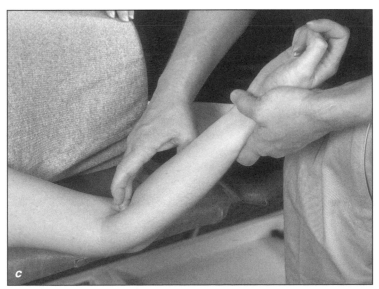

■ **Figure 18.4** Supinator pain-referral patterns *(a–b)*, myofascial release *(c)*, and ice-and-stretch *(d)*.

WRIST AND FINGER MOVERS

It may seem odd to discuss wrist and finger muscles in the elbow chapter, but the long wrist and finger muscles also act on the elbow because they insert proximal to the elbow joint. Although their main function is in the distal upper extremity, the location of their proximal insertion necessitates attention to these muscles in the context of the elbow.

Wrist Extensors and Brachioradialis

Although the extensor carpi radialis rarely has active trigger points, the other muscles here are often activated with lateral epicondylitis. The radial extensors refer pain to the lateral epicondyle, to the hand's dorsum, and in the anatomical snuffbox area (figure 18.5, b and c). The ulnar extensors refer pain to the posterior ulnar wrist (figure 18.5a). The brachioradialis refers pain to the lateral epicondyle, to the thumb's web space, and less often along its muscle belly (figure 18.5d). Trigger point release is performed with the patient in sitting and the forearm supported in partial flexion and full pronation. The trigger points can be treated with either direct pressure (figure 18.5, e–g) or a pincher grasp (figure 18.5h).

Ice-and-stretch is performed with the patient supine or sitting and a support placed under the elbow. For the wrist extensors, the elbow is placed on stretch in an extended position, forearm pronated and wrist flexed as the ice strokes are swept from just above the elbow downward along the posterior forearm and past the wrist (figure 18.5i). For the brachioradialis, the stretch and ice sweeps are similar except that the wrist is placed in flexion with ulnar deviation and forearm pronation (figure 18.5j).

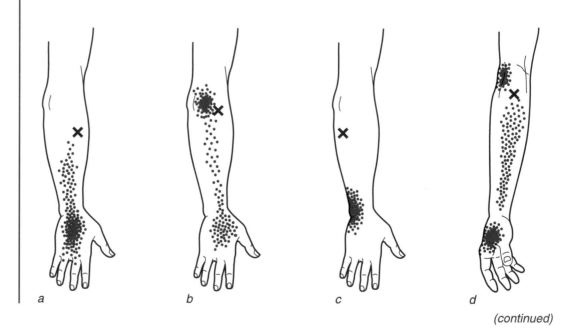

a   b   c   d

(continued)

∎ **Figure 18.5**   Brachioradialis and wrist extensor myofascial release: pain referral patterns for extensor carpi radialis brevis *(a)*, extensor carpi radialis longus *(b)*, extensor carpi ulnaris *(c)*, brachioradialis *(d)*. Trigger point release of extensor carpi radialis longus *(e)*, extensor carpi radialis brevis *(f)*, extensor carpi ulnaris *(g)*, brachioradialis using pincher grasp *(h)*. Ice-and-stretch of wrist extensor *(i)*, brachioradialis *(j)*.

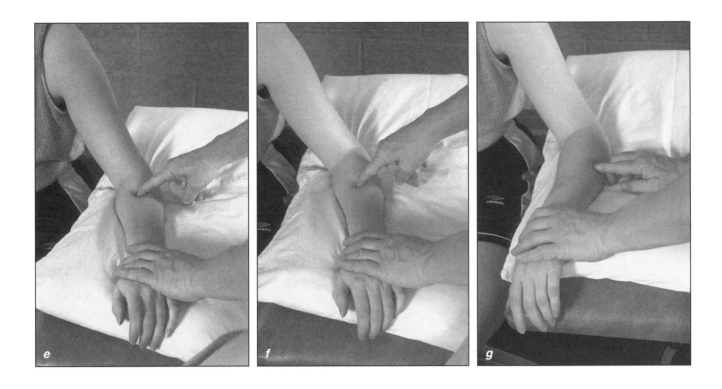

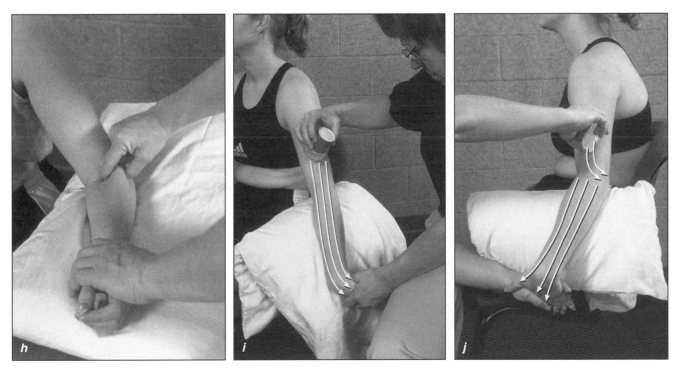

■ **Figure 18.5** *(continued)*

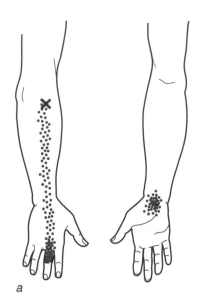
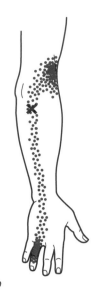
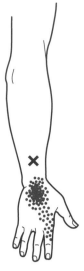

a b c

Finger Extensors

These muscles can refer pain during injuries such as lateral epicondylitis. They refer pain down the forearm along the back of the hand and to the fingers they move (figure 18.6, a–c). The lateral epicondyle is a common pain-referral site. Pain and stiffness of the fingers and hand can also be present even though the source of pain is more proximal.

Trigger point release is performed with the elbow in flexion, the forearm pro-nated, and the wrist flexed. The middle-finger extensor trigger point is located about 3 to 4 cm (1.2–1.6 in.) distally from the radial head and can be treated with direct pressure or a pincher grasp (figure 18.6d). The ring- and little-finger extensor trigger points are located deep and are lateral to the extensor carpi ulnaris. The extensor indicis trigger point is distal on the forearm between the radius and ulna.

Ice-and-stretch is applied with the forearm supported, the elbow extended, and the wrist and fingers flexed as ice is swept distally from the muscle's proximal insertion on the lateral epicondyle toward the fingers (figure 18.6e).

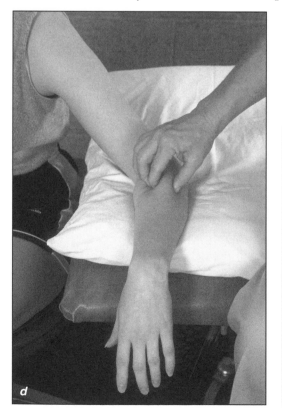

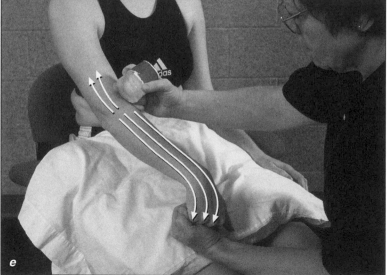

■ **Figure 18.6** Finger extensor myofascial release: *(a)* middle-finger extensor, *(b)* ring-finger extensor, *(c)* extensor indicis, *(d)* trigger point release, *(e)* ice-and-stretch.

Finger and Wrist Flexors, and Pronator Teres

The finger flexors refer into and beyond the end of the digits they move. The wrist flexors refer to the side of the wrist they flex, and the pronator teres refers to the radial wrist with overflow along the radial aspect of the anterior forearm and into the base of the thumb (figure 18.7, a–e).

Trigger point release is performed with the forearm supported and in supination. The wrist should be in a relaxed extension position. Deep pressure is applied to the trigger point areas (figure 18.7f).

Ice-and-stretch is applied with the patient sitting or supine. The forearm is supported in supination, and the elbow is extended. Ice strokes are swept from proximal to the medial epicondyle distally along the anterior forearm to the wrist, and into the digit being treated, as an extension stretch is applied to the wrist and fingers (figure 18.7g).

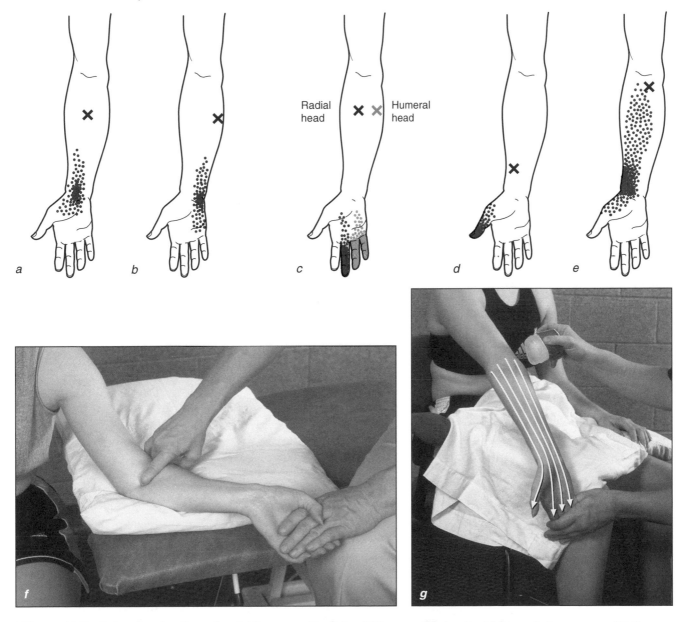

∎ **Figure 18.7**   Pain referral patterns for: *(a)* flexor carpi radialis, *(b)* flexor carpi ulnaris, *(c)* flexor digitorum superficialis (dark = radial head, light = humeral head), *(d)* flexor pollicus longus, *(e)* pronator teres. Pronator teres, and wrist and finger flexor trigger point release about 3 cm distal and slightly lateral to the medial epicondyle, *(f)* and ice-and-stretch *(g)*.

CROSS-FRICTION MASSAGE

This technique is usually performed over the lateral or medial epicondyle as part of the treatment for tendinitis. The area of tenderness is isolated with a finger or thumb pad. Pressure over the area is maintained while deep friction is applied to the area. The finger or thumb moves the overlying soft tissue against the underlying bone in a direction perpendicular to the fiber direction: Figure 18.8 shows application over the lateral epicondyle. Sometimes it may be necessary to pull the skin taut with the other hand while applying the cross-friction massage to maintain pressure over an isolated area. Mobile skin and subcutaneous tissue can easily cause the finger or thumb to move off the site.

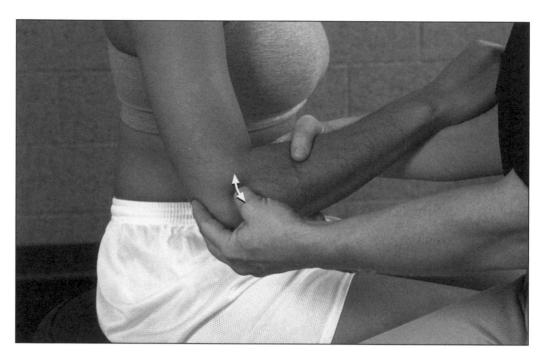

∎ **Figure 18.8**   Transverse friction massage.

JOINT MOBILIZATION

Joint mobilization for the elbow addresses the ulnohumeral joint, the radiohumeral joint, and the proximal radioulnar joint.

The capsular pattern demonstrating capsular tightness in the elbow in flexion is more limited than in extension; supination and pronation are equally limited. A patient who presents with this type of motion loss should be treated with joint mobilization. All three joints are enclosed in one capsule, so capsular restriction can impact all the joints.

If the elbow is very inflamed, initial joint mobilization techniques are mild (grades I and II). Application of more aggressive grades (IIIs and IVs) should be postponed until the inflammation and elbow pain are under control. Aggressive techniques applied too soon may cause additional damage to the sensitive capsule.

Joint mobilization should be performed in the loose-packed position when grades I and II are being applied, and in later stages during the initial applications of the more aggressive grades. This maximizes the effects of the mobilization techniques without aggravating the joint.

During joint mobilization, the sport rehabilitation specialist should always use good body mechanics. The hand applying the force should be positioned as close to the joint as possible. You need to remember the principles of glide, roll, and spin so that you apply forces properly to achieve the desired movement. Both the radial head and ulna are concave surfaces and move on a convex capitulum and convex trochlea, respectively, so force mobilization applications are in the same direction as the restricted movement. In the proximal radioulnar joint, however, the force is applied in the direction opposite the restricted movement because the convex-concare rule applies at this point.

The joint mobilization techniques presented here are the most commonly used techniques for the elbow. As with any joint mobilization procedure, it is important to visualize the joint surfaces and apply the mobilization force parallel to the surface. You must respect precautions and contraindications, and you must consider the healing-tissue time line and strength of new tissue when deciding whether to apply joint mobilization and how much force to use. The elbow's anterior capsule relationship with the brachialis presents unique problems and must be approached cautiously. As always, application of joint mobilization to hypermobile joints is contraindicated. Improper technique, incorrect force application, excessive force, and inappropriate timing of application can all result in unnecessary injury or damage to the joint's structures. You must be aware of the appropriateness or inappropriateness of accessory and physiological joint mobilization application before you decide to use the techniques. If you are unsure, it is better to refrain from using joint mobilization.

ULNOHUMERAL JOINT

This joint is also referred to as the humeroulnar joint. Although the elbow has three joints, the ulnohumeral joint is often considered the primary joint. Even though all three joints lie within the same capsule, joint mobilization for each joint can produce significant range-of-motion gains.

Joint Distraction

This technique can be used with oscillation in grades I and II. Grade III most often uses sustained distraction. This technique is used for pain relief and relaxation in the lower grades (I and II) and to increase flexion and extension in the higher grades (III and IV). The patient lies supine with the elbow flexed to 70° and the forearm in slight supination. The patient's wrist rests against the sport rehabilitation specialist's shoulder. The humerus is fixated with a stabilization strap, with the help of an assistant or the sport rehabilitation specialist's hand. The sport rehabilitation specialist's hands are placed on top of each other around the proximal forearm near the elbow joint, or one hand is used if the other hand is stabilizing the patient's arm. The sport rehabilitation specialist applies a distraction force around the humeral axis by leaning backward (figure 18.9).

Medial Glide

This technique is used to improve elbow flexion. The patient sits or stands, and the sport rehabilitation specialist faces and stands alongside the patient. The patient's forearm is positioned midway between supination and pronation and placed along the sport rehabilitation specialist's rib cage. The sport rehabilitation specialist's stabilizing hand's thenar eminence is placed against the patient's

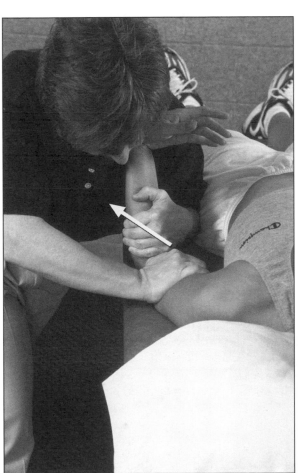

Figure 18.9 Ulnohumeral joint distraction mobilization.

medial epicondyle while the mobilizing hand applies a sustained 10 s pressure against the radius to create a medial glide of the forearm against the arm (figure 18.10). The pressure against the medial elbow may cause discomfort or injury to the ulnar nerve and must be applied with caution.

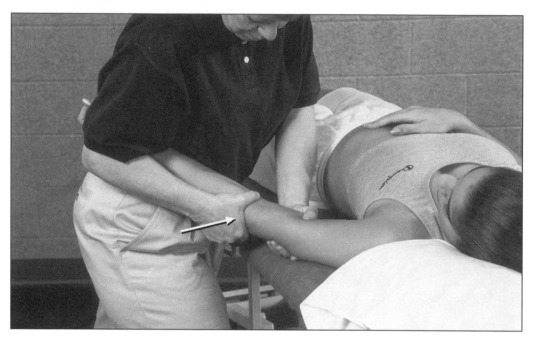

■ **Figure 18.10**   Medial ulnohumeral glide mobilization.

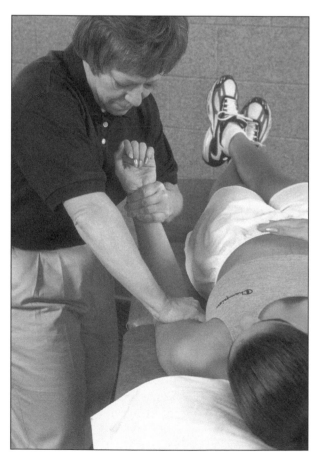

■ **Figure 18.11**   Radiohumeral distraction mobilization.

RADIOHUMERAL JOINT

This joint is also referred to as the humeroradial joint. The radiohumeral joint lies lateral to the ulnohumeral joint and should not be ignored when elbow capsular restriction is present. Mobilization of this specific joint can make significant differences in overall elbow mobility.

Distraction

This technique is used to improve elbow extension and radial motion. The patient lies supine or sits in a chair with the arm slightly abducted and supported on the table. The elbow is flexed and the forearm is supinated. The sport rehabilitation specialist stabilizes the arm with a hand on the distal humerus and the index finger palpating the radiohumeral joint space. The mobilizing hand is placed around the distal radius but not on the distal ulna. The mobilization force is applied when the sport rehabilitation specialist laterally bends his or her trunk away from the patient's arm (figure 18.11). A traction force can be simultaneously applied to the joint.

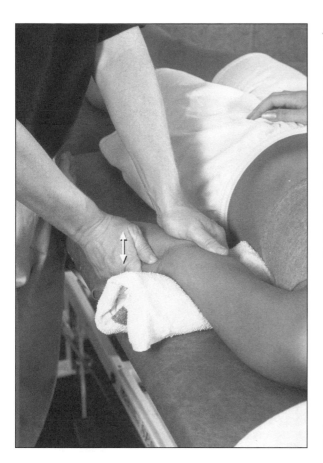

Anterior and Posterior Glides

The anterior glide is also known as a volar glide and increases flexion. The posterior glide, also known as a dorsal glide, increases extension. The patient lies supine with the arm supported on a towel roll on the table. The forearm is supinated, and the elbow is extended as far as possible. The sport rehabilitation specialist places the stabilizing hand on the medial distal humerus and the mobilizing hand on the proximal radius, with the fingers on the posterior aspect and the thenar eminence on the anterior aspect. To create an anterior glide, the thenar eminence moves the radial head posteriorly. To create a posterior glide, the fingers pull the radial head in a posterior-to-anterior direction (figure 18.12).

Figure 18.12 Radiohumeral anterior-posterior/posterior-anterior mobilization.

PROXIMAL RADIOULNAR JOINT

Although this joint is not actually part of the elbow's flexion-extension joint, the fact that it lies within the same capsule with the other two elbow joints means that it should be considered part of the elbow. In fact, restriction of this joint can impact overall elbow movement and therefore should not be ignored.

Ventral Glide

This technique is used to improve supination. The patient is in sitting or supine with the arm supported on the table. The elbow is flexed and the forearm is supinated about 35°. The sport rehabilitation specialist faces the patient. The distal humerus and proximal ulna are stabilized by the medial hand, and the mobilizing hand is wrapped around the radial head with the thenar eminence on the anterior aspect. A downward pressure is exerted from the sport rehabilitation specialist's shoulder to move the radial head posteriorly (figure 18.13).

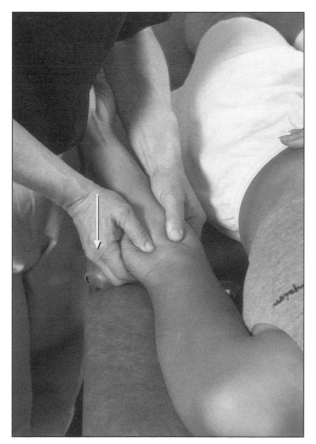

Figure 18.13 Radioulnar ventral glide mobilization.

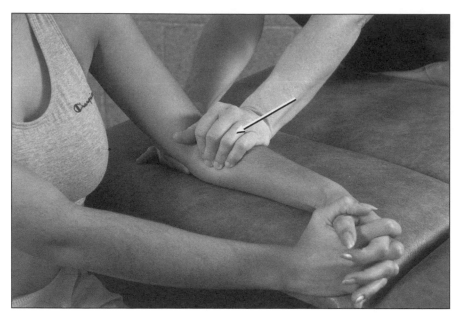

Dorsal Glide

This technique is used to improve pronation. The patient is sitting in a chair or supine with the forearm supported on the table. The elbow is flexed and the forearm is pronated slightly. The stabilizing hand is placed around the medial proximal forearm, and the mobilizing hand is placed around the head of the radius with the palm on the dorsal surface and the fingers anteriorly positioned. The radial head is moved with a posterior-to-anterior force, using primarily the heel of the hand (figure 18.14).

∎ **Figure 18.14** Radioulnar dorsal glide mobilization.

FLEXIBILITY EXERCISES

Normal flexibility of the elbow is restored through use of prolonged stretches including equipment stretches, as well as active and assisted stretching.

The best way to achieve normal elbow flexibility is to prevent loss of motion. Means of doing this include the use of continuous passive motion (CPM) machines, early mobilization following injury, and abbreviated periods of immobilization when appropriate. In cases of loss of motion, a variety of methods can be used to regain normal motion. The elbow heals as other areas of the body do, producing collagen that becomes scar tissue. As the collagen matures, stretching techniques and forces must change to affect the collagen arrangement. Short, active stretches can be used early to improve motion, but more prolonged stretches are necessary later when the collagen matures. These principles and guidelines are discussed in chapters 2 and 5.

PROLONGED STRETCHES

Prolonged stretches to the elbow must be applied with caution. Light forces are applied so as not to disrupt the anterior capsule and still provide greater motion of the joint. They are used only after active stretches have not been successful in restoring elbow motion.

Night Splints

In cases in which motion gains are either difficult to achieve or are slower than normal, a night splint can provide prolonged, low-level forces to effectively increase connective tissue lengthening. The patient wears the brace while sleeping, usually not during the day because the brace prevents the individual from using the arm. The force and angle of the brace can be adjusted to meet the individual patient's needs. It may take a couple of nights for the patient to adjust to the brace; but continued wear, if tolerated, can be beneficial in restoring range of motion.

Equipment Stretches

Although they are not as long as the night-splint stretches, the stretches described in this section are considered prolonged stretches. The mere fact that they use equipment makes it more likely that application may be too aggressive. You must be careful to use less force than you think is needed, because the longer duration of the stretch has a significantly greater impact on tissues than a brief stretch using the same force. Rather than applying too much force and creating capsular damage, you should begin with a force lighter than you think necessary and increase it if the results and patient sensation feedback indicate that this is appropriate.

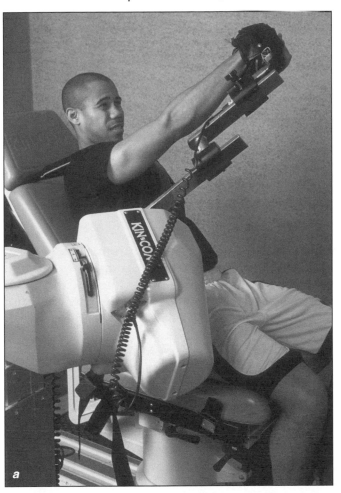

Flexion-Extension Stretches

Often a variety of machines are readily available in the clinic to provide a prolonged stretch. These can be applied for at least 10 to 15 min and longer, if the patient is able to tolerate them. A few pounds of force is applied while the shoulder is stabilized. As discussed earlier, the elbow is unique in that a muscle belly crosses the joint and can complicate attempts to regain lost motion in the joint. You must be careful not to apply too much force and over-stretch the soft tissue to cause more scar-tissue formation. The recommendation is to apply no more than 1.8 kg (4 lb) of force to a stretch to increase flexion range of motion. An isokinetic machine can be used to position the elbow on stretch in either flexion or extension with the speed set at zero to maintain the desired angle (figure 18.15a). An Isoquad exercise unit can also be used to apply a prolonged stretch. If neither of these machines is available, the patient can use free weights in the supine position: a 4.5-kg (10-lb) weight at the shoulder to prevent the shoulder from elevating off the table, and a 1.8-kg (4-lb) weight attached to the wrist. The distal arm should have a towel roll under it to protect the elbow from excessive posterior pressure on the table (figure 18.15b).

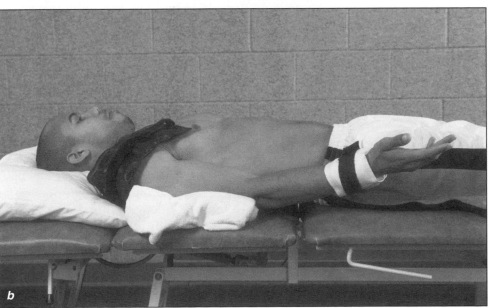

▌Figure 18.15
Flexion-extension equipment stretches: *(a)* using an isometric machine set at zero speed to produce a prolonged stretch, *(b)* using free-weight equipment to apply a prolonged stretch with 4.5 kg (10 lb) at the shoulder to stabilize it, and no more than 1.8 kg (4 lb) at the wrist to produce the stretch.

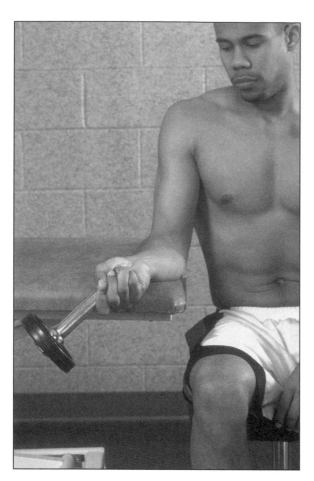

Figure 18.16   Supination equipment stretches.

Pronation-Supination Stretches

A weighted bar can be used to increase either supination or pronation. The patient sits with the elbow supported on a table; the elbow is positioned directly under the shoulder. A bar, wand, or broom handle is held in the patient's hand with the forearm positioned at end range in either supination or pronation (figure 18.16). A more effective stretch is produced if the bar is held in position with an elastic Velcro strap wrapped around the hand and bar; this permits muscle relaxation to improve the stretch results. The position is maintained for at least 5 min.

ACTIVE STRETCHES

Active stretches are performed by the patient throughout the day. They do not require a great deal of equipment so are convenient and easy to apply. Active stretches can affect both muscle and joint structures.

Elbow Flexor Stretch

This exercise stretches the elbow flexors and anterior joint to increase extension. The patient sits or lies supine and places the uninvolved forearm across the abdomen to put the dorsum of the hand just above the involved posterior elbow. With the forearm supinated, the involved elbow is allowed to relax into extension and kept in this position for several minutes. This exercise can be easily performed throughout the day while the patient is sitting. Common substitutions for this stretch that patients should avoid include scapular protraction, forward trunk lean, and shoulder extension.

Elbow Extensor Stretch

This exercise stretches the triceps and posterior joint to increase flexion. The patient grasps the involved forearm with the uninvolved hand. The elbow is stabilized next to the side or on a tabletop. The patient attempts to pull the involved forearm toward the shoulder with the uninvolved hand (figure 18.17). This stretch can be made more effective and more comfortable if a rolled-up towel or pad is placed in the antecubital fossa; the pad provides a distraction on the joint during the stretch. The stretch is held and repeated several times. The most common error for this exercise is shoulder extension and scapular retraction.

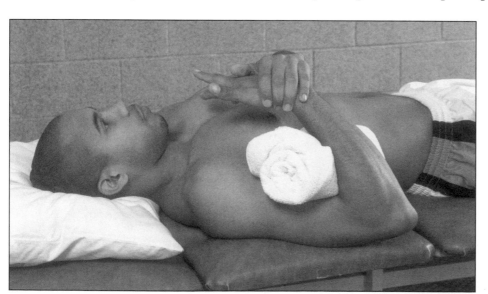

Figure 18.17   The elbow extensor stretch can be performed in supine or sitting

Supinator Stretch

This exercise increases pronation and stretches the supinators. The patient sits with the elbow flexed to 90° and stabilized at the side. The forearm is positioned in as much supination as possible. The uninvolved hand is placed in an underhand grasp

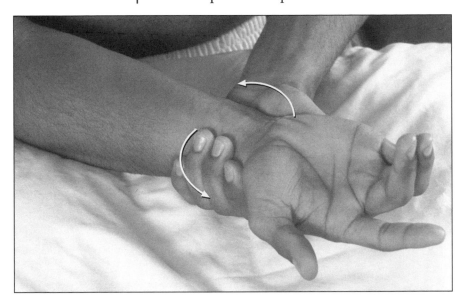

on the distal forearm so that the finger pads are on the volar aspect of the radius and the base of the hand is on the dorsal aspect of the ulna. The finger pads pull the radius downward as the base of the hand pushes the ulna upward (figure 18.18). The most common error in this stretch is movement inward by the elbow, and trunk lean toward the arm. The arm should be placed securely against the ribs to prevent movement during the stretch.

■ **Figure 18.18** Supinator stretch.

Pronator Stretch

This stretch increases supination by stretching the pronators. The patient sits with the elbow stabilized at the side and flexed to 90°. The forearm is actively positioned in as much pronation as possible. The patient grasps the distal forearm with the

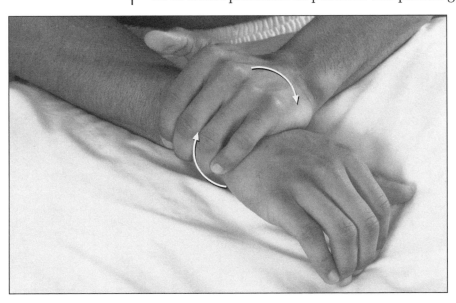

uninvolved hand in an overhand grasp by placing the finger pads around the ventral aspect of the ulna and the base of the hand on the dorsal aspect of the radius. The finger pads are pulled upward as the base of the hand is pushed downward (figure 18.19). A common error for this exercise is elbow movement away from the side as the shoulder abducts, and trunk lean away from the arm. The elbow must remain in contact with the lateral trunk.

■ **Figure 18.19** Pronator stretch.

ASSISTED STRETCHES

The sport rehabilitation specialist should apply stretch to the anterior joint cautiously. Overstretching this area can result in more adhesions or myositis ossificans. Contract-relax-stretch techniques with active contraction of the antagonists can be used with assistive stretches.

Elbow Flexion-Extension

These exercises are performed in sitting or supine, with the sport rehabilitation specialist supporting and stabilizing the elbow. The sport rehabilitation specialist's other hand is placed on the wrist. The stretch to increase flexion is applied by the sport rehabilitation specialist's hand at the patient's wrist, with the patient's hand moving toward his or her shoulder. Placing the sport rehabilitation specialist's other hand or a rolled-up towel in the antecubital fossa provides joint distraction to make the stretch more comfortable and more effective. This exercise should be performed in supination and pronation and can be controlled by the sport rehabilitation specialist's distal hand on the patient's wrist. If not properly stabilized, the shoulder can elevate to give a false impression of improved range of movement. The long head of the triceps can be stretched with the patient in sitting. The elbow is flexed by the sport rehabilitation specialist's hand on the distal forearm. The shoulder is then flexed overhead by the other hand on the patient's elbow (figure 18.20a).

To increase extension, the sport rehabilitation specialist applies the stretch by supporting the elbow and guiding the shoulder into hyperextension as the elbow is extended (figure 18.20b). This stretches the biceps and other anterior elbow structures. The shoulder should not protract during the stretch. The biceps is stretched when the forearm is in pronation, but the stretch should also be applied in supination.

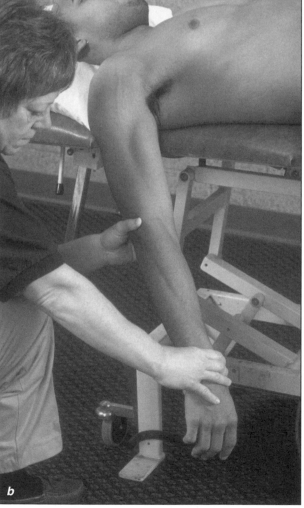

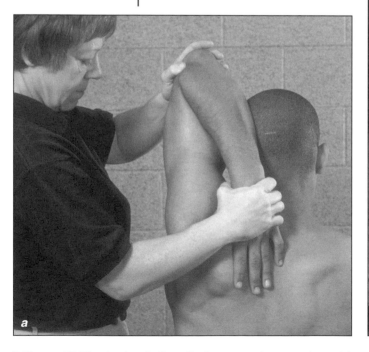

∎ **Figure 18.20** Assisted elbow flexion-extension stretches: *(a)* stretch for long head of the triceps, *(b)* stretch for the biceps.

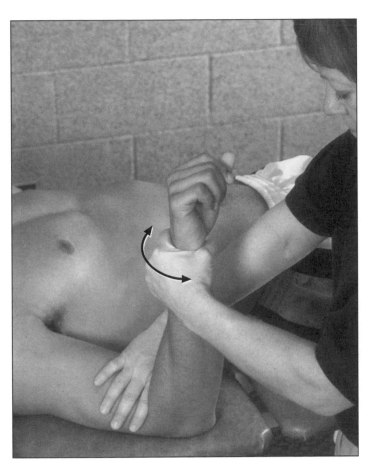

Supination-Pronation Stretches

These stretches should be performed with the elbow flexed and extended. The patient can be sitting or supine. The sport rehabilitation specialist places the stabilizing hand on the distal arm, and the other hand grasps the wrist and supports the hand. The radius is rolled around the ulna, with overpressure applied at the end of each range in supination and pronation (figure 18.21). The arm must be stabilized so that the shoulder is not allowed to abduct or adduct. The distal hand placement should be on the distal forearm, not the hand, so that the stretch occurs at the radioulnar joints, avoiding a twisting of the hand.

❚ Figure 18.21 Assisted supinator-pronator stretches.

STRENGTHENING EXERCISES

Strengthening exercises for the elbow use isometric resistance, manual resistance, straight-plane resistance, plyometrics, carryover shoulder exercises, and isokinetics in a careful progression.

As with other joints, the most basic elbow strengthening exercises include isometrics. Isotonics in straight-plane motions advance to diagonal-plane motions before plyometric exercises become a part of the strength progression. The final part of the therapeutic exercise program includes the functional exercises before the patient's return to sport participation.

ISOMETRIC RESISTANCE EXERCISES

The patient can perform the following resistance exercises independently and frequently throughout the day. Each repetition is held for 6 s. The patient should demonstrate correct execution of the exercises before performing them independently.

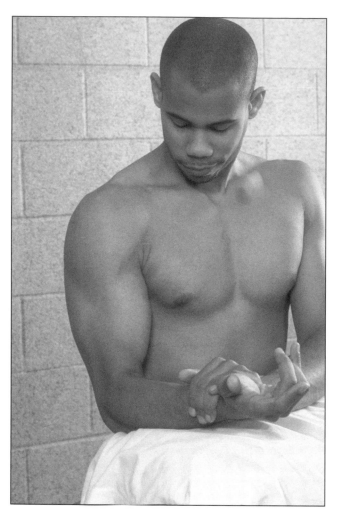

Figure 18.22 Isometric flexion.

Elbow Flexion

The involved elbow is flexed, and the patient's other hand is placed on the distal forearm. The patient attempts to move the elbow into flexion while using the opposing hand to resist the movement (figure 18.22). This exercise should be performed in supination and pronation and in neutral, as well as at several different angles of elbow flexion.

Elbow Extension

For this exercise the resistance is applied to the distal forearm as the patient attempts to extend the elbow. This exercise should be performed at several different positions in the range of motion.

MANUAL-RESISTANCE EXERCISES

Straight-plane manual resistance is provided by the sport rehabilitation specialist. It is important that the elbow moves through the full range of motion. The movement should be smooth, so the sport rehabilitation specialist needs to alter the resistance force according to changes in the patient's strength as the elbow moves through the range of motion. If an area of weakness is present, the sport rehabilitation specialist can offer an isometric resistance at that point in the motion before proceeding through the remaining motion; if an isometric is used, the patient should be informed in advance of the change. You can use manual resistance early and throughout the rehabilitation program, because you can easily alter the resistance to meet the resistance needs and still respect healing-tissue precautions.

Elbow Flexion-Extension

The best position for strengthening exercises is with the forearm in an antigravity position. This utilizes the weight of the forearm as additional resistance. For elbow flexion the patient is sitting or supine. Supine position is preferred because the elbow is more easily stabilized and able to go through a full range of motion. The sport rehabilitation specialist stabilizes the shoulder with one hand and resists elbow flexion with the other hand over the distal forearm (figure 18.23a). To resist primarily the biceps, the forearm is supinated. To eliminate the biceps and resist the brachialis, the forearm is pronated. To resist primarily the brachioradialis, the forearm is in neutral. Common errors with this exercise include shoulder flexion, shoulder shrugging, and scapular retraction.

Elbow extension is performed with the patient prone to maximize gravity's effect at end-range extension. The arm is abducted and supported on the table, with the forearm hanging over the side. A towel support is placed under the distal arm to elevate that arm to a level position on the table. The sport rehabilitation specialist stabilizes the arm with one hand and provides resistance to elbow extension at the distal forearm with the other (figure 18.23b). This exercise can also be performed with the patient in sitting with the shoulder fully elevated and the elbow overhead. This position provides maximal gravity resistance in the middle of the range of motion. A common substitution is scapular protraction.

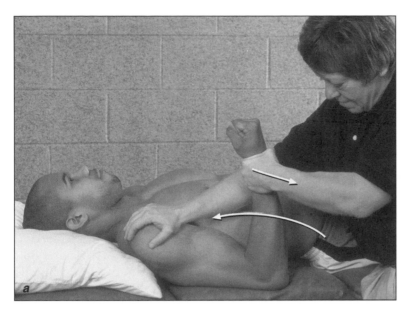

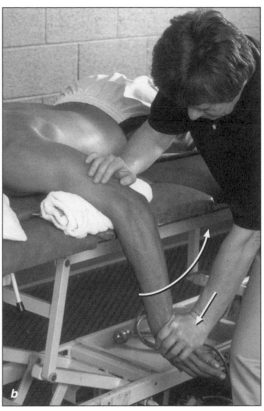

■ **Figure 18.23** Manual resistance: *(a)* resisted elbow flexion in supination, *(b)* resisted elbow extension.

Supination-Pronation

This exercise can be performed with the patient sitting or supine. The elbow is flexed to 90°, and the sport rehabilitation specialist places both hands around the patient's distal forearm. As the patient supinates, the sport rehabilitation specialist provides resistance to the movement. Resistance is reversed for pronation (figure 18.24). The elbow should be held to the patient's side to prevent shoulder abduction with pronation and adduction with supination.

STRAIGHT-PLANE RESISTED EXERCISES

It is important for the patient to perform these exercises through a full range of motion in a slow and controlled manner.

Flexion

Depending on the forearm position, the biceps, brachialis, and/or brachioradialis are strengthened. Supination emphasizes the biceps, pronation emphasizes the brachialis, and neutral works the brachioradialis.

■ **Figure 18.24** Manual resistance to supination and pronation.

The patient stands with the uninvolved hand behind the involved distal arm just above the elbow. The weight is held in the hand in a supinated, pronated, or neutral position as the patient slowly flexes the elbow (figure 18.25a). In this position the maximum resistance occurs at midrange. The hand is held behind the elbow to stabilize the arm and prevent use of the shoulder to lift the weight, the most common substitution in this exercise. Another substitution is to heft the weight up with a sudden shrug movement of the shoulder or the use of momentum. If this occurs, lower the resistance.

An alternative position is with the shoulder flexed to 90° and the arm supported to maintain this position while the elbow is flexed against resistance (figure 18.25b). This position provides maximum resistance in the beginning of the exercise.

This exercise can also be performed with rubber tubing or pulleys. The pulley or tubing is positioned low, near the ground, if maximum resistance is to occur at midrange. Changing the anchor position changes the point in the motion at which maximum resistance occurs. Refer to chapter 7 for additional information on joint positions and maximum resistance. It is important to stabilize the arm by placing the opposite hand behind the upper arm as seen in figure 18.25c.

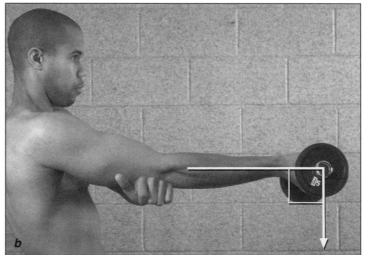

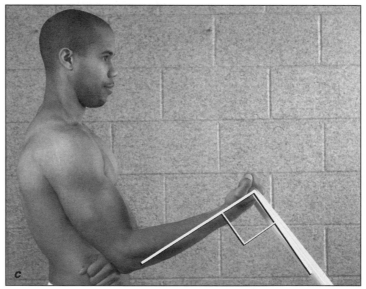

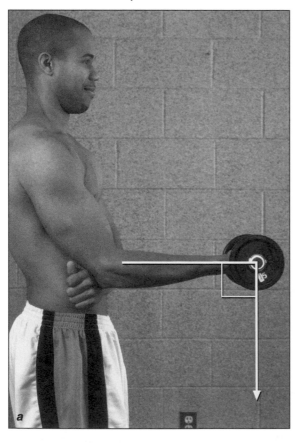

■ **Figure 18.25** Elbow flexion: *(a)* maximum resistance occurs at 90° elbow flexion, *(b)* maximum resistance occurs at the start of elbow flexion, *(c)* maximum resistance can change in the ROM, depending on where the rubber band or pulley is positioned relative to elbow motion.

Extension

This exercise strengthens the triceps and anconeus. To provide maximum resistance at midrange, the exercise is performed with the shoulder elevated overhead so that the elbow is directly over the shoulder. The arm is kept in position with support from the opposite hand (figure 18.26a). If the long head of the triceps is to be emphasized less, the exercise can be performed with the patient supine (figure 18.26b).

To emphasize resistance at end range, the patient leans over at the waist or lies prone on a table. The elbow is extended alongside the body (figure 18.26c). A common substitution is shoulder extension.

Equipment such as the latissimus pull-down bar can also be used to strengthen elbow extensors. The patient positions the bar so that the elbows are at the sides and flexed. Maintaining arm position, the patient lowers the bar by extending the elbows (figure 18.26d).

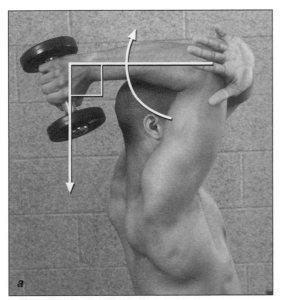
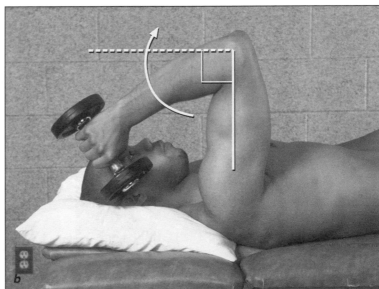
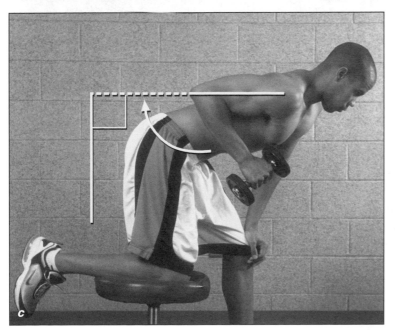
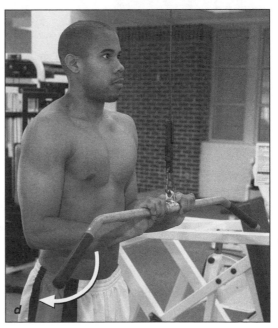

▌Figure 18.26 Elbow extension: *(a–b)* maximum resistance occurs at 90°, *(c)* maximum resistance occurs at end range, *(d)* using the latissimus pull-down bar to strengthen triceps.

Supination

This exercise is performed with the patient sitting and the forearm supported over the end of a table. A weighted bar is held at one end with the forearm in pronation. The patient rotates the bar upward until the bar is pointing toward the ceiling for a concentric exercise (18.27a). To do an eccentric exercise, the patient continues the motion until the palm is completely turned up (figure 18.27b). Common errors with this exercise include letting the weight fall rather than controlling its movement and speed, shoulder adduction, and elbow extension.

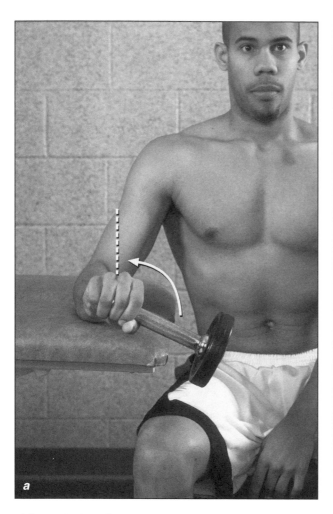 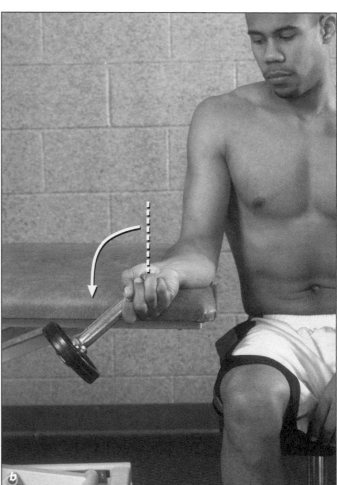

▌**Figure 18.27**   Supination: *(a)* concentric, *(b)* eccentric.

Pronation

In this exercise, the patient is seated as for the supination exercise just described. The patient begins with the hand in full supination and rotates the bar into pronation to the midposition for a concentric exercise, continuing on to full pronation for an eccentric exercise. Substitutions for this exercise include shoulder abduction and elbow flexion. The weight should be controlled throughout the range of motion.

It is incorrect to use a dumbbell to perform this exercise, because one end of the dumbbell will act as a counterbalance force for the other, making the exercise ineffective.

PLYOMETRIC EXERCISES

Once he or she has achieved good strength in straight-plane exercises, the patient progresses to diagonal-plane activities. These are more strenuous in that they demand simultaneous muscle performance in multiple planes, continued control of the extremity, and accuracy of performance. These exercises serve as a transition phase and prepare the elbow and its supporting structures and active components for the next phase, functional activities.

CARRYOVER SHOULDER EXERCISES

Many of the closed kinetic chain exercises discussed in chapter 17 are appropriate for the elbow. Instead of repeating details here, I suggest that you refer to chapter 17 for a listing and for information about progression of these exercises. The push-up, seated push-up, Swiss-ball weight-bearing exercises, rhythmic stabilization activities, and distal movement stabilization exercises are all appropriate for the elbow.

Rubber tubing diagonal patterns in D1 and D2 flexion and extension can incorporate elbow movements or flexion or extension, or can maintain a stationary elbow position throughout the patterns. Which pattern to use depends on the patient's sport. For example, a pitcher or tennis player should use D2 flexion and extension patterns, because those patterns most closely mimic the motions in those sports. A breaststroke swimmer, on the other hand, should use D1 flexion and extension patterns.

Unstable-surface activities as discussed in chapter 17 are recommended for middle-phase elbow rehabilitation. Resisted movements using the treadmill or stair machine, and medicine-ball exercises and their progressions, are also applicable for elbow therapeutic exercise progressions.

ISOKINETICS

Isokinetic equipment is used initially in straight-plane exercises with stabilization and isolation of desired motions. Elbow flexion-extension and forearm pronation-supination can all be performed on the equipment. As the patient progresses, diagonal patterns can be used as a progression into more-functional exercises.

FUNCTIONAL ACTIVITIES

Functional activities for the elbow, progressing in distances, forces, and speeds, prepare the patient for return to sport participation.

Once the patient is able to meet the challenge of plyometric exercises, functional activities are the next logical step and the final preparation before one allows a full return to sport competition. Many of the functional programs discussed in chapters 10 and 17 can be used very appropriately for the elbow. Of course, specific applications depend on the patient's sport and position within the sport.

Functional exercises should include warm-up and cool-down activities. Overhead sport progressions should begin with easy activities at diminished distances, forces, and speeds and should gradually increase only one component at a time until the patient performs all activities at normal performance levels. Increases should occur no more often than every third exercise session to permit adequate adaptation to increased stress levels. If a patient experiences pain with any increase, he or she should return to the previous level of exercises for an additional three days before attempting to try the next level again.

Rather than repeating programs that have already been described, I suggest that you refer to chapters 10 and 17 for details on programs, their progressions, and the precautions that guide those progressions.

SPECIAL REHABILITATION APPLICATIONS

Common elbow injuries that warrant special considerations in therapeutic exercise program design are epicondylitis, Little League elbow, sprains, ulnar nerve injury, dislocation, and post-arthroscopy conditions.

We will now look at rehabilitation programs for some of the more common elbow injuries. For each injury, specific aspects unique to that injury and the rehabilitation program for that injury are presented. These discussions are followed by a case study for you to solve that will enable you to apply your new knowledge of elbow rehabilitation.

EPICONDYLITIS

Epicondylitis or tendinitis is commonly seen in the elbow. As discussed in chapter 15, among the most important aspects of treatment of these conditions are discovering and correcting the cause of the problem. If you do not correct the cause of the injury, the risk of its recurring is very high. Because the elbow sits on either side of two long lever arms, it can be susceptible to tendinitis, especially when the forces applied are exaggerated because of poor technique.

Program Considerations

Lateral epicondylitis is often referred to as tennis elbow, and medial epicondylitis is commonly known as golfer's elbow. These both come under the general heading of tendinitis and usually result from cumulative trauma. Lateral epicondylitis most commonly involves the extensor carpi radialis brevis. It is the result of various improper techniques on the tennis backhand, including hitting the ball too late or flipping the wrist into extension. Medial epicondylitis is seen in golfers who throw the club down with the back arm to hack at the ball rather than moving the club through with the trunk and front arm. Tennis players who hit a forearm stroke with the elbow ahead of the racket and gymnasts who bear weight on hyperextended elbows are also subject to medial epicondylitis.

In either tennis elbow or golfer's elbow, the patient experiences a gradual onset of epicondyle pain. It may begin with pain only after activity. Then it may progress to some pain at the start of activity that resolves as the activity continues but returns after activity. Eventually, pain occurs with daily activities and then at rest. Grasping objects and shaking hands are painful. Extending the wrist against resistance in lateral epicondylitis and flexing the wrist against resistance in medial epicondylitis are painful. The pain is localized to the epicondyle, but if left untreated can extend into the muscle bellies of the forearm. Pronation or supination activities can become painful. Grip strength weakens, as does wrist flexion or extension for medial and lateral epicondylitis, respectively. Pain can restrict full range of motion of the wrist, especially when it is combined with elbow extension.

As with other tendinitis treatments, the cause of the injury must be determined and corrected to diminish the risk of reinjury. The inflammation must be treated and deficiencies rehabilitated. Modalities such as ultrasound, phonophoresis, and iontophoresis are commonly used for these conditions. Cross-friction massage to the tender epicondylar areas is used to reduce tissue adhesions and increase local circulation. Loss of flexibility and weakness are often secondary occurrences with epicondylitis. Elbow, wrist, and finger flexion and extension, as well as forearm supination and pronation, should be returned to normal ranges of motion through a variety of flexibility exercises. If the joint mobility is restricted, mobilization techniques are indicated. End-range stretches and mobilizations should not be aggressive, especially in the early rehabilitation phases when inflammation is significant. Patients who have been long-term participants in tennis or throwing sports may have developed flexion contractures and valgus deformities. These may result from repetitive microtears, scarring, and ossification of the flexor muscles and anterior capsule or hypertrophic bone changes (Ellenbecker and Mattalino 1997). In the presence of these ossification changes, attempts to stretch the elbow are frustrating and are not advised. During the early rehabilitation phase, stretching exercises should be active and within the patient's comfort range.

In the middle rehabilitation phase, if normal range of motion is still lacking, mobilization should be initiated. If a bony end-feel is palpated at less than normal extension, the patient may have structural changes that prohibit full extension. If the end-feel is capsular, however, joint mobilization techniques are indicated. Joint mobility of the wrist, forearm, and elbow is a consideration for epicondylitis treatment because muscles originating on the epicondyle affect wrist and forearm movement. If the muscles are not moved through their full range of motion, loss of mobility can occur. Specific wrist mobilizations and flexibility exercises are discussed in chapter 19. In addition to mobilization techniques, active assistive and passive stretching exercises can be used to improve wrist, forearm, and elbow motion in this phase.

Strengthening includes isometrics, eccentrics, concentrics, and plyometrics that are provided in a progression. Chapter 15 contains information on the rationale for and progression of exercises in the treatment of tendinitis. Isometrics should be used in the early rehabilitation phase if the tendons are very inflamed and other exercises are too painful. Effective strengthening exercises for tendinitis include an eccentric exercise program (Curwin and Stanish 1984). This starts with submaximal eccentric exercises using weights or rubber tubing and progresses to more aggressive use of heavier weights with increased speeds as tolerated by the injury. In the early rehabilita-tion phase, the patient should begin shoulder and trunk exercises to maintain conditioning levels in these areas.

Middle-phase rehabilitation includes the use of diagonal motions, increased resistance, and more functional patterns of movement to prepare the injury for plyometric exercises. Many exercises in this phase are those listed in the shoulder rehabilitation program in chapter 17. Motions begin in a slow and controlled manner and progress to faster movements while the patient maintains control of the arm throughout the motion. Closed kinetic chain exercises and neuromuscular facilitation exercises are used in this phase. Isokinetic exercises, first in straight planes and then in diagonal planes, are suitable in this phase. Isokinetic exercises should be at higher speeds and should emphasize muscle endurance. In later stages of the middle phase, the patient can use the isokinetic equipment to perform full-body initiated and diagonal activities that mimic sport motions. All exercises should remain pain free with no associated postexercise discomfort.

Plyometrics in the final phases of rehabilitation emphasize functional movements that prepare the patient for functional exercises before returning to full sport participation. These exercises are discussed in chapter 17. The progression is the same as that presented for the shoulder, beginning with easier plyometrics and advancing to higher-speed, more resistive plyometrics as the injured segment adapts and the patient is able to tolerate increased stresses. It is during this phase that the isokinetic exercises are performed in functional patterns, using total-body performance positions. They should mimic sport patterns of movement as closely as possible.

Functional activities are individually determined and are based on the patient's sport and position within the sport. Guidelines for functional activity progressions are universal and are based on the patient's response to the exercises. As a rule, increases occur no more frequently than every third day. Only one parameter is increased at one time. In other words, if a pitcher increases throwing distance on a particular day, speed of the throw is not changed on the same day. In fact, it may be prudent to reduce the speed when increasing distance and to gradually build up the throwing speed to the levels that were being attained before the distance increase. If the patient experiences pain with any increase, he or she returns to the immediately preceding program level for another three sessions before advancing.

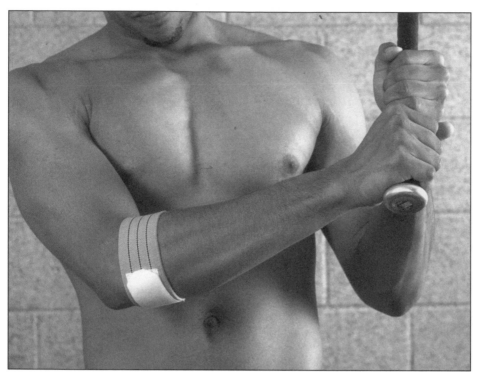

■ **Figure 18.28**   Counterforce brace.

Bracing can assist the patient in pain-free performance. A counter-force brace is approximately 5 cm (2 in.) wide or slightly larger and is made of nonelastic strapping, usually secured with Velcro (figure 18.28). Its purpose is to reduce wrist extensor activity and disperse the stresses applied to the extensor tendons (Groppel and Nirschl 1986). The brace should be worn during the treatment phase and also when the patient returns to competition.

Before the racket-sport patient begins functional activities prior to returning to competition, his or her equipment should be examined for appropriateness. Racket weight, stiffness, and size should be evaluated. A heavy racket requires greater strength, energy expenditure, and muscle endurance. A stiff racket allows the patient to exert greater power on the ball, but it also absorbs less impact stress and transfers the unabsorbed stress to the patient's arm. A tightly strung racket also increases impact-stress transfer to the arm, so a patient returning to participation may be advised to reduce the string tension of the racket slightly. This combination of a less stiff racket and less string tension permits more force absorption in the racket because the ball is in contact with the racket longer (Newton's second law of motion). As the impact force is spread out over a longer period of time, it is reduced.

Grip size is another factor that requires assessment before the patient uses a racket. A grip that is too small can increase the strength requirements, add stress to the epicondyles, and increase fatigue of the forearm muscles. You determine proper size by measuring the distance from the tip of the ring finger to the proximal palmar crease (Nirschl 1977) (figure 18.29).

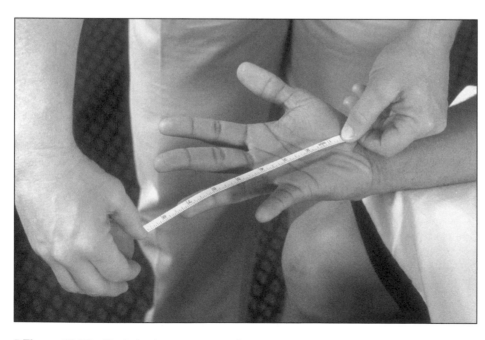

■ **Figure 18.29**   Racket-grip measurement.

Occasionally, surgery is necessary to completely resolve more persistent cases of epicondylitis. In lateral epicondylitis, the extensor carpi radialis brevis tendon is detached from the lateral epicondyle, and debridement of the area is the common procedure. Medial surgical release commonly involves the pronator teres and flexor carpi ulnaris tendons.

Postoperative rehabilitation includes the use of an elbow immobilizer immediately after surgery and continuing for about one week. The brace may be continued for occasional support when the elbow gets fatigued, for up to three weeks postoperatively. Active range-of-motion exercises for the wrist and fingers can start after surgery, although the patient will probably not want to begin these until at least the second postoperative day. Gentle active and active assistive range of motion of the elbow can begin around day 5. By the third week the patient should have full range of motion.

At two weeks, active exercise against gravity without resistance can begin, as can squeezing a soft ball. Pronation and supination motion exercises for the elbow and wrist, as well as flexion and extension motion exercises, should continue.

By three weeks, low-resistance, low-repetition exercises can start with isometrics and straight-plane exercises. Full motion should be present by this time. The patient progresses as tolerated into higher-repetition exercises before moving into heavier weights.

Diagonal-plane exercises can begin at four to eight weeks, depending on the patient's pain tolerance and strength. Once the patient displays good strength and control without pain in diagonal motions, it is appropriate to begin plyometrics.

By three to four months, the patient can begin functional activities if there is no pain with plyometrics and if normal strength, muscle endurance, and flexibility are present. Patients undergoing medial epicondylar releases may not be able to return to full sport participation for five to six months, and those undergoing lateral epicondylar releases may return to sport four to five months postoperatively.

Case Study

A 24-year-old, right-hand-dominant female tennis player has been playing with tennis elbow for the past six months. It started when she bought a new Kevlar tennis racket and began attempting to put a topspin on her serve. The condition has advanced to a level such that she now has pain throughout her game; she is not playing well any more, has a difficult time opening doors and turning the key over to start her car, and is unable to carry her gym bag in the right hand. The forearm feels stiff most of the time. Examination reveals tenderness over the lateral epicondyle extending into the proximal forearm along the radial wrist extensors. Resisted wrist extension is weak and painful. Grip strength measured with a grip dynamometer on the right is 15.8 kg (35 lb) and painful compared to the pain-free left grip strength of 34 kg (75 lb). Her wrist flexion range of motion is limited to 45° because of pain. There is no restriction of joint accessory movements. Passive elbow extension increases the wrist flexion pain.

Questions for Analysis

1. What will your first treatment session include?

2. What are your initial treatment goals?

3. What will be your instructions to the patient in the first treatment?

4. How do you plan to increase her range of motion?

5. Outline your program for strengthening the wrist and identify the guidelines you will use.

6. What suggestions regarding equipment will you make to the patient?

7. Describe a functional activity progression for the patient and identify the criteria you will use to determine when she is ready to return to full participation in tennis.

LITTLE LEAGUE ELBOW

Little League elbow is another type of inflammation of the elbow, but it is unique because it occurs only in youngsters. Its name comes from the population it is most frequently seen in, pitchers of Little League baseball. It has been a common enough problem that youth league governing bodies have attempted to regulate pitching in this population, but the problem remains. Special issues surrounding this injury are presented before a case study is provided for you to solve.

Program Considerations

Little league elbow is unique to the preadolescent population. It involves a number of conditions that have the common thread of elbow pathology as a result of pitching. The most common site of pathology is the medial elbow because of the excessive traction forces applied to the medial epicondyle epiphyseal plate during acceleration. Curves and breaking pitches increase the demands on wrist flexion and pronation, increasing the medial epicondyle stresses. Injury to the inherently weak epiphyseal plate may begin as an inflammation and can progress to an avulsion of the plate with repetitive trauma. In severe cases, osteochondritis dissecans of the radioulnar joint can occur.

Less frequently, the lateral, anterior, or posterior elbow is affected by excessive stresses applied during throwing. The pronator teres increases stresses laterally during extreme pronation, and increased hyperextension forces on follow-through can increase anterior and posterior joint stresses.

In the more common medial Little League elbow, the athlete experiences progressive medial elbow pain with activity, pain with end motion finger and wrist extension, tenderness to medial epicondyle palpation, and pain and weakness with resisted wrist and finger flexion. Swelling, and, in more advanced cases, ecchymosis, can be present over the medial epicondyle.

Common causes for little league elbow are improper warm-up or lack of warm-up, improper or insufficient conditioning, poor pitching mechanics, inadequate rest, pitching too many innings, and the use of curves and breaking-ball pitches. It is recommended that adequate conditioning programs and proper warm-up and cool-down procedures be included in a team's program, and that adherence to Little League baseball pitching rules be enforced in practices as well as games. Those rules include permitting an adolescent to pitch no more than six innings and mandating rest three days between pitching rotations. Patients should avoid those activities that produce little league elbow. If an injury occurs, it becomes even more important for the patient to adhere to recommendations that minimize elbow stresses.

If growth plate damage is evident with the injury, the individual should be advised to stop pitching for the rest of the baseball season. Early-phase treatment for little league elbow includes rest, ice, and in advanced cases, immobilization. Active range-of-motion exercises to tolerance are encouraged. Passive stretches should be avoided. Because of the age of the patient, using heavy weights is not advisable because these could aggravate sensitive growth plates. Exercises are neither as aggressive nor as intensive as they are for older patients, but the program should follow the same progression. This progression emphasizes range of motion and calming of the inflammation in the initial rehabilitation phase, with advancement to a progressive strengthening program before functional activities begin. Valgus stress should be avoided until it does not cause pain. A gradual progression to throwing occurs when the patient is pain free and has full range of motion and normal muscle strength and muscle endurance.

Case Study

A nine-year-old baseball pitcher is in the middle of his season. For the past month he has experienced progressive medial elbow pain on his left throwing elbow. He is the team's top pitcher and usually pitches three days a week. An invitational tournament his team is competing in is planned for next weekend, and he wants to pitch. His parents are reluctant to allow him to do so, but they want your opinion. He has full range of motion of the elbow, but wrist extension is painful in the last 10°. Resisted pronation and wrist flexion are weak and painful. The medial epicondyle is tender to palpation and edematous.

Questions for Analysis

1. What will be your recommendation to the patient regarding the weekend invitational tournament?

2. What will be your recommendations on future pitching?

3. What treatment procedure will you recommend he follow to reduce the pain and inflammation?

4. What will be your instructions about exercises he should perform?

5. How much information will you give the patient's parents?

SPRAINS

Sprains in the elbow most commonly occur as hyperextension sprains. Capsular injury of the elbow can be frustrating if not treated correctly at the very beginning. Special considerations relating to this type of injury are presented followed by a case study.

Program Considerations

The most common sprains in the elbow occur as a hyperextension injury or a medial collateral ligament sprain. A hyperextension sprain can occur when a football opponent runs into and past an outstretched blocking arm or when a gymnast does a handstand. Any sudden valgus force such as a sidearm throw by a shortstop, or a wrench of the elbow by a wrestling opponent, can also cause a sprain. In a hyperextension injury, the anterior capsule is injured; but in a medial collateral stress injury, the medial collateral ligament (MCL), the primary stabilizing unit for the elbow, is injured.

Hyperextension injuries cause pain in the anterior joint and can also cause a bone contusion and pain in the olecranon or olecranon fossa. Medial collateral ligament sprains have medial joint pain. A support brace may be used during the first couple of weeks following injury. Initial rehabilitation includes treatment to relieve pain and swelling. Cross-friction massage to adherent ligamentous structures can also relieve pain but should not be performed within the first 7 to 10 days following injury. Active and active assistive range of motion are used in the early phase, along with mild straight-plane strengthening exercises. Pain during activity should be avoided. Strengthening exercises should include the biceps and triceps, as well as wrist and finger flexors and extensors, and forearm pronators and supinators. Following hyperextension injuries, the biceps, brachialis, brachioradialis, and supinator play an important role in providing dynamic stability anteriorly, and the triceps and biceps co-contract to provide weight-bearing stability. Following MCL sprains, the supinators can assist in stability. Resistance to the flexor carpi ulnaris may aggravate the MCL in early rehabilitation and should be deferred until the middle rehabilitation phase. By the middle phase, full range of motion of the elbow should be present. Strengthening exercise for the flexor carpi ulnaris in wrist flexion and ulnar deviation should be instituted if it did not begin before. Straight-plane exercises continue, but resistance and repetition levels can increase. Eccentric and concentric exercises are used. By the end of the middle phase, diagonal-plane movements can begin with proprioceptive neuromuscular facilitation stabilization activities and closed kinetic chain exercises; rubber tubing can be added as long as the stresses do not cause pain either during or after the exercise. Isokinetics are appropriate, beginning with straight-plane movement and progressing to diagonal planes of movement.

In the late phase, plyometric exercises begin. These are the same exercises as those described for epicondylitis. Functional planes of movement are used during these exercises. The patient should be able to maintain good joint stability during all activities. The goals in this phase are to prepare the injury site for functional activities.

Instability of the elbow occurs primarily in tears of the MCL. In these cases, surgical repair may be required. Postoperative rehabilitation depends on the surgical technique used. If the ligament lacks any viable tissue, a reconstruction is performed using an autogeneous graft and the flexor/pronator tendon group is detached. This requires a longer postoperative rehabilitation process than when the ligament contains viable tissue and can be salvaged without detaching the flexor/pronator mass.

Following surgery, the elbow is locked at 90° in an adjustable elbow flexion splint for the first week. During this time, the patient can perform active wrist and finger motion exercises. Submaximal isometric exercises for the biceps and the shoulder can occur as long as the patient avoids shoulder external rotation, which would increase valgus elbow stress. The patient can also squeeze a ball.

By the end of the second week, the brace is placed at −30° extension and 100° flexion. Submaximal wrist and elbow isometrics can start after the second week. The patient should attempt to move the elbow in the range of motion allowed by the brace. Each week the brace is adjusted to increase motion in both flexion and extension until it is set to full motion by the sixth week. The patient attempts to increase active movement within the expanded available range of motion.

After three weeks, a gradual progression of strength exercises can be added to the program. These include exercises such as wrist and elbow flexion and extension, as well as forearm pronation and supination, against mild resistance. Beginning proprioception exercises for joint-position sense with eyes closed is appropriate, but valgus stress to the elbow should be avoided. Proprioceptive exercises that avoid valgus stresses can advance as tolerated. Shoulder exercises with the exception of external-rotation motions are performed as well. External rotation can start after the sixth week. Concentric, eccentric, and mild isokinetics can be used in straight-plane movements. Co-contraction exercises for the biceps and triceps can be started if valgus stress is avoided. Closed kinetic chain exercises and other stabilization exercises are permissible once the patient has strength and control of the elbow.

Full range of motion should be present by week 6 to 8. The muscles providing dynamic stability—the biceps, pronators, and wrist flexors—are important for assisting the MCL and should be well strengthened. After the sixth week, diagonal movements can begin if adequate strength and control without pain are present in the elbow. Work on proprioceptive neuromuscular facilitation patterns, rubber tubing exercises, more aggressive stabilization exercises, and diagonal isokinetics at high speeds can all be started at this time.

In the final phase, plyometrics begin, after week 9. As with other plyometric activities, these begin with lower-stress activities at reduced speeds and resistance, and then increase to higher speeds and place additional stress on the elbow. Medicine balls, push-up progressions, and functional isokinetic motions are included.

Functional exercises can begin in week 10 to 14. The timing depends on the patient's response to the exercises and the patient's sport. A pitcher may need to wait longer before beginning throwing activities because of the higher elbow stresses in pitching compared with those in a less intense sport, such as golf. The progression of functional activities and the precautions to observe are the same as for other injuries. Following MCL reconstruction surgery, it is common for a patient to return to full sport participation by week 22 to 26. These figures are based on averages, and you must always remember that time lines vary from one patient to another.

Case Study

A 30-year-old right-handed golfer injured his right elbow when he hit a divot and tore his ulnar collateral ligament. He attempted to continue playing through the season, but pain persisted. The elbow became unstable, and he underwent a medial collateral reconstruction. The surgery was 10 days ago, and he has been instructed by the surgeon to begin rehabilitation. The elbow is in a functional brace that is locked at −30° extension and 100° flexion. Supination is to neutral. Your examination reveals mild discoloration still present in the forearm and distal upper arm medially. There is spasm in the upper trapezius and biceps. Active range of motion out of the brace is 60° from extension to 100° into flexion. Wrist extensors have 4/5 strength, the shoulder grossly has 4−/5 strength, the biceps and triceps are also 4−/5, and the wrist flexors are 3−/5. There are active trigger points in the forearm on the flexor and extensor surfaces.

Questions for Analysis

1. What will your first treatment session include?
2. What precautions will you give the patient?
3. When will you start pronation and supination motion activities?
4. What strengthening exercises will you include in the first week, and how will you advance them?
5. At what motion limits will you set the brace in week 5?
6. When will you start shoulder external-rotation exercises?
7. What functional-exercise program will you will establish for the patient, and when will you start it?

ULNAR NERVE INJURY

Injury to the ulnar nerve can occur in any sport but seems most prevalent in throwing sports such as baseball (pitching). The most frequent cause in this population is incorrect mechanics. This injury is treated with both operative and nonoperative techniques. Considerations in therapeutic exercise for both treatments are presented here.

Program Considerations

Repetitive overhand throwing activities, especially in patients whose shoulder external rotation in the cocking phase is reduced, places excessive stress on the medial elbow structures. The ulnar nerve can become stretched, mechanically irritated, or even subluxed out of its sulcus. Adjacent soft-tissue structures can also compress the nerve. The patient commonly complains of fourth- and fifth-digit numbness or tingling and posteromedial elbow pain. Nonoperative treatment includes initial treatments to reduce the inflammation and pain. Exercises used to improve range of motion and strength are similar to those for other elbow injuries. Mobilization can be performed if the joint is hypomobile. Strength exercises are initially low-resistance, high-repetition loads in straight-plane motions. Muscles for all shoulder, elbow, wrist, and forearm motions should be strengthened. If shoulder inflexibility, shoulder weakness, or poor athletic technique is contributing to the elbow injury, it must be corrected. Initial exercises should not place valgus stress on the elbow. As the strength increases, valgus stress is applied gradually. The final phases of the program include a progression from diagonal motions to plyometrics to functional activities before return to full sport participation.

When operative repair is necessary for a subluxating or dislocating ulnar nerve, the surgical technique most commonly used is the creation of fascial slings to support the ulnar nerve along with an anterior transposition of the nerve. Postoperatively, the elbow is placed in a hinged elbow brace that is positioned at 90° flexion for two weeks. After the first week, the brace is positioned at –30° to –15° extension and 100° to 120° flexion. The brace is discontinued by the third week. By about the sixth week, the patient should have full range of motion in all planes. Gentle gripping using a foam ball starts during the first week along with isometric exercises for the shoulder. Active range-of-motion exercises for pronation, supination, and wrist and finger flexion and extension are also included.

By week 2, isometrics for the elbow and wrist can begin. The splint can be removed for the patient to perform active and passive range-of-motion exercises. Early proprioceptive exercises for position sense are started. Mild manual-resistance exercises and light weights can be used for the wrist. By the third week, resistance exercises for the wrist, forearm, and elbow can include low-resistance, high-repetition exercises in all planes. Exercises are started in straight-plane motions and progress to diagonal planes as the strength and control improve.

By the eighth week, plyometrics can start with their normal progression from low-load, controlled movement to increased loads with higher speeds of movement. Functional activities can begin at week 10 to 12 with full return to sport participation usually seen after week 12 to 16.

Case Study

A 19-year-old right-handed volleyball frontline player suffered a subluxed ulnar nerve at the end of the season. She underwent an ulnar nerve transplantation two days ago. The surgeon wants her to begin her rehabilitation program today. She has a posterior splint set at 90°. She has some pain over the surgical site, but nothing significant. There is some tension in the upper trapezius muscle, and it is tender to palpation. Wrist extension and supination movements cause some medial elbow pain at the end range. Wrist flexion motion is lacking about 10°, and the patient reports that the wrist feels weak and sore from the surgery. Pronation is also weak. Shoulder flexion is lacking about 10°, external rotation is lacking about 20°, and there is some weakness in the rotator cuff.

Questions for Analysis
1. What will your first treatment session include?
2. What home exercises will you give the patient?
3. What exercises will the program include for the next three weeks?
4. Outline a functional-exercise program that the patient will use when she is ready for functional activities.

DISLOCATION

When an elbow dislocation occurs, there is no doubt about it because the deformity is obvious. If there has been no vascular compromise and surgery is not required, a therapeutic exercise program can follow the course described next. As is assumed with any therapeutic exercise program, modalities to relieve pain and swelling and to promote healing are applied before and even during the early stages of the therapeutic exercise program.

Program Considerations

Elbow dislocations occur primarily posteriorly and follow sudden hyperextension and abduction force applications. The injury is obvious because of the deformity.

The elbow should be placed in a posterior immobilizing splint at 90° for about a week. Active wrist and shoulder motion in the splint is desirable. Isometric exercises to the elbow and mild resistive exercises to the wrist can be used initially. The patient can squeeze a ball throughout the day. After about five days, the splint can be removed for gentle active range of motion to tolerance in all elbow and forearm planes. Passive motion is avoided.

After the first week, the splint is removed but used as needed when fatigue occurs. After two weeks, the splint is discarded and active range-of-motion exercises are continued. Mild resistive exercises to the elbow with emphasis on high repetitions and low resistance begin. Straight-plane exercises are used initially and advance to diagonal-plane exercises when the patient demonstrates good control, strength, and coordination. By week 6 the patient should have full range of motion in all planes. Joint mobilization can be started by week 4 to 6 if needed.

Strength exercises progress in the same way as for other elbow injuries from isometric to isotonic to isokinetic. Emphasis is on strengthening the elbow flexors to provide dynamic stabilization against hyperextension. Resistive exercises begin in straight planes and progress to diagonal planes, to plyometrics, and finally to functional activities by week 8 to 10. A hyperextension brace may be necessary to offer the patient additional protection against hyperextension forces. It may take the patient 16 to 26 weeks to return to full sport participation.

Case Study

A 20-year-old right-handed gymnast fell off the balance beam and landed on her left hyperextended elbow, dislocating the elbow, five days ago. Surgery was not necessary, but the orthopedist has placed the elbow in a 90° splint and wants you to begin rehabilitation on it today. Elbow range of motion is −50° extension to 100° flexion. Supination is 10°, and pronation is 20°. Edema and ecchymosis surround the elbow and extend into the mid-forearm and mid upper arm. Spasm is present in the biceps, triceps, and upper trapezius. Strength is difficult to test in the elbow because the patient complains of pain and offers minimal resistance to resisted elbow flexion and extension. Wrist movements demonstrate 4/5 strength, and grip strength is 75% compared to that on the right. Shoulder strength overall is 4+/5.

Questions for Analysis

1. What will your first treatment session include?
2. What instructions for home exercises will you give the patient?
3. What exercises will you include as part of the first week's treatment program?
4. What are your goals for the first week?
5. What will be your progression of flexibility and strength exercises?
6. What functional-exercise program will you include for rehabilitation?

ARTHROSCOPY

Although arthroscopic surgery is less complicated than an open procedure and leads to less tissue damage, respect for tissue healing is still warranted. As the therapeutic exercise program begins, the sport rehabilitation specialist must not lose sight of the fact that the patient has had surgery and that tissue healing is ongoing.

Program Considerations

The most common arthroscopic procedure performed on the elbow is debridement of synovitis and removal of loose bodies. Postoperative rehabilitation following this procedure is more accelerated than with open procedures, because less damage and insult have occurred. The arm is often placed in a sling for one or two days (or three days if the pain warrants it) following the surgery. In addition to pain and edema control, initial treatment includes active and mild passive range of motion and joint mobilization for pain modulation. Shoulder and wrist range-of-motion exercises are also performed. Gripping exercises can also be used in the first two or three postoperative days.

Full range of motion should be possible by the third postoperative day. The sling can be discarded, and mild resistive exercises to the elbow can begin. If debridement has occurred in the posterior elbow, it may be uncomfortable for the patient to perform end-range flexion-extension exercises. These should be performed in straight planes within a pain-free range of motion, especially during the first three to four weeks. Shoulder strengthening and wrist and forearm strengthening are also performed within pain-free limits. Proprioception exercises begin within the first week.

By week 3 to 4, the patient begins the middle rehabilitation phase; isokinetic exercises can begin in straight planes, advancing as indicated to diagonal planes. Rubber tubing and other eccentric exercises can begin. Diagonal planes with resistive exercises can be used once good strength and control are seen in straight-plane exercises.

Plyometric exercises can begin once the patient shows good control and strength in diagonal-plane activities. This can be as early as the third week but may not be possible until the fifth or sixth week, depending on the patient's response to the surgery and exercises. Functional activities begin once plyometric exercises are completed and the patient is pain free and has full range of motion and normal strength. By around week 8, the patient may be ready to return to full sport participa-tion once all functional-activity progressions have been completed.

Case Study

A 35-year-old, right-handed, recreational baseball pitcher underwent arthroscopic removal of loose bodies from the posterior elbow yesterday. The surgeon wants him to begin rehabilitation today. The patient reports mild postoperative pain, but nothing unusual. He is wearing an arm sling, but he has been told he can remove it throughout the day. There is swelling around the surgical site. The dressing does not indicate any unusual postoperative drainage. The elbow range of motion is −30° extension and 100° flexion. Pronation is 70° and supination is 50°. Wrist flexion and extension are each 60°. There is some spasm in the triceps. Manual muscle testing reveals 4−/5 strength in the biceps and triceps with some tenderness to triceps resistance, 4−/5 wrist flexion and extension without pain, and 4/5 strength throughout the shoulder.

Questions for Analysis

1. What will your first treatment be?

2. What instructions will you give the patient before he leaves today?

3. Outline your expected progression of exercises for the next two weeks. What guidelines will you use to determine when the patient should begin a progressive throwing program?

4. What will you tell him when he asks you how soon he can get back to playing baseball?

SUMMARY

1. *Discuss why overstretching the elbow should be avoided, especially during the inflammation phase of healing.*

The brachialis inserts onto the elbow's anterior superior capsule; adhesions occur relatively easily in the elbow; and the anterior capsule is relatively thin and can be easily damaged with aggressive stretching, resulting in additional scarring.

2. *Describe the convex-concave rules for the various elbow joints.*

The radial head and ulna both are concave surfaces and move on a convex capitulum and convex trochlea, respectively, so force applications are in the same direction as the restricted movement. In the proximal radioulnar joint, the force is applied in the direction opposite the restricted movement because this joint is a convex surface moving on a concave surface.

3. *Identify the loose-packed positions for the elbow joints.*

As outlined in table 6.3, the loose-packed position for the humeroulnar joint is 70° elbow flexion and 10° supination. The loose-packed position for the humeroradial joint is full elbow extension with full supination. The radioulnar joint's loose-packed position is 70° elbow flexion with 35° supination.

4. *Identify three soft-tissue mobilization techniques for the elbow.*

Cross-friction is used for the biceps tendon; trigger point release is used for the brachialis; and trigger point release is used for the triceps.

5. *List three joint mobilizations for the elbow.*

Distraction of the ulnohumeral joint is used for general relaxation and pain relief; posterior glide of the radiohumeral joint is used to increase extension; and ventral glide of the radioulnar joint is used for increasing supination.

6. *Explain three strengthening exercises for the elbow and their purpose.*

Elbow flexion in a supinated position for primarily increasing strength of the biceps, elbow flexion in pronation for primarily strengthening brachialis, and elbow flexion in neutral for primarily strengthening brachioradialis.

7. *Discuss the general progression of strengthening exercises for the elbow.*

Range of motion begins with cautious active motion and incorporates low-intensity, long-term stretches only if active exercises cannot restore range of motion. Isometric strengthening exercises are followed by light-resistance exercises and then more-intense strengthening exercises as strength increases. Eccentric exercises are preceded by concentric exercises, using careful stabilization to isolate the correct muscles. Shoulder and wrist exercises are included in the program. Exercises are performed initially in straight plane and advanced to diagonal plane as strength and control improve. Plyometric exercises are added after strength and motion are adequate, and functional activities that prepare the patient for return to sport are the last exercises included.

8. *Outline a therapeutic exercise program for epicondylitis.*

Basic to any tendinitis program is discovering the underlying cause and correcting it. Pain, edema, and inflammation relief with modalities is initiated before therapeutic exercises. Soft-tissue mobilizations such as friction massage and myofascial release are used for soft-tissue-related restrictions and pain, and joint mobilization is used with capsular pattern losses of motion. Active range-of-motion exercises can be performed during the soft-tissue and joint mobilization applications. Isometric and manual resistance in straight-plane exercises are followed by greater-resistance and diagonal-plane activities as strength progresses. Plyometric exercises with medicine balls and rubber resistance are followed by functional activities that begin at low resistance and low intensity and progress as the patient's control and execution improve.

9. *Indicate precautions that should be considered in a Little League elbow therapeutic exercise program.*

   If growth-plate damage is evident when an injury occurs, the patient should be advised to stop pitching for the rest of the baseball season. Active range-of-motion exercises (only to tolerance) are encouraged. Passive stretches should be avoided. Use of heavy weights is not advisable, because this could aggravate sensitive growth plates. Exercises should be neither as aggressive nor as intensive as they are for older patients. Valgus stress should be avoided until it does not cause pain.

10. *List precautions for a therapeutic exercise program following an ulnar nerve transposition.*

    Tissue healing must be respected. Exercises begin more slowly than they do with nonoperative treatment for nerve injuries. Straight-plane exercises precede diagonal-plane exercises. While the elbow is in a postoperative sling, handgrip exercises can be used to start early strengthening. Active exercises should be used for stretching. Gentle cross-friction massage should be used only after three weeks if a loss of range of motion persists.

11. *Explain the differences in rehabilitation programs for an arthroscopic debridement and a medial collateral reconstruction.*

    Because the medial collateral reconstruction is an open procedure, rehabilitation is a much slower process than with some alternative procedures. The period of immobilization is longer, and exercises are less aggressive in the early stages of the program. Loss of motion is a more significant factor, so motion and mobility activities are more prominent in the early phases.

CRITICAL THINKING QUESTIONS

1. Rita is faced with a probable Little League elbow tendinitis in the opening scenario. What other possible diagnoses could Pat have? What tests should Rita perform to determine what the problem is? What recommendations should she make to Mr. Skully for care? What precautions should Rita take in making recommendations to him?

2. How does the rehabilitation program for an elbow differ for a dislocation as compared to a sprain? How are the precautions different? Is the progression of exercises different, and if so, how?

3. Can you identify the differences between a medial and a lateral epicondylitis? What structures are affected? How are the mechanisms of injury different? Would the rehabilitation programs be different? If so, how?

REFERENCES

Curwin, S., and W.D. Stanish. 1984. *Tendinitis: Its etiology and treatment.* Lexington, MA: Heath.

Donkers, M.J., An, K.N., Chaos, E.Y., and B.F. Moray. 1993. Hand position affects elbow joint load during push-up exercise. *Journal of Biomechanics* 26:625–632.

Ellenbecker, T.S., and E.G. Mattalino. 1997. *The elbow in sport.* Champaign, IL: Human Kinetics.

Feltner, M., and J. Dapena. 1986. Dynamics of the shoulder and elbow joints of the throwing arm during a baseball pitch. *International Journal of Sport Biomechanics* 2:235–259.

Groppel, J.L., and R.P. Nirschl. 1986. A mechanical and electromyographical analysis of the effects of various joint counterforce braces on the tennis player. *American Journal of Sports Medicine* 14:195–200.

Kibler, W.B. 1995. Pathophysiology of overload injuries around the elbow. *Clinics in Sports Medicine* 14:447–457.

Mero, A., Komi, T.V., Korjus, T., Navarro, E., and R.J. Gregor. 1994. Body segment contributions to javelin throwing during final thrust phase. *Journal of Applied Biomechanics* 10:166–177.

Nirschl, R.P. 1977. Tennis elbow. *Primary Care* 4:367–382.

Travell, J.G., and D.G. Simons. 1983. *Myofascial pain and dysfunction. The trigger point manual.* Vol. 1. Baltimore: Williams & Wilkins.

SUGGESTED READING

Adriani, E., Luziatelli, S., and P.P. Mariani. 1993. Medial instability of the elbow: Surgical management and rehabilitation. *Journal of Sports Traumatology and Related Research* 15:45–52.

Andrews, J.R., and J.A. Whiteside. 1993. Common elbow problems in the athlete. *Journal of Orthopaedic and Sports Physical Therapy* 17:289–295.

Barker, C. 1988. Evaluation, treatment, and rehabilitation involving a submuscular transposition of the ulnar nerve at the elbow. *Athletic Training* 23:10–12.

Ellenbecker, T.S. 1995. Rehabilitation of shoulder and elbow injuries in tennis players. *Clinics in Sports Medicine* 14:87–104.

Jobe, F.W., and G. Nuber. 1986. Throwing injuries of the elbow. *Clinics in Sports Medicine* 5:621–636.

Lee, D.G. 1986. "Tennis elbow": A manual therapist's perspective. *Journal of Orthopaedic and Sports Physical Therapy* 8:134–142.

Morris, M., Jobe, F.W., Perry, J., Pink, M., and B.S. Healy. 1989. Electromyographic analysis of elbow function in tennis players. *American Journal of Sports Medicine* 17:241–247.

Ollivierre, C.O., and R.P. Nirschl. 1996. Tennis elbow. Current concepts of treatment and rehabilitation. *Sports Medicine* 22:133–139.

Sisto, D.J., Jobe, F.W., Moynes, D.R., and D.J. Antonelli. 1987. An electromyographic analysis of the elbow in pitching. *American Journal of Sports Medicine* 15:260–263.

Stroyan, M., and K.E. Wilk. 1993. The functional anatomy of the elbow complex. *Journal of Orthopaedic and Sports Physical Therapy* 17:279–288.

Werner, S.L., Fleisig, G.S., Dillman, C.J., and J.R. Andrews. 1993. Biomechanics of the elbow during baseball pitching. *Journal of Orthopaedic and Sports Physical Therapy* 17:274–278.

Wilk, K.E., Arrigo, C., and J.R. Andrews. 1993. Rehabilitation of the elbow in the throwing athlete. *Journal of Orthopaedic and Sports Physical Therapy* 17:305–317.

CHAPTER NINETEEN

Wrist and Hand

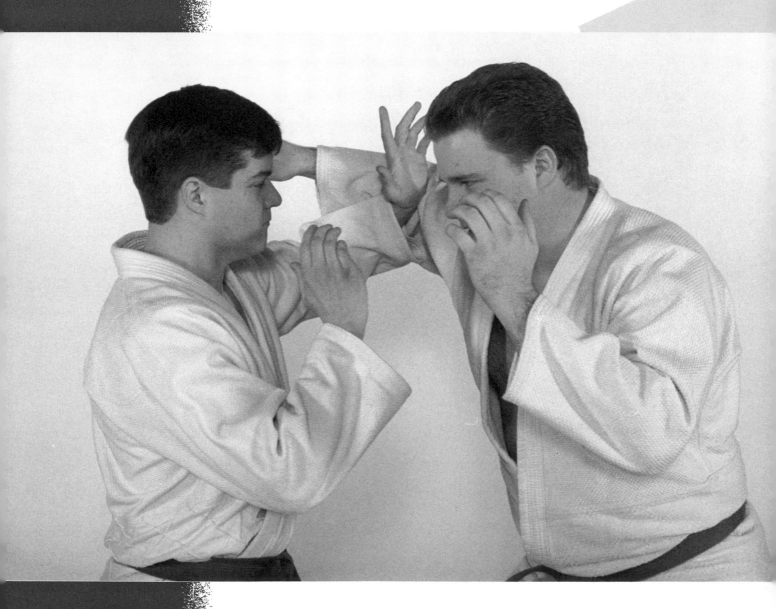

OBJECTIVES

After completing this chapter, you should be able to do the following:

1. Explain the pulley system of the fingers.

2. Explain why reducing edema in the hand is important.

3. Discuss the trimuscular system of the hand and explain its importance to hand function.

4. Identify the precision pinches and power grips of the hand.

5. Explain the difference between static and dynamic splints.

6. Identify what motion is increased with carpal radial glide joint mobilization.

7. Explain the force application sequence to improve long finger flexor and extensor motion.

8. Explain how the intrinsic stretches differ from the extrinsic stretches.

9. Discuss the difference in gliding exercises for the flexor profundus and superficialis tendons.

10. Present the differences between long flexor and long extensor tendons.

11. Explain what procedures should be used to eliminate an extensor lag of a distal phalanx.

12. Identify the early signs of RSD.

Three weeks ago Carlos was playing soccer with his friends when he was tripped and fell, landing on his outstretched hands. His right hand was severely cut by a piece of broken glass hidden in the grass. The surgeon repaired his lacerated long finger flexor tendons and placed the hand in an extension-restricted splint, but now wants Steve Jones to begin the rehabilitation process on the hand.

Steve has had experience with repaired tendons and appreciates the precautions he must consider, especially because the repair is only three weeks old. He is concerned about the adhesions that have begun to form between the flexor superficialis and profundus tendons and other soft tissue in the anterior finger region, and the impact they might have on the finger's hood mechanism. If that is harmed, the intrinsic muscles can be affected, which will impair the hand's function; so Steve understands he has to proceed cautiously, yet effectively, with Carlos's rehabilitation program.

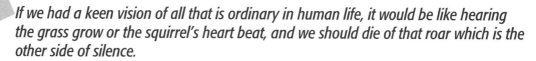

If we had a keen vision of all that is ordinary in human life, it would be like hearing the grass grow or the squirrel's heart beat, and we should die of that roar which is the other side of silence.

George Eliot, *Middlemarch*

Although we use our hands daily for hundreds of activities, not thinking of this as anything beyond the ordinary, if we reflect on the hand at all we realize that it is an extremely complex structure and vital to our daily tasks. Many health care professionals have little concern for finger and hand injuries, but these can be among the most devastating injuries if not properly cared for, if only because the hand has such an important role in everyday activities. In addition, the hand is much more complex than many think, and a seemingly minimal imbalance in the hand can cause profound effects on its abilities. Before we can discuss rehabilitation techniques for the wrist and hand, we must review their unique function and structure. It is important to gain an understanding of the wrist's and hand's structure and function, because they play a vital role in the techniques and applications of therapeutic exercises in a rehabilitation program.

Many texts have been written on the anatomy, biomechanics, and function of the wrist and hand. We will be only skimming the surface of this body of knowledge. A complete investigation of the hand's structure and function is beyond the scope of this chapter, but information vital to establishing a safe and appropriate rehabilitation program for the wrist and hand is presented. I refer you to the suggested reading at the end of this chapter for additional information.

This chapter includes structural and functional information that you will need to create an appropriate rehabilitation program for wrist and hand injuries. A presentation of soft-tissue and joint mobilization techniques includes information organized similarly to that in previous chapters. The exercises presented are limited to flexibility, strengthening, and coordination exercises for the wrist and hand. You should realize, however, that the wrist is intimately connected to the elbow and closely associated with the shoulder, so a therapeutic exercise program should also include activities for these areas. Specific injuries commonly seen in the wrist and hand are discussed, along with rehabilitation programs used to treat these injuries.

GENERAL REHABILITATION CONSIDERATIONS

The hand's many special characteristics include its skeletal structure, its tendon sheaths and pulleys, its fascia and ligaments, and two categories of muscles. Edema is an important consideration in the hand, as are the tendon zones, tendon excursion, the various ways the hand is used, and splinting principles.

The wrist and hand are a complex unit composed of 29 bones, more than 30 tendinous insertions, and an involved neurological system that is vital to the unit's function. Twenty-five percent of the entire body's pacinian corpuscles' sensory endings are located in the hands. The hand's many compactly arranged muscles, including nine for the thumb and seven for the index finger alone, hint at the complexity of its function. The thumb and index finger are used primarily for fine activities requiring dexterity, whereas the middle, ring, and little fingers act primarily as a stabilizing vise for grasping activities. It is important that all of the structures within the hand work in a balanced, coordinated manner for the hand to function optimally.

SKELETAL STRUCTURE

Three flexion arches are formed by the bones of the wrist and hand, proximal and distal transverse arches and a longitudinal arch. The proximal and distal transverse arches are formed by the carpals and metacarpals, respectively. The longitudinal arch runs from the carpals out to the ends of the fingers (figure 19.1). These arches form an equiangular spiral that provides for tremendous adaptation in grasping activities. If these equiangular structures are impaired because of joint restriction or muscle weakness, the hand loses its adaptability.

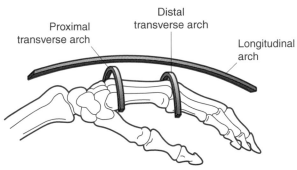

■ **Figure 19.1** Hand arches.

Reprinted from Fess and Philips 1987.

The concave radius joins with the convex proximal carpal row to form the wrist joint. This joint has motions of flexion, extension, abduction, and adduction. Adduction is commonly referred to as **ulnar deviation** or *ulnar flexion*, and abduction is referred to as **radial deviation** or *radial flexion*. These four motions are combined to produce circumduction of the wrist. The distal ulna and radius are supported by the distal radioulnar ligament and the interosseous membrane, and allow forearm supination and pronation movement along with the proximal radioulnar joint. Restricted mobility at either joint prevents full supination-pronation motion.

The carpal bones also form several joints with each other, and the distal row forms the carpometacarpal joints with the metacarpals. The intercarpal joints are irregular in structure and are strongly held in place by ligaments, making it difficult to dislocate any carpal. The carpometacarpal joints are for the most part saddle joints that permit various degrees of flexion, extension, abduction, and adduction of the metacarpals. The thumb and fourth and fifth metacarpals also rotate to provide opposition of the thumb and little finger and grasping by the hand.

The metacarpophalangeal (MCP) joints are formed by the convex metacarpals and concave proximal phalanges. The interphalangeal (IP) joints are named as either proximal (PIP) or distal (DIP) interphalangeal joints. Collateral ligaments provide stability to these joints.

FASCIA AND LIGAMENTS

In addition to the ligaments connecting and supporting the joints throughout the wrist and hand, there are several other static structures that add support to the area. The thick palmar fascia has two layers, the superficial and deep layers. The superficial layer, an extension of the flexor retinaculum (transverse carpal ligament) and the palmaris longus tendon when it is present, expands over the volar hand and runs into each of the fingers. The deep layer covers the floor of the palm and runs between the thenar and hypothenar eminences. The fascia on the dorsum of the hand is in two layers as well but is not as thick as the palmar fascia. The palmar fascia serves to cushion and protect the hand's structures and to assist in maintaining the hand's concavity.

The flexor and extensor tendons are held in place by retinacula positioned throughout the wrist and hand. At the wrist, the flexor tendons are kept from bowstringing away from the wrist by the transverse carpal ligament. This ligament forms the roof of the carpal tunnel and maintains all of the finger flexor tendons except the palmaris longus and flexor carpi ulnaris, the nerves, and the arteries in the carpal tunnel. The extensor retinaculum on the dorsal wrist keeps the extensor tendons from bowstringing away from the wrist.

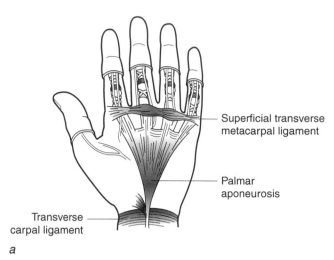

Superficial transverse metacarpal ligament

Palmar aponeurosis

Transverse carpal ligament

a

An extracapsular ligament, the transverse metacarpal ligament, connects the volar plate of one metatarsal head to the volar plate of its adjacent metatarsal heads (figure 19.2). This ligament is important in maintaining the distal transverse arch, and its normal flexibility is vital to hand functions such as prehensile grip and grasping activities. There are several fascial restraints in the digits that maintain alignment of the tendons in the fingers and also provide the pulley system for the tendons.

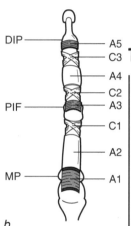

DIP — A5
— C3
— A4
— C2
PIF — A3
— C1
— A2
MP — A1

b

▌**Figure 19.2**
Palmar soft-tissue elements *(a)* and flexor tendon pulley system *(b)*.

TENDON SHEATHS AND PULLEYS

The flexor tendons are surrounded by a complex system of sheaths that serve to protect and nourish the tendons. The sheath system of the extensor tendons is not as elaborate; the extensor tendons are enclosed in sheaths at the wrist when they travel under the extensor retinaculum, but otherwise they are extrasynovial. The flexor sheaths begin proximal to the wrist and extend to the distal digits.

There is an elaborate pulley system on the flexor aspect of the fingers. This is a series of fibrous tunnels that extends from the metacarpal head of each digit to the insertion of the distal finger flexor tendons. These pulleys are similar to the hoops along a fishing rod, positioned to keep the fishing line in place as it travels along the pole. There are five annular pulleys and three cruciate pulleys along the fingers (figure 19.2). Disruption of the key pulleys can cause bowstringing of the flexor tendons. The pulleys that are key to preventing bowstringing are A2 and A4 (Doyle and Blythe 1975). When the pulley system of any finger is disrupted, the mechanical advantage of the tendon is impaired and normal function is lost.

MUSCLES

Hand muscles are divided into two categories, extrinsic and intrinsic. **Extrinsic muscles** originate outside the hand whereas **intrinsic muscles** originate and terminate within the hand. There are 20 extrinsic muscles and 19 intrinsic muscles. The extrinsic muscles are attached to the long tendons. The thenar eminence contains the four intrinsic muscles of the thumb, and the hypothenar eminence contains the three intrinsic muscles of the fifth finger. If the hand is to operate well and avoid deformity following an injury, a balanced system between the intrinsic and extrinsic muscles must be present.

The long finger extensors run to the second through fifth fingers. At the distal metacarpal area they are connected by the juncturae tendinum, a fibrous band that limits independent motion of the extensor tendons. The extensor tendons are connected to the proximal phalanx by sagittal bands that attach on the volar plate to keep the extensor tendons from bowstringing and also transmit the extensor tendons' extension force to the metacarpophalangeal joints. Distal to the MCP joints, the extensor tendons split into three segments: the central slip, which attaches to the

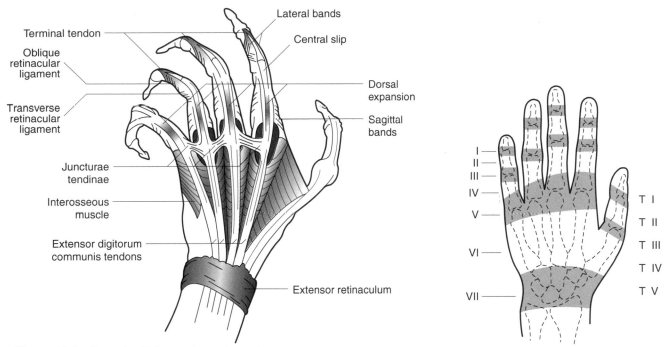

∎Figure 19.3   Dorsal soft-tissue elements and zones.

Extensor tendon zones from Leinert, Schepel, and Gill 1981.

base of the middle phalanx, and two lateral bands that insert when they rejoin at the distal phalanx (figure 19.3).

The long finger flexors include the flexor digitorum sublimis (FDS) and the flexor digitorum profundus (FDP). Both tendons pass deep in the hand. The FDS flexes the PIP joint. Each FDS tendon has its own separate muscle belly, so each can operate independently of the other. Each sublimis tendon splits before it attaches to the base of the middle phalanx and permits the deeper FDP tendon to emerge and attach to the distal phalanx (figure 19.4). The tendons of the FDP, unlike those of the FDS, do not possess separate muscle bellies, so distal phalanx flexion of the fingers cannot be isolated in their movements.

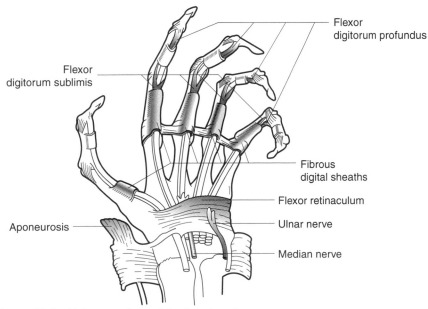

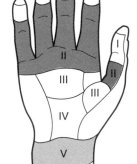

∎Figure 19.4   Palmar surface of the hand and zones.

Flexor tendon zones from American Society for Surgery of the Hand 1983.

Whereas the long finger muscles are used for gross-motor activity, the intrinsic muscles are used for fine-motor activities. They control the more intricate movements of the fingers. The lumbricals and interossei have unique attachments and arrangements with the long flexor and extensor tendons and the ligaments of the fingers. The lumbricals originate from the deep flexor tendons in the palm and insert on the extensor tendon expansion. This unique arrangement allows the lumbricals to function as MCP flexors and IP extensors because their line of force is anterior to the MCP joint, causing flexion at this joint and their line of force is posterior to the IP joint, resulting in IP extension. The dorsal and palmar interossei are responsible for finger abduction and adduction, respectively. Because they are more superficial than the lumbricals, they can be palpated.

EDEMA

Skin covering the volar hand is thick, inelastic, and hairless and is attached to the palmar fascia to allow for grasping objects without their slipping out of the hand. The dorsal skin is elastic, mobile, and easily separated from the underlying fascia to permit skin mobility during grasping activities. Because the dorsal skin is loose and pliable compared to the volar skin, edema frequently accumulates in the dorsum of the hand. Pooled edema rich in proteins easily leads to contractures. Excessive swelling on the back of the hand can cause the hand arches to collapse anteriorly and adduct the thumb. Excessive swelling also requires a greater excursion of the skin to flex the hand. If the skin is already stretched because of the edema, the hand's ability to move the fingers through their full motion is impaired because the skin extensibility is already used by the edema. Fibrous tissue formation secondary to prolonged edema can cause reduced mobility and function of the hand.

Efforts by the sport rehabilitation specialist to reduce early edema are crucial. A circumferential gauge can be used to determine edema of the hand and fingers (figure 19.5). A string wrapped around the finger or hand and then measured for its length can also be used. Compressive dressings, elevation, ice, and compressive machines, as well as other modalities, can be used to reduce edema formation and reduce disability secondary to edema effects.

TENDON ZONES

The flexor and extensor surfaces of the hand are divided into zones. Each zone has characteristics that are unique and that impact both the physician's surgical approach and the sport rehabilitation specialist's rehabilitation approach. For this reason we consider them briefly here. There are five flexor and seven extensor zones of the wrist, hand, and four medial digits. The thumb has three flexor and five extensor zones.

Flexor Tendon Zones

Zone V begins in the forearm at the musculotendinous junction of the extrinsic muscles and goes to the wrist

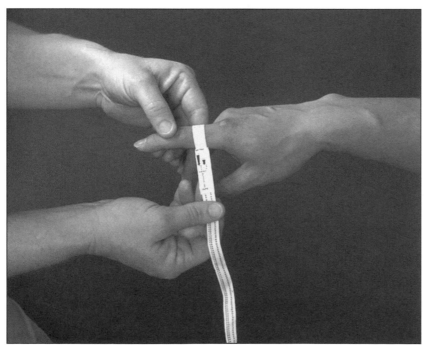

∎ Figure 19.5 Circumferential gauge.

(figure 19.4). The tendons are surrounded by loose tendon sheaths called paratenons. Injured tendons can become adherent to the paratenon and surrounding soft-tissue structures. Following injury in this area, the sport rehabilitation specialist must prevent adhesions or restore normal gliding of tendons if they do occur.

Zone IV is at the wrist. This is the location of the carpal tunnel, the site of carpal tunnel syndrome. Because of the proximity of several tendons, nerves, and blood vessels, adhesions between tendons are a common problem following surgery or injury. The sport rehabilitation specialist must be aware of these problems and prevent them.

Zone III is in the palm after the flexor tendons leave the carpal tunnel. This is where the lumbricals attach to the FDP tendons. Because the extrinsic tendons have more room, they often heal without difficulty or complications. The intrinsic muscles, however, can have adhesions and contractures from prolonged flexor positioning of the palm. Gentle passive range-of-motion (ROM) exercises for the intrinsics can help prevent these complications.

Zone II is from the distal palmar crease, where the synovial sheaths begin, to the middle phalanx where the split slips of the FDS insert on the phalanx and near where the FDP traverses anteriorly from below the sublimis. This is the site of the flexor tendon sheaths. Injuries to the tendons in this region can result in adhesions of the tendons to their sheaths, or adhesions between the sublimis and profundus, and loss of motion. This is a particular concern if any of the pulleys are damaged, especially A2 and A4. These complications can seriously inhibit normal tendon gliding and prevent full restoration of function. This area has been called "no man's land" because of the inhibition of normal function after injury or surgery to this area, but more recent advances in surgical techniques permit improved function following surgery. This topic is discussed more thoroughly in the tendon injury section of this chapter.

Zone I is the area of the DIP joint. The only tendon involved here is the FDP as it inserts on the distal phalanx. Tendons are commonly ruptured from this location. These injuries require careful rehabilitation, because complications such as poor tendon gliding, contractures, and repair failures can occur.

The thumb zones include T I, T II, and T III. These zones are comparable to zones I, II, and III, respectively, of the fingers. Tendon injuries in these zones do not carry with them as strong a risk of adhesions, because the only tendon enclosed in a sheath is the flexor pollicis longus.

Extensor Tendon Zones

Zone VII is located at the wrist joints (figure 19.3). This area contains both wrist extensors and extrinsic finger extensors. The tendons in this area have synovial sheaths, are close together, and are covered by the dorsal retinaculum. This can be an area of adhesion formation after injury or immobilization. If an injury in this area involves only the wrist extensors, the wrist is the only joint in need of immobilization and should be positioned in approximately 45° of extension. However, if the long finger extensors are also involved, the wrist and MCP joints should both be positioned in extension. Because of the synovial sheaths in this area, the problems in rehabilitation of extensor zone VII are similar to those seen in flexor zone II (Evans 1989). The sport rehabilitation specialist must be cognizant of the risks of losing tendon gliding capabilities and should take steps to prevent and treat this complication. Tendon adhesions can cause loss of normal tendon gliding, can reduce wrist motion and strength, and can result in tendinitis. The treatment program, consisting of splinting and mobilization, is discussed later in this chapter.

Zones V and VI are from the hand distal to the extensor sheaths in the region of the CMC joints to distal of the MCP joints at the start of the extensor hood. Extensor tendons and sheaths can adhere to other surrounding soft-tissue structures, especially because they are close to the skin. Edema formation in the hand is usually seen in this area more predominantly than in the palmar aspect and should be controlled by the sport rehabilitation specialist. Control of edema will help reduce the risk of adhesion formation. Wrist immobilization for this area is approximately 45° extension at the wrist with the MCP and IP joints at 0° extension. Zones III and IV include the proximal phalanx and the PIP joints. When injuries occur to the extrinsic extensor tendon's central slip, what results is a **boutonniere deformity** where the PIP is positioned in flexion and the DIP in extension with the unbalanced pull of the intact lateral bands (see figure 19.60 on p. 749). Although stiffness of the PIP joint with loss of joint motion is a complication, immobilization of the digit is necessary, as discussed later in this chapter.

Zones I and II include the middle phalanx and the DIP joints. Ruptures of the distal tendon insertion resulting in mallet deformities occur commonly in this region. If untreated, a **mallet deformity** may lead to a **swan-neck deformity**, in which the PIP joint is hyperextended and the DIP joint is flexed. This occurs in the presence of a lax volar plate as the extensor mechanism slides proximally without its anchor at the distal phalanx. Splinting, and in some cases surgery, is necessary to correct this injury. Care must be taken during this time to guard against an extensor lag and local ischemia. Treatment of this injury is discussed in detail later. The thumb zones coincide with the zones of the finger, and injuries to those zones can be treated similarly to the corresponding finger zones. T I and T II coincide with zones I and II of the fingers. Zones T III and T IV coincide with zones V and VI of the fingers. Zone T V, like zone VII of the fingers, can suffer adhesions following injury. Web-space contracture, extensor pollicis longus adhesions, and reduced excursion of the thumb are common problems that the sport rehabilitation specialist must avoid.

EXCURSIONS

For the hand to close into a fist, a large **excursion** of the extensor tendons and dorsal surface of the hand and wrist must be possible. Adhesions can restrict this necessary mobility and reduce hand function. For this reason, early controlled passive motion of tendon injuries is vital to restoring full hand function. Care must be taken to maintain good tendon glide without risking tendon rupture.

As a tendon glides within its sheath, the adhesions are stretched. The normal excursion of a tendon is variable from one finger to another and is a matter of some dispute. The most commonly repeated values are based on the work of Bunnell reported by Boyes (1970) (table 19.1). The significance of these numbers for rehabilitation is twofold: They indicate how much excursion must be restored following injury or immobilization, and how much each healing tendon can move during immobilization without incurring damage. Based on Bunnell's work, it has been determined that a safe tendon-glide excursion of 5 mm would permit sufficient motion to minimize deleterious immobilization effects without endangering the extensor tendon (Duran and Houser 1975). Five millimeters of motion changes in terms of degrees from finger to finger, depending on the full arc of motion available (Evans and Burkhalter 1986). Table 19.2 lists the degrees of motion permitted with 5 mm (.2 in.) of movement for each digit at the MCP joint. These degrees, which become important in splint design when one is deciding the MCP angle of the splint for hand position after tendon repair, are discussed later. These excursions are also important for understanding the limitations of motion permitted in the early rehabilitation process to allow tendon gliding motion without causing tendon disruption.

USE OF THE HAND

The hand is a trimuscular system that uses the three muscle groups, the extrinsic flexors, the extrinsic extensors, and the intrinsic muscles, to provide balanced, controlled

Table 19.1   Extensor Tendon Excursions

| | Extensor digitorum communis | | | | Extensor pollicus longus |
	Index	Long	Ring	Small	
Total	54 mm	55 mm	55 mm	35 mm	58 mm
Wrist	38 mm	41 mm	39 mm	20 mm	33 mm
MCP	15 mm	16 mm	11 mm	12 mm	7 mm
PIP	2 mm	3 mm	3 mm	2 mm	—
DIP	0	0	0	0	—
IP	—	—	—	—	8 mm

Adapted, by permission, from J.H. Boyes, 1970, *Bunnell's surgery of the hand* (Philadelphia: Lippincott). Copyright by Lippincott, Williams & Wilkins.

Table 19.2   Excursion of Extensor Digitorum Communis at the MCP Joint

Index finger	28.3°
Middle finger	27.5°
Ring finger	40.9°
Little finger	38.3°

Reprinted from Evans and Burkhalter 1986.

function. If any of these muscle groups does not function normally because of either weakness or loss of mobility, balance is lost and the hand is not be able to work in its normal capacity.

Because of the hand's complex system of joints and muscles, uses of the hand as a tool are numerous. The hand can be used to transmit force or to provide movement to produce a desired effect. About 20% of its responsibility involves force transmission (Bowers and Tribuzi 1992). This force transmission occurs through power grips, also known as palmar grips, including the clenched fist, the cylinder grasp, the spherical grasp, and the hook (figure 19.6). In these grasps, the thumb is positioned in opposition to the other fingers to permit a firm grasp on an object. The majority of daily hand activities involve these palmar grips. Because palmar grasping is so vital to hand function, the hand is most commonly splinted in a palmar position with the thumb in slight opposition, facing the other fingers.

The rest of the time, the hand provides movement to accomplish intricate tasks. These tasks include many activities, such as typing, sewing, or writing. They also include prehensile, or grip, activities in which the thumb and finger muscles co-contract to produce a desired activity. The three pinches are the digital prehension pinch (also known as 3 jaw chuck), the lateral prehension pinch, and the tip-to-tip prehension pinch (figure 19.7). The digital prehension pinch is used to handle and maneuver small tools in intricate activities. The lateral prehension pinch places the thumb tip against the side of the index finger and is used to grasp objects such as a key or book. The tip-to-tip prehension pinch uses thumb opposition to position the tip of the thumb facing the tip of another finger. It is used most often to pick up small objects.

In the precision pinches, the fingers are flexed and abducted at the MCP joints with some opposition present. The movements involved in precision activities vary in excursion and number of digits involved, but usually include the motions of flexion and rotation with ulnar deviation. Unless the object being manipulated is heavy or

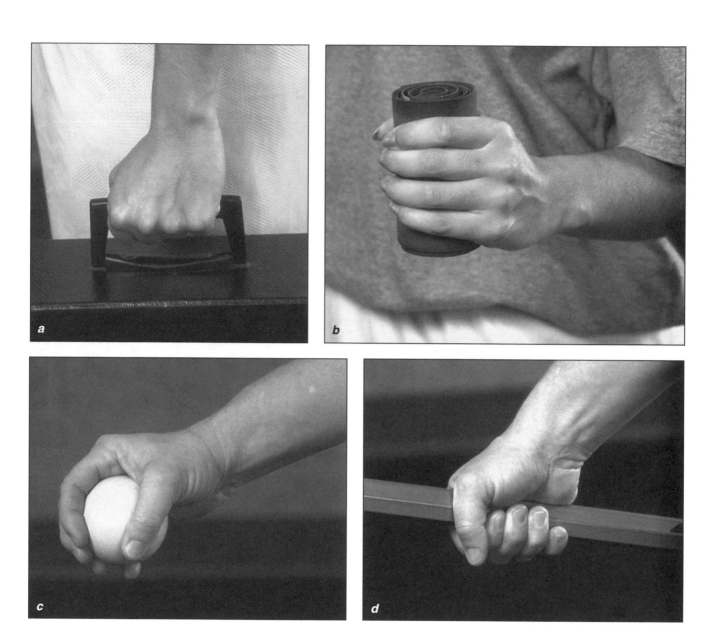

Figure 19.6 Power grips: *(a)* hook, *(b)* cylinder, *(c)* spherical., *(d)* fist

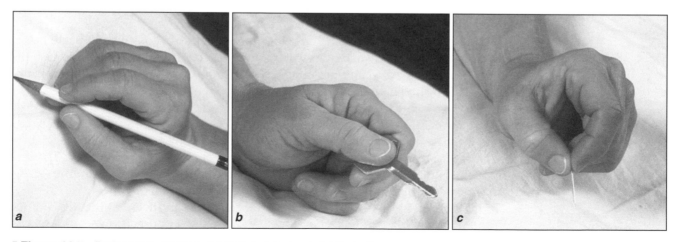

Figure 19.7 Prehension pinches: *(a)* digital, *(b)* lateral, *(c)* tip-to-tip.

large, primarily the radial digits are involved in precision activities. The power grips use the ulnar aspect of the hand to grasp the object and deliver the power and stability while the radial aspect of the hand provides the precision for the activity. Golf presents an example of this utilization of the power grip. In a power grip, the fingers flex and rotate and move into ulnar deviation so that the fingertips point toward the thenar eminence to hold the object in the hand and stabilize the thumb in abduction.

All these motions and grips must be restored to the injured hand. The sport rehabilitation specialist accomplishes this through awareness of the component motions these activities require, restoration of joint mobility, attainment of normal tendon glide, and balance of strength and flexibility.

SPLINTING

Splinting is commonly used in the treatment of hand injuries. Splints are either static or dynamic. **Static splints** are used to restrict motion to support and protect the hand, and **dynamic splints** are used to increase motion of the hand. The aim in using splints is either to prevent damage and maintain balance or to improve balance. Splints are based on a three-point pressure system whereby two points of application are on one side of the hand, wrist, or forearm; and the fulcrum, or other point of application, is on the opposite side (figure 19.8). This system should be familiar because it was presented as a force system in chapter 3.

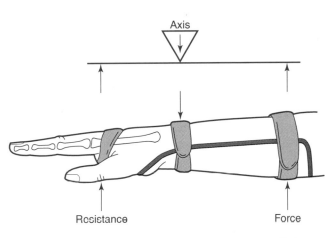

▌Figure 19.8 Three-point pressure system for splinting.

Splints are applied for varying amounts of time, depending on the structure injured, the repair, the adjacent structures and their influence on the injured tissue, and healing of the injured tissue. Splints may be applied during the day for periods of 3 to 8 weeks. Frequently, patients continue to use a night splint after they have reduced or discontinued splint use during the day. Use of night splints may continue for 10 to 12 weeks postinjury. It is not unusual for complex injuries to advance from one splint to a less restrictive splint during the day before removal of any day support is permitted.

Static Splints

Static splints do not have any moving parts (figure 19.9). They immobilize a joint to protect it from movement that would be deleterious. Periods of immobilization are frequently indicated following injury, and the static splint can prevent movement to allow scar-tissue formation to restore joint stability. If a joint has lost its mobility, a static splint places the joint on stretch by applying a low-level prolonged stretch and thus improving joint mobility. A static splint can also be designed to maintain ROM gains resulting from other rehabilitation techniques; this is called a **static progressive splint**.

Although there are some exceptions, most often the hand is placed in a functional

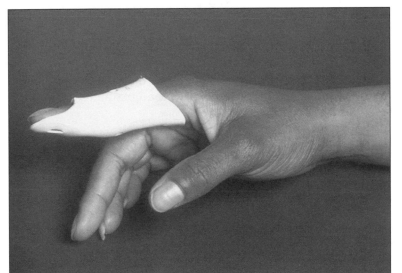

▌Figure 19.9 Static tendon splint to restrict ROM.

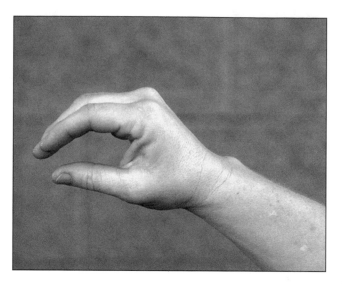

Figure 19.10   Position of hand immobilization.

position with the wrist in slight extension, the fingers slightly flexed at the MCP and IP joints, and the thumb in slight opposition to the other fingers (figure 19.10). Only as many joints as necessary are immobilized so that mobility of the unaffected joints is optimized.

Dynamic Splints

Dynamic splints incorporate a system of movement through the use of springs, rubber bands, or other elastic elements. These splints are designed to produce passive or passive assistive motion in one line of pull and active resistive motion in the opposite direction. Dynamic splints can promote mobility by providing a continual, low-level stretch force to a joint. They are used when the patient lacks normal motion and is unable to achieve the desired mobility independently. The patient should be able to perceive the stretch force applied with the splint but should not find it painful. Because the splint is worn for a prolonged period of time to effect scar-tissue remodeling, the force applied is low. These splints are usually worn at night so that they do not interfere with hand function during the day. The duration it is worn depends on the patient's tolerance, but the longer the splint is in place, the more successful the results are. As the joint's ROM increases, adjustments in the splint are necessary.

Dynamic splints are frequently used following tendon surgery to permit protected, guided movement of the tendon to maintain the tendon glide without risking tendon rupture. The splint permits the appropriate degree of tendon motion based on the numbers presented in table 19.2. The tendon is held in its shortened position by rubber bands, and the splint keeps the opposing tendon from moving the digit beyond the designated degree of movement. The opposing tendon must work against the force of the rubber band to move the finger in the direction permitted, and the rubber band passively returns the finger to the resting position.

When splints are designed for the hand, fit, design, and purpose must be considerations. The purpose will determine what type of splint is used. The fit is individually determined based on the hand size and dimensions. The design is based on a combination of fit, purpose, and precautions.

Precautions in splint design are primarily two: friction and pressure. Whether a splint is static or dynamic, friction can occur between the splint and the skin. When a splint does not fit correctly, it will move from its intended position and cause friction and irritation. A splint should be held firmly, yet comfortably, in position by its straps and other structures. Splints usually require periodic adjustments for maintenance of proper alignment and reduction of friction.

Pressure is particularly a problem when the brace is placed over bony prominences. The hand's most susceptible areas are the ulnar and radial styloid processes, pisiform, base of the fifth metacarpal, and metacarpal heads. Padding over these susceptible areas can be applied during brace construction and removed when the brace is worn to prevent pressure. If padding or relief is added after the brace is made, it may change the alignment and intended force application of the brace.

The patient's skin should be routinely checked for redness and signs of pressure or friction. Adjustments may be necessary as the patient's condition changes. Wrist and hand splint construction can be complicated, depending on the injury. In complex cases, an occupational therapist, orthopedic technician, or other hand specialist typically constructs the splint. In these cases, the sport rehabilitation specialist plays an important role in reporting on the patient's tolerance of the splint and can reinforce wear compliance.

SOFT-TISSUE MOBILIZATION

Soft-tissue mobilization techniques used for the extrinsic and the intrinsic muscles of the hand include trigger point release and ice-and-stretch techniques.

Although soft-tissue treatment of many of the intrinsic muscles of the wrist and hand is discussed in chapter 18, other treatments have yet to be introduced. The soft-tissue mobilization techniques in this chapter are limited to trigger point release and ice-and-stretch techniques based on the work of Travell and Simons (1983). The pain-referral patterns and information presented here are also based on their work.

EXTRINSIC MUSCLES

Although there are several extrinsic muscles of the wrist and hand, they are grossly divided into two groups: flexors and extensors. The palmaris longus is described separately from the other flexors because its pain referral is different from theirs.

Palmaris Longus

The palmaris longus refers pain into the palm, but not the digits, and to a lesser extent along the distal anterior forearm. Because it inserts superficially, the pain is usually a prickly superficial sensation rather than the deep sensation of most muscle pain-referral patterns. The trigger point is a palpable band that is located in the medial aspect of the proximal anterior forearm as seen in figure 19.11a.

Trigger point release of this muscle is performed by placing direct pressure over the trigger point location or rolling across the band (figure 19.11b).

Ice-and-stretch is applied with the muscle on stretch. The elbow is supported on a padded surface while the fingers and wrist are extended. The ice is applied in parallel sweeps from the medial elbow along the medial forearm and into the palm as the elbow and fingers are passively moved into extension (figure 19.11c).

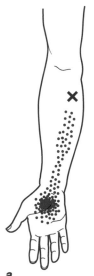
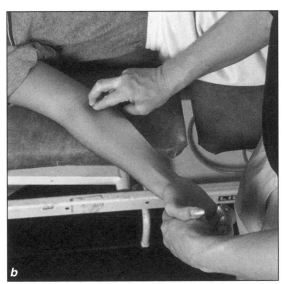
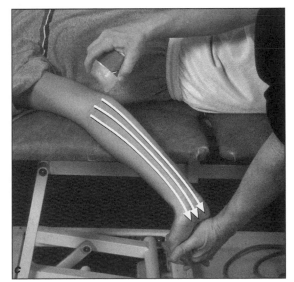

■ **Figure 19.11** Palmaris longus: *(a)* pain-referral pattern, *(b)* trigger point release, *(c)* ice-and-stretch.

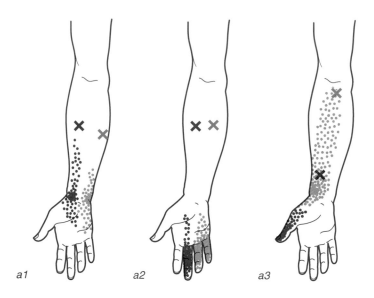

Pronator Teres, and Wrist and Long Finger Flexors

The wrist flexors and pronator teres refer pain into the wrist: the flexor carpi ulnaris to the ulnar aspect, the flexor carpi radialis to the radial aspect, and the pronator teres to the radial wrist. The long finger and thumb flexors refer pain into the digits they activate and extend the sensation of pain shooting out beyond the end of the digits (figure 19.12a). Pain patterns between the finger flexor sublimis and profundus have not been differentiated.

Trigger points are located within the forearm near the midbelly portion of each muscle. The exception is the flexor pollicis longus, whose trigger point is located on the distal forearm. Trigger point release is applied with the specific muscle in a relaxed position. Each muscle is treated with direct pressure over the tender trigger point until the discomfort subsides. Each trigger point elicits a local twitch response and produces a pain-referral pattern.

Ice-and-stretch is applied with the muscle on stretch and a support under the elbow (figure 19.12, b–c). The ice sweeps are made from the medial elbow downward to the specific digit being treated.

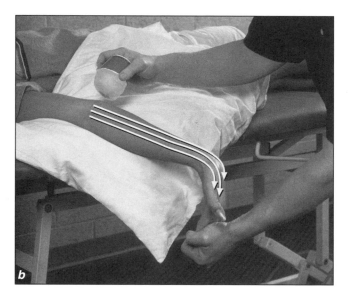
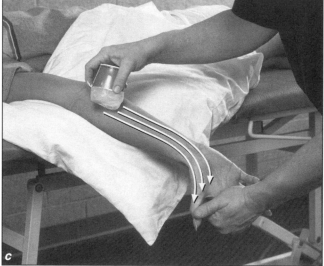

■ **Figure 19.12** Pronator teres, wrist and finger flexors: *(a)* pain-referral patterns, *(a1)* dark = flexor carpi radialis, light = flexor carpi ulnaris; *(a2)* dark = long finger flexors radial head, light = long finger flexors humeral head; *(a3)* dark = flexor pollicus longus, light = pronator teres, *(b)* ice-and-stretch to wrist and finger flexors, *(c)* ice-and-stretch to flexor pollicus longus and pronator teres.

Long Finger Extensors

In contrast with the long finger flexors, the long extensors refer pain into their digits short of the last phalanx. The pain is referred along the posterior forearm, with the primary pain occurring into the digit. The middle finger extensor can also refer to the lateral epicondyle. The extensor indicis refers to the ulnar wrist and into the dorsum of the hand but not the digit (figure 19.13,a–d). The trigger points are located in the belly of each muscle.

Extensor tendon trigger points are easily located as they produce a twitch response, especially the tendon to the long finger. It is located about 3 to 4 cm (about 7.5–10 in.) distal and dorsal to the radial head. Because the little- and ring-finger fibers are the deeper fibers of the muscle, they are more difficult to palpate but produce a twitch response when located. Deep pressure applied over these trigger points while the muscle is relaxed diminishes the discomfort (figure 19.13e).

Ice-and-stretch is performed with the forearm supported and the elbow extended. Ice sweeps, made from the elbow, move distally to the fingers with the wrist and fingers placed on stretch (figure 19.13f). If pain is referred to the lateral epicondyle, ice sweeps upward toward the epicondyle are also performed.

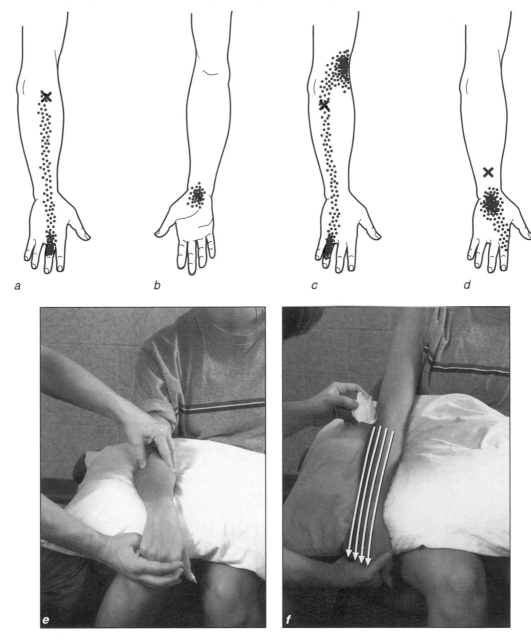

a *b* *c* *d*

e *f*

■ Figure 19.13 Long finger extensors: pain-referral patterns for middle-finger extensor *(a–b)*, ring-finger extensor *(c)*, extensor indicis *(d)*; *(e)* trigger point release; *(f)* ice-and-stretch.

INTRINSIC MUSCLES

The intrinsic muscles are divided into three groups based on where they function: (1) at the thumb, (2) at the little finger, and (3) at the other finger muscles—the interossei and lumbricals. The thumb muscles lie within the thenar eminence, and the little finger muscles lie within the hypothenar eminence. Between these two prominences lie the interossei and lumbricals.

Thumb Muscles

The adductor pollicis refers pain to the base of the thumb, and the opponens pollicis refers pain to the radial volar wrist and along the palmar aspect of the thumb (figure 19.14, a–c). Each trigger point is near the middle aspect of the muscle belly.

Trigger point release of each muscle is applied with the muscle relaxed and pressure over the trigger point until a release is palpated or the discomfort diminishes (figure 19.14d).

Ice-and-stretch is applied with the muscle on stretch. The sweeps are applied across the thenar eminence and over the thumb (figure 19.14e).

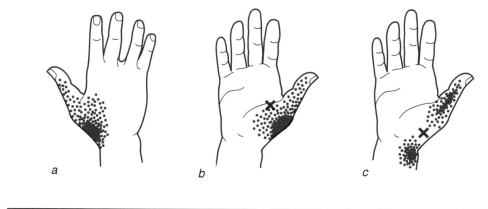

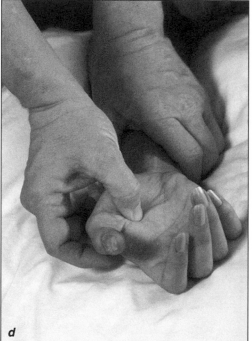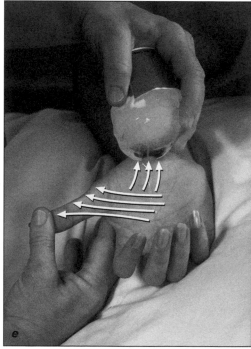

∎ **Figure 19.14** Thumb intrinsics: pain-referral patterns for adductor pollicis *(a–b)*, opponens pollicus *(c)*; *(d)* trigger point release to adductor pollicus; *(e)* ice-and-stretch.

Interossei and Abductor Digiti Minimi

The dorsal interossei produce a strong pain referral along the radial side of the index finger, especially at the DIP joint. The other interossei refer pain along the side of the digit to which they attach (figure 19.15, a–d).

Trigger points can be palpated and treated using a pincher grip with the patient's fingers spread to move the metacarpals apart. While applying pressure on the dorsal surface, the sport rehabilitation specialist applies counterpressure on the palmar surface.

Ice-and-stretch is applied with the patient relaxed and the forearm supported. Only the first dorsal interossei can be reached with ice-and-stretch. With the thumb in abduction, the index finger is adducted toward the middle finger as an ice sweep is performed from proximal to the wrist and along the index finger (figure 19.15e).

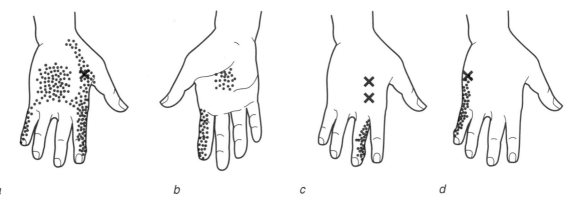

a   b   c   d

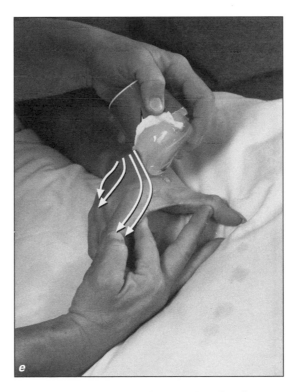

■ **Figure 19.15** Interossei and abductor digiti minimi: pain-referral patterns for first dorsal interosseus *(a–b)*, second dorsal interosseus *(c)*, abductor digiti minimi *(d); (e)* ice-and-stretch.

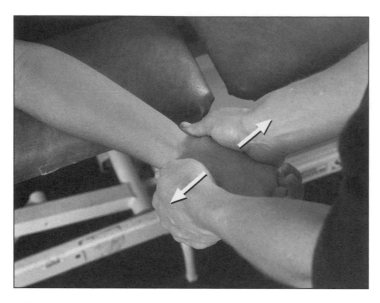

I Figure 19.16   Palmar myofascial release.

Palmar Fascia

This myofascial technique is used to mobilize palmar fascia and the wrist retinaculum. The patient sits facing the sport rehabilitation specialist or lies supine with the forearm resting comfortably on the table. With the patient's hand in a palm-up position, the sport rehabilitation specialist grasps the patient's hand with the thumbs adjacent to each other over the base of the wrist and the fingers wrapped around the hand with the finger pads on the dorsum of the wrist. (figure 19.16). The sport rehabilitation specialist applies a lateral traction of the palmar soft tissue with his or her thumbs and their thenar eminences, as an upward force is applied by the finger pads on the wrist's dorsum.

JOINT MOBILIZATION

Various joint mobilization techniques are used to improve movement in the distal radioulnar joint, the wrist joint, and the carpometacarpal joints.

Most of the joint mobilization techniques discussed here are for joint accessory movements. They are based primarily on Maitland's (1991) work. There are certainly more movements available, but the movements discussed here are the techniques commonly used to improve joint mobility of the distal forearm, wrist, hand, and fingers.

DISTAL RADIOULNAR JOINT

As with any elbow injury, both the proximal and distal radioulnar joints should be assessed for restricted mobility. If any restriction is present, they should be mobilized according to restrictive findings.

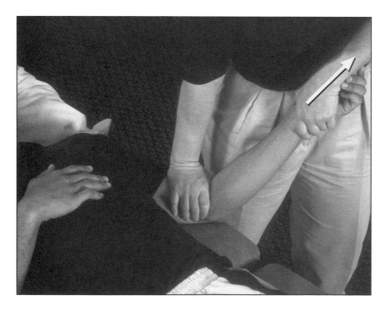

I Figure 19.17   Joint mobilization: radioulnar longitudinal distraction.

Longitudinal Traction

This is an accessory movement that is used to distract both the proximal and distal radioulnar joints. It can be performed in any position of elbow flexion or extension and any position of forearm supination or pronation. The most excursion for this occurs in a midposition of both flexion-extension and pronation-supination (Maitland 1991). This technique is often performed at the end range of the restricted movement.

The patient is positioned comfortably in either sitting or supine. The sport rehabilitation specialist faces the patient and places the stabilizing hand just proximal to the patient's elbow, with the hand's web space wrapped around the arm and the mobilizing hand wrapped around the anterior wrist (figure 19.17). The forearm of the mobilizing arm is in line with the patient's forearm. After the soft tissue's slack is taken up, either an oscillating longitudinal pull or a sustained traction is applied with the mobilizing arm.

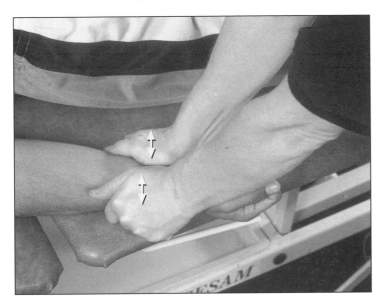

∎ Figure 19.18   Joint mobilization: distal radioulnar AP and PA glides.

Anteroposterior and Posteroanterior Glides

This mobilization technique is used to improve radioulnar mobility in supination and pronation. The sport rehabilitation specialist uses one hand to grasp the ulnar head and the other to grasp the radial head. The pad on one thenar eminence is used to apply the anteroposterior (AP) force on one bone; the fingers of the opposite hand, on the patient's posterior forearm, are used to apply the posteroanterior (PA) force on the other bone (figure 19.18). The vertical forces applied by the two hands should be equal in timing and degree. An AP force on the radius with a PA force on the ulna increases supination, and an AP force on the ulna with a PA force on the radius increases pronation.

WRIST JOINT

Wrist mobilizations are performed with the patient in a comfortable position, either sitting or supine. The sport rehabilitation specialist is sitting or standing. A towel roll is placed under the patient's distal forearm with the wrist over the table edge.

Joint Traction

This maneuver is for general mobilization of the wrist. The forearm is in a comfortable position of pronation, and the wrist is in neutral. The sport rehabilitation specialist stabilizes the distal forearm with one hand around the radial and ulnar styloids and places the mobilizing hand over the distal carpal row. A traction force in a longitudinal direction is applied with the mobilizing hand (figure 19.19). The force can be either a sustained application or a traction oscillation.

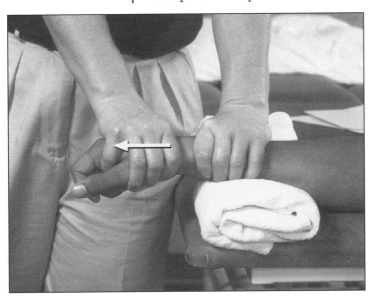

∎ Figure 19.19   Joint mobilization: wrist traction.

Dorsal Glide

This is a general maneuver used to increase wrist flexion. With the patient's forearm in pronation and the wrist in neutral, the sport rehabilitation specialist places the stabilizing hand over the radial and ulnar styloids and the mobilizing hand over the distal carpal row. An AP mobilizing force is applied by the distal, mobilizing hand (figure 19.20). The force should be applied at an angle parallel to the wrist joint.

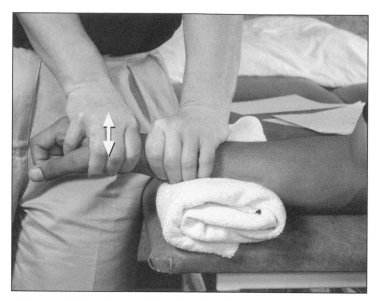

■ **Figure 19.20** Joint mobilization: dorsal and volar glides of the wrist.

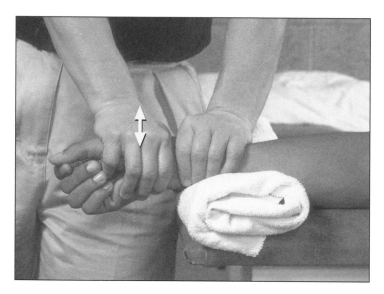

■ **Figure 19.21** Joint mobilization: radial and ulnar glides of the wrist.

Volar Glide

This is a general maneuver used to increase wrist extension. With the patient's forearm in pronation and the wrist in neutral, the sport rehabilitation specialist places the stabilizing hand over the radial and ulnar styloids and the mobilizing hand over the distal carpal row. Then a PA force is applied by the distal, mobilizing hand (figure 19.20). The force should be applied at an angle parallel to the wrist joint.

Radial Glide

This is a general technique used to increase ulnar deviation. The patient's forearm is positioned with the ulnar side upward and the wrist in neutral. The sport rehabilitation specialist places the stabilizing hand over the radial and ulnar styloids and the mobilizing hand over the distal carpal rows (figure 19.21). A vertically downward mobilizing force is applied by the mobilizing hand.

Ulnar Glide

This is a general technique used to increase radial deviation. The patient's forearm is positioned with the radial side upward and the wrist in neutral. The sport rehabilitation specialist places the stabilizing hand over the radial and ulnar styloids and the mobilizing hand over the distal carpal rows (figure 19.21). A vertically downward mobilizing force is applied by the mobilizing hand.

Specific Carpal Glides

Each of the carpals in the proximal and distal rows can be mobilized with each other and with the radius and ulna to improve flexion or extension motion in the wrist. Sometimes when individual carpal joints are restricted, individual joint mobilization techniques are necessary. The concave-convex rule applies to these joints, so it is important to know the joint's configuration before deciding whether a PA or an AP mobilization force is appropriate (figure 19.22).

The radius and ulna are concave surfaces, and the proximal carpal row provides the convex surfaces for the radiocarpal and ulnocarpal joints. To increase extension in the radiocarpal joints, the carpals are glided in a volar (anterior) direction. To increase flexion in the radiocarpal joints, the radius is glided in a volar direction. The ulnocarpal joint is mobilized by gliding the ulna in an anterior direction to unlock the articular disk that can obstruct wrist motion.

In the radial intercarpal joints, the convex scaphoid joins with the concave trapezium and trapezoid; this means that flexion is increased with a volar glide of the trapezium and trapezoid on a fixed scaphoid, and extension is increased with a volar glide of the scaphoid on the distal carpal row. Because the capitate is the convex

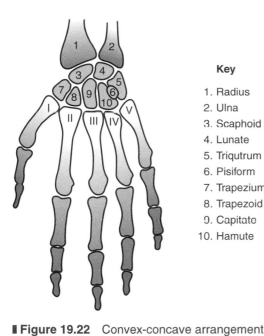

Key

1. Radius
2. Ulna
3. Scaphoid
4. Lunate
5. Triqutrum
6. Pisiform
7. Trapezium
8. Trapezoid
9. Capitate
10. Hamute

■ **Figure 19.22** Convex-concave arrangement of carpal bones.

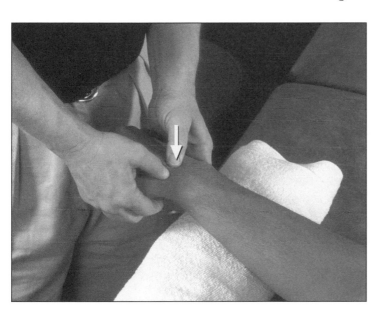

■ **Figure 19.23** Joint mobilization: specific carpal glides.

surface and the lunate is the concave surface of the capitate-lunate joint, flexion is increased by a volar glide of the lunate on the fixed capitate, and extension is increased by stabilizing the proximal lunate and performing a volar glide of the distal capitate.

The mobilization techniques for each of these joints are similar. The forearm is unsupported so that the weight of the arm can provide a slight traction force on the joints. In each case, mobilization is performed using a pinch grasp with both the stabilizing and mobilizing hands with the thumbs on the dorsum of the pronated wrist. The stabilizing finger and thumb grasp the bone that is to remain stationary, and the mobilizing finger and thumb grasp the bone to be mobilized (figure 19.23). Because the joints are small, the sport rehabilitation specialist's thumbs are nearly in contact with each other. The thumbs are used to apply a vertical downward force in a volar direction.

CARPOMETACARPAL JOINTS

For the finger and thumb carpometacarpal (CMC) joints, hand placements for stabilization and mobilization are similar. The stabilizing hand is placed in a thumb-and-index-finger pinch grasp over the carpal bone, and the mobilizing hand is placed in a similar grasp around the base of the metacarpal. Some distraction is applied to the joint while the mobilizing force is simultaneously applied. It is important to be careful not to squeeze the carpal but still grasp it firmly enough to provide adequate mobilization force. Because the CMC joints have a convex carpal and a concave meta-carpal, flexion is increased with a volar (PA) glide of the distal segment, and extension is increased with a dorsal (AP) glide of the distal segment of the joint.

Finger Carpometacarpal Joints

Loss of mobility in these joints can restrict the individual's ability to make a fist and can reduce grip capabilities. Joint mobilization is often required to restore motion in these joints. Some of the most common techniques are presented here.

Joint Traction
This technique is used to relieve pain and provide a general increase in mobility. The carpal is stabilized, and the metacarpal is pulled in the direction of its long axis (figure 19.24).

Carpometacarpal Anteroposterior Glide
This technique is used to increase extension. The patient's hand is positioned in supination. The sport rehabilitation specialist stabilizes the patient's carpal with the thumb and index finger of one hand, then places the thumb and index finger of the other hand over the metacarpal to be treated, with the thumb on the volar surface (figure 19.25). A downward force is applied by the thumb on the metacarpal in a direction vertical to the joint surface.

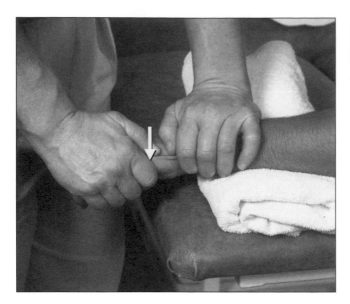

■ **Figure 19.24**   Joint mobilization: CMC distraction.

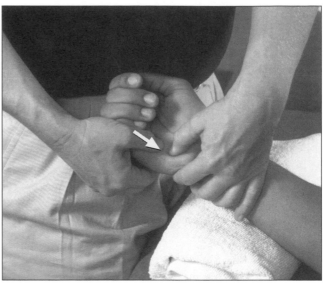

■ **Figure 19.25**   Joint mobilization: CMC AP glide joint mobilization.

Carpometacarpal Posteroanterior Glide

This technique is used to increase flexion. With the patient's hand in pronation, the sport rehabilitation specialist's grasps are similar to those described for AP glides except that the thumbs are placed on the dorsal surface and the fingers are placed on the volar surface (figure 19.26). A dorsal force glide is applied to the metacarpal. If mobilizing the radial side, the sport rehabilitation specialist's fingers grasp around the first web space of the patient's hand. If mobilizing the ulnar hand, the sport rehabilitation specialist grasps the ulnar border of the hand.

Metacarpophalangeal Joint Rotation

Rotation of the MCP joints is an accessory movement that is necessary for full joint motion. If the finger is lacking the last few degrees of motion or the hand cannot make a complete fist, it may be that rotation of the MCP is limited. The MCP is positioned in 90° flexion. A distraction is applied to the joint as the distal segment of the joint is rotated medially and laterally (figure 19.27).

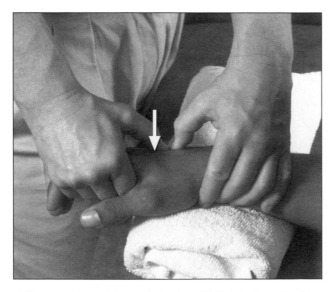

■ **Figure 19.26**   Joint mobilization: CMC PA (dorsal) glide.

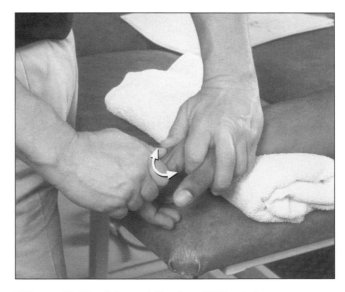

■ **Figure 19.27**   Joint mobilization: MCP rotation.

Thumb Carpometacarpal Joint

As with carpometacarpal techniques for fingers 2 through 5, mobilization of the thumb is applied with the stabilizing hand using a thumb-and-index-finger pinch grasp over the carpal bone and the mobilizing hand placed around the metacarpal bone, close to the joint margin.

Carpometacarpal Traction

This technique is similar to the traction technique for the CMC joints of the fingers. The radial carpals are stabilized while a traction force is applied to the thumb metacarpal.

Carpometacarpal Posteroanterior Glide

This technique is used to increase extension. The sport rehabilitation specialist stabilizes the trapezium and trapezoid at the proximal aspect of the joint, using the thumb and index finger of one hand; he or she holds the patient's first metacarpal with the opposite thumb along the posterior aspect, and the index finger around the anterior aspect. The sport rehabilitation specialist creates slight traction and applies a PA glide to the metacarpal using his or her thumb on its posterior surface (figure 19.28).

Carpometacarpal Anteroposterior Glide

This technique is used to increase flexion mobility. The sport rehabilitation specialist's hand placement is the same as for the PA glide, but the force is applied by the index finger on the volar surface of the metacarpal.

Carpometacarpal Ulnar Glide

Because the thumb's CMC joint is a saddle joint, it is convex at its proximal joint surface and concave at its distal joint surface for abduction-adduction movements. Mobilization for these movements is opposite to the direction of movement.

An ulnar glide increases abduction motion. With the forearm, wrist, and thumb positioned in neutral and the proximal aspect of the joint stabilized with the thumb and index finger of one hand, the sport rehabilitation specialist grasps the metacarpal with the other hand as shown in figure 19.29, and applies a downward force that is perpendicular to the joint surface.

METACARPOPHALANGEAL AND INTERPHALANGEAL JOINTS

The configuration of each of these joints is similar, so the mobilization techniques are similar. Each mobilization described can be used on any of these joints. Traction is applied during each mobilization technique to make the technique more comfortable and produce better results. The grasps should be firm enough to administer the mobilization force effectively but not tight enough to cause discomfort.

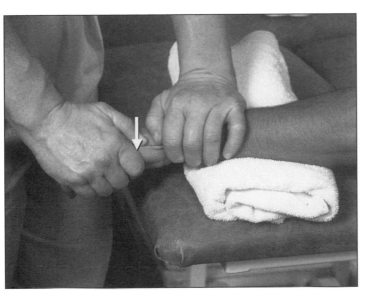

Figure 19.28 Joint mobilization: thumb CMC PA glide.

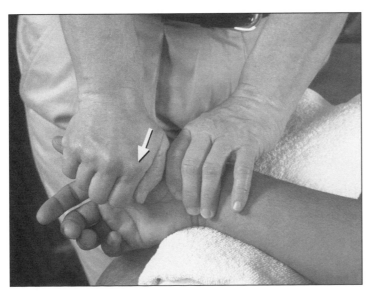

Figure 19.29 Joint mobilization: thumb CMC ulnar glide.

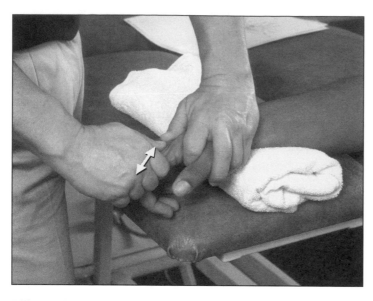

■ **Figure 19.30**   Joint mobilization: MCP distraction.

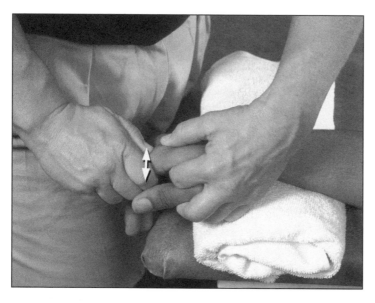

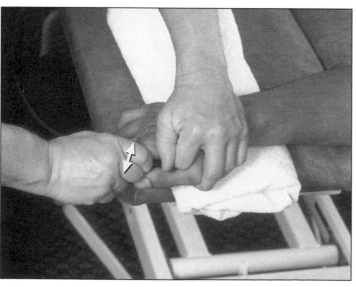

■ **Figure 19.32**   Joint mobilization: MCP lateral glides.

Traction

The proximal aspect of the joint is grasped with one hand while the distal aspect of the joint is grasped by the index finger and thumb of the other hand (figure 19.30). The joint is positioned in slight flexion in a loose-packed position. A traction force in line with the longitudinal axis is applied to the joint.

Rotation

The proximal aspect of the joint is grasped with a lateral pinch of the thumb and index finger. The joint is in some flexion, and a mild traction force is applied by the mobilizing hand before medial and lateral rotation is applied.

Posteroanterior Glides and Anteroposterior Glides

Because the joints are a concave surface moving on a convex surface, the mobilization force is in the same direction of movement. To increase extension, an AP mobilization force is applied. Flexion is increased with a PA mobilization. The proximal aspect of the joint is stabilized while the distal aspect receives traction and a PA force or AP force (figure 19.31).

■ **Figure 19.31**   Joint mobilization: MCP AP and PA glides.

Lateral Glides

Lateral glides are used to increase abduction and adduction of the MCP and IP joints. These are accessory movements that permit full joint motion. A radial or ulnar glide force is applied to the distal aspect of the joint, depending on the finger and movement desired (figure 19.32).

FLEXIBILITY EXERCISES

Flexibility exercises for the hand are used to stretch the joints and ligaments, the extrinsic muscles, and the intrinsic muscles.

Range-of-motion exercises are divided into those for the intrinsic muscles and those for the extrinsic muscles. The two groups require different considerations for correct stretch application. Because extrinsic muscles can cross multiple joints, the sport rehabilitation specialist must know these muscle insertion locations to apply appropriate stretches. Each joint the muscle crosses must be placed on stretch to produce optimal ROM changes, but the force should be applied precisely and in sequence from the most distal to the most proximal joint. When one joint is stretched, the other joints must be stabilized. If the proximal joint is not stabilized, the stretch force and surrounding tissue tension can cause the proximal joint to extend rather than flex. The force applied should be a slow, gentle, and sustained stretch to avoid incorrect stretch application or excessive force that can damage the small hand and finger structures.

One finger should be stretched at a time. Joint mobilization is used before stretching so that the stretch of soft-tissue structures is more effective. If joint motion is restricted by extrinsic tightness, each joint is placed on stretch in the sequence just described to affect extrinsic structures but not intrinsic muscles. If it is restricted by intrinsic tightness, the distal joint is stretched and the proximal joint is placed in the opposite direction in order to eliminate the stretch on extrinsic muscles and apply the intended stretch to the intrinsic muscles. For example, when the PIP joint is placed in flexion and the MCP joint is placed in extension, the intrinsic muscles are stretched and the extrinsic muscles are not; but when the PIP and MCP joints are placed in flexion, the extrinsic muscles are stretched but the intrinsics are not. When both structures have limited flexibility, stretching exercises in both positions will be necessary.

JOINTS AND LIGAMENTS

As already mentioned, mobilization techniques—both accessory and physiological techniques—should be applied before joints are stretched. The accessory techniques are those already discussed, including motions that are not actively possible but that must take place for full motion to occur. These should be applied before the physiological motions. The physiological motions are those that can be actively produced, such as joint flexion and extension. Techniques used to produce the physiological motions are often referred to as stretching exercises.

Only one joint is stretched at a time. The other joints are positioned in neutral and kept relaxed to reduce soft-tissue tension on the joint being treated. When you are applying a stretch force, the distal portion of the distal arm of the joint being stretched is the location of the stretch force. You need to be careful, however, to apply the force on the distal arm and not on the next distal joint. For example, when stretching a PIP joint, your force is on the distal portion of the middle phalanx, not on the DIP joint or the distal phalanx. Proper stabilization of the proximal phalanx must also occur for the stretch application to be correct (figure 19.33).

Abduction movements are crucial to maintaining vital web space flexibility of the thumb and MCP extension movement of the fingers. Abduction of the fingers can assist in stretching the MCP collateral ligaments. Soft tissue of the web space is stretched with thumb abduction. These movements can be performed actively and passively. Passive movements can be performed by the sport rehabilitation specialist or the patient. The patient can stretch the finger MCPs by intertwining the fingers of the two hands together as in a praying position. The thumb's web space can be stretched by actively abducting the thumb or applying an abduction force at the CMC joint. Care must be taken not to apply the force on the MCP joint. The patient can also stretch the thumb's web space by placing the hand over the top of the knee, with the fingers separated from the thumb, and applying a downward force from the shoulder to push the hand on the knee (figure 19.34).

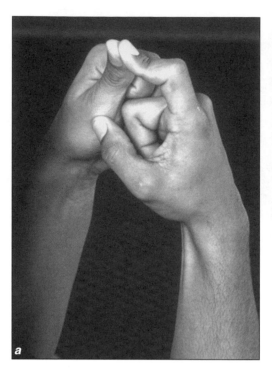
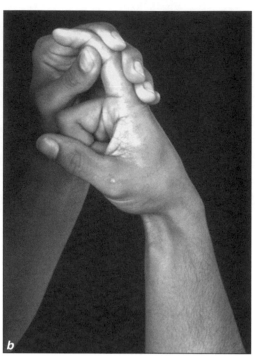

▌Figure 19.33
Stretch force application. *(a)* Incorrect: force is applied on the digit's distal segment. *(b)* Correct: force is applied at the distal joint first, then moves one joint at a time to the most proximal joint.

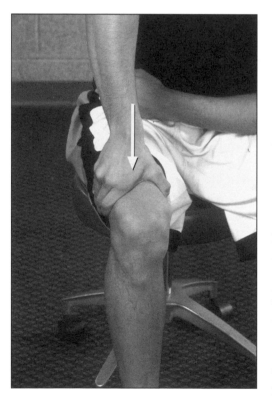

▌Figure 19.34 Thumb abduction stretch.

As mentioned earlier, the CMC and intermetacarpal joints form the palmar arches that are vital to hand formation and function. The second and third metacarpals, which have little mobility, form the peak of the palmar arches. The fourth, and especially the fifth, meta-carpals move into flexion as the hand is formed into a fist; this motion is crucial to normal hand function and permits a firm grasp. The sport rehabilitation specialist can stretch these joints by placing his or her thumbs in the palm of the patient's hand and his or her fingers on the dorsum over the metacarpals. The thumbs are stabilizers as the fingers roll the metacarpals around the thumbs (figure 19.35). The palmar fascia can be stretched using the technique demonstrated in figure 19.16.

Wrist joint stretches are utilized with the fingers relaxed and the force applied proximal to the MCP joints. The patient can apply the stretches passively in all wrist motions (figure 19.36).

The distal radioulnar joint stretches are the same as those for the proximal radioulnar joint. These are discussed in chapter 18 and are shown in figures 18.19 and 18.20. The stretch is applied at the distal radioulnar joint. The hand is not included in the stretch.

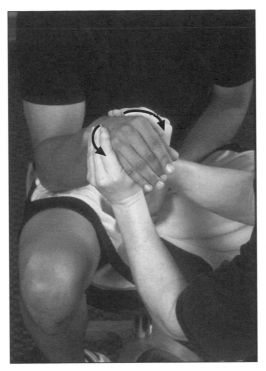

Figure 19.35 Range of motion of CMC and intermetacarpal joints.

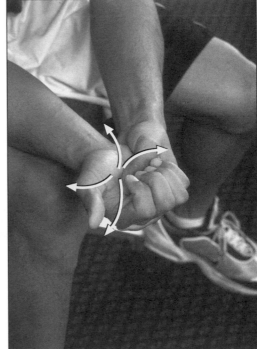

Figure 19.36 Wrist stretches.

The oblique retinacular ligament acts on the IP joints similarly to the way the intrinsics act on the MCP and PIP joints. When the PIP joint is flexed, it extends the DIP joint. If passive DIP flexion is more with the PIP joint flexed than with the PIP extended, the oblique retinacular ligament is restricted. Tightness limits DIP flexion particularly during PIP extension. To stretch this ligament, the PIP joint is passively maintained in extension while the DIP joint is stretched into flexion.

EXTRINSIC MUSCLES

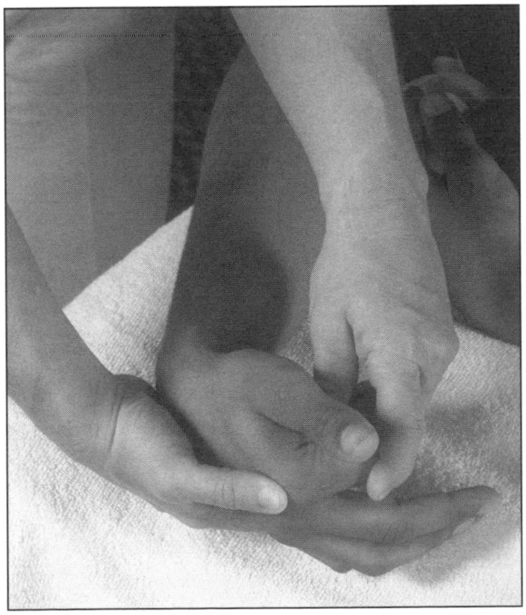

As mentioned previously, the stretch applied to extrinsics begins with the distal joint and proceeds in sequence distally to proximally until full length of the muscle is attained. The force is applied slowly and deliberately without excessive stress to the structures. Contract-relax-stretch techniques can improve results of the stretch because of reflex inhibition. Application of a slight traction force on the joints makes the stretch more comfortable by reducing compressive forces on the joints.

Because of the easy accessibility of the hand and wrist joints and the relatively small force required to stretch them, the patient can learn proper stretching techniques and can apply them frequently throughout the day.

Stretching for both the extrinsic extensors and extrinsic flexors starts distally and moves proximally. For example, improving flexion motion involves beginning at the DIP joint and stabilizing the PIP joint as the DIP is brought into flexion. The DIP joint is moved to its end position before the PIP joint is moved into flexion. The MCP joint is then moved into flexion while the IP joints are held in their flexed positions. Finally, the wrist is brought into flexion to its end range with the finger maintained in its fully flexed position. Stretch to increase flexion

Figure 19.37 Extrinsic finger extensor stretch. In sequence: DIP, PIP, MCP, wrist, elbow.

is seen in figure 19.37. Stretches to increase flexion and extension of the extrinsic muscles are each applied in both elbow flexion and extension. The patient should feel a stretch on the forearm.

Wrist stretches should be applied with the fingers on stretch, because the long finger muscles can also influence wrist mobility. To increase wrist extension motion, the patient extends the fingers first and then moves the wrist into extension (figure 19.38a). As with stretches to the fingers, the wrist should be stretched with the elbow in flexion and in extension. The stretch should be felt on the anterior forearm.

A slow sustained stretch is applied to the finger and wrist extensors to increase wrist flexion. The stretch begins at the fingers and is applied last to the wrist (figure 19.38b). The stretch should be applied with the elbow flexed and extended until a stretch on the posterior forearm is felt.

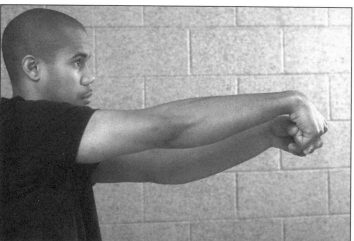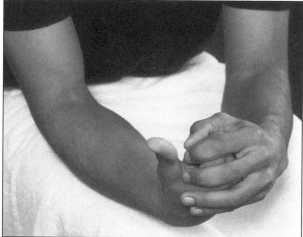

■ **Figure 19.38** Independent stretches to increase wrist extension (a) and wrist flexion (b).

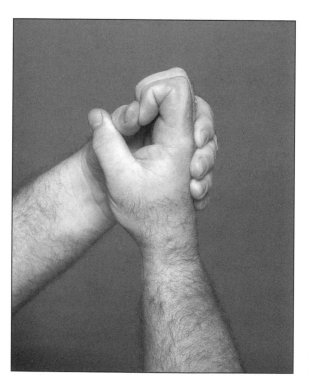

INTRINSIC MUSCLES

Because the lumbricals and interossei flex the MCP joint and extend the IP joints, the stretch is applied in the opposite direction of their movement. The IP joints are maintained in a flexed position while a stretch to increase MCP extension is applied (figure 19.39). The wrist should be stabilized in neutral during this activity to prevent extrinsic muscle influences on the stretch.

■ **Figure 19.39** Intrinsic stretch: IPs are flexed, MCP is extended, wrist is in neutral.

STRENGTHENING EXERCISES

Strengthening exercises are used to restore normal glide of the hand's flexor and extensor tendons; and a large variety of resistive exercises promote strength of the wrist extensors, ulnar and radial flexors, and supinators and pronators.

During periods of immobilization, isometric exercises can be used for all wrist and hand muscles. Active exercises are good for maintaining motion and early strengthening. As the patient progresses, various equipment including weights, putty, and rubber bands can be used in the therapeutic exercise program. In the early stages, the muscles may fatigue quickly, so the patient must be cautioned against overdoing it, causing undue stress. Concentric exercises, rather than eccentric exercises, for the fingers are the primary emphasis, because little functional hand activity is eccentric.

TENDON GLIDE EXERCISES

When restriction of normal tendon glide occurs because of adhesions of tendons or their sheaths, you must restore the normal tendon glide if full motion is to be achieved. When adhesions occur, they can occur anywhere along the tendon and can restrict tendon motion proximally and distally to the point of adhesion. Friction massage assists in reducing adhesions of superficial tendons, and exercises improve mobility of both superficial and deep tendons. Muscle activity aids in restoring proximal glide of the tendon. Active and passive exercises and splinting can restore distal glide of the tendon. Because active exercises can restore both proximal and distal tendon glide, it is advisable to use these whenever possible. The effectiveness of these exercises, however, is limited by the muscle's strength and endurance. Passive stretching and massage may be key to improving tendon glide when these parameters are restricted.

Flexor Tendons

Gliding exercises for the long flexor tendons necessitate differentiating between the profundus and superficialis. You must isolate each tendon to facilitate gliding, because adhesions between the tendons restrict gliding. To show whether or not the tendons are gliding properly, the patient maintains extension of the MCP joint while flexing the PIP joints. With the fingers in this position, the sport rehabilitation specialist passively extends the DIP joint and should meet no resistance. If there is no resistance, it is normal and only the superficialis is being used. If the patient maintains this position with contraction of both muscles, normal tendon gliding is restricted. In this situation, the MCP and PIP joints are stabilized in flexion while the patient attempts to flex and extend the DIP (figure 19.40a). To isolate the superficialis, the proximal phalanx is stabilized and the PIP joint is flexed and extended: either one digit is stabilized at a time as shown in figure 19.40b, or all digits except the one being treated are stabilized. In this exercise the other IP joints are maintained in extension while the digit of interest is flexed Because the profundus tendons all originate from the same muscle belly, it is easy to eliminate profundus activity by restriction of movement of the other digits (figure 19.40c).

There are three functional flexor tendon gliding exercises that belong in a therapeutic exercise program when flexor tendon gliding is restricted. Keeping the MCP extended and flexing the IPs enhances gliding between the two longer finger flexor tendons (figure 19.41a). This is known as the hook position. The fist formation with the IP and MCP joints in flexion produces gliding of the profundus tendon within its sheath (figure 19.41b), and the position with the MCP and PIP joints flexed and the DIP joints extended (modified fist) provides optimal gliding of the superficialis tendons in their sheath (figure 19.41c).

Flexor pollicis longus gliding exercises are performed in a similar manner by moving the IP and MCP joints through a full range of flexion and extension. These exercises are initially performed with the wrist in neutral, but as the patient progresses, the wrist should be moved into flexion with finger flexion and into extension with finger extension.

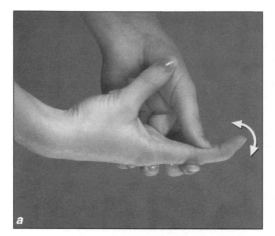

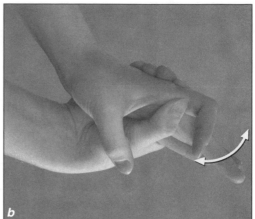

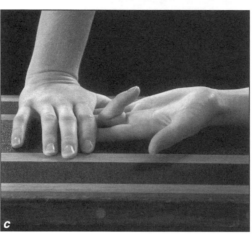

Figure 19.40 Isolation of tendons for gliding exercises: (a) flexor digitorum profundus, (b) flexor digitorum superficialis, (c) elimination of flexor digitorum profundus activity.

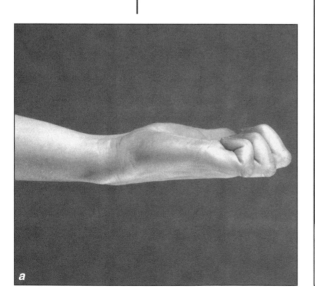

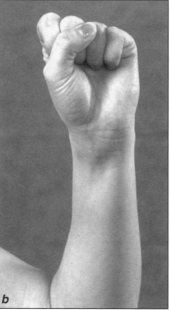

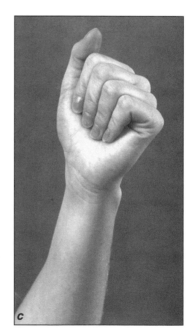

Figure 19.41 Flexor tendon gliding exercises: (a) Hook enhances gliding between FDS and FDP. (b) Fist enhances gliding of FDP. (c) Modified fist enhances gliding of FDS.

Extensor Tendons

Because the extensor tendons are flatter and wider than their flexor counterparts and because they have an intimate relationship with the intrinsic muscle system, they are more susceptible to adhesions. Adhesions can cause an extensor lag of the finger. If full extension occurs passively but not actively, adhesions may be the cause. This is particularly true if the digit's passive flexion is also limited, because the adhesion restricts full tendon excursion during a stretch. Care must be taken in stretching the extensor tendons following tendon repairs or fractures. The sport rehabilitation specialist must keep a close eye on increases in the extensor lag throughout the stretching process. If the extensor lag increases, it may be that the tendon is actually elongating or tearing from its attachment. Emphasizing the use of active exercises for reducing extensor lag rather than passive forces to increase flexion motion helps to minimize this risk.

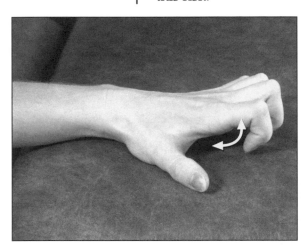

Figure 19.42 Extrinsic extensor gliding exercises: Keeping the IPs in flexion, the MCPs are moved into flexion and extension.

If an extensor lag is present at the MCP joint because of an adhesion, the adhesion is of the extensor digitorum communis (EDC) tendon. This tendon is the only extensor of the MCP joint. A gliding exercise for the EDC is performed by moving the hand from a hook to a fist formation as seen in figure 19.42. The MCP joint is moved from flexion to extension while the IP joints are kept in flexion to eliminate the intrinsic muscles. If the patient has difficulty maintaining flexion of the IP joints during this exercise, he or she can facilitate the activity by grasping a drinking straw or pencil in the fingers while moving the MCP joints. Wrist flexion and extension should also be added to the exercise when it is easy to perform with the wrist in neutral.

If the extensor lag occurs at either IP joint, it is the result of adhesions within the extensor mechanism and can include both intrinsic and extrinsic structures—the interossei, lumbricals, and EDC. To isolate the intrinsic muscles and facilitate their movement of IP extension, the MCP should be stabilized in flexion (figure 19.43a). As this exercise becomes easier, the MCP joint should be moved into extension. The most difficult position for this exercise is with the hand flat on a table and the proximal phalanx stabilized; in this position the patient attempts to lift the middle and distal phalanxes off the table (figure 19.43b).

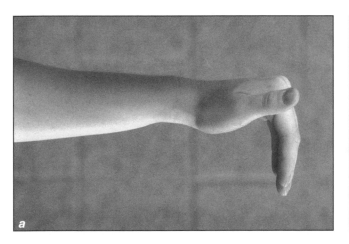 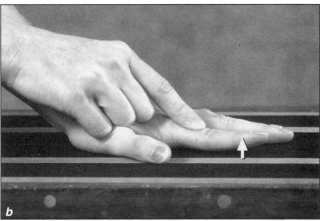

Figure 19.43 Extensor gliding exercises. (a) Intrinsic: MCP flexion with IPs in extension. (b) Terminal extension: IP extension with MCP in extension.

RESISTIVE EXERCISES

There are many variations for resistive exercises for the wrist and hand. Specific exercises are limited only by the sport rehabilitation specialist's imagination. A few of the more commonly used resistive exercises are outlined here. Common substitution patterns for the exercise are also listed. You should correct any errors in technique.

Wrist Extension

This exercise is used to increase the strength of the wrist extensors. The forearm rests on a tabletop in pronation with the hand over the end of the table. The patient lifts a dumbbell, moving through a full ROM from wrist flexion to wrist extension (figure 19.44). The forearm must stay in contact with the tabletop throughout the exercise; it may be necessary to stabilize the forearm with a hand across the proximal forearm. Substitutions seen in this exercise include flexing the elbow and moving the weight through a partial ROM.

Wrist Flexion

This exercise strengthens the wrist flexors. The patient sits next to a table with the forearm resting on the table in supination and the hand over the end of the table. He or she moves a dumbbell weight through a full ROM from wrist extension to flexion (figure 19.45). Substitutions for this exercise include flexing the elbow and moving the wrist through a partial ROM.

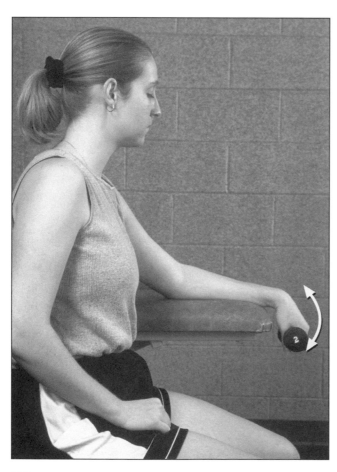

■ **Figure 19.44** Wrist extension resistance exercise.

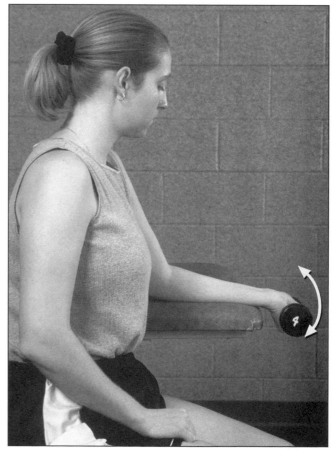

■ **Figure 19.45** Wrist flexion resistance exercise.

Ulnar and Radial Deviation

These exercises strengthen ulnar and radial flexors. To strengthen the ulnar flexors, a bar with a weighted end is placed in the hand, with the weight on the ulnar side. The patient stands with the elbow extended. The patient moves the wrist into ulnar deviation, lifting the weight as high as possible (figure 19.46a). He or she should maintain a firm grasp on the bar so that the wrist rather than the fingers is used to produce the motion. In addition to finger movement, shoulder extension is a common substitution.

To strengthen radial flexors, the patient's position remains the same, but the weighted bar is positioned with the weight on the radial aspect of the hand. The weight is lifted upward as high as possible toward the thumb (figure 19.46b). The patient must maintain a firm grasp to produce the motion from the wrist and not the fingers. Elbow flexion is a common substitution for this exercise.

Pronation and Supination

These exercises are demonstrated in chapter 18, figure 18.25. They can also be used to provide additional eccentric activity through the use of rubber tubing. The rubber tubing is attached to a handle or weighted bar and anchored to the side of the table. To provide eccentric resistance to the supinators, the bar is positioned with the rubber tubing attached to the side of the table opposite the injured wrist. The bar is passively positioned with the forearm in supination. The patient then controls the bar as the rubber tubing pulls the forearm into pronation (figure 19.47a).

Eccentric resistance for the pronators is provided with the rubber tubing anchored to the table on the same side as the injured wrist. The bar is passively positioned with the forearm in pronation; and as the rubber tubing pulls the bar, the patient controls the supination motion of the forearm (figure 19.47b).

During each exercise, the forearm must remain stable on the tabletop, and no substitution by shoulder abduction or adduction is allowed.

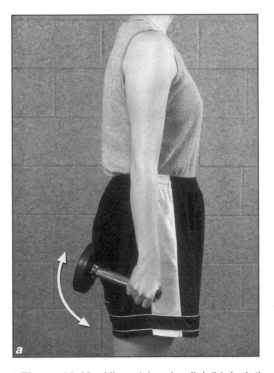 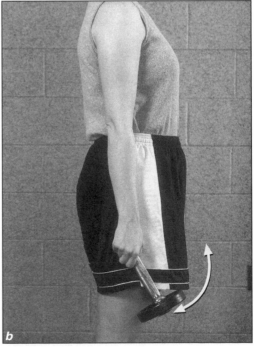

■ **Figure 19.46**   Ulnar *(a)* and radial *(b)* deviation resistance exercise.

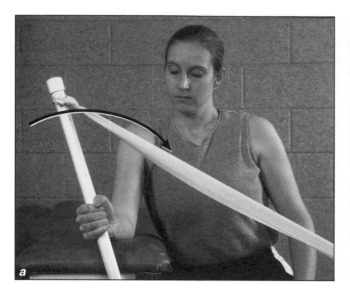 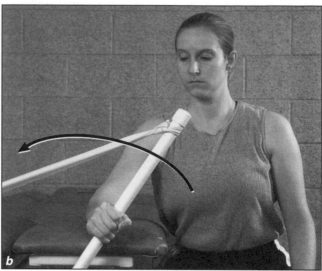

❚ Figure 19.47   Eccentric supination *(a)* and pronation *(b)* resistance exercises.

Putty Exercises

A number of putty exercises can be incorporated into a program that the patient can perform at home or on road trips with the team. The putty comes in a variety of resistances, indicated by different colors, and can be switched as the patient's strength improves. Some putty uses the addition of chips to increase resistance. Different colors can be used for different exercises to offer optimal resistance for each exercise. The patient can perform wrist flexion and extension by grasping the putty with the uninvolved hand and pulling on the putty with the involved hand (figure 19.48, a and b). The same precautions for substitutions apply as with the dumbbell exercises. Ulnar and radial deviation motions can also be resisted with putty. For ulnar deviation the patient places the hands together, index finger and thumb of one hand in contact with the other hand. With only wrist movement, he or she separates the hands as the wrists move into ulnar deviation (figure 19.48c). For radial deviation, the patient positions the little finger of the involved hand on top of the thumb of the other hand. The putty is formed into a tube shape and is grasped by both hands. Stabilizing the uninvolved hand and the involved forearm and elbow, the patient moves the involved wrist into radial deviation. To perform pronation and supination, the patient uses the stabilizing hand to hold the putty while the involved forearm moves into supination and pronation as it grasps the putty (figure 19.48d). Supination-pronation motion should be limited to the forearm; no elbow motion is permitted.

A number of finger exercises can be designed using putty of different strengths to provide a progressive resistive program. These are discussed next.

Grip Exercises

Grips using putty for resistance with the entire hand (spherical) (figure 19.49a), the thumb and index finger (hook) (figure 19.49b), and the thumb and fingers (cylinder) (figure 19.49c) address power-grip strengthening. The putty selected should provide enough resistance to make the exercise challenging but also be light enough to allow a full ROM. The hand is positioned as shown, and the putty is squeezed. It is then reshaped, and the exercise is repeated.

Patients can also perform precision grips using resistive putty (figure 19.50). The patient should do these exercises with each phalanx in slight flexion. The IP joints should not be extended. Precision-grip exercises can also be performed with

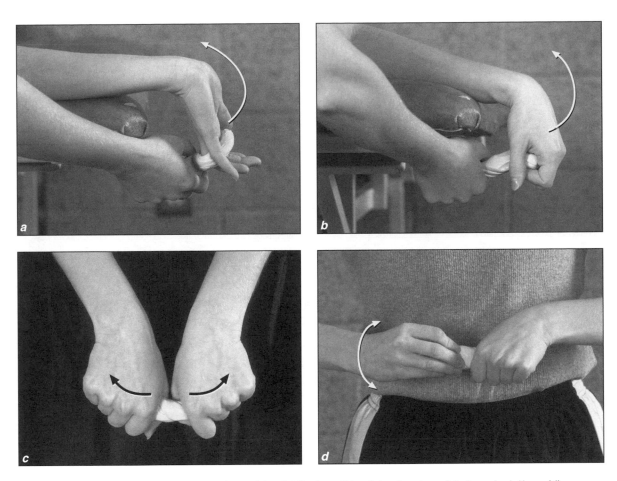

Figure 19.48 Theraputty wrist exercises: *(a)* wrist flexion, *(b)* wrist extension, *(c)* ulnar deviation, *(d)* supination-pronation.

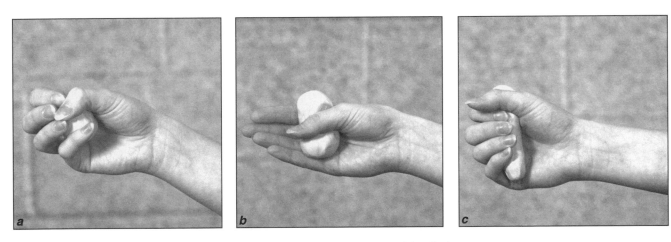

Figure 19.49 Theraputty power-grip exercises: *(a)* spherical, *(b)* hook, *(c)* cylinder.

clothespins. Wrapping rubber bands around the end of the clothespin provides additional resistance. As with the putty exercises, the patient should grasp the clothespins with the IP joints in slight flexion. Extension of any IP joint should not be permitted.

Flexion exercises can be performed against manual resistance, rubber bands, putty, or other objects. You can adjust these exercises according to the availability of your equipment.

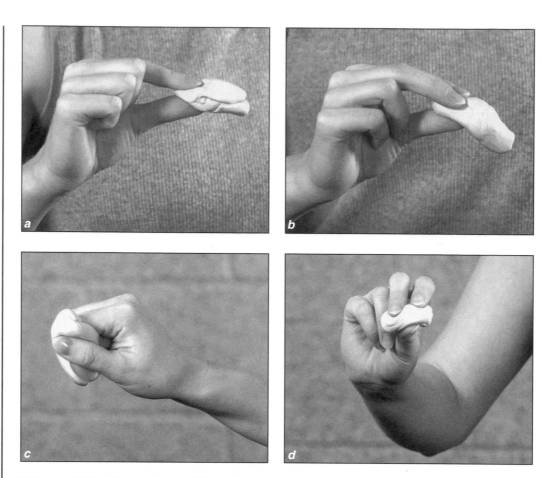

■ **Figure 19.50**   Theraputty precision-grip exercises: *(a)* tip-to-tip, *(b)* digital prehension, *(c)* lateral prehension, *(d)* three-prong chuck.

Opposition Exercise

Gross finger-opposition strengthening exercise is shown in figure 19.51. The putty begins in a pancake on a tabletop (figure 19.51a). The patient places all the finger pads on the putty and pulls the finger pads together to pull the putty up into a cone shape (figure 19.51b). The intrinsic muscles are worked if the IP joints are kept in extension during the exercise. The extrinsics are worked if the IP joints are flexed during the exercise.

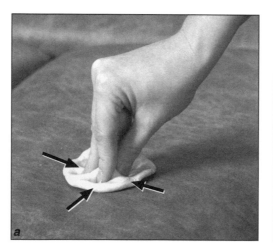
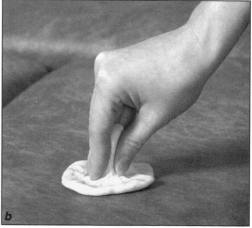

■ **Figure 19.51**   Gross opposition exercise for the intrinsic muscles: a cone should be formed in the middle as the patient repeats the exercise *(b)*.

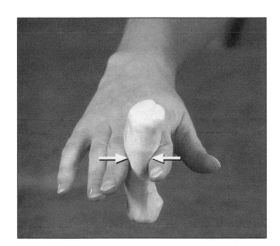

Adduction

The patient can place the putty between any two fingers or between the index finger and the thumb; he or she then pulls the fingers together (figure 19.52). The IP and MCP joints should remain extended.

Finger Extension, and Thumb and Finger Abduction

Using either putty or a rubber band, the patient places the item around the fingers and thumb and spreads these as far apart as possible (figure 19.53). Depending on the direction of movement, the abductors or extensors will be worked. This exercise can be used either on the entire group or on individual fingers.

▌**Figure 19.52**   Finger adduction exercise.

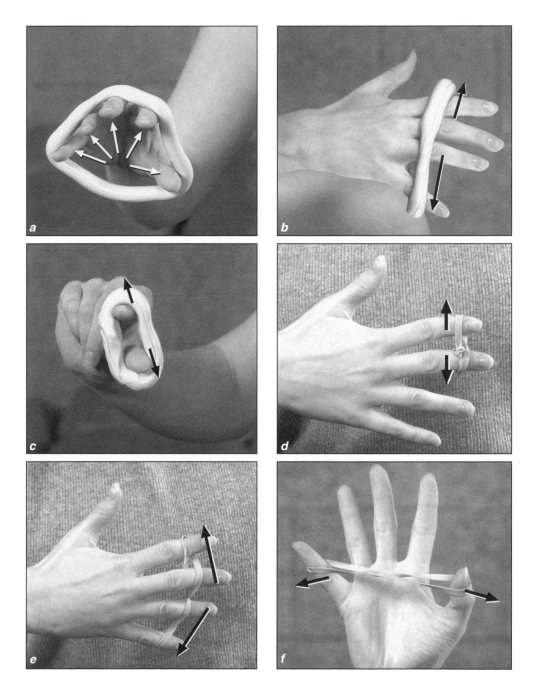

▌**Figure 19.53**
(a) Multiple-finger and thumb extension with putty, (b) finger abduction with putty, (c) index-finger and thumb extension with putty, (d) two-finger abduction with rubber band, (e) multiple-finger abduction with rubber band, (f) thumb and fifth-finger abduction with rubber band.

Extensor Lag Exercises

To use the putty to strengthen the intrinsics, the patient places the putty on a table-top. With the palm facing down and the MCP and IP joints flexed, the fingers push outward against the putty as the fingers move into extension (figure 19.54a).

A medicine ball, pushed while the MCP joints remain in flexion and the IP joints move from flexion into extension, will also provide resistance to the intrinsic muscles (figure 19.54b). This exercise becomes more challenging with the use of a heavier ball or with an increase in the surface friction.

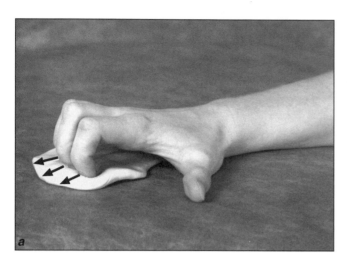 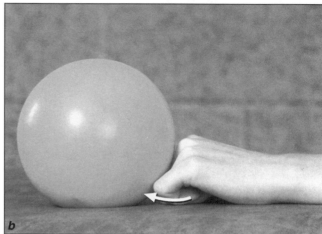

■ **Figure 19.54**   Extensor lag exercises: *(a)* with putty, *(b)* with medicine ball.

ISOKINETIC EXERCISES

As with other isokinetic protocols, wrist-strengthening exercises progress from straight plane to more functional diagonal planes. Fast and slow speeds are used to enhance strength and muscle endurance. Exercises should remain pain free.

PLYOMETRIC EXERCISES

In addition to plyometric exercises that are also used for the shoulder and elbow, plyometrics for the hand include activities using a medicine ball and isokinetic activities.

Many of the plyometric exercises for the shoulder and elbow are also used for the wrist and hand. A couple of additional exercises can be used for the hand. For specific information on the plyometric exercises for the shoulder and elbow, refer to chapters 17 and 18.

BALL DROP AND CATCH

This exercise uses a medicine ball small enough to be grasped in one hand. The patient stands with the arm outstretched in front and the hand positioned palm down. He or she grasps the medicine ball in the hand and allows it to drop, then immediately retrieves the ball before it reaches the floor by grasping with the hand in the palm-down position. As the exercise becomes easier, a heavier ball is selected. The patient should grasp the ball with all the fingers.

OTHER PLYOMETRIC ACTIVITIES

Numerous other activities can be used as plyometric exercises for the hand. Some of these are bouncing a medicine ball against the wall or incline trampoline, boxing against a medicine bag, plyometric push-ups, and volleyball passes with a medicine ball.

FUNCTIONAL ACTIVITIES

The great range of uses for the hand in sports means that the sport rehabilitation specialist working with a hand injury must understand the particular demands of each patient's sport and position.

Because the hand has wide variation of function, it is nearly impossible to define functional activities for the hand. Specific demands for functional activities are determined by the demands of the patient's sport and the position the patient plays within the sport. A football quarterback's demands for hand function differ from those for the football lineman. The golfer's demands for hand function vary greatly from the basketball player's. The range of demands can include varying grips, varying positions, rapid or slow movements, sustained or changing grips, and forceful or light grasping. The sport rehabilitation specialist must understand the demands of each patient's sport and position and outline a functional exercise progression based on those requirements.

SPECIAL REHABILITATION APPLICATIONS

Among the more common types of injuries to the hand are fractures, dislocations and sprains, overuse injuries including carpal tunnel syndrome, and tendon injuries. The sport rehabilitation specialist also encounters reflex sympathetic dystrophy of the hand.

Because the hand is so complex, with many structures in close contact with each other, an injury to one area or tissue can impact adjacent tissues and other segments within the wrist and hand. The sport rehabilitation specialist must be cognizant of this, must be keenly aware of the possibility of secondary involvement of other segments, and must do everything possible to attempt to prevent these complications.

Some of the more common injuries requiring rehabilitation are addressed here. Although tendon rupture and repairs are not often seen in sport injuries, the rehabilitation programs for them are outlined here, because the sport rehabilitation specialist must take additional precautions when they do occur and necessitate a rehabilitation program.

FRACTURES

There are many bones in the wrist and hand. Which bone is fractured has a great impact on the rehabilitation process. This section presents some general concepts, applicable to all fractures, before addressing specific fractures. Although there are exceptions, a fracture is generally immobilized in a position so that the ligaments of the joints are placed on some stretch. This helps reduce the risk of contractures. Immobilization is often maintained for two to three weeks unless the fracture is unstable, displaced, or comminuted. Fractures that are unstable are often corrected with **open reduction and internal fixation (ORIF)**, followed by immobilization. Open reduction and internal fixation is advantageous when the fracture is unstable, because it provides needed stability. However, because of the disruption of blood flow and increased soft-tissue damage that occurs with ORIF, healing time can be delayed.

Splints used to immobilize fractures affect only as many joints as necessary to maintain good fracture alignment. Joints proximal and distal to the fracture site, and not included in the splint immobilization, should be moved through their ranges of motion regularly.

Distal Forearm and Wrist Fractures

The most common distal forearm fracture is the **Colles fracture**. The distal radius proximal to the wrist is fractured and is displaced dorsally. A **Smith's fracture** also involves the radius, but the distal radius fragment displaces palmarly. Surgical repair is common with Smith's fractures but does not take place as often with a Colles fracture. A **Barton's fracture** occurs at the radial articular region and results in wrist subluxation as well as the fracture. While the Colles and Smith's fractures are most often the result of falling on an outstretched hand, the Barton's fracture occurs with a sudden violent wrist extension and pronation. The likelihood of its being unstable makes the need for ORIF highly probable.

As with all fractures, whether treated with open or closed reduction, management of pain and edema is the goal of early rehabilitation. Coban wrap is useful for controlling edema in the fingers and hand. Isotoner gloves are also used to reduce edema once the wrist is out of the cast. Modalities are useful in controlling pain as well as edema. Early rehabilitation includes the use of active range-of-motion (AROM) exercises of the uninvolved joints. These exercises will encourage good tendon gliding, reduce edema, and relieve joint stiffness.

Immobilization casts or splints used for these fractures should permit full MCP flexion motion and full thumb opposition. Active range-of-motion exercises for the extrinsic finger muscles and the intrinsics should be permitted while the patient is in the brace or cast. The patient should be able to perform three exercises: MCP joint full flexion with IP extension, MCP joint extension with full IP flexion, MCP joint full flexion combined with IP joint full flexion.

It should be possible for AROM to come close to passive range-of-motion (PROM) excursion. If full PROM is significantly greater than full AROM, the muscle may be atrophied and may lack sufficient strength, or the tendon is being restricted by adhesions, or both influences may be present. Active exercises, electrical stimulation, friction massage in regions where it is appropriate, proprioceptive neuromuscular facilitation, or biofeedback can be used to restore active motion while the wrist is immobilized.

It is common for distal radial fractures to be immobilized four to six weeks. Once immobilization is discontinued, the patient should attempt to regain full wrist motion and long tendon mobility. Joint mobilization with active stretches is used. Grades I and II joint mobilization can be used to relieve pain. Grades III and IV joint mobilizations are not incorporated into the program until the fracture is healed enough to withstand that stress. Range of motion in all planes should be emphasized. Many rehabilitation specialists do not address radial and ulnar deviation, but these must be restored if the patient is to have full wrist function.

Isometric strengthening exercises can be used while the wrist is immobilized. Once the cast or splint is removed, the patient can begin low-resistance, low-repetition isotonic activities, progressing to higher repetitions and resistance as tolerated. If pain or swelling increases with exercises, the exercises are too aggressive and should be reduced in intensity or number of repetitions.

Once strength gains are substantial, the patient begins functional activities. Specific functional activities are determined by the patient's sport and position. Tennis has different requirements for the wrist than golf does, and golf and baseball differ in their demands. The sport rehabilitation specialist should be aware of the demands of the patient's sport and design a functional program that will lead the patient to an appropriate return to that sport.

Carpal and Metacarpal Fractures

The carpal most frequently fractured is the scaphoid. Because of the bones' variability in blood supply, healing time is extremely varied, from 4 to 20 weeks, and depends primarily on the location and type of fracture. The area remains immobilized until radiography demonstrates signs of healing.

Edema control should be aggressive, and the patient should perform ROM of the uninvolved segments of the shoulder, elbow, and hand immediately and continually throughout the immobilization period. Pain should be avoided with these exercises.

Once the cast or splint is removed, ROM for the thumb should begin. These exercises should be active. If joint mobility is restricted in a capsular pattern, joint mobilization should be added to the program. The patient should perform active exercises with the proximal joint stabilized passively to ensure correct movement of the digit.

The hook of the hamate and the pisiform can incur fractures from impact with a baseball bat, golf club, or racket or from a fall on an outstretched arm. Because they are not often unstable, these fractures heal well most of the time with cast immobilization for six to eight weeks. As with other fractures in this area, ROM exercises for the shoulder, elbow, and other hand joints are routine while the splint is on, and restoration of full ROM for all joints should be the goal following cast removal. If pain occurs with hand and wrist activity following cast removal, a protective splint may be used at night and throughout the day to relieve the stress of motion and use. Progression of flexibility exercises should continue until full motion is achieved.

Joint mobilization of restricted metacarpal and carpal joints should be used to provide full physiological and accessory movements that are necessary for full hand and wrist function. Strengthening exercises are initiated when the cast is removed. Grip exercises are used early, because they help to mobilize the metacarpals and to restore the normal palmar arches. Wrist strengthening is also incorporated. The patient is weaned from the splint as pain and edema subside and motion and strength are restored.

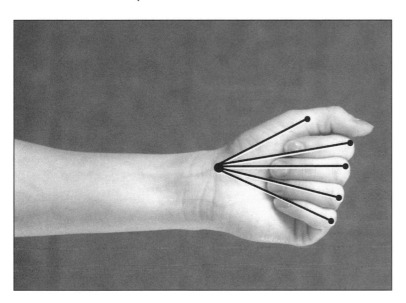

❚ Figure 19.55 Finger alignment with MCP and PIP flexion.

Because the neck of the metacarpal is the weakest aspect of the bone, it is the most frequent site of metacarpal fractures. These fractures most commonly occur in the fourth and fifth metacarpals. Fractures here result primarily from compressive forces like those that occur when a fist is used to administer a direct blow. For this reason they are referred to as boxer's fractures. The alignment of the fingers determines whether the fracture can be treated with immobilization or whether it requires an ORIF. Normal oblique flexion of the digits with the MCP and PIP joints flexed causes an alignment of the digits such that they point toward the scaphoid tubercle (figure 19.55). If the angulation of the digit is off by more than 20° to 30°, an ORIF may be necessary.

Two to four weeks of immobilization may be necessary for carpal and metacarpal fractures. Range-of-motion exercises while the cast is on are recommended for the uninvolved areas. Once the cast is removed, ROM exercises for the entire hand and wrist begin immediately. Active range-of-motion exercises are used for the metacarpal joints, and passive and active-motion exercises are used for the digits. This helps to reduce tendon adhesions. Intrinsic and extrinsic ROM exercises should be incorporated. Support for the metacarpals during finger ROM exercises should be provided either manually or with a splint. As with other fractures, once the fracture is well healed the patient progresses to PROM exercises to all areas, then to resistive exercises, and then to functional exercises. Joint mobilization can also be used to increase joint mobility in restricted segments. Resistive exercises begin with light weights and progress to heavier weights and more repetitions, using pain and edema as guidelines for advancing the patient.

A **Bennett's fracture** involves the first metacarpal. Because the thumb is responsible for at least 50% of hand function, appropriate management and treatment of thumb injuries are crucial. Proper angulation must be ensured with either closed or open reduction to ultimately permit good function of the thumb. The immobilization period is often four weeks. During that time, efforts to control edema and pain are important. The sport rehabilitation specialist should be aware that adhesions may occur in the first web space and should take steps to maintain appropriate web spacing during immobilization. If the web space is reduced, full thumb motion is restricted. Removal of the cast allows initiation of AROM exercises. Once union of the fracture site is observed on X ray, usually about 6 to 8 weeks postinjury, PROM exercises can be used to regain motion. If PROM is significantly more than AROM, it is likely that tendon adhesions are present. Friction massage, electrical stimulation, and active and passive ROM exercises assist in restoring tendon glide. Dynamic splinting may be necessary when full ROM is not restored by 8 to 10 weeks. As with other fractures, resistive exercises begin after healing is apparent. Strengthening exercises should include both fine-tuned and grasping activities and should also incorporate associated segments that have become weakened secondary to reduced use of the hand.

Phalangeal Fractures

Because of the long finger tendon forces, fractures of the proximal and middle phalanges often result in displacement and instability. Proximal phalanx fractures occur because of falls or direct blows to the phalanx, most often in the thumb and index finger. Middle phalanx fractures are not as common; these result from a crush injury such as occurs when a baseball player's hand is stepped on. Distal phalanx fractures are common; these account for half of hand fractures. Proximal phalanx fractures typically result in flexion of the proximal bone segment from the pull of the interossei and extension of the distal segment because of the long extensor tendon's pull (figure 19.56). This fracture is reduced and immobilized with either open or closed reduction; the use of external wires is common. If the fracture is stable, buddy taping the fingers can immobilize the fracture and still permit tendon movement to reduce tendon gliding problems.

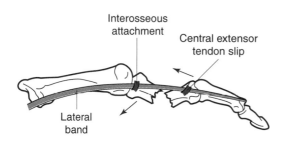

▌Figure 19.56   Forces affecting proximal phalanx fracture.

If the fracture is stable, motion exercises can begin as early as the first to second week. If the fracture is displaced, motion is usually started three to four weeks postinjury. Finger fractures are seldom immobilized for more than four weeks because of the deleterious effects of prolonged immobilization on surrounding soft-tissue structures.

One of the greatest complications of phalangeal immobilization is adhesions of tendons, causing restriction of normal tendon gliding. Adhesions of the extensor tendon can result in an extensor lag and limited IP flexion. Adhesions of the long flexor tendons also prevent full extension. Scar massage can be used to limit adhesions and to treat them if they occur. Exercises that restrain specific motions to isolate tendon function can reduce tendon adhesions. For example, if the FDP is restricted, the MCP and PIP joints are positioned passively in flexion and blocked from moving while the DIP is moved into flexion and extension (figure 19.57).

Once the fracture is healed sufficiently to be stable, more aggressive PROM exercises and joint mobilization can be used to improve ROM. Dynamic splints can provide a continual low-level stress to tight structures. One can also apply tape to position digits into a stretch position (figure 19.58). These techniques should be used for 15 to 20 min periods throughout the day, as tolerated, to improve scar-tissue mobility and ROM. Caution is necessary in the application of forces with prolonged stretching, especially to

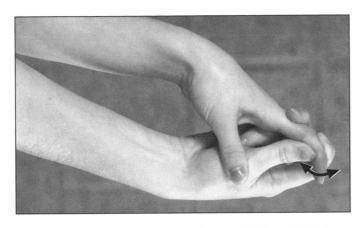

Figure 19.57 Restraining exercise: the MCP and PIP joints are restrained while the DIP is moved.

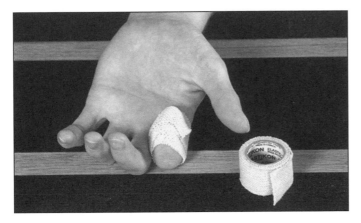

Figure 19.58 Aggressive techniques to increase ROM: tape is applied to increase IP joint flexion range of motion.

the extensor tendons, because it is relatively easy to overstretch the flat, broad extensor tendon. The end result with an overstretch of the extensor tendon is an extensor lag. If an extensor lag develops, an extension splint is required to correct it.

Stretching exercises should involve both intrinsic and extrinsic muscles. Intrinsic exercises are performed with the IP joints in flexion, and the MCP joints moving from flexion to extension, as seen in figure 19.39. Extrinsic muscles are stretched with the IP and MCP joints in various combinations of flexion and extension. Refer to figures 19.37 and 19.41 for these exercises.

Once the patient has achieved ROM, resistive exercises, including those using therapeutic putty and rubber bands and other exercises listed earlier, are necessary to restore full strength of the long finger flexors and extensors and the intrinsics. Wrist, elbow, and shoulder strength deficits should also be treated. Exercises begin with light resistance, increasing as the patient progresses. Exercises should emphasize full tendon and joint function that permit normal movement.

Case Study

A 21-year-old hockey forward suffered a fracture of the neck of the fourth MCP when he was involved in a fight during a game and hit an opponent. The hand was casted for two weeks and then placed in a splint that could be removed for his rehabilitation activities. The fracture is stable, so the physician wants to wean him from the splint over the next two weeks. The initial examination reveals some swelling in the hand and fingers. Wrist flexion is 50° and wrist extension is 65°. Ulnar deviation and radial deviation are 10°. Supination is 70° and pronation is 90°. MCP flexion is 45°, PIP flexion is 80°, and DIP flexion is 60°. The patient is unable to make a complete fist. The MCP and IP joints can extend passively to 0°. He is unable to simultaneously flex the MCP and extend the IP joints.

Questions for Analysis

1. What do you suspect this patient's primary problems are?
2. What will be included in your first three treatment sessions with him, assuming no regression with your treatments?
3. What will your initial goals during the first week be for him?
4. What precautions must you be aware of in treating him?
5. Describe three home exercises you will give this patient at the time of your first treatment.
6. List four strengthening exercises you will use with him.
7. What functional exercises will you incorporate into his rehabilitation program before he returns to hockey?

DISLOCATIONS AND SPRAINS

Because dislocations are a severe form of sprain, these two types of injuries are addressed together here. A **dislocation,** the most severe type of **sprain,** is immobilized for longer periods of time than a sprain. Dislocations and sprains occur primarily in the IP joints, and more commonly in the PIP than the DIP joints. A term commonly used for a finger sprain is "jammed finger." Sprains usually occur in ball-handling sports when the ball hits the end of the finger.

Program Considerations

When a dislocation occurs, the joint's supporting structures—the radial and ulnar collateral ligaments and the volar plate—have been damaged either individually or in any combination. Fractures can frequently accompany dislocations. If the dislocation is unstable, surgical repair using either a Kirschner wire or pin is often the standard course of treatment. This is accompanied by a postoperative cast or splint for three to five weeks. The wire or pin may be removed after three weeks, although use of the splint may continue. Removal of the splint for performing gentle active and passive PIP extension can be initiated with the surgeon's approval. Exercises include activities that permit tendon gliding while protecting the injured joint. A gradually progressive program of strengthening exercises starts at six to eight weeks once the patient has achieved full motion.

If the dislocation is stable, the finger is immobilized similar to the way it is with an unstable dislocation, with the PIP joint in 20° to 40° of flexion to permit maximal collateral ligament length and to control edema. Efforts should be made to control edema and pain even before motion exercises are started. In 7 to 10 days, AROM is initiated to prevent tendon gliding restrictions. These exercises are restricted by blocking individual joints. They should promote distal and proximal tendon gliding and emphasize both intrinsic and extrinsic muscles. Splinting is often discontinued after three weeks, with buddy taping applied to continue to protect the joint. Full active extension should be achieved within six to eight weeks. Resistive exercises can begin at around eight weeks.

Case Study

A 16-year-old, right-handed volleyball setter suffered a dislocated dominant-hand middle finger three weeks ago. The finger has been in a partial flexion splint for the past three weeks. The physician has instructed the patient to tape the finger to her ring finger throughout the day except when in rehabilitation. She has been moving the wrist and MCP joint, but the finger has been immobilized since the injury. The edema is gone, but the finger is stiff in the IP joints. Passive DIP extension/flexion is −15/30°, and PIP extension/flexion is −30/50°.

Active DIP extension/flexion is −20/25°, and PIP extension/flexion is −40/50°. The patient is unable to make a complete fist because the middle finger does not flex into the palm. Her grip strength measurement is 13.6 kg (30 lb) on the right and 31.7 kg (70 lb) on the left. There is tenderness over the PIP collateral ligaments, especially on the radial side.

Questions for Analysis

1. What will your first treatment goals be for this patient today?

2. What will you attempt to accomplish in the next three treatments? How will you accomplish those goals?

3. What precautions should you consider in the treatments?

4. What are two exercises you will send home with the patient today?

5. What strengthening exercises will you use?

6. What functional activities will you eventually include in her therapeutic exercise program?

OVERUSE INJURIES

The two most common overuse injuries of the wrist and hand are **carpal tunnel syndrome** and **De Quervain's disease**. Overuse is the term commonly used to describe these injuries, because trauma is produced over a period of time and applied at a greater rate than the structures can accommodate. Microscopic injury results and the structure is unable to rebuild before additional stress is applied. This creates an inflammatory response. If insult to the tissues continues, a chronic inflammatory response occurs and scar tissue develops, making the injury more difficult to manage. These injuries can be frustrating and challenging for the sport rehabilitation specialist, especially when the patient has failed to seek treatment until the injury has become advanced. The key to successful treatment is early intervention and correction of the causes.

Carpal Tunnel Syndrome

This is also known as *median nerve compression syndrome*. The median nerve is compressed as it passes under the transverse carpal ligament and through the carpal tunnel. Compression of the median nerve results in loss of sensation over its distribution in the hand, as well as weakness and pain. Pain occurs primarily at night, when the wrist is placed in flexion while the patient sleeps. Prolonged flexion positioning of the wrist causes compression on the nerve and venous congestion, and thus pain. This problem often results from prolonged or repeated wrist extension positioning during daily activities. A gymnast with weak wrists who performs on the bars with the wrists in hyperextension can develop carpal tunnel syndrome.

If carpal tunnel syndrome occurs bilaterally, the cervical region should be investigated as the possible source of the problem. Cervical radiculopathy is a differential diagnosis that should be ruled out for any upper-extremity injury not specifically related to an incident. Obtaining an accurate history is key to correctly determining the cause of the patient's symptoms. If passively placing the neck in a quadrant position (extension with lateral flexion and rotation to the involved side) reproduces the patient's symptoms, cervical radiculopathy cannot be ruled out; further evaluation of the neck is necessary.

When treatment begins early, it can often succeed in relieving symptoms. Use of a splint to position the wrist in neutral, especially at night, is helpful in reducing median nerve compression and night pain. Modalities can be used to relieve the inflammation. Ice, contrast baths, phonophoresis, iontophoresis, or electrical stimulation can be helpful. Flexibility exercises for the wrist and long finger flexors, restriction of those activities aggravating the condition, and remedy of incorrect techniques all assist in relieving the pain. Strengthening exercises for all wrist, thumb, and finger movements—beginning with isometrics and advancing to isotonics, eccentric exercises, and concentric exercises—should progress when the inflammation is under control. Endurance, speed, and coordination all should be included in the progression of exercises.

If conservative treatment does not resolve the patient's carpal tunnel syndrome, surgical intervention for release of the transverse carpal ligament may be necessary. Gentle AROM may begin within three to seven days postoperatively. Once the sutures are removed, scar-tissue management and desensitization through massage and soft-tissue mobilization can begin. The patient can start doing progressive resistive exercises when tolerated. The progression of exercises follows a course similar to that discussed earlier for other wrist injuries.

De Quervain's Disease

De Quervain's tendinitis affects the first dorsal compartment and involves the abductor pollicis longus and the extensor pollicis brevis. These tendons travel together in the same synovial sheath in the first compartment and pass around the bony radial styloid process, a site of friction for the tendons. Repetitive stress and inflammation from friction of these tendons occur with activities such as weight training and rowing.

As with carpal tunnel syndrome, modalities can be useful conservative treatment for relief of the inflammation. A spica splint is used to place the wrist in 15° of extension. The thumb is positioned in abduction, with the MCP joint in 10° flexion to put the affected tendons on slack. Although the splint is worn continually, it should be removed throughout the day for AROM exercises for the wrist and thumb. The patient should perform active range of motion of the fingers throughout the day.

Once pain and edema are reduced, mild strengthening and endurance activities can begin. The patient is gradually weaned from the splint during this stage. Gross- and fine-pinch activities, wrist and finger exercises, and endurance and coordination exercises should be a part of the strengthening program.

For surgical cases in which conservative treatment failed to resolve the injury, AROM exercises begin two to three days postoperatively to promote tendon gliding and prevent loss of motion. The wrist may be in a splint for about one week, but the patient removes it frequently during the day for ROM exercises. Pain and edema are controlled with various modalities, elevation, and active motion. The thumb should move in all its planes through full active motion. Thumb motion exercises should also include wrist motion.

Once the sutures are removed and the scar is healed, scar-tissue desensitization and softening can begin with massage. Strengthening exercise progression, which can begin after 7 to 10 days, follows the same procedure as for other wrist injuries.

Case Study

A 24-year-old crew team member underwent a surgical release of his right-nondominant first dorsal compartment three days ago. He has just seen the physician, who has removed the surgical dressing and instructed him to begin exercising the wrist and thumb. The physician has given the patient a splint to wear throughout the day except during treatments. Some swelling and tenderness are present over the scar. The wrist has good motion, but the thumb moves 10° at the MCP joint and 30° at the IP joint. There is some tenderness to radial deviation, but the patient has full motion.

Questions for Analysis

1. What will your treatment today include?
2. What instructions will you give the patient for home treatment?
3. What precautions must be considered?
4. What kind of ROM exercises will you give him?
5. When will you start working on strength, and what will the first strengthening exercises include?
6. What functional exercises will you advance the patient to before he returns to competition?

TENDON INJURIES

Tendon gliding exercises have already been presented. These are important exercises to perform following any injury to the hand, because adhesions to either flexor or extensor tendons cause significant loss of motion and hand function. In addition, the sport rehabilitation specialist must have knowledge and understanding of the specific differences between flexor and extensor tendons to apply proper rehabilitation techniques to injuries affecting hand tendons.

Special Tendon Considerations

Although the biochemical structures of the hand's flexor and extensor tendons are similar, several differences govern variations in the rehabilitation of flexor and extensor tendon injuries. Some of the differences have already been mentioned. Among the more obvious differences is the presence of the strong pulley system for the flexor tendons versus the absence of any pulleys for the extensor tendons. The majority of the length of the flexor tendons is enclosed in sheaths, but the extensor tendons are primarily extrasynovial.

Normally, finger flexion strength is significantly greater than finger extension strength. The flexors require greater strength for activities such as grasping, propelling, and catching objects than the extensors require for opening the hand. When an injury occurs to an extensor tendon, care must be taken to prevent the stronger flexor muscles from overpowering and causing further damage to the weakened extensor tendon.

The extensor tendons are flatter and thinner than the flexor tendons; therefore overall they have less tensile strength than the larger-diameter, thicker flexor tendons. When the fingers flex into the hand, the extensor tendons undergo significant lengthening. These factors make the extensor tendon susceptible to stretch or rupture, especially when in a weakened condition following an injury.

Although the extensor tendons are not surrounded with tendon sheaths like the flexor tendons, both are at risk for adhesion formation with immobilization. Loss of extension motion can be more functionally debilitating than flexion motion loss (Stewart 1992). Because of the intricate relationship between the extensor tendons and the intrinsic muscles, loss of mobility of the extensor tendons can have a significant impact on the function of the interossei and lumbricals and can hamper the intrinsic and extrinsic muscle balance necessary for normal hand function.

Tendon ruptures and lacerations are the most common tendon injuries of the hand. The ruptures usually result from impact avulsions such as occur when a player's hand is hit with a baseball bat. Lacerations can result from cleats, contact with sharp objects hidden in the grass, and accidents in archery and many other sports. The timing of rehabilitation is crucial to the success of the rehabilitation. Careful application of rehabilitative techniques is important to achieving desired end results. Recent advances in rehabilitation following tendon repair have improved results and reduced the risk of tendon adhesions. New approaches to postoperative tendon repair include the use of early controlled motion during the first weeks after surgery rather than the more traditional three weeks or more of immobilization. Because of the relative fragility of extensor tendons, early controlled motion was first used primarily with flexor tendon injuries; but more recently, early controlled motion has proven successful with extensor tendon injuries as well. At present, most believe that early controlled motion is advantageous for both flexor and extensor hand tendons; however, there must remain a fine balance between the proper amount of motion for allowing tendon gliding, and too much motion, which causes elongation or rupture of fragile tendon tissue during the early healing phases. The sport rehabilitation specialist must feel free to coordinate a patient's rehabilitation program with a hand specialist if necessary.

Early controlled motion includes passive movement of the repaired tendon. The initial goal of early motion is to promote tendon gliding and good tendon healing simultaneously. The ultimate goal is to produce a good surgical and rehabilitative result. Areas of the hand, such as no man's land, that were previously approached with caution and misgiving because of poor surgical results can be successfully and effectively repaired using early controlled motion.

Early controlled motion is achieved using a splint that is applied approximately three days postoperatively. The splint is designed to limit flexion if an extensor tendon has been repaired and to limit extension if a flexor tendon has been repaired. The angles of the splints are based on the 5-mm rule discussed earlier in the context of excursion of tendons during finger motion. The splints include a passive elastic force that pulls the fingers passively in the direction of the repaired tendon's pull. For example, an extensor tendon repair splint is constructed to block MCP joint flexion at 30° for the index and middle fingers, MCP joint flexion at 38° for the ring and small fingers, and extension of the IP joints with the wrist at about 40°. An elastic system, attached to the fingers, passively extends the fingers so that active motion of the tendon is not required to pull the finger into a resting position after it has flexed.

Conversely, a flexor tendon repair is placed in a dorsal splint with the wrist in about 20° flexion, the MPs in about 40° to 50° of flexion, and the IPs in extension. An elastic system is attached to the distal finger to pull the digit passively into flexion so as not to stress the newly repaired flexor tendon.

It is necessary to take care with both these splints so that the tension of the rubber band is sufficient to permit passive flexion or extension of the digits, yet not strong enough to promote a contracture because the tension is too much for the opposing tendon to overcome.

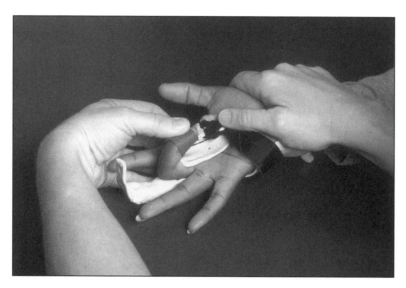

∎ Figure 19.59   Passive range of motion in a splint.

While the repaired flexor tendon finger is in the splint, the IP joints are passively flexed frequently throughout the day (figure 19.59). The patient performs finger extension actively to return the finger to the splint surface. Also, so that a splinted tendon-repair finger moves frequently within the splint, have the patient extend the fingers against the rubber bands on the flexor surface and allow the bands to passively return the fingers to the resting position, throughout the day.

Tendon glide and careful avoidance of adhesions are the primary concerns during the early stages of postoperative rehabilitation. Extensor tendon repairs have the additional problem of possible extensor lag development. The sport rehabilitation specialist must be aware of these conditions and take steps to provide good care while protecting against these complications. Observation of joint mobility is necessary for assessing the presence of these potentially debilitating conditions. You must differentiate between capsular restriction and tendon adhesions when the patient's motion is less than normal. One way to do this is to assess the digit's ROM at the individual joints and the quantity of motion with all joints involved. For example, if the patient is able to fully extend the wrist and MCP, PIP, and DIP joints of a digit one at a time while the other digit's joints are positioned in flexion, but unable to fully extend them all at once, the joint capsules have good mobility, but the tendon is probably restricted.

Once sutures are removed, scar-tissue management and desensitization can begin with massage. The patient can be instructed to perform this technique frequently throughout the day. This will help reduce the risk of tendon adhesions, because the tendons lie so close to the surface in the hand and fingers.

When to begin strengthening exercises for repaired tendons is a point of controversy. If a tendon is adherent, strengthening exercises begin earlier than if it glides well. Strength exercises initially are light strengthening exercises, starting at four to five weeks postoperatively (Stewart 1992). Other determining factors include the type of tendon (extensor or flexor) and the zone in which the repair is located.

Flexor Tendons

Active range of motion begins at three to six weeks for flexor tendons. If there is good flexion movement, in terms of quality, not necessarily quantity, gentle active motion can begin. Blocking exercises that limit motion at the proximal joint while emphasizing the distal joint can be used during this phase. Placing the wrist in extension during finger flexion and in flexion during finger extension motions, permit the desired motion without placing undue stress on the tendons.

Tendon glide must be present before the patient can advance to resistive exercises. The patient's readiness is assessed using observation skills and the techniques already described to ascertain fluidity of movement and restriction of mobility. As a rule, if the patient is unable to passively simultaneously extend the wrist and MCP and IP joints, tendon gliding is restricted and needs to be treated before strengthening exercises begin.

Although some advocate the initiation of mild strengthening at four weeks postoperatively, the more typical time to begin strengthening is seven to eight weeks after surgery. To some extent, this time line depends on the location of the repair. Zone V repairs heal quickly because of their blood supply; patients with these repairs can begin isolated AROM exercises by the third week and mild strengthening by the fifth week. Flexor digitorum sublimis tendons can withstand resistive exercises sooner than the FDP tendon.

Mild strengthening exercises include isometrics with gradual buildup to maximum output, grasping exercises, prehension activities, and use of the hand in daily activities as long as the patient does not lift or hold any heavy objects. Repetitions should begin low and should increase over the next couple of weeks. Progression of resistance is slow, with careful attention to the deleterious effects of too rapid a progression: pain, swelling, and stiffness.

The therapeutic exercise program continues to progress, with increases in strength, muscle endurance, and coordination, as the patient tolerates. The normal progression to functional exercises and return to activities occurs within 12 weeks.

Extensor Tendons

The most common extensor avulsion tendon rupture is the mallet finger, in which the distal attachment of the extensor tendon is torn—usually when the digit is hit on the end and forced into sudden flexion. This rupture is frequently not surgically repaired but rather placed in a splint that maintains the DIP in 0° extension. Placing it in hyperextension risks local ischemia of the region. After six to eight weeks, the splint is removed and the digit is exercised with AROM, emphasizing full extension movement. Flexion exercises are active only and are gentle so that an extensor lag does not form as a result of overstretching the new connective tissue on the extensor tendon. If a lag develops, the digit must be placed in the splint once again for another couple of weeks before the patient resumes exercises.

Extensor tendon injuries in zones III and IV cause what is known as a boutonniere deformity (figure 19.60). The cause, a disruption of the long extensor tendon's central slip, affects other structures within the extensor mechanism. The transverse retinacular ligament and the triangular ligament stretch with repeated motion of the digit without balance of the digit's forces. This causes

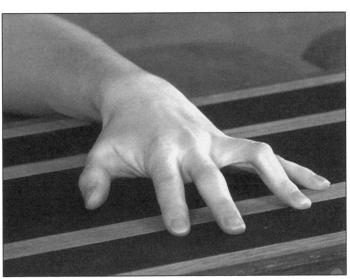

■ **Figure 19.60**   Boutonniere deformity.

an extensor lag at the PIP joint. When the lag occurs, the lateral bands of the extensor tendon move anteriorly to change the angle of pull of the intrinsics and create a hyperextension force at the DIP joint.

Treatment usually includes immobilization with extension of the PIP joint. Surgical repair of the central slip and lateral bands is occasionally required. The splint is commonly applied for six weeks, with isometric exercises beginning at three weeks while the digit is in the splint. The finger is taken out of the splint for gentle flexion AROM exercises at three to six weeks. To prevent tendon rupture, extension should be assisted. Early protective motion using a splint similar to the early protective extension splint, mentioned previously, can be used at three weeks.

When initiated, active exercises should stress active extension, isolating joint movement by blocking the proximal joints and advancing into combined joint extension movements. Passive stretching into flexion should be avoided for seven to eight weeks. Care must be taken throughout the therapeutic exercise process to avoid an extensor lag and flexor contractures. The sport rehabilitation specialist must monitor continuously for these problems.

Mild resistive extension exercises start at 8 to 10 weeks and progress as with flexor tendon injuries.

Extensor tendon injuries in zones V, VI, and VII vary from those in the other zones because they are not impacted by the extensor mechanism. Extraneous forces and deformity are less of a problem, so motion can begin earlier.

A splint is applied for three weeks immediately after injury or repair; the wearer is then weaned from it over the next two weeks. The wrist is maintained in about 30° to 45° extension with the MCPs and IPs in 0° extension. As with other tendon injuries, extensor lag and tendon adhesions must be prevented.

Gentle active motion can begin at three weeks with blocking exercises. Wrist extension and MCP flexion-extension with the IPs in extension, as well as hook exercises, are good tendon gliding exercises. At four weeks, full extension exercises for individual fingers begin; and at five or six weeks the hand exercises advance from a hook to a full fist. Resisted exercises and full stretch exercises begin after six weeks, progressing as with other hand therapeutic exercise programs.

Case Study

A 16-year-old softball catcher suffered a mallet deformity of her dominant right-hand ring finger in a game three weeks ago. It has been in a splint for the past three weeks. The doctor wants the patient to begin active exercises today and wants her to continue to wear the splint but to remove it for her treatments. Your initial examination reveals the following ring-finger flexion/extension measurements: MCP 90°/0°, PIP 90°/0°, DIP 15°/−10°. When the patient simultaneously extends the wrist and finger, the DIP is at −20°. Grip strength measures 13.6 kg (30 lb) on the right and 34 kg (75 lb) on the left. Wrist extension is 4/5. Both ulnar and radial deviation have normal motion and strength. Wrist flexion is 4/5, finger flexion is 4/5, MCP extension is 4−/5, and finger abduction is 4−/5.

Questions for Analysis

1. What will your first treatment include?

2. What instructions will you give the patient for home exercises?

3. What precautions must you consider in her treatments?

4. What determining factors will you use to decide when she should begin her strengthening exercises?

5. List three strengthening exercises and explain why you have selected them.

6. Identify three functional exercises and indicate your guidelines for beginning these.

REFLEX SYMPATHETIC DYSTROPHY

Reflex sympathetic dystrophy (RSD) more commonly involves the upper extremity than the lower extremity. It can occur as the result of an injury in any part of the extremity, but the symptoms are most apparent in the hand. When it originates from a shoulder injury, it is sometimes referred to as *shoulder-hand syndrome*. It is an extremely difficult problem to treat.

Program Considerations

Reflex sympathetic dystrophy is believed to occur because of some reflex sympathetic response to an injury. Characteristic complaints include pain disproportionate to the degree of injury, stiffness that is exaggerated in relation to the expected response to the injury, edema in the hand, cyanotic discoloration with redness around the MCP and PIP joints, coldness, and excessive sweating in the hand. The edema is initially soft and pitting, but with time it becomes brawny and hard. X rays can reveal bone demineralization. The skin appears tight and shiny because of immobilization and poor nutrition to the tissues. The patient tends to hold and protect the hand, moving the extremity little.

The most important aspect of treatment of RSD is early intervention. It is important to stop the sympathetic reflex cycle. The physician may attempt to select from a variety of medications or try a stellate ganglion block. The sport rehabilitation specialist can use a variety of techniques but must keep in mind that each patient with RSD may respond differently to these techniques.

Modalities can include a variety of methods such as various heat modalities to increase blood flow, reduce stiffness, and increase tissue extensibility for improved mobility. Heat, however, can sometimes cause increased edema. Electrical modalities, including high-voltage galvanic stimulation, transcutaneous electrical nerve stimulation, and functional electrical stimulation, can help reduce edema, decrease pain, and promote muscle activity, respectively. If tolerated, massage can be beneficial when pitting edema is present. It should be applied before exercise to maximize the effects of the exercise. Reduced edema can improve ROM and allow a greater excursion of muscle activity.

Splinting can be useful in preventing contractures. The wrist and hand are placed in a functional position with the wrist in slight extension, the MCP joints in midflexion, and the IP joints in extension. Continuous passive motion machines for the wrist and hand can also be useful in preventing contractures in the hand.

Exercises should be light and active. Exercise that is more than gentle often aggravates the patient's pain and increases stiffness. Low-repetition, active exercises are used to tolerance. These should include isolated joint motion and gross activities such as hook-grip, full-fist, and prehensile motions.

Passive motion and joint mobilization should not begin until the patient's pain is decreased. If pain intensifies, the exercises should return to previous levels of therapeutic activity. A gradual progression based on patient tolerance should include increased endurance exercises, strengthening, and functional activities.

Case Study

An 18-year-old female gymnast was referred to you four weeks after incurring a hand injury. Your evaluation reveals pitting edema throughout the hand. The skin is red and shiny, with increased redness over the MCP and PIP joints. Active range-of-motion measurements of the fingers' extension/flexion were the following: thumb MCP –10°/25°, IP –15°/20°; finger MCP –25°/50°; index PIP –20°/50°; middle PIP –30°/50°; ring –15°/60°; little –20°/50°; and all DIPs fixed at –20° extension. Wrist flexion is 30° and extension is 20°. The patient reports tenderness to light touch over the entire surface of the hand. The skin is cool and clammy to the touch.

Questions for Analysis

1. What are your initial goals for this patient?
2. What will your first treatment include?
3. What exercises will you initiate?
4. What instructions will you give the patient?

SUMMARY

1. *Explain the pulley system of the fingers.*

   There is an elaborate pulley system on the flexor aspect of the fingers—a fibrous tunnel that extends from the metacarpal head of each digit to the insertion of the distal finger flexor tendons. These pulleys are similar to the hoops along a fishing rod, positioned to keep the fishing line in place as it travels along the pole. There are five annular pulleys and three cruciate pulleys along each finger. Disruption of the key pulleys can cause bowstringing of the flexor tendons. The key pulleys preventing bowstringing are A2 and A4. When the pulley system of any finger is disrupted, the mechanical advantage of the tendon is impaired and normal function is lost.

2. *Explain why reducing edema in the hand is important.*

   Because the dorsal skin is loose and pliable compared to the volar skin, edema frequently accumulates in the dorsum of the hand. Pooled edema rich in proteins easily leads to contractures. Excessive swelling on the back of the hand can cause the hand arches to collapse anteriorly and adduct the thumb. Excessive swelling also requires a greater excursion of the skin for the person to flex the hand. If the skin is already stretched because of the edema, the hand's ability to move the fingers through their full motion is impaired. Fibrous tissue formation secondary to the presence of prolonged edema can cause reduced mobility and function of the hand.

3. *Discuss the trimuscular system of the hand and explain why it is important to hand function.*

   Three muscle groups compose the trimuscular system of the hand—the extrinsic flexors, the extrinsic extensors, and the intrinsic muscles—and provide for balanced, controlled hand function. If any of these groups is not allowed to function normally, because of either weakness or loss of mobility, balance is lost and the hand is not able to work in its normal capacity.

4. *Identify and explain the importance of the precision and power grips of the hand.*

   The power grips, also known as palmar grips, include the clenched fist, the cylinder grasp, the spherical grasp, and the hook. In these grasps, the thumb is positioned in opposition to the other fingers to permit a firm grasp on an object. The majority of daily hand activities involve these palmar grips. Because palmar grasping is so vital to hand function, the hand is most commonly splinted in a palmar position with the thumb in slight opposition, facing the other fingers. The precision or prehensile grips include the digital prehension grip, the lateral prehension grip, and the tip-to-tip prehension grip. These movements include fine-tuned activities such as typing, sewing, or writing. These prehensile activities occur when the thumb and finger muscles co-contract to produce an activity requiring precision.

5. *Explain the difference between static and dynamic splints.*

Overall, the aim of splints is either to prevent damage and maintain balance or to improve balance. Static splints restrict motion to support and protect the hand. Dynamic splints are used to increase motion of the hand. Splints are based on a three-point pressure system whereby two points of application are on one side of the hand, wrist, or forearm and the other point of application is on the opposite side.

6. *Identify what motion is increased with carpal radial glide joint mobilization.*

A carpal radial glide is used to improve ulnar flexion of the wrist.

7. *Explain the force application sequence for improving long finger flexor or extensor motion.*

The basic application sequence is the same for flexors and extensors. If the distal phalanx has limited flexion motion, the proximal joint is stabilized as the distal joint (DIP) is moved into flexion; then the PIP joint is moved into flexion as the MCP joint is stabilized while the DIP's flexed position is maintained. The MCP joint is then moved into flexion as the wrist is stabilized and the IP joints are kept in their flexion positions. Finally, the wrist is gradually moved into flexion. The stretch should be performed in both elbow flexion and elbow extension, and the forces applied gradually until the patient feels a stretch in the forearm.

8. *Explain how the intrinsic stretches differ from the extrinsic stretches.*

Because the lumbricals and interossei flex the MCP joints and extend the IP joints, the stretch is applied in the opposite direction of their function or direction of motion. The IP joints are maintained in a flexed position while a stretch is applied to increase MCP extension. The wrist should be stabilized in neutral during this activity to prevent extrinsic muscle influences on the stretch.

9. *Discuss the difference in gliding exercises for the flexor profundus and superficialis tendons.*

Three exercises for flexor tendon gliding include (1) keeping the MCP extended and flexing the IPs to enhance gliding between the two longer finger flexor tendons, (2) forming a fist with the IP and MCP joints in flexion to produce gliding of the profundus tendon within its sheath, and (3) positioning the MCP and PIP joints in flexion and extending the DIP joints. Flexor pollicis longus gliding exercises are performed in a similar manner by moving the IP and MCP joints through a full range of flexion and extension. These exercises are initially performed with the wrist in neutral; but as the patient progresses, the wrist should be moved into flexion with finger flexion and into extension with finger extension. A gliding exercise for the EDC is performed by moving the hand from a hook to a fist formation. The MCP joint is moved from flexion to extension while the IP joints are kept in flexion to eliminate the intrinsic muscles. If the patient has difficulty maintaining flexion of the IP joints during this activity, he or she can grasp a drinking straw or pencil in the fingers while moving the MCP joints. Wrist flexion and extension should also be added to the exercise when it is easy for the patient to perform the exercise with the wrist in neutral.

10. *Present the differences between long flexor and long extensor tendons.*

    Among the more obvious differences is the presence of the strong pulley system for the flexor tendons versus the absence of any pulleys for the extensor tendons. The majority of the length of the flexor tendons is enclosed in sheaths, but the extensor tendons are primarily extrasynovial. Finger flexion strength is significantly greater than finger extension strength. The extensor tendons are flatter and thinner than the flexor tendons; for this reason they have less overall tensile strength than the larger-diameter, thicker flexor tendons. When the fingers close into the hand, the extensor tendons undergo significant lengthening. The flexor tendons are surrounded with tendon sheaths and risk loss of tendon glide and formation of adhesions with immobilization. Loss of extensor motion can be more functionally debilitating than flexion motion loss.

11. *Explain what procedures should be used to eliminate an extensor lag of a distal phalanx.*

    A gliding exercise for the EDC can be used to reduce adhesions that may be causing an extensor lag and is described in the answer to question 9. If the extensor lag occurs at either IP joint, it is the result of adhesions within the extensor mechanism and can include both intrinsic and extrinsic structures, the interossei, lumbricals, and EDC. To isolate the intrinsic muscles and facilitate their movement into IP extension, the MCP should be stabilized in flexion. As this exercise becomes easier, the MCP joint should be moved into extension. In the most difficult position for this exercise, the hand is flat on a table and the proximal phalanx stabilized, and the patient attempts to extend the distal phalanx off the table.

12. *Identify the early signs of RSD.*

    Early complaints include pain disproportionate to the degree of injury, stiffness that is exaggerated in relation to the expected response to the injury, pitting edema in the hand, cyanotic discoloration with redness around the MCP and PIP joints, coldness, and excessive sweating in the hand.

CRITICAL THINKING QUESTIONS

1. Why do you suspect that tendinitis and overuse injuries are common in the hand and wrist? On the basis of the anatomy and the causes of overuse injuries, what sports would you suspect would have a higher-than-average incidence of overuse injuries of the hand and wrist, and why? Given this, what efforts can be made to prevent these injuries in these sports?

2. If a patient suffers a scaphoid fracture, how long would you expect him or her to complain of pain? If the wrist pain continues for several weeks beyond your expectations, what would you suspect is the reason? What would you do in this situation?

3. In the opening scenario, what test did Steve use to determine that adhesions were forming between the flexor digitorum superficialis and profundus? What specific techniques would you use to reduce these adhesions? What exercises and home program would you give Carlos to help create more mobility between the tissues? How would the adhesions interfere with hand function by affecting the intrinsic muscles?

4. If a mallet finger injury begins to lose active extension after having started rehabilitation exercises, what would you suspect is the cause? How would you remedy the situation to restore active extension?

REFERENCES

Bowers, W.H., and S.M. Tribuzi. 1992. Functional anatomy. In *Concepts in hand rehabilitation*, ed. B.G. Stanley and S.M. Tribuzi. Philadelphia: Davis.

Boyes, J.H. 1970. *Bunnell's surgery of the hand.* Philadelphia: Lippincott.

Doyle, J.R., and W.F. Blythe. 1975. The finger flexor tendon sheaths and pulleys. Anatomy and reconstruction. In *A.A.O.S.: Symposium on tendon surgery of the hand.* St. Louis: Mosby.

Duran, R.J., and R.G. Houser. 1975. Controlled passive motion following flexor tendon repair in zones 2 and 3. In *A.A.O.S. Symposium on tendon surgery of the hand.* St. Louis: Mosby.

Evans, R.B. 1989. Clinical application of controlled stress to the healing extensor tendon: A review of 112 cases. *Physical Therapy* 69:1041–1049.

Evans, R.B., and W.E. Burkhalter. 1986. A study of the dynamic anatomy of extensor tendons and implications for treatment. *Journal of Hand Surgery (Am)* 11:774–779.

Maitland, G.D. 1991. *Peripheral manipulation.* Boston; London: Butterworth-Heinemann.

Stewart, K.M. 1992. Tendon injuries. In *Concepts in hand rehabilitation*, ed. B.G. Stanley and S.M. Tribuzi. Philadelphia: Davis.

Travell, J.G., and D.G. Simons. 1983. *Myofascial pain and dysfunction. The trigger point manual.* Vol. 1. Baltimore: Williams and Wilkins.

SUGGESTED READING

Brunet, M.E., Haddad, R.J., Sanchez, J., and E. Leonard. 1984. How I manage sprained finger in athletes. *Physician and Sportmedicine* 12:99–108.

Burnett, W.R. 1992. Rehabilitation techniques for ligament injuries of the hand. *Hand Clinics* 8:803–815.

Clemens, S., and B. Foss-Campbell. 1993. Rehabilitation following traumatic hand injury: Hand therapists' perspective. Part 1: Acute phase of hand rehabilitation. *Plastic Surgical Nursing* 13:129–139.

Dovelle, S., and P.K. Heeter. 1985. Early controlled mobilization following extensor tendon repair in zone V-VI of the hand: Preliminary report. *Contemporary Orthopaedics* 11:41–44.

Evans, R.B., and D.E. Thompson. 1992. An analysis of factors that support early active short arc motion of the repaired central slip. *Journal of Hand Therapy* 5:187–201.

Halikis, M.N., and J. Taleisnik. 1996. Soft-tissue injuries of the wrist. *Clinics in Sports Medicine* 15:235–259.

Hunter, J.M., Schneider, L.H., Mackin, E.J., and A.D. Callahan, eds. 1990. *Rehabilitation of the Hand. Surgery and Therapy.* St. Louis: Mosby.

Kleinert, H.E., and C. Verdan. 1983. Report of the committee on tendon injuries. *Journal of Hand Surgery (Am)* 7:794–798.

Levine, W.R. 1992. Rehabilitation techniques for ligament injuries of the wrist. *Hand Clinics* 8:669–677.

May, E.J., Silfverskiold, K.L., and C.J. Sollerman. 1992. Controlled mobilization after flexor tendon repair in zone II: A prospective comparison of three methods. *Journal of Hand Surgery* 5:942–952.

Wadsworth, C.T. 1983. Clinical anatomy and mechanics of the wrist and hand. *Journal of Orthopaedic and Sports Physical Therapy* 4:206–216.

Wehbe, M.A. 1996. Early motion after hand and wrist reconstruction. *Hand Clinics* 12:25–29.

Zimmerman, G.R. 1994. Carpal tunnel syndrome. *Journal of Athletic Training* 29:22–30.

CHAPTER TWENTY

Foot, Ankle, and Lower Leg

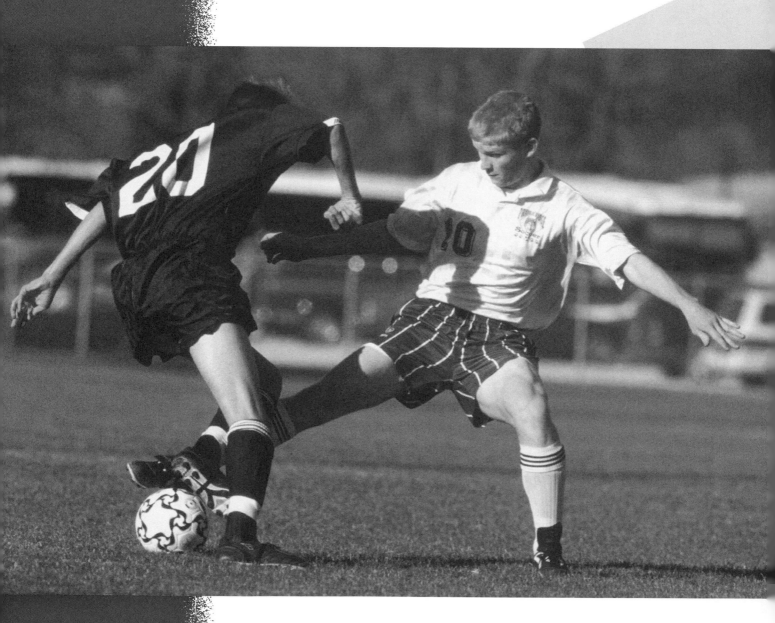

OBJECTIVES

After completing this chapter, you should be able to do the following:

1. Discuss normal foot mechanics in ambulation.

2. Identify two foot deformities and discuss their impact on athletic injury.

3. Describe the primary structures of a shoe.

4. List the important factors in shoe considerations for a pes cavus foot.

5. Outline key factors in an orthotic evaluation.

6. Explain one joint mobilization technique for improving ankle dorsiflexion.

7. List three stretching exercises for the ankle and lower leg, including one that is not mentioned in the text.

8. Identify three strengthening exercises for the ankle and lower leg.

9. Explain three agility exercises.

10. Describe three functional exercises for the lower extremity.

11. Provide an example of a therapeutic exercise program progression for an ankle sprain.

After two months of persistent heel pain, cross country runner Troy felt he could no longer hope the pain would go away on its own and decided to seek care for it. After Bob Pamaloo had performed his evaluation, he informed Troy that the problem was plantar fasciitis.

Bob concluded from his evaluation that Troy had a few problems that were contributing to the plantar fasciitis. His excessive pronation would have to be corrected with orthotics; the tight hip rotators were causing altered knee alignment that contributed to increased torsional stress on the plantar fascia and would have to be stretched and corrected, as would the tightness in the iliotibial band and Achilles. The muscle imbalance in Troy's quads and hamstrings was another possible contributing factor that would be resolved with strengthening activities. Bob also explained to Troy that not only were his shoes too worn to wear running; they also did not have the proper construction for his foot needs. Although there were several problems, Bob was optimistic that they were all correctable with proper rehabilitation and changes in footwear so that Troy would be able to resume his normal running program.

I find the greatest thing in this world, not so much where we stand, as in what direction we are moving.

Johann W. Goethe, 1749–1832, poet, dramatist

The foot and ankle are complex structures that impact the entire lower leg, because they form the base that moves the rest of the body from one location to another. Injuries in these areas can affect the efficiency and effectiveness of body propulsion, the primary function of the lower extremities.

Injuries to the foot and ankle are common in sport. A key responsibility of the sport rehabilitation specialist is to use his or her skill and knowledge of the foot and ankle to provide the patient with an appropriate and efficient recovery program that will permit a full return to sport participation.

The foot, ankle, and lower leg, like the hand, wrist, and forearm, are complex structures composed of many bones, joints, and muscles. There are 26 bones and 33 joints in the foot, ankle, and lower leg, along with several intrinsic and extrinsic muscles. These structures are divided into segments within the foot, ankle, and lower leg; each segment forms integral relationships with the other segments within the area as well as with more proximal segments such as the knee, hip, and back. There is evidence to demonstrate the direct impact that foot position and mechanics have on the knee (Tiberio 1987; Klingman, Liaos, and Hardin 1997; Powers, Maffucci, and Hampton 1995) and other more distal segments (Massie and Spiker 1990). It is important, then, that you have knowledge of the structure and function of the distal lower extremity so that the rehabilitation program you establish will return the patient to full function without applying additional stresses to more proximal segments.

This chapter outlines the basic structure of the lower leg, ankle, and foot as it pertains to the normal function of those segments as well as the more proximal segments. We will pay specific attention to concepts that directly relate to rehabilitation following injury. The second half of the chapter addresses specific injuries most commonly seen in the lower leg, ankle, and foot, along with case studies.

GENERAL REHABILITATION CONSIDERATIONS

Normal foot mechanics in ambulation depends on the correct timing and coordination of the motions of many joints and the extrinsic and intrinsic muscles of the lower leg and foot. Subtalar motion and position also influence movement of the lower extremity.

Before discussing the foot and ankle, we need to define some of the more common terms used to describe these body segments. These terms are often misused, so establishing definitions helps to ensure common understanding.

TERMINOLOGY

One possible reason for confusion about terms relating to the foot may be that the foot is not in the same plane as the rest of the body: the foot is at a 90° angle to the leg. Another possible reason is that the foot seldom moves in cardinal, or straight, planes; many of the joints are multiplanar. As a point of reference, ankle and foot motions in the cardinal planes (frontal, sagittal, and transverse) and multiplanes are defined here.

Pronation is a multiplanar rotational motion that occurs in the subtalar and transverse tarsal joints and is the combination of dorsiflexion, abduction, and eversion. This motion is sometimes incorrectly referred to as eversion. A common foot deformity occurs when an unstable subtalar joint causes pronation to occur for a longer period of time than is normal during ambulation. This is commonly referred to as prolonged pronation or excessive pronation. **Dorsiflexion** is the sagittal plane movement in which the ankle joint angle is decreased as the dorsal foot is moved upward toward the anterior surface of the lower leg. **Abduction** is the transverse plane movement of the foot in which the lateral foot is moved away from the midline. **Inversion** is a frontal plane movement in which the plantar foot rotates inward so that the medial border is lifted upward.

Supination is a multiplanar rotational motion that includes plantar flexion, adduction, and inversion. This combined motion is sometimes incorrectly referred to as inversion. **Plantar flexion** is the sagittal plane motion in which the foot moves downward and the dorsal foot moves away from the anterior surface of the lower leg. **Adduction** is the transverse plane movement of the foot in which the medial foot is moved toward the midline. **Eversion** is a frontal plane movement in which the plantar foot rotates outward so that the lateral border is lifted upward. These straight-plane motions of adduction-abduction, inversion-eversion, and dorsiflexion-plantar flexion occur in open chain activities (figure 20.1). In closed chain activities, the combined motions of pronation and supination occur, not the cardinal plane motions. Along with pronation and supination in the closed kinetic chain, associated motions take place further up the chain. With pronation, the lower leg internally rotates, the knee flexes, and the hip flexes and internally rotates. Conversely, with supination, the lower leg externally rotates; the knee extends; and the hip extends, abducts, and externally rotates. Because supination and pronation occur in the subtalar joint, the subtalar joint is instrumental in foot motion and in control of the other joints. For example, if the subtalar joint in the closed kinetic chain is positioned in pronation, the lower leg will internally rotate, the knee will flex, and the hip will internally rotate and flex. If the subtalar joint stays in pronation when it should be in supination during ambulation, injuries can result in either the foot or more proximal segments, especially if those segments are forced to be in an abnormal position because of the pronation in the subtalar joint. These injuries are discussed later in this chapter.

LOWER LEG, FOOT, AND ANKLE JOINTS

Specifics of gait analysis are discussed in chapter 12. Reviewing that chapter may help you understand some additional concepts presented here. The first structure to hit the ground in walking is the calcaneus. It, along with the talus, forms the subtalar

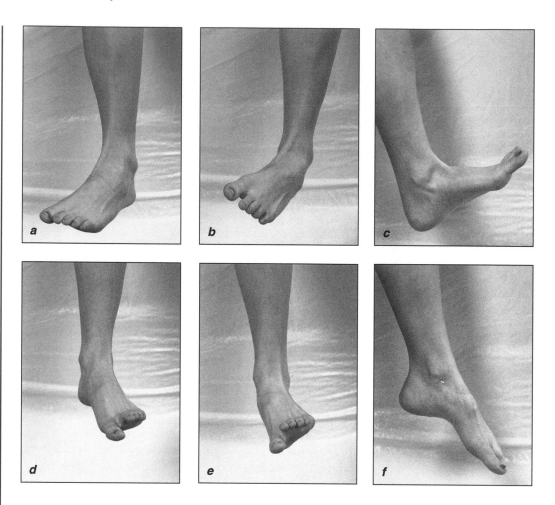

Figure 20.1 Foot planar motions: *(a)* adduction, *(b)* inversion, *(c)* dorsiflexion, *(d)* abduction, *(e)* eversion, *(f)* plantar flexion.

joint; and the talus along with the tibia and fibula forms the talocrural joint. Normal function of these two joints permits us to land the foot on the ground and adapt to variations in ground topography while maintaining a steady gait. Although the talocrural joint is actually the ankle joint, both of these joints are often thought of as the ankle. These two joints are responsible for a number of ankle motions. The talocrural joint moves primarily in dorsiflexion and plantar flexion. The subtalar joint is responsible for pronation and supination. Pronation and its component motions cause the foot to convert from a rigid lever to a mobile adapter to accommodate for uneven surfaces. Supination causes the foot articulations to become more rigid and provide for power transfer to permit appropriate force application needed for propulsion in ambulation. As mentioned in chapter 12, these motions must occur at specific times for gait to be normal.

The talocrural joint is a mortise joint, with a convex talar dome in contact with a concave tibial mortise. The lateral malleolus is posterior and distal to the medial malleolus. This arrangement allows more inversion and eversion to occur in the subtalar joint, and also causes plantar flexion to occur more in a posterolateral direction and dorsiflexion to occur more in an anteromedial direction. As the ankle goes into plantar flexion, the talus moves anteriorly so that the posterior, narrower aspect of the talus sits in the mortise joint. This can contribute to instability of the ankle in plantar flexion and is one reason that women wearing high-heeled shoes, and athletes landing from a jump with the foot in plantar flexion, are especially susceptible to ankle sprains. Conversely, the most stable close-packed position for the talus is with the ankle in dorsiflexion when the wider anterior talus is wedged up into the mortise joint. During dorsiflexion, the fibula glides superiorly and rotates laterally;

and in plantar flexion, it moves inferiorly and rotates medially. If these fibular motions are not present, full ankle dorsiflexion and plantar flexion cannot occur. Distal to the talocrural and subtalar joints are the midtarsal joints, a combination of the talonavicular and calcaneocuboid articulations. Their position is determined by the subtalar joint position; the midtarsal joints become locked during supination and unlocked during pronation. Movements of the midtarsal joints closely follow movements of the subtalar and talocrural joints. During supination, the navicular and cuboid bones move medially and inferiorly, and during pronation they move laterally and superiorly.

The tarsometatarsal joints are divided into five rays. The first ray is the joint between the first metatarsal and the medial cuneiform. Although the first ray has triplanar motion, its movements are generally referred to as plantar flexion and dorsiflexion. Movement of the first ray occurs equally in plantar flexion and dorsiflexion, with each movement equivalent to about a thumb's width of motion. The second ray includes the joint between the second metatarsal and the middle cuneiform, the third ray includes the third metatarsal and the lateral cuneiform, the fourth ray is the fourth metatarsal alone, and the fifth ray is the fifth metatarsal alone.

Metatarsophalangeal (MTP) joints permit flexion-extension, abduction-adduction, and accessory rotation and dorsal-plantar glides. The interphalangeal (IP) joints, which are hinge joints, permit flexion and extension with accessory rotation and dorsal-plantar glides. The first MTP joint must have about 65° of hyperextension for toe roll-off during gait.

MUSCLE FUNCTION

There are 12 extrinsic muscles and 11 intrinsic muscles of the lower leg and foot. The extrinsic muscles are divided into four compartments or groups: anterior, lateral, posterior superficial, and posterior deep (figure 20.2). The anterior compartment muscles cross the ankle joint anteriorly and provide for dorsiflexion, and lateral and posterior compartment muscles cross the ankle posteriorly and are plantar flexors (figure 20.3). The muscles that have the greatest mechanical advantage to produce inversion and eversion because of their positions are the anterior and posterior tibialis medially and the peroneals laterally.

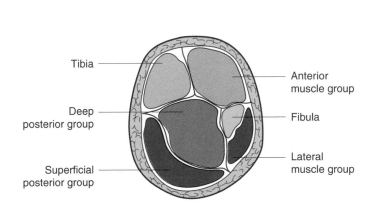

■ **Figure 20.2** Cross section of the lower-leg muscle compartments.

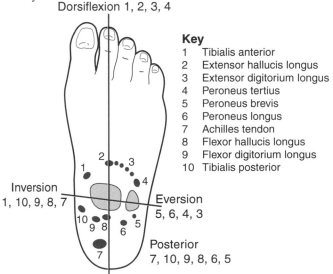

■ **Figure 20.3** Ankle motions. The vertical axis divides muscles that provide inversion and eversion, whereas the horizontal axis divides dorsiflexors from plantar flexors. Muscles are listed in order of their mechanical advantage for motion.

The posterior lower leg has a superficial and a deep compartment; the two compartments are separated by deep fascia, the intermuscular septum. The superficial group includes the large plantar flexors, the soleus, gastrocnemius, and plantaris. The deep posterior muscles originate from the same location as the anterior compartment muscles but traverse posteriorly.

The intrinsic foot muscles are contained within the foot itself. Their purpose is to provide stability to the toes, tarsometatarsal joints, and midfoot while extrinsic muscles move the joints. They attempt to keep the toes on the ground until toe-off during gait and convert the toes to rigid beams for propulsion in gait. These muscles are weakened with ankle injuries and must be rehabilitated along with the extrinsic muscles. In a foot that is unstable, such as a foot that is hypermobile or one that has excessive pronation, the intrinsics are required to work far beyond normal expectations. Excessive sweating of the foot and consequent foot odor are evidence of intrinsic muscle overactivity.

FOOT ARCHES

There are three arches of the foot, the medial and lateral longitudinal arches and the transverse arch. These arches are formed by the architecture of the tarsals and their arrangement with each other, the ligaments, and the supporting muscles. The primary tensile supporting structure for the longitudinal arches is the plantar fascia; the transverse arch is supported by the peroneus longus. These arches protect the underlying blood vessels and nerves and provide an efficient system of support for the body's weight. If the arches are unable to maintain a normal configuration, an imbalance is created, and abnormal stresses applied to the foot can cause injury. The normal alignment of the longitudinal arches is determined through use of the Feiss line test. In non-weight bearing, a line is drawn from tip of the medial malleolus to the first metatarsal head. This line should cross over the navicular tubercle. In weight bearing, the navicular tubercle should remain on the line or slightly below it.

SUBTALAR NEUTRAL POSITION

Because the subtalar joint has a significant impact on the entire lower extremity, the sport rehabilitation specialist must know what normal subtalar motion and position are to be able to assess and treat an abnormal subtalar joint.

Subtalar neutral is the position in which the talus is equally palpable from its medial or its lateral aspect within the subtalar joint. It is at this point that the talus and navicular are most congruent and the alignment of the subtalar bones is optimal. Subtalar neutral should be assessed in both weight bearing and non-weight bearing (Lattanza, Gray, and Kantner 1988). In non-weight bearing, the patient lies prone with the opposite leg flexed at the hip and knee and the hip in abduction and external rotation to stabilize the pelvis. With the patient's foot and distal lower leg to be examined over the edge of the table, the sport rehabilitation specialist places a thumb and index finger on the medial and lateral aspects of the talus. The sport rehabilitation specialist locates the medial aspect, in a depression slightly inferior and anterior to the medial malleolus and just proximal to the navicular, using the thumb. He or she locates the lateral aspect, anterior to the lateral malleolus, using the index finger (figure 20.4). As the talus is palpated with one hand, the other hand grasps the fourth and fifth metatarsal heads and moves the foot into dorsiflexion until resistance is

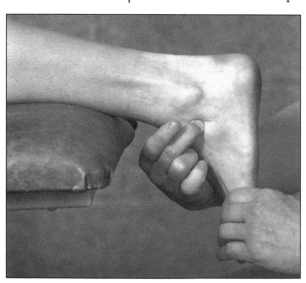

▮ Figure 20.4   Subtalar neutral positioning.

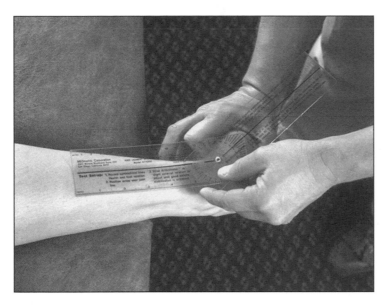

■ **Figure 20.5** Measurement of subtalar range of motion. Lines bisecting the calcaneous and lower leg are used to define subtalar or rearfoot inversion and eversion range of motion.

felt. In this position, the forefoot is in pronated and supinated to invert and evert the rearfoot. When the forefoot is supinated, the talus is inverted so that the lateral border can be palpated; and when the forefoot is pronated, the talus is everted so that the medial border can be palpated. The foot is rocked back and forth in the two directions with progressively smaller arcs until the talus is centrally positioned and cannot be palpated on either the medial or the lateral aspect or is palpated equally on each side. If subtalar neutral is being palpated in weight bearing, the patient is asked to raise and lower the longitudinal arch to rotate the forefoot until subtalar neutral is determined.

Once subtalar neutral is determined, range of motion of the rearfoot based on calcaneal position can be assessed. Normal rearfoot motion is 30° with one third in eversion and two thirds in inversion. A perpendicular line bisecting the posterior calcaneus and a line bisecting the posterior tibia are used as reference points. The calcaneus is passively moved into eversion and inversion, and measurements are taken at the end range of each position (figure 20.5).

COMMON STRUCTURAL DEFORMITIES

Pes cavus and planus, hallux valgus, tibial torsion, tibial varum, and rearfoot and forefoot varus and valgus are among the common structural deformities of the foot and lower leg.

Although the deformities we will consider are not injuries but structural deviations, they can often lead to injuries. Athletic activity imposes greater-than-normal forces on the foot and thereby exaggerates the impact of a deformity. The sport rehabilitation specialist must be familiar with these deformities and their impact on the patient to provide appropriate treatment programs.

PES CAVUS

In **pes cavus**, the foot has an abnormally high longitudinal arch (figure 20.6). The navicular tubercle is above the Feiss line in both weight bearing and non-weight bearing. This is a rigid foot with limited stress-absorption abilities. The foot does not pronate as it should to absorb impact stresses, so the forces are transmitted up the leg. Pes cavus feet can lead to fallen transverse arches, hammertoes or claw toes, corns, stress fractures, and other overuse injuries.

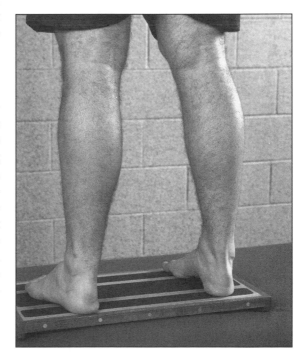

■ **Figure 20.6** Pes cavus.

PES PLANUS

In **pes planus**, the foot has an abnormally low longitudinal arch (figure 20.7). A rigid pes planus has the navicular tubercle below the Feiss line in both weight bearing and non-weight bearing. A flexible pes planus foot has the navicular tubercle below the Feiss line in weight bearing but on the Feiss line during non-weight bearing.

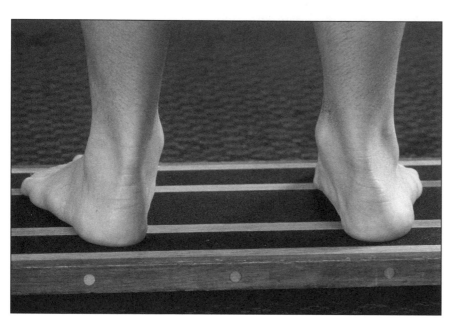

Figure 20.7 Pes planus.

Either rigid or flexible pes planus can lead to injuries in athletes. During weight bearing, the foot is unable to form a rigid lever for efficiency of propulsion and remains in a pronated position when it should be supinated. This imposes additional stresses on more proximal leg segments. During heel-off and just before toe-off, the lower leg and hip are externally rotating, a motion in conflict with pronation, so torque forces become exaggerated. This is especially true at the knee, particularly at the patellofemoral joint. The condition also places torsion on the plantar fascia and Achilles tendon, because they should be supinating but are pronating. Common terms for the foot with pes planus are pronated foot, flatfoot, and pancake arch.

HALLUX VALGUS

This condition is also known as a bunion. **Hallux valgus** is present when the first MTP joint is greater than 10° in valgus with the first toe pointed laterally toward the other toes (figure 20.8). The condition is most commonly seen in a pes planus foot. With the foot in pronation and the lower leg externally rotated, the force at toe-off is transmitted though the medial aspect of the first ray. This increases medial joint stress. The first ray deviates medially, and the phalanx deviates laterally.

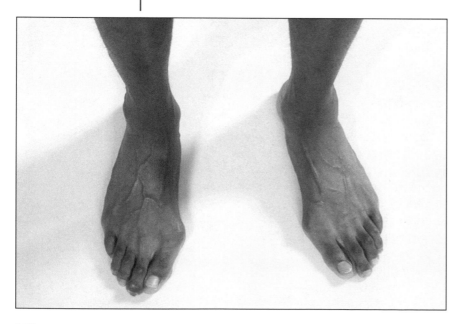

Figure 20.8 Hallux valgus.

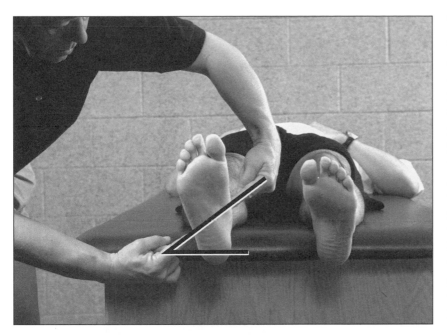

Figure 20.9 Measuring tibial torsion: tibial torsion is the angle formed between the line through the malleoli and the plane of the tabletop when the femoral condyles on the table and the patella are facing the ceiling.

TIBIAL TORSION

Tibial torsion is present when the tibia is rotated on its long axis. Normally, the midline of the patella is in line with the first- and second-toe web space. In tibial torsion, the foot is rotated laterally to the patella's midline. One can quantify this with the patient supine and the medial and lateral femoral condyles in the transverse plane and the patella facing the ceiling. The sport rehabilitation specialist measures the angle between the plane of the table and the line between the medial and lateral malleolus (figure 20.9). Normal value is 15°, with a normal range of 2° to 3° in either direction.

Patients with tibial torsion experience increased stress to the knee. Because the tibia is externally rotated relative to the patella, an increased torque is applied to the patellar tendon. External rotation of the tibia can also be related to prolonged pronation, lateral thigh tightness, and altered patellofemoral alignment.

TIBIAL VARUM

Tibial varum is present when the distal tibia is closer to the midline than the proximal tibia. This can be measured with the patient in standing. With the patient's feet shoulder-width apart, the sport rehabilitation specialist places the goniometer's stationary arm on the floor and the movable arm along a posterior line bisecting the distal tibia (figure 20.10). The movable arm should be vertical.

Tibial varum is usually accompanied by genu varum and coxa valgus. This deformity places above-normal stress on the knee, Achilles, and hip.

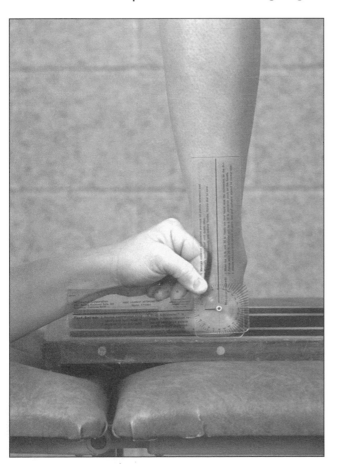

Figure 20.10 Measuring tibial varum: the line bisecting the lower leg should be vertical if normal tibial alignment is present.

REARFOOT VARUS AND VALGUS

The rearfoot is composed of the talus and calcaneus, and its alignment is sometimes referred to as subtalar varus and valgus. Its alignment is determined by the position of the calcaneus relative to that of the posterior lower leg. Rearfoot varus (figure 20.11b) is present when the calcaneus is inverted relative to the posterior bisection of the lower leg. Rearfoot valgus is present when the calcaneus is everted relative to the tibia (figure 20.11c). The source of rearfoot varus is difficult to ascertain: it may be within the talus, the calcaneus, or both.

Rearfoot varus should be assessed in both a relaxed standing position and a subtalar neutral position. Ideally, the results should be the same in the two positions. In a foot that has compensated for the deformity, the calcaneus is perpendicular to the floor in neutral and everted in resting standing. If a foot is uncompensated, the calcaneus remains in eversion in both positions, but the amount of eversion is less in neutral.

With rearfoot varus, the foot remains partially or fully pronated until heel-off during the weight-bearing phase of gait. More pronation than normal must occur to get the inverted heel to the ground. Once the foot is off the ground, the calcaneus rapidly supinates to catch up to the position it should be in at heel strike. This causes a medial heel-whip, which you can see as the patient ambulates when you observe from the rear.

Because the rearfoot does not supinate, hypermobility of the forefoot occurs, and the first ray is unable to get fully stabilized for propulsion. This causes transferal of increased shear and loading forces to the second metatarsal head, and sometimes to the third and fourth metatarsal heads. This in turn causes calluses predominantly over the second metatarsal head and secondarily over the third and fourth metatarsal heads (figure 20.11a). The rearfoot position is important to recognize because it is a key determining factor for the rest of the foot and has a significant impact on the knee and hip.

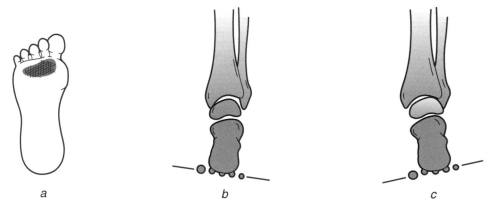

a   *b*   *c*

▌**Figure 20.11**   Varus and valgus rearfoot deformities: *(a)* callus pattern for compensated subtalar varus, *(b)* varus, *(c)* valgus.

FOREFOOT VARUS AND VALGUS

A forefoot varus is an inversion deformity of the midtarsal joint. It is identified through comparison of the plane of the five metatarsal heads with the perpendicular line of the calcaneal bisection. For this assessment, the patient is in prone and the rearfoot is placed and maintained in subtalar neutral. The forefoot is loaded on the fifth metatarsal head, and the foot is passively moved into dorsiflexion. In the normal forefoot, the line in the plane of the metatarsals and the line bisecting the calcaneous are perpendicular to each other (figure 20.12b). In forefoot varus, the medial forefoot is higher than the lateral side (inverted) (figure 20.12a). A related condition is first-ray dorsiflexion.

In compensated forefoot varus, the subtalar joint is pronated to allow the medial toes to get to the ground. This calcaneal pronation occurs at a time when the joint should be starting to supinate. The rearfoot is unable to supinate in time for heel-off and toe-off because the forefoot is still in contact with the ground, forcing the rearfoot to remain pronated. A slight heel-whip may be seen at heel-off; but it usually is ineffective, because the deformity in the forefoot causing the compensation is still in contact with the ground.

With the calcaneus in pronation throughout propulsion, the body's weight is distributed more medially than normal, and the midtarsal joint becomes hypermobile. This causes the first ray to become unstable and incapable of carrying its propulsive load. The weight and force are then transferred to the second and third metatarsal heads, where callus formations appear as a result of this increased shear and force stress. Because the body's weight is more medially distributed than normal, the foot abducts and a callus forms on the medial hallux from shearing stresses as the body moves over this aspect of the hallux (figure 20.12d).

If the forefoot varus is uncompensated, the individual stays on the lateral aspect of the foot and is unable to pronate as much as he or she should normally. The forefoot varus does not permit the rearfoot to pronate in relaxed standing, so the calcaneus may appear either erect or slightly inverted. Callus formation in this case occurs over the lateral aspect of the foot and over the fifth metatarsal head, because rotation occurs off the fifth metatarsal head and weight bearing is primarily over the lateral foot (figure 20.12e). The rotation is secondary to the rearfoot's failure to go through a full excursion of supination, thereby limiting lower-leg external rotation; the body attempts to abduct the foot so that the tibia can tilt to evert the foot to get the propulsive forces delivered from the medial foot, as close to the first metatarsal as possible.

Forefoot valgus is the opposite condition. The metatarsal head line is higher on the lateral side than on the medial side (everted) (figure 20.12c). A related condition is first-ray plantar flexion. If the first ray is rigid with little available mobility, during ambulation the first ray will hit the ground too early and the peroneus longus will assist by moving the weight more medially to transfer weight to the other foot. In a very rigid first ray, the fifth ray's ability to get to the ground is limited because the foot supinates too early in the mid-weight-bearing phase. With the forefoot in extreme valgus because of the rigid first ray, the forefoot inversion on the rearfoot is severely limited. The rearfoot then attempts to compensate by supinating during midstance. This causes the fifth ray to hit the ground suddenly and undergo increased loading before heel-off. This, in turn, causes the lateral foot to become unstable; and to compensate, the rearfoot moves into pronation at heel-off. The pronation imposes increased shearing forces on the forefoot. Because of the increased shearing forces and the increased time the first ray spends on the ground, there is usually a large callus buildup over the medial first metatarsal head. There is also a callus over the fifth metatarsal head because of the increased friction (figure 20.12f).

On the other hand, if the first ray is mobile, the rearfoot will pronate normally, and no problems should become evident because motion will occur fairly normally. A large callus forms over the first metatarsal head because of the prolonged contact of the first ray with the ground and its plantar-flexed position (figure 20.12g).

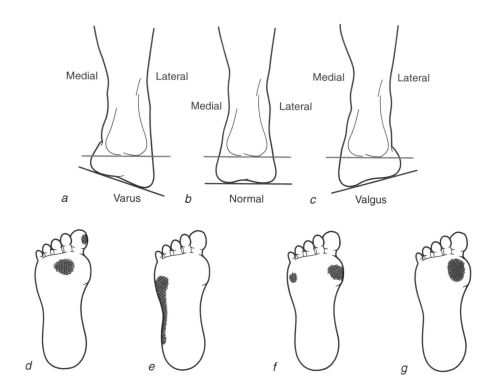

■ **Figure 20.12** Forefoot alignment—varus and valgus deformities: *(a)* forefoot varus alignment relative to rearfoot, *(b)* normal forefoot and rearfoot alignment, *(c)* forefoot valgus, *(d)* callus pattern for compensated forefoot varus, *(e)* uncompensated forefoot varus, *(f)* callus pattern for compensated forefoot valgus with a rigid first ray, *(g)* compensated forefoot valgus and rearfoot varus with a flexible first ray.

ORTHOTIC TREATMENT FOR FOOT DEFORMITIES

Orthotic devices for the correction of foot deformities are either premade or custom made. The orthotist relies on a number of patient characteristics to design an orthotic device that fits that patient.

Normal foot mechanics during ambulation includes pronation immediately after heel strike and continuing through 25% of the stance phase. During midstance, the rearfoot moves to a neutral position with the calcaneus erect and all the metatarsal heads in contact with the ground. From that point until toe-off, the rearfoot continues its progression in supination in preparation for converting the foot from a mobile adapter to a rigid lever for propulsion. If the patient's foot does not function in this manner, increased stresses are applied to segments within the foot or leg. The purpose of foot orthotics is to make the abnormal foot's function closer to that of a normal foot, thereby reducing the abnormal stresses imposed on the foot and leg. Although not all patients have correct foot alignment and function, many patients who have poor alignment do not have symptoms of pathology. For these asymptomatic patients, orthotics may not be indicated. Foot orthotics are used to correct or support symptomatic rearfoot and/or forefoot malalignments thereby reducing abnormal stress and improve the patient's mechanical efficiency.

PREMADE ORTHOTICS

Several types of orthotics are available. The type a patient uses depends on that person's specific needs. There are premade orthotics and custom-made orthotics. Premade orthotics, the off-the-shelf variety, are less expensive than custom orthotics and in some situations may meet the patient's needs. These include items such as heel cushions that assist in shock absorption at heel strike and that can also alter heel position if varus or valgus wedges are attached to them. A variety of pads and inserts can assist in reducing stress on specific areas of the foot. These items include metatarsal pads, arch cookies, heel pads, and other supportive devices. Premade arch supports can help support pes planus feet and feet with excessive pronation. Full-length insoles can replace the regular inner liners in shoes and further add to shock absorption.

CUSTOM ORTHOTICS

Custom orthotics are built to satisfy the individual's specific needs, either to absorb stress or to correct alignment. Some of the more common types of orthotics are briefly described next.

Three Types of Orthotics

Custom orthotics are either accommodating or functional and are of three basic types: rigid, semirigid, and soft. The more rigid the orthotic, the more exact the fit must be in order for the device to be effective. Soft orthotics, often made of a soft polyethylene foam, are used for cavus or rigid feet to provide stress absorption. They are known as accommodative; they do not so much correct mechanics as accommodate and attempt to relieve symptoms by reducing stresses without altering the foot position.

Most athletic orthotics are of the semirigid variety. They contain a rigid shell, usually made of acrylic plastic or thermoplastic polymer, with a soft covering. These are functional orthotics but may also have accommodating aspects. Their purpose is to change the position of the rearfoot or forefoot (or both) to provide optimal alignment, reduce shear stresses, reduce shock, and stabilize and support the foot joints. The shell has either intrinsic or extrinsic posts to correct the deformities. These posts are either in the rearfoot or forefoot, depending on the correction needed. Extrinsic posts can be made from a variety of materials with varying densities, including ethyl vinyl acetate (EVA), polyethylene, crepe rubber, and polyplastic (figure 20.13).

Specialty orthotic devices can also be constructed for specific sport needs of the patient. Special orthotics can be designed to accommodate for the stresses applied in aerobics by providing more control for loading on the anterior foot. Cycling orthotics must be lightweight and must provide control for the anterior foot, which bears the weight during cycling. A low-profile orthotic can be designed to conform to special footwear such as ski boots, soccer shoes, and track racing shoes.

Three Impression Methods

The three most common methods of taking foot impressions are to use plaster casts, foam boxes, and wax. With the plaster cast method, the patient is prone as he or she would be if you were finding subtalar neutral. A traditional plaster cast using one layer of plaster splints is applied to the plantar foot. While the plaster dries, the foot is passively maintained in a subtalar neutral position. This method is the most useful when the orthotic is to be functional. Although the procedure can be messy, the molds are durable after they dry and can be taken or sent to an orthotics lab without being damaged.

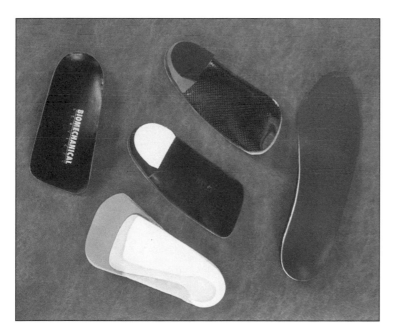

■ **Figure 20.13** Custom orthotics are made from a variety of substances and are rigid, semirigid, and soft.

With the foam-box method, the patient's foot is pushed into a box of foam material much like that used by florists. The foot is actively maintained as close to subtalar neutral as possible. This is not an accurate method to use for flexible feet because it can be difficult for a patient with a flexible foot to maintain subtalar neutral. A foam box impression is most commonly used for an accommodative orthotic device, or devices that do not require a precision fit.

Orthotic Evaluation

In addition to impression molds of the feet, assessment of various patient characteristics is necessary for an orthotic to be designed to fit accurately. Information that the orthotist needs includes the following:

1. **The patient's height and weight.** Some materials have limited ability to withstand stresses beyond specific weights, so the patient's size determines the material used for the orthotic.

2. **The patient's type of sport and activity level.** Different orthotics are designed to withstand different stresses, so the orthotist will use information about the patient's sport participation to decide on the specific construction of the orthotic. For example, a soccer player will use a low-profile device that fits in the shoe and absorbs shock during quick running starts and stops.

3. **The patient's medical history.** Surgery, neuromuscular deficiencies, and other medical abnormalities can alter the body's ability to tolerate changes. For example, an open reduction and internal fixation (ORIF) of the ankle may cause soft-tissue adhesions that affect the patient's ability to tolerate a great deal of change in rearfoot position.

4. **The patient's primary and secondary complaints.** These are what you are trying to relieve by providing the orthotic.

5. **The calcaneal position in relaxed standing and in subtalar neutral standing.** These positions indicate whether the subtalar deviation is accommodated or not.

6. **The appearance of the arches in weight bearing and non-weight bearing.** This indicates whether or not rearfoot and possible forefoot accommodation is occurring.

7. **The toe positions.** These are good indicators of rearfoot deformities. For example, hallux valgus is an indication of excessive pronation, and hammertoes are an indication of pes cavus.

8. **The knee positions.** Knee positions can contribute significantly to foot deformities. For example, genu varus and valgus can increase pronation.

9. **Tibial varum.** If this value is beyond 18°, it is abnormal. Tibial varum also adds to foot-deformity stresses and can increase pronation.

10. **First-ray positions.** This is determined in subtalar neutral with the ankle dorsiflexed. These positions are significant in that they demonstrate forefoot varus or valgus.

11. **Subtalar mobility.** Normal subtalar motion is 30° with a 2 to 1 ratio of inversion to eversion. Subtalar mobility is determined using the method described earlier. If the total motion is less than 30°, limited rearfoot mobility that can cause forefoot accommodation or changes is present. If motion is less than 30° and there is no forefoot accomodation, a rigid foot may be present. Subtalar mobility of greater than 30° indicates an unstable foot that is in pronation more than it should be.

12. **Midtarsal mobility.** This is a subjective assessment of midfoot mobility. With the rearfoot locked in subtalar neutral, the forefoot is supinated and pronated. Normal mobility should allow full but not excessive motion. This is a difficult motion to assess until you have performed the maneuver many times to obtain an impression of what is loose, what is normal, and what is restricted.

13. **First metatarsal mobility.** This is the flexibility of the first ray. As mentioned previously, the first ray should move about one thumb's width each in plantar flexion and in dorsiflexion. If it moves well in one direction but not the other, it is semirigid. If it is limited in both directions, it is rigid.

14. **Hallux dorsiflexion.** The hallux should have 60° to 65° of dorsiflexion for normal ambulation. Patients with a lower value may have problems such as sesamoiditis, plantar fasciitis, or tendinitis. An adjustment in the orthotic may be necessary if the patient's motion is less than 60°.

15. **Ankle dorsiflexion.** This is measured in subtalar neutral with passive pressure applied to the ankle into dorsiflexion. Normal dorsiflexion needed for ambulation is 10°. If the ankle does not have this motion, pronation may occur to compensate and to allow the patient the mobility needed. An adjustment in the orthotic to relieve the stress on the Achilles and plantar fascia may be necessary if the patient lacks full ankle dorsiflexion.

16. **Location of corns and calluses.** This is important in that corns and calluses are indicators of accommodating or non-accommodating forefoot and rearfoot deformities.

BIOMECHANICAL
S E R V I C E S

1050 Central Ave., Suite D. Brea, CA 92821

(714) 990-5932

Acct. No.:_____

Practitioner's Name: _____

Address: _____

Telephone: _____

Date: _____

_____

Patient Name: _____ Gender: _____ Age: _____ ① Weight: _____ Height: _____

Shoe Size: _____ Shoe Style: _____ Heel Height: _____

② Sport/Activity Level: _____ Previous Orthotic Therapy _____

③ Medical History (Neuromotor, structural, surgical) _____

_____

_____

_____

Primary complaint: _____

④ _____

Other complaints: (Knee/hip/back)

_____

_____

_____

⑤ **Calcaneal stance position:**

(Resting/relaxed)

Left ❑ Inverted ❑ Rectus ❑ Everted

Right ❑ Inverted ❑ Rectus ❑ Everted

(Neutral subtalar)

Left ❑ Inverted ❑ Rectus ❑ Everted

Right ❑ Inverted ❑ Rectus ❑ Everted

⑥ **Foot appearance:**

(weight-bearing arch)

Left ❑ High ❑ Med ❑ Low

Right ❑ High ❑ Med ❑ Low

(non-weight-bearing arch)

Left ❑ High ❑ Med ❑ Low

Right ❑ High ❑ Med ❑ Low

⑦ **Toe positions:**

Left ❑ Straight ❑ Contracted

   ❑ Subluxed ❑ HAV

Right ❑ Straight ❑ Contracted

   ❑ Subluxed ❑ HAV

⑧ **Knee positions:**

Left ❑ Genu Varum ❑ Straight

   ❑ Genu Valgum

Right ❑ Genu Varum ❑ Straight

   ❑ Genu Valgum

⑨ **Tibial Varum (if any):**

Degrees Right _____ Left _____

Short leg (if any):

Left/right _____ MM/inches

⑩ **First metatarsal ray position:**

Left ❑ Normal ❑ Plantar flexed

   ❑ Dorsiflexed

Right ❑ Normal ❑ Plantar flexed

   ❑ Dorsiflexed

⑪ **Range of motion:**

Subtalar:

Left ❑ Restricted ❑ Loose

   ❑ Within normal limits

Right ❑ Restricted ❑ Loose

   ❑ Within normal limits

⑫ Midtarsal:

Left ❑ Restricted ❑ Loose

   ❑ Within normal limits

Right ❑ Restricted ❑ Loose

   ❑ Within normal limits

⑬ First metatarsal segment:

Left ❑ Flexible ❑ Semi-rigid

   ❑ Rigid

Right ❑ Flexible ❑ Semi-rigid

   ❑ Rigid

⑭ Hallux dorsiflexion:

Left ❑ 65° ❑ 25°

   ❑ 45° ❑ None

Right ❑ 65° ❑ 25°

   ❑ 45° ❑ None

⑮ Ankle dorsiflexion:

Left ❑ 10° ❑ 5–6°

   ❑ 7–8° ❑ 3–4° or less

Right ❑ 10° ❑ 5–6°

   ❑ 7–8° ❑ 3–4° or less

Area of pain:

⑯

Corns/calluses:

R   L

Your diagnosis:

_____

_____

_____

_____

_____

Courtesy of Biomechanical Services.

The wax method uses warm wax sheets that are molded to the plantar surface of the foot. The rearfoot is maintained in subtalar neutral as the wax cools and hardens. This method is not used if the impressions are to be sent elsewhere, because it is not easy to transport them and the wax melts in heat and cracks in cold weather. The method can be used if the orthotics are to be constructed in-house.

The firmer the orthotic, the less error is tolerated in the fit. Rigid orthotics require the most precision in creating the foot's impression. The softer orthotics tolerate a larger margin of error in the impressions from which they are made. If a semirigid orthotic is desired, an accurate impression should be used.

DETERMINING PROPER FOOTWEAR FOR PATIENTS

To help a patient select a shoe, the sport rehabilitation specialist must understand shoe structure, note the wear pattern on the patient's current shoes, ascertain the patient's injury history, understand how a shoe should fit, and consider the purpose the shoe will be used for.

One of the most frequently asked questions regarding footwear is "What's the best shoe?" There is not a single best shoe. The best shoe is the one that meets the individual's needs. There are many athletic shoes to choose from and new models are released every six months; it is more important for the sport rehabilitation specialist to be aware of general functional concepts and purposes of shoe components than it is to have knowledge of specific models. He or she can select a shoe on the basis of this general information as it applies to specific models.

Shoes have many functions, including protecting the foot's skin and other soft-tissue structures, providing traction for improved propulsion, reducing shock impact during propulsion activities, increasing foot stability, and accommodating or correcting foot deformities. Companies emphasize style characteristics and fashion trends to increase the popularity of shoes. Ultimately, a shoe should be chosen on the basis of structure and function, not color, style, or name.

SHOE STRUCTURE

All shoes have the same basic structure consisting of an upper and a lower section. The upper section of an athletic shoe includes the vamp, toe box, saddle, collar, insole board, sock liner, and heel counter. The lower section includes the outsole, wedge, and midsole (figure 20.14). The **vamp**, which covers the toes and forefoot, includes the toe box. Running shoes whose vamp is made of nylon or another type of fabric usually have a mudguard around the rim of the toe box. The **toe box**, which varies in width and height from one style and company to another, functions to retain the shape of the shoe's forefoot and to provide room for the toes. The **saddle**, the midsection of the shoe along the longitudinal arch, is usually reinforced to provide support to the midfoot. The **heel counter** is an important stabilizer for the rearfoot. A foxing, an additional piece in many athletic shoes, further reinforces the rearfoot to assist in maintaining the counter's shape. The medial aspect of the counter is sometimes extended forward to resist pronation. The **collar** is the top rim of the shoe, often padded to reduce friction on the Achilles. Sometimes it is angled inward slightly to provide a snugger fit around the ankle. The **insole board** lies between the upper and lower segments of the shoe and serves as the attachment for the two segments. A **sock liner** on top of the insole board is used for shock absorption and friction reduction. The sock liner may be either glued into the shoe or just inserted in it.

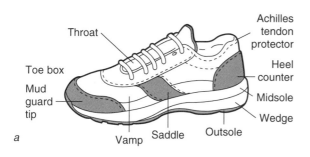

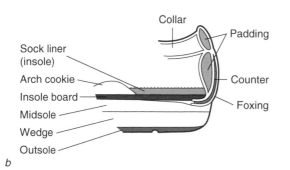

■ Figure 20.14 Shoe anatomy: *(a)* upper section, *(b)* lower section.

The **outsole** is the portion of the lower segment of the shoe that is in contact with the ground. This is composed of a durable material and has a variety of designs of ripples, waves, and nubs. The **midsole** and wedge are made of a variety of substances including EVA, gas-filled or gel-filled chambers, and polyurethane. These sections provide shock attenuation, stability, and control. They can include wedges to provide stability, varying densities to reduce pronation, and special materials to reduce impact stresses.

The **last** is an important component of a shoe. It is the insole board and is made of a firm substance and determines the shoe's shape, size, style, and fit. The most common types of last are the straight last and the curved last (figure 20.15). The straight last, which can be bisected lengthwise into two equal parts, offers the foot the most medial support and is recommended for pronators. Curved lasts are flared inward to varying degrees. These provide the least amount of medial support and should be avoided by patients who excessively pronate. A curve-lasted shoe is generally more flexible than a straight-lasted shoe. Construction of the shoe around the last involves attaching the outsole and midsole to the bottom of the last and attaching the heel counter, toe box, and upper section of the shoe to the top of the last.

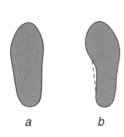

■ **Figure 20.15** Shoe last: *(a)* straight, *(b)* curved. Last determines the shoe's shape, size, style, and fit.

A last is either a board last, a slip last, or a combination last. You can easily see the last by removing the sock liner. A board last is made of a cardboard or cardboard-like material that provides for a stiff sole and thus adds to the stability to the foot. A slip-lasted shoe looks like a moccasin, with the upper section stitched along its bottom to the last. This shoe is appropriate for a more rigid foot and offers more flexibility than a board-lasted shoe. A combination last has a board-lasted rearfoot and a slip-lasted forefoot. This type of last is designed to offer rearfoot stability and forefoot flexibility, as well as ease of shoe bend to reduce stresses on the plantar fascia and Achilles during heel-off and toe-off.

SHOE WEAR

An examination of the patient's worn shoes can give clues to foot deformities, helping the sport rehabilitation specialist guide the patient toward the most appropriate shoe. If the heel counter and medial heel are collapsed to the medial side of the shoe, the patient excessively pronates. A medial wedge, or increased density of the medial wedge or midsole, along with a strong heel counter will provide increased stability. This patient should use a board-lasted shoe.

If the lateral heel counter of the worn shoe is moved laterally, the patient has a rigid foot and needs a shoe with a slip last, a lot of cushion but no medial wedge, and a firm heel counter.

If the patient's hallux has a blackened toenail, the toe box may not be deep enough. If the hallux is wearing through the upper section of the shoe, the patient may have a rigid first ray and require increased shock absorption in the forefoot. The forefoot of the shoe should also be flexible, bending easily with light pressure on the sole.

Although shoe wear is a good indicator of deformities, a shoe that has noticeable wear is one that should be replaced. The life of a shoe depends on the patient, the frequency of participation, and the surfaces the patient plays the sport on. Footwear varies greatly in longevity. It is important, however, that the shoe be replaced once a wear pattern is seen. A worn shoe changes the mechanics and stresses applied to the foot and can magnify any structural deformity.

INJURY HISTORY

A profile of the patient's injury history also aids in determining the correct shoe for that person. For example, if the patient has a history of Achilles tendinitis, the cause may be either excessive pronation or tightness in the Achilles. This patient should find a shoe that has good heel-counter stability, a straight board or combination last, good forefoot flexibility, and a higher-than-normal elevation in the wedge to relieve Achilles stress.

If the patient has a history of knee pain, excessive pronation may be the cause. A board-lasted shoe with good rearfoot control and a firm heel counter is appropriate for this patient. Plantar fasciitis is also related to excessive pronation, so a similar shoe would be appropriate for a patient with a history of plantar fasciitis.

PROPER SHOE FIT

Once the specific needs of the patient have been determined, the shoe must be fit properly. Shoe size is most easily determined using the **Brannock measuring device** found in shoe stores (figure 20.16). This determines the width and length of the shoe. A good heel fit is critical for an athletic shoe. The shoe should fit snugly to provide adequate support for the rearfoot. There should be approximately one thumb's width between the end of the longest toe and the end of the shoe. The toe box should have adequate depth and width for the forefoot and toes. The bend in the vamp should coincide with the bend of the patient's forefoot. A good heel counter should feel firm and have little give when it is squeezed. The vamp should bend easily when you grasp the heel and try to bend the shoe by applying pressure with the index finger of your other hand. If a shoe is board lasted, it should be difficult to wring the shoe and produce much motion when stabilizing the heel and rotating the vamp.

Shoes should be evaluated to make sure that the heel counter is perpendicular to the sole, the sole is parallel to the floor, and the last is the same on the right as on the left shoe. It is also important to ascertain that there are no abnormalities in stitching, construction, or angle from one shoe to the other. Because there is no quality control in shoe manufacturing, errors in production are not uncommon. A construction error can cause an injury or aggravate any structural deformity.

Patients should try on shoes in the store, wearing socks of the same type and thickness as those they will use with the shoes. An individual should be able to give shoes a good trial in the store on a treadmill or track or be able to run outside before purchasing them. It is best to try shoes on in the later part of the day when foot volume is greater than in the morning. Because foot size may vary from right to left, it is advisable to try on both shoes, properly laced. It is a good idea to try on a variety of shoes and compare comfort and fit. The patient should be sure to ask about the store's return policy. The store should stand behind the product and permit exchanges if someone who has tried a shoe at home finds that it does not meet specific needs or is uncomfortable.

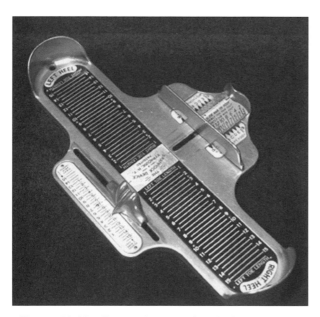

■ **Figure 20.16**   Brannock measuring device.

SHOE TYPES

Because different sports place different stresses on the foot, the requirements for an athletic shoe differ among sports. There are as many types of shoes as there are sports. It is not advisable for a patient to wear a shoe intended for use in one sport for a second sport. The shoe is not designed to meet the demands of another sport.

Tennis Shoes

Tennis involves sudden stops and changes in direction and many lateral movements, so safe tennis participation requires good medial and lateral support to protect the lateral ligaments and peroneals. Because most tennis is played on a variety of outdoor surfaces, the outsole should be durable; the material should be able to adapt to differing playing surfaces and allow some sliding on the court. A toe guard or reinforcement over the medial toes will prolong the life of the shoe and protect it against toe drag on the serve. In a shoe appropriate for tennis, the heel and toe are almost in the same plane, whereas a running shoe has an elevated heel to reduce stress on the Achilles. Because placing the foot in a plantar-flexed position makes the ankle susceptible to inversion sprains and because tennis involves lateral movements, a tennis shoe is flat.

Running Shoes

In addition to the elevated heel, a running shoe should be flexible so that the foot does not have to work excessively to bend the shoe during heel-off. The shoe should have good cushion in the rear and forefoot yet provide stability to the heel.

Aerobics Shoes

Aerobics shoes should have good forefoot cushioning, and many have additional cushioning in the sock liner. A reinforced toe box supports the forefoot primarily during forefoot-impact activities. The forefoot should have good flexibility to allow the foot to bend easily during aerobic activities; in many shoes this flexibility comes from flex bars cut into the sole. There should be good rearfoot stability with a good heel counter for adequate ankle support during medial and lateral activities. Stability is necessary for the multidirectional movements in aerobics. Stability straps in the midfoot region can provide medial-lateral stability in the midsole and the upper section. In some shoes, a mid-height upper section provides added medial-lateral support without interfering with plantar flexion-dorsiflexion. Aerobic shoes come in leather and synthetic materials; synthetic material is usually lighter and does not absorb as much moisture as the leather.

Volleyball Shoes

Volleyball shoes must meet the demands of sudden stops, starts, jumps, and lateral moves. The shoe should not have an elevation to the heel but should have a durable outsole, good medial-lateral stability, and sufficient traction; it should be lightweight and flexible enough not to contribute to fatigue. Stabilizing straps add medial-lateral support and forefoot stability. A gum-rubber sole increases traction and durability. Additional leather guards prolong the life of the shoe by protecting the toes from excessive wear during drag.

Basketball Shoes

Basketball shoes must provide cushion during jumps, stability during quick stops and starts and changes in direction, and ease of foot-bend during running. Mid- and high-top shoes provide medial-lateral support, as do the forefoot support straps and sole design. A good heel counter also provides stability. Flex joints in the sole of the forefoot facilitate bending, and the midsole is composed of a shock-absorbing substance such as EVA. Basketball court surfaces are rough on the outsole, so a basketball shoe should have a stitched rubber outsole with a reinforced toe region.

Soccer Shoes

A soccer shoe should have a flexible sole to permit ease in dorsiflexion-plantar flexion motion of the ankle. The cleats should be placed in areas that do not promote undue pressure on or irritation of the foot; rearfoot cleat placement should be around the perimeter to avoid heel irritation. Cleats vary according to the surface the patient plays on. Short cleats are appropriate for hard turf, whereas long cleats are suitable for softer surfaces such as wet grass.

Walking Shoes

Walking shoes have many of the same characteristics as running shoes. The heel is slightly raised, but not as much as in a running shoe, and a firm heel counter provides for rearfoot and impact stability. The forefoot, which is usually more flexible, has a rocker bottom to provide efficiency and to lessen energy requirements during heel strike and rolling from heel-off to toe-off. The shank portion of the midsole is usually stiffer in a walking shoe to provide for better medial-lateral stability. Selection of a walking shoe should be based on the type of walking the patient performs. Olympic walkers require flexibility for economy of movement; off-trail walkers need stability and traction for uneven surfaces; and power and fitness walkers need stability and cushioning.

Mountaineering Shoes

Requirements for mountaineering shoes vary according to the specific activity involved. Hiking, climbing, and high-altitude climbing each place different demands on the feet and so require different shoes.

Hiking is one of the most popular mountaineering sports. A hiking shoe should provide stability and should have a good heel counter and midsole for medial-lateral support. Hiking shoes should be waterproof or water resistant and should have a very durable outsole. The outsole should have good traction for uneven and rough terrain. The upper section should be mid to high for rough terrain and mid to low for easy terrain. A hiking shoe needs to be lightweight and comfortable; it should not have pressure points and should not need to be broken in.

Cross-Training Shoes

Cross-training shoes are designed to meet the needs of individuals involved in multiple activities. The goal is to meet all the needs of all the people all the time. The problem is that these shoes usually do not meet any specific need most of the time. There are various styles of shoes in this category. A person who wants a cross-training shoe should select the shoe that meets the demands of the activity he or she participates in most of the time.

LACING PATTERNS

Some shoes, especially running shoes, have multiple eyelets that the wearer can select from when lacing the shoe. These allow the use of a variety of lacing patterns to meet specific needs. Alternative lacing patterns can add to the support the shoe provides or accommodate for some deformities. A person who has a narrow foot should use the eyelets farthest from the tongue of the shoe, which will pull the sides of the shoe more closely together (figure 20.17a). People with wide feet should use the eyelets closest to the tongue (figure 20.17b).

Women often have the problem of a wide forefoot and a narrower heel than is accounted for in the construction of a shoe. They can accommodate for this by using two laces, one for the lower eyelets and the other for the higher eyelets, and tying the upper lace more tightly to support the heel (figure 20.17c).

Patients with high arches should avoid lacing a shoe in the traditional crisscross pattern but instead should use a straight-across pattern (figure 20.17d).

People with toe problems can obtain some relief by using the laces to lift up the forefoot of the shoe. As the shoe is tied, the lace that goes through the eyelet nearest the problem toe is brought directly to an eyelet at the top of the shoe. Pulling on this lace lifts up part of the forefoot (figure 20.17e).

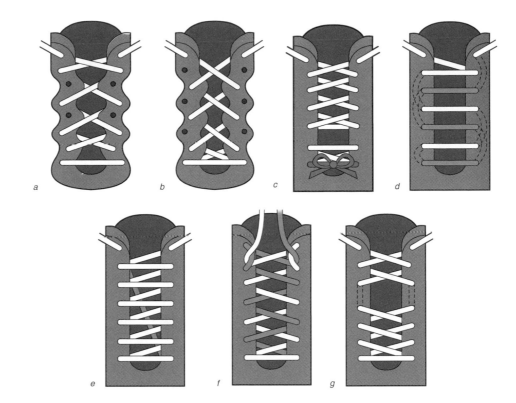

■ **Figure 20.17**   Shoe-lacing patterns for *(a)* narrow feet, *(b)* wide feet, *(c)* wide forefoot and narrow heel (using two laces), *(d)* high arches, *(e)* toe problems, *(f)* heel blisters, *(g)* dorsal foot bump.

Reprinted, by permission, from C. Frey, April 1998, "Common shoe lacing patterns." Retrieved August 17, 2000 from the World Wide Web: **www.wcsportsmed.com/lacing/htm**. Copyright 1998 by Carol Frey, MD.

Heel blisters are often caused by friction of the shoe over the heel. The wearer can decrease the friction by securing the heel more firmly in the shoe using a loop-through technique at the top of the shoe as seen in figure 20.17f. The lace should be pulled tighter at the top of the shoe than at the bottom.

A bump on the top of the foot can be painful with regular-lacing-pattern pressure. To relieve pressure on the top of the foot, don't cross the laces; instead, keep the laces on the same side of the shoe and skip the eyelet at the painful level (figure 20.17g).

SOFT-TISSUE MOBILIZATION

Soft-tissue mobilization is used to treat common myofascial pain referred from the lower leg and foot. Treatment is applied to superficial intrinsic foot muscles, deep intrinsic foot muscles, and several muscles extrinsic to the foot.

As with the upper extremity, pain and referred pain in the lower extremity can come from several sources. Sciatica is a common pain-referral source in the lower extremity, with symptoms extending anywhere from the back to the toes. Before the sport rehabilitation specialist treats a pain locale, he or she must identify the source. If the source is myofascially based, soft-tissue mobilization techniques can be effective in relieving the pain. The areas discussed here are common myofascial pain-referral patterns from the muscles of the lower leg and foot. These pain-referral patterns and the treatments presented are based on the work of Travell and Simons (1992). The following sections deal with identification of trigger points and pain-referral patterns for the muscles and then present trigger point release and ice-and-stretch techniques. Remember that ice-and-stretch applications are repeated several times. The procedure is to apply the ice during the passive stretch and then to perform active shortening and repeated stretches. After the ice-and-stretch application, the patient should actively move the muscle through its full range of motion several times.

SUPERFICIAL INTRINSIC FOOT MUSCLES

These muscles include the extensor digitorum brevis, extensor hallucis brevis, abductor hallucis, flexor digitorum brevis, and abductor digiti minimi. These muscles generally refer pain over the muscle site with a small degree of radiation that remains locally in the foot. The intrinsic toe extensors refer to the dorsum of the foot in the area of their muscle bellies (figure 20.18a). The abductor hallucis brevis refers to the medial heel with some radiation into the medial arch (figure 20.18b). The abductor digiti minimi refers pain along the fifth metatarsal's plantar aspect (figure 20.18c); the short toe flexors refer pain to the second through fourth metatarsal heads (figure 20.18d).

Deep pressure is applied to relieve the trigger point (figure 20.18, e–f). A local twitch is not commonly seen, but the patient may demonstrate a jump response to pressure over the trigger point. Ice-and-stretch is applied with the patient in a comfortable position. For application to the toe extensors, the foot is plantar flexed and the toes moved passively into flexion as the ice strokes are brought from the anterior lower leg along the foot's dorsum to the toes (figure 20.18g). For ice-and-stretch to the abductors and intrinsic toe flexors, the ankle can remain in a neutral position. The abductor hallucis and intrinsic toe flexors are positioned in flexion while the ice is stroked from the plantar heel toward the toes (figure 20.18, h–j).

The patient can perform self-massage techniques using a tennis or golf ball, a ridged vegetable can, or a rolling pin. In sitting, the patient places the plantar foot on top of the object being used and applies pressure downward on the knee while rolling the foot back and forth over the object (figure 20.19).

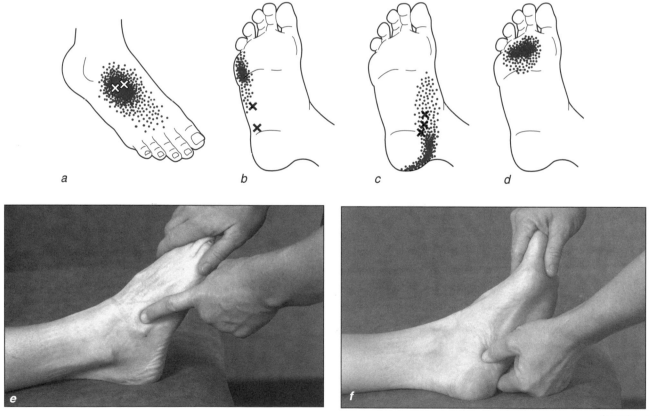

(continued)

■ **Figure 20.18** Superficial intrinsic muscle pain-referral patterns: *(a)* extensor digitorum brevis and extensor hallucis brevis, *(b)* abductor digiti minimi, *(c)* abductor hallucis, *(d)* flexor digitorum brevis. Trigger point release of extensor digitorum brevis *(e)* and abductor hallucis *(f)*. Ice-and-stretch for intrinsic toe extensors *(g)*, flexor digitorum brevis *(h)*, abductor hallucis *(i)*, flexor hallucis brevis *(j)*.

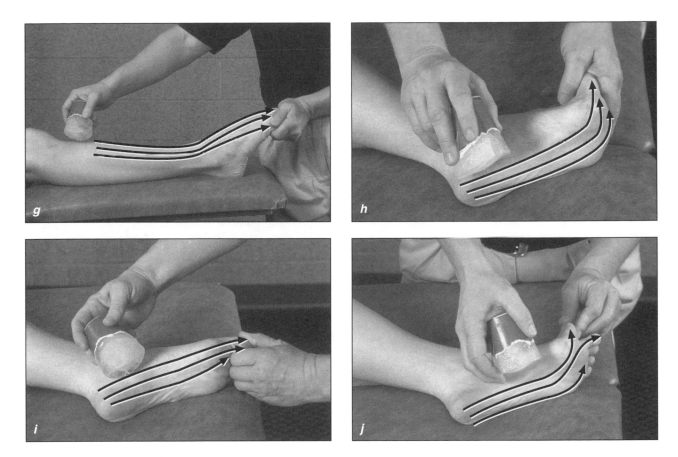

▌Figure 20.18   (continued).

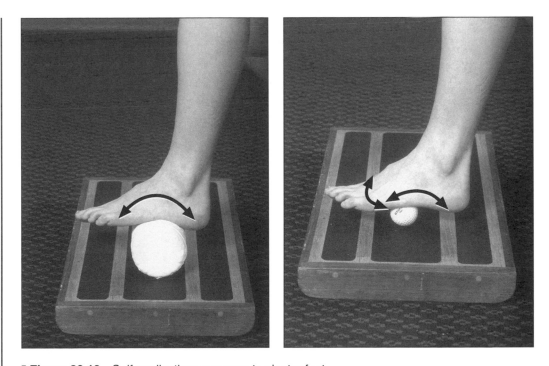

▌Figure 20.19   Self-application: massage to plantar foot.

DEEP INTRINSIC FOOT MUSCLES

These muscles include the quadratus plantae, lumbricals, flexor hallucis brevis, adductor hallucis, flexor digiti minimi brevis, and interossei. Like the pain-referral pattern of the superficial group, the pain-referral pattern of these muscles is primarily localized and over the region of their trigger points (figure 20.20, a–d). The quadratus plantae refers pain to the heel; the flexor hallucis brevis refers pain to the plantar and medial aspect of the head of the first metatarsal. The adductor hallucis refers pain to the ball of the foot; the interossei refer pain to the corresponding digit and along the dorsal and ventral aspects of the distal portion of the metatarsal to which they attach. The pain patterns of the lumbricals and flexor digiti minimi have not been determined.

Because these muscles lie deep to the plantar aponeurosis, long tendons, and superficial intrinsic muscles, deep palpation is required to affect them. Direct pressure over the trigger point is effective in releasing the painful trigger point (figure 20.20e).

The deep intrinsic muscles most amenable to ice-and-stretch techniques are the flexor hallucis brevis and the adductor hallucis. These muscles are treated with the ankle in neutral and the hallux hyperextended as sweeps are made from the heel toward the toe (figure 20.20f).

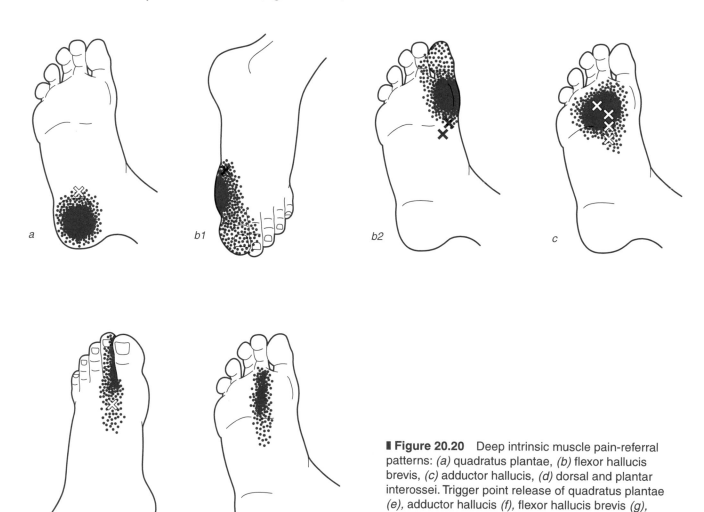

a   *b1*   *b2*   *c*

d1   *d2*

▌Figure 20.20 Deep intrinsic muscle pain-referral patterns: *(a)* quadratus plantae, *(b)* flexor hallucis brevis, *(c)* adductor hallucis, *(d)* dorsal and plantar interossei. Trigger point release of quadratus plantae *(e)*, adductor hallucis *(f)*, flexor hallucis brevis *(g)*, interossei and lumbricals *(h)*. Ice-and-stretch to intrinsic flexor muscles *(i)*.

(continued)

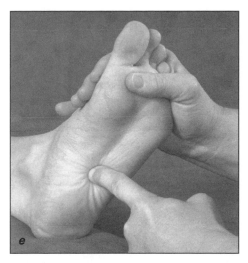
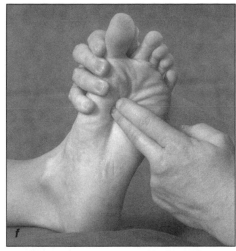
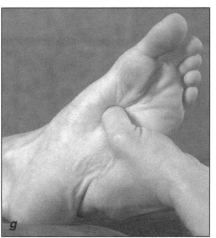
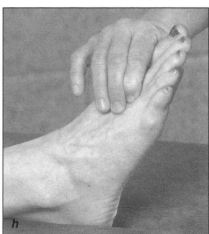
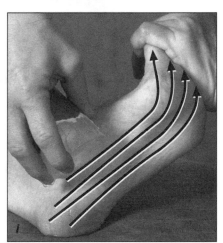

■ **Figure 20.20** *(continued).*

EXTRINSIC MUSCLES

As in the upper extremity, several extrinsic muscles function in the foot and ankle. They are presented here according to the lower-leg compartments they lie in, moving from anterior to lateral and posterior.

Tibialis Anterior

The tibialis anterior refers pain to the anteromedial ankle and over the dorsal and medial big toe (figure 20.21a). It can occasionally refer pain along the anterior shin.

Trigger point release is performed with flat palpation of the trigger point that is located at the border of the proximal and middle third of the anterior lower leg near the tibial ridge (figure 20.21b). The area is tender to palpation, and a taut band can be palpated. A local twitch response may be elicited with snapping palpation of the trigger point. Direct pressure to the patient's tolerance relaxes the band and relieves the pain.

Ice-and-stretch is applied as the foot is plantar flexed and pronated; ice sweeps are made from the knee distally toward the foot (figure 20.21c).

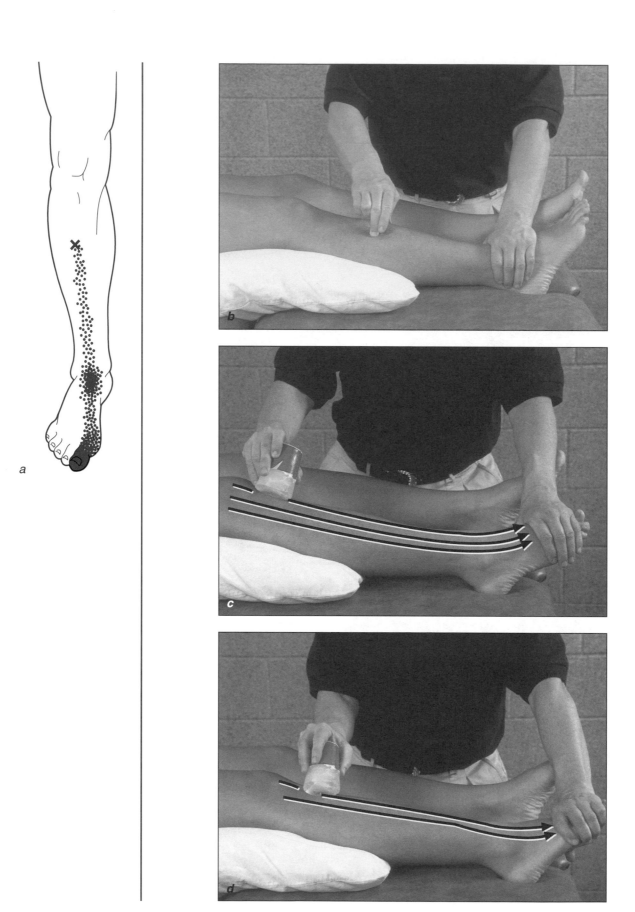

■ Figure 20.21 Tibialis anterior: *(a)* pain-referral pattern, *(b)* trigger point release, *(c)* ice-and-stretch in plantar flexion, *(d)* ice-and-stretch in plantar flexion with pronation added.

Peroneals

The peroneus longus and brevis refer pain to the lateral malleolus and proximally and distally to it (figure 20.22a). The longus pain may also spill over to the middle lateral lower leg. The peroneus tertius refers pain to the anterolateral ankle and into the lateral heel.

Snapping palpation of the peroneus longus elicits a local twitch response that produces ankle plantar flexion and eversion. Its trigger point is located about 2 to 4 cm (0.8–1.6 in.) distal to the fibular head near the shaft of the fibula (figure 20.22b). The peroneus brevis trigger point is located at the juncture of the middle and distal thirds of the lower leg. The peroneus tertius trigger points are just anterior and distal to those of the peroneus brevis.

Ice-and-stretch is applied to the peroneus longus and brevis with a passive stretch of the ankle into inversion and dorsiflexion while proximal-to-distal sweeps of ice are made along the lateral lower leg. To treat the peroneus tertius, the sport rehabilitation specialist performs a plantar-flexion and inversion stretch and applies ice more anteriorly on the distal lower leg (figure 20.22c).

Gastrocnemius

This muscle has four trigger points with different referral patterns. They can refer pain to the medial arch with spillover into the medial calf (figure 20.23a1), close to the medial border of the medial gastrocnemius head (figure 20.23a2), close to the lateral border of the lateral gastrocnemius head (figure 20.23a3), and slightly more distal on the lateral head of the gastrocnemius (figure 20.23a4). Nocturnal cramps are often associated with these trigger points.

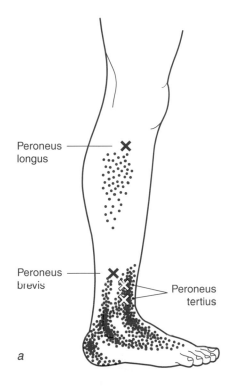

Peroneus longus

Peroneus brevis

Peroneus tertius

a

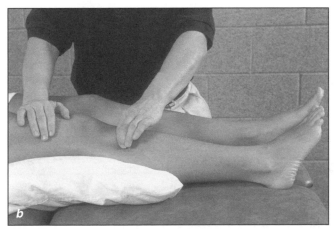

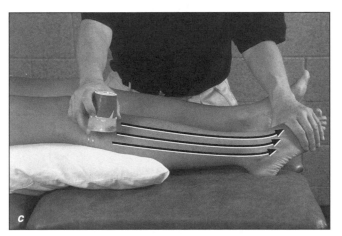

■ **Figure 20.22**   Peroneal pain patterns *(a)*, trigger point release to peroneus longus *(b)*, and ice-and-stretch for peroneus tertius *(c)*.

Trigger point release using deep pressure can be performed with the patient either lying or kneeling (figure 20.23b). Either a flat thumb pressure or a pincher grasp can be used. If the muscle is taut, a flat pressure is easier and more comfortable to administer.

Ice-and-stretch is applied with the patient in prone and the foot over the edge of the table. While the sport rehabilitation specialist uses his or her knee to dorsiflex the ankle with pressure over the ball of the patient's foot, he or she applies ice from above the knee in a distal direction toward the plantar foot (figure 20.23c).

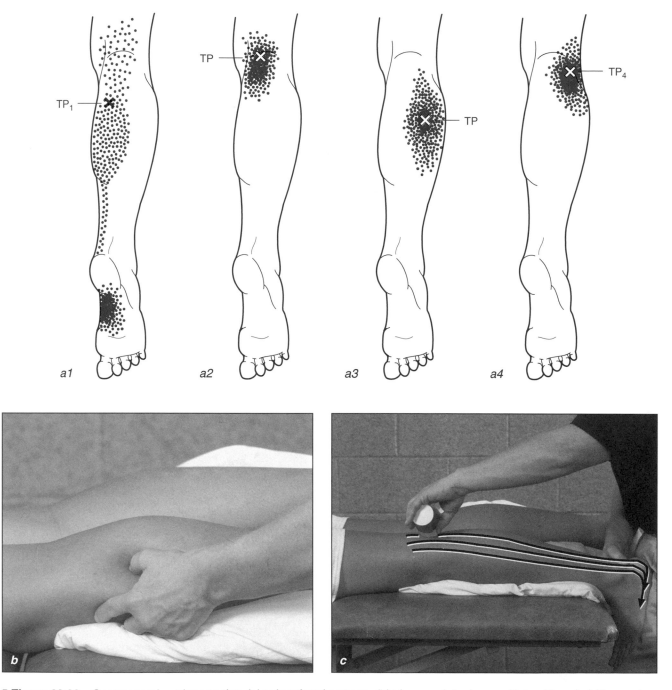

∎ Figure 20.23   Gastrocnemius trigger point: *(a)* pain referral pattern, *(b)* trigger point release of lateral head, *(c)* ice-and-stretch.

Soleus

The most common site of pain referral of the soleus is into the posterior and plantar heel area and into the distal Achilles. The soleus occasionally refers pain into the upper calf and rarely into the ipsilateral sacroiliac joint (figure 20.24a).

Trigger point release uses either a pincher or flat-pressure application. The patient can be either in prone with the knee flexed to keep the gastrocnemius slack (figure 20.24b) or in a kneeling position. The distal trigger points are located just medial and distal to the gastrocnemius muscle belly bulge. Direct pressure to the patient's tolerance is applied until the muscle becomes relaxed and the pain subsides.

Ice-and-stretch is performed with the knee in flexion. The patient can be kneeling or prone (figure 20.24c). As the ankle is passively dorsiflexed, the ice is swept from proximal to distal across the posterior lower leg and into the plantar foot.

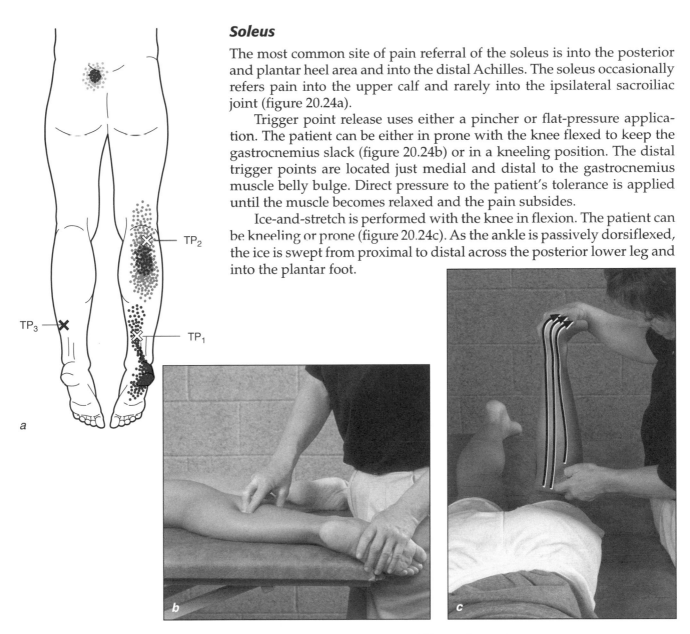

■ **Figure 20.24** Soleus: *(a)* pain-referral pattern, *(b)* trigger point release, *(c)* ice-and-stretch.

Tibialis Posterior

Trigger point activation of this muscle makes it painful for the patient to run or walk on uneven surfaces when the muscle's activity is increased for providing additional stabilization for the foot. The pain can refer into the Achilles tendon with spillover into the midcalf proximally and the heel, instep, and plantar foot and toes distally (figure 20.25a).

Because the tibialis posterior is the deepest muscle of the lower leg, it is not possible to make direct contact with it through deep pressure. Deep pressure to more superficial muscles can be used to apply indirect pressure. The sport rehabilitation specialist presses deeply between the soleus and the medial border of the posterior tibia (figure 20.25b). Ice-and-stretch is applied with the patient prone and the foot over the edge of the table. The ankle is stretched into dorsiflexion and eversion as the ice sweeps begin at the posterior knee and extend distally into the plantar foot (figure 20.25c).

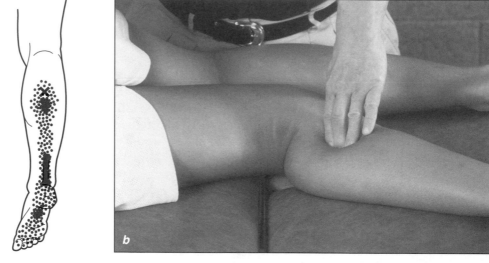

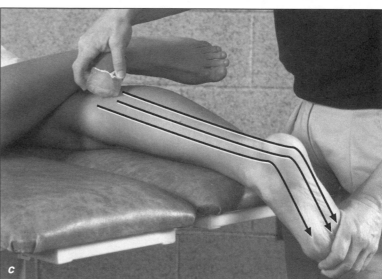

Figure 20.25   Tibialis posterior: *(a)* pain-referral pattern, *(b)* trigger point release (medial approach), *(c)* ice-and-stretch.

Long Toe Extensors

These muscles include the extensor digitorum longus and the extensor hallucis longus. Trigger points can cause night cramps in the toe extensors. The most common pain-referral pattern for these muscles is along the anterior ankle, along the dorsum of the foot over the metatarsals, and extending distally into the toes and proximally into the distal lower leg (figure 20.26a).

Trigger point release is performed on the extensor digitorum longus through application of pressure over the muscle about 8 cm (3 in.) distal and slightly anterior of the fibular head (figure 20.26b). Trigger point release for the extensor hallucis longus is applied anterior of the fibula at the location of the juncture of the middle and distal thirds of the lower leg (figure 20.26c).

Ice-and-stretch is applied with the patient supine. The ankle and toes are passively plantar flexed with pressure on the distal toes while ice sweeps are applied from the anterior and lateral proximal lower leg distally over the ankle and foot to the toes (figure 20.26d).

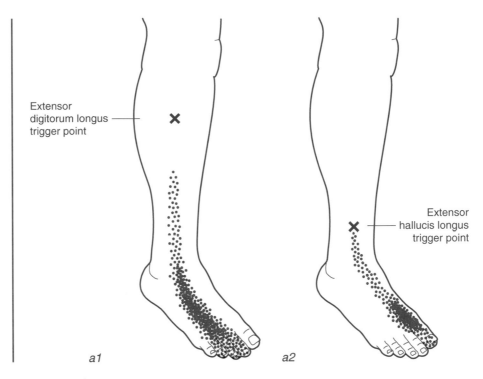

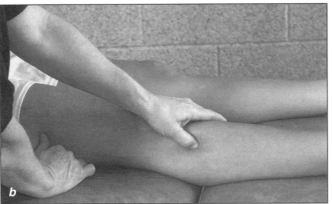

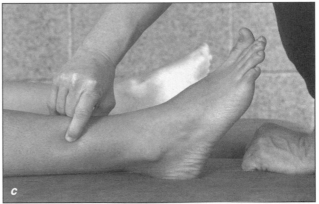

■ **Figure 20.26** Long toe extensors: *(a)* pain-referral patterns, *(b)* trigger point release of extensor digitorum longus, *(c)* trigger point release of extensor hallucis longus, *(d)* ice-and-stretch.

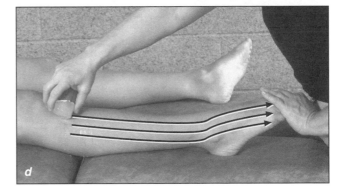

Long Toe Flexors

The most common symptom reported with active trigger points of the long toe flexors is pain in the feet during walking. The referral pain pattern for the flexor digitorum longus is into the sole of the forefoot with occasional spillover into the toes and medial calf (figure 20.27a1). The flexor hallucis longus refers pain to the plantar great toe and into the first metatarsal head (figure 20.27a2).

For trigger point release, the patient is in side-lying on the involved side with the knee flexed and the ankle in a relaxed plantar-flexed position. Using a flat-pressure technique, the sport rehabilitation specialist applies pressure on the medial proximal lower leg between the tibia and gastrocnemius-soleus complex (figure 20.27b). Once the gastrocnemius is pushed posteriorly, pressure is applied downward and then laterally. The flexor hallucis longus is treated with the patient in prone; deep pressure is applied through the soleus lateral to the midline and at the juncture of the middle and lower thirds of the lower leg (figure 20.27c).

Ice-and-stretch is performed with the patient prone and the knee passively flexed. As the ankle is passively dorsiflexed and everted and the toes are extended, ice sweeps are applied from the proximal calf along the medial ankle into the plantar foot to the toes (figure 20.27d).

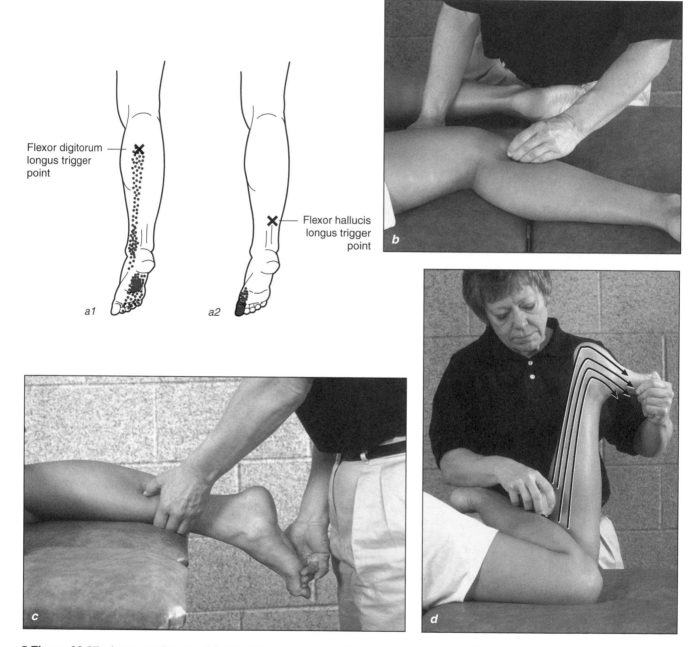

▮ **Figure 20.27**   Long toe flexors: *(a)* pain-referral pattern, *(b)* trigger point release of flexor digitorum longus, *(c)* trigger point release of flexor hallucis longus, *(d)* ice-and-stretch.

DEEP-TISSUE MASSAGE

The sport rehabilitation specialist uses deep-tissue massage of the foot and ankle to promote tissue flexibility and improve range of motion. Patients can perform self-massage on foot intrinsic muscles.

Soft-tissue restriction often occurs after a patient has experienced excessive edema or immobilization of the ankle, foot, or lower leg. Either the prolonged presence of edema or reduced tissue mobility can result in adhesions. Releasing the adhesions permits good tissue flexibility and aids in restoration of normal range of motion. Deep-tissue massage techniques, discussed in chapter 6, can be useful in accomplishing these goals. Review the discussion of proper application of these massage techniques before using them. The patient can perform deep massage to foot intrinsic muscles that are in spasm or that have myofascial tightness. Sitting in a chair, the patient places the bare foot on the side of a ribbed fruit or vegetable can positioned on the floor. Applying some downward force on the knee with the hands, the patient rolls the foot back and forth over the can to provide a self-massage.

JOINT MOBILIZATION

Joint mobilizations—glides or oscillations—are used to reduce pain and swelling or to improve mobility in many joints in the ankle.

Joint mobilization is often necessary in the ankle, especially after periods of immobilization. The techniques can be either repeated sustained glides or oscillations. In more restricted joints, sustained glides may be more effective than oscillations. Oscillation may be more comfortable for the patient and is frequently used in distractions to aid in reduction of swelling and pain (grades I and II). More aggressive grades (III and IV) are used to improve mobility.

To determine whether joint mobilization for mobility is indicated, the sport rehabilitation specialist assesses the joint's capsular pattern and motion loss and also compares the involved with the uninvolved segment. The normal capsular pattern for the talocrural joint is more limitation of plantar flexion than of dorsiflexion; in the subtalar joint, inversion is more limited than eversion. The great toe's MTP and all the toes' IP joints have capsular patterns of more limitation of extension than flexion. Refer to chapter 6 for this information and for details on close-packed and loose-packed positions for these joints.

As with other joints, precautions and contraindications should be respected. Body mechanics, force-direction application, and amount of force should be proper in all techniques. The hands should be as close to the joint as possible, with one hand acting as the stabilizing hand and the other applying the mobilization force. The convex-concave rule determines the direction of the mobilization force. That is, when a convex surface is moved on a concave surface, the force is applied in the direction opposite than that of the bone's movement; when a concave surface is moved on a convex surface, the force is applied in the same direction as the bone's movement. Many of the mobilization techniques in this chapter are based on Maitland's (1991) work.

TIBIOFIBULAR JOINT

The tibia and fibula articulate with each other proximally in the distal knee region and distally at the ankle mortise joint. Both proximal and distal articulations must have restored movement for ankle motion to be normal.

Superior Tibiofibular Joint

Mobilization of the superior tibiofibular joint should accompany any restricted movement of the distal tibiofibular joint. Normal mobility of this joint allows the fibular head to move anteriorly during knee flexion and posteriorly during knee extension. Mobilization glides for this joint include anterior-posterior (AP) and posterior-anterior (PA) movements of the fibular head. These can be performed either separately or in one continuous motion from full anterior to full posterior positions. Assessment of the joint's mobility, though, should be performed in one direction at a time.

The patient can be either supine with the knee flexed and the foot flat on the table, or sitting with the lower leg over the table's edge and with the sport rehabilitation specialist stabilizing the distal lower leg between his or her knees. The sport rehabilitation specialist's medial hand stabilizes the tibia, and the lateral hand grasps the fibular head with the thumb pad anteriorly and the index and middle fingers posteriorly (figure 20.28a). Compression of the peroneal nerve behind the fibula should be avoided. The lateral hand glides the fibular head anteriorly and posteriorly.

When each movement is performed individually, the patient is positioned to provide the sport rehabilitation specialist the best mechanical advantage and ease of force application. For an AP mobilization force, the patient is positioned supine with the knee in extension. The tibia is stabilized with the medial hand over the proximal tibia, and the lateral hand's fleshy aspect of the thenar eminence over the fibular head and proximal fibula to act as the mobilizing hand. A vertical downward force is applied by the mobilizing hand against the fibular head to produce a posterior glide of the fibula (figure 20.28b).

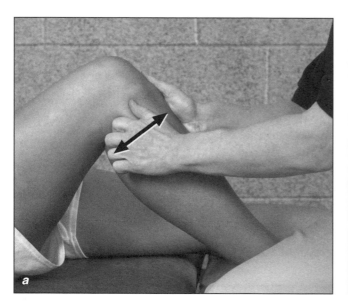 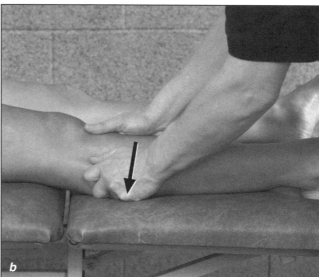

∎ Figure 20.28   Proximal tibiofibular joint mobilization: *(a)* AP-PA mobilization *(b)* posterior glide.

PA mobilization of the proximal tibiofibular joint is performed with the patient in side-lying. The weight of the leg stabilizes the tibia while the sport rehabilitation specialist's distal hand stabilizes the middle lower leg. The mobilizing hand applies an anterior glide with the pad of the wrist against the fibular head.

Inferior Tibiofibular Joint

During dorsiflexion, the distal fibula moves superiorly from the tibia and rotates medially. During plantar flexion, the distal fibula moves in the opposite directions. Normal ankle motion depends on good fibular mobility. Restriction of joint play between the fibula and tibia may require fibular mobilization in both AP and PA directions to restore normal motion.

An AP glide is performed with the patient supine. The sport rehabilitation specialist places the medial hand over the medial malleolus to stabilize the tibia and places the thenar eminence of the lateral hand over the lateral malleolus and distal fibula. A posterior glide is performed using a vertical movement of the lateral hand (figure 20.29).

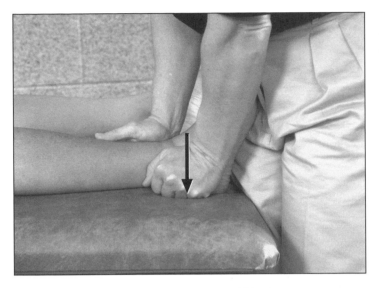

Figure 20.29 Distal tibiofibular joint mobilization.

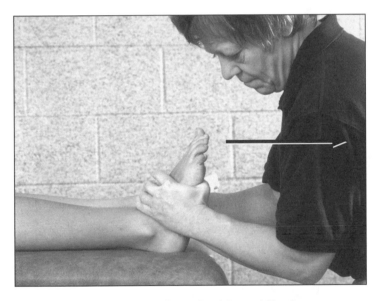

Figure 20.30 Talocrural distraction joint mobilization.

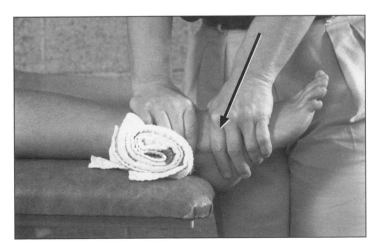

Figure 20.31 Talocrural posterior glide joint mobilization.

A PA glide is performed with the patient prone and the distal lower leg over the edge of the table. The base of the lateral hand is placed over the lateral malleolus while the medial hand stabilizes the distal tibia. The anterior force is applied perpendicular to the plane of the distal tibiofibular joint.

TALOCRURAL JOINT

There are several joints throughout the ankle and foot. The talocrural joint is the true ankle joint, allowing flexion and extension motion. The next sections present some of the most common joint mobilization techniques for this joint.

Distraction

Distraction movement is used to increase general joint play in the ankle joint and can also be used with lower grades of mobilization to relieve pain.

The patient is supine with the leg extended. The sport rehabilitation specialist faces the foot and grasps the foot's dorsum with both hands, intertwining or overlapping the fingers of the two hands on top of the foot and placing the thumbs on the plantar aspect (figure 20.30). The sport rehabilitation specialist leans backward to apply a distraction force.

Anterior Glide

This technique is used to increase ankle plantar flexion. It is also known as a ventral glide or PA movement.

With the patient prone and his or her foot comfortably over the end of the table, the sport rehabilitation specialist places a pad or rolled towel for comfort under the distal lower leg. The stabilizing hand is placed on the anterior lower leg just above the malleoli, and the mobilizing hand cups the talus and calcaneus. The talus and calcaneus are glided anteriorly with downward force applied by the mobilizing hand.

Posterior Glide

This technique is used to increase dorsiflexion and is also known as a dorsal glide or AP glide.

The patient is in supine with the knee extended; the sport rehabilitation specialist faces the foot. The stabilizing hand is placed anteriorly around the distal lower leg, and the mobilizing hand is placed around the proximal foot with the thumb and index finger in contact with the malleoli. The talus is glided posteriorly in the plane of the joint (figure 20.31).

Alternative Technique for Dorsiflexion

An alternative technique for gaining dorsiflexion utilizes a mobilization strap. With the patient standing in a forward-backward stride position on a table, and a mobilization strap secured around the distal tibia and fibula and the sport rehabilitation specialist's hips, the sport rehabilitation specialist places the web of the thumb and index finger around the anterior ankle joint. The belt is used to stabilize the ankle. With the knee partially flexed, the sport rehabilitation specialist uses the hips to pull the strap forward (figure 20.32).

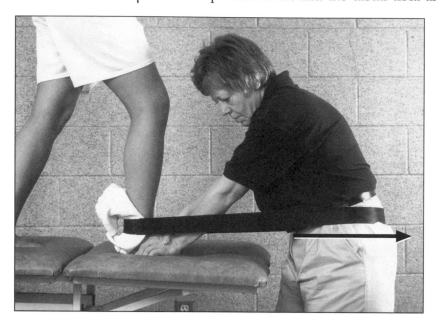

∎ Figure 20.32 Alternative AP talocrural glide joint mobilization.

SUBTALAR JOINT

Although the talocrural joint is the true ankle joint, the subtalar joint is often incorrectly thought of as the ankle joint also. This joint allows inversion and eversion movements to permit ambulation on uneven surfaces without injury. Some, but not all, mobilization techniques for the subtalar joint are presented here. Hand positions for some of these techniques, such as distraction, are subtly different from those for talocrural mobilization but nonetheless important.

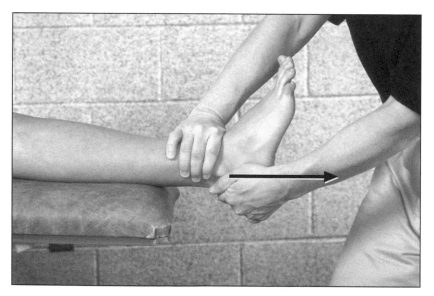

Distraction

This technique is used to reduce pain and to improve general mobility. The patient is supine with the foot over the end of the table, and the sport rehabilitation specialist faces the foot. The stabilizing hand grasps the talus anteriorly, and the mobilizing hand cups the posterior calcaneus (figure 20.33). The calcaneus is pulled distally from the long axis of the leg.

∎ Figure 20.33 Subtalar joint distraction joint mobilization.

Medial Glide

This technique is used to increase eversion. With the patient side-lying on the uninvolved side and the involved ankle off the end of the table, a towel roll is placed under the distal lower leg. The distal lower leg is stabilized with the cephalic hand over the lateral lower leg, and the caudal hand is positioned with its heel on the lateral calcaneus and the fingers on the plantar surface (figure 20.34). A medial glide in a downward direction is applied to the calcaneus.

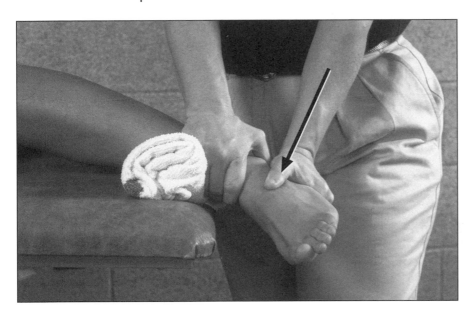

Figure 20.34 Subtalar joint medial glide joint mobilization.

Lateral Glide

This maneuver is used to increase subtalar inversion. With the patient in side-lying on the involved side, the foot over the end of the table, and the distal lower leg supported with a towel, the sport rehabilitation specialist stabilizes the lower leg with the cephalic hand over the medial distal lower leg. The mobilizing hand is placed with the heel of the hand over the medial calcaneus and the fingers on the plantar aspect (figure 20.35). A lateral glide is applied, with the force directly downward and parallel to the joint surface.

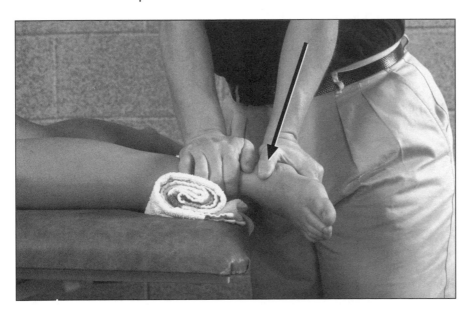

Figure 20.35 Subtalar joint lateral glide joint mobilization.

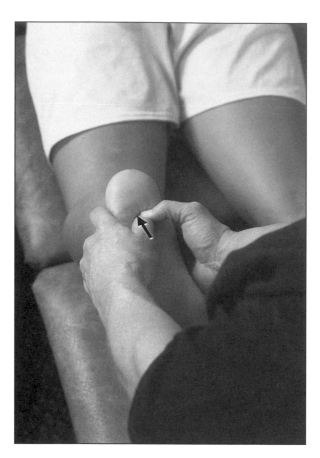

INTERTARSAL JOINTS

These mobilizations can be performed on all midtarsal joints, including the talonavicular, calcaneocuboid, and naviculocuneiform.

Anterior Glide

This technique increases midfoot plantar flexion. With the patient prone, the sport rehabilitation specialist grasps the midfoot with one thumb, reinforced by the other thumb, over the bone to be mobilized. The forefoot is stabilized with the hands while the thumbs are used to provide a PA movement of the bone (figure 20.36).

Figure 20.36 Anterior glide intertarsal joint mobilization.

Posterior Glide

This technique is used to increase midfoot dorsiflexion. With the patient supine, the sport rehabilitation specialist stabilizes the rearfoot with one hand, and places the thumb of the other hand on the dorsum and the fingers on the plantar aspect of the bone to be mobilized. The mobilizing hand applies an AP movement in the plane of the joint surface (figure 20.37).

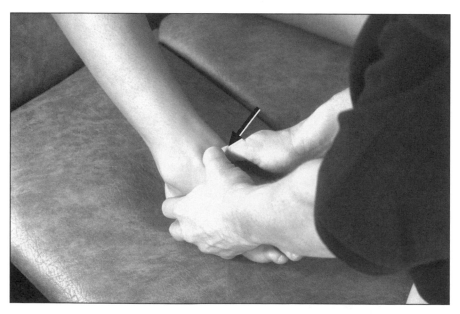

Figure 20.37 Intertarsal posterior glide joint mobilization.

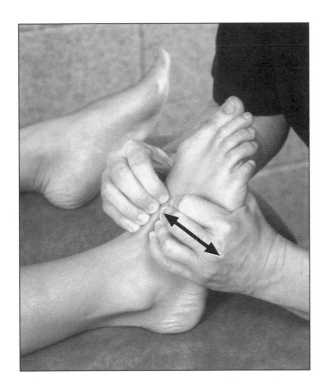

INTERMETATARSAL JOINTS

Anterior and posterior glides can increase intermetatarsal mobility. The sport rehabilitation specialist stabilizes one metatarsal and grasps the adjacent one, with the thumb on the dorsum and the fingers on the plantar aspect. An AP-PA force is applied to the metatarsal (figure 20.38). A gross AP and PA glide can also be applied to the intertarsal joints: the proximal tarsal row is stabilized, and the distal row is mobilized in either an anterior or a posterior direction.

▌Figure 20.38   Intermetatarsal glide joint mobilization.

TARSOMETATARSAL, METATARSOPHALANGEAL, AND INTERPHALANGEAL JOINTS

Many of the basic hand positions and force applications are the same for these joints, so they are grouped together. You must realize, however, that specific finger and hand positions vary according to the particular joint being mobilized.

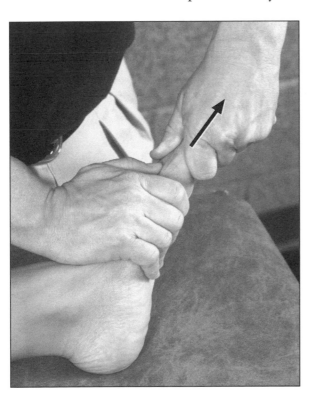

Distraction

Distraction is a general technique that can enhance general joint mobility and relaxation. The phalanx is grasped with the thumb and fingers while the metatarsal is stabilized with the opposite hand (figure 20.39). A distraction force is applied to the phalanx.

Anterior and Posterior Glides

Anterior glides increase toe extension at the MTP and IP joints, and posterior glides increase toe flexion at the MTP and IP joints. For the MTP and tarsometatarsal joints, the metatarsal is stabilized with one hand while the mobilizing hand grasps the proximal phalanx and applies an AP-PA glide. Slight traction can be simultaneously applied to provide more comfort for the patient. For the IP joints, the proximal phalanx is stabilized while the mobilizing force is applied to the adjacent distal phalanx.

▌Figure 20.39   Metatarsophalangeal distraction joint mobilization.

FLEXIBILITY EXERCISES

There are many flexibility exercises for the ankle, foot, and lower leg. Among those often used are gastrocnemius, soleus, and Achilles stretches; ankle exercises the patient can do throughout the day; and BAPS board exercises.

The following sections present certainly not all flexibility exercises but rather some of the more commonly used techniques for improving ankle, foot, and lower-leg flexibility. As with most exercises, the sport rehabilitation specialist must have a knowledge of the body's mechanics, the muscle's function, and appropriate application of forces to design an effective flexibility exercise program.

Although there are some exceptions, the active flexibility exercises are held for 15 to 20 s and repeated four to five times. If the patient has less-than-normal flexibility, he or she should repeat the exercises frequently throughout the day.

GASTROCNEMIUS STRETCH

Because the gastrocnemius extends from above the knee to the calcaneous, both the knee and ankle joints must be placed on stretch to effectively stretch the muscle.

Standing Position

This stretch is performed with the patient in a straddle position with the leg to be stretched behind the opposite leg. The patient places his or her body weight on the arms, which are supported on the wall and on the front foot while the back leg remains extended at the knee. The heel should remain in contact with the floor; the hip should be forward of the knee; and the foot should be in a straight line or the toes slightly turned inward (figure 20.40). Common substitutions are allowing the midfoot to collapse by turning the foot outward, lifting the heel off the floor, bending the knee, or moving the hips posteriorly.

Sitting Position

If the patient is non-weight bearing, he or she can use this gastrocnemius stretch to increase flexibility until weight bearing is permissible.

With the patient in a long sitting position, a stretch strap or towel is hooked around the forefoot. Keeping the knee straight, the patient pulls on the strap to dorsiflex the ankle. Additional stretch can be applied with active contraction of the ankle dorsiflexors. Common substitutions in this exercise are hip rotation and foot pronation.

SOLEUS STRETCH

Because the soleus does not cross the knee joint, to isolate this muscle the stretch should be applied with the knee flexed. This eliminates the stretch on the gastrocnemius and isolates the stretch to the soleus. As with the gastrocnemius stretch, this stretch can be performed in weight bearing or non-weight bearing.

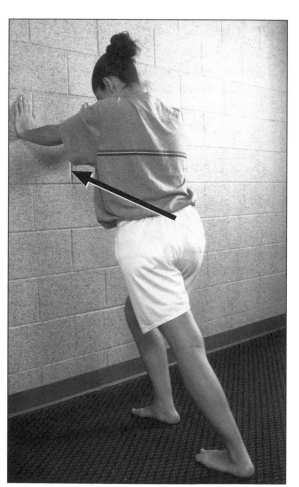

▌Figure 20.40   Gastrocnemius stretch in standing.

Standing Position

In the standing position, the patient is in a position similar to that described for the gastrocnemius. With the involved leg behind the uninvolved leg, he or she keeps the foot flat on the floor with the foot turned slightly inward, then slowly flexes the knee until a stretch is felt in the calf (figure 20.41). Common substitutions are outward rotation of the foot, knee valgus positioning, and posterior movement of the hip as the knee is flexed.

Sitting Position

A soleus stretch, if partial weight bearing is allowed, can be performed with the patient in sitting and the feet on the floor. The forefoot is on a $\frac{1}{2}$ foam roller, and the heel is off (figure 20.42a). The patient attempts to push the heel to the floor, feeling the stretch in the distal calf.

Using a stretch strap in sitting, the patient positions the involved leg with slight knee flexion. The strap is placed around the forefoot, and the patient pulls the strap to dorsiflex the foot while maintaining the knee in the same position (figure 20.42b). As with the gastrocnemius stretch in this position, additional stretch can be applied with the simultaneous activation of the ankle dorsiflexors. Common substitutions include increasing knee flexion rather than ankle dorsiflexion and placing the strap too proximal on the foot to apply an effective stretch force.

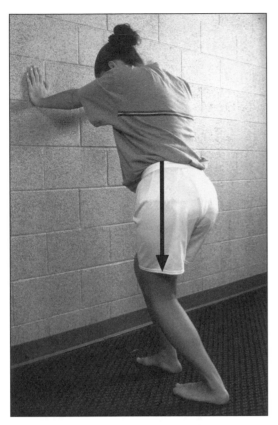

Figure 20.41   Soleus stretch in standing.

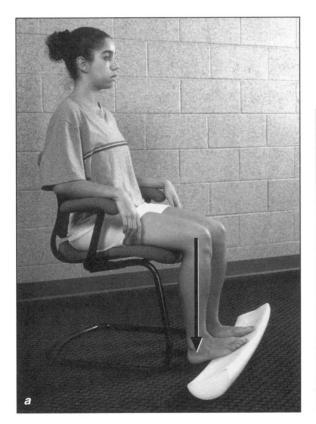
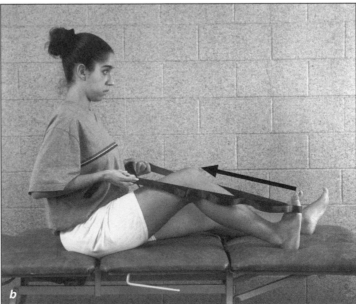

Figure 20.42   Soleus stretch in sitting: (a) with $\frac{1}{2}$ foam roller, (b) with stretch strap.

ACHILLES STRETCH

If the Achilles is the tight structure, a prolonged stretch is most effective for increasing motion. Because of the connective-tissue structure of the thick Achilles tendon, short-term stretches do not change its length. To perform a prolonged stretch, the patient stands with the back to a wall. The feet are positioned either on an incline (figure 20.43a) or on the edge of a book (figure 20.43b), with the heel no more than 2.5 cm (1 in.) from the wall. A towel roll is placed between the posterior knees and the wall to prevent knee hyperextension. The patient stands in this position for a prolonged period, at least 5 min and as much as 20 min if tolerable. It is useful to place a chair next to the patient so that he or she can place the hands on the back of the chair for stabilization and support. Once the stretch is released, the patient commonly feels a stiffness in the posterior calf or ankle area, but this should subside quickly. Common substitutions are standing with the feet in pronation, standing too far away from the wall, and hyperextension of the knees.

Some people attempt to stretch the Achilles or gastrocnemius on the edge of a step. This is ineffective because the very muscle that is being stretched is contracting to maintain balance.

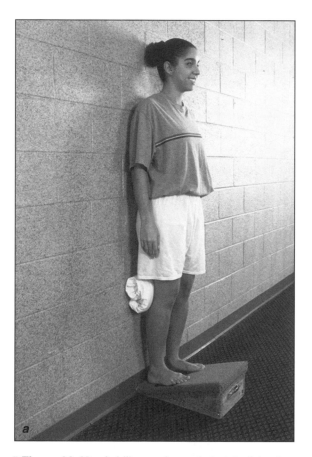 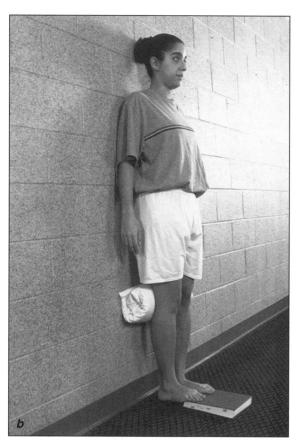

▌Figure 20.43   Achilles prolonged stretch: *(a)* using an incline, *(b)* using a book. A towel roll should be placed behind the knees to prevent knee hyperextension.

DORSIFLEXOR STRETCH

Ankles lacking full plantar flexion can be stretched with the patient sitting on the heels. With very tight ankles, full weight bearing onto the ankles in this position may be too uncomfortable. The recommendation is that the patient lean forward on the hands and push the hips back toward the heels as tolerated. Eventually, if there are no knee injuries, he or she should be able to sit fully on the ankles. In this position, the anterior ankles should be flat on the floor (figure 20.44). A less aggressive stretch can be performed in standing, using a foam roller. The patient places the dorsum of the foot on the foam roller on the floor and pushes the ankle downward toward the floor.

ANKLE PUMPS, ALPHABET, AND TOE EXERCISES

General active exercises that the patient can perform independently throughout the day to increase ankle motion include ankle pumps and the alphabet. Leaving the heel on the floor for ankle pumps, the patient taps the foot up and down, going as high as possible each time he or she raises the foot. In another active-motion exercise, the patient spells the alphabet with the toes and foot while keeping the heel on the floor. These exercises can also be performed with the ankle elevated and can be useful in reducing edema. Patients can perform active toe motions, including curling, extending, abduction, and adduction, throughout the day.

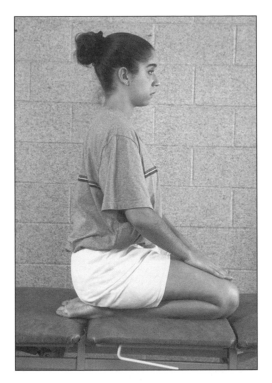

Figure 20.44 Ankle dorsiflexor stretch, sitting. If the patient has a history of knee problems, this position should be avoided.

BAPS BOARD

The BAPS board, or Biomechanical Ankle Proprioception System, is used to increase ankle flexibility and can also be used for strengthening. It consists of a board, or platform, and a variety of sizes of half-balls to which the platform is attached. The size of half-ball selected for an exercise depends on the patient's range of motion and the goal of the exercise. Patients may begin by sitting in a chair and placing the involved foot on the board to perform active range-of-motion exercises. They can advance to weight bearing on two legs and then weight bearing on only the involved extremity to do full range-of-motion exercises for the ankle (figure 20.45). Once the patient has

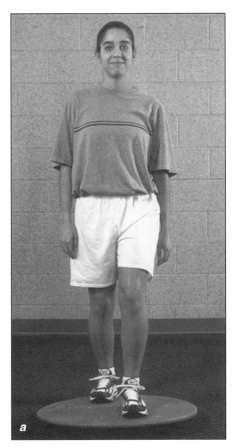
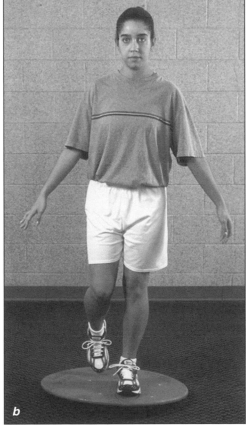

Figure 20.45 BAPS board: (a) double-leg support, (b) single-leg support.

attained full range of motion and control on the BAPS board, you can add weights to the board to provide resistance to specific muscle groups. You can also use the board as a proprioception exercise device by having the patient single-leg stand on the involved limb and slowly perform controlled isolated motions of inversion-eversion or plantar flexion-dorsiflexion.

ADDITIONAL ACTIVE-MOTION EXERCISES

Cardiovascular exercises that can be used to improve ankle range of motion while simultaneously contributing to cardiovascular fitness include exercises on the stationary bike and the cross-country ski machine (figure 20.46). Both machines facilitate range of motion of the ankle, especially when the patient has received careful instruction in proper exercise execution. You should teach the patient ankling on the bike: dorsiflexing the ankle on leg lift and plantar flexing the ankle on the downstroke. On the cross-country ski machine, the patient should attempt to push off from the posterior leg by lifting the heel, and bearing weight on the ball of the foot before pulling the leg and ankle forward and upward.

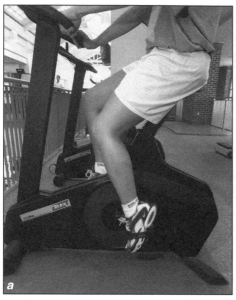 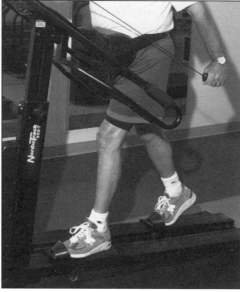

■ **Figure 20.46** Other ankle range-of-motion exercises: *(a)* on stationary bike, *(b)* on cross-country skier.

STRENGTHENING EXERCISES

Strengthening activities for the foot and ankle include isometrics, rubber tubing activities, exercises specifically for the toes, body-weight resistance for the ankle and foot, and resistance with equipment.

Strengthening exercises that can be used earliest in a rehabilitation program include isometrics. The patient can perform these even while the foot is in a cast or immobilizer. Normal progression is to isotonics and isokinetics. Isotonic exercises include those using rubber tubing, free weights, machine weights, and body resistance. Isokinetic exercises usually do not start until the patient's foot and ankle have sufficient strength to control isotonic activities.

ISOMETRICS

Isometrics are held at the maximum contraction for 6 s, with a slow buildup and release of the force so that the total contraction is about 10 s long. No movement is produced.

Inversion

Sitting with the inside of the foot against a table leg, the patient pushes the foot into the table leg, attempting to invert the foot. The foot should not move, and the patient should feel the muscles working on the inside of the leg. Common substitutions for this exercise are hip adduction, hip rotation, and tibial rotation.

Eversion

Sitting with the outside of the foot against a wall or table leg, the patient pushes the foot into the wall or table leg, attempting to evert the foot. The patient should feel

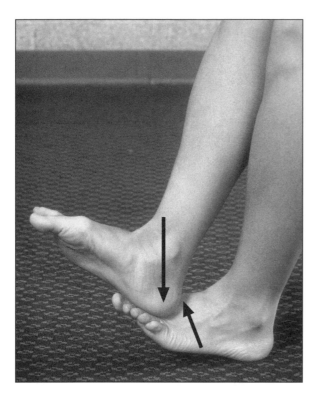

Figure 20.47   Isometric exercise for dorsiflexion.

the lateral leg muscles working. Common substitutions include hip abduction, hip rotation, and tibial rotation.

Dorsiflexion

Sitting with the uninvolved heel on top of the involved foot, the patient pushes the involved foot upward against the top foot, attempting to dorsiflex the ankle (figure 20.47). The patient should feel the anterior lower-leg muscles working. Common substitutions include hip flexion and foot eversion.

RUBBER TUBING EXERCISES

Because the various ankle muscle groups have different strengths, you must evaluate the patient's strength for each exercise before determining which rubber tubing resistance is most appropriate for obtaining the desired results from the resistive exercise. Normally, ankle plantar flexors are the strongest, and ankle everters are the weakest. Injured ankles have reduced levels of strength in all motions, but most of the time, the proportional stregth remains close to normal. In other words, even though a patient's ankle has less-than-normal strength, the plantar flexors are still the strongest muscle group and the ankle everters the weakest. These exercises can also be performed with either manual resistance or pulleys.

Eversion

This exercise strengthens ankle everters. The patient sits in a chair, with the tubing around the forefoot and anchored to a table leg near the uninvolved leg. The ankle begins in inversion and is moved against the tubing into a full range of eversion (figure 20.48a). The most common substitutions for this exercise are hip abduction and rotation. To reduce this, you should instruct the patient in the proper technique and caution against moving the knee. Placing the hands on either side of the knee to stabilize the thigh also reduces substitutions. The patient can also perform this exercise in a long sitting position, but it is more difficult to stabilize the thigh and avoid hip substitutions in this position (figure 20.48b).

Inversion

This exercise is used to strengthen ankle inverters. The patient sits in a chair with the tubing around the forefoot and anchored to a table leg near the involved side. He or she starts with the ankle in full eversion and moves it into a full range of motion to end-range inversion (figure 20.48c). Hip adduction and rotation are the most common substitutions in this exercise.

Dorsiflexion

This exercise strengthens the ankle dorsiflexors. The patient sits with the tubing around the forefoot and anchored to a table leg, which the patient faces (figure 20.48d). The patient pulls the foot toward the shin, dorsiflexing the ankle. The most common substitution is knee flexion.

Plantar Flexion

This exercise can be used to strengthen plantar flexors if the patient is non-weight bearing. The patient is in a long sitting position with the tubing around the plantar foot and grasped in both hands (figure 20.48e). Maintaining a firm tension on the tubing and starting with the foot in full dorsiflexion, the patient pushes the foot against the tubing to move the ankle into full plantar flexion.

This exercise can also be performed with the knee in flexion and the patient sitting on a table with his or her lower leg hanging off the table. In this position, plantar-flexion motion isolates and strengthens the soleus muscle.

If the patient has good strength in the early ranges of plantar flexion but is unable to stand in full plantar flexion, the tubing can be used to facilitate strength in the weak part of the motion. To do this, the patient places the foot in the weak range of motion and positions the tubing around the plantar foot. While the patient maintains the ankle position, he or she increases tension on the tubing by pulling on it with the arms to provide the resistance in the weak position. Maintaining good tension on the tubing, the patient slowly dorsiflexes the ankle to facilitate an eccentric contraction of the plantar flexors. This technique can be used to isolate weak positions in the other motions as well.

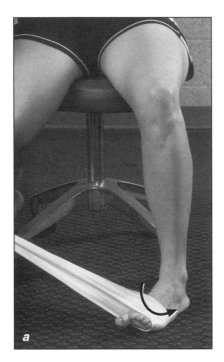
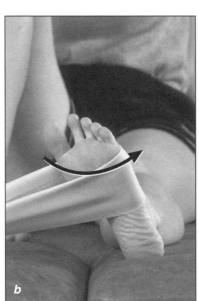
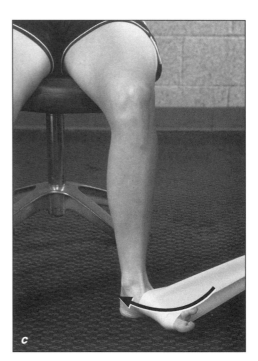
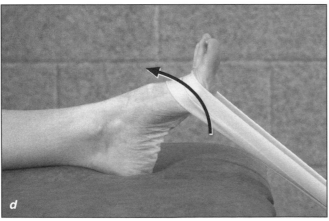
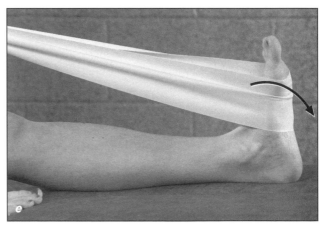

∎ **Figure 20.48** Tubing exercises: *(a)* eversion, *(b)* eversion in long sitting, *(c)* inversion, *(d)* dorsiflexion, *(e)* plantar flexion.

TOE EXERCISES

Strengthening toe muscles helps to restore optimal foot function. Both intrinsic and extrinsic toe muscles are strengthened with these exercises. The long toe muscles can also add support to the ankle.

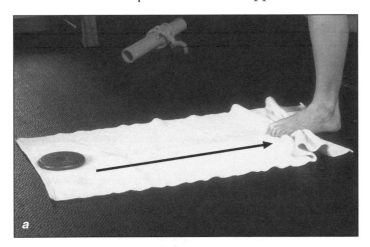

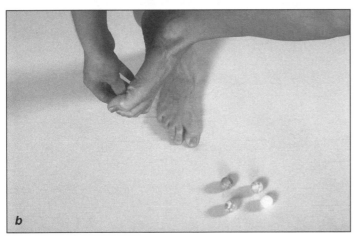

▌Figure 20.49   Toe exercises: *(a)* towel roll, *(b)* marble pickup.

Towel Roll

This exercise strengthens primarily intrinsic muscles but also strengthens long toe flexors. The patient sits on a chair with a towel placed on the floor in front of the chair. Without shoes or socks, the patient uses the toes to curl the towel toward him- or herself (figure 20.49a). Resistance can be provided by placing a weight at the end of the towel, using a wet towel, or using newspaper. A common substitution is knee flexion motion. The thigh and lower leg should not move during the exercise.

Marble Pickup

This exercise strengthens extrinsic and intrinsic toe flexors and can also help to facilitate ankle inverters or everters. The patient uses the toes to pick up marbles that have been placed on the floor. The marbles are placed in the hand on the same side to facilitate eversion and in the hand on the opposite side to facilitate inversion (figure 20.49b). Objects such as a pencil, pieces of paper, or a towel can be used in place of the marbles.

BODY-WEIGHT RESISTANCE EXERCISES

Exercises for both the gastrocnemius and soleus are necessary for complete restoration of strength. Exercises already mentioned for the long toe extensors also help to strengthen the posterior muscles. Body weight is an excellent form of resistance that strengthens many body segments, including the ankle and foot.

Heel Raises

This exercise strengthens the calf muscles. With feet about shoulder-width apart, the patient rises up on the toes as high as possible and then returns to feet flat on the floor. This exercise is more difficult when performed on an incline (figure 20.50) or on the edge of a stair, and also when it is performed on only the involved leg. Common substitutions include using the hamstrings by flexing the knees during the heel raise, moving the body forward or rocking rather than moving straight upward, and placing most of the body weight on the uninvolved leg rather than equally distributing the weight over both legs.

Weigh-Scale Exercise

If the patient has difficulty bearing weight on the involved extremity, or is apprehensive about transferring weight onto that side, a weigh scale is an effective tool for teaching weight transfer and for helping the individual gain confidence in the involved extremity as well as improving strength.

This exercise uses a balance weight scale and a platform of height equal to that of the scale's foot plate. The platform is placed next to the scale. The patient stands with the uninvolved extremity on the platform and the involved extremity on the scale, and initially stands with most weight on the uninvolved leg (figure 20.51). The scale balance is moved to a desired weight for the exercise. The patient is instructed to transfer enough weight to the involved side to move the balance arm to the top of the scale and then maintain the balance arm in the up position while performing a heel raise. As the patient's strength improves, the weight on the scale is increased until the patient is able to perform a single-leg heel raise with full body weight.

This exercise is also good for weight-transfer instruction for gait training. The technique is similar, but the instruction is to move weight from the left to the right lower extremity. The scale weight is increased as the patient improves in ability to transfer weight properly.

Toe Raise

This exercise increases strength of the ankle dorsiflexors. The patient stands on an incline with the heel on the higher aspect of the incline. Keeping the heels in contact with the incline, he or she lifts the toes and forefoot upward and off the incline (figure 20.52). If this exercise is too difficult, the patient can start by performing the exercise on the floor. Use of the incline requires the muscle to work through a greater range of motion and increases the difficulty of the exercise. Common substitutions include hip flexion and body sway. For optimal results, correct improper execution.

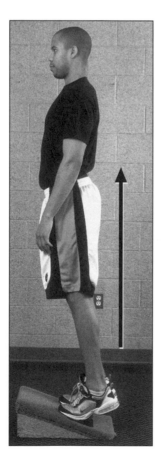

Figure 20.50 Heel raise on an incline.

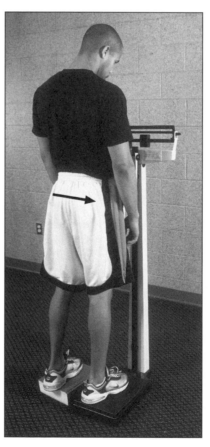

Figure 20.51 Weigh-scale exercises can be used to teach weight transfer and to increase strength of the involved extremity.

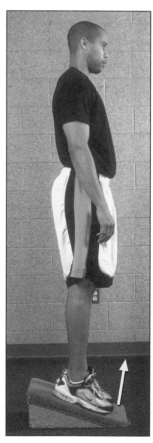

Figure 20.52 Toe raise on a incline.

EQUIPMENT RESISTANCE

In addition to body weight, several kinds of equipment can be used to strengthen the ankle and foot. Presented here are a few of the possibilities.

Free Weights

Cuff weights can be used in strengthening exercises for ankle inversion, eversion, and dorsiflexion. The patient, placed in an antigravity position with the cuff weight wrapped around the midfoot, moves the ankle through a full range of motion. For dorsiflexion, the position is sitting (figure 20.53a). For inversion and eversion, the position is side-lying on the involved side and on the uninvolved side, respectively (figure 20.53b).

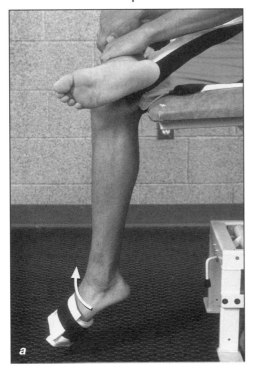
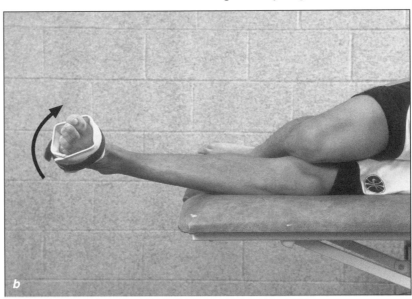

Figure 20.53 Cuff-weight exercises: *(a)* dorsiflexion, *(b)* inversion. The weight should be lifted through a full range of motion.

Machine Weights

Calf raises in the standing and seated positions using machines strengthen the calf muscles. Standing calf raises can be performed on machines designed specifically for that exercise, or on machines such as an upright press or bench press that can be modified for use as a calf-raise machine. A seated heel-raise exercise to isolate the soleus muscle can be performed on a hamstring-curl machine.

Placing an incline under the foot in the seated heel raise, or having the patient on a step in the standing heel raise, increases the difficulty of the exercise, because these modifications require the muscle to move through a greater range of motion.

PROPRIOCEPTIVE EXERCISES

Proprioception is an important part of any ankle rehabilitation program. Proprioceptive exercises for posture and balance help improve ankle stability.

Proprioception is key for kinesthesia and balance control. Research shows that deficits in these areas exist following ankle sprains, especially chronic ankle sprains (Forkin et al. 1996; Lofvenberg et al. 1995). Posture and balance, important factors in controlling ankle stability, can be improved with rehabilitation (Leanderson et al. 1996; Bernier and Perrin 1998). It is important, then, to include proprioception exercises in an ankle rehabilitation program. If a patient is non-weight bearing, early kinesthetic exercises can include mirroring activities with the two ankles, with the patient's eyes closed. The alphabet exercise mentioned earlier can also help improve kinesthetic awareness.

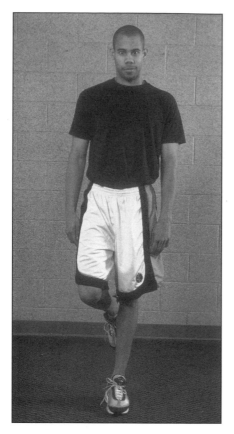

Figure 20.54 Stork stand.

Once the patient is weight bearing, additional proprioceptive exercises can be incorporated into the program. One of the beginning weight-bearing exercises is the stork stand. The patient stands on the involved extremity while attempting to maintain balance for 30 s (figure 20.54). Having accomplished this, the individual performs the exercise with eyes closed to eliminate the visual component of balance. The next level is to have the patient stork stand on an unstable surface, such as a trampoline, a foam roller, or a $\frac{1}{2}$ roller (figure 20.55).

To progress to more advanced balance activities, the patient either attempts to maintain balance while performing another activity with another body part, so that concentration on balance is diverted, or performs additional activity with the lower extremity while maintaining balance. For example, a football reciever or softball or baseball player can catch a medicine ball while balancing on a foam roller or trampoline. The ball is thrown at different levels and to different sides of the body so that the patient must move to reach for it and still maintain balance. If the patient is a basketball player, bouncing a ball while maintaining balance on an unstable surface is a good activity (figure 20.56a). Setting a volleyball while stork standing on an uneven surface diverts the volleyball player's conscious effort from balance to enhance autonomic responses for balance.

Various kinds of balance boards can be either made or purchased. Wobble boards, circle boards, BAPS boards, and balance boards can all be used for balance work. A board placed on top of a PVC pipe is a simple balance board. In an exercise with this type of board the patient attempts to keep the ends of the board off the floor (figure 20.56b). This exercise becomes more difficult if the patient rolls the board side to side, still keeping the ends of the board off the floor, or if smaller pipes are used so that the ends of the board are closer to the floor.

Once the patient demonstrates good balance, he or she can advance to more complex exercises that require a combination of balance, agility, control, coordination, and strength. These exercises include activities with equipment such as the Fitter, tubing, slide board, and boxes. The Fitter and slide board are used to develop eccentric and concentric strength and proprioception of the intrinsic and extrinsic muscles (figure 20.57a). They can also assist in cardiovascular development. With tubing attached to the waist, the patient begins with left-to-right lateral or forward-backward jumps and

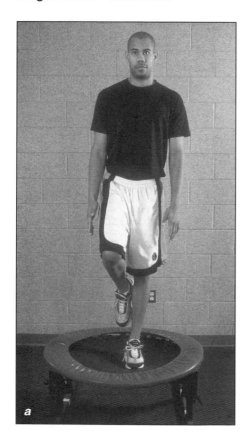
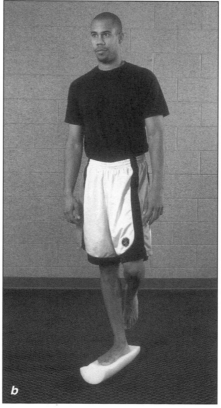

Figure 20.55 Advanced stork-stand exercises: *(a)* on trampoline, *(b)* on foam roller.

progresses to single-leg lateral and forward-backward jumps (figure 20.57b). Tubing exercises facilitate concentric strength, eccentric strength, power, control, coordination, and agility.

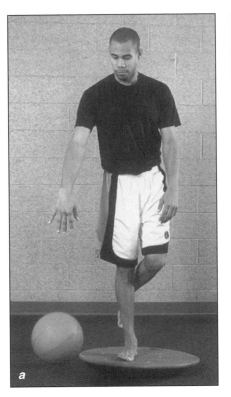
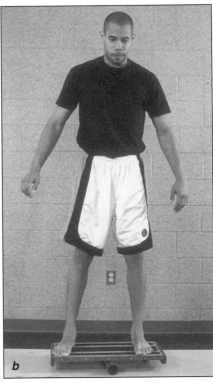

■ **Figure 20.56**   Advanced balance exercises: *(a)* sports activity on unstable surface, *(b)* balance board.

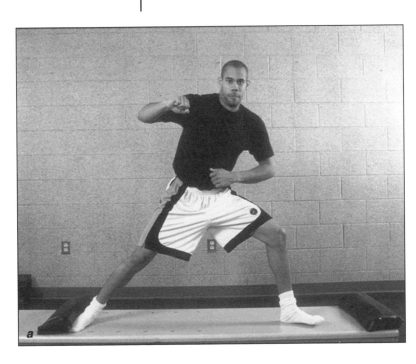
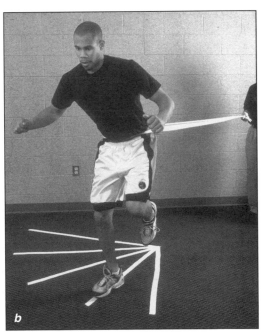

■ **Figure 20.57**   Agility exercises: *(a)* slide board, *(b)* tubing exercise—lateral, left-to-right activity.

Box activities are used as plyometric exercises to promote power and agility. Patients can perform various exercises created and designed by the sport rehabilitation specialist. Generic examples of these activities include rapid lateral jumping (figure 20.58a), rapid front-to-side agility step-ups (figure 20.58b), and multidirectional-change jumps (figure 20.58, c–d).

Plyometric jumps can advance to lateral high jumps (figure 20.58e) and box drop-jumps. For additional suggestions on plyometric exercises for the lower extremities, refer to chapter 9.

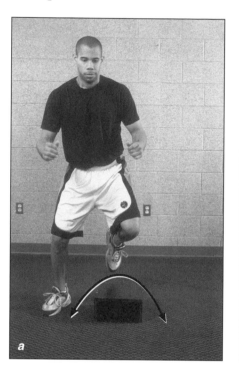

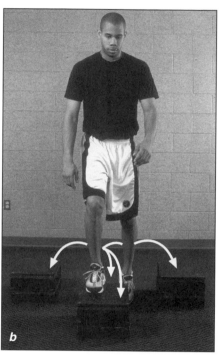

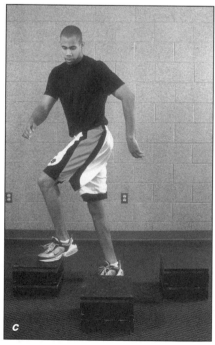

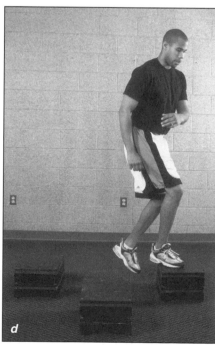

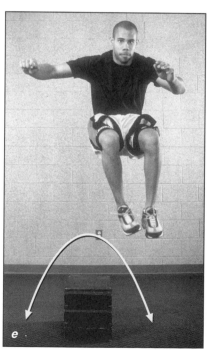

■ **Figure 20.58**   Plyometric box activities: *(a)* jump-over side-to-side, *(b)* alternate jumps side-to-front-to-side, *(c–d)* rapid sequencing from one box to another, *(e)* lateral high jumps.

TREADMILL ACTIVITIES

The treadmill can be used for more than gait analysis, walking, and running. It can be used to identify subtle differences between the involved and the uninvolved extremity during running. Besides using the treadmill to visually observe walking and running mechanics, you can use it as an auditory tool for defining running abnormalities. Listening to the foot hit the treadmill becomes a comparative tool; if the patient's feet do not sound the same at impact, it is likely that the individual has a difference in gait between the involved and uninvolved extremity. Increasing the speed of the treadmill will also reveal differences in stride, gait, and weight transfer that you may not see at slower speeds.

The treadmill can also be used for facilitation, range-of-motion, strength, agility, and coordination exercises. Walking backward on a treadmill—retro walking (figure 20.59a)—has been shown to increase range of motion and muscle activity demands on the knee and ankle (Cipriani, Armstrong, and Gaul 1995). In retro walking, ankle dorsiflexion needs are increased, greater eccentric activity is required of the gastrocnemius, and the anterior tibialis also is more active. Many believe that these increased demands aid in facilitating the kinesthetic system and that they improve lower-extremity proprioception. Varying the speed of the treadmill alters demands on the muscles.

Agility and coordination exercises on the treadmill include activities such as slides and cariocas going to both the left and the right (figure 20.59b). The patient may start with sets of 30 s bouts in each direction and then increase the time on each bout or increase the number of repetitions as improvement occurs. Requiring the patient to make a more rapid change from left side to right side increases the agility demands of the exercise. Placing the treadmill on an incline or increasing the speed also increases the difficulty.

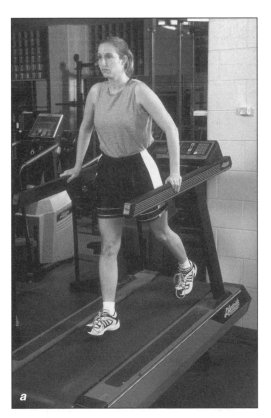 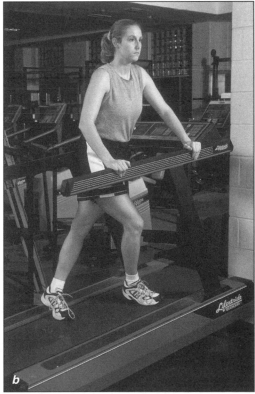

∎ **Figure 20.59** Treadmill activities: *(a)* retro walking on an incline, *(b)* carioca on an incline.

HOPPING ACTIVITIES

Hopping exercises are often a necessary part of an ankle rehabilitation program because many athletic events include some type of hopping or jumping. These exercises can begin on a soft, force-absorbing surface such as a trampoline or mat and then advance to the patient's normal playing-field surface. Many different combinations of hopping activities are possible. Which specific patterns to select may depend on the patient's sport requirements, the injured ankle's deficiencies, and general conditioning demands. Some patterns are box hops, side-to-side hops, forward-backward hops, cross-pattern hops, high hops, long hops, zigzag hops, and circular hops. Some of these are presented as suggestions in figure 20.60. Patients may begin with two-legged hops and advance to one-legged hops. They may also alternate legs or perform hops in combinations, such as two on the left and then two on the right, or two on the injured side and then one on the uninjured side.

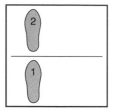

Forward-backward hop: Hop forward and backward between two quadrants.

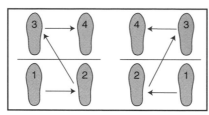

Cross-pattern hop: Hop in an X pattern.

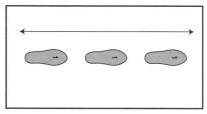

Straight-line hop: Hop forward and then backward along a 15- to 20-ft line.

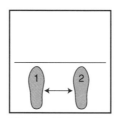

Side-to-side hop: Hop laterally between two quadrants.

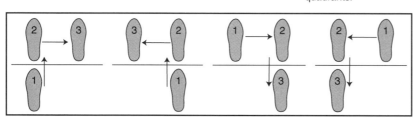

Triangular hop: Hop within three different quadrants. There are four triangles, each requiring a different diagonal hop.

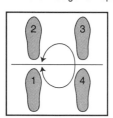

Circular hop: Hop from square to square in a circular pattern. Sets are performed clockwise and counterclockwise.

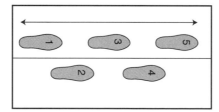

Zigzag hop: Hop from side to side across a 15- to 20-ft line while moving forward and then backward.

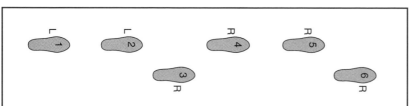

Mixed patterns: Various combination hop patterns can be used, such as two on the injured (i.e., left) side and one on the uninjured (i.e., right) side.

▌ Figure 20.60 Suggestions for hopping patterns. You can design a number of hopping patterns, limited only by your imagination.

FUNCTIONAL EXERCISES

By the end of the rehabilitation program, a patient with a foot or ankle injury must be able to perform functional activities—for example, zigzag runs and 90° cuts to the left and right—without hesitation, smoothly, and efficiently.

As the patient nears reentry into full sport participation, functional exercises must become a part of the complete rehabilitation program so that the patient's return is smooth and uneventful. As mentioned throughout this book, functional activities should mimic the patient's sport requirements. These functional activities are also a reliable means of final evaluation of the patient's ability to perform accurately and safely within the sport (Bolgla and Keskula 1997).

Functional activities vary somewhat from sport to sport, but many running sports entail many of the same functional activities. These include activities such as single, double, or triple hops; zigzag runs with rapid changes in direction; backward running; sprinting; running circles in clockwise, counterclockwise, backward, and forward directions; 90° cuts to the left and to the right; and running figure 8s. The patient should be able to perform the exercises without hesitation, smoothly in both directions and without favoring the involved extremity, and rapidly and efficiently.

Functional exercises should also encompass sport-specific drills and skill activities that are unique to the demands of the patient's sport and position within the sport. These activities vary greatly from one sport to another. You must have an appreciation and understanding of these activities so that you can incorporate correct drills and exercises into the final phase of the patient's rehabilitation program.

SPECIAL REHABILITATION APPLICATIONS

The sport rehabilitation specialist sees a number of common foot and ankle injuries that call for specific approaches within the therapeutic exercise program. Some of these injuries are sprains and dislocations, Achilles tendon injuries, shinsplints, compartment syndromes, a variety of foot injuries, and fractures.

This section deals with specific injuries to the foot and ankle. Injuries to the lower leg, especially the ankle, are among the most common injuries in sport. Some—certainly not all—of the more frequently seen injuries are discussed in the following sections.

ANKLE SPRAIN OR DISLOCATION

An ankle dislocation is on the same continuum as an ankle sprain, so we will consider these two injuries together. As with other sprains, the severity determines the rate of rehabilitation progression and the time when various therapeutic exercises can begin. The more extensive the injury and the consequent tissue damage, the less aggressive the program can be, especially in the initial stages. It is important for the sport rehabilitation specialist to understand concepts and time lines and to assess the severity of the injury before proceeding with a rehabilitation program. It is just as crucial to observe the injured ankle's reaction to prior treatments and to design a program that appropriately stresses the injured ankle without causing additional damage.

Discoloration is the result of bleeding in the area. It is generally a sign of the severity of the sprain as well. If no discoloration occurs, the sprain is likely to be mild or first degree, and the patient's other symptoms should be consistent with this assessment. If discoloration occurs, at least a second-degree sprain is present. Instability indicates a possible third-degree sprain of at least one ligament. Rehabilitation for second- and third-degree sprains proceeds more slowly than that for first-degree sprains. A first-degree ankle sprain may restrict the patient from sport participation for no more than one week, with return to full participation in two to three weeks; but a second-degree sprain may restrict the patient from participation for three weeks and full participation for four to six weeks. Third-degree ankle sprains vary widely in recovery times, which may depend, at least, on the course of treatment provided (Konradsen, Holmer, and Sondergaard 1991). Third-degree sprains can take as little as six weeks or as much as three or more months to improve before the patient can return to full sport participation.

Third-degree sprains and dislocations can be treated either conservatively with rehabilitation or with surgery and rehabilitation. The choice is often made according to the patient's objective and subjective findings, age, level of sport participation, and surgeon's preference. Ankle instabilities are often surgically repaired. Studies show that early rehabilitation with controlled weight bearing in a boot, with early active-motion and therapeutic exercise, yields better results than the more conservative approach of prolonged casting with a slower initiation of rehabilitation (Konradsen, Holmer, and Sondergaard 1991; Glascoe et al. 1999).

The patient's ability to recover from an ankle sprain is dependent on the history of prior injuries. Multiple episodes of ankle sprains may result in an unstable ankle, making the rehabilitation process more complex and more difficult. The sport rehabilitation specialist must obtain an accurate history from the patient before instituting a therapeutic exercise program, because a prior history of ankle sprains can alter the program progression and anticipated results.

Chronic ankle sprains also affect other factors. One of these is additional scar tissue with probable adhesions that limits joint mobility and soft-tissue mobility. Repeated ankle sprains can result in chronic muscle weakness and reduced kinesthetic awareness, making the ankle susceptible to additional injury (Garn and Newton 1988). Chronic ankle sprains may also lead to compensatory changes with alterations in gait, strength, and flexibility, reducing the mechanical effectiveness of the ankle and foot. Because of these additional factors, chronic ankle sprains require more time to properly rehabilitate and achieve an appropriate recovery status (Seto and Brewster 1994).

Most ankle sprains are inversion sprains. The specific ankle ligaments and structures involved and the severity of the injury depend on the mechanical forces applied and the angle of stress application. Ankle sprains may also involve other structures; for example, there may be an avulsion fracture of the malleoli, peroneal strains or dislocations, or other tendon injuries. Of the ankle ligaments, the anterior talofibular is the most commonly injured ligament, and the calcaneofibular is the next most commonly injured ligament.

Occasionally, the tibiofibular ligament is injured. This ligament injury deserves careful consideration. The function of the tibiofibular ligament is to hold the tibia and fibula in alignment and formation of the ankle mortise joint. When weight is borne on the extremity, the force tends to spread the two bones apart. If the tibiofibular ligament is injured, repetitive stress with weight bearing can inhibit the healing process. If this ligament is injured, the patient should be placed in non-weight bearing or partial weight bearing on crutches to ambulate pain free until full weight bearing does not cause pain. If this is not done, the ligament can develop chronic inflammation and can become difficult to treat successfully.

More-typical ankle sprains permit weight bearing to tolerance. The rule of thumb is that if the patient is able to ambulate without limping, crutches are not required; however, if pain or dysfunction causes an abnormal gait, crutches with either partial or non-weight bearing are used. In most cases, weight bearing can be partial, to tolerance.

Control of edema and pain is the first priority, as with any injury in a rehabilitation program. Common methods of reducing edema and pain include the use of ice and modalities along with strapping or bracing. Active range-of-motion exercises can be instituted early, usually within the first three days, to restore ankle range of motion. Joint mobilization and soft-tissue mobilization techniques are used as indicated and on the basis of the assessment before treatment. With chronic sprains, it is common to observe scar-tissue adhesions in the joints and surrounding tissue. Sometimes intertarsal and metatarsal joints become restricted, especially if the patient has been using an immobilizer boot or a cast.

Non-weight-bearing exercises can be used early in the therapeutic exercise program for strengthening. These include isometric exercises, aquatic exercises, and manual resistance. The BAPS board in a seated position can be used during partial weight-bearing periods.

Ankle inversion-eversion strength is key to ankle stability. Exercises for muscles controlling these movements must certainly be included among therapeutic exercises for a sprained ankle. Isometrics, manual resistance, pulleys, tubing, and aquatic exercises can all provide good strengthening activities for these groups. Closed kinetic chain exercises for inversion and eversion movements make strengthening of these motions more functional and enhance proprioceptive gains.

Once full weight bearing is pain free, gait training and closed kinetic chain exercises can be used to produce additional strength and coordination. Balance activities can progress from stork standing on the floor to stork standing on a $\frac{1}{2}$ foam roller, trampoline, or other unstable surface. Initial closed chain strengthening exercises begin with low resistance, repetitions, and sets, and increase to more resistance, repetitions, and sets as the patient progresses. Early closed chain activities are performed slowly and in a controlled manner, but as the patient gains strength and control of the ankle, quicker movements requiring greater control and strength are added. This places demands on strength as well as the balance, coordination, and agility systems. When the patient has pain-free full motion and approximately 90% strength, plyometrics can be incorporated into the program. The final phase includes functional activities before return to full sport participation.

Case Study

A 16-year-old volleyball hitter jumped up for a hit and landed on another player's foot three days ago, causing an inversion sprain to the right ankle. She felt a pop and had immediate swelling. She was unable to bear weight on the ankle at the time. X rays were negative, but the patient was placed on crutches, with weight bearing to tolerance. Ice, elevation, and taping have been applied periodically for the past three days, but the patient comes to you today to start her rehabilitation program. She denies any previous ankle injury. So far she has performed only alphabet exercises because it is too painful for her to do anything else. She can bear about 11 kg (25 lb) of weight on the foot in standing before she complains of pain in the lateral ankle and above the ankle joint. Her pain is located over the anterior talofibular, anterior tibiofibular, and calcaneofibular joints, with most of the pain over the first two ligaments. She has moderate swelling of the ankle, foot, and toes, with ecchymosis over the midfoot to the toes. She is able to wiggle her toes through about 50% normal motion. Her ankle range of motion is −10° dorsiflexion with pain, 45° plantar flexion, 10° inversion with pain, and 10° eversion. Her ankle strength is restricted by pain on dorsiflexion and inversion. She is unable to bear weight on the foot so that you cannot assess antigravity strength of the calf, but you are easily able to overcome plantar flexion with manual resistance. Eversion is 4/5. Joint mobility is normal. Soft-tissue mobility is limited by the edema present, but you are unable to palpate any abnormal soft-tissue restriction.

Questions for Analysis

1. What are your goals for today's treatment?

2. What treatment will you provide for the patient today?

3. What home instructions will you give her?

4. What precautions will you give her?

5. What will be your guidelines for deciding when she can begin resistive weight-bearing exercises?

6. List three agility exercises that you will include in the patient's program when she is able to do them.

7. What will your functional testing include before her return to full sport participation?

Throughout the progression, you must watch for signs of increased inflammatory response indicating that too much stress is being applied to the ankle. These signs include postexercise swelling, and pain either during or after the exercises. If these signs are present, you should reduce the severity of the program for one to three days before advancing the patient to the next level of exercise difficulty.

It is advisable to have the patient refrain from wearing a protective brace during therapeutic exercises, but he or she may choose to use a supportive ankle device before returning to full sport participation. During therapeutic exercises the patient performs activities under controlled circumstances and in a restricted environment so risk of injury is reduced; but on returning to participation, he or she performs in an unpredictable environment, which creates an increased risk of injuring scar tissue that has less-than-maximum tensile strength. Because it may take a year or more for the tensile strength of injured tissue to achieve maximal levels, it is advisable for the patient to have the additional protection of ankle supports. A number of studies have demonstrated increased ankle stability with these devices (Sitler et al. 1994; Gross et al. 1987; Rovere et al. 1988; Kimura et al. 1987).

PERONEAL TENDON DISLOCATION

Peroneal tendon dislocations can often be overlooked, probably because they frequently occur in conjunction with other injuries. For this reason, they are also frustrating to treat unless discovered through the use of good evaluation techniques.

Peroneal tendon dislocation occurs most commonly through two mechanisms, ankle dorsiflexion with active peroneal contraction, and an inversion sprain (Baumhauer, Shereff, and Gould 1997). In an inversion ankle sprain, the peroneal tendons are most susceptible to dislocation with the ankle in 15° to 25° of plantar flexion. This position places the tendons in a tenuous position along the distal fibula. If an inversion ankle sprain occurs with the ankle in less than 15° plantar flexion, the peroneal retinaculum can be stretched, leading to instability of the peroneal tendons. Skiers are commonly subjected to these injuries. If the ankle is in more than 25° of plantar flexion, the peroneal tendons move into a deep-seated position posterior to the fibular head and are stable in that position with little chance of dislocation.

Peroneal dislocations are usually self-reduced once the ankle is in a nonstressed position. The patient typically complains of a painful, snapping sensation in the posterolateral ankle with walking or ankle circumduction. Swelling along the tendon is sometimes observable. Treatment includes controlling the inflammation with modalities. Stabilization of the tendons with taping and pad support can sometimes help to relieve the subluxation episodes. If conservative treatment fails to prevent recurrent dislocations, surgical repair may be necessary.

Postoperative care includes soft-tissue massage around the surgical site to reduce soft-tissue adhesions in the area once the sutures have been removed. Joint mobilization techniques should be used in areas that demonstrate restricted joint mobility. Active range of motion is permitted anywhere from 10 to 21 days postoperatively. Ankle plantar flexion and eversion are motions that cause the least disruption of the tendons and can take place passively relatively early in the program.

Once weight bearing is permitted, the exercises and progression mentioned earlier for other ankle and lower-leg injuries can begin. A weigh-scale weight-bearing progression can be useful in helping the patient gain confidence in the injured extremity. Balance activities once the patient is fully weight bearing can begin with a stork stand and progress to more difficult exercises as strength and control are achieved. Strengthening exercises can begin with isometrics and progress to isotonics using techniques such as manual resistance, pulleys or tubing, and progressive standing heel raises. Other lower-extremity muscle groups in the hip and knee should be strengthened as well, because they have likely diminished in strength following the injury and surgery.

Case Study

A 20-year-old tennis player was downhill skiing during winter break with his family. While he was maneuvering to the right, he fell forward and dislocated his left peroneus longus tendon. The injury was surgically repaired. The lower leg was placed in an immobilizer boot, and the patient was non-weight bearing for two weeks. He is now able to partial weight bear to 75% on the left and is to start rehabilitation. He presents to you today still non-weight bearing on the left. He admits that he is fearful of bearing weight on the leg. His hip and knee strength is grossly 4/5. Ankle dorsiflexion and inversion are 3/5, and ankle eversion is 2+/5. His ankle range of motion is −5° dorsiflexion, 40° plantar flexion, 0° inversion, and 5° eversion. Joint mobility is moderately restricted in the subtalar and intertarsal joints. The calcaneocuboid and cuboid-metatarsal joints are also restricted. Soft-tissue mobility around the surgical scar, along the lateral foot, and into the posterior ankle is moderately limited. There is mild to moderate swelling around the ankle.

Questions for Analysis

1. What are the patient's primary deficiencies?

2. What will your first treatment today include?

3. What will your goals for today's treatment be?

4. What instructions will you give the patient today before he goes home?

5. What do you expect to accomplish in the next two weeks of treatments?

6. List precautions that you must respect at this point in the rehabilitation program.

7. List three strengthening exercises that you will use when the ankle is ready, and explain their progression.

8. What agility exercises will you eventually include in the therapeutic exercise program?

When the patient has achieved full range of motion and adequate strength for control, balance exercises during dynamic activities can begin, and the patient can then progress to agility exercises. Agility exercises on boxes, jumping with tubing resistance, and lateral movements are the final agility activities before functional activities.

ACHILLES TENDON INJURIES

The most common injuries to the Achilles tendon are a rupture and tendinitis. Either injury can be debilitating and can restrict the patient from a rapid return to sport participation. The sport rehabilitation specialist's proper management of each injury is key to a safe and prompt return.

Tendinitis

If not treated correctly, tendinitis can be a frustrating and prolonged condition. Causes must be addressed and the inflammation brought under control before therapeutic exercises can be started.

Achilles tendinitis is usually a gradual-onset injury that originates secondary to overuse. Overuse of the Achilles tendon occurs when the tendon undergoes excessive stresses without sufficient time between stress applications to adjust to those stress levels. Excessive stress can be the result of cumulative forces caused by inherently poor foot mechanics, increased conditioning sessions, improper surfaces and playing fields, inadequate or improper footwear, weakness, or inflexibility. As with other tendinitis conditions, it is necessary to correct the fundamental causative factor or factors in order for there to be complete recovery with reduced risk of reinjury.

A foot with excessive pronation increases Achilles tendon stress. The Achilles tendon's normal configuration has a medial spiral rotation from its origin in the gastrocnemius-soleus complex, where it begins as a flat, fan-shaped tendon, to its insertion on the calcaneus where it ends as a rounded cord (figure 20.61). This spiral

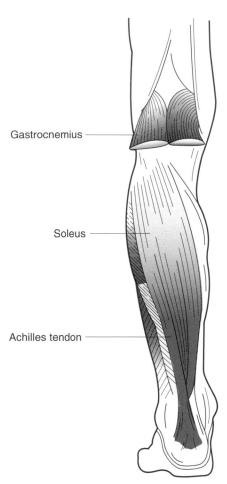

Gastrocnemius

Soleus

Achilles tendon

Figure 20.61   Achilles tendon.

rotation begins about 12 to 15 cm (4.7–5.9 in.) above its insertion (Curwin and Stanish 1984). This twist of the tendon is an area of stress concentration, especially 2 to 5 cm (0.8–1.9 in.) above its calcaneal insertion where the rotation is at its greatest. This is coupled with the fact that this region is also an area of reduced circulation within the tendon. This site is the most common location for tendinitis in the Achilles.

With the calcaneus in eversion, the Achilles tendon suffers an additional torque force. Tightness in the Achilles causes even more pronation to occur. If pronation is prolonged into the phase of heel-off and beyond, when the foot should be inverting, a wringing of the tendon occurs, increasing stress to the Achilles at its most vulnerable site. In cases of repetitive stress and prolonged tendinitis, a nodule of scar tissue from microscopic tears can often be palpated on the tendon 2 to 5 cm (0.8–1.9 in.) above its calcaneal insertion. The nodule is usually larger and more tender on the medial aspect, where the tendon incurs more stress.

As with other cases of tendinitis, the patient's history typically includes a gradual progression of pain. The pain begins as tenderness that occurs during running but that goes away if the individual continues running. Gradually, pain persists longer and longer into the run until it continues after running and even during simple daily activities such as walking. Stiffness can occur after periods of inactivity or sitting. Eventually, pain is present with rest.

Common signs are reduced ankle dorsiflexion; tenderness along the Achilles, especially 2 to 5 cm (0.8–1.9 in.) above the calcaneal insertion where a nodule can be palpated; possible swelling; possible weakness; possible crepitus to palpation; and pain with unilateral hopping.

Treatment includes initially correcting the cause and reducing the inflammation. If the cause is excessive pronation, orthotics may be necessary. A low-dye strapping technique to stabilize the calcaneus and reduce pronation can be used either alone or in combination with heel cups or medial heel wedges to assess the effectiveness of orthotics. Use of commercially available arch supports can also determine whether custom orthotics may be necessary. Inflexibility, weakness, scar-tissue adhesions and joint immobility from previous injuries, and alterations in footwear should all be assessed and corrected as necessary. A good history must include inquiries regarding recent changes in conditioning or workout sessions that may have overstressed the tendon. Changes in surfaces, for example when an individual goes from flat surfaces to hills or from soft to hard surfaces, may also be a contributing factor that must be corrected.

In extreme cases it may be necessary to have the patient temporarily cease the aggravating activity until the inflammation is under control. Anti-inflammatory techniques include the use of various modalities, such as ultrasound, phonophoresis, iontophoresis, electrical stimulation, ice, and others presented in Denegar's (2000) *Therapeutic Modalities for Athletic Injuries.* Cross-friction massage over the nodule and other areas of soft-tissue restriction can help to mobilize the adherent scar tissue to reduce pain and improve soft-tissue mobility.

Therapeutic exercises must include stretching and flexibility activities for restricted areas. Hamstring and hip muscle tightness can influence Achilles flexibility and should be evaluated and corrected as needed. Gastrocnemius and soleus tightness should also be addressed with the flexibility exercises presented earlier.

You should initiate strengthening exercises cautiously because it is important to avoid exacerbation of the pain. Weight-bearing strengthening exercises can begin when the patient reports pain at around 5/10. Before that, theraband exercises for ankle inversion, eversion, and dorsiflexion strength are appropriate. The patient can perform theraband exercises for ankle plantar flexion through a full, pain-free range of motion. Weight-bearing Achilles exercises can include heel raises on a supine or seated leg press, standing heel raises beginning on a flat surface and progressing to an incline, and heel raises with weights. Once weight-bearing exercises have begun, the patient can do eccentric heel raises beginning with a slow heel-drop on the floor and progressing from a medium speed on the floor, to a fast speed on the floor, to a slow speed on an incline, to a medium speed on an incline, and finally to a rapid heel-drop on an incline with three sets of 15 to 25. Other exercises for the lower extremity include squats, lunges, and knee flexion strengthening exercises as tolerated. When the patient's pain level is 8/10, agility exercises are suitable. Plyometrics start once the patient is pain free. At no time throughout the therapeutic exercise program should any exercise increase Achilles pain. If any progression results in Achilles pain, the patient should return to previous levels of activity for another one or two treatments until he or she is able to progress to the next level without pain.

Once the patient is able to perform plyometric exercises well and without pain, functional activities are the last step before full return to sport participation. Throughout the program, the patient must communicate to the sport rehabilitation specialist any changes in Achilles pain and the response to treatment. You must respect the patient's pain and realize that each person will respond differently to an exercise progression. The key to the success of the program is correcting the underlying causes of the Achilles tendinitis and getting the inflammation under control before the patient advances in the program.

Retrocalcaneal bursitis is often mistaken for Achilles tendinitis. Bursitis occurs over the posterior aspect of the calcaneus where the bursa is located. This is an unusual location for Achilles tendinitis to occur, so a patient presenting with complaints of pain in this area should be assessed for bursitis as well as tendinitis. A **pump bump** is frequently present because a heel-whip occurs as the calcaneus is moved toward supination after being positioned in pronation longer than it should be during late stance and heel-off. The bursa becomes irritated with friction against the shoe's heel counter, especially with a heel-whip. Treatment includes symptomatic relief of the inflammation along with correction of the cause of the bursitis. In addition to excessive pronation, other causative factors of bursitis include tight Achilles, tight plantar fascia, and poor shoes.

Case Study

A 24-year-old, male recreational runner reports to you with complaints of pain in the right lower leg just above the ankle. He reports that about two months ago while he was running, he stepped off a curb and rolled his right ankle but continued running. The ankle swelled slightly but did not require him to cut back on his running program. He did not think much about it because it did not seem to cause any problems. This patient usually runs about 8 km (5 miles) once a day but has recently increased running to twice a day in preparation for an upcoming marathon. Because the marathon course is hilly, he has recently made it a point to run at least one steep hill during his workouts. When the pain began he would continue running, and the pain would go away; but it soon lingered longer into the run until it now is present throughout the run and has forced him to reduce his mileage. He has pain after prolonged sitting, while climbing stairs, and while walking barefoot. He reports that he feels a creaking in the back of his ankle when he walks. He does a few stretches but usually does not have time after his run to do any stretch more than once, holding each stretch for 20 s.

Your examination reveals that dorsiflexion in subtalar neutral is −5°. The calcaneus inversion-eversion motion is a total of 35°, and the midfoot is loose when you lock the rearfoot and passively invert and evert the midfoot. Strength for heel raise in weight bearing is slightly less than normal, with pain occurring after about eight repetitions. There is a tender nodule about 3 cm (1.2 in.) above the base of the heel on the Achilles tendon. The nodule is significant in size, protruding about 2 mm medially and 1 mm laterally on the Achilles tendon. You can feel crepitus in the tendon as you passively dorsiflex and plantar flex the ankle.

Questions for Analysis

1. How do you think the ankle rollover incident has affected the Achilles tendon injury?
2. How will you describe for the patient the probable causes for his Achilles tendon injury?
3. What will your advice be regarding his workout program?
4. Describe what your first treatment session with the patient will include.
5. What home exercises will you give him?
6. What factors will you consider in deciding when to begin strengthening exercises?
7. What will you tell the patient when he asks you how long this will take to resolve?

Achilles Rupture

Treatment programs for Achilles ruptures have become less conservative in recent years, primarily because of the poor results seen with delayed rehabilitation. This section presents a program of treatment and then a case study for you to solve.

An Achilles rupture most commonly occurs in athletes in the fourth and fifth decades of life. In younger athletes, a rupture occurs when the foot is anchored and the patient is thrust forward to produce a sudden stretch on the tendon. A typical history for the older patient includes an incident in which the patient was running or cutting and felt as though he or she had been shot in the leg. A younger athlete may be in a football pileup with one player on top of his foot and then be pushed forward by another player who comes into the pileup. A pop can be felt or heard. The pain is usually intense, and the patient is unable to walk on the leg. Passively squeezing a normal calf muscle causes a plantar-flexion movement of the ankle, but this does not occur with a torn Achilles tendon.

Surgical repair, either open or subcutaneous, most recently has been the treatment of choice. Conservative care with immobilization often lends itself to poor results, especially in the athletic population. Following repair, the lower leg is placed either in a series of progressively reduced plantar-flexion casts or, more commonly, in a hinged ankle walking boot with ankle immobilization. The boot is initially positioned in plantar flexion and gradually positioned to neutral. The patient may be non-weight bearing initially and progress to partial weight bearing before weight bearing as tolerated is allowed.

Initial treatments include cardiovascular conditioning and exercises for the uninvolved lower-extremity segments and other body segments. Isometric exercises in the immobilization boot can be encouraged, but the patient should be instructed to perform a slow buildup to maximum with a maximal hold and a gradual release of muscle tension. Once the surgeon permits treatment to the involved segment, this should initially involve efforts to reduce edema and scar-tissue adhesions. Soft-tissue massage and mobilization, along with joint mobilization, often begin early to assist in restoring flexibility and range of motion. Active and passive range-of-motion exercises and strengthening exercises for ankle inverters, everters, dorsiflexors, and plantar flexors begin in non-weight bearing and progress as tolerated to partial and then full weight bearing. Use of the theraband for ankle motions once the patient is out of the boot assists in promoting strength. When the patient is permitted partial weight bearing, he or she can begin to use the BAPS board in sitting. Other activities can include exercise on a stationary bike, the towel-roll exercise, and marble pickups for extrinsic and intrinsic muscles. Plantar foot massage with a ribbed can, golf ball, or rolling pin is also appropriate during this time.

If the patient is on crutches, it is best to encourage a correct heel-toe gait. If the patient acquires bad habits on crutches, they may extend into full weight bearing and become difficult to correct. Gait training is a necessary part of the therapeutic exercise program once the patient is fully weight bearing.

Patients are typically reluctant to bear weight on the involved extremity once they are permitted full weight bearing without the boot. Weight transfer from the uninvolved to the involved extremity through the use of the weigh scale, with progressive increases in the weight placed on the scale, is a good way to help the patient develop confidence in weight bearing on the involved leg. The scale can also be used to control and increase resistance in heel-raise exercises. This can be an especially significant exercise if the surgeon is permitting limited weight bearing on the extremity. The scale exercise can also be used in full-weight-bearing exercise, and can be used for monitoring and recording increases in the patient's ability to bear weight on the involved leg through a full range of motion.

When the patient is able to bear full weight on the involved extremity, stork-standing exercises can improve balance and proprioception. Additional strength activities should include exercises for the entire lower extremity because it is likely that with inactivity, an antalgic gait, and surgery, the entire lower extremity is weaker than normal. These exercises can involve activities such as resisted hip exercises and knee exercises, as well as weight-bearing exercises such as squats and lunges. These exercises are discussed in chapters 21 and 22. Other activities include step exercises, balance and agility exercises, and eventually plyometric exercises as described earlier in this chapter. Functional exercises are part of the final phase of the rehabilitation program and are specific to the patient's sport.

During the early phase of the program, manual-resistance exercises for the hip and knee are feasible even when the lower leg is immobilized. Manual resistance to the ankle can begin once the immobilization brace or cast is off. Weight-bearing exercises are gradually increased in the program as the patient tolerates them. Initially, the resistance and repetitions are low, and emphasis should be on correct technique and proper execution. The patient may tolerate increased repetitions better than increased resistance in the early days of therapeutic exercise.

Resistance exercise beyond body weight is frequently added to the program around 8 to 12 weeks postoperatively. Once the patient has 10° to 15° of dorsiflexion, usually toward the end of the second month or the beginning of the third, jogging activities can begin. Straight jogging on a flat surface is permitted until the patient is up to 3.2 km (2 miles). After that, agility drills are appropriate.

Progression of the strengthening exercises is determined by tissue healing times, the patient's flexibility and mobility, and his or her tolerance. Pain and swelling are the primary signs to avoid with any exercise. It is desirable to achieve muscle fatigue without causing pain or swelling with strengthening exercises. Exercise stress is gradually increased, and the response to any increase in exercise stress—either increased difficulty in an exercise or the addition of new exercises—must be carefully monitored. You must rely on your own observational skills, as well as on the patient's reports of the Achilles response to changes in therapeutic exercises, to gauge the effectiveness of the program. These factors dictate alterations.

Case Study

Two weeks ago, a 45-year-old male tennis player was running to return a drop shot when he suddenly felt as though he had been shot in the left calf. He had intense pain and was unable to stand or walk. He was taken to the emergency room, placed on crutches, given ice, and instructed to follow up with an orthopedic surgeon.

He underwent surgical repair for a ruptured Achilles tendon 10 days ago. His surgeon wants him to begin his rehabilitation program today. He has a walking boot fixed at 10° plantar flexion and is permitted partial weight bearing to 50%. He is apprehensive about putting weight on the left leg and continues to walk non-weight bearing on the left. He does not have much pain in the Achilles because he is not moving it much. Although the surgical scar is well healed, there is moderate swelling throughout the foot and distal lower leg. His active ankle movement is 30° plantar flexion and −15° dorsiflexion. Inversion-eversion is stiff and 20°. Joint mobility of the tarsals and metatarsals is restricted overall at about 50% normal mobility. Strength of the hip and knee is 4–/5; ankle dorsiflexion, inversion, and eversion are 3/5; and plantar flexion is 2/5. Palpation reveals myofascial tenderness with soft-tissue restriction throughout the calf muscles and the presence of adhesions in the dorsum of the foot and around the ankle. The surgical site has moderate adhesions of the scar to underlying soft tissue.

Questions for Analysis

1. How will you outline for the patient the general course of treatment progression?

2. What are your short-term goals with this patient, and when would you expect to achieve them?

3. What will your treatment include today?

4. What instructions will you give him today for a home program?

5. How aggressive will you be with your treatments during the next two weeks?

6. When will you begin strengthening exercises, and what will they initially include?

7. List three agility exercises you will give the patient when he is able to perform them, before he progresses to functional exercises.

Other Tendinitis

Although several tendons in the foot, ankle, and lower leg can develop tendinitis, the most common sites are the tibialis posterior and the peroneal tendons. These tendons become inflamed most often because of overuse secondary to excessive pronation combined with increased mileage on hard surfaces.

The tibialis posterior works eccentrically to decelerate subtalar pronation and internal rotation of the tibia at heel strike, and concentrically as a supinator and inverter of the subtalar joint and external rotator of the tibia during stance. The peroneus longus and brevis work as pronators of the subtalar joint and as plantar flexors and everters of the first ray during the non-weight-bearing phase of gait. During midstance and heel-off, they evert the foot to transfer weight from the lateral to the medial foot. These lateral and medial muscles both act as stabilizers of the foot during weight bearing. The tibialis posterior stabilizes the midtarsal joint, and the peroneus longus stabilizes the first ray to accept the load as it is transferred from the lateral to the medial foot at heel-off. When the foot is pronated longer than it should be in weight bearing, excessive loads are placed on these tendons. If the excessive load from changes in workouts, poor shoes, or ungiving surfaces causes breakdown that the tendon insufficiently recovers from before the next workout, tendinitis can occur.

Tibialis posterior tendinitis results in pain in the posteromedial ankle region and/or into the tendon's insertion site on the navicular and surrounding tarsals. Peroneal tendinitis pain, located in the posterolateral ankle region, can run along the tendon on the lateral foot.

As with Achilles tendinitis, it is crucial for the sport rehabilitation specialist to identify the causes if a treatment program is to have lasting effects. Once you have identified the causes, you can take steps to alleviate them. If the injury is not severe, it may be possible for the patient to continue sport participation once the causes have been corrected. In severe cases it may be necessary for the patient to refrain from sport participation until the inflammation is alleviated.

Initial treatment includes the use of anti-inflammatory modalities that have been discussed previously. The patient should be instructed in proper stretching exercises for tight areas. These may often include structures adjacent to the injured area. For example, a tight iliotibial band or piriformis may impact the tibialis posterior tendinitis, making it necessary to include stretches for these structures in the therapeutic exercise program.

Strengthening activities once the inflammation is under control include those exercises discussed previously. The patient should do concentric and eccentric exercises for all ankle muscles, especially those deficient in strength or endurance, as well as the injured structures. Antigravity positioning using weights, rubber tubing, or manual resistance for inverters and everters provides additional resistance to those muscles. Marble pickups with placement of the marbles in the ipsilateral or contralateral hand, lateral towel roll, and inversion-eversion on a BAPS board or wobble board are important exercises for peroneal and tibialis posterior tendons. Balance activities provide stress to lateral ankle tendons. The Fitter and rolling balance board can also be used for lateral ankle-stressing exercises. Resistive exercises for ankle dorsiflexors and plantar flexors should also be included.

Agility exercises and functional exercises are the same as for other injuries; you should add these to the program once the inflammation is gone and the patient is pain free with activity.

Case Study

A 16-year-old, female cross country runner presents to you with a two-month history of medial ankle pain. She does not remember injuring the ankle. The pain was tolerable, even though it has increased in duration during her workouts, until this past week, when she began increasing the intensity of her workouts in preparation for the start of the cross country competitive season. The pain is now present throughout her workouts and does not go away when she stops running as it had in the past. She has pain if she stands too long and when she walks. She reports that she has been meaning to buy new running shoes because the ones she wears now are worn out, but she thought she would wait until she saw you to ask your advice on what to buy.

Your examination reveals ankle dorsiflexion in subtalar neutral to 0°, plantar flexion to 55°, and inversion-eversion to 30°. The midfoot is loose with the rearfoot locked. In non-weight bearing, the patient has a normal arch, but in weight bearing the navicular is close to the floor and the calcaneus is everted. In walking, the calcaneus never inverts to a vertical position. The patient's shoes are collapsed medially in the heel. Palpation reveals tenderness under the navicular and running along the tibialis posterior tendon posterior and superior to the ankle.

Questions for Analysis

1. What will your first treatment today include?
2. What will you give the patient today for a home program?
3. Do you think she will need orthotics, and if so, why?
4. What will your recommendations be on shoe selection?
5. What are your short-term goals, and what is your best estimate on when to anticipate reaching them?
6. What are your criteria for when to begin strengthening exercises?
7. List three agility exercises you will include when appropriate.
8. What functional activities will you include in the patient's program?
9. What will your criteria be for her return to normal running activities?

SHINSPLINTS

Shinsplints are also known as medial tibial stress syndrome. This is a stress-reaction inflammation of the periosteal and musculotendinous fascial junctions. The pain is located in the middle and distal third of the lower leg. The pain may vary in intensity, from pain that resolves after running to pain that interferes with daily activities.

This condition is usually seen in distance runners and is commonly caused by training errors coupled with improper or poor shoes and a tight Achilles (Kohn 1997). Treatment includes correction of the causes along with reduced activity until symptoms are under control. In addition, modalities should be used to relieve the inflammation. Stretching of the Achilles and other tight structures should be performed throughout the day. Soft-tissue release through deep-tissue massage can be useful in relieving adhesions that occur and that add to the patient's pain.

If shinsplints occur on the lateral lower leg, the cause is usually an overuse inflammatory reaction of the tibialis anterior and extensor digitorum communis, compounded by excessive pronation, hill running, poor shoes, or training errors. This condition is usually relieved with changes in shoes, training methods, and orthotics.

Athletes may experience lateral lower-leg pain at the outset of preseason conditioning if they have not maintained an appropriate activity level up to that time. In these cases, the pain should resolve with time as the patient becomes conditioned. Ice-and-stretch can provide symptomatic relief in the short term. If symptoms continue beyond normal expectations, the patient should be referred to the physician to rule out anterior compartment syndrome.

Case Study

An 18-year-old, male sprinter presents to you with complaints of lateral and anterior lower leg pain that began about one week ago. He has started training for the track season and is distance running to create a cardiovascular base. He reports that he had this pain last year but it went away after a couple of weeks, so he didn't think too much about it; however, this year, his first year as an intercollegiate athlete, the pain seems more intense. He likes the team's shoes, which he started wearing when he began training this year; he had never used the brand before.

Your examination reveals tightness in the Achilles with ankle dorsiflexion to 0°. Hamstring range of motion is 65° in a straight-leg raise. His new shoes have a stiff sole. He is tender to palpation of the tibialis anterior.

Questions for Analysis

1. What will your first treatment today include?

2. What will you give the patient for a home program?

3. What will be your recommendations regarding his shoes?

4. What will be your recommendations regarding his workouts?

5. What are your short-term goals for him?

6. List three exercises you will include in his program.

COMPARTMENT SYNDROMES

There are various degrees of **compartment syndromes**, ranging from slight discomfort to emergency situations. Increased pressure within the lower-leg compartments can be an irritating problem at the least and possibly a dangerous situation.

The four compartments of the lower leg are divided by thick, inelastic fascial coverings. The fascia creates unyielding walls that enclose the muscles in each compartment. If volume changes occur in a compartment, there is no room for expansion, and pressure builds up within the compartment. If pressure persists, a compromise of tissue, vascular, and neural structures can result. Although any of the compartments can experience compartment syndrome, the most commonly affected one is the anterior compartment.

An increase in compartment volume is commonly the result of edema from intense activity or the result of an injury, such as a crush injury or fracture, that causes bleeding and soft-tissue swelling. Activity-induced compartment syndrome is usually chronic, whereas injury-induced compartment syndrome is acute. The acute condition results from an increase in arterial flow from the injury, with a reduction in venous return because of pressure on the vessels, and leads to ischemic pain and tissue death if it persists.

The patient complains of intense pain that is not relieved by any treatment or positioning and of pain with passive plantar flexion. Palpation of the area reveals a hardness and tension of the soft tissues. As the condition advances, the distal pulses are diminished, and neurological changes can be observed.

Because tissue life is being threatened, this is considered a medical emergency and must be referred to the physician immediately. A surgical fasciotomy is usually performed to release the pressure.

In chronic compartment syndrome, the symptoms are different in some ways and similar in others. The patient has recurrent, usually bilateral, lower-leg pain and tightness in the compartment during activity, but the symptoms subside with rest. Edema and tenderness can be palpated, and some patients also experience paresthesia. This occurs because arterial flow from increased muscle activity is greater than the capillary perfusion rate. The local blood flow is restricted—much like cars in a rush-hour traffic jam. Many fast-moving cars are suddenly forced to slow down because the number of vehicles is beyond the capacity of the road to handle them all at one time. Once the number of vehicles on the road decreases, the traffic moves smoothly again.

In some chronic cases, fasciotomy for compartment release can be avoided with conservative treatment. Conservative treatment includes lower-leg-stretching exercises and strengthening exercises for balanced strength among all muscle groups. The patient should work out on softer surfaces and wear running shoes that absorb shock. Orthotics that reduce shock may also be helpful.

Patients who undergo fasciotomy may be placed on crutches, non-weight bearing, for 7 to 10 days. Isometric and active range-of-motion exercises can begin within a week of surgery. Once the wound is healed, aquatic exercises are useful for gaining range of motion and strength. Myofascial release and massage for soft-tissue mobility, joint mobilization if indicated following immobilization, and gait training may all be necessary if the patient shows deficiencies on the initial assessment. Once the patient is fully weight bearing, closed kinetic chain exercises can begin with a progression of the resistive exercises discussed previously. Rubber tubing exercises can be used before full-weight-bearing activities. At four to six weeks, treadmill and stair-climber exercises can begin if the patient has shown strength and flexibility gains.

Return to running activities is commonly slower in posterior compartment releases than in anterior compartment releases. Return to running activities proceeds slowly on the basis of the patient's symptoms and the healing progression. Jogging is the initial speed, which progresses to slow running, then to fast running before return to normal speeds. Initial jogging distances may be no more than 0.8 km (0.5) miles with a gradual progression to 3.2 to 4.8 km (2–3 miles) before the patient has permission to return to former running distances. Running should be on soft, flat surfaces before the patient progresses to hill running.

Case Study

A 16-year-old, female cross country runner fractured her right tibia in a motor-vehicle accident five years ago. The leg was in a cast for two months before the patient underwent a rehabilitation program. One month ago she was competing in a cross country race and began experiencing right shin and foot numbness and burning. After that she continued to experience the same symptoms during her workouts. She underwent an anterior and a posterior compartment release and removal of extensive scar tissue two weeks ago. The surgeon wants her to begin rehabilitation today.

She is partially weight bearing on crutches, but the surgeon has instructed her to ambulate without the crutches in the next couple of days. She admits that she lacks the confidence to get rid of the crutches. Your assessment reveals well-healed surgical scars anteriorly and posteriorly on the lower leg. You note the presence of mild edema and stiffness to passive range of motion, but the patient has no pain. Dorsiflexion is –5°; plantar flexion is 35°. Inversion-eversion is 30°. Palpation reveals mild soft-tissue restriction around the surgical scars and moderate tissue restriction in the calf and anterior lower leg.

Questions for Analysis

1. What are your goals for the patient's first treatment with you today?
2. What modalities will you use, if any, and why?
3. What exercises will you initiate today?
4. What home program and instructions will you give the patient before she leaves today?
5. What are your goals for her for the next two weeks, and how will you attempt to accomplish them?
6. What specific activities will you have the patient perform the first day she is on a treadmill?
7. Outline a progressive running program that you will give the patient when she is ready to begin running.

FOOT INJURIES

A number of common and some unusual foot problems can arise in the athletic population. Some of the more commonly seen conditions are presented here.

Plantar Fasciitis

Of all foot injuries, plantar fasciitis is among the most common in athletics. Its cause can be any number of factors, and you must recognize and correct the cause to correct the problem and reduce the risk of reinjury.

The thick aponeurosis that covers the plantar foot from the calcaneus to the MTP joints is the plantar fascia. It is a thick connective tissue structure that protects the structures in the plantar foot, provides flexibility for shock absorption, and creates a windlass mechanism that transforms the foot into a rigid lever for transferring propulsion forces during push-off. It can become irritated when subjected to abnormal stress, usually during running activities. Patients in any sport involving these activities can be susceptible to plantar fasciitis. High arches and excessive pronation can both be culprits that increase normal stress loads and lead to plantar fasciitis. These inherent structural stresses are usually combined with other factors such as increased workout levels, poor shoes, restricted dorsiflexion from tight Achilles or calf muscles, restricted great-toe dorsiflexion, and workouts on hard surfaces.

The most classic symptom of plantar fasciitis is heel pain with weight bearing when the person arises in the morning, as well as after prolonged sitting, that decreases with continued walking. In more severe cases, pain can occur at rest and extend into the midarch region. The pain is usually unilateral. X rays often reveal a heel spur; however, the source of pain is not the heel spur but the soft tissue that is inflamed because of the irritation and stress it is experiencing. Repetitive stresses applied to the plantar fascia at its origin on the calcaneus commonly result in the development of exostosis at the location where the fascia attaches.

Treatment must include correction of the underlying causes. This frequently involves flexibility exercises for tight structures, proper shoe selection, orthotics if needed to correct abnormal foot structure, changes in conditioning, and changes in workout surfaces. Treatment must also include modalities to relieve the inflammation. Occasionally, the physician may opt for a cortisone injection into the inflamed area. Alternative methods that may provide relief to the inflamed tissues include using a heel cup with strapping techniques, applying a low-dye strapping technique to the arch to reduce the stress on the plantar fascia, putting heel lifts in the shoes to reduce the stress from a tight Achilles tendon, and providing a heel cup to increase calcaneal stability and provide a cushion to the plantar calcaneus. Stretching of the Achilles and calf must be performed soon in the program so that the heel lift can be discarded as soon as possible; prolonged use of the heel lift can encourage tightness and prevent restoration of full motion. Calf stretching must be performed with the ankle in subtalar neutral so that the foot does not collapse and give a false impression of stretching the calf. Stretching of the plantar fascia and great toe can be performed with the ankle in dorsiflexion and the great toe in hyperextension. Massage with golf balls, a rolling pin, or a ribbed can may provide additional relief.

If orthotics seem necessary, before they are provided the sport rehabilitation specialist should attempt temporary orthotic relief to assess whether an orthotic can achieve the desired result. If either a temporary orthotic or a low-dye strapping technique provides significant relief, this is a good indication that a permanent orthotic is needed.

Once the inflammation is under control and flexibility exercises have been provided, the patient should begin strengthening exercises for the ankle inverters and the intrinsic and extrinsic toe flexors. These muscles can assist in supporting the arch and plantar fascia. Marble pickups with deposit into the opposite hand and towel-roll, heel raise, and resisted inversion exercises are all appropriate for plantar fasciitis.

Only in extreme cases will the patient have to refrain from sport participation. Pain is normally the limiting factor; but because the fascia is inflamed, it is susceptible to tears, especially during sudden acceleration or push-off movements. If a rupture of the plantar fascia occurs, pain and swelling will prevent the patient from ambulating normally. A stiff-soled shoe or partial weight bearing on crutches for three to seven days may be necessary. Treatment for a plantar fascia rupture follows a course similar to that for plantar fasciitis. Inflammation control, flexibility exercises, and the usual progression to strengthening, coordination, agility, and functional activities are normal program components.

Case Study

A 19-year-old basketball player has developed right plantar fasciitis over the past month. The pain is present when he gets up in the morning and when he stands after sitting in class for an hour. He is able to perform his workouts without any difficulty, but he has noticed that the pain is worse the morning after a particularly hard workout. Your examination reveals higher-than-normal arches of both feet. Ankle dorsiflexion in subtalar neutral is −5°. Great-toe hyperextension is 50°. There is tenderness to pressure over the plantar medial calcaneus where the plantar fascia inserts. Shoe wear is excessive on the lateral aspect of the shoe.

Questions for Analysis

1. What will your first treatment include?

2. What home exercises will you give the patient before he leaves today?

3. What accommodations will you place in his shoes or on his feet?

4. What strengthening exercises will you give him, and when will you give them?

5. If you decide that the patient needs orthotics, what specifications will you want in them?

Tarsal Tunnel Syndrome

The **tarsal tunnel** is formed by the medial malleolus, calcaneous, talus, and deltoid ligament's posterior aspect. Tarsal tunnel syndrome is an entrapment of the posterior tibial nerve as it passes under the flexor retinaculum posterior to the medial malleolus along with the tendons of the tibialis posterior, flexor digitorum longus, and flexor hallucis longus (figure 20.62). Excessive pronation, especially with improper shoes, can cause increased tension on the flexor retinaculum to increase compression on the nerve. Dancers, especially tap dancers who wear rigid shoes and sustain high-impact forces, are susceptible to tarsal tunnel syndrome. Swelling from trauma or tendinitis can also cause tarsal tunnel syndrome. Symptoms during weight bearing include a burning pain, tingling, and numbness in the medial and plantar foot. Tinel's sign is often positive. Toe flexor and abductor hallucis weakness and decreased ability to plantar flex and invert the foot can be noted in more advanced cases.

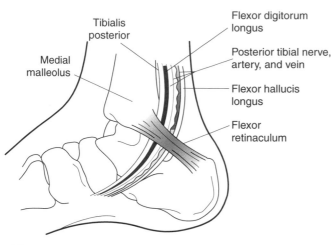

Figure 20.62   Tarsal tunnel.

Only severe cases require cessation of activities or surgery. Most cases can be treated conservatively. Treatment entails orthotics to reduce pronation and reduce posterior tibial nerve irritation, modalities such as phonophoresis or iontophoresis to diminish inflammation, and therapeutic exercises to resolve weakness. Properly fitted shoes and anti-inflammatory medications are also useful. Flexibility exercises and soft-tissue mobilization for release of adhesions can also be beneficial for pain relief. If shoe compression on the medial foot contributes to the problem, use of padding for nerve relief can reduce symptoms.

Cases requiring surgical release of the retinaculum may necessitate either a walking boot or a non-weight-bearing posterior splint for about 2 weeks postoperatively. A normal therapeutic exercise progression is followed by jogging at around 6 to 8 weeks and return to full sport participation at around 10 to 12 weeks following surgery.

Sesamoiditis

The two sesamoids under the first metatarsal head function to enhance the windlass mechanism of the foot for increased propulsion and to disperse the weight-bearing forces. A sesamoiditis does not actually involve the sesamoids but rather the soft tissue surrounding the bones. Restriction of soft tissue around the sesamoids, a tight Achilles tendon, plantar-flexed first ray, reduced great-toe hyperextension motion, and a restricted midfoot are underlying causes of sesamoiditis. Occasionally, cleat misplacement on shoes can increase pressure on the sesamoids and cause soft-tissue inflammation. Hyperextension of 65° is required for walking and running activities. Less hyperextension than that can increase forces imposed on the sesamoid region during propulsion.

The patient complains of pain with running, especially during push-off. The pain is located over the first metatarsal head. Standing heel raises with pressure over the first metatarsal head are painful, as is passive dorsiflexion of the great toe. Palpation reveals tenderness of the sesamoids.

Treatment includes relieving the inflammation and correcting the underlying cause. Flexibility exercises to correct tight structures is vital. Soft-tissue mobilization is usually necessary, because the soft tissue becomes adherent around the sesamoids and further restricts great-toe hyperextension motion. A pad or orthotic with a cutout for the first ray and with an extension pad to the second metatarsal head and toe can help to reduce stress on the sesamoids. Placing the foot in a rigid-soled shoe also limits the stress applied to the sesamoids.

This injury is self-limiting and does not usually require cessation of activity. Modification of shoe wear, correction of the causes, and modifications in activity usually will allow the patient to continue some level of participation.

Turf Toe

Turf toe is a hyperextension injury to the first MTP joint that occurs when the phalanx is jammed into the metatarsal. Improperly fitting shoes and high acceleration forces are common accompanying factors.

Symptoms include tenderness, swelling, and reduced range of motion of the great toe. Rehabilitation includes modalities to reduce the swelling and pain, scar-tissue mobilization, and active range-of-motion exercises. Ankle dorsiflexion with toe flexion-extension can be performed in a whirlpool initially and then in weight bearing as tolerated. Joint mobilizations, initially in grades I and II for pain relief but later in grades III and IV for joint mobility, are included. Strengthening exercises including closed kinetic chain activities and progressing to jumping and plyometric exercises are added as the patient tolerates them.

Shoe fit should be appropriate before the patient is allowed to return to participation. A rigid toe box and plantar-flexion positioning of the first ray with strapping or padding can be useful in reducing pain when the patient returns to the sport.

Case Study

An 18-year-old, male college freshman sprinter had a plantar wart removed from the medial aspect of the ball of his left foot five years ago. Recently the ball of the foot has become progressively painful during running. He does not remember any injury to the foot recently. Your examination reveals an area of swelling with hard scar tissue around the first metatarsal head. His great-toe hyperextension is 45°. He complains of pain when you attempt to hyperextend the toe beyond that point. He is unable to stand on his toes without pain. His ankle dorsiflexion in subtalar neutral is −5°. Mobilization of the sesamoids is difficult, with mobility about 50% compared to that of the right foot. The patient reports pain when you attempt to mobilize the sesamoids with medial-lateral and superior-inferior glides.

Questions for Analysis

1. What is your assessment of the cause of the patient's pain?
2. What will your treatment for him today include?
3. What modifications will you place on his foot or in his shoe that will permit him to continue his workout program?
4. What instructions will you give the patient for his workout tomorrow and for his home program?
5. How will your treatment program change as he improves over the next few weeks?

FRACTURES

The primary concern with a fracture in a young patient is that it may include the growth plates. If this occurs, further development and bone growth can be severely impaired. Stress fractures and acute fractures are more common than one might think. Each is treated differently; programs and considerations related to these fractures are outlined here.

Fractures can occur in any of the lower-leg, ankle, or foot bones. Stress fractures result from repetitive stress to the tibia and metatarsal bones, whereas acute fractures result from sudden application of excessive forces. In younger patients, epiphyseal plate fractures can occur, especially in the distal fibula and tibia. Acute fractures vary greatly in their presentation and according to how the forces are applied. Lateral stresses to the ankle can result in malleolar fractures; compression forces from jumping can cause talus, tibia, and metatarsal fractures; crush injuries from having the foot stepped on can cause metatarsal and phalangeal fractures; other phalangeal fractures can occur as a result of stubbing a toe; and torsional stresses can cause fractures of the tibia and foot.

Phalangeal fractures are painful but seldom casted. The fractured phalanx is commonly buddy taped to an adjacent toe. Metatarsal fractures of the second, third, and fourth metatarsals are commonly placed in a wooden shoe to restrict movement during ambulation. Crutches are sometimes needed if the patient is unable to ambulate normally. Fractures of the first metatarsal require special attention because this is a major weight-bearing bone. Fifth metatarsal fractures also deserve special attention because they can cause problems that linger, depending on the fracture's location. Tarsal fractures can be interarticular and involve interarticular ligamentous damage. If the fracture is displaced, surgery is usually indicated. Ankle fractures are often surgically repaired, because even minimal displacement of fragments produces better results than conservative management (Thigpen 1983). Fractures in young patients should be referred to an orthopedic surgeon because epiphyseal injuries can impair normal bone growth.

Because the tibia, talus, calcaneus, and first ray are the primary weight-bearing structures of the foot and lower leg, fractures to these bones require immobilization and non-weight bearing. The fibula is a non-weight-bearing bone, so walking boots or walking casts are usually used for fractures of this bone. Displaced fractures are surgically repaired whereas nondisplaced fractures may be immobilized with or without surgery.

Immobilization for fractures of the lower leg, ankle, or foot must include immobilization of the ankle. Following immobilization, limited joint mobility is most often the greatest debilitating factor. The greater the damage, the more extensive the scar-tissue formation. The risk of increased formation of scar tissue is greater with a greater and more prolonged presence of edema. Immobilization and soft-tissue edema with subsequent scar-tissue adhesions combine to produce restricted joint mobility of the ankle and surrounding joints. Normal mobility of these joints must be restored to make full balance of function possible. If one joint is restricted, an adjacent joint suffers additional stress as it attempts to compensate for the lost mobility of the restricted joint. Over time, the increased stress can lead to tissue breakdown and injury.

In addition, the immobilization time required for fracture healing leads to capsular restriction, muscle weakness, balance and proprioception loss, and muscle endurance deficits. Joint motion and soft-tissue mobility must be emphasized in early rehabilitation, because the window of opportunity for regaining these elements is narrower than for the other factors. As scar tissue matures, the opportunity to impact changes in its length diminishes. If prolonged immobilization and extensive scar-tissue formation have occurred, prolonged stretches to affect more mature scar tissue may be necessary to increase mobility of shortened tissue or adherent collagen.

The typical duration of immobilization is three to six weeks. This may vary for stress fractures and surgically repaired fractures. Stress fractures are not frequently casted, but activity is reduced to relieve the stress and permit healing to occur. Fractures that undergo ORIF can usually advance to weight bearing sooner than conservatively treated fractures. Patients with fractures that involve the primary weight-bearing bones generally advance to weight bearing with more caution, and full weight bearing is delayed.

Joint mobilization and soft-tissue mobilization techniques are initiated as soon as safely possible. Modalities, such as heat or ultrasound, applied before mobilization techniques can be useful in preparing soft tissue and achieving better treatment results. Massage is useful in relieving edema. Deep-tissue massage, friction massage, and myofascial techniques are used to improve soft-tissue mobility.

Joint mobilization techniques for pain relief and joint mobility are often used in combination, beginning and ending with grade II mobilizations for pain relief. If a joint is very tender, grade III and IV techniques may not be possible until pain is under control. Active stretches, passive stretches, and contract-relax-stretch techniques are useful in increasing motion of both joint and soft-tissue structures.

Immobilization and periods of altered weight bearing necessitate gait-training instructions once the patient is able to resume full weight bearing. During partial weight bearing it is important to instruct the patient in a normal heel-toe gait to encourage proper gait patterning in preparation for full weight bearing. Once the patient is permitted to bear full weight on the extremity, pre-gait instruction, including weight-transfer activities and normal stride re-education, is usually needed.

Closed kinetic chain exercises for strengthening, as well as static balance activities such as stork standing, can begin when full weight bearing is permitted. Therapeutic exercises proceed in the manner discussed earlier in this chapter. Advancement follows a logical progression from light to heavier weights, reduced to increased repetitions, static to dynamic balance and agility exercises, and simple to complex activities until the patient advances to plyometric exercises and finally to functional activities before returning to full activity.

The rate of progression is determined by the tissue-healing time line, the tissue's response to stresses, and the individual's ability to tolerate the therapeutic exercise progression. Functional testing before return to sport participation must mimic demands that the patient will encounter during his or her sport performance. Once all the parameters are improved and the patient passes all the functional tests, without any difference in performance from left to right lower extremity, he or she may resume full sport participation. Depending on the extent of the injury, the time of immobilization, the age of the patient, and initial joint and soft-tissue restriction following immobilization, three to six months is considered a reasonable amount of time before the patient is able to resume sport participation.

Case Study

A 16-year-old wrestler sustained a left ankle lateral malleolar fracture during a wrestling match. He underwent an ORIF the following day and was placed on crutches, non-weight bearing for two weeks before advancing to partial weight bearing. It is now four weeks after the surgery and the patient is not yet full weight bearing, although the surgeon has instructed him to begin weight bearing to tolerance and to advance to weight bearing without the crutches. The patient admits to you that he is apprehensive about putting weight on the leg for fear of breaking it again. The lower leg had been placed in a cast following surgery until yesterday, when it was removed.

On examination, the patient's ankle has $-10°$ dorsiflexion, $30°$ plantar flexion, $0°$ eversion, and $5°$ inversion. Ankle strength in these directions is 2+/5 in the available ranges of motion. His hip and knee ranges of motion are normal, but strength is 4–/5 for all of the muscle groups. The surgical scar is well healed, but sloughing skin is present around the ankle and there are dry scabs over the wound. Palpation reveals stiffness of soft tissue around the ankle and into the foot. The foot is mildly enlarged, but there is no pitting edema. Joint mobility of the ankle joints is restricted to no more than 30% of normal, and the intertarsal and metatarsal joints are restricted to 50% normal mobility.

Questions for Analysis

1. What are your goals for today's treatment session?

2. What home program will you send with the patient today?

3. The patient wants to attend a wrestling camp in 10 weeks; what will you tell him when he asks whether he will be able to attend the camp?

4. List your long- and short-term goals for the patient for the next six weeks.

5. What will be your criteria for advancing him to closed kinetic chain exercises?

6. List three closed kinetic exercises that you will give the patient the first day these types of exercises are in his program.

7. List three non-weight-bearing exercises that you will give him in the next week.

8. List three agility exercises you will use in the patient's program and the criteria he must meet before they are used.

SUMMARY

1. *Discuss normal foot mechanics in ambulation.*

   The first structure to hit the ground during ambulation is the calcaneus. It, along with the talus, forms the subtalar joint; and the talus, along with the tibia and fibula, forms the talocrural joint. Normal function of these two joints permits us to land the foot on the ground and adapt to variations in ground topography and stresses while maintaining a steady gait. The talocrural joint moves primarily in dorsiflexion and plantar flexion. The subtalar joint is responsible for pronation and supination. Pronation and its component motions cause the foot to convert to a mobile adapter for accommodation to uneven surfaces. Supination causes the foot articulations to become more rigid and provide for power transfer to permit appropriate force distribution needed for propulsion in ambulation. As the ankle goes into plantar flexion, the talus moves anteriorly so that the posterior, narrower aspect of the talus sits in the mortise joint. During dorsiflexion, the fibula glides superiorly and rotates laterally; and in plantar flexion, it moves inferiorly and rotates medially. In addition to the talocrural and subtalar joints, the more distal tarsal bones of the foot form the midtarsal joint. This joint's movements closely follow the subtalar and talocrural joint movements. During supination, the navicular and cuboid bones move medially and inferiorly; during pronation they move laterally and superiorly. The first-ray movement occurs in plantar flexion and dorsiflexion and is equal in each direction, with each equal to about a thumb's width of motion. The second ray includes the joint between the second metatarsal and middle cuneiform; the third ray includes the third metatarsal and the lateral cuneiform; the fourth ray is the fourth metatarsal alone; and the fifth ray is the fifth metatarsal alone. Metatarsophalangeal joints permit flexion-extension, abduction-adduction, and accessory rotation and dorsal-plantar glides. The IP joints, which are hinge joints, permit flexion and extension with accessory rotation and dorsal-plantar glides. The first MTP joint must have about 60° to 65° of hyperextension for toe roll-off during gait.

2. *Identify two foot deformities and discuss their impact on athletic injury.*

   Pes cavus, a rigid foot, makes force absorption of the foot more limited, causing forces to be absorbed farther up the closed chain and thus risking injury to other structures. Pes planus, or flatfoot, causes the foot to move inefficiently, requiring more effort from, and subsequently applying more stress to, other structures. It also changes the mechanics of the lower leg, increasing stresses applied to structures such as the Achilles, patella, and hip.

3. *Describe the primary structures of a shoe.*

   A shoe's main components include an upper and a lower section. The upper section includes the vamp, toe box, saddle, collar, insole board, sock liner, and heel counter. The lower section includes the outsole, wedge, and midsole. The vamp covers the toes and forefoot and includes the toe box. The toe box varies in width and height and functions to retain the shape of the shoe's forefoot and provide room for the toes. The saddle is the midsection of the shoe along the longitudinal arch, which is usually reinforced to assist in supporting the midfoot. The heel counter is an important stabilizer for the rearfoot. A foxing is an additional piece often seen in athletic shoes that further reinforces the rearfoot to assist in maintaining the counter's shape. The medial aspect of the counter is sometimes extended forward to resist pronation. The collar, the top rim of the shoe, is often padded to reduce friction on the Achilles. The insole board lies between the upper and lower segments and serves as the attachment for the two segments. A sock liner on top of the insole board is used for shock absorption and friction reduction for the foot.

4. *List the important factors in shoe considerations for a pes cavus foot.*

   Because a pes cavus foot is rigid and has limited stress-absorption capabilities, a shoe for someone with this deformity should have as much force absorption as possible. Factors such as a soft midsole, a curved last, and flexibility should be standards in a shoe for a rigid foot.

5. *Outline key factors in an orthotic evaluation.*

   (1) The patient's height and weight; (2) type of sport and activity level of the patient; (3) medical history; (4) the patient's primary and secondary complaints; (5) the calcaneal position in relaxed standing and in subtalar neutral standing; (6) the appearance of the arches in weight bearing and non-weight bearing; (7) toe positions; (8) knee positions; (9) tibial varum; (10) first-ray positions; (11) subtalar mobility; (12) midtarsal mobility; (13) first-metatarsal mobility; (14) hallux dorsiflexion; (15) ankle dorsiflexion; and (16) location of corns and calluses. This last factor is important because corns and calluses are indicators of accommodating or non-accommodating forefoot and rearfoot deformities.

6. *Explain one joint mobilization technique for improving ankle dorsiflexion.*

   A dorsal glide can be used: The stabilizing hand is placed anteriorly around the distal lower leg, and the mobilizing hand is placed around the proximal foot with the thumb and index finger in contact with the malleoli. The talus is glided posteriorly in the plane of the joint.

7. *List three stretching exercises for the ankle and lower leg, including one that is not mentioned in the text.*

   Some stretches for these structures are the standing gastrocnemius stretch, the seated soleus stretch with a strap, and standing sideways on an incline board with the ankle positioned in inversion.

8. *Identify three strengthening exercises for the ankle and lower leg.*

   Exercises for strengthening the ankle and lower leg include calf raises, toe raises, and eversion in side-lying with a weight attached to the ankle.

9. *Explain three agility exercises.*

For agility the patient can do lateral jumps, zigzag runs, and rapid change-of-direction maneuvers performed on command.

10. *Describe three functional exercises for the lower extremity.*

Some functional exercises for the lower extremity are side-to-side sprints; run, stop and jump exercises; and running and stopping while bouncing a basketball.

11. *Provide an example of a therapeutic exercise program progression for an ankle sprain.*

Initial treatment includes modalities for edema and pain relief and reduction of inflammation. Joint mobilization and soft-tissue mobilization may be necessary if those structures are impaired in their normal movement. Active and passive range-of-motion exercises are accompanied by mild strengthening exercises, such as isometrics, manual resistance, and rubber band exercises. If the patient has been non-weight bearing, it may be necessary to use exercises with a weight scale to reintroduce the concept of weight bearing on the extremity as a prelude to gait training. Body-weight resistance exercises and machine-weight resistance exercises are then included. Balance and proprioception exercises begin with simple stork standing and progress to standing on unstable surfaces, then moving on one leg. Once strength, flexibility, and balance are restored, plyometric and then functional activities are used before return to participation.

CRITICAL THINKING QUESTIONS

1. Explain how Bob concluded that Troy's plantar fasciitis was being caused by his pronation, hip tightness, and knee and tibial malalignments. Why would he suspect that Troy's thigh muscle imbalance was also contributing to the plantar fasciitis? What shoe characteristics should Troy look for when he buys his next running shoes?

2. If a patient had a leg-length discrepancy but no other major structural problems, would you expect to see an abnormal wear pattern on the bottom of his or her shoes? If so, what?

3. Using the repaired-Achilles case study (pp. 819–820) what would you include in an aquatic exercise program for this patient for range of motion, strength, and cardio-vascular conditioning? When could you begin his aquatic program?

REFERENCES

Baumhauer, J., Shereff, M., and J. Gould. 1997. Ankle pain in runners. In *Running injuries*, ed. G.N. Guten. Philadelphia: Saunders.

Bernier, J.N., and D.H. Perrin. 1998. Effect of coordination training on proprioception of the functionally unstable ankle. *Journal of Orthopaedic and Sports Physical Therapy* 27:264–275.

Bolgla, L.A., and D.R. Keskula. 1997. Reliability of lower extremity functional performance tests. *Journal of Orthopaedic and Sports Physical Therapy* 26:138–142.

Cipriani, D.J., Armstrong, C.W., and S. Gaul. 1995. Backward walking at three levels of treadmill inclination: An electromyographic and kinematic analysis. *Journal of Orthopaedic and Sports Physical Therapy* 22:95–102.

Curwin, S., and W. Stanish. 1984. *Tendinitis: Its etiology and treatment.* Lexington, MA: Heath.

Denegar, C. 2000. *Therapeutic modalities for athletic injuries.* Champaign, IL: Human Kinetics.

Forkin, D.M., Koczur, C., Battle, R., and R.A. Newton. 1996. Evaluation of kinesthetic deficits indicative of balance control in gymnasts with unilateral chronic ankle sprains. *Journal of Orthopaedic and Sports Physical Therapy* 23:245–250.

Garn, S.N., and R.A. Newton. 1988. Kinesthetic awareness in subjects with multiple ankle sprains. *Physical Therapy* 68:1667–1671.

Glascoe, W.M., Allen, M.K., Awtry, B.F., and H.J. Yack. 1999. Weight-bearing immobilization and early exercise treatment following a grade II lateral ankle sprain. *Journal of Orthopaedic and Sports Physical Therapy* 29:394–399.

Gross, M.T., Bradshaw, M.K., Ventry, L.C., and K.H. Weller. 1987. Comparison of support provided by ankle taping and semirigid orthosis. *Journal of Orthopaedic and Sports Physical Therapy* 9:33–39.

Kimura, I.F., Nawoczenski, D.A., Epler, M., and M.G. Owen. 1987. Effect of the AirStirrup in controlling ankle inversion stress. *Journal of Orthopaedic and Sports Physical Therapy* 9:190–193.

Klingman, R.E., Liaos, S.M., and K.M. Hardin. 1997. The effect of subtalar joint posting on patellar glide position in subjects with excessive rearfoot pronation. *Journal of Orthopaedic and Sports Physical Therapy* 25:185–191.

Kohn, H.S. 1997. Shin pain and compartment syndromes in running. In *Running injuries*, ed. G.N. Guten. Philadelphia: Saunders.

Konradsen, L., Holmer, P., and Sondergaard, L. 1991. Early mobilizing treatment for grade III ankle ligament injuries. *Foot & Ankle* 12:69–73.

Lattanza, L., Gray, G.W., and R.M. Kantner. 1988. Closed versus open kinetic chain measurements of subtalar joint eversion: Implications for clinical practice. *Journal of Orthopaedic and Sports Physical Therapy* 9:310–314.

Leanderson, J., Eriksson, E., Nilsson, C., and A. Wykman. 1996. Proprioception in classical ballet dancers. *American Journal of Sports Medicine* 24:370–374.

Lofvenberg, R., Karrholm, J., Sundelin, G., and O. Ahlgren. 1995. Prolonged reaction time in patients with chronic lateral instability of the ankle. *American Journal of Sports Medicine* 23:414–417.

Maitland, G.D. 1991. *Peripheral manipulation.* Boston; London: Butterworth-Heinemann.

Massie, D.L., and J.C. Spiker. 1990. *Foot biomechanics and the relationship to rehabilitation of lower extremity injuries.* Berryville, VA: Forum Medicum.

Powers, C.M., Maffucci, R., and S. Hampton. 1995. Rearfoot posture in subjects with patellofemoral pain. *Journal of Orthopaedic and Sports Physical Therapy* 22:155–160.

Rovere, G.D., Clarke, T.J., Yates, C.S., and K. Burley. 1988. Retrospective comparison of taping and ankle stabilizers in preventing ankle injuries. *American Journal of Sports Medicine* 16:228–233.

Seto, J.L., and C.E. Brewster. 1994. Treatment approaches following foot and ankle injury. *Clinics in Sports Medicine* 13:695–719.

Sitler, M., Ryan, J., Wheeler, B., McBride, J., Arciero, R., Anderson, J., and M.B. Horodyski. 1994. The efficacy of a semirigid ankle stabilizer to reduce acute ankle injuries in basketball. *American Journal of Sports Medicine* 22:454–461.

Thigpen, C.M. 1983. Early management of fractures of the foot and ankle. *Current concepts in trauma care* 6:4–8.

Tiberio, D. 1987. The effect of excessive subtalar joint pronation on patellofemoral mechanics: A theoretical model. *Journal of Orthopaedic and Sports Physical Therapy* 9:160–165.

Travell, J.G., and D.G. Simons. 1992. *Myofascial pain and dysfunction. The trigger point manual.* Vol. 2. Baltimore: Williams & Wilkins.

SUGGESTED READING

Batt, M.E. 1995. Shin splints—a review of terminology. *Clinical Journal of Sports Medicine* 5:53–57.

Janisse, D.J. 1994. Indications and prescriptions for orthoses in sports. *Orthopedic Clinics of North America* 25:95–107.

Loudin, J.K., and S.L. Bell. 1996. The foot and ankle: An overview of arthrokinematics and selected joint techniques. *Journal of Athletic Training* 31:173–178.

Mascaro, T.B., and L.E. Swanson. 1994. Rehabilitation of the foot and ankle. *Orthopedic Clinics of North America* 25:147–160.

McPoil, T.G. 1988. Footwear. *Physical Therapy* 68:1857–1865.

Reynolds, N.L., and T.W. Worrell. 1991. Chronic Achilles peritendinitis: Etiology, pathophysiology, and treatment. *Journal of Orthopaedic and Sports Physical Therapy* 13:171–176.

CHAPTER TWENTY-ONE

Knee and Thigh

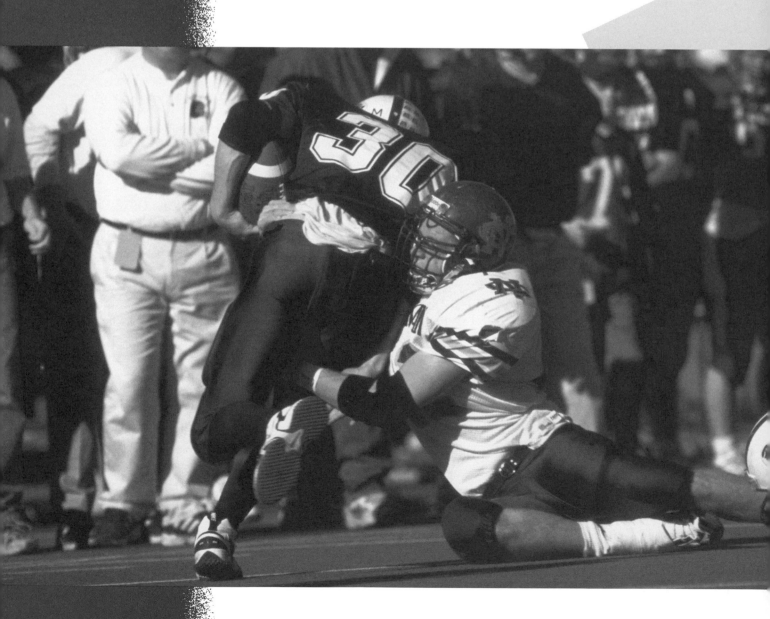

OBJECTIVES

After completing this chapter, you should be able to do the following:

1. Discuss the relationship and alignment between the patella and femur.

2. Identify postinjury factors that influence strength output.

3. Define quadriceps extensor lag and explain its significance.

4. Outline a general progression of rehabilitation for a knee.

5. Identify three soft-tissue mobilization techniques for the knee.

6. Identify three joint mobilization techniques for the knee, and their purpose.

7. Explain three flexibility exercises for the knee, and identify the structures they affect.

8. Explain three proprioception/balance exercises for the knee.

9. Identify three functional activities.

10. Identify three factors that influence PFD.

Three mornings a week Cory and his friends play a game of basketball at the university gym before going to work. It was their way of having fun and getting exercise at the same time. They have been following this routine since they were in their mid-30s, about 10 years ago.

About two weeks ago their routine was suddenly disrupted. Cory jumped to retrieve a rebound and landed in severe pain. He felt as if someone had shot him in the thigh. Several hours later he underwent a quadriceps tendon repair and was placed on crutches. Today he had his first rehabilitation appointment with Susan Scott.

After Susan completed her evaluation, she explained to Cory what she saw as primary problems and discussed how she thought they could best resolve those problems. Cory agreed with her and realized that this was not going to be an easy or short process, but he was willing to work with her to get back onto the basketball court. He liked Susan's approach and appreciated the way she was able to explain things better than the doctor did, so he could understand them. He knew she would work him hard; but he also knew that if he wanted to play basketball again, he would have to work hard, and he was eager to start.

Although Susan explained to Cory that it would not be an easy process and would require him to be committed and consistent in his approach to his rehabilitation, she also knew that the tissue's healing process had to be respected. Because it was only two weeks since he had had the surgery, stress to the newly formed tissue was important, but too much stress could be detrimental. The proper amount of stress to the patellar tendon was important, but she could also start Cory with more aggressive exercises on the hip and ankle and not stress the patellar tendon. She sensed that Cory was the type of person who was eager and willing to work hard but would also understand precautions if he knew about them. As with all her patients, she would keep him well informed throughout his program about what he should and should not be doing and why.

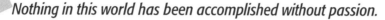

Nothing in this world has been accomplished without passion.

George W. Hegel, German philosopher, 1770–1831

Passion and a quest for understanding drive the accumulation of knowledge that makes us all better sport rehabilitation specialists. Perhaps one of the most passionately pursued orthopedic topics is the knee. A tremendous amount of research has provided us with a wealth of knowledge on the knee. There is still a plethora of information to be gleaned about the knee; but in the past several years, investigators have given us new insights and information regarding knee biomechanics, improved surgical procedures, and optimal rehabilitation techniques.

This chapter deals with thigh and knee injuries. Thigh injuries could just as easily have been considered along with the hip in the next chapter. Indeed, I will refer you from one chapter to the other, because there is an intimate relationship between the thigh and knee and the thigh and hip. I have placed most thigh injuries in this chapter because the knee comes before the hip in the text, and it will be easier for you to understand this and the next chapter if you receive information about therapeutic exercise programs for the thigh here. Thigh injuries that impact primarily the hip are presented in chapter 22.

As with the other chapters in part IV, this one begins with general information that impacts therapeutic exercise programs for knee and thigh injuries. This information is vital if the sport rehabilitation specialist is to design and establish an appropriate therapeutic exercise program for the various injuries of the knee and thigh. This chapter presents specific therapeutic exercise techniques, including soft-tissue and joint mobilization and exercises for flexibility, strength, and coordination. Recommendations for functional activities before the patient's return to full sport participation are also included. The final section of the chapter discusses rehabilitation programs for specific injuries commonly seen in the knee and thigh.

Controversy continues on the best surgical repair technique and the most appropriate postoperative and postinjury methods of rehabilitation for the knee. Over the past several years, treatment of knee injuries and postoperative care have changed dramatically. The trend has shifted from conservative care, including cast immobilization and non-weight bearing for six weeks following surgery or serious injury, to weight bearing to tolerance with hinged-splint immobilization. Although cast immobilization is rare today, many surgeons choose to remain conservative while others prefer a more accelerated approach. It is important for the sport rehabilitation specialist to work with the physician to provide a successful rehabilitation outcome for the patient. Both the physician's and the sport rehabilitation specialist's protocols for rehabilitation of knee and thigh injuries should be based on the severity of the injury, the structure injured, and the tissue healing time line. If there is to be an error, as with any rehabilitation program, it should be on the side of caution. Knowledge of these factors, common sense, keen observation skills, and good judgment are essential to the sport rehabilitation specialist if proper guidance and execution of a patient's therapeutic exercise program are to lead to a successful end.

GENERAL REHABILITATION CONSIDERATIONS

The knee encompasses two major joints, the tibiofemoral joint and the patellofemoral joint. The knee also contains a joint capsule, ligaments, menisci, and muscles. A therapeutic exercise program must take into account the knee's unique structure, as well as a number of biomechanical and physiological characteristics specific to the knee.

The knee is one of the most frequently injured joints in athletics. The forces applied to it during running, twisting, and impact in sport activities are complicated by the fact that there are two long lever arms on either end of the joint, making it a joint that is susceptible to injury-causing stresses. For as shallow a joint as the knee is, complete dislocation is surprisingly rare. This may be so because of the strong static and dynamic structures that surround the joint. The ligaments and muscles of the knee give the joint a sound structure that requires tremendous forces to produce an injury. The more common knee injuries seen in athletics are discussed later in this chapter. This section deals with the structures unique to the knee that serve to support and protect the joint but are impacted when injury occurs.

KNEE STRUCTURE

Although at first glance the knee appears to be a relatively simple joint, it is actually a complex structure involving several factors that influence its function. When balance is lacking in structure or function, the knee becomes susceptible to injury. An understanding of the knee's structures and the ways they influence one another is basic to the ability to develop a therapeutic exercise program for any injury of the knee.

Tibiofemoral Joint

The knee joint is actually two joints, the tibiofemoral joint and the patellofemoral joint. The tibiofemoral joint has a concave tibia platform attached to a convex humerus. This means that during joint mobilization, the concave tibia moves on the convex femur in the same direction as the physiological movement of the joint. In other words, a posterior glide produces flexion and an anterior glide produces extension.

Capsule

The knee joint is the largest joint of the body and is surrounded by a capsule that aids in joint stability by merging with the collateral ligaments. The capsule also distributes the synovial fluid around the joint during movement and merges with many of the knee's bursae. If the joint capsule is restricted, a capsular pattern becomes apparent. The knee's capsular pattern is restriction of flexion more than of extension. The joint is in a loose-packed position when it is in about 20° to 25° of flexion and in a fully close-packed position in full extension with external tibial rotation.

Ligaments

The collateral ligaments provide for protection and stability of medial and lateral or valgus and varus stress. The medial collateral ligament (MCL) is attached to the medial meniscus. This arrangement may be one reason the medial meniscus is often injured with MCL sprains. In addition to providing protection against valgus stresses, it helps to restrict external rotation of the tibia on the femur. The lateral collateral ligament (LCL) is not attached to the lateral meniscus and is taut during internal rotation of the tibia on the femur, and also when the knee incurs varus stress. Because valgus stress from lateral forces is more frequently applied to the knee than varus stresses, the MCL is the more frequently injured of these two ligaments.

The anterior and posterior cruciate ligaments (ACL and PCL, respectively) are structures unique to the knee. Their position within the knee joint allows them to provide distinctive anterior-posterior stability to the knee. The ligaments also provide the knee with rotational stability. Fibers of each ligament are taut throughout the knee's range of motion. Injury to either ligament can cause instability within the knee that can be disabling to an athlete.

The ACL and PCL are enclosed within a synovial membrane that provides the ligaments with their primary blood supply. If a partial tear of either ligament occurs, the synovial membrane can become disrupted as well, compromising the ligament's vascular supply. If this happens, dehiscence or erosion of the ligament can eventually result.

The ACL is the most commonly injured knee ligament. It protects the knee from anterior translation of the tibia on the femur. The PCL is not as frequently injured because it is much stronger. It serves primarily to restrict knee hyperextension and posterior tibial displacement of the tibia on the femur.

Rotational stresses at the knee are restrained by all the ligaments. The cruciate ligaments twist and become taut during internal rotation. The collateral ligaments become taut to provide stability during external rotation. Rotation is a primary motion of the knee in both weight bearing and non-weight bearing. In weight bearing the femur rotates on the tibia, and in non-weight bearing the tibia rotates on the femur. Injury mechanisms that produce excessive rotational forces can cause damage to more than one ligament and can result in joint instability.

The knee's joint capsule and intra-articular structures, including the ACL, contain various neuroreceptors that provide the neural system with position-afferent information from the knee. We know that the ACL contains afferent mechanoreceptors that impact the knee's stability. The joint capsule has mechanoreceptors (Ruffini endings) that are sensitive to pressure and deformation (Freeman and Wyke 1967). Injury to the knee's ligamentous structures can damage these receptors, impairing proprioception. Therapeutic exercise programs must include proprioception facilitative techniques to restore the deficiencies resulting from interarticular knee injuries.

Although each ligament has its own responsibility in supporting and protecting the knee, ligaments also provide assistive support to other ligaments. These protective designs are referred to as *primary* and *secondary restraint*. As an example, the ACL is the primary restraint protecting the knee against tibial anterior translation; but if it is injured, other structures such as the capsule, other ligaments, and dynamic structures act as secondary restraints to continue to protect the joint. Sometimes the secondary structures are able to assume the responsibilities of providing normal stability to the joint and sometimes they fall short. Instability caused by ACL or PCL insufficiencies is often minimally supported by secondary structures (Butler, Noyes, and Grood 1980).

Meniscus

The medial and lateral meniscus serve to cushion the joint, deepen the socket, increase joint congruity to better distribute weight-bearing forces, assist in joint lubrication, and provide stability. These structures are commonly referred to as cartilage, although this is a misnomer. These structures are primarily fibrocartilage (hence the name), but this is certainly not their only component. The knee joint also has articular cartilage, so the term "cartilage" is not only erroneous but sometimes confusing, especially to the athlete who has injured articular cartilage, not meniscus. Of the two menisci, the medial meniscus is the more frequently injured. It is attached to the MCL, the ACL, and the semimembranosus. This arrangement is believed to be one cause for the greater frequency of injury to the medial meniscus. Even though the lateral meniscus is not attached to the LCL but does connect to the popliteus and PCL, it has more freedom of movement and is not impacted by collateral ligament positioning and stresses.

When the knee moves sagittally in flexion and extension, the menisci follow the tibial movements. During flexion the menisci are pulled posteriorly via the semimembranosus and popliteus, and during extension they are pulled anteriorly by the meniscopatellar ligaments. During rotation the menisci follow the movements of the femur. When the knee moves from extension to flexion, the femur slides posteriorly on the tibia so that in a squat or flexed position, the weight is borne primarily by the posterior aspect of the menisci, whereas in extension the femur is primarily on the anterior menisci. Compressive forces absorbed by the menisci are up to 50% to 60% of the knee's loads. When the knee is at 90° flexion and the primary force is applied at the posterior aspect of the joint, the meniscal load increases to 85% of the total knee joint compressive forces (Ahmed and Burke 1983). Meniscal posterior horn tears seem to be primarily degenerative tears, whereas anterior horn and lateral tears are often traumatic events. Posterior degenerative tears may be related to the increased forces absorbed by the menisci in flexion, as well as to the repetitive activity imposed on the menisci during squatting and other positional activities. On the other hand, acute tears occur most often during a running or cutting maneuver, when the knee is near extension.

The menisci are avascular except for roughly their peripheral 25%. This has a significant impact on conservative and surgical intervention following injury of the meniscus. This topic is discussed later in the chapter.

Screw Home Mechanism

The knee joint is a modified hinge joint. This means that although it is similar to a hinge joint, permitting movement in one plane, the bony segments are not entirely and purely congruent throughout. Because the medial aspect of the joint is larger and extends slightly more distally than the lateral side, when the knee moves into extension during weight bearing the tibia rotates laterally as the medial femoral condyle rotates on the medial tibial plateau. This mechanism, called the screw home mechanism, occurs in the last 30° of extension. It affords the joint greater stability than a pure hinge-joint arrangement would because it provides a kind of locking. The popliteus is responsible for unlocking the knee during movement from full extension into flexion. It does this by laterally rotating the femoral condyles with its medial tibial insertion anchored in weight bearing. In non-weight bearing, the popliteus unlocks the knee as it medially rotates the tibia with its proximal insertion stabilized.

Patellofemoral Joint

The patella, the largest sesamoid bone in the body, sits within the femoral groove. Its loose-packed position is knee extension, and its close-packed position is knee flexion. The patella serves to increase the lever-arm length of the quadriceps tendon, adds to the cosmesis of the knee joint, and protects the knee from anterior blows. It is a site of common knee pain and dysfunction.

The patella is surrounded by the quadriceps tendon and its medial and lateral expansions. The tendon attachment from the patella to the tibial tubercle is sometimes referred to as the patellar ligament because it travels from bone to bone. This structure is also called the patellar tendon.

Patellar stability is the result of static and dynamic structures. The greatest bony contributor to patellar stability is the femoral sulcus formed by the medial and higher-ridged lateral epicondyles within which the patella sits. Ligamentous stability from the patellofemoral and patellotibial joints assists in providing static restraints. Active restraints from the quadriceps provide the greatest dynamic stability. Indirect secondary dynamic support is provided by the pes anserine group and the biceps femoris with their control of tibial rotation. Tibial rotation changes the tibial tubercle position and can alter stability provided by the patellar tendon.

Patellar alignment is assessed in static and dynamic positions. The patella is assessed in long sitting for abnormalities in resting. Position of the patella during contraction of the quadriceps in long sitting and in weight bearing is also assessed, because patellar movement in open and closed kinetic chain conditions may be different. A closed kinetic chain position can change the patellar alignment because other factors, such as hip rotation and foot pronation, alter the way the patella moves when the quadriceps contract.

Superior Tibiofibular Joint

This joint is not actually a joint of the knee because it is distal to the knee joint, but it can impact the ankle and knee joints. There are no physiological movements in this joint, but it must have full accessory motion for full ankle range of motion to occur. Reduced tibiofibulor joint mobility can cause lateral knee pain by restricting soft-tissue mobility in the region.

Muscles

The quadriceps and hamstrings have been the most widely addressed muscles because of their prominence in knee control. Both groups also impact the hip, and because they do, positioning of the hip must always be a consideration when one is exercising the muscles at the knee.

The quadriceps provide the most dynamic restraint for the knee. The rectus femoris is the quadricep component that also assists in hip flexion. Hip positioning determines where in the motion the rectus femoris is most contributory at the knee. In supine straight-leg raising, it works throughout the motion; but in sitting, it works only in terminal extension (Close 1964).

Because of the angle of their pull and tendon insertions, the hamstrings also produce tibial rotation. The biceps femoris produces tibial lateral rotation, and the semimembranosus and semitendinosus produce tibial medial rotation. They provide dynamic secondary restraints to assist the ACL, and in ACL-deficient knees they must be trained to become more prominent stabilizers.

Rehabilitation of isolated hamstring muscles should include the additional movements of rotation along with hip extension and knee flexion. Eccentric and concentric activities for all motions would most appropriately strengthen the hamstrings throughout all their functions.

BIOMECHANICAL AND PHYSIOLOGICAL CONCEPTS

An appreciation of biomechanical and physiological concepts helps the sport rehabilitation specialist understand the significance of specific therapeutic exercise applications for various knee injuries, as well as the indications and precautions.

Patellofemoral and Tibiofemoral Relationship

When the knee extends, the patella glides superiorly and inferiorly during knee flexion for a total excursion of 5 to 7 cm (2.0–2.8 in.). The patella must glide freely for full knee motion to be possible.

In a normal knee, the patella's inferior pole is at the knee joint's margin and rests on the supratrochlear fat pad. A patella that lies superior to this position is called **patella alta,** and one that is inferior to the normal position is called **patella baja.** Either position restricts full range of motion of the knee. Injuries of the patellor tendon, including ACL reconstructions utilizing the quadriceps tendon, may develop patella baja. Injuries such as repaired quadriceps ruptures are susceptible to developing patella alta. Patella baja or alta requires aggressive patellar mobilization and soft-tissue-stretching techniques. These techniques are discussed in detail later.

The patella glides in the femoral groove and makes contact with the femoral groove. When contact between the two segments is made, compressive forces are applied to the posterior patella. These compressive loads can reach up to 10 times body weight during daily activities (Brownstein et al. 1988). In full extension, the patella rests on the fat pad and is not in contact with the sulcus. The area of contact between the posterior patella and femoral groove migrates from the inferior pole to the superior aspect as the knee moves from about 10° to 20° of flexion to 90°. The area of contact is fairly uniform across the breadth of the patella. Once the knee approaches the end of flexion, however, the contact is on the odd facet medially and the lateral-superior aspect of the patella until the patella rests on the top of the lateral condyle in full flexion (figure 21.1).

Of significance with this change in points of contact between the patella and femur is the fact that as the knee moves into flexion, the amount of contact pressure and area of contact both increase. **Contact pressure** is a ratio between the patellofemoral joint reaction force and the contact area. **Joint reaction force** is a compressive force equivalent to the resultant vector force (of the patellofemoral quadriceps and patellar tendon forces) that is perpendicular to the patellar contact surface. Stress to the patellofemoral joint is the force per area of contact. In a closed kinetic chain activity, the joint reaction forces and the area of contact both increase as the knee moves from extension to 90°; but the force applied is greater than the area of contact, so joint stress increases as the knee moves into flexion to 90°. As the knee moves from 90° toward 120°, the force decreases and the surface area of contact remains the same, so the stress decreases. The greatest compressive forces occur in the 60° to 90° positions (Huberti and Hayes 1984; Steinkamp et al. 1993). If a patella is not in good alignment within the femoral groove, the congruency between the two bones is altered, so compressive forces are distributed over a smaller area. This may be one reason why malalignment of the patella results in increased pain and irritation of the patellofemoral joint.

In an open kinetic chain activity, the joint stress is lowest at 90° and greatest at 0°. Although there may be some individual variations, open kinetic chain exercises are least irritating when performed from 60° to 90°, while closed kinetic chain exercises cause the least patellofemoral joint irritation in the ranges of 0° to 30° and greater than 90° (Grelsamer and Klein 1998).

During closed kinetic chain activities such as walking, patellofemoral compressive forces of about one-half body weight are produced, while stair climbing produces about three times body weight and squatting produces compressive forces of over seven times body weight (Reilly and Martens 1972). During open kinetic chain activities the amount of compressive force changes with the type of activity and the angle at which it occurs. If knee extension is performed with a weight attached to the

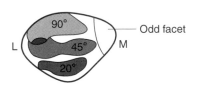

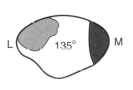

■ **Figure 21.1**
Patellofemoral contact patterns.

From Goodfellow, Hungerford, and Zindel 1976.

end of the extremity, compressive forces reach their peak at 35° to 40°; but if the force is applied by a machine arm at right angles to the ankle such as in an N-K table or isokinetic machine, the peak compressive forces occur at 90° and decrease as the knee extends (Reilly and Martens 1972). On the basis of mathematical formulas, it has been estimated that isokinetic exercises reach a peak patellofemoral compressive force of about five times body weight (Kaufman et al. 1991).

Many functional activities are performed in the 0° to 40° range of motion. It is important when you are treating patients with patellofemoral pain to avoid painful arcs of motion. As a general rule, closed kinetic chain exercises from 0° to 30° flexion provide less lateral patellar motion and less patellofemoral stress than open kinetic chain exercises, and open chain exercises in positions greater than 50° flexion are less stressful (Doucette and Child 1996; Steinkamp et al. 1993).

These numbers may seem confusing, but you need to understand their significance when treating patients with patellofemoral stress injuries. Several points are important to remember. The most patellofemoral stress in open chain exercises occurs in the first 30° of motion, and the least amount of stress occurs in the range of 60° to 90°. The least patellofemoral stress in closed chain activities occurs in the first 30° of motion, and the greatest amount of stress occurs in the range of 60° to 90°. Because there is no contact between the femur and patella in 0° to 10°, it should be safe to strengthen in this range with any exercise (Steinkamp 1993). The more inflamed the patellofemoral joint is, the more limited are the ranges of motion you can use to strengthen the quadriceps pain free. Because the patella does not make contact with the femur until about 20° of flexion, very irritated patellofemoral joints may tolerate motion only in the first 20° of flexion. Squatting exercises and full range-of-motion exercises with weight boots or cuff weights attached to the ankle should be avoided until later in the treatment program when the inflammation is reduced and strength is improved enough for the patellofemoral joint to tolerate the greater stresses of these activities. It is logical to include a slow progression in range of motion as symptoms decrease and strength increases. If you use isokinetic exercises, avoid going into the 90° range of motion where peak patellocompressive forces are produced. Shortening the lever-arm length on weight machines can reduce the compressive forces.

Q-Angle

Q-angle is the angle that is formed by a line from the anterior superior iliac spine to the middle patella and a line from the middle patella to the tibial tubercle (figure 21.2). Lower normal Q-angle measurement is 10°. Upper normal values, which vary for men and women because of the differences in pelvic structure, are 12° and 15°, respectively. The Q-angle can change from non-weight bearing to weight bearing, because tibial rotation changes the Q-angle. If the patient has pronation in weight bearing, the tibia is internally rotated and increases the Q-angle. If the leg externally rotates, the Q-angle decreases. A weak vastus medialis oblique (VMO) can also increase the Q-angle.

In the past, many thought the Q-angle key to patellofemoral alignment and symptoms. Because it can change with functional activities, unless it is profoundly excessive its significance is not considered as great as in the past. The Q-angle should be assessed for gross abnormalities in non-weight bearing and for changes in standing, however, because it may be one of several contributing factors in patellofemoral pain syndromes. It may not be a primary cause of patellofemoral pain syndromes, as was once believed, but it can contribute to the syndrome, especially if it increases during functional activities.

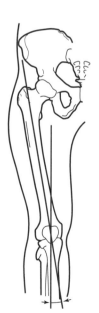

■ **Figure 21.2**
Measuring Q-angle.

Lower-Leg Alignment

As mentioned earlier, excessive rearfoot pronation influences the patella's alignment because it increases tibial rotation and changes the quadriceps tendon pull on the patella. There are other lower-extremity alignments that you should evaluate during a knee examination because alterations from normal can increase stress levels of various knee structures. For example, increased hip internal rotation, squinting patellae, genu recurvatum, patella alta, tibial varum, internal tibial rotation, and compensatory pronation are malalignments that can contribute to patellofemoral pain. Because the lower extremity is a closed kinetic chain during most of its functions, malalignment in one segment results in compensatory changes in another segment. Changes at the hip or at the foot cause compensatory alterations and increased stress in the knee. Compensatory pronation and hip internal rotation with resulting internal tibial rotation are two malalignment problems that should be investigated in patients with patellofemoral pain.

Factors Influencing Postinjury Strength

Obviously, injury and surgery weaken the knee muscles. Other factors, however, influence knee strength and function. Some are not often considered, but all impact knee function and are important for that reason.

These factors—edema, pain, and abnormal ambulation—lead to impaired muscle function. Reduced function leads to atrophy and weakness of the muscle. Muscle weakness leads to reduced function and control of the body segment. The sport rehabilitation specialist must pay attention to these factors when assessing a patient before initiating a therapeutic exercise program.

Edema

One of the important goals of first-aid treatment of athletic injuries is minimization of edema. Once edema forms, efforts should be made to relieve it as quickly as possible. One reason this is a priority is that edema causes an inhibition of quadriceps function. Studies have demonstrated that swelling in the knee joint causes a reflex shutdown of the quadriceps (deAndrade, Grant, and Dixon 1965). Other researchers have injected plasma or saline in small quantities (20–30 ml) into normal knees and found a profound inhibition of quadriceps activity to levels 60% below normal (Young, Stokes, and Iles 1987; Spencer, Hayes, and Alexander 1984). As fluid quantity increases, quadriceps activity decreases.

Pain

It is commonly understood that pain causes a reflex inhibition of muscle activity. Pain affects both the autonomic and the conscious pathways. The reflex response in the presence of pain is to withdraw. The conscious response is to refrain from activity that produces pain. If pain persists following an injury, the patient's ability to perform active muscle contraction is impaired. Use of electrical stimulation and other modalities to control pain before therapeutic exercise may result in improved strength-output levels during exercises. This can ultimately reduce the patient's rehabilitation time by enhancing strength gains.

Ambulation

Normal ambulation utilizes the right and left lower extremity equally, applying weight-bearing and propulsive forces equally on the two extremities. When a patient sustains a lower-extremity injury that causes him or her to favor the extremity, weakness results. An unequal gait produces less-than-normal stresses on the extremity as the patient spends less weight-bearing time on the leg and applies less stress to it. An antalgic gait produces weakness not only in the injured segment but throughout the entire lower extremity. Therefore it is important to assess the total lower extremity following an injury and to correct secondary weaknesses that develop in the extremity's noninjured segments.

REHABILITATION CONCEPTS

In addition to the routine rehabilitation concepts guiding development of a therapeutic exercise program, special factors enter into knee rehabilitation. The sport rehabilitation specialist must address them all if a rehabilitation program is to be successful. The following sections deal with the special factors that have the most influence.

Extensor Lag

Questions that have elicited particular interest are what types of resistive knee exercises optimally strengthen the quadriceps and which quadriceps muscle works at what time within the knee's range of motion. The condition in which full passive motion is present but active extension is incomplete is an **extensor lag.** Two deficiencies are typically present after a knee injury: VMO atrophy and an extensor lag. Because the two problems frequently appear concurrently, a clinical presumption has been that the extensor lag is the result of VMO insufficiency. The VMO's oblique fiber insertion has tended to support this presumption. Research has shown, however, that the VMO does not exert any more effort than any of the other quadriceps muscles during terminal extension (Lieb and Perry 1971). Muscle fiber atrophy is more prominent in the VMO, but the reason is unclear. The atrophy may be apparent not because it is greater in the VMO than in the other quadriceps muscles, but because the fascial covering of the muscle is thinner over the oblique fibers of the vastus medialis than in the rest of the quadriceps group. On the other hand, it may be true that VMO atrophy occurs more readily because the VMO is unable to perform its function as a patellar medial stabilizer as effectively as the other quadriceps muscles perform their task as knee extensor. Research evidence to confirm either suspicion is lacking.

Terminal extension is difficult for a weakened quadriceps to achieve. Some researchers hold that because of its fiber alignment, the function of the VMO is to maintain medial patellar alignment, providing dynamic restraint for the patella (Witvrouw et al. 1996). If this is the case, an extensor lag may occur not because the VMO is deficient, but because the force required of the quadriceps to produce the last 15° of extension is twice as great as for the other ranges of knee motion (Grood et al. 1984). The quadriceps muscles' loss of mechanical advantage (decreased lever-arm length) as the knee approaches its end range means that a much greater muscular effort is needed to complete the movement.

Some of the open kinetic chain exercises most often used to strengthen the knee are the quad set, the straight-leg raise, and the short-arc quad. Among these, the quad set is the most effective in producing total quadriceps activity (Gough and Ladley 1971). The rectus femoris works more during the straight-leg raise and the short-arc quad. Vastus medialis activity is most apparent during a quad set. As would be expected, quadriceps muscles work more during a knee extension exercise than during a straight-leg raise (Knight, Martin, and Londeree 1979). Open kinetic chain exercises are an important tool in restoring isolated quadriceps strength, so these exercises are key elements in a therapeutic exercise program for a patient with isolated quadriceps weakness.

Open and Closed Kinetic Chain Exercises

Open and closed kinetic chain exercises have been the subject of debate in knee rehabilitation, especially ACL rehabilitation, for the past several years. Most recently, the type of exercise most widely advocated for ACL injuries has been closed kinetic chain exercise. This is because research demonstrates a reduction in anterior shear stress and ACL strain in weight-bearing activities that are performed in 0° to 60°. The least amount of anterior displacement in an anterior cruciate-deficient knee during a closed chain exercise occurs at 60°, while the greatest displacement in an open chain exercise occurs at 30° (Jenkins et al. 1997). It has been assumed that closed kinetic chain exercises recruit a co-contraction of hamstrings and quadriceps to provide stability; but this has yet to be substantiated through research, and recent studies have indicated that it may not always be the case. For example, investigators

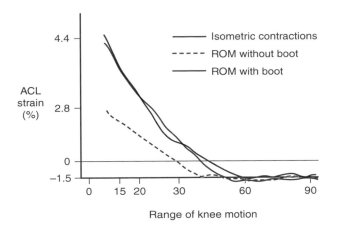

▌Figure 21.3 ACL strain with open kinetic chain activities.

Adapted from Beynnon et al. 1995.

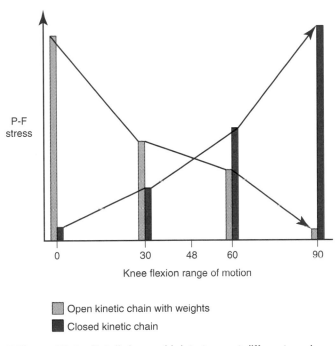

■ Open kinetic chain with weights
■ Closed kinetic chain

▌Figure 21.4 Patellofemoral joint stress at different angles.

Adapted from Steinkamp et al. 1993.

have demonstrated that the lateral step-up exercise, thought to recruit hamstrings and quadriceps, recruits the vastus lateralis and vastus medialis components of the quadriceps significantly but does little to recruit the hamstrings (Worrell, Crisp, and LaRosa 1998). Joint compressive forces in closed kinetic chain exercises may be responsible for reducing the shearing forces and anterior translation that occur in open kinetic chain activities (Isear, Erikson, and Worrell 1997). Additional investigations are needed before judgment on this topic can be final.

In an open kinetic chain exercise as indicated in figure 21.3, less anterior shear stress is applied to the ACL in knee extension resistive exercises from 60° to 90° flexion, and more is applied in terminal-extension ranges of motion (Beynnon et al. 1995). The greatest shear stress to the ACL occurs in 0° to 40° flexion. The quandary for the sport rehabilitation specialist is that 30° is the best position for quadriceps strengthening but puts the greatest strain on the ACL. Less strain is applied to the ACL in closed kinetic chain, but increased stress is applied to the patellofemoral joint in closed kinetic chain activities beyond about 50° flexion (figure 21.4) This can create a dilemma regarding patients who have undergone ACL reconstructions and have patellofemoral pain. Closed kinetic chain activities are less stressful for an ACL injury, but many patients with patellofemoral pain have difficulty performing closed kinetic chain exercises because of the pain.

Shear Stress

Aside from open kinetic chain activities, factors that also influence tibiofemoral shear stress include joint angle, location of the applied resistance, and the speed of the exercise. Peak shear stress occurs in the joint at around 28° to 14° flexion. This may be one reason open chain exercises create their greatest shear force in 15° to 30°. Outside force that is applied more distally on the leg produces greater shear force than more proximally applied force. Manual resistance, especially in the early phases of therapeutic exercise, should be applied just distal to the knee joint to reduce shear-force applications. This is also true for exercise-machine arms used in open chain exercises.

Isokinetic exercise is not used until the later phases of rehabilitation because it is open chain; its lever arm can be shortened but still applies significant shear stresses. When isokinetic exercise is first used, the slower speeds should be avoided because slower speeds produce a greater torque to increase anterior tibial displacement and ACL strain.

Bracing

Perhaps more than any other joint, the knee is a frequent site for sport braces. There are three types of braces: prophylactic, rehabilitative, and functional. The prophylactic brace is used to prevent or reduce the severity of an injury, the rehabilitative brace restricts motion of an injured joint, and a functional brace improves stability of an unstable joint. A functional brace can also be a prophylactic brace.

There are custom-made braces and off-the-shelf braces. Custom-made braces, which are more expensive, can cost several hundred dollars or more. Off-the-shelf braces are similar in construction to the custom-made braces but come in generic sizes, usually ranging from extra small to extra large.

Braces are most often used for ACL injuries. Braces provide anterior stability during low-stress loads but have not shown adequate stability during more functional athletic load applications. Subjective reports often indicate a sense of security and improved performance when exercising with a brace as compared to exercising without one. Braces do seem to provide some proprioceptive feedback, and may be of value for this reason.

Patients who have patellofemoral pain often use knee sleeves. Once again, the proprioceptive benefit as reflected in subjective reports of decreased pain may be the primary advantage. The sleeves do not alter patellar glide or protect the knee from external stress. But one cannot dismiss the psychological benefits of increased confidence and assurance that using a sleeve may give the patient.

Program Progression

Rate of progression of a knee therapeutic exercise program is dictated primarily by tissue healing and the injury's response to exercise. Parameters of range of motion, strength and endurance, balance and agility, and functional performance are advanced as with therapeutic exercise programs for other body segments. Careful observation by the sport rehabilitation specialist, as well as reliance on the patient for accurate communication regarding responses to exercise, is essential for a steady progression within a therapeutic exercise program.

Flexibility exercises, joint mobilization, and soft-tissue mobilization are all techniques that improve range of motion and flexibility. Strength and endurance exercises encompass a variety of activities that advance from static to dynamic and from isometric to isotonic to isokinetic. The method of advancing strength depends on the timing of the program, the patient's response, availability of equipment, and the sport rehabilitation specialist's preference. Isometric exercises are used more often when rehabilitation is in its early phases, when the knee is immobilized, when range-of-motion exercises are too painful for the patient, and when the aim is to isolate weak ranges of motion. In most cases a combination of open and closed kinetic chain exercises is beneficial.

Balance and agility exercises begin with double-support weight-bearing activities and progress to single-limb static balancing on a stable surface. Initial double-support activities might be as simple as gait training with correct weight transfer from the right to the left leg. From there the activities advance to single-limb stance on a stable surface then on an unstable surface. Balance activities can begin at a low level when the patient is able to bear weight on the extremity. Once the patient is able to place total body weight on the injured extremity, single-limb stance activities can begin. For these the patient must be able to correctly shift weight without trunk lean onto the involved extremity. A trunk lean not only does not permit accurate body-weight transfer onto the extremity, but it also promotes bad weight-bearing habits that can become difficult to overcome.

Agility activities advance from balance and coordination exercises. Prerequisites to a patient's progressing to agility exercises are an intact neuromuscular response system, and strength and motion sufficient to return the body's center of gravity to within its base of support when balance is disturbed (Wegener, Kisner, and Nichols 1997). Agility exercises also demand appropriate coordination and muscle power, so they are the next logical step in the rehabilitation progression before functional activities. Agility exercises are dynamic; they may begin with no-impact activities and progress to high-impact activities. The lower-level agility exercises are unidirectional, and more advanced agility exercises are multidirectional. Agility activities begin at reduced speeds and advance to full speed as the patient progresses.

When adding a new agility exercise to a program, it is beneficial to include it early in the exercise session before the patient becomes fatigued. There is evidence to demonstrate that fatigue reduces the knee's proprioceptive function (Lattanzio et al. 1997). An agility activity requires proprioceptive feedback for proper execution. If fatigue reduces proprioceptive function, the execution will not be as good as it should be, and the application is undesirable because of the risk of engramming an incorrect execution.

Once the patient has mastered the agility exercises, the final step—functional activities—prepares the individual physically and psychologically for return to full sport participation. The program can advance to this phase when there is no evidence of pain or edema postexercise and when the injured knee has full range of motion, near-normal strength, and good balance. As with other therapeutic exercise programs, functional activities include specific sport-related drills that mimic the patient's sport activities. They are designed to come as close to normal sport participation demands as possible. They may begin at reduced stress levels, but as the patient's skills and confidence return, the stress of the activity is akin to the stress he or she will experience on returning to full participation.

The functional assessment to determine the patient's readiness for return to sport participation should mimic the sport activities. The sport rehabilitation specialist should assess the patient for accurate execution, ability to use both lower extremities equally, without hesitation to use the involved extremity or inclination to favor it, and confidence in performance.

SOFT-TISSUE MOBILIZATION

Soft-tissue mobilization for knee injuries addresses pain referred from the quadriceps, the hip adductors, the hamstrings, the popliteus, and the tensor fascia lata. Deep-tissue massage is typically for the quadriceps tendon and the iliotibial band.

Pain in the soft tissue surrounding the knee can result from injury to the local tissue or to distant tissue. The foot and hip can refer pain into the knee. Sciatica can also occur as knee pain without leg or back pain. You should assess these areas as possible sources of knee pain if there has been no frank injury. With injuries that might have involved other segments, assessment of these segments is also indicated. You must make a differential diagnosis to eliminate other sources of pain to provide appropriate rehabilitative care for the patient.

Muscles surrounding the knee have specific pain-referral patterns. They can refer pain if they are injured, if they have associated soft-tissue adhesions with restrictions of normal tissue mobility, or if they suffer loss of flexibility and are subjected to increased stress during activity. Trigger points become active with abnormal or excessive stress application. These issues are discussed in chapter 6.

Soft-tissue mobilization techniques discussed in this chapter include the common pain-referral patterns and trigger point release techniques identified and advanced by Travell and Simons (1992), deep-tissue massage for relief of scar-tissue adhesions, and cross-friction massage for tendinitis treatment. You should review chapter 6 for information on other soft-tissue mobilization techniques, such as effleurage for edema.

Hip muscles that cross the knee joint or impact knee movement are discussed here. Other hip muscles are addressed in chapter 22.

QUADRICEPS

For the most part, soft-tissue referral pain in the anterior aspect of the knee and thigh originates from the anterior thigh and hip muscles.

The pain-referral pattern for the quadriceps covers the anterior thigh and knee. The rectus femoris and vastus medialis are the only quadriceps muscles referring into the anterior knee. The vastus lateralis refers to the posterolateral knee. The vastus lateralis also refers pain anywhere along the lateral thigh to the knee and sometimes into the posterior knee. Proximal thigh pain caused by the vastus lateralis can make sleeping on that side uncomfortable. Rectus femoris pain is usually described as a deep thigh ache, especially at night. Referred pain from the vastus medialis can sometimes cause buckling of the knee. The vastus intermedius refers into the midthigh and the upper thigh (figure 21.5a).

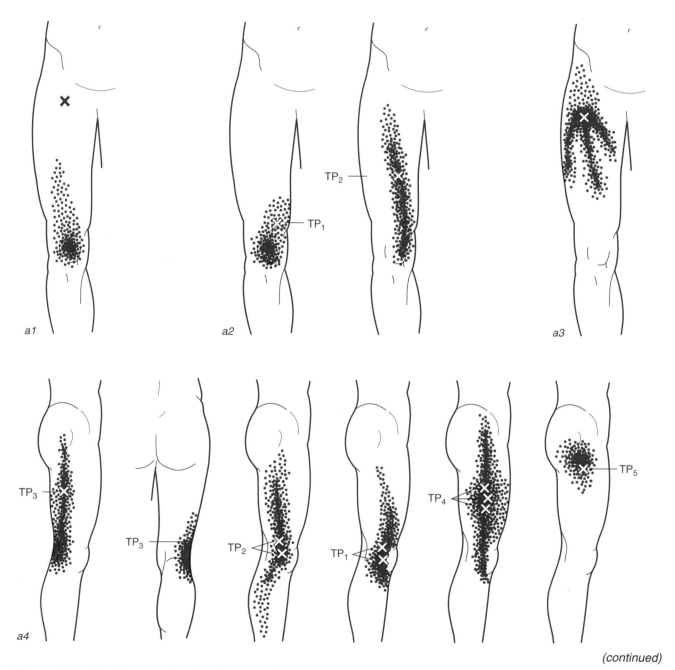

(continued)

▌Figure 21.5 Quadriceps: pain-referral patterns for the rectus femoris *(a1)*, the vastus medialis *(a2)*, the vastus intermedius *(a3)*, and the vastus lateralis *(a4)*.

You can provide trigger point release either by using finger-pad pressure or by grasping the taut band. The vastus medialis is usually treated with a finger pad technique. The hip and knee are in partial flexion and hip external rotation, supported for comfort. The distal trigger points are more often tender than the proximal trigger points. The distal trigger points are at the muscle's medial distal border, whereas the proximal trigger points are in the midthigh region of the muscle's medial border. The rectus femoris trigger point is inferior to the ASIS, just distal to the inguinal ligament. The vastus intermedius cannot be palpated directly but can be located lateral and deep to the rectus femoris proximally. The vastus lateralis has multiple trigger points located in taut bands along the muscle and can be treated with finger-pad pressure (figure 21.5b).

Ice-and-stretch treatment is performed with the patient side-lying or supine for the rectus femoris and supine for the other quadriceps muscles. The hip is extended and the knee flexed for treatment to the rectus femoris with ice sweeps from proximal to distal along the muscle. For treatment to the vastus medialis, the hip is externally rotated and flexed and the knee is flexed as the ice is swept from the medial superior thigh to below the knee. Ice-and-stretch for the vastus intermedius and vastus lateralis is performed with a stretch moving the knee into flexion as the ice is swept from the hip to below the knee.

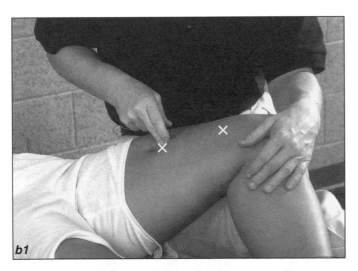

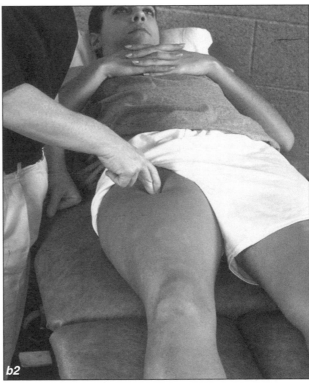

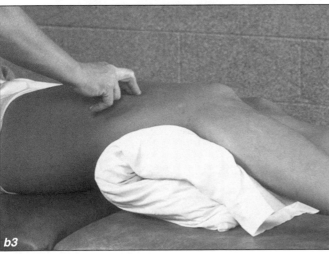

∎ **Figure 21.5** *(continued)* Quadriceps: trigger point release for vastus medialis *(b1)*, vastus intermedius *(b2)*, and vastus lateralis *(b3)*.

HIP ADDUCTORS

The adductor longus and brevis refer pain deep into the groin, the anteromedial upper thigh, and the upper medial knee. The adductor magnus refers deep pain into the groin and distally over the anteromedial thigh. The gracilis referral pain is a superficial, hot, stinging pain along the inside of the thigh (figure 21.6a). The trigger points are located along each muscle belly.

Trigger point release is performed with the patient supine with the hip and knee flexed and the hip externally rotated and abducted. A pillow placed beneath the thigh provides comfort. A pincher grasp or flat pressure with the finger pads can be used (figure 21.6b). The adductor longus and brevis trigger points are located high in the groin. The adductor magnus and gracilis trigger points can be located in the middle third of the inner thigh. The adductor magnus trigger points can also be located beneath the gracilis and hamstrings posteriorly.

Ice-and-stretch is applied with the patient supine and the thigh abducted and externally rotated and the knee flexed. Ice sweeps for the adductor magnus are applied from the knee proceeding proximally along the length of the muscle to the groin (figure 21.6c). The stretch is applied, moving the hip into abduction and flexion. Ice-and-stretch for the adductor magnus and brevis is performed with the patient's hip abducted and externally ro-

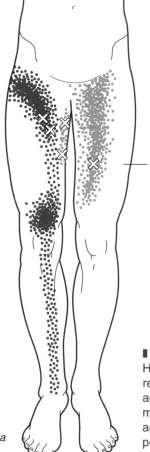
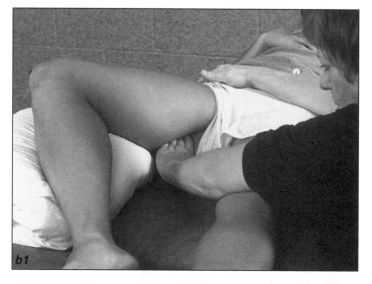

▌Figure 21.6
Hip adductors: *(a)* pain-referral patterns, dark = adductor longus and brevis, medium = gracilis, light = adductor magnus; trigger point release for adductor magnus *(b1)*, anterior longus and brevis *(b2)*, adductor longus *(b3)*. Ice-and-stretch for adductor longus and brevis *(c1)*, adductor magnus *(c2)*.

TrP₁

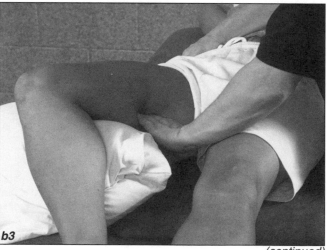

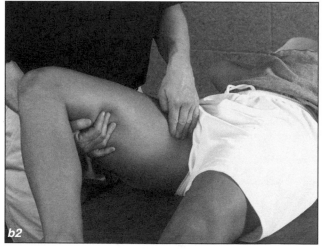

(continued)

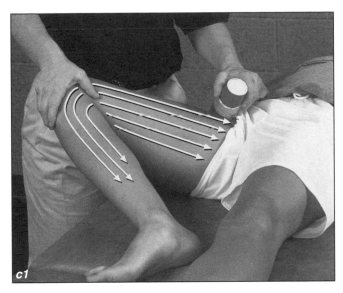 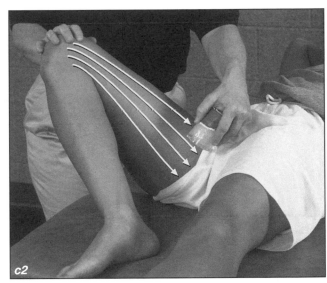

∎ **Figure 21.6** *(continued)*

tated and the knee flexed with the foot against the opposite thigh. As the ice sweeps are moved from the knee and along the inner thigh to the groin, the muscle is stretched, moving the hip into as much flexion and abduction as tolerated (figure 21.7c). The gracilis muscle technique is similar to the hamstring technique with the knee straight.

HAMSTRINGS

Pain referred from the hamstrings occurs in the gluteal fold and posterior knee with overflow along the muscle and into the distal medial calf (figure 21.7a). The semimembranosus and semitendinosus pain is often described as a sharp pain, whereas referred pain from the biceps femoris is more often a deep ache. Trigger points are located in the middle third of the muscles.

Trigger point release can be performed with the patient supine (for medial hamstrings only), side-lying, or prone, with the knee partially flexed to relax the hamstrings. Either a pincher grasp or flat pressure can be used for the medial hamstrings, but the lateral hamstrings are best approached with a flat pressure (figure 21.7b). A twitch response is usually seen with trigger point contact on the medial hamstrings. The trigger points are located in the middle third of the muscles.

Ice-and-stretch of the hamstrings is performed with the patient supine and the opposite leg in extension. The involved leg is supported at the ankle by the sport rehabilitation specialist. The initial distal-to-proximal ice sweeps are performed with the leg abducted to release the adductor magnus. Once the leg is abducted as far as possible, the sweeps move in a proximal to distal direction while the leg is moved into flexion and adduction while the knee is maintained in extension (figure 21.7c).

Biceps femoris (both heads)

Semitendinosus

Semimembranosus

(continued)

a

∎ **Figure 21.7** Hamstrings: pain-referral patterns. Dark = medial hamstrings, light = lateral hamstrings.

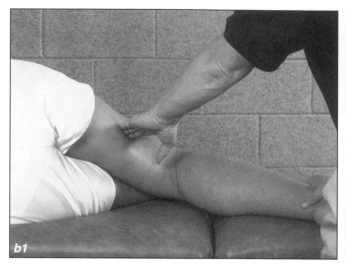

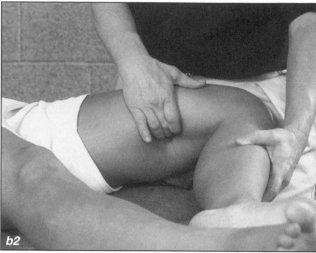

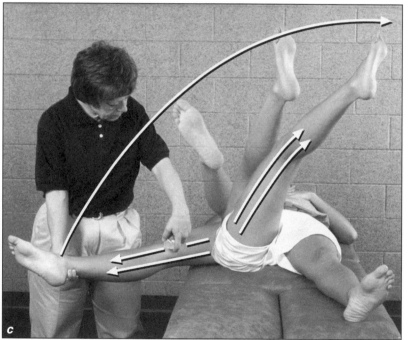

I Figure 21.7
(continued) Trigger point release: for lateral hamstrings *(b1)*, medial hamstrings *(b2)*; ice-and-stretch *(c)*.

POPLITEUS

The pain-referral pattern of the popliteus muscle (figure 21.8a) is commonly reported as posterior knee pain during activities such as running, walking down stairs and hills, and squatting.

Trigger point release is performed with the patient side-lying or prone with the knee partially flexed and the ankle plantar flexed. A flat pressure is applied in a downward and anterior direction medial to the medial head of the gastrocnemius between it and the semitendinosus (figure 21.8b).

Ice-and-stretch is performed with the patient prone. Ice sweeps begin distally and move along the muscle's path in a proximal direction as the leg is externally rotated and the knee extended but not locked (figure 21.8c).

TENSOR FASCIA LATA

The tensor fascia lata refers a deep pain in the anterolateral hip from the greater trochanter and can extend as far as the knee (figure 21.9a). The pain can sometimes mimic trochanteric bursitis, making it painful to lie on the side or to run.

Trigger point release is performed with the patient supine and the knee supported in slight flexion to relax the muscle. A flat palpation of the muscle is performed distal to the anterior superior iliac spine and medial and proximal to the greater trochanter (figure 21.9b).

Ice-and-stretch is performed with the patient side-lying, the involved leg on top. The sport rehabilitation specialist supports the leg under the distal thigh and applies the ice sweeps from the anterolateral thigh distally and laterally to above the knee. The stretch is applied by stabilizing the pelvis and lowering the thigh as it is moved into external rotation (figure 21.9c).

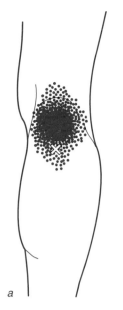

a

■ Figure 21.8 Popliteus: *(a)* pain-referral pattern, *(b)* trigger point release, *(c)* ice-and-stretch.

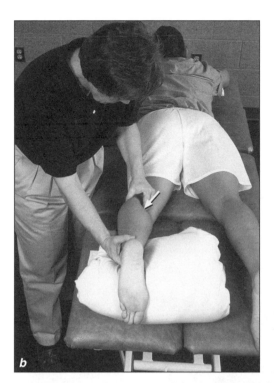

b

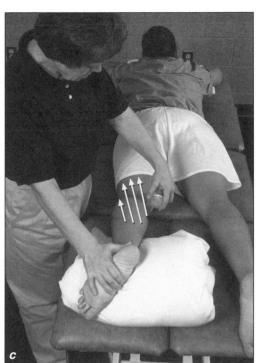

c

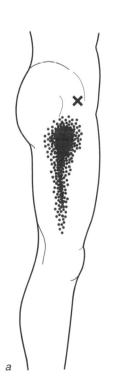

a

■ Figure 21.9 Tensor fascia lata: *(a)* pain-referral pattern, *(b)* trigger point release, *(c)* ice-and-stretch. ● = greater trochanter, ■ = ASIS.

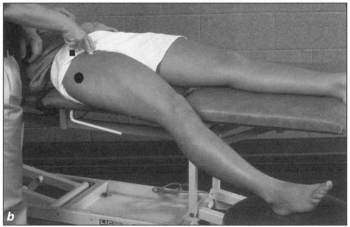

b

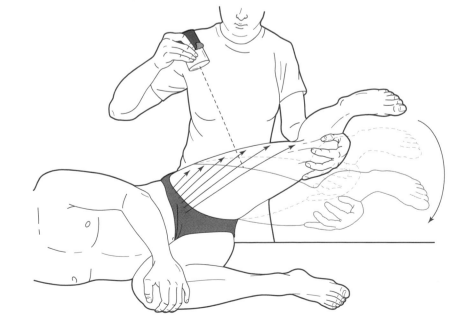

c

DEEP-TISSUE MASSAGE

Two areas of the knee and thigh typically require deep-tissue massage, the quadriceps tendon and the iliotibial band (ITB). When the quadriceps tendon becomes inflamed, cross-friction massage is frequently used to relieve scar-tissue adhesions that can occur secondarily to the inflammation. The tendon fibers are cross-frictioned in the manner described in chapter 6. Because the tendon fibers run vertically from the patella to the tibial tuberosity, the cross-friction technique is applied horizontally across the fibers.

Cross-friction massage can be used on surgical sears to prevent adhesions of skin to underlying structures. Even the portal sites of arthroscopy should be assessed and treated as needed to prevent adhesions and promote good tissue mobility following surgery.

The tensor fascia lata is a frequent site of adhesions, especially following injury or the use of prolonged poor biomechanics such as seen with genu valgus. These areas along the ITB are relieved by deep-tissue massage. The sport rehabilitation specialist flexes the metacarpophalangeal and proximal interphalangeal joints so that the finger pads rest in the palm. With a closed hand in this position, the sport rehabilitation specialist uses posterior surfaces of the middle and distal phalanx to apply pressure while guiding the hand

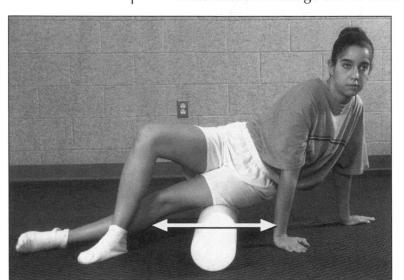

■ Figure 21.10
Iliotibial band foam-roller self-massage.

along the patient's lateral thigh from the knee moving toward the hip. Soft-tissue restrictions can be palpated as "sticking points" as the hand moves along the lateral thigh. The sport rehabilitation specialist repeats the massage strokes several times, spending additional time on the more-restricted regions. As the restriction releases, tissue mobility is less inhibited and the patient reports less tenderness with the massage.

In an alternative technique, the patient can apply self-massage using a foam roller. The patient lies on the involved side, with the weight on both hands and the thigh on the foam roller (figure 21.10). He or she rolls from knee to thigh on the foam roller, spending more time on the areas that are tender and restricted. Normally, this should not produce tenderness, but it will in an ITB that has areas of soft-tissue restriction.

The foam roller can also be used to massage the quadriceps muscle if it becomes restricted from immobilization or injury (figure 21.11). The patient lies prone with weight on both forearms and with the anterior thighs on the foam roller. He or she uses the arms to move the roller from the hips to the knees, spending more time over the tender sites.

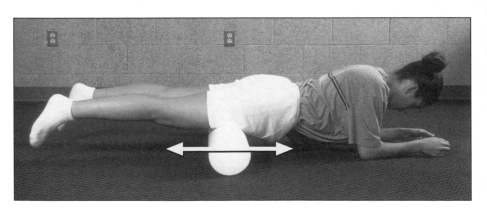

■ Figure 21.11   Quadriceps foam-roller massage.

JOINT MOBILIZATION

Joint mobilization techniques for the knee include anterior glides for extension, posterior glides for flexion, and rotational glides for terminal flexion and extension.

Injury, surgery, edema, and immobilization can lead to reduced joint mobility involving the patellofemoral joint, tibiofemoral joint, and proximal tibiofibular joint. Although the tibiofibular joint is not actually part of the knee, if it develops reduced mobility it can refer pain to the knee and affect ankle mobility. For this reason, you should assess the tibiofibular joint for mobility along with the knee joints before establishing a therapeutic exercise program.

SUPERIOR TIBIOFIBULAR JOINT

Anterior and posterior glides are the mobilization techniques used for this joint. With the patient's knee and hip flexed and the foot resting on the tabletop, the sport rehabilitation specialist grasps the head of the fibula with the pads of the thumbs anteriorly and the index and middle fingers posteriorly. The fibular head is moved anteriorly and then posteriorly (figure 21.12). The weight of the leg stabilizes the lower leg.

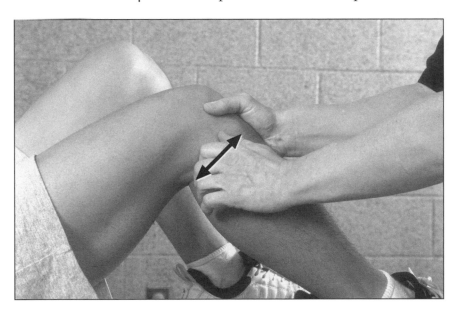

Figure 21.12 Joint mobilization: superior tibiofibular anterior and posterior glides.

PATELLOFEMORAL MOBILIZATIONS

Patellar mobility is necessary for full knee flexion-extension motion and tibial rotation.

Lateral Glide

The patient lies supine, and a rolled towel is placed under the knee for knee support. The sport rehabilitation specialist places both thumb pads on the medial surface of the patella. The thumbs move the patella laterally (figure 21.13a). Care must be taken to apply a lateral force, not a compressive force, on the patella.

Medial Glide

With the patient and the knee in the same position as just described, depending on which side of the treatment table the sport rehabilitation specialist is standing on, the sport rehabilitation specialist places the thumbs or fingertips on the lateral aspect of the patella and moves the patella in a medial direction (figure 21.13b). Compression of the patella into the femur should be avoided.

Inferior Glide

The patient and knee are in the position described for lateral glides. The sport rehabilitation specialist places a thumb and index finger around the superior rim of the patella. Being careful not to compress the patella on the femur, the sport rehabilitation specialist glides the patella distally in an inferior direction (figure 21.13c).

Superior Glide

With the patient in the position described for lateral glides, the sport rehabilitation specialist places a thumb and index finger around the inferior rim of the patella. A cephalic force is exerted on the patella (figure 21.13d). Compression of the patella on the femur should be avoided.

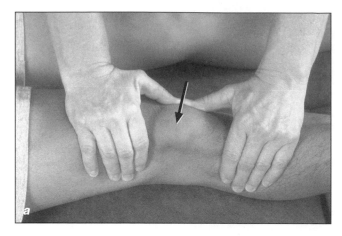
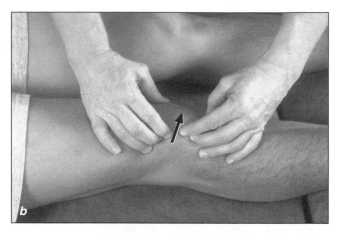
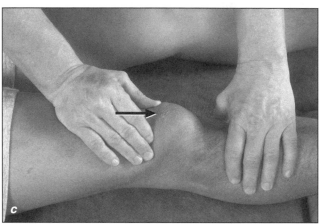
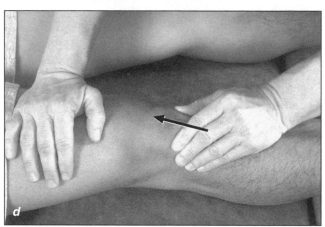

■ **Figure 21.13** Patellofemoral joint mobilization: *(a)* lateral glide, *(b)* medial glide, *(c)* inferior glide, *(d)* superior glide.

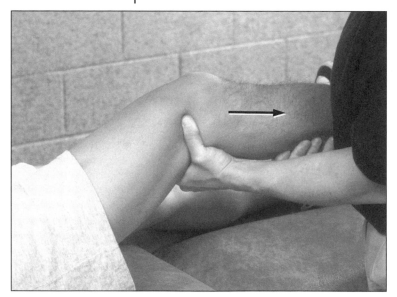

■ **Figure 21.14**
Joint mobilization: tibiofemoral distraction.

TIBIOFEMORAL MOBILIZATIONS

This is the joint most often mobilized to improve range of motion in the knee. Although the patellofemoral joint also can affect total range of motion, this joint has the greatest impact. For this reason, tibiofemoral mobilization techniques are outlined here.

Distraction

Distraction is a mobilization technique used for general restriction. The patient is prone with the knee supported by the sport rehabilitation specialist. The knee is partially flexed. The femur is stabilized with one hand proximal to the knee, and the mobilizing hand is placed above the ankle joint. The tibia is pulled distally by the mobilizing hand while the stabilizing hand secures the thigh (figure 21.14).

Anterior Glide

An anterior glide of the tibia is used to increase knee extension. This technique is performed with the patient prone. The knee is flexed with the thigh supported on the table and the patient's lower leg resting on the sport rehabilitation specialist's shoulder. A pad under the thigh will make the position more comfortable for the patient and align the thigh more appropriately for the glide. The patient's distal lower leg is supported on the sport rehabilitation specialist's shoulder. The sport rehabilitation specialist clasps his or her hands around the proximal lower leg near the knee and glides the tibia anteriorly on the femur (figure 21.15). The glide force must be parallel to the plane of the joint surface, so as the knee bends, the angle of the glide force changes. Before applying the mobilization force, the sport rehabilitation specialist must take note of how the joint is positioned and must apply the force accordingly. The hamstrings should remain relaxed to produce the most effective results.

An alternative posterior-to-anterior mobilization technique is performed with the patient prone and the sport rehabilitation specialist supporting the tibia with the knee in 30° flexion. An anterior force is applied by the mobilizing hand just distal to the knee joint.

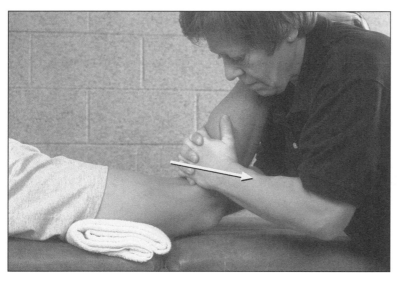

∎ Figure 21.15 Joint mobilization: tibio-femoral anterior glide.

Posterior Glide

A posterior glide of the tibia is used to increase knee flexion motion. The thigh is stabilized with the patient supine and a pad under the knee to position it in slight flexion. The sport rehabilitation specialist places the heels of his or her hands on the anterior proximal tibia and applies a posterior glide parallel to the joint surface (figure 21.16). In an alternative position, the patient is in sitting with the knee over the edge of the table and the thigh supported by a towel roll under the distal thigh. The sport rehabilitation specialist applies a posterior glide at the tibial condyles.

Rotational Glides

If the patient is lacking the last few degrees of flexion or extension, it may be that the femur and tibia are not rotating properly. To gain those last few degrees of motion, you can mobilize the tibial condyles unilaterally.

Anterior Glide, Medial Condyle

This maneuver is used to gain tibial external rotation and knee extension. The patient is prone with a pad placed under the anterior thigh. The knee is flexed and supported by the sport rehabilitation specialist's stabilizing hand. The heel of the mobilizing hand is placed over the medial tibial plateau, and a posterior-anterior (PA) glide is applied (figure 21.17).

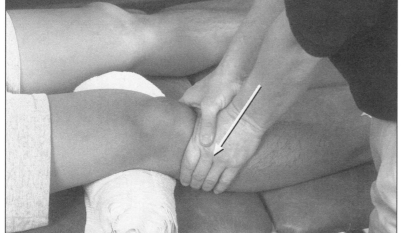

∎ Figure 21.16 Joint mobilization: tibio-femoral posterior glide.

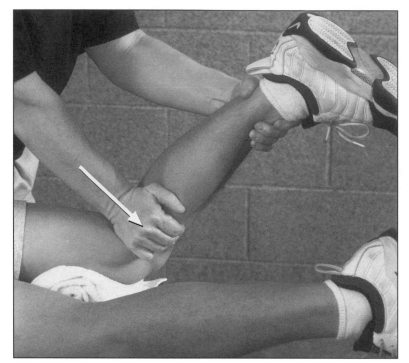

■ **Figure 21.17**   Joint mobilization: medial tibial condyle anterior glide.

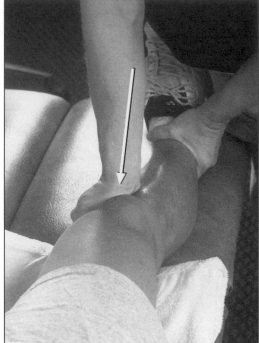

■ **Figure 21.18**   Joint mobilization: medial tibial condyle posterior glide.

Posterior Glide, Medial Condyle

This technique is used to gain tibial internal rotation and knee flexion. The patient is supine with a pad under the distal femur. The sport rehabilitation specialist applies an anterior-posterior (AP) glide with the heel of the hand on the medial tibial plateau (figure 21.18).

If the sport rehabilitation specialist applies the mobilizing force to the femur rather than to the tibia in AP glides or to the opposite side of the tibia in rotational glides, the opposite motions are influenced. For example, on an anterior glide of the tibia, the motion affected is knee extension. However, if the femur receives the anterior glide, knee flexion is the motion affected. So, too, if a posterior glide is applied to the lateral tibial condyle rather than to the medial tibial condyle, gains are seen in external rotation and extension; and if an anterior glide is applied to the lateral rather than to the medial tibial condyle, internal rotation and knee flexion are affected.

FLEXIBILITY EXERCISES

Flexibility exercises for the knee include prolonged extension and flexion stretches, as well as active stretches for the quadriceps and hamstrings.

Flexibility exercises for the knee can be active or passive. The specific techniques used depend on the type of tissue being stretched. If scar tissue is being stretched, the technique also depends on the age of the scar tissue. Recent scar tissue may be effectively stretched with active and short-term stretches. Scar tissue that is very adherent and is well into the remodeling phase of healing requires a combination of scar-tissue massage to loosen adhesions and long-term stretches to affect the tissue's plastic element.

Following surgical repair of the knee, orthopedic surgeons frequently have the patient's knee placed in a continuous passive motion (CPM) machine or begin early active motion. Although not used as frequently as they were a few years ago, CPMs are beneficial in reducing pain and edema and encouraging restoration of range of motion. One should not assume, however, that the CPM will restore full knee motion. You must assess the patient's knee motion at the time of the initial examination and frequently throughout the rehabilitation process.

The exercises presented here are divided into prolonged and active stretches. The active stretches include some exercises that use assistive equipment and some that require only the patient's active motion. During active stretches it is important for the patient to contract the opposing muscle whenever possible to enhance relaxation of the muscle being stretched and achieve a more effective stretch.

PROLONGED STRETCHES

These stretches are used when scar tissue that is limiting motion is mature or is becoming mature, and a short-term stretch would be ineffective.

When using prolonged stretches, the sport rehabilitation specialist must inform the patient that the knee will feel stiff once the stretch is removed but that the stiffness sensation should resolve within a few minutes. It may be difficult for the patient to take the first few steps after standing up. A prolonged stretch is more effective the longer it is applied. At first the patient may not feel that a stretch is being applied, but as time passes he or she will feel the stretch. A patient may not be able to tolerate a stretch for more than 5 or 10 min initially. If this is the case, and a weight is being used, the stretch weight should be decreased or removed to make a longer stretch tolerable. As the patient adjusts to the stretch, either the weight can be increased or the time can be lengthened; but the time should not be reduced. If an increased weight necessitates less time on the stretch, it is better to reduce the weight and permit a longer time on the stretch.

Prolonged Extension Stretch

These exercises are used to increase knee extension. They are performed in two positions, prone and long sitting. The prone stretch can also increase rectus femoris length. The patient lies prone with the foot over the end of the table. A pad is placed under the thigh for patella comfort (figure 21.19). The patient relaxes the leg and maintains this position for at least 10 to 15 min. A weight on the ankle will increase the stretch force, but the weight should start light and increase only as the patient tolerates. If the hip flexes during the stretch, a stabilization strap across the hip and thigh may be necessary. You can increase the rectus femoris stretch by having the patient lie on the elbows to increase hip extension.

The other prolonged extension stretch is in the long sitting position. The leg is extended. A towel roll can be placed under the heel to lift the calf off the tabletop. A weight is applied to the thigh (figure 21.20). The patient can easily perform this stretch independently at home by placing the foot on top of another chair or a coffee table and applying a weight on the thigh for a specified amount of time. The sport rehabilitation specialist must instruct the patient not to externally rotate the leg. Applying hot packs before and during the stretch may permit a greater tolerance for the stretch.

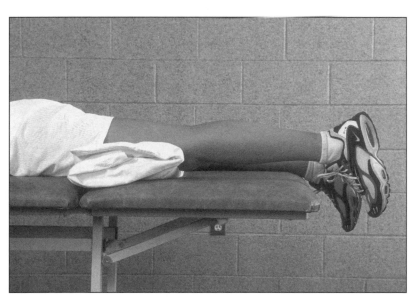

Figure 21.19 Prolonged extension stretch in prone.

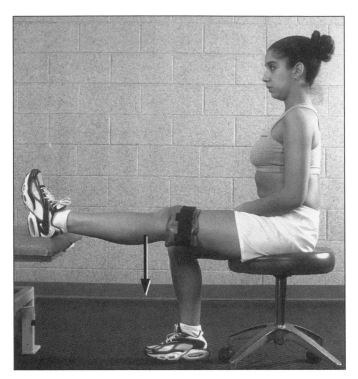

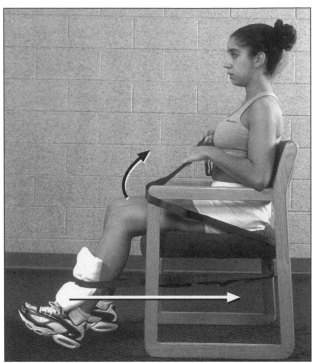

■ **Figure 21.20** Prolonged extension stretch in long sitting.

■ **Figure 21.21** Prolonged knee flexion with rope system.

Prolonged Flexion Stretch

The position used for this stretch depends on how much restriction of knee flexion movement is present. If restriction is severe, the patient can be instructed to lie supine on a bed with a chair back against the bed. A pad is placed on the top of the chair back, and the posterior knee is positioned on top of the pad. The patient is instructed to relax the thigh and allow the leg to drop down, relaxong in this position for 10 to 15 min, if tolerable. Placing a weight around the ankle will increase the stretch force.

Using a rope-and-pulley system, the patient can perform a prolonged flexion stretch in sitting (figure 21.21). The rope is anchored to the back chair leg. The rope is attached around the patient's ankle and controlled by the patient's pulling on the rope. The patient is instructed to pull the leg back to a point that feels tight but not painful. He or she holds this position for several minutes before attempting to increase flexion. The exercise is repeated several times for a total of 10 to 15 min.

ACTIVE STRETCHES

A number of exercises are used to gain knee flexibility. The important point to remember for each stretch is to position the muscle so it is not working during the stretch. A hamstring stretch that many athletes use, standing and bending over to touch the floor, is a good example of what not to do. The hamstrings are used to hold the body upright; attempting to stretch the muscle in this position is futile because the muscle has to contract to maintain balance.

Active stretches can be repeated several times throughout the day. As discussed previously, a 20 s hold for about four repetitions is advocated. When possible, the opposing muscle should contract to produce a more effective stretch on the intended muscle.

Quadriceps Stretches

The quadriceps can be stretched using several different methods. Factors such as weight-bearing status, tolerance, agility, and balance ability determine which exercise is used. Listed here are a few examples.

Wall Slides

This exercise is used very early in the therapeutic exercise program when the patient does not have good muscular control of the joint, when the joint is painful, and when motion is significantly restricted because of pain, swelling, or recent immobilization.

The patient lies supine with the buttocks about 60 cm (2 ft) from the wall. A towel is placed between the foot and the wall, with the foot on the wall. The patient slides the foot down the wall, bending the knee as far as possible (figure 21.22). The foot, knee, and hip should remain in alignment with each other throughout the motion. The uninvolved leg assists in returning the foot to the starting position. As motion improves, the buttocks are moved closer to the wall. If the patient is able to tolerate more movement, he or she can encourage more flexion by using the uninvolved leg to push on the top of the involved leg at the ankle.

Seated Knee Flexion

Once the patient has about 50° of flexion, he or she can perform stretches in sitting using the uninvolved leg to move the involved leg into greater flexion. With the foot flat on the floor and the uninvolved foot across the involved ankle, the patient uses the uninvolved leg to push the involved leg back as far as possible (figure 21.23). The knee must remain aligned with the foot and hip. This exercise can be performed throughout the day during sitting.

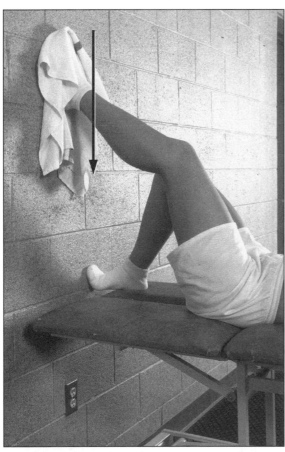

■ **Figure 21.22** Wall slides.

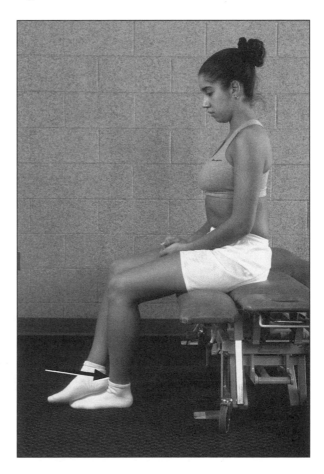

■ **Figure 21.23** Seated knee flexion.

Standing Knee Flexion

Patients can perform this exercise once they have achieved near-normal flexibility. Standing near a table or wall to use as support, the patient grasps the foot behind the back and pulls it toward the buttocks. The body should remain in an upright position with the hips forward to include the rectus femoris in the stretch (figure 21.24).

If the patient is unable to reach the foot because of insufficient flexibility, he or she can use a stretch strap in standing. The strap is wrapped around the ankle and grasped behind the back. The strap is pulled to move the foot toward the buttock. An erect posture must be maintained for this exercise.

Stationary Bike

Once the patient has about 90° flexion and is allowed at least partial weight bearing, a stationary bike can be used to facilitate greater motion. With the feet secured on the foot pedals, the patient uses the uninvolved leg to guide and control the involved leg during pedaling. It is best to begin with a backward motion, because it is easier to achieve a full circle going backward than it is forward. Once the patient is moving the pedals smoothly in reverse, he or she can do forward cycling. The height of the seat should be such that at the bottom of the crank position, the knee is near full extension (figure 21.25). The patient may tend to shift from side to side at the hips as he or she attempts to move the crank through its full cycle, but this should be discouraged.

Hamstring Stretches

Hamstring stretches can be performed in a variety of positions. The important consideration in positioning the patient is that the muscle remains relaxed throughout the exercise. If the muscle works to maintain the position, the stretch will be ineffective.

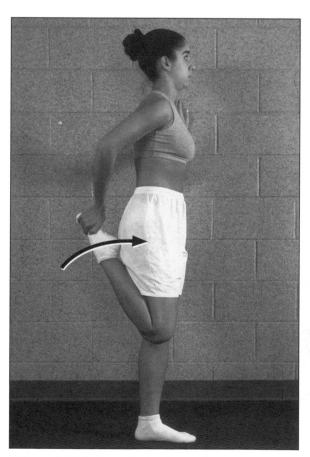

∎ Figure 21.24   Knee flexion in standing.

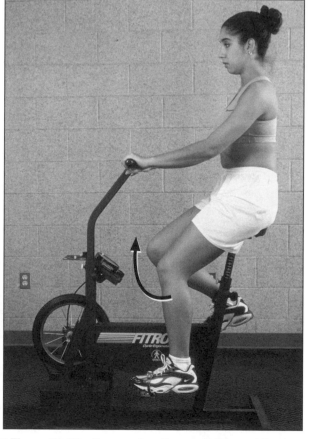

∎ Figure 21.25   Range of motion on stationary bike.

Supine Stretches

Supine stretches ensure relaxation of the hamstrings, because the quadriceps are used to extend the knee during these exercises.

The patient lies supine with the uninvolved leg extended. The involved leg is brought toward the chest, and the hands are clasped behind the thigh. The knee is then extended as far as possible so that a stretch is felt behind the knee or in the thigh (figure 21.26). The opposite leg is kept in extension to stabilize the pelvis so that the ischial tuberosity does not roll upward and reduce the effectiveness of the stretch on the hamstrings.

A stretch strap can be used around the foot if it is too difficult for the patient to reach the thigh. Another alternative is to have the patient lie supine in a doorway with the involved leg extended into the doorway and the involved foot on the wall (figure 21.27). The stretch is released by bending the knee. As the patient's flexibility increases, the buttocks are moved closer to the door frame.

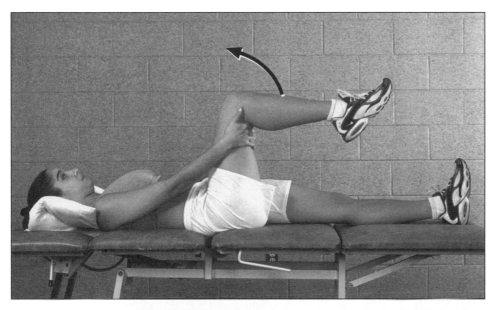

▌Figure 21.26 Hamstring stretch, supine.

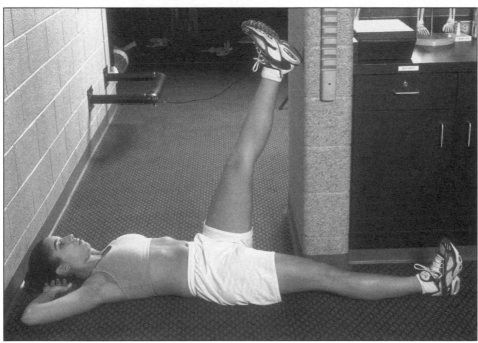

▌Figure 21.27 Hamstring stretch in doorway.

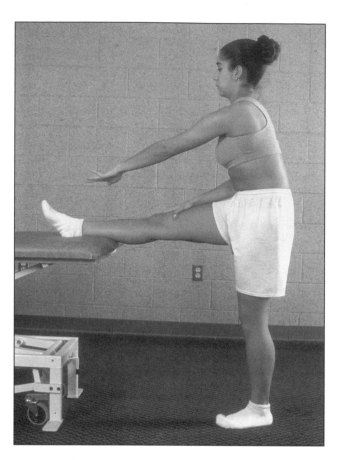

Standing Stretch

Standing hamstring stretches assure stabilization of the pelvis because the supporting leg remains in extension during the stretch. The height of the surface that the involved leg is placed on depends on the patient's flexibility. In very tight hamstrings, it may be best to begin the stretch with the foot on a footstool or chair seat. The standing leg is positioned with the foot facing forward. The involved knee is kept extended during the stretch, with the foot facing the ceiling. The patient bends forward from the hips, not the back, and attempts to reach toward the toes with the opposite hand (figure 21.28). Reaching forward with the same hand allows trunk rotation. The back should remain straight during the stretch.

As the patient's flexibility improves, the height of the supporting object can be raised. If flexibility is normal, an individual should be able to touch the toes of the leg elevated to hip height with the opposite hand. The patient should not bounce during this exercise. Contraction of the quadriceps improves the flexibility during the stretch.

▌**Figure 21.28**   Hamstring stretch in standing.

STRENGTHENING EXERCISES

Patients with knee injuries perform many kinds of strengthening exercises, including isometrics, non-weight-bearing isotonics, weight-bearing resistive exercises, machine exercises, and isokinetic exercises.

Strengthening exercises can begin early in a therapeutic exercise program even if the knee is immobilized and weight bearing is not permitted. Isometrics can be used to retard muscle atrophy. Once active motion is permitted, isotonic activities against gravity can progress to exercises against resistance in the form of free weights, manual resistance, machine resistance, body weight when weight bearing is permitted, and isokinetic exercises.

The sport rehabilitation specialist must bear in mind that both hip and ankle muscles cross the knee joint and must also be strengthened if they show weakness. The hip and lateral thigh muscles act as stabilizers for the knee and are important for knee control. Trunk muscles also are important for knee stability and must not be neglected. Although exercises for the trunk, hip, and ankle are not discussed here, they should be part of a total therapeutic exercise program for a patient with a knee injury.

Strengthening exercises should not cause pain or swelling either during or after the exercise. The sport rehabilitation specialist must solicit reliable feedback from the patient about the knee's response to exercises in the therapeutic exercise program, especially during the initial treatment phase and whenever there are increases in the program. Increased pain and swelling are indications that the exercises are too severe for the knee to tolerate. In the presence of these signs, the exercises should be reduced in intensity or severity. It is important not to provide too many new exercises that stress the same tissue at one time, because if the patient returns for the next treatment session with increased edema and/or pain, it is too difficult to assess which exercise caused the inflammatory response. In the early stages of a therapeutic exercise program when the sport rehabilitation specialist wants to move the rehabilitation process along but not overstress tissue, it is better to provide a balance of exercises that include perhaps only one or two strengthening exercises for various deficient areas rather than emphasizing only the quadriceps or only the hamstrings. For example, the first treatment session's strengthening exercises may include short-arc quads; manual resistance to hip abduction, adduction, and extension; and hamstring curls. In this case, if the patient returns with increased anterior knee pain, it is likely that the short-arc quads caused the irritation. If the patient had received short-arc quad exercises along with full-arc quad and standing squat exercises, it would be difficult to determine the cause of the new pain. Once the knee's reaction to stress has been established, it is easier to decide what exercises are likely to be tolerated; but in the beginning it is safer to add exercises cautiously.

ISOMETRICS

Instructions on isometric exercises should emphasize a gradual buildup of the muscle contraction to a maximum level, a hold at the maximum level for 5 to 6 s, and then a gradual decline to full relaxation before the next repetition. A sudden contraction to maximal levels can cause discomfort and yields a less-than-optimal result. You should also instruct the patient to repeat the exercise in at least sets of 10 several times throughout the day.

Quad Set

This exercise strengthens the quadriceps. Perhaps the earliest exercise used to strengthen the quads, it can begin in the recovery room following surgery. With the patient supine, the uninvolved knee flexed with the foot flat on the tabletop, and the involved knee straight with the patella facing the ceiling, the patient pushes the back of the knee down onto the tabletop. Placing the hand on the quad to feel for muscle tightening helps facilitate a contraction. If the patient is unable to feel a contraction, have the individual perform the exercise with the uninvolved leg to feel a normal contraction before performing the isometric with the involved knee.

If the patient is still unable to facilitate a quad contraction, you can lift the heel of the involved leg off the table about 15 cm (6 in.) and instruct the patient to hold this position as you reduce hand support. You should not completely remove your hand, though, because the patient will probably not be able to hold the position independently.

If the patient has difficulty producing a quad set in supine, he or she can use an alternative position. In prone with a rolled towel under the ankle (figure 21.29), the patient attempts to push the ankle into the towel roll, facilitating quadriceps activation. Electrical stimulation can also be useful for quadriceps facilitation if the patient is unable to produce a good quad contraction with an active exercise.

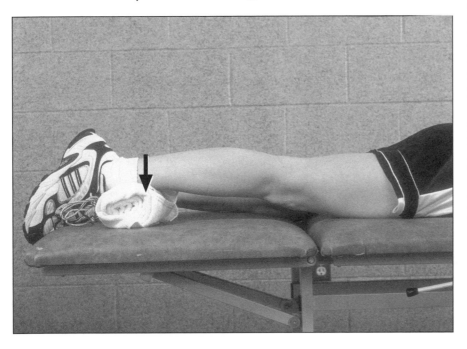

■ **Figure 21.29** Quad set, prone.

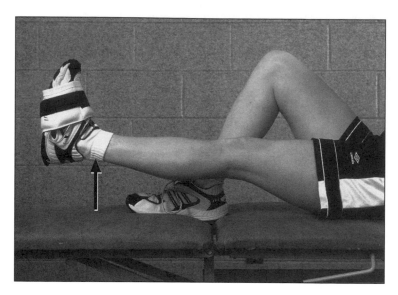

■ Figure 21.30
Straight-leg raise.

Straight-Leg Raise

The straight-leg raise is a hip exercise; but because it requires the quadriceps to hold the knee in extension it is essentially an isometric exercise for the quadriceps, with the exception of the rectus femoris, which also acts at the hip.

The patient is supine with the uninvolved leg flexed and the involved leg extended. The patient first contracts the quadriceps muscle, then raises the involved leg off the table about 20 cm (8 in.) and holds the leg at that level for about 5 s (figure 21.30). The leg is then slowly lowered, and the quadriceps muscle is not relaxed until the leg is on the table.

The exercise becomes more difficult if the patient is in a long sitting position rather than supine. It also is more difficult if the hip is externally rotated during the lift rather than in a neutral position. Weights can also be used to increase the difficulty of the exercise.

Hamstring Sets

This isometric exercise assists in maintaining hamstring strength. With the patient supine, the uninvolved leg extended, and the involved knee partially flexed, the patient pushes the heel into the table. No movement is produced. This exercise can be repeated at different knee joint angles.

NON-WEIGHT-BEARING ISOTONIC EXERCISES

Strengthening can begin early in the therapeutic exercise program even though the patient is non-weight bearing or partial weight bearing. Open kinetic chain exercises can be useful at this stage of the program.

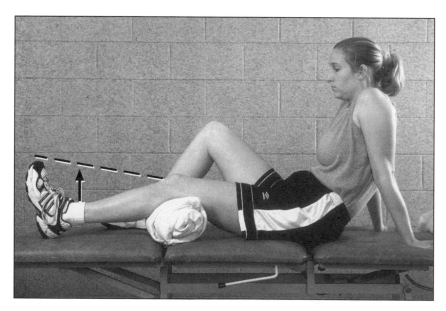

■ Figure 21.31   Short-arc quad exercise.

Short-Arc Quad Exercise

This exercise is a terminal-extension exercise to strengthen the quadriceps in the final degrees of knee extension. This exercise applies a significant stress to the ACL. Therefore it is not an exercise that should be used early in an ACL injury or reconstruction.

A towel roll is placed under the knee to position the knee in partial flexion. The patient is supine to utilize the rectus femoris or sitting to increase the difficulty of the exercise. With the uninvolved knee flexed, the involved knee is straightened, held in full extension, and then returned to the starting position (figure 21.31). The patient can be instructed to hold the position in full extension for

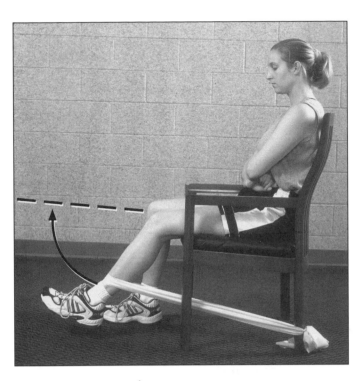

Figure 21.32 Full-arc quad exercise.

about 5 s. A weight or manual resistance can be applied to the ankle to increase the difficulty of the exercise. The size of the towel roll can vary, depending on how much of an arc you want the patient to go through.

Full-Arc Quad Exercise

This exercise strengthens the quadriceps muscle. The patellofemoral joint may be painful during this exercise; this is especially the case during the range of motion from 100° to 60° of flexion, because these positions place more joint reaction force on the patellofemoral joint. However, the ACL is not stressed as greatly during the 100° to 60° of motion, so this exercise is appropriate as long as the motion is within this range.

The patient sits in a chair or on the edge of a table with the knees over the edge. The foot is lifted slowly upward to straighten the knee (figure 21.32). Manual resistance, ankle weights, or rubber band resistance can be used to increase the exercise's difficulty.

This exercise can be used in partial ranges of motion. If necessary, the sport rehabilitation specialist can restrict motion manually to limit the patient's ability to extend or flex beyond a desired range; or an object such as a chair or bench can be used to block motion. Pain should not result either during or after this or any strength exercise.

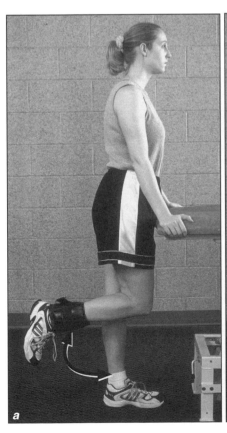

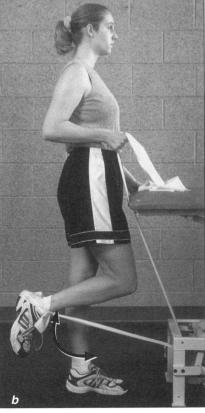

Hamstring Curls

These exercises are used to increase hamstring strength. The patient lies prone with the foot over the edge of the table and the knee in full extension. The knee is flexed against gravity, manual resistance, a cuff weight, or rubber tubing. In standing, the patient is supported by the non-involved extremity and the hands. The involved knee is flexed as far as possible. Gravity, cuff weights, manual resistance, or rubber tubing can be used to provide resistance (figure 21.33).

These two positions for the hamstring provide maximum resistance curl in different parts of the

Figure 21.33 Hamstring curl: *(a)* with cuff weight, *(b)* with rubber band resistance.

range of motion, so both positions can be used in a program. Maximal resistance in the prone exercise occurs in the beginning of the motion, in which the muscle is strongest, but the standing exercise provides maximum resistance at the end of the motion, wherein the muscle is at its physiologically weakest position.

WEIGHT-BEARING RESISTIVE EXERCISES

Once the patient is able to bear weight on the injured knee, weight-transfer activities and gait training may be necessary if the individual has been on crutches, has been non-weight bearing or partial weight bearing, or demonstrates a poor gait pattern. These activities, discussed in chapter 20, include weight-transfer exercises on a scale, gait-training activities, and use of a mirror for facilitation of weight transfer and proper gait.

Reciprocal Training

Machines such as a stationary bike, a treadmill for gait training, a step machine, or a ski machine can be useful once weight bearing is permitted. The stationary bike produces less tibiofemoral force stress than walking and is appropriate for strengthening and cardiovascular conditioning. Step machines used with controlled degrees of knee motion, and the ski machine, facilitate strength, motion, reciprocal motion between the right and lower extremities, and cardiovascular conditioning.

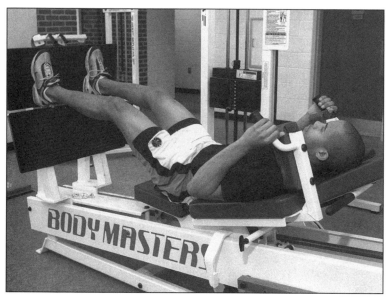

■ **Figure 21.34**
Platform leg press.

Platform Leg Press

Platform leg-press machines come in a variety of models and can be used in a variety of ways to exercise the quads. They are all closed kinetic chain units on which the feet remain stationary and the platform on which the body rests is moved by leg force. The most traditional method of machine use is with the patient supine and the involved foot on the platform. The patient pushes against the platform to move the sled away from the foot. The patient may initially use two legs and progress to a single-leg press (figure 21.34). Pre-selected and adjusted rubber bands or weights are used to vary the resistance. Ankle plantar flexion at the end of the motion can be added to provide ankle resistance. To reduce patello-femoral stress, the foot should be positioned on the platform so that the knee is flexed no more than 90° in the starting position. The knee should remain in alignment with the hip and ankle throughout the movement.

In the supine position, you can add resistive concentric and increased eccentric activity by having the patient push off the platform and catch him- or herself as the feet return to the platform. The speed of this exercise depends on the force with which the patient pushes off the platform and the amount of resistance used.

If the patient is in a tripod position on elbows and knees with the involved foot on the platform, the foot should be placed high on the platform to facilitate the quads and hip extensors. In this position, the patient can perform a slow and controlled motion as well as a rapid push-off and eccentric catch; however, the faster speed is more difficult and should be used only after the patient has demonstrated proficiency with the slower exercise.

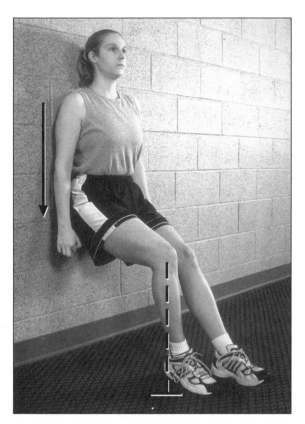

Figure 21.35   Wall squat.

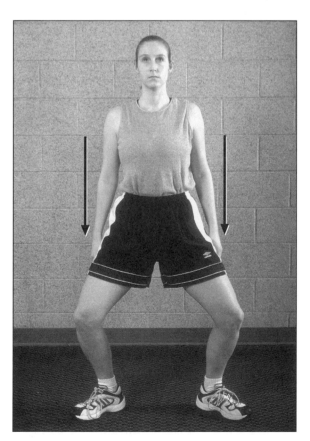

Wall Squats

This exercise strengthens the quads. The patient stands with the back to the wall and the feet out in front. He or she squats to bend at the hips and knees, but the knees should remain over the ankles so that the lower leg does not go beyond a perpendicular line to the floor. If the knee is flexed more than 90°, patellofemoral stress increases and pain may result. The deeper the squat, the farther away from the wall the feet should start so that from the wall the knee is never flexed more than 90°. Placing a ball between the knees is thought to increase response from the vastus medialis, but this theory has recently been challenged (Mirzabelgi et al. 1999).

The patient can hold this position in an isometric for several seconds or move up and down without pausing in the low position. A Swiss ball can be placed between the wall and the patient if repetitions without an isometric hold are used.

Common errors with this exercise include positioning the feet too close to the wall so that flexion goes beyond 90°, placing more weight on the uninvolved extremity, and hiking the hip so that the knee does not flex as much. If the patient is reluctant to bear weight equally on left and right extremities, a small platform placed under the uninvolved foot can facilitate increased weight bearing on the involved extremity.

You can advance this exercise by increasing the repetitions or sets, increasing the depth of the squat (as long as the knee does not move in front of the ankle), or having the patient perform the exercise with one leg only (figure 21.35).

Plié

This exercise strengthens the quads, especially the VMO. The patient stands with the feet in a wide stance with the hips and feet turned outward about 45°. The buttocks are squeezed as the patient slowly bends the knees, keeping the knees in line with the second toe (figure 21.36). The back should remain straight, so as the patient flexes the knees and hips, the trunk leans forward; the pelvis should not be allowed to move into a posterior tilt.

Common errors with this exercise include not aligning the knees over the second toes, causing the knees to move into a valgus position, not keeping the weight evenly distributed over right and left legs, and not keeping the back straight.

Figure 21.36   Plié.

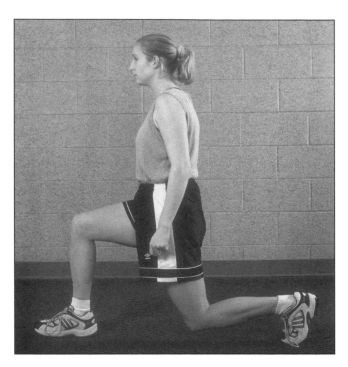

Figure 21.37 Lunge.

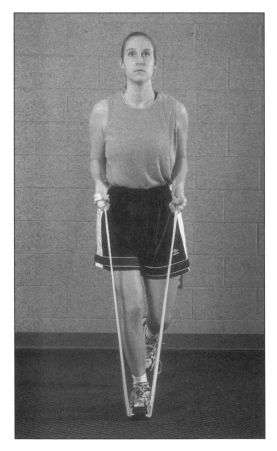

Figure 21.38 Mini-squat on one leg.

Lunge

This exercise strengthens the hip extensors and quads. The patient stands with the feet in a forward-backward stance with the involved leg in front. The quadriceps and buttocks are tightened, and the weight is shifted to the front leg as the patient bends the knee (figure 21.37). The knee should remain in line with the second toe, and the arch should be lifted as weight is placed on the extremity. This position can be held for several seconds and then repeated.

Common errors are to allow the arch to fall and the knee to move into a valgus position. The knee should not move forward ahead of the foot. The lower leg should remain at an angle no more than perpendicular to the floor.

Mini-Squats

This exercise strengthens the quads and buttock muscles. The patient stands with feet shoulder-width apart and toes turned slightly outward. Keeping the weight equally distributed, the patient squats to a comfortable position, maintaining the knees in alignment with the second toes. In a progression of this exercise, the patient grasps tubing that is anchored under the feet to increase concentric resistance. Holding weights in the hands increases eccentric and concentric resistance. Performing the exercise on only one leg increases the difficulty (figure 21.38).

The back remains straight as the patient squats, so the hips flex and move posteriorly and the pelvis remains in neutral throughout the exercise. Common errors are valgus movement of the knees, trunk flexion, and hip hiking on the involved side to reduce knee flexion. If genu valgus is noted, the patient should be instructed to keep the knees over the second toe and to arch the foot; trunk flexion is corrected with verbal cueing for a straight back and instructions to push the hips back and to keep the chest up; hip hiking is corrected with instructions to bend the knee more and keep the hips level.

Step Exercises

The patient should not attempt these exercises until he or she is able to bear weight on the involved extremity in a single-leg stance position. Proper weight transfer is also a prerequisite for these exercises. The step height may begin at a low level, around 10 cm (4 in.) and increase to 20 cm (8 in.) as the patient gains strength and knee control. The sport rehabilitation specialist should observe for exercise execution and should correct errors as needed. The patient should perform the exercise slowly and in a controlled manner. As with other weight-bearing resistive exercises, the knee should remain in line with the second toe throughout. The knee should achieve extension at the top of the exercise, but it should not lock. During initial performance of these exercises, patients often demonstrate poor knee control evidenced by wobbling of the knee as the individual raises and

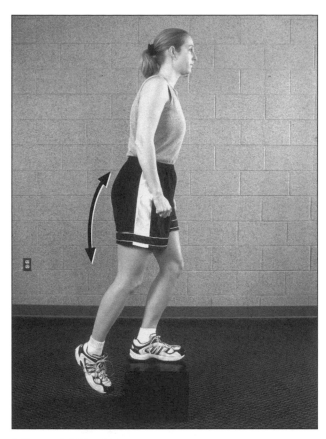

▌ Figure 21.39   Step-up.

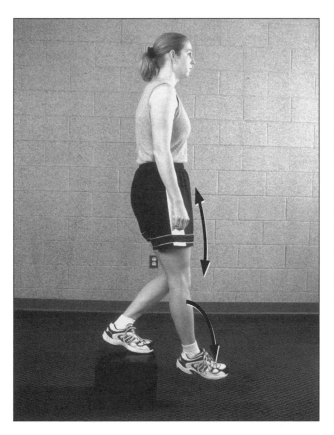

lowers body weight. With gains in strength, the knee movement becomes steady with no lateral knee movement.

Common errors for these exercises include bending at the hip and trunk to reduce the amount of quadriceps activity required, locking the knee in the extension position to reduce the need for muscular control, hip hiking to reduce the amount of knee flexion motion in the lowered position, jerking up and dropping down rather than maintaining a smooth and controlled motion throughout the exercise, moving the knee into a valgus position and flattening the foot arch, and pushing off with the uninvolved leg. Usually, corrections for these errors require verbal cueing and placing the patient in front of a mirror to provide visual feedback during the exercise. If pushing off with the uninvolved leg, dropping down and jerking up, and trunk and hip flexion are not corrected with these cues, the height of the step may be preventing the patient from correcting the errors and it may be necessary to use a lower step.

You can advance these exercises by increasing the numbers of repetitions and sets, increasing the depth of the step, and adding weights to the hands.

Step-Up

This exercise strengthens the quads. The patient stands facing a step with the involved leg on the step. The patient shifts the weight to the involved leg and moves the uninvolved leg up onto the step, being careful not to push off with the uninvolved leg (figure 21.39). He or she then returns to the starting position.

Step-Down

This exercise strengthens the quads and gluteal muscles. It stresses the knee more than the step-up exercise does because the patient is moving forward on the leg and the knee must move in front of the foot. If the exercise causes knee pain, it can be performed on a lower step; but if pain occurs on the lower step, the exercise should be deferred until knee control and strength increase. The patient stands on a step and slowly lowers the uninvolved leg to the floor so that the heel touches the floor first (figure 21.40). The patient then lifts the body backward, up to the starting position, while the uninvolved toes remain off the ground.

▌ Figure 21.40   Step-down.

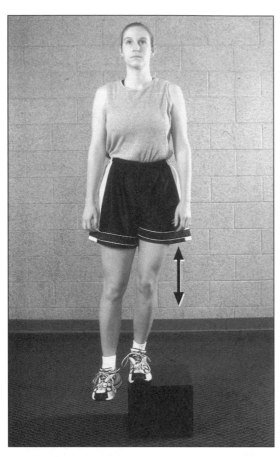

■ **Figure 21.41**   Lateral step-up.

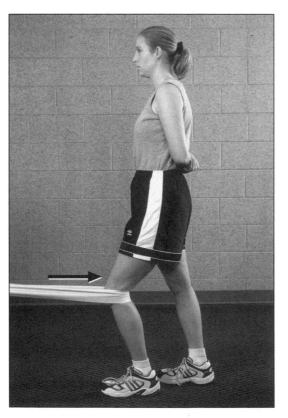

Lateral Step-Up

This exercise strengthens the quads and isolates the quads more than the other step exercises do. The patient stands sideways on a step, with the involved leg on the step and the uninvolved leg on the ground. The patient lifts the body weight up to the step by tightening the quads and gluteals (figure 21.41). Keeping the toe of the uninvolved leg up so that it does not touch the floor, the patient slowly lowers the uninvolved heel to the floor.

You can provide additional overload by requiring the patient to step away from the step to abduct the uninvolved leg when it is lowered.

Sit-to-Stand

This exercise strengthens the quadriceps and can increase strength in the midranges of motion. The patient sits in a chair with both feet on the floor under the knees. Without using arms for assistance, the patient moves in a slow and controlled manner from the sitting position to standing and then returns to the chair. The knees should remain in line with the second toes; weight should be equally distributed over right and left legs; and the back should remain straight with the pelvis in neutral. Once the patient performs this exercise easily, he or she can advance to a single-leg exercise. In this exercise, the uninvolved leg is positioned with the heel on the floor and in front of the involved leg, which remains back, as during the double-leg exercise.

Common errors in this exercise include shifting the weight to the uninvolved side, bending the trunk, jerking up, and dropping down into the chair. Correction techniques are verbal cueing, using a mirror for visual feedback, or using a higher chair and later advancing to a lower chair as strength improves.

Terminal Extension

This exercise is used to increase weight-bearing strength in the terminal-extension range. A rubber band is anchored around a stable object such as an upright bar, door jamb, or table leg. It is placed around the posterior knee. A pad or towel roll between the knee and band will enhance comfort. The patient stands facing the door jamb or table with the knee slightly flexed to 30° to 45°, weight on the involved extremity, and the band taut. The quadriceps muscle is tightened to straighten but not lock the knee (figure 21.42). The position is held for up to 5 s and then slowly released and repeated several times.

Common substitutions for this exercise include rotating the hips, bending the trunk, and flexing the hips.

■ **Figure 21.42**   Terminal extension.

MACHINE EXERCISES

A number of machine and weight exercises are available for strengthening the knee. Some units vary in features or style from one brand to another but have underlying similarities and exercise the same muscles or muscle groups. Available equipment varies from one facility to another according to budget, space, and staff preferences. Whatever equipment is used, it is imperative for the sport rehabilitation specialist to be familiar with the machine, with the instructions for use and the indications, and with the precautions and dangers before using it with patients. The following sections describe exercises with a few of the more commonly used machines.

Knee Extension

This machine should be used with caution. I do not often use it because of its potential for injury to the patellofemoral joint and ACL. It provides an open kinetic chain exercise that produces patellofemoral compression in the early portion of motion and places shear stress on the ACL in the later portion of the motion. It is essential that you use this machine cautiously, if at all, and in limited degrees of motion.

I mention the knee extension unit here not because I advocate its use, but because many facilities have such a unit and therefore it is important for the sport rehabilitation specialist to be aware of it, of how to use it, and of its dangers.

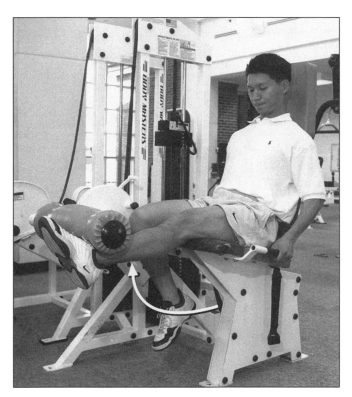

■ **Figure 21.43**   Machine knee extension.

The patient sits with the feet anchored around a weighted bar. To facilitate the rectus femoris, the patient should incline backward with the weight on the hands behind the hips. The individual then extends the knees (figure 21.43). If pain is produced with the machine, it should not be used.

Machine Leg Press

The machine leg press unit strengthens the quads and calf and gluteal muscles. The patient sits (or lies supine) with the feet on a platform. The patient pushes the platform with the feet either to move the foot platform or to move the body away from the platform, depending on the machine (figure 21.44). The patient can perform the exercise with either both legs or one leg. The exercise should be performed slowly and in a controlled manner through a full range of motion.

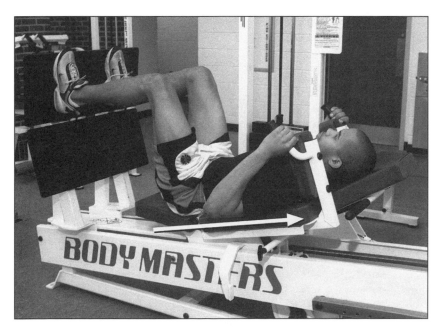

■ **Figure 21.44**   Machine leg press.

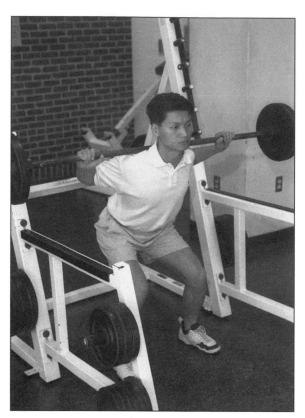

▌Figure 21.45
Squat.

Squat

This exercise strengthens the quads and hip extensors. It is an advanced exercise that patients should not have in their therapeutic exercise programs until they have demonstrated good strength and knee control with the step exercises and other closed chain activities previously outlined.

With the feet about shoulder-width apart, the weight is placed on the patient's shoulders. Keeping the back straight, the patient squats to no more than a 90° angle at the hips and knees (figure 21.45). The knees should remain in line with the second toe. Although the figure demonstrates the exercise with a barbell, the exercise can also be performed with adaptable machines such as a bench-press or heel-raise unit.

Hamstring Curl

This exercise strengthens the hamstrings. Depending on the machine, the patient may lie prone, stand, or sit on the unit with the machine secured around the posterior ankle. The knee begins in an extended position, and the patient flexes the knee (figure 21.46).

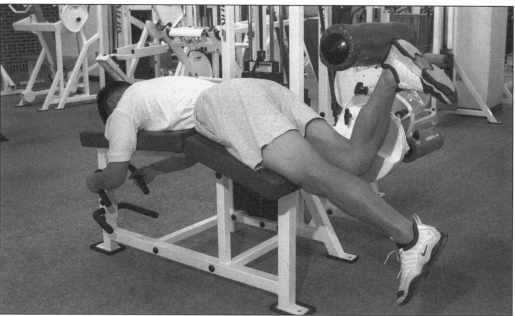

▌Figure 21.46
Machine hamstring curl.

ISOKINETIC EXERCISES

Isokinetic exercises for the quads and hamstrings usually begin after the patient has demonstrated control in isotonic exercises. Hamstrings and quads can be exercised isokinetically, isometrically, or eccentrically on isokinetic machines. If facilitation of the rectus femoris is desired, the seat back should be reclined to extend the hip (figure 21.47). The hamstrings can be exercised in a seated position to maximize output at the knee or in prone.

PROPRIOCEPTIVE EXERCISES

A rehabilitation program for a patient with a knee injury includes a progression of proprioceptive exercises aimed at restoring balance, agility, and coordination.

Balance, agility, and coordination must be restored following knee injury or surgery, just as with other segments. Proprioception is the element basic to these parameters. Early proprioceptive exercises before weight bearing can include a variety of activities. For example, with eyes closed the patient can move the involved knee to mimic the uninvolved knee's position, or with eyes closed can position the knee at a designated angle. With the latter activity, the sport rehabilitation specialist measures the angle to determine the patient's ability to produce the desired angle.

Weight-bearing proprioceptive exercises are similar to those for the ankle as discussed in chapter 20. The patient performs stork standing on the floor with eyes open (figure 21.48a) and then eyes closed before advancing to stork standing on unstable surfaces such as the BAPS board (figure 21.48b), trampoline (figure 21.48c), or foam rollers.

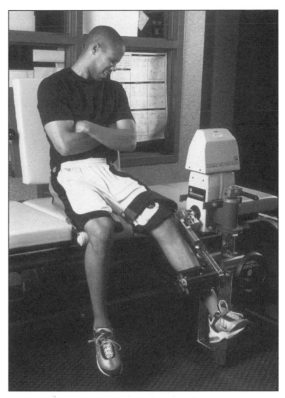

■ **Figure 21.47** Isokinetic exercises.

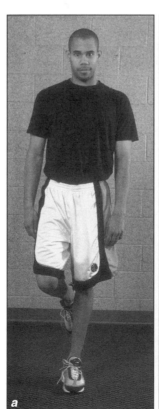
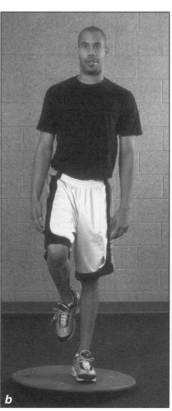
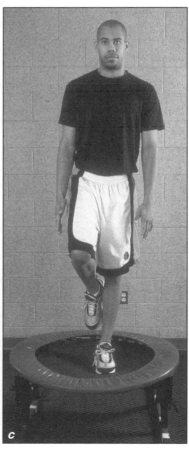

■ **Figure 21.48**
Stork-standing balance progression: (a) on ground, (b) on BAPS, (c) on trampoline.

The next progression is to make the balance activity more challenging and to facilitate change in the activity from a conscious to a subconscious activity. To accomplish this you can have the patient perform a distracting activity while maintaining balance on an unstable surface. For example, the patient can stand on a foam roller while using an upper-extremity device such as a B.O.I.N.G., Body Blade, or other device (figure 21.49). Another example is shown in figure 20.56a.

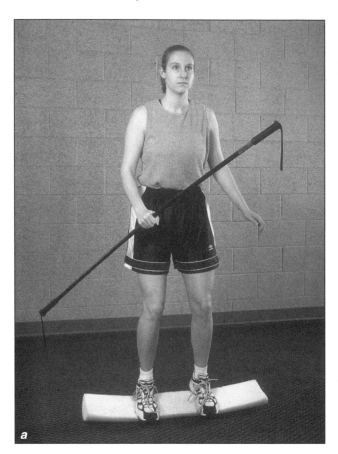 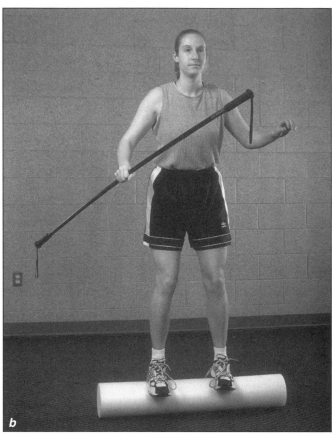

■ **Figure 21.49**   Advanced- and beginning-level distracting balance activities: *(a)* on ½ foam roller, *(b)* on foam roller.

Other balance and proprioceptive exercises include activities on balance boards, the Fitter, and slide boards. Activities that develop agility, coordination, and balance include jumping activities against rubber tubing with both legs and then with just the involved extremity; treadmill activities such as retro walking, side shuffle, and cariocas; and bilateral and unilateral hopping and jumping activities. Plyometric exercises with boxes develop agility and power in preparation for functional exercises. These advanced proprioceptive exercises are discussed in chapter 20 and shown in figure 20.58.

FUNCTIONAL EXERCISES

Functional exercises for the knee, which are similar to those for the ankle, use hopping, running, and cutting as well as sport-specific drill and skill activities.

Many of the functional exercises used for the knee are similar to those discussed in chapter 20 for the ankle. The exercises vary more according to the patient's sport than according to the lower-extremity segment injured, because a safe return to full sport participation depends on the entire lower extremity's ability to withstand stresses and perform properly regardless of the segment injured.

Functional activities include single, double, and triple hops; zigzag runs with sudden changes in direction; backward running with sudden changes to forward running; sprinting; running circles in clockwise and counterclockwise directions; 90° cuts to the left and to the right; and sport-specific drill and skill activities. Sport-specific drill and skill activities are dictated by the patient's specific sport and position within the sport. Because running, rapid changes of direction, and reliance on both lower extremities are vital to most sport participation, the running and hopping activities are universal and should be a part of most therapeutic exercise programs. These are discussed in detail in chapters 10 and 20.

Before returning to full sport participation, the patient must undergo an assessment of functional activity performance. This assessment uses many of the functional exercise activities the patient has been performing, and quality of performance is a crucial element. The patient should be able to perform all functional activities without psychological or physical impediment and should demonstrate equal use and performance with both lower extremities.

SPECIAL REHABILITATION APPLICATIONS

Specific injuries to the knee and thigh that require particular types of therapeutic exercise approaches include ligament sprains, collateral ligament sprains, meniscus injuries, patellofemoral injuries, strains and contusions, and bone injuries.

This section deals with specific injuries to the knee and thigh. The more common injuries are discussed.

LIGAMENT SPRAINS

Any ligament in the knee can become injured if the stresses applied are sufficient to overstress the ligament. Depending on the magnitude and direction of the forces applied, a single ligament or multiple structures can incur injury simultaneously. For the sake of simplicity, this discussion focuses primarily on injuries to individual ligaments.

Anterior Cruciate Ligament Sprain

The ACL is the knee ligament that is most frequently sprained. Considerations unique to this ligament are discussed here, then a case study is presented.

Although daily activities apply around 454 N of stress to the ligament, it is able to tolerate up to 1730 N before it ruptures (Dye and Cannon 1988; Markolf et al. 1990). It is in a position of maximum stress when the knee is either at full extension or at 90° flexion. The ACL is most typically injured when the knee suffers a valgus stress with external rotation in a foot-planted position as the athlete decelerates. The athlete is often in a cutting maneuver, and the injury can occur with or without contact with another player. Sudden knee hyperextension with rotation is another mechanism of ACL injury.

When contact with another player occurs, the ACL is frequently only one of the structures injured. The MCL or medial meniscus, or both, can be involved along with the ACL when outside contact force is added to the internal stresses of cutting or hyperextension. When more than one structure is injured, the rehabilitation process becomes more complicated because it must address considerations other than those related to the ACL.

The athlete may hear or feel a pop and then experience a giving way of the knee. Swelling occurs within the next 2 to 24 h, but is not apparent immediately.

Once an individual sustains an ACL injury, the decision about surgery must be made. Factors determining an individual's candidacy for ACL reconstructive surgery include age, activity level, desire to return to sport, and knee instability. Long-term differences between ACL injuries that have been surgically treated and those that have not include arthritic changes, progressive instability, and an alteration in activity level; these changes are more prominent in ACL injuries that have not undergone reconstruction.

If a patient elects to have reconstructive surgery, results are best in terms of motion recovery and return to participation when the surgery is delayed. Studies have demonstrated that surgical repair produces the best results when performed after the inflammation has subsided and full range of motion has been restored (Irrgang et al. 1997).

Over the years, many types of reconstructive surgeries for the ACL have been attempted. Surgical techniques continue to evolve, but currently the two most commonly accepted reconstructive procedures utilize either the patellar tendon or the medial hamstring tendon. The jury remains out on which is more effective and beneficial. The patellar tendon graft technique, which uses the central third of the patellar tendon with bone-plug ends from the patella and tibial tuberosity, is performed partially arthroscopically and also involves either one or two surgical incisions. Advocates of the patellar tendon graft point out that it is a graft using bone blocks so it necessitates less healing time before return to sport participation. The patellar tendon graft reconstruction allows immediate weight-bearing and allows therapeutic exercises two to three days following surgery. The rehabilitation time is three to six months. Advocates are also quick to point out that hamstring tendon graft reconstructions do not permit running for six months. In addition, because the fixation is not bone to bone, it has a more tenuous attachment site with greater risk of failure. Because of the weaker fixation, the rehabilitation program for the hamstring tendon graft begins later and the therapeutic exercise progression must be more conservative.

The semitendinosus and gracilis are used for the hamstring tendon procedure, which is a combined open and arthroscopic procedure. Advocates of the hamstring tendon graft procedure present the case that subjects who receive hamstring tendon grafts have fewer donor-site complications and regain quadriceps strength faster (Brown, Steiner, and Carson 1993). Donor-site problems seen with quadriceps tendon autografts include common complaints of patellofemoral pain or patellar tendinitis and, more rarely, problems of patellar tendon rupture and patellar fracture. There are pros and cons to both procedures. The physician's choice may depend on the patient's history and the physician's personal preference. The central-third patella tendon graft has a high tensile strength, stiffness, and fixation strength, while the hamstring tendon grafts have a lower surgical morbidity during the harvesting (Brown, Steiner, and Carson 1993). If the ACL-deficient knee is chronic, a patellar tendon graft may be more successful because of its greater stiffness and the probable laxity that has developed in the knee's secondary restraining structures. If the patient has a history of patellar tendinitis, patellofemoral pain, or patellar dislocations or has a failed patellar tendon ACL reconstruction, he or she is a likely candidate for the hamstring tendon graft.

Rehabilitation following ACL reconstruction follows two schools of thought, one for delay and the other for acceleration. Some advocate using the accelerated program with competitive and serious recreational athletes and the more conservative program with less serious recreational athletes (Wilk et al. 1999). The primary differences between the two programs relate to the timing of weight-bearing and therapeutic exercises. Those in the delayed-program camp are concerned about the vulnerability of new tissue and feel that stressing the tissue too soon will risk detachment at the graft site, compromise the graft, and render the joint unstable. A delayed protocol includes touchdown weight bearing for the first four weeks postoperatively, knee extension motion limited by a locked brace to around 15° and full motion not permitted until week 4, and refraining from closed kinetic chain exercises for the first six to eight weeks. Running is restricted until about the fifth month, with full return to sport occurring six to nine months following surgery.

Those advocating the accelerated program for ACL reconstructions believe that there are few complications from the surgery with early weight-bearing and therapeutic exercise applications and that stability is not threatened with the accelerated protocol. Weight bearing is to tolerance immediately postoperatively. The patient may wear a brace, but it does not restrict knee range of motion. Within a week postoperatively, closed kinetic chain exercises are used, with return to sport participation in five to six months.

Histologically, the ACL graft undergoes necrosis and remodeling once it is transplanted. Initially it is avascular, but revascularization occurs at 8 to 10 weeks and is completed around 16 weeks postoperatively. It is around 4 to 8 weeks that cellular proliferation into the graft site takes place. Because of proliferation and remodeling, it takes about 8 weeks for a graft to firmly attach to bone. Before this time, the graft is at risk of rupture. Once the graft is secure, it is safer to apply strain to the reconstructed site. A gradual progression of tissue remodeling occurs especially during the first 26 weeks, maturing the graft site and allowing it to manage progressively greater applied stresses. It may take at least a year for the graft to appear histologically normal, but it does not ever regain normal tensile strength. Although it is known that the graft strength is reduced, especially during the first few months following surgery, precise load-tolerance levels have not been determined. This means that the sport rehabilitation specialist must proceed cautiously, use common sense, rely on available knowledge and on the patient's reports of the knee's response to treatment, and observe carefully to determine therapeutic exercise applications.

When you are designing a specific ACL rehabilitation program for a patient who has undergone reconstructive surgery, key considerations must include the type of graft and fixation used, the type of surgery performed, the surgeon's rehabilitation preferences, and other injuries present. Although the timing is different for exercises in delayed and accelerated programs, the exercises and the progression are essentially the same.

Two program timing progressions are provided here as examples of a delayed and an accelerated ACL program. In actuality, a patient's program may be accelerated or delayed or may be a combination of the two programs. Communication with the physician regarding the patient's progression is crucial to a safe and successful rehabilitation program.

In an accelerated program, the patient ambulates with crutches, weight bearing to tolerance with full knee extension permitted. Two days postoperatively, passive knee extension to 0°, active hip exercises including straight-leg raises, and ankle range-of-motion exercises begin. The patient may wear a knee brace, but it is set at 0° extension. Although CPMs are used infrequently, one may be used in conjunction with electrical stimulation to the quadriceps. By the end of the first week, the patient should have 90° range of motion with full extension.

During the second week, active range-of-motion exercises for the knee begin, as do patellar mobilization and soft-tissue mobilization. By the end of the second week, the patient should be ambulating without crutches, but he or she continues to use the brace. Gait training may be necessary. Some physicians discontinue the brace during the third week, whereas others continue it for about six weeks, with removal only for showers and passive exercises. Closed kinetic activities such as mini-squats and stationary-bike exercises with minimal tension are used during the second week. Hamstring curls, toe raises, and range of motion to 105° are included at this time.

By the third week, the patient can exercise in the pool, can add other exercise equipment, such as the ski machine and the stepper with no more than a 10-cm (4-in.) step, and can leg press through a range of motion that is limited to 60°. The patient can do stork standing if weight transfer in ambulation is correct. By the end of the first month, the patient should have flexion to about 115° and full extension.

Tibiofemoral joint mobilizations should be used if capsular tightness is evident. None of the exercises should increase pain or edema or give the patient the sensation of increased knee laxity.

During weeks 6 to 8, if there has been no increase in swelling and the patient has full active extension and flexion to 115° to 120° and good isometric quadriceps strength, he or she can begin ambulation without the brace. Step-up exercises on a 15-cm (6-in.) step, active knee extensions in 100° to 60° ranges of motion, and a treadmill walking program are implemented during this time. Research has demonstrated that a treadmill set at an incline slightly greater than 12% reduces ACL strain and patellofemoral strain but recruits greater quadriceps activity, and thus may be beneficial for ACL and patellofemoral rehabilitation programs (Lange et al. 1996).

During the weeks leading up to the third month, the exercises that the patient has done so far continue, progressing as tolerated and in the absence of unwanted signs of pain and edema. By the third to fourth month, the patient can begin jogging and then progress to running and sprinting. During this time the patient advances to agility drills, plyometrics, and sport-specific activities, provided that strength is about 80% that of the uninvolved leg, full range of motion is present, and proprioception is good in static and dynamic balance activities.

During the fifth to sixth month, the program continues with strengthening and flexibility exercises and advances to more functional activities as the patient prepares to return to full sport participation. Because the physician often relies on the sport rehabilitation specialist for the information needed to determine readiness to return to full sport participation, an appropriate assessment is necessary. Before returning, the patient must pass all aspects of the functional assessment; have full motion, strength, and normal proprioception; and be pain free without edema postexercise.

A delayed program has the same progression, but at a slower rate. Weight bearing progresses from non-weight bearing during the first two weeks, to toe-touch weight bearing during the third through sixth weeks, to full weight bearing during the sixth through eighth weeks. Patellar mobilization is started during week 2, and electrical stimulation and modalities for pain and edema modulation can begin during the first week. During the first week, stretching exercises for the hamstrings, gastrocmemius, ITB, and quads can begin along with straight-leg raises and quad sets. Cardiovascular activities are limited to an upper-body ergometer or unilateral stationary cycling without the involved leg.

Other exercises are not added until week 5 to 6, when the patient can begin to do hamstring curls, hip exercises, and stationary-bike exercise. Leg-press-machine exercise with restrictions in motion of 10° extension to around 60° to 70° flexion can also start. Pre-gait activities that include weight shifting and proprioceptive exercises begin at this time.

Once the patient is full weight bearing, mini-squats, toe raises, wall sits, BAPS activities, and an aquatic program can be added. Active knee extensions from 90° to 30° are added as well. These exercises continue to progress as the patient is able to tolerate them, without increases in swelling or pain, throughout the program. At week 9 to 10, treadmill walking, stepper-machine exercises, and ski-machine activities can begin.

Jogging progressing to straight running is not permitted until about six months postoperatively. Cutting and lateral movements are permitted after the sixth month. A progression of plyometrics, agility exercises, and functional activities is gradually incorporated into the program.

During the 8th through 12th month, once the patient has passed the same assessment tests as in the accelerated program, return to full sport participation is permitted.

Patients who sustain partial ACL tears or who opt not to have surgery must undergo a therapeutic exercise program to rehabilitate the injured knee. The emphasis for these patients is on hamstring strengthening and use of the hamstrings to act as a secondary stabilizer for the ACL-deficient knee. A brace is usually used for three to six weeks, with partial weight bearing advancing to full weight bearing over the first three weeks. The brace may be restricted to 15° extension and 90° flexion and advance to 0° extension by week 3 to 5. During the first two to four weeks, the exercises include quad sets, hip exercises including straight-leg raises, knee flexion range-of-motion exercises, and hamstring curls. Patellar mobilization is performed. Electrical stimulation for quadriceps facilitation and pain- and edema-modulating modalities are also used.

During weeks 3 to 4 the brace is removed for range-of-motion exercises, co-contraction activities for the hamstrings and quadriceps, resisted hamstring curls, stationary-bike exercise, and other closed chain exercises such as mini-squats and stork standing to begin. The patient can perform pool exercises and exercises emphasizing hamstring function.

By week 6, active extension to 0° is started, and step-up exercises and other previously mentioned strengthening exercises are used. A walking treadmill program also begins. A derotational brace is used during weight-bearing activities.

By week 8 to 10, jogging begins, progressing to running and sprinting. Once the patient is able to sprint, he or she can perform lateral activities. Agility exercises, plyometrics, and functional activities then progress as previously outlined.

Recovery from ACL reconstruction can be a slow process. In a prospective study, patients who underwent ACL reconstruction took anywhere from one to two years to regain full muscle function and pain relief (Risberg et al. 1999). The sport rehabilitation specialist must be careful always to consider the tissue healing time line and to coordinate intensity levels of therapeutic exercises with the time line. Optimal results are most likely to occur if these factors are respected.

Case Study

A 16-year-old, male soccer forward suffered a right ACL injury that was repaired last week. His physician instructed him in straight-leg-raise exercises and quad sets before discharging him from the hospital, but now the physician wants the patient to begin rehabilitation using an accelerated program. The patient is using crutches and bearing about 50% of his weight on the right lower extremity. He has a rehabilitative brace on the leg, with the knee joint set at 0° extension and 90° flexion. He is allowed to remove the brace for passive activities only. The knee has minor edema and some ecchymosis around the knee and into the proximal lower leg. The surgical repair was a patellar tendon transfer; the patient has two scars, one over the patellar tendon and one over the distal lateral thigh, in addition to portal scars from the arthroscopy. The surgical scars are healing well but still have sutures that will be removed next week. There are some soft-tissue adhesions around the knee, especially surrounding the surgical sites and the patellar pouch areas. The patient reports only minor postoperative pain. Patellar mobility is about 50% normal in all planes, but the patient does not report pain with movement. Alignment of the patella is normal, without the presence of patella alta or baja. The patient is able to perform a straight-leg raise but is unable to tolerate any resistance to the motion. Hip adduction is 3+/5, hip abduction is 4–/5, and hip extension is 4–/5. He reports some pain with attempts at full weight bearing but admits that he is very apprehensive about putting full weight on the leg.

Questions for Analysis

1. What will your first treatment for this patient include today?
2. What will your goals for this first treatment today be?
3. What pre-gait activities will you use to encourage the patient to put more weight on the right lower extremity?
4. What instructions will you give him before he leaves today?

5. What exercises will you include in his program over the next two weeks?

6. Over the next six weeks, what exercises will you assign, and what will be your criteria for advancing the exercises during that time?

7. How long do you expect the patient's program to take, assuming that he follows a program without complications or problems?

8. When will you have him start on a treadmill, and what will be your first exercise on it?

9. Outline a progression from the treadmill to a full running program.

10. List four exercises you will include in the patient's functional activities program.

11. Describe the functional tests you will use before the patient is allowed back to full sport participation.

Posterior Cruciate Ligament Sprain

PCL injuries are not as frequently surgically repaired as ACL injuries. Necessary special considerations for this ligament are discussed here, then case study is presented.

PCL injuries occur less often than ACL injuries. The common mechanisms of injury are either hyperextension of the knee or forced hyperflexion of the knee with the foot planted. Although reconstructions using the semitendinosus, middle third of the patellar tendon, or the medial gastrocnemius are occasionally performed, most often injury management is nonoperative with emphasis on rehabilitation. Surgical repair is performed if the knee is unstable or if other ligaments have been injured as well as the PCL.

PCL-deficient knees do not generally feel unstable unless the person is walking down an incline, because the PCL protects the tibia from posterior displacement on the femur (or anterior femoral displacement on the tibia). Most patients are able to return to full sport participation following an appropriate rehabilitation program without surgical reconstruction.

The initial goals of rehabilitation are to resolve the inflammation and restore range of motion. Once the inflammation is under control, important goals are restoration of strength, control, and normal function. Modalities for modulation of pain and edema along with electrical stimulation for muscular facilitation are used initially. Range-of-motion exercises include active knee extension and passive flexion. Active hamstring exercises should be avoided because they produce posterior translation of the tibia on the femur. Strong gastrocnemius contractions should also be avoided beyond 30° of knee flexion because of the translational stress applied to the joint and stress added to the PCL (Durselen, Claes, and Kiefer 1995).

Open kinetic chain exercises can provide good isolated strengthening for the quadriceps as long as patellofemoral pain is avoided. If patellofemoral pain occurs, the exercises should be modified to avoid the pain. Modifications can include changing the degrees of motion and angles of the exercise, reducing the resistance, reducing the lever arm of the applied resistance, and using low weights with higher repetitions. These exercises include quad sets, straight-leg raises, and quad range-of-motion exercises. Crutches are used in weight bearing to tolerance with gradual progression to weight bearing without assistive devices. A closed kinetic chain exercise in terminal extension with rubber tubing can be used to strengthen the hamstrings and produce minimal posterior tibial translation (see figure 21.42). The hamstrings can also be strengthened in an open kinetic chain exercise for the hip extensors if the patient keeps the knee extended to reduce the posterior tibial shear stress.

Once the patient has progressed to full weight bearing, other closed kinetic chain exercises can begin. Proprioception exercises should emphasize recruiting the quadriceps for posterior translation control, first in static positions and advancing through dynamic activities. The program can progress from treadmill walking to jogging, running, increased weights, agility exercises, plyometrics (stressing deceleration activities, pivoting, lateral movements, and jumping), and functional activities. Knee control for posterior tibial translation should be emphasized throughout the program.

PCL injuries that are surgically reconstructed are immobilized with a brace that is locked in 0° extension for four weeks and is worn for a total of six to eight weeks, with free range of motion permitted in the last two weeks of wear. The brace is removed after the first week for passive exercises only. The lower leg is supported in long sitting to prevent a posterior sag of the tibia on the femur. During the first week, quad sets, straight-leg raises, and short-arc quad (SAQ) exercises are started. Patellar mobilization is performed. Hip extension and knee flexion activities are avoided during the first three weeks, but hip adduction and abduction exercises can be used with resistance applied proximally on the leg.

After six to eight weeks, once the patient has no extensor lag and demonstrates good control and a normal gait, the crutches and brace can be discontinued. Closed kinetic chain activities during this time include exercises to 45° flexion. Hip extension with the knee in extension, exercise on the stationary bike with toe-clips to reduce hamstring activity, balance activities, and proprioceptive exercises are also started once the patient is full weight bearing.

The patient gradually progresses to the treadmill, ski machine, stepper, and to running activities. The progression is the same as for the ACL program, with advancement to agility, plyometrics, and functional activities. The patient is able to return to full sport participation after 9 to 12 months, depending on the individual patient's response to the program.

Case Study

Last week an 18-year-old, female volleyball player injured the left posterior cruciate when landing hyperflexed after hitting a ball. The physician will not perform surgery, because the knee is not unstable. He wants you to begin the rehabilitation process with the patient today.

Your examination reveals moderate edema around the knee. The patient has a brace and is able to bear partial weight on the left leg. Her range of motion out of the brace is 30° extension and 60° flexion. Her patellar mobility is limited by about 75%, but her knee is too flexed for you to decide whether the restriction is attributable to the knee position or to reduced patellar mobility. She has pain at 6/10. Although there is edema around the knee with some discoloration, the soft tissue feels tight from the edema pressure. Her strength is 4–/5 in hip flexors and abductors and 3+/5 in hip extensors, adductors, and quads. You have deferred hamstring testing because of the PCL injury.

Questions for Analysis

1. What will your first treatment with the patient today include?

2. What instructions will you give her to do at home?

3. What exercises will you include in today's session?

4. Outline your expected time line for beginning hamstring exercises, walking on a treadmill, and stationary cycling. Will you use pool exercises with the patient? If you will use the pool, list three exercises.

5. List four agility exercises and functional skill activities you will include in the last phases of her therapeutic exercise program.

6. List the functional tests you will use to determine when the patient is ready to return to full sport participation.

COLLATERAL LIGAMENT SPRAINS

The MCL can be injured by itself or in combination with other knee structures. Collateral ligament injury treatment is different from protocols for cruciate ligament treatment.

Medial collateral ligaments are more frequently injured than LCLs. An MCL injury occurs as the result of a valgus stress, and an LCL injury results from a varus stress to the knee. Medial collateral ligament injuries are rarely surgically repaired except when instability results from a combination of ACL and MCL tears. In those situations, the MCL may or may not be repaired even if the ACL is repaired.

The rehabilitation programs are similar for MCL and LCL injuries. Initial treatment includes modalities for pain and swelling modulation. The current philosophy in treating isolated collateral ligament injuries is to use bracing or support in conjunction with an early therapeutic exercise program (Reider 1996). The patient's injured knee is placed in a functional or rehabilitative brace, and the knee is limited to 0° extension and 90° flexion to control ligament stress and still allow motion. The brace is worn for three to six weeks; and crutches, with either non-weight bearing or weight bearing to tolerance, are used for two to four weeks. During this time, active range-of-motion exercises, isometric exercises to retard quad and hamstring atrophy, and hip and ankle exercises are used. Patellar mobilization may be necessary if the joint becomes stiff. Cross-friction massage to soft tissues can be helpful in promoting healing and preventing adhesions. In 7 to 10 days, pool exercises are useful for range of motion and strength. After about two weeks, the stationary bike can be used if the knee has about 105° of flexion. Before that time, the patient can use the bike as a means of increasing range of motion.

A combination of open and closed kinetic chain exercises is used to increase hamstring and quadriceps strength. These exercises follow the progression outlined for cruciate ligament injuries and must not produce patellofemoral pain or increase collateral ligament pain. Once the patient is ambulating in full weight bearing, stork standing and other balance activities can begin. Walking on the treadmill with progression to jogging occurs once a normal walking gait has been achieved. Jogging then progresses to running and sprinting as long as pain and edema are avoided.

If full motion is not achieved by around week 5 or 6, joint mobilization techniques and prolonged stretches may be required. The patient progresses in strength and agility exercises as long as there are no deleterious signs. The program advances from agility and plyometrics to functional activities. A functional knee brace is often used before and after return to sport. The collateral ligament brace does not require the rotational stability that an ACL brace does, but it should have medial and lateral upright supports to control valgus and varus stress.

The rate at which the patient progresses depends on the individual's tolerance and the severity of the injury. Return to normal function can occur in as few as three to four weeks or can take as long as two to three months.

Case Study

A 17-year-old, male gymnast suffered a grade II sprain of his right MCL during a rings dismount three days ago. The physician wants him started on a rehabilitation program. For the past three days he has received ice, elevation, compression, and electrical stimulation for edema control. He is on crutches with a hinged brace set at 0° and 90°. He is bearing about 75% of his body weight on the right leg when he ambulates. There is moderate swelling with tenderness to palpation along the MCL. His hip and hamstring strength is grossly 4/5. He has an extensor lag of 15°. He reports mild pain unless he attempts to bend the knee past 60°; then the pain level becomes moderate. Patellar mobility is normal.

Questions for Analysis

1. What will your first treatment for this patient today include?

2. What home program will you give him before he leaves your facility today?

3. Outline the exercise program you will have the patient perform for the next week. How will you determine his progression?

4. List three open kinetic chain and three closed kinetic chain exercises you will have him perform within the next two weeks, and list them in the order that you will assign them.

5. What agility exercises will you include in his program?

6. What plyometric exercises will you use?

7. Describe the functional activities you will use in your assessment to determine when the patient is ready to return to full sport participation.

MENISCUS INJURIES

Among all the rehabilitation programs for knee injuries, the rehabilitation program for meniscal injuries has seen the greatest changes over the past 15 to 20 years. Current trends in treatment allow for a more rapid return to participation than in the past, with reduced deleterious effects.

Surgical treatment of meniscal injuries has evolved over the past several years. Arthrotomies for complete removal of damaged meniscus have been replaced by arthroscopic procedures for partial removal of torn segments, repair, and allograft replacements.

Isolated injury to the medial meniscus does not result in instability to the knee, but if a meniscal tear is combined with an ACL rupture, the knee becomes unstable. Isolated meniscal tears tend to be degenerative tears, whereas meniscal tears that accompany ACL injuries are more likely to be acute (Shelbourne et al. 1996). A stable knee with a meniscal injury may not be a candidate for a meniscal repair, but an unstable knee will become more unstable if the meniscus is removed or partially removed. Knees that undergo a meniscal repair with an ACL repair do better than with an isolated meniscal repair (Tenuta and Arciero 1994).

Lateral meniscal repairs and lateral meniscectomies have a greater success rate than medial meniscal repairs. One may presume that the higher success rate of lateral meniscectomies and their lower impact on ACL-deficient knees is attributable to the lower amount of rotation on the lateral knee and the smaller attachment the lateral meniscus has to the knee.

Meniscal repairs must have a viable blood supply to be successful. The peripheral rim of the menisci have a blood supply, but the majority of the inner substance is avascular. The blood supply can reach inward as far as 6 mm (about 0.25 in). Tears that occur over the outer third of the meniscus have the best healing capabilities. Tears that extend inward farther than the blood supply do not do well with meniscal repair procedures. Surgeon's preferences regarding the width of the meniscal tears that do well with repairs are variable, and range from 2 mm to 6 mm (Scott, Jolly, and Henning 1986; Stone, Frewin, and Gonzales 1990). Up to 20% of all meniscal tears are reparable. Meniscal repair is advantageous over meniscectomy because the meniscus remains, and there is consistent evidence that even partial meniscectomy leads to osteoarthritic changes in the joint. The rehabilitation process, however, is significantly longer for a meniscal repair than for a meniscectomy. Whereas a rehabilitation program for a meniscectomy generally requires four to six weeks, a patient is often restricted from sport participation after a meniscal repair for four to six months.

The patient who has a medial meniscus and ACL injury that both require surgical repair is a difficult case for the surgeon and sport rehabilitation specialist. Meniscal repairs do better if performed as soon after the injury as possible. Following the meniscal repair, the postoperative care is conservative, with non-weight bearing and limited motion for up to six to eight weeks. On the other hand, the ACL repair is most successful when delayed until after the inflammation is resolved and with immediate postoperative partial to full weight bearing and motion.

Traditionally, the postoperative care for meniscal repairs has been conservative, but accelerated programs have been used more recently (Barber 1994). There is much controversy about use of an accelerated program for meniscal repairs. The conservative protocol guards the repair by using limited motion and weight bearing to reduce the shearing forces applied to the repair. The accelerated program limits the time on crutches and uses partial weight bearing and active motion in the early stage to apply appropriate stresses to healing tissue and prevent unwanted loss of motion and patellofemoral pain problems. The sport rehabilitation specialist must communicate with the physician to create a feasible rehabilitation program for the patient who has received a meniscal repair.

A conservative postoperative meniscal repair program includes placing the patient on crutches, non-weight bearing on the involved leg for six to eight weeks. Toe-touch weight bearing is sometimes allowed after two weeks, with slowly progressive increases in weight bearing to full weight bearing at six to eight weeks. A rehabilitative brace is used to keep the knee in a flexed position for about six weeks after surgery. During this time of immobilization, the patient can perform hip and ankle exercises. Manual resistance to the hip should be applied above the knee to prevent stress on the knee joint. Once the brace is removed, patellar mobilization, and after six to eight weeks tibiofemoral joint mobilizations, can be used. Active range of motion and a progressive strengthening program begin after the brace is removed. Crutches are discarded when the patient is able to walk normally and has adequate quad strength to control the knee. Pivoting and acceleration-deceleration activities are not allowed for four to six months after surgery. From then on, the patient progresses to functional activities before returning to sport.

In an accelerated program, weight bearing is allowed as the patient tolerates it, but the patient uses crutches until he or she is able to walk normally. Range-of-motion exercises are used during the first postoperative week. Quad sets and straight-leg raises also begin during the first two weeks. The goal during the first few weeks is to achieve full range of motion without increased edema in the knee. By the end of week 2 to 3, the patient should be able to ambulate normally without crutches.

In week 2 to 4, the patient can use pool exercises, closed kinetic chain exercises including those on a stationary bike, mini-squats, and a walking treadmill program. By week 6 to 8, isokinetic exercises are suitable. Jogging progressing to running is added before lateral and pivoting movements are allowed. By that time the patient should have about 80% quad strength. The progression then follows that outlined for the ACL programs, with return to sport participation at 10 to 12 weeks post-operatively.

If the meniscus is not reparable, an arthroscopic partial meniscectomy is often the surgery of choice if the patient continues to experience knee locking or giving way following the injury. The patient may be placed on crutches immediately post-operatively because of reflex inhibition of muscle activity subsequent to surgery and edema. Weight bearing is to tolerance with the expectation that the patient will be able to walk without assistance in the next few postoperative days as the pain and edema subside and knee control improves. Quad sets and straight-leg-raise exercises can begin immediately postoperatively, but often the patient has difficulty with these exercises on the first day because of reflex inhibition. Electrical stimulation can aid the quadriceps in regaining function. A combination of open and closed kinetic chain exercises is used within the first two to three days after surgery. Gait-training and weight-transfer activities may be necessary if the patient demonstrates an abnormal gait. Wall slides for range of motion, ankle pumps, hip exercises, and hamstring stretches can begin on the first or second day. Mini-squats, wall squats, step-ups and step-downs on a small step, standing terminal extensions, stationary-bike exercise, tubing exercises, and use of free weights can all start at this time as the patient tolerates. Once the patient is able to transfer weight appropriately onto the involved leg, static balance activities are used to increase proprioception, advancing to dynamic balance activities.

By the second week, step-up exercises can usually be tolerated. Lunges can be added at this time. The slide board, ski machine, and stepper can also be used. A jogging program is started by week 3 to 5, progressing to running as the patient responds to the stresses appropriately without increased swelling or pain.

Isokinetic, agility, plyometric, and functional activities are the last progressions before the patient's return to full sport participation. These are added to the program once the patient has good control with adequate strength and coordination. Although the timing varies from one patient to another, these activities are usually added around week 5 to 6, with full return to participation within six to eight weeks postoperatively.

Rarely, the surgeon may opt to perform an autograft meniscus transplant. Transplantations can be performed arthroscopically or with an open procedure. Sutures with bone plugs at either end of the meniscus are used as the anchors for the graft (figure 21.50). Postoperative care guidelines have been primarily reported as case studies (Fritz, Irrgang, and Harner 1996). Program progression, as with other conditions, is based on a combination of tissue healing and knowledge of stresses and loads applied to the menisci.

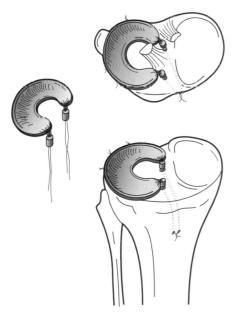

Rehabilitation for meniscal transplants involves non-weight bearing or partial weight bearing on the involved extremity for six weeks. Continuous passive-motion and range-of-motion exercises are used immediately postoperatively, with flexion limited to 90°. The patient wears a brace to maintain the knee in extension when not exercising in order to reduce the shear stress on the graft for about six weeks. Patellar mobilization techniques can be used to maintain good patellar mobility while the patient is in the brace. Treatment goals in the first six weeks are to control the inflammation, maintain full knee extension, minimize quadriceps atrophy, and protect the graft.

After six weeks, gait training without the brace begins, as do closed kinetic chain exercises from full extension up to 60° flexion. As mentioned earlier, compressive loads on the menisci increase to 85% of those for the entire knee at 90° flexion; so flexion greater than 60° is avoided in the closed kinetic chain, but motion to 90° is permissible in an open kinetic chain motion. Continued protection of the graft with normal gait and increased motion and strength becomes a goal as the program progresses for the next six weeks. Closed chain exercises include toe raises, mini-squats, wall sits, leg presses, and step-ups. Open chain exercises include range-of-motion exercises, hip exercises, and pool activities. Standing balance activities begin at this time. Progression continues as the patient tolerates and as he or she shows no signs of unwanted stress.

Figure 21.50
Meniscal transplant.

Rehabilitation progression for a meniscal transplant procedure follows that for most other programs but at a slower rate. Once the patient has adequate strength, range of motion, and coordination to control the knee, agility, plyometric, and functional activities proceed. Full return to sport participation may take around 8 to 10 months or longer.

Case Study

A 20-year-old male ice hockey forward experienced a left knee meniscal tear. He underwent an arthroscopic partial meniscectomy yesterday and comes to you today to begin his rehabilitation program. He is walking without crutches, but he has an antalgic gait on the left leg. He reports mild pain and a sensation of tightness around the knee. Your examination reveals swelling of 2.5 cm (1 in.) around the knee. The patient's active range of motion is −15° extension and 90° flexion. Passive range of motion is 0° extension and 100° flexion. He is able to perform a straight-leg raise but cannot tolerate resistance in the motion. Other hip motions are 4/5. Hamstring strength is 4−/5. The patella is slightly restricted in mobility.

Questions for Analysis

1. What will your first treatment with the patient include today?

2. What will you give him as home exercises and instructions before he leaves today?

3. What are your goals with him for the first week of treatment?

4. Preseason hockey practice begins in two months. What will you tell the patient when he asks you whether he will be ready by then?

5. When do you expect him to be able to begin squats with weights?

6. What will you say when the patient asks you why he cannot straighten the knee when he could before the surgery?

7. Present a progression of proprioceptive exercises that you will have in this program. Discuss the progression of agility exercises you will use. List the functional activities you will include in the final phase of the patient's program.

PATELLOFEMORAL INJURIES

Patellofemoral injuries can be complex injuries and frustratingly slow to respond to treatment. Several factors may contribute to patellofemoral injuries, especially those that are nontraumatic. This section deals with the injuries that are most frequently seen.

Patellar Dislocations and Subluxation

Patellar instability is more frequently seen in women than in men. This is thought to be the result of an increased Q-angle secondary to a wider pelvis, which increases the lateral vector force on the patella. Other predisposing factors include a shallow lateral femoral condyle or posterior patella, an improper position of the patella, and a weak VMO, especially if it is combined with tight or strong lateral structures.

The mechanism for injury is lateral rotation of the thigh with knee flexion on a planted foot. If the patella is subluxed, it often relocates independently. A frank dislocation may or may not relocate on its own. First-time dislocations may not relocate, but recurrent ones often do without assistance. Pain and edema are severe.

Treatment includes use of crutches with weight bearing to tolerance. An immobilizer brace may be initially used with progression to a functional brace to stabilize the patella. Therapeutic exercise progresses to the patient's tolerance. Electrical stimulation to the quadriceps and modalities for pain and edema control are applied in the early phase of a rehabilitation program, usually in the first two weeks. Increases in pain and edema are avoided throughout the program. Patellofemoral pain can be produced at any time, but especially in the early phases of rehabilitation when the area is still inflamed from the initial insult. All exercises should be pain free. If an exercise produces pain, it should be delayed until the patient is able to perform it without pain.

Exercises begin in an extended and short-arc pain-free position with a progression into a greater arc of motion as strength gains and pain permit. Exercises are a combination of open and closed kinetic chain. Program emphasis should be on VMO strength and patellar control during activities. As strength and knee control improve, exercises progress to more rapid activities until functional speeds are possible with good patellar control.

Lower-extremity alignment should be assessed in standing and walking, because pronation can increase the risk of patellar instability and can be corrected with orthotics.

The duration of a rehabilitation program depends on whether the dislocation or subluxation is a first-time event or a recurring injury. Recovery in an acute subluxation/dislocation can take more time than for a recurring injury. An average expected recovery period is 4 to 10 weeks, with that for recurrent injuries on the shorter side and that for first-time injuries more toward the end of the range.

Patella Plica Syndrome

Plicae are residual synovial folds that persist into adult life and can become symptomatic secondary to a persistent synovitis and resulting loss of normal elasticity (Galloway and Jokl 1990). A secondary synovitis can result from the presence of loose bodies, meniscal tears, instability, or chondromalacia. The plica as an extension of the synovium becomes inflamed. In persistent cases, the plica becomes fibrotic and can be palpated as a firm, inelastic band, usually on the medial aspect of the knee.

Conservative treatment includes modalities and medication to relieve the inflammation, hamstring stretching, and quadriceps strengthening. If conservative measures do not relieve the patient's pain, arthroscopic excision of the plicae may be necessary.

Rehabilitation following surgical excision follows a course similar to that for an arthroscopic partial meniscectomy. Therapeutic exercises can begin on the day of surgery and progress according to the patient's tolerance. The patient should be able to return to sport participation within three to six weeks after surgery if the post-operative course is normal.

Osgood-Schlatter Disease

In spite of its name, **Osgood-Schlatter disease** is not a disease but a mechanical disruption of the patellar tendon insertion site on the tibial tuberosity. It is an avulsion, an avascular necrosis, or an epiphysitis of the tibial tuberosity. It is most commonly seen in active adolescents, often after a recent growth spurt. A direct impact such as a fall on the tibial tuberosity can also cause the injury. The signs and symptoms are similar to those of a patellar tendinitis, with pain during activities such as running or jumping. Stiffness and edema can also be present.

Treatment for this condition has changed over the years. Cast immobilization used to be the preferred method of treatment, but current treatment focuses on activity modification. An enlargement of the tibial tuberosity occurs, and only in extreme cases is this surgically excised. Patients can derive benefits from modalities for modulation of inflammation, pain and edema; stretching exercises for the hamstrings, ITB, and gastrocnemius; strengthening exercises to the quadriceps; and cross-friction massage to the patellar tendon. The injury is self-limiting in that the patient's activities are constrained by pain. Activity to tolerance is generally allowed once the inflammation has subsided.

Patellofemoral Syndrome

Syndromes of the patellofemoral joint can be caused by many different factors, individually or in combination. The term for this frustrating injury, "syndrome," demonstrates that the medical community has been unable to identify one specific etiology.

Mechanism

Patellofemoral pain is a common complaint among athletes as well as among those who do not participate in athletics. Anterior knee pain has been classified under various headings including chondromalacia patellae, patellofemoral stress syndrome, patellofemoral pain syndrome, extensor mechanism malalignment syndrome, runner's knee, and patellofemoral malalignment syndrome. *Chondromalacia* is a term that was used in the past to describe anterior knee pain. Chondromalacia refers to a specific injury that involves softening and degeneration of the patella's posterior articular cartilage and it is not an accurate diagnosis for most anterior knee pain conditions. The most commonly used terms today to describe anterior knee pain include patellofemoral pain syndrome (PFPS) or patellofemoral stress syndrome (PFSS).

Signs and Symptoms

Typical signs and symptoms of PFPS, regardless of the terminology, include stiffness after prolonged sitting, pain with activities such as stair climbing and running, and pain after activity. Crepitus is usually present. The patient may experience a giving way of the knee because of reflex inhibition secondary to pain, especially on stairs or ramps. Swelling is usually mild, but the posterior surface of the patella is tender to palpation.

Underlying Factors

PFPS is anterior knee pain and inflammation caused by abnormal stresses applied to the knee's extensor mechanism. Several underlying conditions can lead to PFPS. Patellofemoral pain syndrome can result from direct trauma to the patella, but is more often the result of cumulative stresses in the presence of additional contributing factors, both extrinsic and intrinsic to the joint itself. These factors include tightness in the ITB, hamstrings, and gastrocnemius; weakness in the VMO or imbalance of strength between the VMO and vastus lateralis; excessive pronation; increased Q-angle; knee hyperextension; and patellar alignment. You must evaluate each of these elements when examining the patient with PFPS, because correction of or compensation for these malalignments must occur if the PFPS is to be resolved.

Normal function of all body segments relies on a balance of the surrounding structures. This balance includes adequate flexibility and proper strength so that forces are adequately and appropriately directed to produce the desired motion and force applications. If hamstring, gastrocnemius, ITB, or lateral connective tissue structures are tight, they apply an imbalance of forces on the knee. Tight hamstrings increase the need for knee flexion during activities and increase compressive forces on the patella anteriorly. The need for increased knee flexion during ambulation in turn necessitates increased dorsiflexion to clear the toe. Normally 10° dorsiflexion is necessary for ambulation; but if the gastrocnemius does not permit this motion or if the hamstrings increase the need for additional dorsiflexion but it is not available, the foot pronates in an attempt to increase flexibility. Excessive pronation necessitates tibial internal rotation, which increases the knee's valgus stress. A tight ITB pulls the patella laterally as the band moves posteriorly during knee flexion. In cases of severe distal tightness of the ITB, the patella can become positioned to tilt laterally because of the ITB's lateral pull.

If either the VMO is weak or an imbalance is present between the VMO and the vastus lateralis, the patella moves laterally during quadriceps contractions. This permits the patella's lateral rim to ride more on the lateral femoral condyle than in the intercondylar groove, where it normally glides during knee motion. If the vastus lateralis is tight, the lateral pull during quadriceps contractions is exaggerated. Repetitive gliding against the condyle leads to inflammation of the patella's articular surface.

If the knee is in hyperextension, the inferior pole of the patella is frequently tilted inward. This causes the patella to push into the fat pad in full extension, and to glide with an inferior tilt during knee motion, altering the relationship between the patella and femoral groove. The patella has increased contact inferiorly as it glides in the groove, increasing stresses at the inferior pole.

Patellar Orientation

Patellar orientation and alignment should be examined in a relaxed long sitting or supine position, and in closed chain positions in both static and dynamic conditions. Patellar alignment varies from one patient to another; it can also be different from left to right knee in the same individual. In a relaxed open chain position with the knee in full extension and the femur in parallel alignment with the examination tabletop, the sport rehabilitation specialist should assess the patellar alignment in various planes. He or she should assess for the presence of a lateral glide, lateral tilt, inferior tilt, and rotation. In full extension, the patella should rest slightly lateral to the center of the knee with the inferior pole at the knee's joint margin. If the patella's position is more than a few millimeters to the lateral aspect, it has a lateral glide. A medial glide is rare. When a finger is placed on the medial and lateral poles of the patella, they should be in the same plane; if the lateral finger is lower than the medial finger, the patella has a lateral tilt. A medial tilt is rare. When a finger is placed on the superior patella pole and another is placed on the inferior patellar pole, they should be in the same plane; if the distal finger sits deeper than the proximal finger, the patella has an inferior tilt or posterior tilt. This is referred to as an AP tilt. The superior medial and lateral poles should be in the same plane; if the lateral pole lies more superiorly on the knee and the medial pole lies more inferiorly, the patella is laterally rotated. If the medial pole lies more inferiorly, the patella is medially rotated. A lateral rotation is more common than a medial rotation. These patellar positions are demonstrated in figure 21.51.

The patella's tracking pattern should be assessed in non-weight bearing. With the patient contracting the quadriceps in full knee extension, the sport rehabilitation specialist observes the patella for its movement. Normal movement is 8 to 10 mm superiorly, with some lateral motion. If lateral structures are tight or the VMO is weak, the patella will move more laterally with the lateral component occurring sooner in the

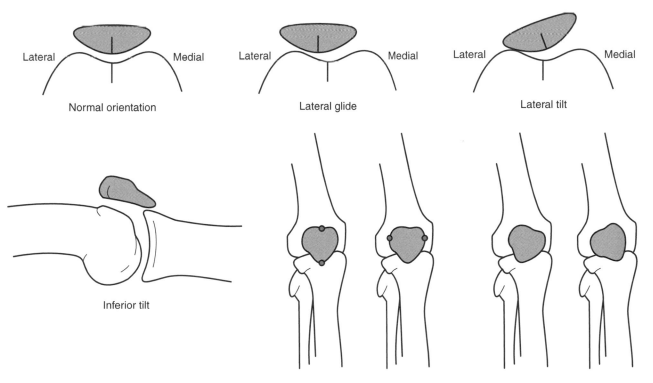

I Figure 21.51 Patellar orientation.

motion. During knee movement into flexion, the patella migrates medially as the Q-angle decreases and the patella becomes centered in the trochlea.

Alignment should also be observed in standing, and movement of the patella should be observed while the patient performs an activity such as a lunge or step-down movements. Changes in patellar alignment and glide during weight bearing can indicate various influential factors that should be corrected, such as pronation, weakness, incorrect firing patterns, and tightness.

Corrections

Common surgical procedures to treat patellofemoral pain and patellofemoral malalignment in the past included a lateral release in which the lateral retinaculum was cut, or an advancement of the tibial tubercle into a better alignment. It has been demonstrated, however, that patients with PFD have better results with nonsurgical management that consists primarily of exercise (Karlsson, Thomee, and Sward 1996).

Assessment of the underlying causes dictates what is included in the treatment program. Orthotics may be needed if pronation is present; flexibility exercises and soft-tissue mobilization techniques are necessary if tightness and adhesions exist; muscle re-education for timing of contractions is necessary for imbalance in timing of activity or strength between the VMO and vastus lateralis; and strengthening exercises, especially for the VMO, are needed with all patellofemoral pain regardless of cause, because pain causes an inhibition reflex and weakens the quadriceps.

Patellar Taping Technique

A technique developed by Jenny McConnell, an Australian physiotherapist, uses a combination of taping to the patella and exercises to correct patellofemoral alignment and reduce pain. Although McConnell's theory is that the taping corrects patellar alignment, recent studies have shown conflicting results on the efficacy of patellar taping. Some have demonstrated that no change occurs (Kowall et al. 1996) whereas others have demonstrated that a reduction in pain or alignment does occur with the tape (Somes et al. 1997; Worrell et al. 1998). These studies, however, did point out that the effects of taping were limited. Patellar position changed only at 10° of knee flexion (Worrell et al. 1998), and no change occurred in the open chain position (Somes et al. 1997). Empirical evidence persists to support the theory that McConnell taping reduces pain in spite of the limited research to substantiate these claims. It has been speculated that the tape may provide neural inhibition through neurosensory afferent stimulation of the large A fibers (Bockrath et al. 1993).

Research has shown that patellar taping facilitates a quicker response of the VMO during step-up activities and delays the onset of vastus lateralis response while increasing the onset of VMO response during a step-down exercise (Gilleard, McConnell, and Parsons 1998). It has yet to be determined whether this change in muscle response results from improved muscle response secondary to pain reduction or neurosensory facilitation.

Patellar Tape Applications

When more than one malalignment is present and one of them is a posterior tilt, the posterior tilt is corrected first; otherwise, the greatest malalignment is corrected first. The tapes used for patellar taping are Cover-Roll, used as a hypoallergenic cloth undertape to protect the skin, and Leukotape, used to guide patellar alignment. The tape should improve the patient's symptoms immediately. To evaluate its effectiveness, the patient should perform an activity that reproduces the pain such as a step-down and assess the pain level. After the tape is applied, the patient repeats the activity to reassess the pain level. Although the pain may or may not completely resolve, it will be significantly reduced with the tape application in 50% of the cases (Bockrath et al. 1993). If no change in pain is perceived, the correction tape should be reapplied in a different sequence. The tape can be worn for extended periods of time

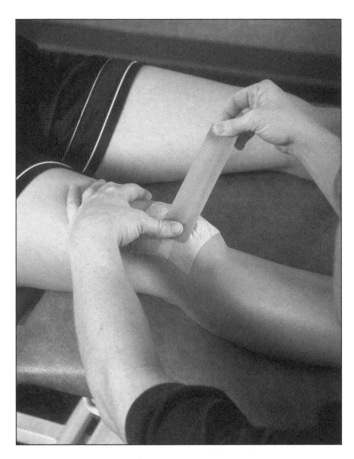

Figure 21.52
Lateral glide
correction.

to effect a low-load, long-term stretch on soft tissues. It is worn 23 h a day with an hour off, usually after a shower, to relieve skin stress. With a reduction in pain, an increase in VMO facilitation and quadriceps strengthening can occur. The tape can get wet without any effect on its adhesion, but over time it loses its effectiveness. The top tape strip can be readjusted if it loosens. If taping proves effective, the patient can be instructed in tape application, removal, and skin care so that he or she can reapply the tape daily until symptoms subside. As VMO strength and timing improve and pain decreases, the patient is weaned from the tape.

The cloth undertape is applied smoothly to the skin over the patella, and the correction tape is applied with force to correct patellar position. The tape is usually applied with the knee in extension. If pain occurs during the middle range of a squat, the tape can be applied with the knee positioned in the painful range of flexion. The quadriceps must remain relaxed during any McConnell tape application.

To correct a lateral glide, the correction tape is applied from lateral to the lateral border of the patella with a medial pull on the tape over the medial femoral condyle (figure 21.52). The soft tissue over the medial femoral condyle is lifted toward the patella manually to create a fold in the skin on the medial side and provide a better pull of the tape. A couple of strips of correction tape may be necessary. Each strip should create a larger soft-tissue crease.

To correct for a lateral tilt, a strip of tape is firmly anchored at the middle of the patella and pulled firmly toward the medial femoral condyle so that the lateral patellar border is lifted to move the patella level with the anterior femoral plane (figure 21.53). The soft tissue is lifted on the medial aspect to provide a better result.

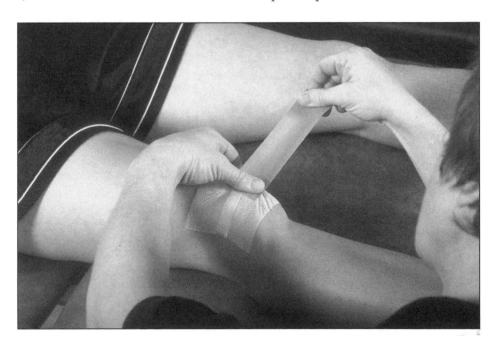

Figure 21.53
Lateral tilt correction.

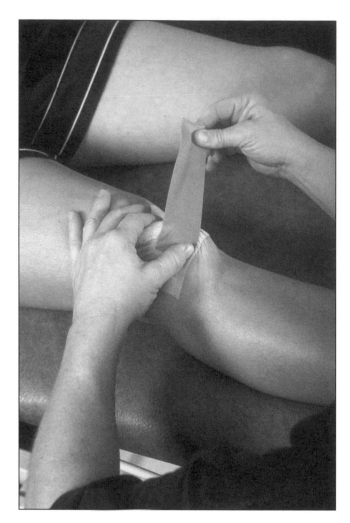

■ Figure 21.54   Lateral rotation correction.

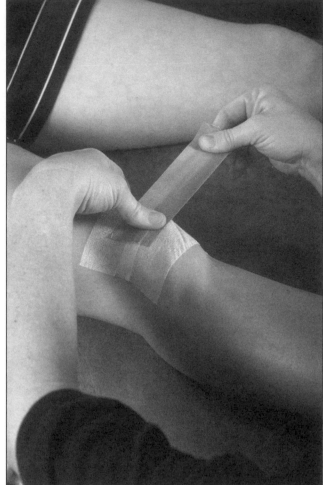

■ Figure 21.55   Inferior tilt correction.

To correct a lateral rotation alignment, the tape is anchored on the inferior patellar pole. The patella is manually rotated in correct alignment while the tape is pulled upward and medially (figure 21.54).

If present, a posterior or inferior tilt is corrected first to reduce infrapatellar fat-pad irritation with other tape corrections. A posterior tilt is usually corrected in combination with a lateral tilt or lateral glide. The tape is applied over the superior half of the patella to lift the inferior pole up and away from the fat pad (figure 21.55).

Skin irritation can occur with the use of taping. To minimize this risk, the tape should be removed carefully; an adhesive remover should be used after the tape has been taken off, and the skin should be carefully cleansed and conditioned with a moisturizer when the tape is not in use. If a small area of skin breakdown occurs, it should be covered with a protective dressing or, if possible, the tape should be averted from the area. If the breakdown area is too large, use of the tape should be discontinued until the skin heals. If an allergic reaction occurs, the tape should be discontinued.

Soft-Tissue Mobility

Soft-tissue adhesions and tightness along the distal ITB and into the lateral retinaculum often play a role in patellar malalignment. These structures should be treated with deep-tissue massage and stretching. Deep-tissue massage can be applied by the sport rehabilitation specialist with the flat side of a closed fist, with pressure

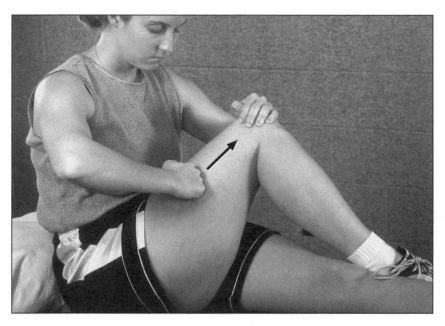

Figure 21.56
Iliotibial band massage.

delivered over the posterior middle and distal phalanges, as was discussed earlier in this chapter in the "Deep-Tissue Massage" section. The patient can also use a foam roller to perform self-massage techniques (figure 21.10). The patient can perform manual massage techniques over the distal lateral thigh throughout the day while sitting (figure 21.56).

The patient should receive instructions for stretching exercises for all tight muscle groups and should perform them throughout the day. The muscle groups commonly included are the hamstrings, gastrocnemius, and tensor fascia lata.

Additional Therapeutic Exercises

Therapeutic exercise is a vital part of the total rehabilitation program for patellofemoral pain. Stretching and strengthening exercises can alter patellar tracking to establish a more correct alignment (Doucette and Goble 1992). Because muscle imbalance can play a role in PFPS, it is logical to assume that improvement in muscle balances can impact improvement in this condition.

Lower-limb alignment and mechanics have a direct impact on the patellofemoral joint. Muscles in distal and proximal segments must be corrected for imbalances along with the knee muscles if patellofemoral pain is to be resolved. Muscles controlling foot pronation, including the posterior tibialis, anterior tibialis, and peroneals, should be strengthened and re-educated for pronation control and foot stability during closed chain activities.

Pelvis stability is important in knee control. Hip muscles and abdominals, especially lower abdominals, play a key role in providing adequate knee control during closed chain activities. Lower abdominal and hip control deficits are often seen in PFPS. Stabilization and strengthening exercises for these groups should be included when deficiencies exist.

Quadriceps strength is primary to a successful rehabilitation program. Electrical stimulation and biofeedback can be used to facilitate quadriceps activation. These electrical modalities are used in open chain exercises such as straight-leg raise and SAQ and in closed chain exercises for concentric and eccentric activity such as walking, step-downs, and lunges. A combination of open and closed chain activities within a pain-free range of motion is part of a total therapeutic exercise program. Patellofemoral taping might be required, especially in the early phases of therapeutic exercise when patellofemoral pain prevents adequate quadriceps activation.

When the patient is able to perform closed chain activities in a slow and controlled manner and without pain, the speed of the activities is increased to challenge muscle recruitment patterns and prepare the patient for agility and functional activities. As the patient gains strength, control, and flexibility, he or she follows a progression of exercises similar to that for other knee injuries, advancing to increased stress and forces, more challenging coordination and agility activities, and finally functional activities. Return to full sport participation is possible once the patient is pain free; has normal flexibility, strength, agility, and power; and is able to demonstrate normal performance of sport-specific activities.

Patellar Tendinitis

Patellar tendinitis can be related to patellofemoral alignment, so the same factors discussed in PFPS should be assessed for patellar tendinitis. Patellar tendinitis is often called jumper's knee because jumping activities are the primary precipitating factor. With the energy absorption that must occur during landing from a jump, jumping on hard surfaces and excessive jump repetitions can overload the tendon beyond its stress-absorbing capabilities. Tissue breakdown then occurs. This stress is exaggerated with muscle imbalances of weakness or tightness or mechanical malalignments such as foot pronation.

Pain occurs in the patellar tendon between the patella and tibial tuberosity. Pressure over the tendon, quadriceps tightening (especially eccentric activity), and stair climbing (especially going down) cause tenderness or pain. There may be slight edema in the area.

Initial rehabilitation goals are to reduce the inflammation and pain. This is accomplished with modalities such as phonophoresis, iontophoresis, ice, and electrical stimulation. Cross-friction massage across the tendon can be useful in promoting healing and reducing soft-tissue adhesions. The sport rehabilitation specialist applies cross-friction to one tender location on the tendon until the pain is reduced or relieved; he or she then moves to another site on the tendon and repeats the procedure until all tender sites have been treated.

Therapeutic exercises should include a combination of flexibility and strength. Stretching exercises for the hamstrings, quadriceps, lateral thigh, and calf muscles are taught to the patient. Strengthening exercises include open chain exercises to isolate the quadriceps and closed chain exercises for functional stresses. They may begin with isometric exercises for the quadriceps and active exercises for the hamstrings, hip, and ankle; but this depends on the patient's tolerance. In some cases the patient tolerates concentric closed chain activity but the eccentric portion of the closed chain exercise is too painful to perform. If this is the case, the exercise should be either postponed until the patient can perform it pain free or modified to eliminate the eccentric phase.

The rate of the program's progression is purely dependent on the patient's response to the exercises. The exercises should be performed pain free. During eccentric exercises, mild pain may occur during the last of three sets, but it should resolve when the exercise is completed. The program for eccentric exercises for tendinitis is outlined in chapter 15.

When the patient is able to perform sport-specific activities without pain or hesitation, return to full sport participation is possible.

Tendon Rupture

Tendon ruptures occur most commonly in people 30 to 50 years old as a result of a sudden quadriceps contraction; the cause is probably a gradual degeneration, although prior complaints of tendinitis are not usual. Tendon ruptures occur more often in males than in females. As with Achilles tendon ruptures, the patient feels as though he has been shot or kicked in the knee. The patient is unable to bear weight on the extremity. The rupture can occur from either the tendon attachment between the patella and tibial tuberosity (patellar tendon rupture) or the tendon between the patella and quadriceps (quadriceps tendon rupture). Complete ruptures are surgically repaired, with the knee kept either locked in extension with a brace or on a CPM. Straight-leg raises, quad sets, and hip exercises are used during the first 10 days to two weeks. Patellar mobilizations are used to maintain patellar mobility. Weight bearing is restricted initially and then advanced to weight bearing as tolerated in the brace. After about three weeks, exercises begin out of the brace and follow a progression similar to that for other surgical repair programs. The period until return to full activity is four to nine months.

Case Study

A 16-year-old, female cross country runner has had left knee pain for the past month. The pain has progressed so that it now interferes with her workouts and occurs during walking. The physician has diagnosed anterior knee pain and wants her to begin rehabilitation. Your examination reveals genu valgus and recurvatum with foot pronation in standing. The patient's running shoes have excessive wear on the lateral posterior heel so that the midsole is evident. The shoes have a sewn curved last. The patient's rearfoot and forefoot have excessive mobility. Straight-leg raise is to 70°; ankle dorsiflexion in rearfoot neutral is 0°. She has a positive Ober's test, and deep palpation reveals tenderness along the distal ITB. Her quadriceps strength is 4–/5, lower abdominal strength is 3/5, and hip extension strength is 4/5. Patellar alignment assessment reveals a posterior and lateral tilt. Patellar tracking in long sitting is lateral. In standing, lateral patellar tracking is less. When the patient performs a step-down exercise, pain is produced, and the knee wobbles. Palpation of the posterior patellar surface reveals tenderness medially and laterally, especially over the inferior aspect.

Questions for Analysis

1. What will your treatment for the patient include today?

2. What instructions will you send her home with today?

3. What will you tell her when she asks what she should do about her workouts?

4. Given her signs, what part of the range of motion would you expect the patient to have the most pain in?

5. List two elements you will use to strengthen the VMO during the first week.

6. What are your short-term and long-term goals for the patient, and when do you expect her to achieve them?

STRAINS AND CONTUSIONS

The severity of a strain determines the length of recovery. Ecchymosis indicates at least a grade II strain and necessitates a longer recovery time than a strain that does not produce discoloration. Ecchymosis is often distal to the site of muscle tear, because gravity pulls the blood caudally.

Lack of normal flexibility, fatigue, incoordination, and a sudden violent contraction or stretch of a contracting muscle are frequent precipitating factors for muscle strains.

Initial treatment goals include relieving inflammation, pain, and spasm. Pulsed ultrasound is effective in promoting the absorption of ecchymosis. Electrical stimulation is useful in relieving pain and spasm. Stretches with activation of the antagonists assist in relieving muscle spasm and regaining range of motion.

If the patient is unable to ambulate normally, assistive devices are used with weight bearing to tolerance. Strength exercises are incorporated into the program as the patient tolerates them. Active range of motion against gravity may be all that is tolerated initially, but progression to resisted open and closed chain exercises occurs within a few days. A variety of activities including proprioceptive neuromuscular facilitation, manual resistance, pool exercises, stationary-bike exercise, co-contraction exercises, and unilateral weight bearing can begin within one to three days once spasm and pain have subsided.

The program is quickly advanced to eccentric and isokinetic exercises. Eccentric exercises are important for muscle strains, because athletic activity places high eccentric demands on lower-extremity muscle groups (Stanton and Purdam 1989). Agility activities requiring more rapid muscle responses are introduced into the program as the patient gains strength, coordination, and balance control. When the patient is able to perform functional and sport-specific activities, he or she is ready to be tested functionally for return to full sport participation.

Hamstrings

Hamstring strains most commonly occur at the musculotendinous junction, either near the ischial tuberosity or more toward the lateral middle of the muscle where the biceps femoris tendon inserts more distally. They often occur during high-speed activities such as sprinting or during sudden changes in muscle activity.

Stretching exercises should begin within two to four days after an injury. Hamstring tightness is often a predisposing factor in strains. After an injury, additional flexibility loss occurs. Appropriately timed deep massage and cross-friction to the injury site promote healing and reduce scar-tissue adhesions that can further restrict hamstring mobility.

Strength exercises start as isometrics and progress to concentrics, and then eccentrics, before transitioning to isokinetics and faster-speed activities.

Quadriceps

The quadriceps are subject to strains, contusions, and other injuries, some severe and others not. The injuries requiring rehabilitation have unique characteristics that are outlined here, then a case study is presented.

Strains

Jumping or sudden changes in direction are activities that often produce quadriceps strains. The treatment course follows the same routine as for hamstring strains. Stretching activities are started on day 2 to 4 and are accompanied initially with isometric exercises. Pool exercises, proprioceptive neuromuscular facilitation, passive stretching, and stationary-bike exercise are used early in the program. Isometric exercises are replaced with isotonic and open and closed chain activities and advance to eccentric activities as tolerated. Isokinetic, agility, plyometric, and functional activities progress as with other knee rehabilitation programs.

Contusions

Contusions occur more commonly in the quadriceps than strains do. Pain and spasm are the most debilitating symptoms, so initial treatment goals are to resolve these conditions and maintain flexibility. Electrical stimulation, pulsed ultrasound, and ice help to relieve spasm and pain. Mild active and passive stretches with contraction of the contralateral muscle are recommended after spasm is relaxed, usually on the second or third day postinjury. A stationary bike can be used to improve range of motion. Pool exercises can also relax the muscle. Pain reflexively inhibits the muscle, so quadriceps strengthening is necessary and can begin when muscle spasm has been relieved. The progression is the same as outlined for other injuries, with the rate of progression based on the patient's response to specific exercises. Recovery with full return to sport participation usually can occur in two to three weeks for moderate and severe contusions.

Myositis ossificans is a condition that results from either a severe direct blow or repetitive blows to the quadriceps that affect the periosteum of the femur and cause non-neoplastic bone formation in the muscle. A painful, rigid mass can be felt through deep palpation of the anterior thigh in the muscle belly. Loss of range of motion accompanies myositis ossificans.

Surgical treatment is indicated for unresolved conditions but is usually not performed until the growth has stabilized, about one year postinjury. Surgical excision before that time can exacerbate the problem. Conservative treatment involves the treatment course outlined for contusions.

Iliotibial Band Syndrome

Iliotibial band syndrome is an overuse syndrome that results from friction between the ITB and the lateral femoral epicondyle. It occurs in middle- and long-distance

Case Study

A 30-year-old male tennis player sprinted to return a ball at the net when he felt a tear in his right hamstring one week ago. He was unable to walk and sought medical attention. The physician has diagnosed a grade II hamstring strain and wants the patient to begin rehabilitation. The patient ambulates with a slight antalgic gait. His knee motion is 115° flexion to −15° extension. Left straight-leg raise is 60°, but the patient states that he has always been tight in his hamstrings. His hamstring strength is 3/5 and painful with resistance. His quadriceps strength, ankle strength, and hip strength are each 4/5. A large area of ecchymosis on the posterior leg is present from the proximal thigh below the gluteal fold to about 10 cm (3.9 in.) distal to the knee. The ecchymotic region is most tender in the darkest area of discoloration along the posterolateral thigh. There is a small indentation with tenderness to palpation about 10 cm distal and 5 cm lateral to the ischial tuberosity.

Questions for Analysis

1. What will you include in today's treatment for the patient?

2. What home program will you give him before he leaves today?

3. What are your short-term goals for him and when do you expect him to achieve them?

4. Outline the course of exercises for this patient for the next two weeks. What functional activities will you include in his program?

5. What will your criteria be for permitting the patient to return to full sport participation?

runners. It is thought to take place at 30° of knee flexion when the ITB is pulled over the lateral femoral epicondyle. This position occurs during running when the tensor fascia lata and gluteus maximus, the muscles attaching to the ITB, are active and are pulling on the band during the initial stance phase (Orchard et al. 1996). During downhill running, more time is spent in flexion, increasing the ITB stress.

Predisposing factors include leg-length discrepancy, increased Q-angle, genu valgus, and foot pronation. Running on hills and increased running distances also causes ITB syndrome.

The patient complains of pain along the ITB (especially over the lateral femoral epicondyle), increased pain with walking or running (especially down hills), edema, and crepitus. Snapping over the lateral femoral epicondyle can sometimes be felt.

Treatment must involve correction of predisposing factors, stretching, and strengthening. Modalities to relieve the inflammation and a workout modification are useful. Running at a faster speed may reduce ITB pain, because during faster running the knee is at more than 30° flexion in the early weight-bearing phase. When pain is relieved, strengthening exercises for deficiencies should proceed with the inclusion of open and closed kinetic chain exercises, concentric and eccentric closed chain activities, and a progression as previously presented for return to full sport participation.

OSSEOUS INJURIES

Fractures of the knee bones can be traumatic or stress related. Femur fractures are not common occurrences, fortunately, but tibial fractures are seen more frequently.

Fractures

Fractures of the knee result from direct blows and impact forces, torsional stresses, or compression loads. A patellar fracture usually occurs as the result of a direct blow, but a tibial fracture occurs most often because of torsional or compression forces. Epiphyseal plate injuries of the proximal tibia or distal femur occur in adolescent patients whose growth plates have not yet matured. Damage to these sites can alter bone growth. Tibial plateau fractures require non-weight bearing for six to eight weeks because of the tibia's major role in weight bearing. Displaced fractures require open reduction and internal fixation (ORIF).

Fractures repaired with ORIF procedures become more stable more quickly and can sometimes undergo a more accelerated therapeutic exercise program.

Chondral fractures and articular cartilage defects occur as a result of trauma to the articular surface, often a direct impact. These lesions occur most often in young adults. The lesions frequently develop into localized joint degeneration. Several treatment options are available for these isolated degenerative changes in the knee. Surgical options involve resurfacing of the chondral defect and commonly include arthroscopic debridement of the chondral surface. This is often accompanied by an abrasion arthroplasty, subchondral drilling, or creation of microfractures to stimulate bleeding to produce scarring that ultimately produces cartilage. Cartilage formation using these techniques is fibrocartilage, not hyaline cartilage, the normal articular cartilage. Fibrocartilage, unlike hyaline cartilage, has poor tolerance for weight-bearing activities.

The most recent advances in cartilage transplant were developed by Swedish physicians (Brittberg et al. 1994). Chondral tissue is harvested from a non-weight-bearing surface of the patient's knee. The harvested cells regenerate chondrocytes in a laboratory until sufficient quantities are available to transplant into the chondral defect. The recent reports indicate that the cartilage graft is hyaline, not fibrocartilage. This procedure is still under study, but cases that have been reported demonstrate favorable results.

Rehabilitation following chondral resurfacing techniques is similar to fracture rehabilitation in that weight bearing is either non-weight bearing or toe-touch weight bearing for six weeks. A brace locked in extension is used during ambulation to reduce shear stress on the lesion site. If debridement is the only procedure performed, weight bearing immediately postoperatively is to tolerance. Electrical stimulation, isometric exercises, and other nonresistive open chain exercises, with the knee in a position that does not stress the articular cartilage lesion site, are permitted during the non-weight-bearing phase. Biofeedback for muscle re-education is useful for quadriceps facilitation and control. The goal during this period is to stimulate chondral formation without applying excessive loads on the lesion site. It is appropriate to add pool exercises in deep water for range of motion after the operative wounds are well healed. Patellar mobilization and soft-tissue mobilization can be used. A stationary bike without resistance can be used after the third week. Active assistive range-of-motion exercises advancing to active range-of-motion exercises can also be used then. By week 3 or 4, the patient should be able to demonstrate good quad control without an extensor lag and should have near-normal range of motion. After the third week, mild resistive pool exercises in deep water are suitable.

After the sixth week, progressive weight bearing with crutches can begin. Crutches are not removed until the patient is able to ambulate normally, has no extensor lag, and has full extension. Pool exercises can progress from the deep to the shallow end with progressive weight bearing. Progressive resistive exercises in the open and closed kinetic chain, using small arcs of motion initially and advancing to larger arcs of motion, start after six weeks. Exercises should remain pain free in all arcs of motion. A ski machine or stepper can also be used. Once the patient is able to ambulate without crutches, treadmill activities can begin. Static balance exercises progress to dynamic balance exercises as tolerated.

A gradual progression from balance to coordination to agility exercises takes place as the patient gains strength and proprioception. Running is allowed at 6 to 8 months postoperatively with return to full sport participation at 7 to 12 months.

Bone-fracture rehabilitation programs follow the same basic progression, but the timing for return to full sport participation is more rapid. A general range of time for return to sport following a fracture is 4 to 8 months. The range varies according to whether the fracture is treated surgically or immobilized, the location and type of fracture, the age of the patient, and the physician's preference.

Osteochondritis Dissecans

Osteochondritis dissecans (OD) is a disease of unknown etiology without related trauma that affects the femoral epiphysis in juvenile OD and the femoral condyle in adult OD. A bone flake in juvenile OD or a bone fragment in adult OD occurs at various sites of the femoral condyle. Juvenile OD occurs in youths under age 15, and adult OD is seen in people over age 15. Symptoms include nonspecific knee pain, point tenderness over the site, and quadriceps atrophy. There is minimal effusion, and the patient may experience catching, locking, or giving way during ambulation.

Treatment for adult OD includes arthroscopic debridement of loose bodies. If the lesion is small, an abrasion arthroplasty or autogenous grafting can also be performed. Treatment for juvenile OD is more conservative, with prolonged rest, three months or more, occasionally with immobilization.

Rehabilitation for juvenile OD must attempt to reverse the deleterious effects of prolonged immobilization and inactivity. Cardiovascular exercise using the upper extremities, and lower-extremity exercises for the uninvolved segments help to maintain conditioning levels. Quad sets, straight-leg raises, and electrical stimulation can assist in retarding atrophy during immobilization.

Range-of-motion exercise, joint and soft-tissue mobilization, and active exercises are used once immobilization is removed. Weight-bearing exercises include weight-transfer activities and gait training. Pool exercises with progressive weight bearing can be used, and activities to restore proprioception using a BAPS board and a balance board, as well as stork standing, are helpful.

Rehabilitation following surgical treatment includes immediate weight bearing unless the lesion is large; in this case, weight bearing may be restricted. A gradual progression of exercises that do not produce pain takes place as with other knee lesions. An expected recovery to full sport participation usually takes about four to six months.

SUMMARY

1. *Discuss the relationship and alignment between the patella and femur.*

   Patellar stability is the result of static and dynamic structures. The bony configuration, with the patella seated within the femoral sulcus formed by the medial and higher-ridged lateral epicondyles, is the greatest bony contributor to patellar stability. Ligamentous stability from the patellofemoral and patellotibial joints assists in providing static restraints. Active restraints occur primarily from the quadriceps. The patella is in various degrees of contact within its groove in the femur during any specific point within the knee's range of motion. A combination of compressive forces and the amount of area of contact determines the patellofemoral joint stress.

2. *Identify postinjury factors that influence strength output.*

   Edema and pain both cause automatic withdrawal of quadriceps activity. An abnormal gait, using the injured extremity less than normal, also results in reduced muscle activity. These factors in combination contribute to further reduction of strength in the injured extremity.

3. *Define quadriceps extensor lag and explain its significance.*

   An extensor lag occurs when full passive motion in knee extension is present but the patient is unable to actively achieve full extension. It is an indication of quadriceps weakness.

4. *Outline a general progression of rehabilitation for a knee.*

   As with other body segments, specific applications depend on specific deficiencies. Modalities are used to relieve pain and edema and to encourage the healing process. Soft-tissue and joint mobilization techniques may be necessary. Range of motion, active and passive, is used to increase motion. Strengthening exercises can be started early in a pain-free range of motion or with isometric exercises. Manual resistance can progress to machine and body-weight resistances, rubber tubing, and isokinetics. Proprioception and balance activities begin with something simple like a stork stand and progress to balance activities on unstable surfaces. Once flexibility, balance, and strength have reached appropriate levels, plyometric exercises, such as target jumping, lateral jumps, box activities, and depth jumps, can be used. Functional activities that mimic the patient's specific sport are the final aspect of the therapeutic exercise program before full participation in the sport is permitted.

5. *Identify three soft-tissue mobilization techniques for the knee.*

   Three such techniques are foam roller myofascial release to the ITB, trigger point release to the quadriceps, and cross-friction massage to the patellar tendon.

6. *Identify three joint mobilization techniques for the knee, and their purpose.*

   Lateral glides of the patella are used for full flexion-extension range of motion of the knee, posterior glide of the tibia on the femur is used to increase flexion, and rotational glides are used to increase terminal flexion and extension of the knee.

7. *Explain three flexibility exercises for the knee and identify the structure they affect.*

   Flexibility exercises include standing knee flexion stretch for the quadriceps with the heel behind the buttocks, standing hamstring stretch with the involved extremity on an elevated surface, and the gastrocnemius stretch with the knee straight.

8. *Explain three proprioceptive/balance exercises for the knee.*

   Exercises for proprioception/balance include stork standing with eyes open and then closed, stork standing on a $\frac{1}{2}$ foam roller, and standing on a foam roller while catching a ball.

9. *Identify three functional activities.*

   Three functional activities are running and cutting while dribbling a basketball, sprinting forward and then backward with rapid changes in direction, and lateral glides with pivots to left and right.

10. *Identify three factors that influence PFPS.*

    Three such factors are weak quadriceps, weak hip and trunk control, and tight hamstrings.

CRITICAL THINKING QUESTIONS

1. In this chapter's opening scenario, how much knee flexion motion would you expect Cory to have after two weeks of immobilization? What kind of motion exercise would he be able to start on his first day of rehabilitation? What strengthening exercises would you give him for his hip and ankle on his first day of rehabilitation? When you would expect him to have full knee motion? When would you start him on passive stretching exercises for his quads? Give your justification for this timetable.

2. When would you begin patellar mobilization on Cory? When would you begin soft-tissue mobilization to the quadriceps repair site? Give your rationale for these timetables.

3. If you had two patients with knee injuries, one with an ACL sprain and the other with an MCL sprain, which one (if either) would you be more cautious with and why? How would their rehabilitation programs differ?

4. If a patient complains of patellar tendinitis, what structures would you investigate for possible causes? What key items would you include in your history questions? Would you use primarily open or closed chain exercises initially, and why?

5. A teenaged patient you have been rehabilitating for weakness following an anterior medial knee contusion continues to complain of pain in the knee even though his strength is improving. How would you approach the problem and what would you suspect?

REFERENCES

Ahmed, A.M., and D.L. Burke. 1983. In vitro measurement of static pressure distribution in synovial joints: I. Tibial surface of the knee. *Journal of Biomedical Engineering* 105:216–225.

Barber, F.A. 1994. Accelerated rehabilitation for meniscus repairs. *Arthroscopy: The Journal of Arthroscopic and Related Surgery* 10:206–210.

Beynnon, B.D., Fleming, B.C., Johnson, R.J., Nichols, C.E., Renstom, P.A., and M.H. Pope. 1995. Anterior cruciate ligament strain behavior during rehabilitation exercises in vivo. *American Journal of Sports Medicine* 23:24–34.

Bockrath, K., Wooden, C., Worrell, T., Ingersoll, C.D., and T. Farr. 1993. Effects of patellar taping on patella position and perceived pain. *Medicine and Science in Sports and Exercise* 25:989–992.

Brittberg, M., Lindahl, A., Nilsson, A., Ohlsson, C., Isaksson, O., and L. Peterson. 1994. Treatment of deep cartilage defects in the knee with autologous chondrocyte transplantation. *New England Journal of Medicine* 331:889–895.

Brown, C.H., Steiner, M.E., and E.W. Carson. 1993. The use of hamstring tendons for anterior cruciate ligament reconstruction. Technique and results. *Clinics in Sports Medicine* 12:723–756.

Brownstein, B., Mangiene, R.E., Noyes, F.R., and S. Kryer. 1988. Anatomy and biomechanics. In *Physical therapy of the knee,* ed. R.E. Mangiene. New York: Churchill Livingstone.

Butler, D.L., Noyes, F.R., and E.S. Grood. 1980. Ligamentous restraints to anterior-posterior drawer in the human knee. *Journal of Bone and Joint Surgery* 62-A:259–270.

Close, J.R. 1964. *Motor function in the lower extremity. Analysis by electronic instrumentation.* Springfield, IL: Charles C Thomas.

deAndrade, J.R., Grant, C., and A.S-J. Dixon. 1965. Joint distension and reflex muscle inhibition in the knee. *Journal of Bone and Joint Surgery* 47-A:313–322.

Doucette, S.A., and D.D. Child. 1996. The effect of open and closed chain exercise and knee joint position on patellar tracking in lateral patellar compression syndrome. *Journal of Orthopaedic and Sports Physical Therapy* 23:104–110.

Doucette, S.A., and E.M. Goble. 1992. The effect of exercise on patellar tracking in lateral patellar compression syndrome. *American Journal of Sports Medicine* 20:434–440.

Durselen, L., Claes, L., and H. Kiefer. 1995. The influence of muscle forces and external loads on cruciate ligament strain. *American Journal of Sports Medicine* 23:129–136.

Dye, S.F., and W.D. Cannon. 1988. Anatomy and biomechanics of the anterior cruciate ligament. *Clinics in Sports Medicine* 7:715–725.

Freeman, M.A., and B. Wyke. 1967. The innervation of the knee joint. An anatomical and histological study in the cat. *Journal of Anatomy* 101:505–532.

Fritz, J.M., Irrgang, J.J., and C.D. Harner. 1996. Rehabilitation following allograft meniscal transplantation: A review of the literature and case study. *Journal of Orthopaedic and Sports Physical Therapy* 24:98–106.

Galloway, M.T., and P. Jokl. 1990. Patella plica syndrome. *Annals of Sports Medicine* 5:34–41.

Gilleard, W., McConnell, J., and D. Parsons. 1998. The effect of patellar taping on the onset of vastus medialis obliquus and vastus lateralis muscle activity in persons with patellofemoral pain. *Physical Therapy* 78:25–32.

Gough, J.V., and G. Ladley. 1971. An investigation into the effectiveness of various forms of quadriceps exercises. *Physiotherapy* 57:356–361.

Grelsamer, R.P, and J.R. Klein. 1998. The biomechanics of the patellofemoral joint. *Journal of Orthopaedic and Sports Physical Therapy* 28:286–298.

Grood, E.S., Suntay, W.J., Noyes, F.R., and D.L. Butler. 1984. Biomechanics of the knee-extension exercise. Effect of cutting the anterior cruciate ligament. *Journal of Bone and Joint Surgery* 66-A:725–734.

Huberti, H.H., and W.C. Hayes. 1984. Patellofemoral contact pressures. The influence of Q-angle and tendofemoral contact. *Journal of Bone and Joint Surgery* 66-A:715–724.

Irrgang, J.J., Harner, C.D., Fu, F.H., Silbey, M.B., and R. DiGiacomo. 1997. Loss of motion following ACL reconstruction: A second look. *Journal of Sport Rehabilitation* 6:213–225.

Isear, J.A. Jr., Erickson, J.C., and T.W. Worrell. 1997. EMG analysis of lower extremity muscle recruitment patterns during an unloaded squat. *Medicine and Science in Sports and Exercise* 29:532–539.

Jenkins, W.L., Munns, S.W., Jayaraman, G., Wertzberger, K.L., and K. Neely. 1997. A measurement of anterior tibial displacement in the closed and open kinetic chain. *Journal of Orthopaedic and Sports Physical Therapy* 25:49–56.

Karlsson, J., Thomee, R., and L. Sward. 1996. Eleven year follow-up of patello-femoral pain syndrome. *Clinical Journal of Sport Medicine* 6:22–26.

Kaufman, K.R., An, K-N., Litchy, W.J., Morrey, B.F., and E.Y.S. Chao. 1991. Dynamic joint forces during knee isokinetic exercise. *American Journal of Sports Medicine* 19:305–316.

Knight, K.L., Martin, J.A., and B.R. Londeree. 1979. EMG comparison of quadriceps femoris activity during knee extension and straight leg raises. *American Journal of Physical Medicine and Rehabilitation* 58:57–67.

Kowall, M.G., Kolk, G., Nuber, G.W., Cassisi, J.E., and S.H. Stern. 1996. Patellar taping in the treatment of patellofemoral pain. A prospective randomized study. *American Journal of Sports Medicine* 24:61–66.

Lange, G.W., Hintermeister, R.A., Schlegel, T., Dillman, C.J., and J.R. Steadman. 1996. Electromyographic and kinematic analysis of graded treadmill walking and the implications for knee rehabilitation. *Journal of Orthopaedic and Sports Physical Therapy* 23:294–301.

Lattanzio, P-J., Petrella, R.J., Sproule, J.R., and P.J. Fowler. 1997. Effects of fatigue on knee proprioception. *Clinical Journal of Sport Medicine* 7:22–27.

Lieb, F.J., and J. Perry. 1971. Quadriceps function. An electromyographic study under isometric conditions. *Journal of Bone and Joint Surgery* 53-A:749–758.

Markolf, K.L., Gorek, J.F., Kabo, J.M., and M.S. Shapiro. 1990. Direct measurement of resultant forces in the anterior cruciate ligament. An in vitro study performed with a new experimental technique. *Journal of Bone and Joint Surgery* 72-A:557–567.

Mirzabelgi, E., Jordan, C., Gronley, J.K., Rockowitz, N.L., and J. Perry. 1999. Isolation of the vastus medialis oblique muscle during exercise. *American Journal of Sports Medicine* 27: 50–53.

Orchard, J.W., Fricker, P.A., Abud, A.T., and B.R. Mason. 1996. Biomechanics of iliotibial band friction syndrome in runners. *American Journal of Sports Medicine* 24:375–379.

Reider, B. 1996. Medial collateral ligament injuries in athletes. *Sports Medicine* 21:147–156.

Reilly, D.T., and M. Martens. 1972. Experimental analysis of the quadriceps muscle force and patellofemoral joint reaction force for various activities. *Acta Orthopaedica Scandinavica* 43:126–137.

Risberg, M.A., Holm, I., Tjomsland, O., Ljunggren, E., and A. Ekeland. 1999. Prospective study of changes in impairments and disabilities after anterior cruciate ligament reconstruction. *Journal of Orthopaedic and Sports Physical Therapy* 29:400–412.

Scott, G.A., Jolly, B.L., and C.E. Henning. 1986. Combined posterior incision and arthroscopic intra-articular repair of the meniscus. *Journal of Bone and Joint Surgery* 68-A:847–861.

Shelbourne, K.D., Patel, D.V., Adsit, W.S., and D.A. Porter. 1996. Rehabilitation after meniscal repair. *Clinics in Sports Medicine* 15:595–612.

Somes, S., Worrell, T.W., Corey, B., and C.D. Ingersoll. 1997. Effects of patellar taping on patellar position in the open and closed kinetic chain: A preliminary study. *Journal of Sport Rehabilitation* 6:299–308.

Spencer, J.D., Hayes, K.C., and I.J. Alexander. 1984. Knee joint effusion and quadriceps reflex inhibition in man. *Archives of Physical Medicine and Rehabilitation* 65:171–177.

Stanton, P., and C. Purdam. 1989. Hamstring injuries in sprinting—the role of eccentric exercise. *Journal of Orthopaedic and Sports Physical Therapy* 17:343–349.

Steinkamp, L.A., Dillongham, M.F., Markel, M.D., Hill, J.A., and K.R. Kaufman. 1993. Biomechanical considerations in patellofemoral joint rehabilitation. *American Journal of Sports Medicine* 21:438–444.

Stone, R.G., Frewin, P.R., and S. Gonzales. 1990. Long-term assessment of arthroscopic meniscus repair: A two- to six-year follow-up study. *Arthroscopy* 6:73–78.

Tenuta, J.J., and R.A. Arciero. 1994. Arthroscopic evaluation of meniscal repairs. Factors that effect healing. *American Journal of Sports Medicine* 22:797–802.

Travell, J.G., and D.G. Simons. 1992. *Myofascial pain and dysfunction. The trigger point manual.* Vol. 2. Baltimore: Williams & Wilkins.

Wegener, L., Kisner, C., and D. Nichols. 1997. Static and dynamic balance responses in persons with bilateral knee osteoarthritis. *Journal of Orthopaedic and Sports Physical Therapy* 25:13–18.

Wilk, K.E., Arrigo, C., Andrews, J.R., and W.G. Clancy Jr., 1999. Rehabilitation after anterior cruciate ligament reconstruction in the female athlete. *Journal of Athletic Training* 34:177–193.

Witvrouw, E., Sneyers, C., Roeland, L., Victor, J., and J. Bellemans. 1996. Reflex response times of vastus medialis oblique and vastus lateralis in normal subjects and in subjects with patellofemoral pain syndrome. *Journal of Orthopaedic and Sports Physical Therapy* 24:160–165.

Worrell, T.W., Crisp, E., and C. LaRosa. 1998. Electromyographic reliability and analysis of selected lower extremity muscles during lateral step-up conditions. *Journal of Athletic Training* 33:156–162.

Worrell, T.W., Ingersoll, C.D., Bockrath-Pugliese, K., and P. Minis. 1998. Effect of patellar taping and bracing on patellar position as determined by MRI in patients with patellofemoral pain. *Journal of Athletic Training.* 33:16–20.

Young, A., Stokes, M., and J.F. Iles. 1987. Effects of joint pathology on muscle. *Clinical Orthopaedics.* 219:21–27.

CHAPTER TWENTY-TWO

Hip

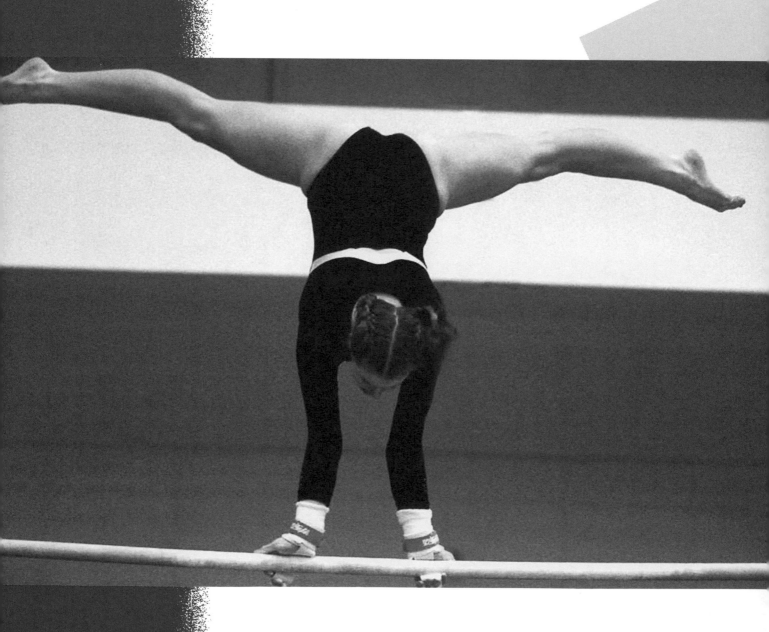

OBJECTIVES

After completing this chapter, you should be able to do the following:

1. Discuss how anteversion and retroversion change lower-extremity mechanics.

2. Explain the mechanical factors involved in gait with hip abductor weakness and explain how a cane assists in normal gait.

3. Identify a joint mobilization technique for the hip and explain its benefit.

4. Identify a flexibility and a strengthening exercise for the hip.

5. Identify a proprioception exercise for the hip and indicate its progression.

6. List precautions for a hip-dislocation rehabilitation program.

Dave has worked with dancers for several years. Having responsibility for the city ballet company's rehabilitation programs, he is quite busy. Over the years he has come to realize that the novice dancers' injuries tend to be acute whereas the experienced dancers' injuries are more often chronic. Although he is able to resolve the acute injuries more quickly, Dave sees the chronic injuries as a challenge—one that he is usually able to meet and resolve, much to his patients' delight.

Dave's current patient, however, has been his greatest challenge yet. Jackson, the lead male dancer in the company, had been bothered with a groin strain for several months before he reported it. It occurred early in the season during rehearsal, and Jackson had dismissed it as minor, not worth treating. But the problem has not gone away, and now that the company is at the peak of the performance season, the injury is aggravated with each performance. Still, Jackson refuses to take any time off to allow the strain to heal.

To accomplish great things, we must not only act but also dream, not only plan but also believe.

Anatole France, 1844–1924, French novelist, literary critic

At the conclusion of this final chapter you will have acquired the tools you need to work as a sport rehabilitation specialist, planning and providing sound therapeutic exercise programs to patients. Having dreams, as well as believing in our ability to make those dreams a reality, is a professional purpose that we should all aspire to. To ascend to new levels of knowledge is a professional goal and responsibility shared by those who have a desire that the profession excel, because individual professional greatness is measured not by what we know but by how we share what we know.

The actions of the sport rehabilitation specialist in hip rehabilitation must be carefully planned if the patient is to return to full sport participation promptly and in accordance with the mutually established goals. The hip joint is secured by a deep socket and is supported by strong muscles. It is an area that experiences repetitive, microtraumatic injuries more frequently than acute, macrotraumatic injuries. Like other segments, this area relies on a balance of muscle flexibility and strength, along with coordination of movement, to maintain an equilibrium of function and health. If the normal length, strength, or function of any element is lost or changed, other elements are impacted and the hip is prone to injury.

The hip is a common site for referral from other sources, so complaints of pain in this area warrant a differential diagnosis before treatment can begin. Because of the various structures that can produce pain in the hip and groin, establishing the source of pain in these areas is not always easy. Hip or groin pain can be secondary to referral from sources such as a lumbar disk disruption, spondylolysis, organ disease, myofascial pain, sacroiliac dysfunction, and the knee. The sport rehabilitation specialist must eliminate these areas as pain sources before he or she can accurately treat the patient. During the initial assessment, if the patient's pain is not reproduced by stress applied to peripheral structures, but is reproduced when stress is applied to the hip, it is likely that the hip is the source of the pain. If there is no change in the patient's condition after four to six sessions or two weeks of treatment, reassessment for other sources of pain is necessary.

This chapter introduces basic concepts the sport rehabilitation specialist must consider for hip-injury rehabilitation, focusing on topics relevant to treatment and to the progression of a therapeutic exercise program. Specific techniques for soft-tissue and joint mobilization and exercises for flexibility, strength, and proprioception are presented. Once the foundation for a therapeutic exercise program has been established, specific injuries commonly seen in the hip are discussed along with program progression for these injuries. Cases are presented in connection with some injury programs to help you conceptualize how a program is put together and advanced for a specific patient.

GENERAL REHABILITATION CONSIDERATIONS

A rehabilitation program for the hip must be based on knowledge of the hip's osseous structures, neural structures, and joint mobility and joint mechanics. The sport rehabilitation specialist must also be familiar with methods of reducing stress in an injured hip.

The hip is a stable joint with extensive range of motion in several planes. The socket is deep and is reinforced with strong ligaments for stability. Strength and motion are important for the hip because it serves as a force transmitter for both lower- and upper-limb activities and provides motion and strength for propulsion in walking and running.

OSSEOUS STRUCTURES

The **acetabulum,** the hip socket, is in an inferior and anterolateral position. The femoral neck forms a 125° angle with the shaft of the femur, as shown in figure 22.1a (Kapandji 1978). An angle greater than 125°, called **coxa valga,** increases pressure into the joint (figure 22.1b); an angle less than 125°, called **coxa vara,** increases stress on the femoral neck (figure 22.1c). The femoral neck is rotated relative to the line of the femur's long axis. Normal alignment places the neck in a line that is 15° anterior to the line of the femur in the adult (figure 22.2). If the angle is greater than 15°, the leg is positioned in internal rotation; this condition is called **anteversion.** If it is less than 15°, **retroversion** occurs to position the leg in external rotation. Anteversion and retroversion alter knee alignment and change the forces acting throughout the entire lower extremity. Anteversion leads to squinting patellae, and/or foot pronation, causing the individual to ambulate with a toe-in gait. Retroversion results in frog-eyed patellae, and/or calcaneal inversion, and causes the person to ambulate with a toe-out gait. Anteversion and coxa valga each make the hip susceptible to dislocation.

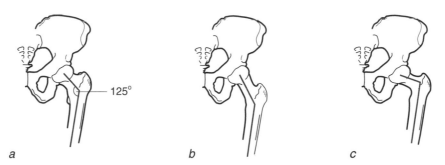

Figure 22.1 Femoral neck angles: *(a)* normal; *(b)* coxa valga—increased angle with increased joint stress; *(c)* coxa vara—decreased angle with increased femoral neck load.

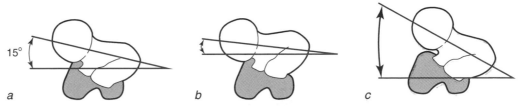

Figure 22.2 Femoral neck alignment with long axis of femur: *(a)* normal, *(b)* retroversion, *(c)* anteversion.

Anteversion is measured with the patient in prone and the knee flexed to 90°. The sport rehabilitation specialist moves the patient's leg into internal rotation until palpation of the greater trochanter reveals that it is parallel to the tabletop (figure 22.3). The hip is then rotated until the tibia is vertical to the table, and the difference between the two positions of the tibia is measured. This value is the degree of anteversion.

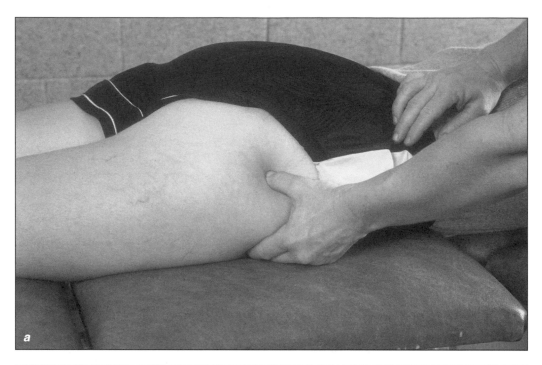

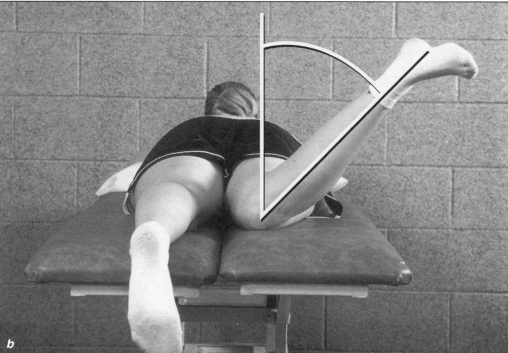

❚ Figure 22.3   Craig's test for femoral anteversion: greater trochanter is positioned parallel to the tabletop *(a)*, and the angle between the lower leg's position in 90° flexion at this point and in a vertical position is measured *(b)*.

NEURAL STRUCTURES

Nerves entering the lower extremity must pass through the hip region. This can lead to nerve irritations when structures around the hip impinge on a nerve. The sciatic nerve passes beneath and occasionally through the piriformis muscle and through the sciatic notch before it travels along the posterior thigh. Entrapment of the nerve in the piriformis region can occur and can cause neural irritation distally.

A sensory branch of the femoral nerve, the lateral femoral cutaneous nerve, travels through the psoas major muscle and then passes under the inguinal ligament near the anterior superior iliac spine (ASIS). Compression of this nerve by the inguinal ligament can cause aching and burning over the tensor fascia lata in the anterolateral thigh where it provides sensory innervation.

The obturator nerve enters the pelvis from the upper lumbar nerve roots and provides sensory and motor innervation to the medial thigh. Entrapment of this nerve can cause medial thigh sensory changes and adductor weakness.

JOINT MOBILITY

The joint configuration is a convex femoral head on a concave acetabulum, so glide of the femur on the pelvis occurs in the direction opposite to movement during open chain motion. The hip's capsular pattern has its most significant restriction of motion in internal rotation. Flexion and abduction are less limited, and extension is less limited than flexion or abduction. External rotation is normal (Cyriax 1975).

The hip joint's close-packed position is full extension, abduction, and internal rotation. The open-packed position is 30° flexion and 30° abduction with slight external rotation.

Key
A = Lever-arm length of hip abductors
B = Lever-arm length of center of gravity

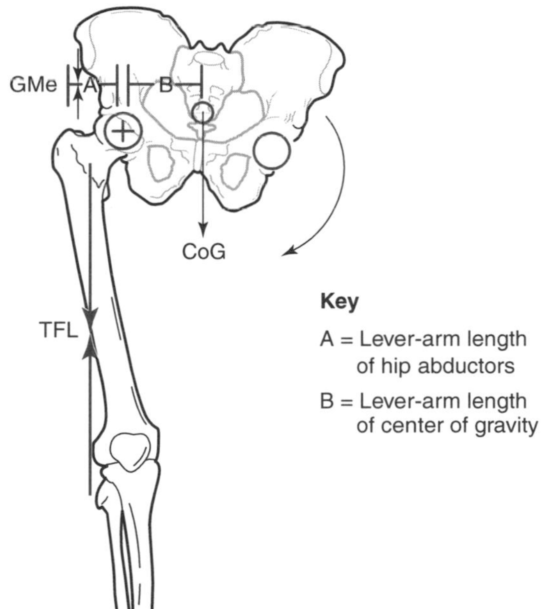

Figure 22.4 Single-leg stance mechanics.

JOINT MECHANICS

Pelvis movement has a direct influence on hip movement because the hip joint socket lies within the pelvic bones. Pelvic motion alters hip positioning, and hip abnormalities affect pelvic posture. An anterior pelvic tilt moves the anterior pelvis closer to the anterior femur, and a posterior pelvic tilt moves the posterior pelvis closer to the posterior femur. This change in position relationships alters the hip so that an anterior pelvic tilt increases hip flexion and a posterior pelvic tilt increases hip extension.

When a person moves from a two-leg to a one-leg stance, the center of gravity must be transferred toward the supporting leg. This places rotatory stress on the weight-bearing hip because gravity's pull on the nonsupporting leg drops the pelvis on that side. To prevent pelvic drop and rotatory forces, the abductors on the weight-bearing leg must work to keep the hips level with each other. The force required of the abductors is significantly greater than the weight of the body, because their lever-arm length is less than that of the center of gravity (figure 22.4). If the abductors are not strong enough to counter the force of gravity that is pulling the non-weight-bearing hip downward and laterally rotating the pelvis, a normal gait is not possible. The patient either drops the non-weight-bearing hip and downwardly rotates the pelvis to the non-weight-bearing side, or tilts the trunk to lurch over the weak hip during stance on the leg so that the center of gravity is closer to the fulcrum, the femoral head. If the center of

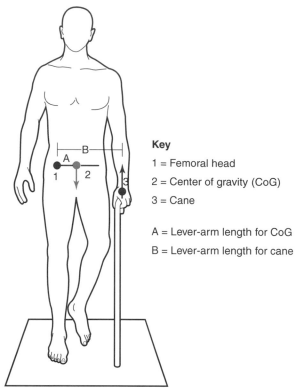

Key

1 = Femoral head

2 = Center of gravity (CoG)

3 = Cane

A = Lever-arm length for CoG

B = Lever-arm length for cane

■ **Figure 22.5** Force application with cane use in ambulation.

gravity is moved far enough laterally to be placed on top of or lateral to the fulcrum, the abductors do not have to work, and the pelvis will not drop.

If a cane is used on the side opposite the weakness, an upward force is transmitted through the cane to counterbalance the downward gravitational force on the same side (figure 22.5). Because the lever arm from the cane to the fulcrum is longer than the center of gravity's lever arm, the force transmitted through the cane is relatively small. Patients who use a cane or a single crutch for ambulation need only apply light pressure on the handle to offset the gravitational pull and produce adequate substitution for the weak abductors.

Leg-length discrepancies can result from actual differences in length or from other unilateral differences such as genu valgus, coxa vara, rotated sacrum, or foot pronation, as well as from soft-tissue differences such as hip flexor tightness, abductor tightness, and muscle imbalances. When one leg is shorter than the other, the pelvis drops on the shorter side, and the trunk bends away from the short leg when weight bearing on the short leg. The greater the discrepancy, the more notable are these compensations. If a leg-length discrepancy is suspected, shoe wear is the most obvious indication that one is present. If there is the possibility of a leg-length discrepancy, the sport rehabilitation specialist should assess all possible causes, because correction or adaptation of the discrepancy may be necessary to alleviate the patient's pain.

Leg-length differences can eventually lead to osteoarthritis of the longer leg. This occurs because in weight bearing, the longer leg is in a position of adducted angulation. This produces increased joint incongruence in which greater weight is borne on the superior lateral aspect of the acetabulum. The weight shift to the shorter leg is caused by a leg-length difference, so increased compressive forces are applied to the hip joint as the abductors on the longer leg increase their exertion to keep the pelvis level.

STRESS-REDUCTION CONCEPTS

One rule of thumb is that if a patient ambulates with an antalgic gait, he or she should use assistive devices until normal ambulation is possible. An abnormal gait may result from pain, inadequate muscle control, or apprehension; and if it continues, additional injury to the hip, back, or other lower-extremity segments can result. When weight bearing is permitted, an assistive device is used only as much as necessary to create a normal gait. As the precipitating factor is resolved, the patient is weaned from the crutches or cane until a normal gait without assistive devices is possible.

Stress can be reduced in the hip by shortening the stride length during walking or running. A smaller stride reduces the force and motion demands on the muscles, tendons, and ligaments. Application of a hip spica wrap can help diminish stride length.

GENERAL REHABILITATION PROCEDURES

Hip-pain complaints without a specific injury can sometimes be difficult to interpret because of the various possible sources. Hip joint pain commonly refers to the groin, the anterior or medial proximal thigh, or the knee. Spinal-based pain can refer to the anterior hip, buttock, or thigh. Sacral pain can refer to the buttock or posterior or lateral thigh. Internal organs and the abdomen can refer pain to the groin. When a patient complains of pain in these areas without a specific history of injury, a differential diagnosis is necessary to eliminate these locations as sources of hip pain. The assessment tests should reproduce the patient's pain complaints for a differential diagnosis.

Pain and inflammation control are the primary goals for initial treatment programs for hip injuries; the means of pain control include anti-inflammatory medication, reduced activity, and modalities. Some hip injuries are self-limiting in that pain is the determining factor with respect to participation. The patient may wish to continue sport participation in this case, because continued activity will not make the condition worse; but the recovery time may need to be longer because irritation is being introduced on a regular basis.

Therapeutic exercises include a progression of stretching or flexibility exercises, strengthening exercises, proprioception activities, and functional activities. When injuries result from predisposing factors rather than acute insult, those factors must be corrected to reduce the risk of recurrence. Flexibility exercises require adequate stabilization of adjacent segments and proper application of the stretch force, because many hip muscles cross more than one joint. Because the hip is so closely aligned with the pelvis, strengthening exercises must include stabilization exercises. Because the hip depends on the back, pelvis, knee, and ankle for its balance and quality of motion, exercises for deficiencies in these segments must be a part of the therapeutic exercise program for the hip.

Return to full sport participation is possible when the patient is pain free with muscle balances intact and when performance of sport-specific activities is normal.

SOFT-TISSUE MOBILIZATION

Soft-tissue mobilization techniques for the hip, including massage, scar-tissue mobilization, and cross-friction mobilization, are directed at the iliopsoas; the gluteus maximus, medius, and minimus; the piriformis; and the pectineus.

Because of the neurological, myofascial, orthopedic, and organ systems that can refer pain into the hip region, it is prudent for the sport rehabilitation specialist to identify any differential diagnosis that may be contributing to hip or groin pain. If myofascia is the expected source of pain, treatment can proceed. If changes in the patient's complaints do not occur with soft-tissue mobilization techniques, it is necessary to reassess for other probable causes.

Soft-tissue mobilization techniques for the hip include deep-tissue massage, scar-tissue mobilization, cross-friction massage, and myofascial release, including trigger point treatments and ice-and-stretch techniques. The myofascial release techniques and pain-referral information presented here are based on the work of Travell and Simons (1992). The quadratus lumborum muscle is discussed in chapter 16; the rectus femoris, hamstrings, adductors, and tensor fascia lata are addressed in chapter 21.

Myofascial techniques include direct pressure with the flat finger or thumb pad or with a pincher grasp of the muscle that is held until the muscle relaxes. If soft-tissue resistance is palpated after the initial application, the technique can be repeated. Ice-and-stretch techniques incorporate ice massage applied in parallel sweeps, usually proximally to distally, with a simultaneous application of manual stretching. The sport rehabilitation specialist repeats this process three to five times, attempting to increase mobility with each application. He or she assists the patient in actively moving the leg to the starting position between bouts of ice-and-stretch. The patient performs several bouts of active motion following ice-and-stretch. Heat can be applied after the ice-and-stretch. Pain should not be produced during the application.

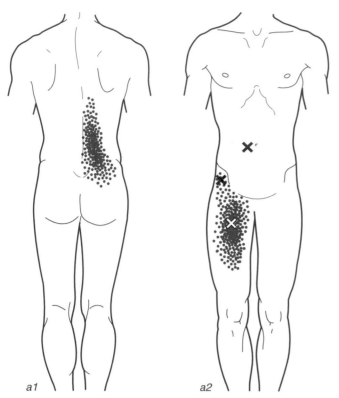

a1   a2

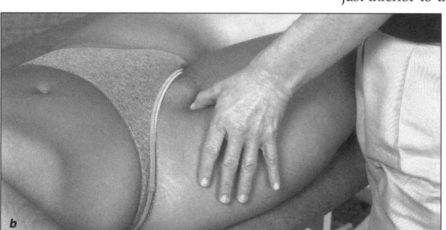

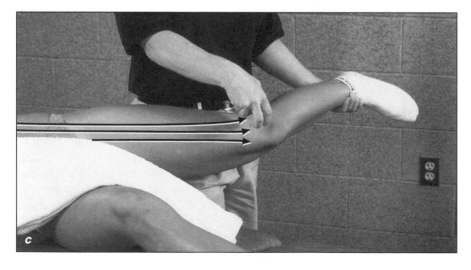

ILIOPSOAS

Pain from the iliopsoas trigger points is noticed particularly during weight bearing but is relieved with non-weight bearing. Pain is referred either throughout the lumbar paraspinal region on the same side as the lesion or into the anterior thigh and groin (figure 22.6a).

Myofascial release to the trigger points is performed using the finger or thumb pads. The patient is supine, with the abdominal muscles relaxed and the hip slightly flexed, abducted, and supported for relaxation. The distal trigger point is located on the lateral wall of the femoral triangle (figure 22.6b). It is important to avoid pressure on the medial side of the muscle, because the femoral nerve is located in this region. Just behind the ASIS and inside the rim of the iliac crest, the middle trigger point can be treated with finger-pad pressure pushing the muscle against the inside rim of the ilium. The third trigger point is more difficult to access because the patient must keep the abdominal muscles relaxed, and this is sometimes difficult to do. The region is lateral or just inferior to the umbilicus on the lateral rim of the rectus abdominis. Direct downward pressure is exerted slowly. Once past the rectus abdominis, the pressure continues downward and medially toward the spine. Depending on the patient's size, the psoas may or may not be directly palpated; but indirect pressure is effective if direct palpation is not possible.

Ice-and-stretch techniques are applied with the patient in side-lying on the unaffected side and the top leg supported by the sport rehabilitation specialist in hip extension (figure 22.6c). Ice sweeps are made from the abdomen downward past the thigh and to the knee, with stretch force applied to increase hip internal rotation. Ice sweeps are finally applied to the low back and posterior hip.

▌**Figure 22.6** Iliopsoas trigger points: *(a)* pain-referral patterns, *(b)* trigger point release on distal trigger point, *(c)* ice-and-stretch.

GLUTEUS MAXIMUS

The gluteus maximus refers pain locally in the buttock region around the sacrum or the gluteal fold above the ischial tuberosity (figure 22.7a). Pain related to this muscle is commonly reported after prolonged sitting, walking uphill, and swimming the freestyle stroke.

Trigger point myofascial release is performed with the patient in side-lying with the involved hip on top. The top thigh is flexed comfortably. Pressure is applied with either a pincher grasp or a finger or thumb pad. A taut band can be palpated in the muscle's middle and distal fibers in the direction of fiber arrangement (figure 22.7b).

Ice-and-stretch is applied with the patient in side-lying and the top hip flexed. The ice sweeps are started at the posterior iliac crest; they move along the muscle fiber direction to the midposterior thigh as stretch is applied to move the hip into flexion (figure 22.7c).

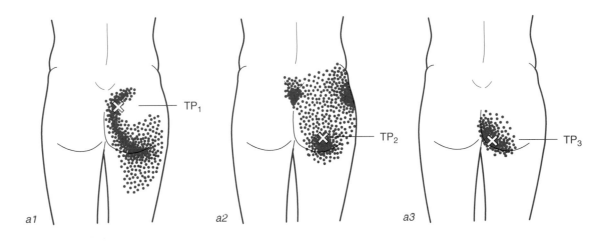

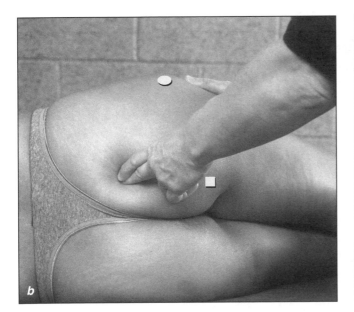
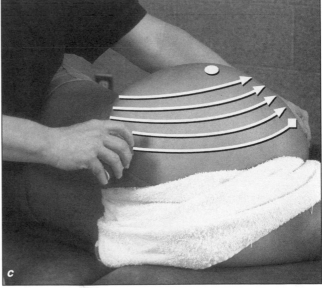

∎ **Figure 22.7** Gluteus maximus trigger points: *(a)* pain-referral patterns, *(b)* trigger point release to superior trigger point, *(c)* ice-and-stretch. ○ = greater trochanter, □ = ischial tuberosity.

GLUTEUS MEDIUS

Pain from the gluteus medius is aggravated with walking, lying supine or side-lying on the affected side, or sitting in a slouched position. The location of pain is along the posterior iliac crest, down the sacrum, and into the lateral posterior gluteal area; and the trigger points are along the iliac crest (figure 22.8a).

Trigger point release is performed with the patient in prone or side-lying; the affected leg is superior, and the hip is flexed and supported with a pillow between the knees (figure 22.8b). Thumb or finger pad pressure of the trigger points against the ilium is used along the iliac crest at the tender sites until their relaxation is palpated.

Ice-and-stretch is applied with the patient side-lying. The hip is in adduction behind the uninvolved leg for stretch to the anterior fibers and in front of the uninvolved leg for stretch to the posterior fibers. Parallel ice sweeps are made from the iliac crest, over the lateral thigh to the knee (figure 22.8c).

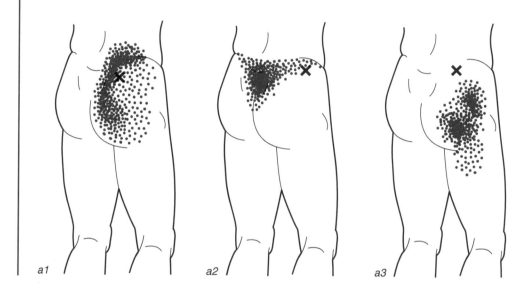

a1   a2   a3

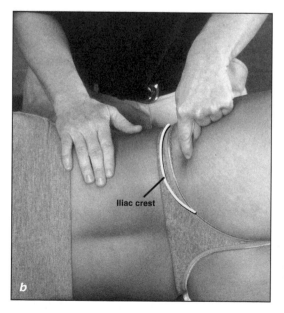

b   Iliac crest

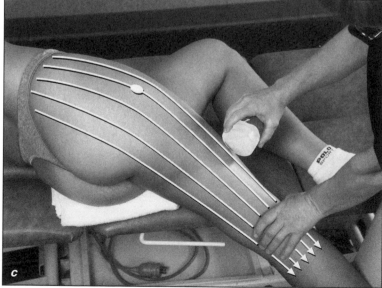

c

▌Figure 22.8   Gluteus medius trigger points: *(a)* pain-referral patterns, *(b)* trigger point release to the posterior trigger point *(a1)*, *(c)* ice-and-stretch. ◯ = greater trochanter.

GLUTEUS MINIMUS

Pain from the gluteus minimus occurs with getting out of a chair and with walking. The pain-referral pattern is over the lower lateral buttock and down the lateral or posterior thigh and into the proximal posterior calf or lateral lower leg to the ankle (figure 22.9a). This can sometimes mimic a sciatic pain pattern, so sciatica should be ruled out.

Trigger point treatment is performed with the patient lying supine for the anterior trigger points, or side-lying on the unaffected side for the posterior trigger points (figure 22.9b). Because the gluteus minimus lies deep to the medius and maximus muscles, deep pressure is required for treatment. The gluteus medius and maximus should be relaxed with supportive pillows for optimal effectiveness. The anterior fibers are palpated just distal to the ASIS on either side of the tensor fascia lata (TFL), deep to the TFL. The TFL is located by resisting hip internal rotation and palpating for the TFL. The posterior trigger points are treated with the hip slightly flexed and adducted. They are located just above the piriformis toward the middle and lateral aspects of the piriformis.

Ice-and-stretch is applied with the patient in side-lying with the buttock close to the end of the table (figure 22.9c). With the hip in adduction and supported by the sport rehabilitation specialist, ice is applied in sweeping strokes

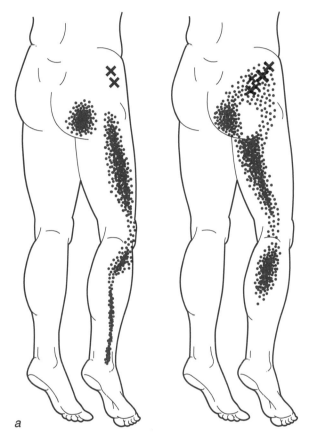

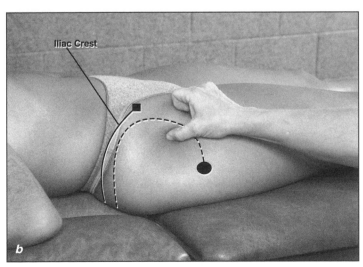

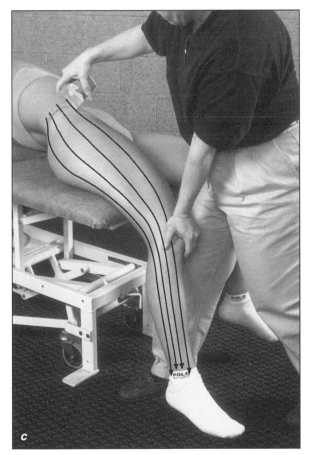

■ **Figure 22.9** Gluteus minimus trigger points: *(a)* pain-referral patterns, *(b)* trigger point release, *(c)* ice-and-stretch.
● = greater trochanter, ■ = ASIS.

from the iliac crest, down the lateral thigh to the lateral lower leg and ankle for the anterior trigger points and along the posterior hip, thigh, and calf for the posterior trigger points. The stretch force is applied with the hip in extension and adduction for the anterior fibers and in 30° flexion and internal rotation for the posterior fibers.

PIRIFORMIS

Activities such as sitting, standing, and walking aggravate myofascial pain of the piriformis. The piriformis refers pain into the sacroiliac area and the posterior hip (figure 22.10a). The pain can also extend into the upper two thirds of the posterior thigh.

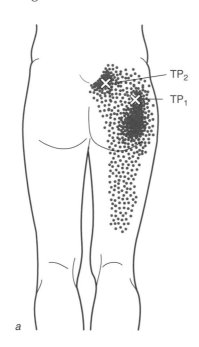

Trigger point release can be performed with the patient prone or side-lying on the uninvolved side (figure 22.10b). A line from the greater trochanter to the superior border of the sciatic foramen is the course of the muscle. Two trigger points are found on this line; one is at the junction of the medial and middle third of the line and the other is at the junction of the middle and lateral third of the line.

Ice-and-stretch is performed with the patient side-lying and the hip in about 90° flexion and adducted in front of the bottom thigh. The patient keeps the thigh anchored with his or her hand at the knee while the sport rehabilitation specialist applies ice sweeps from the sacrum to the lateral hip and down the posterior thigh (figure 22.10c). To apply the stretch at the pelvis, the sport rehabilitation specialist pulls backward on the pelvis while the patient holds the thigh stable.

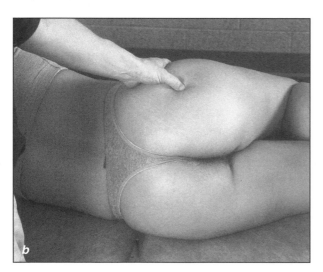

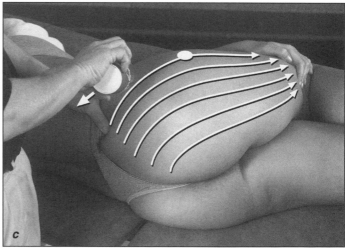

∎ **Figure 22.10** Piriformis trigger points: *(a)* pain-referral patterns, *(b)* trigger point release to lateral trigger point, *(c)* ice-and-stretch. ○ = greater trochanter.

PECTINEUS

The pectineus muscle refers pain deep into the groin just below the inguinal ligament (figure 22.11a).

The trigger point is treated with the patient supine and the hip abducted, slightly flexed, and supported (figure 22.11b). Medial to the femoral artery and inferior to the inguinal ligament, finger-pad pressure is applied to the muscle's trigger point.

Ice-and-stretch is performed with the patient supine, the leg abducted and over the edge of the table (figure 22.11c). The stretch force is applied so that the leg becomes progressively more abducted and moves into extension.

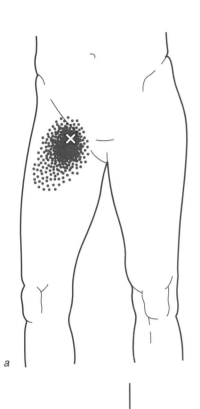

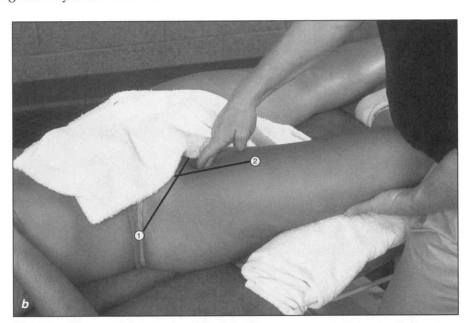

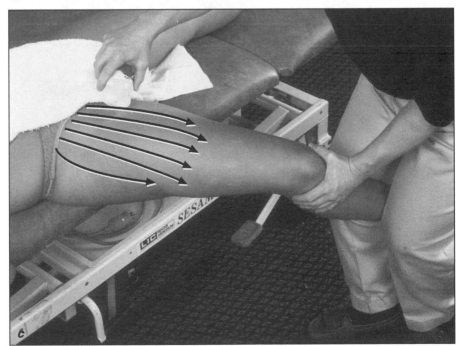

■ **Figure 22.11** Pectineus trigger point: *(a)* pain-referral patterns, *(b)* trigger point release, *(c)* ice-and-stretch. ① = inguinal ligament, ② = femoral artery.

JOINT MOBILIZATION

The sport rehabilitation specialist uses joint mobilization of the hip to improve joint play and general hip mobility, as well as hip flexion, extension, abduction, and rotation. Patients can also apply self-mobilization techniques.

Whereas painful hip joints can benefit from grades I and II mobilization techniques, hip joints that display a capsular pattern of restricted movement can benefit from grades III and IV mobilization techniques. Although not always, oscillating techniques are often used for grades I and II and a sustained force for grades III and IV.

Because the proximal aspect of the hip joint is the pelvis, which is firmly attached to the trunk, there is little need to stabilize the hip joint before mobilization. The weight of the pelvis is sufficient to act as an anchor.

INFERIOR GLIDE

This technique, also referred to as hip distraction, helps the patient regain joint play, which is essential for all hip motions. Distraction is also useful in pain control. A history of knee disorders necessitates using an alternative technique. The patient lies supine while the sport rehabilitation specialist grasps the distal tibia and fibula of the affected leg and places the leg in a loose-packed position. The patient is instructed to relax the hip and thigh muscles while the technique is applied. The sport rehabilitation specialist leans backward, using the body weight to supply the traction force (figure 22.12a).

If the patient has a history of knee disorders, an alternative position for an inferior glide is to have the patient's lower leg over the sport rehabilitation specialist's shoulder. The sport rehabilitation specialist clasps his or her hands around the proximal thigh and applies the inferior glide (figure 22.12b).

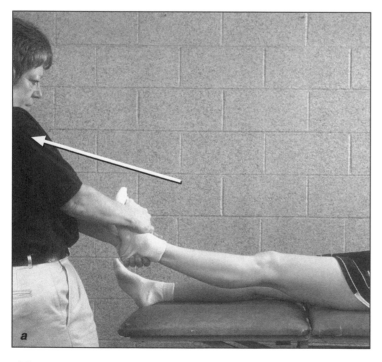
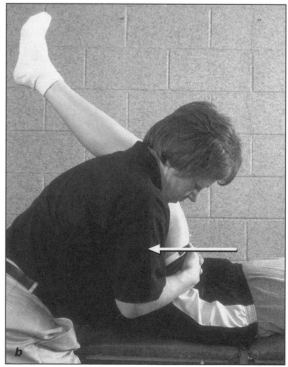

▌ Figure 22.12   Joint mobilization—inferior glide: *(a)* with force applied in knee extension, *(b)* with force applied in knee flexion.

LATERAL GLIDE

Lateral glides are used to promote gains in general hip mobility. The patient lies supine with the sport rehabilitation specialist standing at the side of the affected leg. A strap is secured around the proximal thigh and the sport rehabilitation specialist's hips (figure 22.13a). The sport rehabilitation specialist places the cephalic hand on the lateral pelvis to stabilize it and the caudal hand on the distal thigh. With the patient's thigh in slight flexion, the sport rehabilitation specialist transfers his or her weight from the front leg to the back leg, pushing his or her body against the strap to apply the traction force through the strap. The patient's hip can be placed in various positions of flexion and rotation for application of superior or inferior distractions with the lateral glide (figure 22.13, b and c).

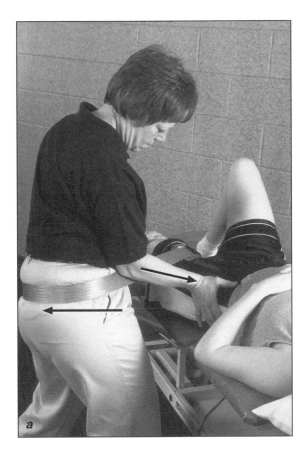

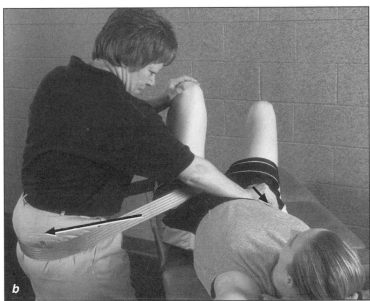

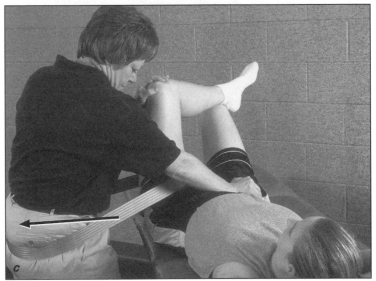

▌Figure 22.13 Joint mobilization—lateral glide: *(a)* with hip in extension, *(b)* with leg in hip flexion and pelvis stabilized at opposite ASIS, *(c)* with hip in flexion and external rotation and pelvis stabilized at opposite ASIS.

POSTERIOR GLIDE

The posterior glide is useful for increasing hip flexion and internal rotation. The patient lies supine with the hip and knee flexed. The degree of hip flexion depends on the technique used. When a belt is used, partial flexion of the joints is necessary, with the belt placed around the distal thigh and secured to the sport rehabilitation specialist's shoulder. The sport rehabilitation specialist places the stabilizing hand under the belt and the mobilizing hand over the anterior proximal thigh. With the elbow kept straight, the sport rehabilitation specialist applies a downward force on the proximal thigh, using his or her legs, while the patient's thigh is kept stable with the belt (figure 22.14a).

An alternative position is with the hip in 90° flexion and about 10° adduction and the knee in full flexion. The sport rehabilitation specialist applies the posterior glide force through the long axis of the femur by leaning his or her body weight into the femur (figure 22.14b). Care must be taken not to apply the mobilizing force through the patella.

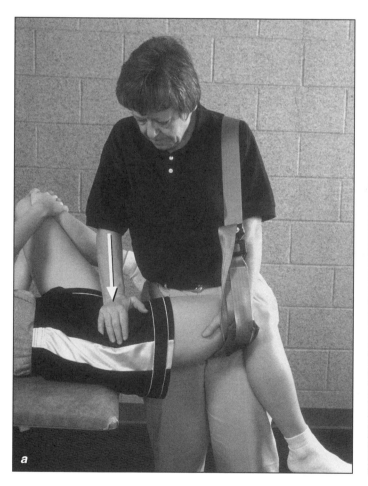
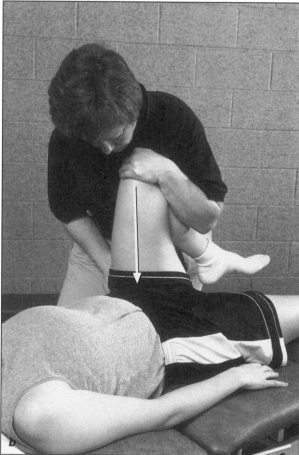

▌Figure 22.14   Joint mobilization—posterior glide: *(a)* with strap, *(b)* large axis.

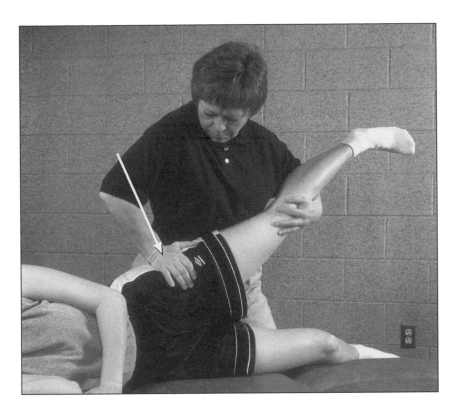

MEDIAL GLIDE

This mobilization technique is used to increase hip abduction and flexion. The patient is in side-lying on the unaffected side while the sport rehabilitation specialist supports the leg at the distal thigh and knee and positions it in slight abduction and flexion (figure 22.15). The sport rehabilitation specialist's mobilizing hand is placed on the proximal thigh, and the mobilizing force is applied downward.

∎ **Figure 22.15**   Joint mobilization: medial glide.

ANTERIOR GLIDE

This technique is used to increase hip extension and external rotation. With the patient prone, the sport rehabilitation specialist supports the distal thigh with the knee flexed, using the stabilizing hand; the mobilizing hand is at the proximal thigh (figure 22.16a). The stabilizing hand keeps the hip positioned in slight extension or

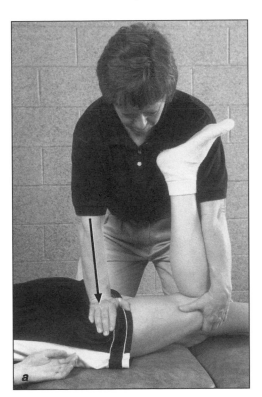

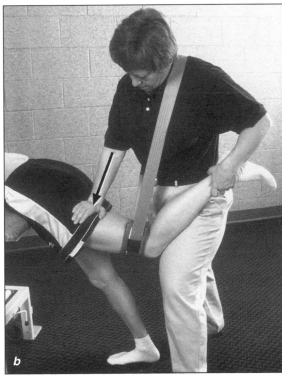

∎ **Figure 22.16**
Joint mobilization—anterior glide: *(a)* prone on table, without strap, *(b)* prone off table, with strap.

neutral while the mobilizing hand applies a downward force through a straight elbow; body weight exerts the force. The hip can be placed in various rotation positions for additional techniques.

In an alternative position, the patient is prone, with the hips on the edge of the table and the noninvolved leg supporting the body weight with its foot on the floor. The sport rehabilitation specialist can either support the patient's distal thigh in one hand or can have a stabilizing strap over the shoulder and wrapped around the distal thigh (figure 22.16b).

SELF-MOBILIZATION

The patient can perform self-distraction using a stretch strap. The patient is supine with the strap anchored around the foot and the anterior hip; the knee and hip are placed in flexed positions, about 90° each (figure 22.17). A pad is placed on the anterior thigh for comfort. Keeping the opposite hip flexed with hands supporting the thigh, the patient pushes the involved foot against the strap, attempting to extend the hip and knee.

In an alternative position, the patient places a weight around the ankle and stands with the foot off a step, allowing gravity to create a distraction force on the hip. The position is maintained for several minutes, as tolerated.

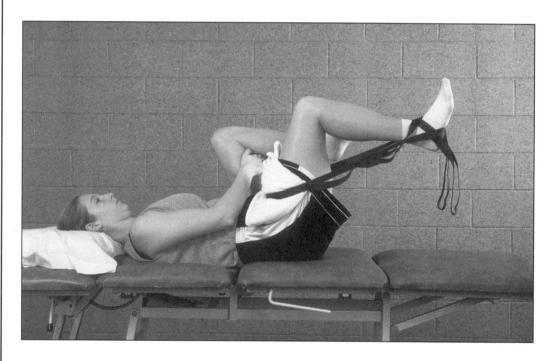

▌Figure 22.17 Joint mobilization: self-mobilization distraction.

FLEXIBILITY EXERCISES

Active stretches and prolonged stretches are used to improve flexibility in the hip's lateral, anterior, medial, and posterior muscles.

Several muscles cross the hip joint, acting not only on the hip but also on the knee, back, and pelvis. One must consider these areas when discussing flexibility exercises. For effective stretching of the hip, these segments must be positioned appropriately.

Active stretches are held for 15 to 20 s and are repeated about four times each. They should be repeated at least three to four times throughout the day. Active contraction of opposing muscles leads to improved results in flexibility exercises by enhancing relaxation of stretched muscle. Enough force is applied to move the muscle to a point at which the patient perceives a stretch without pain. Prolonged stretches are most effective in altering tissue length in scar tissue and connective tissue.

LATERAL MUSCLES

Lateral hip muscles are frequently tight, and impact not only the hip but also the knee. Improper mechanics results, placing additional stress on the hip and knee joints and their structures.

Lower Lumbar Rotation

The lower lumbar muscles are stretched with the patient lying supine. The patient flexes the involved hip and knee and rotates the thigh across the body, keeping the ipsilateral shoulder on the ground. The contralateral hand can be used to apply additional stretch (figure 22.18). The stretch should be felt in the lower back and hip. The more the hip is flexed, the lower the stretch is felt.

The ipsilateral shoulder must be kept on the ground. If necessary, the arm can be extended outward from the side to prevent the shoulder from rising up.

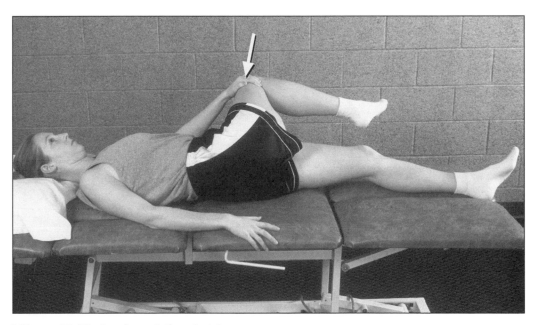

∎ **Figure 22.18**   Lumbar rotation stretch.

Tensor Fascia Lata Stretch

The TFL, in addition to the other hip abductors, can be stretched in standing, sitting, or side-lying. In standing, the patient places the affected side closest to a wall about an arm's-length distance from the wall. The feet are crossed, with the affected leg behind the uninvolved leg. Placing the hand on the wall, the patient pushes the hips toward the wall, keeping both feet on the ground as the hand on the wall provides a push force (figure 22.19a). The patient should not rotate the body or bend the elbow. The stretch should be felt on the outside of the thigh.

In sitting, the patient has the uninvolved leg out straight and the involved leg flexed at the knee and hip; the foot on the involved leg is placed flat on the ground on the outside of the uninvolved knee. The patient uses the hands to pull the involved knee across the body toward the opposite shoulder (figure 22.19b).

In side-lying, the patient lies on the uninvolved leg with the top hip extended and the knee flexed. The top leg is allowed to drop down behind the bottom leg (figure 22.19c). The patient must not rotate the trunk to place the top hip behind the bottom hip. A pad under the bottom hip makes the position more comfortable. This position can be used for a prolonged stretch.

ANTERIOR MUSCLES

Hip flexors include the iliopsoas and rectus femoris. To include the rectus femoris in a stretch, the knee must be flexed. If the knee is extended, the iliopsoas will be the only muscle stretched. Positions for stretching these muscles are standing, kneeling, supine, and prone. In standing, the patient grasps the foot from behind to bring the heel to the buttock while keeping the knee pointing to the floor (figure 22.20a). The back must remain erect in order to prevent iliopsoas shortening, and the knee must be kept pointing to the floor to prevent shortening of the rectus femoris.

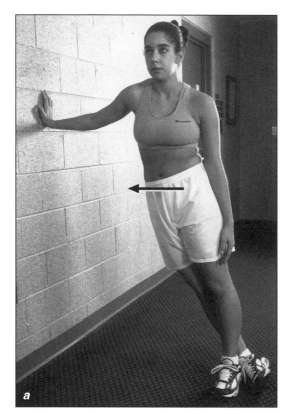

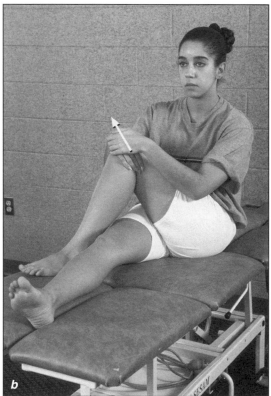

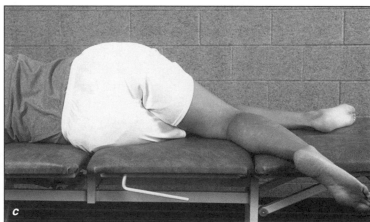

■ **Figure 22.19** Tensor fascia lata stretch:
(a) standing stretch, *(b)* seated stretch, *(c)* sidelying position for prolonged stretch.

In kneeling, the involved leg is the kneeling leg, and the opposite leg bears weight on the foot in front. The patient transfers weight from the back knee to the front foot so that the weight moves in front of the back knee (figure 22.20b). The back should remain erect. The patient can apply additional stretch by attempting to flex the knee, although this can be a difficult maneuver. A pad can be placed under the knee for comfort.

In prone, the patient lies on the edge of a table with the uninvolved foot on the floor and the hip and knee slightly flexed to stabilize the pelvis. A pillow or wedge is placed under the thigh on the table. The patient rests with weight on the elbows. Additional stretch can be applied by increasing the pillow height or flexing the knee. This position can be used for a prolonged stretch (figure 22.20c).

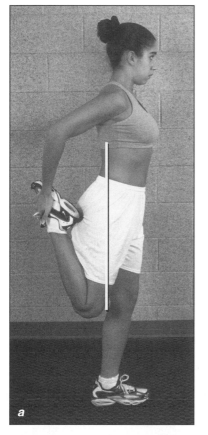

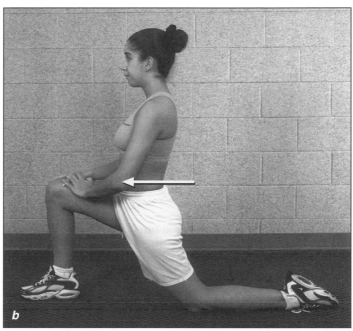

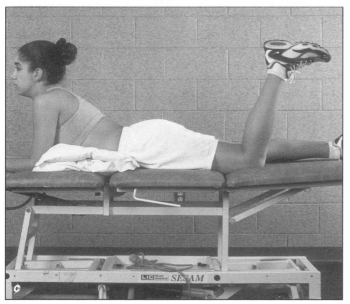

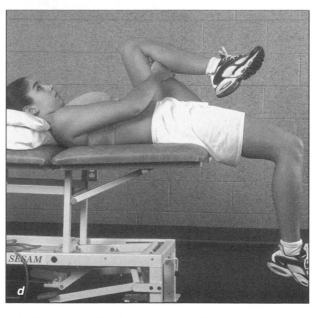

■ **Figure 22.20** Anterior muscle stretch: *(a)* standing hip flexor stretch, *(b)* kneeling hip flexor stretch, *(c)* prone hip flexor stretch, *(d)* supine hip flexor stretch.

In supine, the stretch position is the Thomas hip flexor stretch. The patient lies with the buttocks on the end of the table. The uninvolved leg is flexed at the hip and knee and can be supported by the patient's hands. The involved leg is placed over the edge of the table so that the mid to upper thigh is at the edge (figure 22.20d). Substitutions during this stretch include hip abduction and external rotation. The leg position can be aligned passively by the sport rehabilitation specialist or with use of stabilization straps. This position can be used for a prolonged stretch. Weights can be applied to the ankle for additional stretch force during a prolonged stretch.

MEDIAL MUSCLES

The adductors can be stretched in sitting, standing, or kneeling. The long adductors pass below the knee joint, so they are stretched when the knee is extended; the shorter adductors can be stretched with the knee flexed or extended.

In sitting, the patient flexes and abducts the hips and knees to place the bottom of the feet together. He or she pulls the feet toward the buttocks. In this position, the hands are placed on the ankles, and the forearms are placed along the inner lower legs. A stretch force is applied along the forearms to lower the knees (figure 22.21a). The stretch is felt in the groin. The back should be kept straight, with forward bending originating from hip flexion.

An alternative position is in long sitting with the hips abducted and the knees extended. The patient flexes forward from the hips, keeping the back straight, while placing the weight on the hands to keep the groin muscles relaxed (figure 22.21b). Additional stretch can be provided to the long adductors by rotating to the affected leg and reaching for the toes.

In kneeling, the patient is on the uninvolved knee and places the involved leg in abduction with the knee straight (figure 22.21c). The uninvolved hip is pushed laterally away from the involved leg as the involved leg is pushed downward. A pillow can be placed under the supporting knee for comfort, and the patient can use hand support if needed. The inside border of the involved foot should remain in contact with the floor so that the leg does not rotate.

In standing, the patient stands sideways to a supporting object that is about hip height and places the involved foot on top of the object (figure 22.21d). Keeping the medial border of the foot facing downward, the patient squats on the supporting leg while pushing on the involved lateral thigh. The patient should be cautioned regarding substitutions of hip or pelvis rotation.

POSTERIOR MUSCLES

The hip extensors and external rotators are the posterior muscle groups. The hip extensors include the hamstrings and gluteals; the external rotator of primary concern is the piriformis.

Hip Extensors

The hamstrings are frequently stretched in standing or supine. In standing, the patient places the involved leg on a supporting surface (figure 22.22a). The height is determined by the tightness of the hamstrings: The tighter the hamstrings, the lower the surface. The standing leg should be positioned with the foot facing forward. Keeping the back straight, the patient leans forward from the hips toward the elevated foot. The involved leg should be maintained with the foot facing the ceiling and in good body alignment, not in abduction. Reaching with the opposite hand prevents the pelvis from rotating and lessening the effectiveness of the stretch.

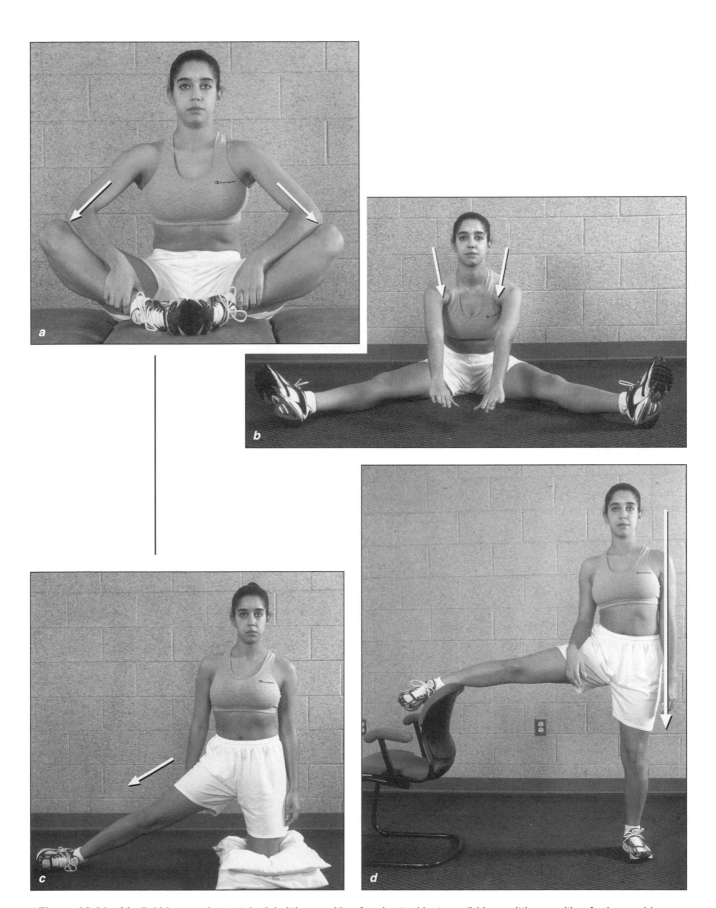

Figure 22.21 Medial hip muscle stretch: *(a)* sitting position for short adductors, *(b)* long-sitting position for long adductors, *(c)* kneeling position, *(d)* standing position.

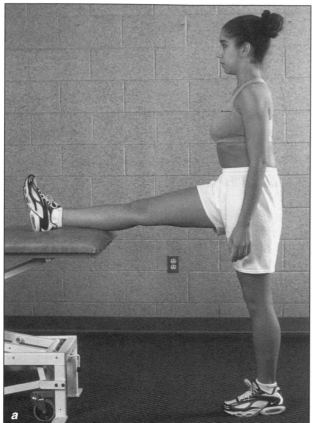

The hamstrings can be stretched in supine with the uninvolved leg in full hip and knee extension. With the involved knee in extension, the patient places his or her hands around the posterior thigh and pulls the leg toward the chest (figure 22.22b). The back should not arch, and the uninvolved knee should not come off the supporting surface. The knee is extended until a stretch is felt.

The gluteals are stretched in a position similar to that for the supine hamstring stretch, with the difference being that the involved knee is flexed and the force pulls the knee toward the chest. The pelvis should not roll posteriorly, and the opposite thigh should not lift off the table (figure 22.22c).

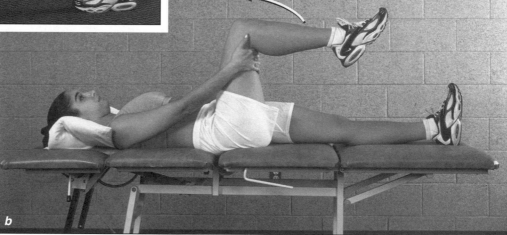

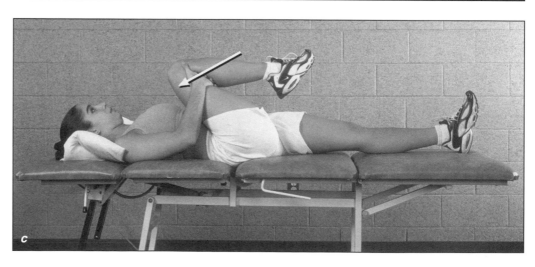

■ **Figure 22.22**
Hip extensor muscle stretches: (a) standing hamstring stretch, (b) supine hamstring stretch, (c) supine gluteal stretch.

Piriformis

The piriformis can be effectively stretched in a supine, standing, or quadruped position. In supine, the patient lies with the knees crossed, the involved leg on top of the uninvolved leg. The knees are brought to the chest, and the patient pulls them, with the involved knee directed toward the opposite shoulder (figure 22.23a).

In a quadruped position, the patient crosses the involved leg under the uninvolved leg and leans the hips backward, keeping the uninvolved knee off the floor and allowing it to move back (figure 22.23b). This permits the involved hip to adduct, flex, and internally rotate. In standing, the patient rests the involved lower leg on a tabletop with the hip in external rotation and flexion. He or she leans forward toward the tabletop to feel the stretch in the hip.

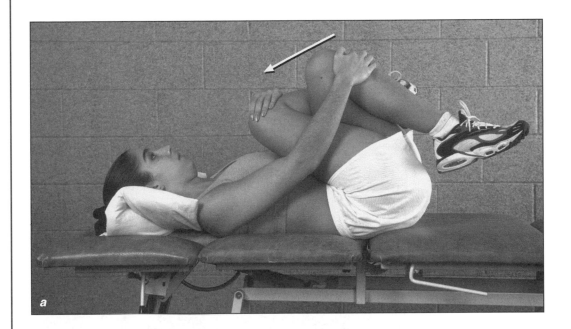

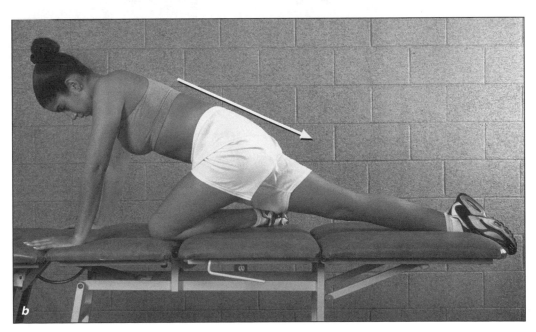

❚ Figure 22.23 Piriformis stretches: *(a)* supine stretch, *(b)* quadruped stretch.

STRENGTHENING EXERCISES

Strengthening exercises for the hip, which are analogous in their progression to those for other body segments, include isometric, body-weight resistance, rubber tubing, machine, free-weight, and Swiss ball activities.

As with other body segments, hip exercises begin with isometrics and can be performed in various joint positions for optimal results. Isotonic exercises include concentric and eccentric exercises; these use gravity as resistance for the least difficult exercise and advance to various other forms of resistance including manual resistance, weight cuffs, rubber tubing, pulleys, and machines. Increased manual resistance and weight-cuff resistance are applied at the ankle. If less resistance is necessary, the same amount of resistance can be placed more proximally on the leg.

The exercises should be performed in a smooth, controlled motion of the hip through a full range of motion. Substitutions of other muscles occur easily in the hip and must be carefully observed and corrected as needed by the sport rehabilitation specialist. Low intensity, high repetition resistance can be replaced with higher loads and fewer repetitions as strength and control improve.

Because the trunk, knee, and ankle are so intimately connected to the hip, strength, motion control and stabilization within all of these segments are vital to hip stability and quality of performance. Exercises to satisfy deficiencies in these areas must be part of a total hip rehabilitation program. As exercises for these segments have been presented in previous chapters, they are not repeated here.

ISOMETRIC EXERCISES

The patient can perform isometrics independently against his or her hand or a stationary object. To perform hip adduction in long or short sitting, the patient places either the hands or a rolled towel between the knees and attempts to push the knees together (figure 22.24a).

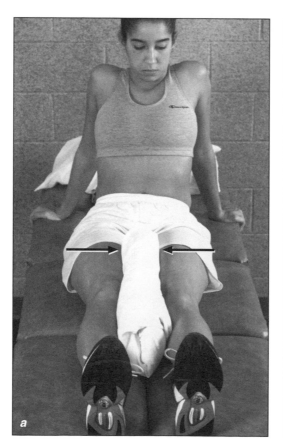
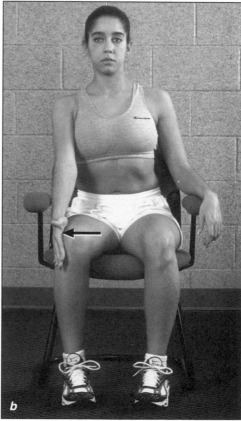

∎ **Figure 22.24**   Isometric hip exercises: *(a)* hip adduction, *(b)* hip abduction.

Hip abduction isometrics are performed in sitting. The patient moves the thigh outward as he or she resists the motion at the knee on the lateral distal thigh (figure 22.24b).

Hip flexion is best performed while sitting in a chair. The patient places a hand on the distal thigh and resists attempts to lift the knee up. The patient should refrain from using the foot to push off the floor.

Hip extension is performed best in supine. The patient squeezes the buttocks to set the gluteals.

All isometric exercises are performed using a buildup to maximal tension. The tension is held for 5 or 6 s and then gradually released to full relaxation before the exercise is repeated. Isometrics are performed several times throughout the day in sets of at least 10 repetitions. They are used early in the rehabilitation program when the muscle is very weak or when range of motion is limited either by immobilization or by restricted mobility.

BODY-WEIGHT RESISTANCE EXERCISES

In a 68-kg (150-lb) patient, the lower extremity weighs about 11 kg (25 lb). This can be substantial resistance for a very weak hip muscle. Weight should not be added to the leg until the patient is able to control the extremity against gravity through a full range of motion.

If the patient is unable to lift the lower extremity against gravity, he or she may need to shorten the lever-arm length of the leg's resistance by flexing the knee to perform the exercise. If antigravity exercises are too difficult for the patient, he or she can perform the same activity in standing; gravity is less in this position, but the muscle is still required to contract and move the leg.

Hip Abduction

With the patient in side-lying on the uninvolved leg, the lower leg is flexed at the hip and knee for stability. The patient keeps the knee and hip extended and lifts the leg against gravity (figure 22.25). Common substitutions in this exercise include rotating the hip, lying more toward the back, and moving the hip into flexion and out of the abduction plane. These substitution patterns should be corrected to prevent either the rotators or the hip flexors from performing the exercise.

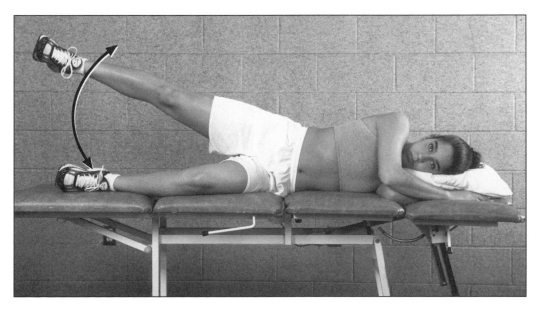

∎ **Figure 22.25**   Isotonic hip abduction exercises.

Hip Adduction

The patient lies on the involved side with the upper leg flexed at the hip and knee and the foot placed in front of the bottom knee. Keeping the involved knee and hip extended, the patient lifts the leg against gravity (figure 22.26a). Common substitutions are rolling toward the back or flexing the hip to permit the hip flexors to perform the exercise. The exercise is more difficult because greater trunk stabilization is required if the patient lifts the top leg into abduction and maintains that position while lifting the bottom leg to meet the top leg (figure 22.26b). An alternative position is with the top leg placed on a supporting object such as the seat of a chair (figure 22.26c).

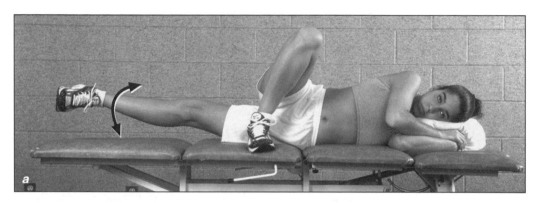

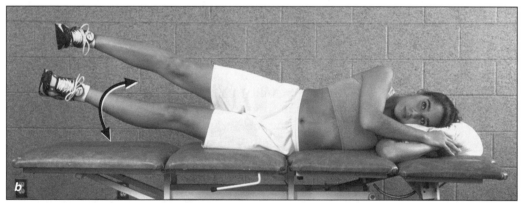

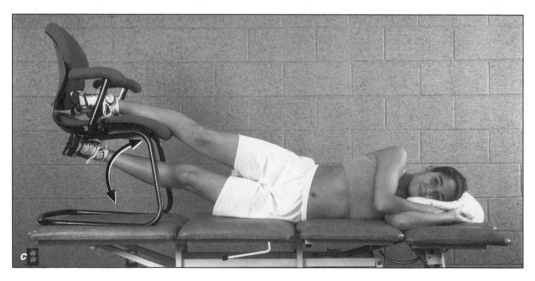

▌Figure 22.26   Isotonic hip adduction exercises: *(a)* without top leg support, *(b)* with additional requirements for trunk stabilization, *(c)* with top leg supported.

Hip Extension

The patient lies in prone with the leg either supported in extension or positioned in flexion. Hip hyperextension is limited to about 15°, so when the patient begins in a fully extended position, the amount of motion the muscles produce is relatively small (figure 22.27a). If the patient lies prone with the leg over the edge of a table, the hip begins in flexion and must travel through a greater range of motion (figure 22.27b). In either position, the patient should squeeze the gluteal muscles while lifting the

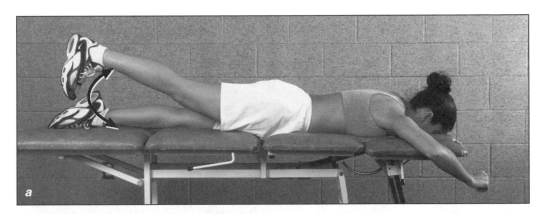

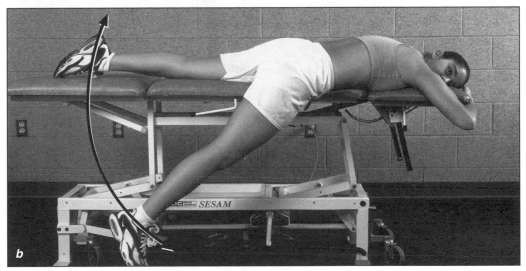

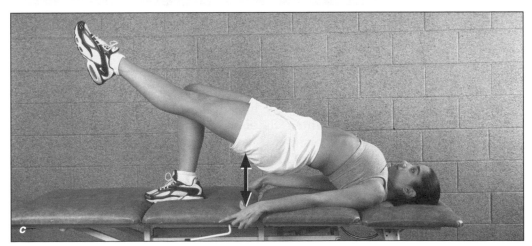

▮ Figure 22.27   Isotonic hip extensor exercises: *(a)* prone on table, *(b)* over table edge, *(c)* supine.

leg and should keep the knee extended to facilitate all hip extensor muscles. If the patient is to isolate the gluteals, the knee should be flexed; but remember that with a shorter lever-arm length, the resistance of the leg is less. Common substitutions for this exercise are hip rotation and trunk rotation.

The patient can also strengthen hip extensors with a bridge exercise. The patient lies supine with the hips and knees flexed and with the feet flat on the floor. The hips are raised so that the hips and trunk form a straight line, and the patient is instructed to hold this position for several seconds. This exercise can be advanced to one-leg support (figure 22.27c). A common substitution is dropping the hips to move them into flexion.

A figure-4 exercise serves the dual purpose of strengthening hip extensors and external rotators. The patient lies prone; the involved leg is flexed at the hip and knee, and the ankle is under the uninvolved thigh. If the patient lacks enough flexibility for the position, he or she should place the involved ankle on top of the uninvolved leg as proximal along the leg as possible. In a figure-4 position, the patient lifts the flexed knee as high as possible (figure 22.28). If the right knee is being lifted, the face should be turned to the left, and vice versa. Typical substitutions for this exercise are hip rotation and trunk rotation.

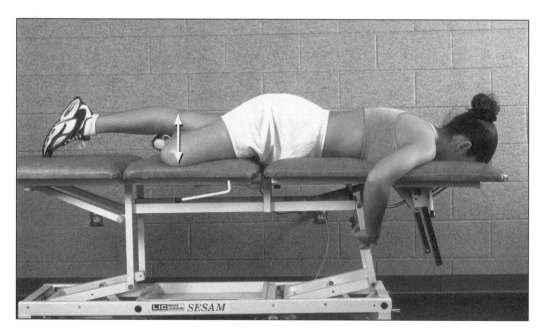

▌Figure 22.28   Figure-4 lift.

Hip Flexion

A straight-leg raise performed in supine strengthens the hip flexors. The uninvolved leg is flexed at the hip and knee, with the foot flat on the supporting surface. The patient tightens the abdominals to prevent the back from arching, tightens the quadriceps to maintain knee extension, and lifts the leg upward toward the ceiling. Rotation and hip abduction should be corrected if the patient attempts substitutions with these activities.

RUBBER TUBING RESISTANCE EXERCISES

Rubber tubing or bands or weighted pulleys can be used progressively once the patient is able to perform antigravity exercises through a full range of motion. In the following descriptions of the exercises, the involved leg is used as the exercising leg, so it is advisable to use upper-body support devices for balance in order to promote better execution.

Rubber tubing exercises can also be performed with the resistance attached to the uninvolved leg so that the involved leg must work to support and stabilize the body during exercises with the uninvolved extremity. When these exercises are used with that goal, the recommendation is to use upper-extremity support objects minimally, or not at all, to facilitate a greater effort from the weight-bearing leg. When the exercises are used for balance and proprioception, they can be executed either as explained here—in straight planes of movement—or in the more challenging diagonal proprioceptive neuromuscular facilitation planes.

If the patient performs the exercise using a substitution pattern, you should correct the execution by providing verbal cueing or by providing visual feedback with a mirror. If substitution continues with these corrections, the resistance may be too much for the patient to control properly, and he or she should use the next-lightest resistance band instead. The motion should be full and should be controlled by the patient throughout the exercise.

Hip Abduction

With the tubing attached to a doorway or table leg, the patient places the tubing around the involved ankle. The patient stands sideways with the uninvolved side closest to the anchor site, takes the slack out of the tubing, tightens the quadriceps and gluteals, and abducts the leg out to the side (figure 22.29). Common substitutions for this exercise include trunk forward lean, side lean to the opposite side, and hip hiking. If verbal and visual cueing do not correct the substitution patterns, a less-resistive band may be necessary. A full range of motion should be possible.

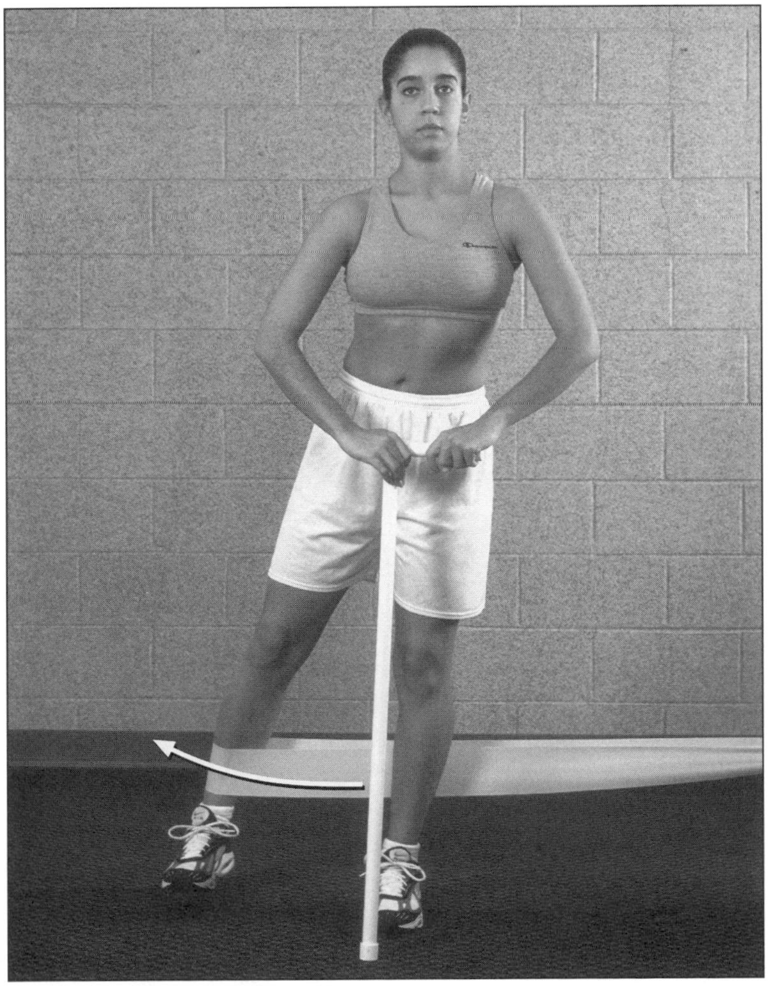

Hip Adduction

With the tubing anchored around a table leg or positioned low on a door frame, the patient places the tubing around the involved ankle and stands sideways from the anchor site with the involved side closest to the anchor site. With the laxity taken out of the tubing, the patient moves the leg across and in front of the uninvolved leg with the knee straight. Common substitutions are rotating the trunk as the leg moves across the body, flexing the hip too far forward, and trunk lean toward the tubing anchor.

Gluteus Medius

For this exercise, short-length tubing is wrapped around both ankles. In standing, the patient tightens the quadriceps and gluteals and extends the involved hip backward and outward to about a 45° angle (figure 22.30a). Placing both hands on a wall

Figure 22.29 Rubber tubing hip abduction.

keeps the patient from substituting trunk forward bend and side-bend away from the involved leg.

An alternative gluteus medius exercise is performed with the patient standing sideways with the uninvolved side about 5 to 10 cm (2–4 in.) from the wall. The uninvolved knee is flexed to 90° and is pressed sideways into the wall. The involved leg is flexed slightly at the knee and should be in line with the ipsilateral shoulder and the second toe (figure 22.30b).

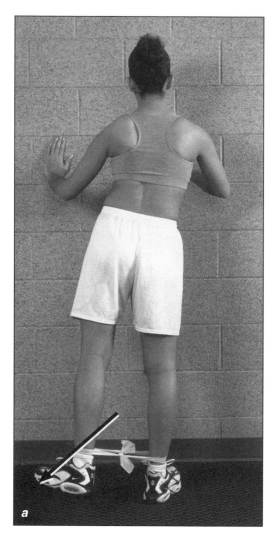
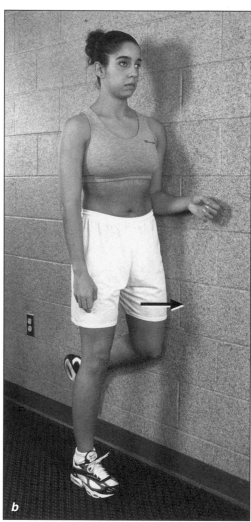

■ **Figure 22.30** Gluteus medius strengthening: *(a)* with short-length theraband, *(b)* the standing leg is the involved leg.

Hip Extension

With the tubing anchored around a table leg or in the low part of a doorjamb, the patient places the tubing around the involved ankle and faces the anchor site. Taking the slack out of the tubing, the patient tightens the quadriceps and gluteals and extends the hip (figure 22.31). Common substitutions that should be corrected include trunk forward lean, hip abduction, and knee flexion.

Hip Flexion

With the tubing anchored around a table leg or low in a doorjamb, the patient stands with the tubing around the involved ankle and his or her back to the anchor site.

After having removed the slack from the tubing, the patient tightens the quadriceps to keep the knee extended and lifts the leg into hip flexion. Common substitutions include backward trunk lean and knee flexion.

Hip Internal Rotation

The tubing is anchored to a door frame about 30 to 45 cm (12–18 in.) from the floor. With the uninvolved side closest to the tubing, the patient lies prone on the floor with the tubing around the involved ankle. The involved knee is flexed to 90°, and the slack is taken out of the tubing. The patient uses the involved leg to pull the tubing away from the anchor site (figure 22.32). Common substitutions to avoid include pelvis rotation and hip extension.

Hip External Rotation

With the tubing anchored as for hip internal rotation, the patient lies prone on the floor with the involved leg closest to the anchor site and the tubing around the involved ankle. With the knee flexed to 90° and the slack taken out of the tubing, the patient pulls the involved lower leg toward and across the uninvolved leg. Substitutions include extending the knee and rotating the hips or pelvis.

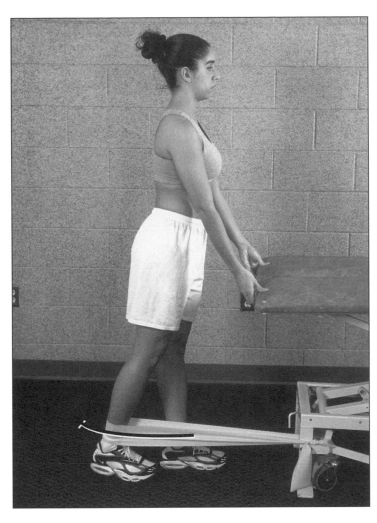

■ **Figure 22.31**   Rubber tubing hip extension.

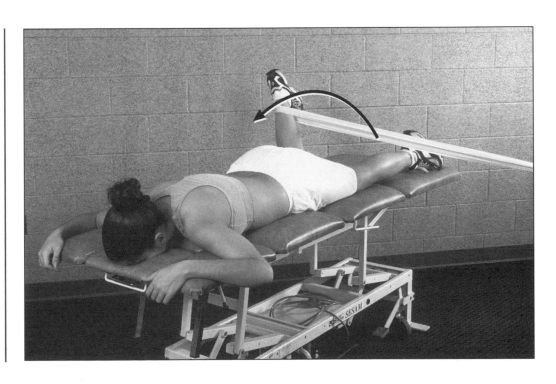

■ **Figure 22.32**
Rubber tubing internal rotation.

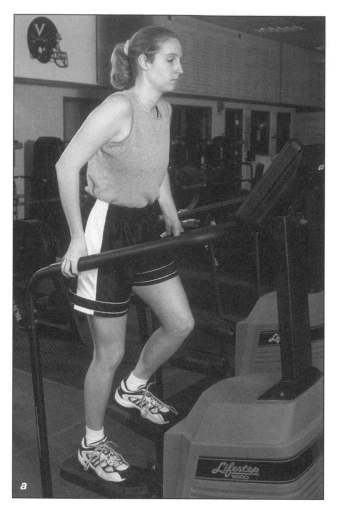

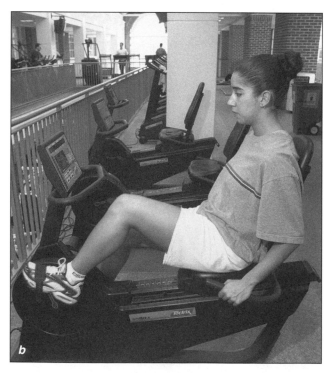

Figure 22.33 Reciprocal machines, such as the step machine (a) or stationary bike (b), can be used to increase strength, ROM, and coordination.

MACHINE AND EQUIPMENT EXERCISES

Many resistive exercises for the hip are the same as those used for the knee as discussed in chapter 21. Some additional exercises are mentioned here, but you should revisit chapter 21 for additional hip exercises. Some of these are step exercises, wall squats, mini-squats, the plié, lunges, sit-to-stand, and leg press machine exercises.

Reciprocal-Exercise Equipment

Reciprocal-exercise equipment can be useful for range-of-motion gains, strengthening, and coordination. These can be used early in strengthening work when the patient may not have antigravity strength but is able to tolerate resistance in an upright posture that does not require full antigravity strength. These exercises include activities on machines such as the step machine, ski machine, or stationary bike (figure 22.33).

Resistance Machines

Resistance machines have a variety of resistance mechanisms, including weights and hydraulic, rubber, and asymmetrical cam systems. They all provide progressive resistance for various exercises. Resistance increments vary from one type of machine to another.

Hip Abduction, Adduction, Extension, and Flexion

Some machines that are on the market offer progressive resistance in individual motions and also allow the user to make alterations so that the machine offers resistance in coronal and sagittal planes of hip motion. In each case the machine isolates a hip motion and does not utilize motion from other joints or other hip motions (figure 22.34). It is essential to give careful instruction in the proper use of these machines. The patient should receive instruction on correct alignment, proper weight that is controlled through the full range of motion, and precise execution without improper substitution.

Recliner Leg Press

There are different models of this design on the market. The machines are closed kinetic chain devices that coordinates hip, knee, and ankle activity. The hip can be exercised in supine with the involved leg placed on the platform so that the knee and hip are at 90° in the starting position. The patient pushes on the leg so that the body moves away from the platform (figure 22.35).

The patient can take an alternative position to further increase hip-extension activity. With the patient in a quadruped position on the machine, the involved leg is placed high on the platform and the patient bears weight on the uninvolved knee and elbows. The patient pushes on the platform to extend the knee and hip.

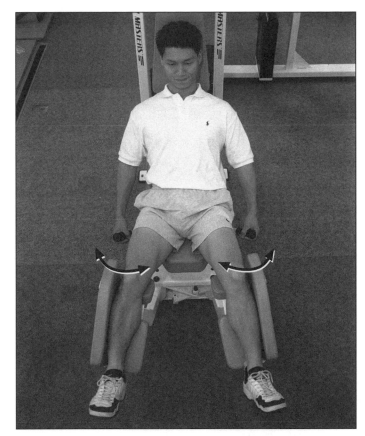

Figure 22.34 Isolated hip-motion exercises.

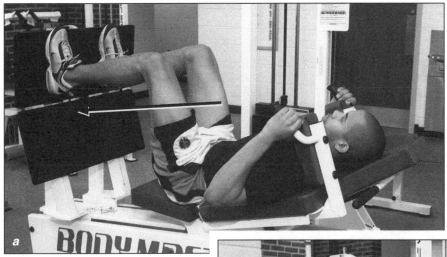

Figure 22.35 Recliner leg press exercises: *(a)* supine position, *(b)* prone position.

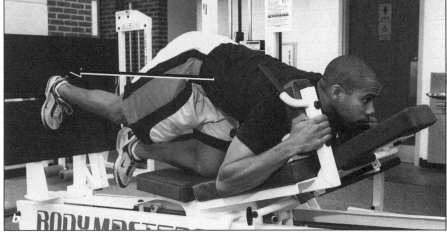

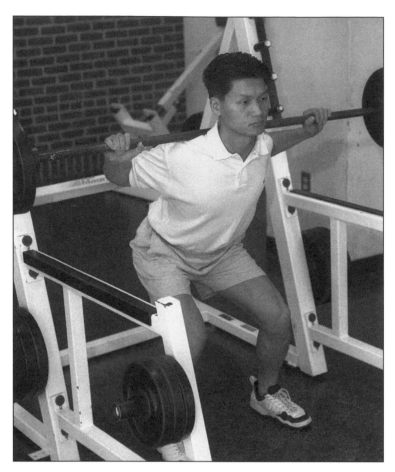

▮ Figure 22.36   Squat exercise with free weights. Correct body alignment should be maintained.

FREE-WEIGHT SQUATS AND SPLIT SQUATS

Barbells and dumbbells can provide resistance to squat and split-squat exercises. The patient should be cautioned to keep good alignment of the knee and back in executing these exercises (figure 22.36). Weights should begin light and progress as the patient demonstrates control and adequate strength.

SWISS BALL EXERCISES

Swiss ball exercises can involve activities such as bridging with leg curls, first with both legs and then with the involved leg only. This exercise facilitates the hip extensors.

Hip flexor exercises on the Swiss ball are performed with the patient's hands on the floor and the lower legs on the ball. The patient pulls the knees toward the chest while maintaining balance on the ball (figure 22.37).

Both of these exercises become more difficult when manual resistance is applied to the movement of the ball: the sport rehabilitation specialist provides friction resistance on the ball while the patient attempts to move the ball.

▮ Figure 22.37
Swiss-ball hip-flexion exercise: With legs on the ball, the knees and hips begin in an extended position. The patient pulls the knees toward the chest to end in the position shown.

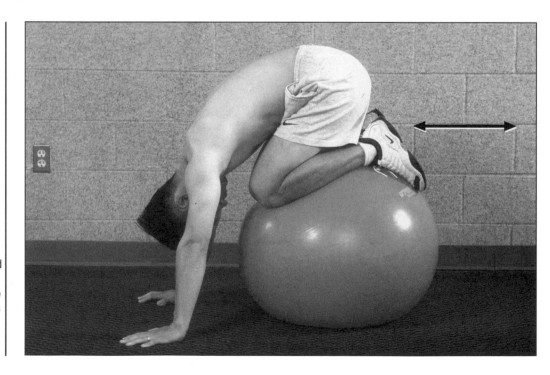

PROPRIOCEPTIVE EXERCISES

Proprioceptive exercises for the hip progress from static balance activities to distracting balance activities, then to agility exercises such as rapid box exercises, and finally to plyometrics.

Balance exercises can begin early in the therapeutic exercise program when the patient is able to bear weight on the extremity. As with other lower-extremity injuries, progression is from weight-transfer activities and gait training to stork standing with eyes open and then eyes closed. Balance begins with static activities and advances to distracting activities in which static balance is challenged while the patient performs other functions and dynamic activities. These can include the tubing exercises performed with the uninvolved leg while the patient balances on the involved leg on the ground or on a $\frac{1}{2}$ foam roller; stork standing on a trampoline or BAPS board while catching or bouncing a ball; and using a balance board or other machine such as a Fitter or slide board.

As balance, proprioception, strength, and coordination improve, the patient progresses to agility exercises that demand higher proprioceptive responses and control. These include resistive weight-transfer activities, exercises entailing increased speed of movement, and finally explosive exercises using jumping and plyometrics.

Agility exercises were introduced in chapters 20 and 21. Some of these are rapid box exercises such as rapid step-up-and-step-down activities, changes in direction from left to center to right box steps, and hopping over boxes.

Rubber tubing can be used to increase resistance of rapid-direction-change exercises. With tubing attached to the waist, the patient can be required to jump to different targets on the floor, change directions of movement, and alternate patterns of jumps. Some of these exercises are detailed in chapter 20.

Plyometric exercises maximize use of the patient's agility, strength, power, and coordination; these begin when the patient has demonstrated good control in rapid agility exercises and has good strength and adequate flexibility to perform the exercises safely.

Plyometric exercises such as drop-and-jump activities, lateral jumps, and cone jumps can all be used for all lower-extremity injuries, including hip injuries. These activities are discussed in chapters 9 and 20.

FUNCTIONAL EXERCISES

The sport rehabilitation specialist selects functional exercises for the hip, when the patient is ready for them, according to the patient's specific sport and position.

A wide variety of functional exercises can be included in hip rehabilitation. The primary factor in determining which ones to use in a hip program is the patient's sport and position within the sport. If the sport includes primarily running activities, then those types of activities are included in the functional program. If the sport includes rapid changes of direction, acceleration, and deceleration, then those are the activities that the functional portion of the program includes. If the patient's sport demands include jumping, pivoting, and backward motions, then those are added to the functional program.

Speed and difficulty of the exercises are at a low level at first and are increased progressively as the patient is able to tolerate the added stress. A continuous progression to activities that precisely mimic the demands of the patient's sport is provided, as long as pain and other deleterious signs are avoided.

The patient may return to full sport participation once he or she is pain free; has normal strength, flexibility, and agility; can perform equally on the left and right lower extremities without hesitating or favoring the involved extremity; and uses both lower extremities normally.

SPECIAL REHABILITATION APPLICATIONS

Among common hip injuries that the sport rehabilitation specialist encounters are muscle-imbalance syndromes, acute soft-tissue injuries, various inflammation conditions, and fractures and dislocation.

Although hip injuries do not occur as often as injuries of the ankle and knee, they can be just as disabling and need proper rehabilitation if the patient is to have a successful return to sport participation. Younger patients whose bones have not matured sustain more growth plate injuries in the hip than they do ligamentous and musculotendinous injuries (Mellman et al. 1996). Some of the more common injuries and dysfunctions of the hip and their rehabilitation are discussed next.

MUSCLE-IMBALANCE SYNDROMES

Many of the soft-tissue injuries around the pelvis, hip, and thigh result from muscle imbalances (Geraci 1994). These syndromes are characterized by tightness of a muscle group and weakness of its antagonist and compensatory muscle firing patterns in adjacent areas. The resulting symptoms typically include pain and reduced function and can cause structural changes. Changes in myofascial tissue are also commonly seen.

Hip Flexor Tightness Syndrome

This problem is common in gymnasts and dancers. Hip flexors are tight, and their antagonists, the hip and lumbar extensors, are weak and inhibited. This imbalance is characterized by an excessive anterior pelvic tilt and lumbar lordosis in standing. Lower lumbar spine dysfunctions including disk degeneration, spondylosis, spondylolysis, or spondylolisthesis can develop. Myofascial restriction is common in the lumbar paraspinals, quadratus lumborum, and latissimus dorsi.

Objective assessment findings demonstrate a positive Thomas test for hip tightness. In prone, assessment of muscle firing in hip extension reveals an asynchronous pattern. Normal firing sequence in prone hip extension is initiated by the hamstrings, sequentially followed by the gluteus maximus, contralateral lumbosacral paraspinals, ipsilateral lumbosacral paraspinals, contralateral thoracolumbar paraspinals, and finally the ipsilateral thoracolumbar paraspinals (Geraci 1994). Excessive scapular muscle firing is seen as a compensation for weak, inhibited extensor muscles.

Treatment of this syndrome requires correction of shortened muscles, myofascial release of restricted soft tissue, correction of posture, strengthening of the weak muscles, and muscle re-education to facilitate correct muscle firing patterns. When the antagonistic muscles are weak secondary to tightening of agonists, lengthening of the tight muscles often has a significant impact on positive strength changes in the antagonists. Pelvic stabilization activities and strengthening lower abdominals for pelvic support provide a base for posture correction. The use of electrical stimulation and instruction in muscle firing sequence patterns, beginning with slow sequences and progressing to more rapid firing sequences and finally to functional activities, can be helpful in muscle re-education.

The patient can usually continue with sport activities during this time, but he or she should be cautioned that sport performance may change as muscle firing patterns change. This can be frustrating for a patient who has adapted specific sport skills to compensate for imbalances.

Piriformis Syndrome

Buttock pain is the most distinguishing symptom of piriformis syndrome. Pain can also radiate distally into the thigh and lower leg, mimicking an S1 nerve root syndrome. It is aggravated by running, standing, or prolonged sitting. Clinical examination reveals tightness of the piriformis that is often accompanied by weakness. When the patient is relaxed in supine, the involved leg is more externally rotated than the contralateral leg. Palpation reveals tenderness, tightness, and soft-tissue restriction in the piriformis muscle. Active trigger points are often the source of pain referral into the lower extremity. Sciatic nerve irritation that occurs as the tight piriformis presses on the nerve can also refer pain into the lower extremity. The 15% of the population whose sciatic nerves pass through the piriformis muscle are more susceptible to this condition as the source of leg pain from piriformis syndrome.

Common causes of piriformis syndrome include sacroiliac dysfunction; leg-length discrepancies; running on canted surfaces, creating a false leg-length difference; and muscle imbalances including tightness of the piriformis, hamstrings, and lateral thigh muscles.

Treatment includes correction of underlying causes, myofascial release and trigger point release techniques, stretching exercises, and strengthening exercises. The patient can usually continue sport participation during treatment of piriformis syndrome. It is a self-limiting condition in that pain dictates the patient's ability to perform.

Case Study

A 25-year-old distance runner presents with complaints of right buttock and posterior thigh pain that has become progressively worse over the past three weeks. He has recently increased his distance from 6.4 to 9.7 km (4–6 miles). The pain occurs about 4.8 km (3 miles) into his run and remains. The patient reports that when he gets up from his desk after sitting for about 45 min, his right buttock is painful until he walks around for a few minutes. He had a back injury about five years ago that was treated, and he has not had any back problems since then. Standing trunk motions do not elicit pain in any direction. When he lies supine on the treatment table, his right leg is externally rotated about 20° more than his left. Placing the hip in 60° flexion, adduction, and internal rotation elicits pain in the right buttock. Straight-leg raising is to 70° and negative for sciatic pain. Palpating the right buttock with the patient in prone reveals tenderness in the midbuttock region to deep pressure. You can feel a tightness in the piriformis. Resisted hip external rotation in this position is painful. Hip rotation is weak.

Questions for Analysis
1. What other tests should you perform to eliminate any other possible cause of the patient's problem?
2. What do you suspect is his problem?
3. What will be your first treatment for him today?
4. What instructions for home treatments will you give him before he leaves today?
5. What will your goals for the first week of treatment include?
6. What will you tell the patient when he asks you if he can continue running?

ACUTE SOFT-TISSUE INJURIES

Injuries in this category include sprains, strains, and contusions. Traumatic bursitis can also come under this heading, but bursitis will be discussed in connection with repetitive stress injuries.

Contusions

Hip contusions are very common in athletics. When they occur along the crest of the ilium, they are called a **hip pointer.** A hip pointer usually does not require rehabilitation unless it is severe and disabling. In these cases the patient experiences a progressive onset of pain within 24 h following the injury as the injured site develops edema and secondary spasm of the muscles that attach to the iliac crest. Ecchymosis is also evident. These injuries involve both hip and abdominal muscles, so activities that elicit complaints of pain include hip motions of flexion and abduction and trunk motions, especially resisted motions. Ambulation is painful, especially long striding and faster speeds.

Treatment includes anti-inflammatory medication and modalities to absorb the ecchymosis, relieve muscle spasm, and encourage healing. The injury is self-limiting, primarily because of the muscle spasm and tenderness from the ecchymosis. Range of motion with the aid of electrical stimulation can be useful in restoring early active mobility and should be encouraged within the first or second day of the injury. Ultrasound is helpful for ecchymotic absorption. Light resistive strengthening exercises should be possible by day 2 or 3, depending on the severity of the injury. Resistive exercises progress in repetitions and resistance as the patient tolerates them.

Recovery depends on the severity of the injury; the quality of initial treatment in controlling the swelling, bleeding, and muscle spasm; and the time point at which rehabilitation begins. With a moderate injury and appropriate care, the patient may return to competition in less than one week, but more severe injuries with delayed care can disable the patient for at least a couple of weeks.

Groin Strain

Groin strains are defined as strains not only to the hip adductors but also to the hip flexors. The iliopsoas, rectus femoris, adductor longus, brevis, magnus, or sartorius may be involved. Most often, an adductor or the iliopsoas is the muscle injured. The muscle is injured when it is brought beyond its normal limits of motion or produces a rapid forceful contraction. Inherent contributing factors include muscle tightness, weakness, or imbalances. The injury is usually at the site of the musculotendinous junction and can be disabling in moderate or severe cases.

The patient has an antalgic gait favoring the injured leg, with an uneven stride cadence, a shortened stride length on the involved side, and reduced knee and hip motion. Muscle spasm, swelling, and tenderness to palpation of the injury site can also be present. Ecchymosis occurs in second- and third-degree sprains.

Assessment of the injured muscle includes resisted muscle activity tests to determine which motion produces the greatest pain response. Hip flexion with knee extension tests the iliopsoas; hip flexion with knee flexion tests the rectus femoris; hip flexion, external rotation, and abduction with resisted knee flexion tests the sartorius; and hip adduction tests the adductors.

Treatment includes anti-inflammatory medication and modalities for pain control and spasm reduction. Electrical stimulation for muscle spasm reduction, along with assistive active range of motion and active range of motion, is used to regain lost range of motion as soon as possible. If the patient displays an antalgic gait, crutches are necessary until he or she demonstrates a normal gait with good control. A hip spica wrap supports the muscle and reduces range of motion during ambulation to make walking more comfortable. Pool exercises and reciprocal-motion machines can be helpful after day 2 or 3. The patient begins with isometric exercises on day 2 or 3, and a gradual, progressive, resistive exercise program starts when the patient is able to move the limb in antigravity positions. Once the patient is able to weight transfer correctly, stork standing and progressive proprioception exercises are used to develop balance and, later, agility. Treadmill activities can begin when the patient walks normally without crutches; these entail first walking and then jogging and finally running. Agility activities on the treadmill can be used when the patient demonstrates good muscle control and range of motion with closed kinetic chain exercises. Soft-tissue massage is helpful in reducing scar-tissue adhesions and stimulating blood flow to encourage healing after day 5 to 10, depending on the injury's severity and the extent of tissue damage.

Resistive tubing jumping, box drills, and lateral movements begin when good dynamic balance and muscle control are present. The patient advances to plyometrics then functional activities prior to his or her return to full sport activity.

Depending on the severity of the injury, the patient's program may span from less than a week to up to several weeks.

Sprains

Ligament sprains in the hip are relatively rare in athletics. The joint is stable because of its deep socket and strong ligamentous support and does not succumb easily to outside forces. Hip ligaments can incur sprains when a violent injury involving severe forces occurs. The hip is placed in a position of combined extreme flexion, abduction, and external rotation or combined extreme flexion, adduction, and internal rotation during these events.

Grades I and II joint mobilizations can relieve joint pain following a sprain. The patient can do pool exercises in small arcs of motion initially, with progression in the size of the arc of motion as the joint responds. Therapeutic exercises for flexibility and strength progress as in other hip rehabilitation programs.

Case Study

A 16-year-old sprinter injured her left hip when she was practicing three days ago. She has continued pain in the proximal inner thigh with some discoloration along the middle aspect of the inner thigh. She is unable to walk normally because of the pain. Your examination reveals hip abduction to 20°, limited by pain. The patient is unable to lift the leg against gravity into adduction. Hip flexion is 4/5 but is not as tender as adduction. The inner thigh area feels tight and is tender to palpation from the middle thigh to the groin.

Questions for Analysis

1. What do you suspect is the patient's injury?
2. What other differential tests will you do?
3. What will her treatment today include?
4. What instructions for home care will you give her today?
5. Outline the progression of therapeutic exercises you will provide for this patient. What modalities will you use with her and why?

INFLAMMATION CONDITIONS

These injuries are overuse based and are the result of repetitive stresses applied at a rate greater than the body's ability to recover. Among the number of conditions that fall into this category are **bursitis, tendinitis,** and **osteitis.**

Bursitis

The most common bursitis in the hip is greater trochanteric bursitis; but other hip bursae, including the ischiogluteal and iliopectineal bursae, are also subject to inflammation.

If the patient's symptoms persist in spite of treatment efforts, other diagnoses must be considered. Additional diagnoses that should be ruled out include lumbar disk injury, facet syndrome, fracture, nerve entrapment, inguinal hernia, abdominal visceral diseases, hip joint disease, and bone tumor. Additional diagnoses for males are testicular torsion and chronic prostatitis.

Greater Trochanteric Bursitis

The greater trochanteric bursa is susceptible to bursitis when the patient's running mechanics increases stress to the bursa because the person has a greater-than-normal adduction angle or is running on a canted surface. Muscle imbalance between adductors and abductors, an increased Q-angle, leg-length discrepancy, and a wider pelvis are also precipitating causes for trochanteric bursitis. Falling on the lateral hip can cause a traumatic bursitis. The patient experiences pain in the lateral hip that can radiate distally down the thigh or proximally into the lateral buttock. There is pain with lying on the involved side and crossing the legs, as well as during running or walking.

The examination reveals tenderness to palpation over the greater trochanter, pain with hip rotation, and tightness of the ITB as demonstrated with a positive Ober's test. Resisted abduction is tender because of the pressure placed on the bursa by the contracting muscles. Passive hip flexion with adduction and internal rotation press the bursa into the greater trochanter and cause tender areas. The patient may stand with the involved leg more abducted or may place more weight on the contralateral leg.

Iliopectineal Bursitis

Dancers and skaters are the athletes who most commonly experience iliopectineal bursitis, although it can occur in most sports. The iliopectineal bursa lies superficially to the anterior acetabulum and deep to the iliopsoas tendon. Sudden flexion-extension activities, especially resisted motions, can aggravate the bursa. The bursa lies adjacent to the femoral nerve and can often irritate the nerve if it becomes inflamed and swollen. Pain occurs with either stretch or contraction of the iliopsoas muscle. The pain is located at the site of the bursa in the inguinal area, but it can also radiate into the hip, anterior thigh, or knee if the femoral nerve is also affected.

Ischiogluteal Bursitis

The ischiogluteal bursa lies between the ischial tuberosity and gluteus maximus. A traumatic bursitis can develop if the patient falls and lands on the buttocks, or it can develop over time consequent to prolonged sitting on hard surfaces or with the legs crossed. Pain is present with hip or trunk flexion, stair climbing, and walking or running. Palpation of the ischial tuberosity with the patient in side-lying reveals localized tenderness with occasional radiation into the hamstrings or hip.

Treatment

Ultrasound and thermal techniques are the modalities most commonly employed for hip bursitis. Anti-inflammatory medications are provided either orally or by injection. Cross-friction massage reduces adhesions and promotes circulation. Therapeutic exercises should include stretching exercises to increase flexibility of tight muscles and strengthening to correct muscle imbalances. Correction of underlying causes such as running mechanics and running surfaces is necessary to reduce the risk of recurrence. The bursitis injury is self-limiting; and although a modification of activity level may be advantageous, total cessation of sport participation is left to the discretion of the sport rehabilitation specialist and/or physician, and depends on factors such as severity of the injury, type of sport, intensity of participation, and correction of mechanics.

Tendinitis

The adductor longus, iliopsoas, and rectus femoris tendons are the most common sites of tendinitis in the hip (Micheli and Coady 1997). Mechanisms of injury relate to overuse and can involve additional factors such as tightness, muscle imbalances, leg-length discrepancy, running on canted surfaces, increasing workloads too quickly, and incorrect mechanics. A gradual onset of pain in the groin (adductor longus) or inguinal area (rectus femoris or iliopsoas) is the primary complaint. The course of tendinitis in the hip follows that of tendinitis in other body segments, with a progression of pain into the patient's workout until daily activities such as walking and stair climbing are painful.

Examination reveals tenderness to palpation of the tendon. Crepitus may be felt. Stretching or resisted contraction can be painful. Flexibility is often reduced. Reduced stride length and hip motion may be present in an antalgic gait.

Treatment follows the same course as for other tendinitis conditions. Anti-inflammatory medications and modalities for pain and inflammation control accompany therapeutic exercises. Stretching exercises and a graduated program of strengthening exercises are used as tolerated. Correction of the underlying causes is necessary. Cross-friction massage on the tendon reduces adhesion formation and promotes circulation. The patient's sport participation may have to be altered during treatment, depending on the severity of the injury.

Osteitis Pubis

Distance runners, race walkers, and soccer players are susceptible to **osteitis pubis.** This is an inflammatory condition of shear stresses caused by either repeated trauma or strain on the symphysis pubis joint. Pain onset is gradual and localized, with occasional radiation to the abdomen or groin. Aggravating activities include pivoting, jumping, sprinting, kicking, and sudden direction changes. Daily activities such as stair climbing are also painful. The patient may ambulate with an abducted gait. Stretching the legs into full abduction is painful, as is resisted adduction.

Treatment includes anti-inflammatory medication, modalities for pain relief, and therapeutic exercises for flexibility and strength as tolerated. The treatment progression follows that of a tendinitis program. This injury is self-limiting, but an initial reduction in normal activity helps to improve the response to treatment efforts.

Rice Krispie Syndromes

Snap, crackle, and pop sounds in the hip, resulting from a variety of factors, occur most commonly in dancers and gymnasts; but they can also occur in athletes in other sports such as skating and running.

The ITB can be the source of snapping in the hip. The snapping occurs when a tight ITB moves across the trochanteric bursa during hip flexion-extension. The condition becomes more noticeable with internal rotation when the band is moved across the bursa. It can cause pain and result in irritation of the trochanteric bursa or the proximal ITB.

Another malady found in dancers is the iliopsoas snap syndrome, which occurs when the hip is in about 45° flexion and moving into extension (Mellman et al. 1996). In this position the iliopsoas snaps against the iliopectineal bursa and anterior ridge of the acetabulum. Tightness of the iliopsoas or an anterior pelvic tilt can be the source of this syndrome, which can cause either bursitis or tendinitis in the area if it persists.

A clicking sound that accompanies pivoting movements may result from a torn acetabular labrum. The pivoting motion of the femur catches the labrum when the hip is in extension. A torn acetabular labrum presents with a sharp pain into the groin or anterior thigh.

Patients with the acetabular click syndrome should be referred to the physician for orthopedic examination. Patients with either iliopsoas or ITB syndrome should learn proper stretching exercises to lengthen shortened structures, should use stabilization techniques for proper pelvic and hip alignment, and should strengthen muscles if imbalances exist. Deep-tissue massage can be used to reduce adhesions, stimulate circulation, and reduce pain.

Case Study

A 16-year-old, male, competitive figure skater has been diagnosed with right iliopectineal bursitis. He has been referred to you by his physician for treatment. The patient presents with tenderness in the inguinal area for the past four weeks. Over that time the pain has increased to the point that it interferes with his practices. He is unable to lift his partner during their practices without intense pain. He also experiences pain throughout the practice, especially when he pivots, jumps, or lands on the right leg. During the past week he has noticed pain extending down the front of the thigh. Your examination reveals pain with resisted hip flexion and stretch into hip extension. The patient has pain and weakness to resisted hip flexion. He has a moderate lumbar lordosis and weakness in the lumbar extensors, and his hip-extension firing-pattern test reveals increased scapular activity with mild to moderate gluteal firing last in the sequence.

Questions for Analysis

1. List other tests for a differential diagnosis that you should perform today.
2. What treatment will you give the patient today?
3. What home instructions will you discuss with him?
4. What will you tell the patient when he asks if he can continue his workouts?
5. Outline your program for the patient for the next two weeks. What functional activities will you include in his program before full return to sport participation?

FRACTURES AND DISLOCATION

Fractures fall into three main categories: traumatic, stress, and growth plate fractures. Traumatic fractures are not commonly seen in athletics because of the great forces required. Stress fractures, however, are more common. Growth plate fractures occur in younger athletes whose epiphyseal plates remain immature.

Traumatic Fractures

The traumatic fractures include avulsion fractures involving an apophysis that a muscle is attached to and non-apophyseal fractures that can include the pelvis or femur. Both types occur as the result of a high-energy violent trauma—the apophyseal fractures because of an internal force, and the non-apophyseal fractures because of an external force.

Avulsion Fractures

Avulsion fractures occur because of a sudden, forceful contraction of a muscle that pulls the apophysis away from the bone. The sites of avulsion fractures are at the origins of the hip's strong muscles. These locations include the ischium, ASIS, anterior inferior iliac spine, lesser trochanter, inferior pubic ramus, and iliac crest—the origin sites for the hamstrings, sartorius, rectus femoris, iliopsoas, adductors, and abdominals, respectively. The greater trochanter rarely is a site of avulsion fractures.

The patient has pain with active movement and attempts to shorten the muscle's motion during ambulation. For example, if the ischium is fractured, the patient ambulates with a shortened stride length and keeps the leg from moving very far in front of the body to reduce stretching and activity of the hamstrings. Resistance against the muscle is more painful than stretching the muscle, but both elicit significant pain responses. The site is very tender to palpation, and edema and discoloration are present.

Treatment depends on the size of avulsion and its location. An open reduction and internal fixation may be necessary but often is not. Crutches with partial weight bearing to tolerance are used for the first three to six weeks until the patient is able to walk normally. Isometric exercises and active range-of-motion exercises, pain free, are used early in the therapeutic exercise program. Modalities for modulation of pain, edema, and muscle spasm are used initially. Strength exercises progress from isometric to isotonic. Pool exercises can be used after the first or second week. Isotonic exercises progress as the patient tolerates them pain free, moving to anti-gravity resistance and weight-resistance activities as tolerated. When the patient is able to bear total body weight on the extremity, he or she can perform stork standing and other static balance activities and then advance to dynamic balance activities and agility exercises. From this point the typical progression is to plyometrics and then to functional exercises before return to full sport participation.

Rehabilitation may take up to three months following an avulsion fracture. The time required for full recovery depends on the site of the fracture, type of treatment (surgical or nonsurgical), and the individual patient's ability to progress.

Non-Avulsion Fractures

Common sites of these fractures include the pelvis, acetabulum, femoral neck, and intertrochanteric femur. Fractures of this type, which are rare in athletics, cause significant pain. Most often they require hospitalization and surgical treatment, especially if the fracture is displaced. The rehabilitation process is prolonged, a minimum of three months. During immobilization or after surgery, isometric exercises are used to reduce muscle atrophy. Other exercises and weight bearing may be delayed in comparison to the timing for avulsion fractures, but the program progression is similar.

Stress Fractures

Stress fractures occur most commonly in patients who suddenly increase their training intensity. This type of fracture is most often seen in distance runners and soccer players. The common sites of stress fractures are the pubic ramus, femoral neck, and subtrochanteric region of the femur. In patients with coxa vara, stress loads placed on the femoral neck may be increased, predisposing these individuals to femoral neck stress fractures.

The patient reports a sharp, deep, localized pain that is aggravated with jumping and running. In the early stages, rest relieves the pain; but as the injury progresses, the pain continues during rest.

Treatment includes correction of the causative factors. Non-weight bearing or partial weight bearing on crutches is used for up to three weeks. Exercises on reciprocal machines such as the stationary bike or upper-body ergometer, pool exercises including deep-water running, and pain-free open kinetic chain exercises can take place early in the program. Hip, knee, ankle, and trunk exercises should be part of the program. As the patient progresses to full weight bearing with a normal gait and without pain, he or she performs progressive closed kinetic chain and proprioception exercises to make additional strength, balance, coordination, and agility gains.

Growth Plate Fractures

Slipped capital femoral epiphysis is a displacement of the femoral head from the femoral neck because of a weakness in the epiphyseal plate. It occurs in boys, ages 10 to 17, and in girls, ages 8 to 15. It is seen in youths who have predisposing factors such as a recent growth spurt, an imbalance of sex hormones and growth hormones, and an overweight or a lanky build. The patient reports an insidious, gradual onset of pain in the groin that can refer to the thigh and knee in chronic slips. Less often the patient experiences an acute slipped capital femoral epiphysis that presents with a sudden onset of pain and disability following a traumatic event. Pain produces an antalgic gait.

Examination reveals restriction of hip internal rotation, abduction, and flexion, with the greatest restriction in internal rotation. During active hip flexion, the hip also moves into external rotation. In a relaxed position, the leg is in greater external rotation than the contralateral limb. Hip abductors are weak.

Possible differential diagnoses with groin, anterior thigh, and knee pain must be investigated. Other possible diagnoses are fracture, tumor, hernias, strains, and contusions. An evaluation of the patient's history, hip motion and motion patterns, pain level, and strength helps the sport rehabilitation specialist determine other possible sources of the patient's pain.

Treatment includes open reduction and internal fixation followed by partial weight bearing for two to six weeks. Isometric exercises immediately postoperatively, followed by open kinetic chain exercises, are used early in the rehabilitation process. Pool exercises after the surgical incision has healed and during partial weight bearing are used to achieve range-of-motion and strength gains. Once full weight bearing is permitted, the patient continues to use the crutches until normal gait and hip control are evident. Stork standing and other proprioception exercises progress as tolerated when unilateral weight-bearing activities are permissible. The therapeutic exercise progression follows that for other fractures once the patient is full weight bearing.

Dislocation

Because the hip joint is deep and the ligaments surrounding it are strong, the hip is rarely dislocated in sport: a large, violent force is required to disrupt the joint. One may see dislocations in high-energy sports with large external force applications such as downhill skiing, soccer, football, and rugby. Rarely are orthopedic injuries considered medical emergencies, but hip dislocations are emergencies because of the risk of arterial damage.

Rehabilitation of hip dislocations follows up to three weeks of bed immobilization. During this time, isometric hip exercises and isotonic exercises for the knee and ankle are used to retard atrophy. Theraband exercises for the ankle and knee can be performed in bed throughout the day. Manual resistance exercises can also be used. Activities that put the hip at risk for redislocation include hip adduction, hip flexion, and trunk forward bending. For this reason, the patient should not cross the legs, sit in a chair with the leg at 90° to the trunk, or bend over from the waist for 12 to 16 weeks postinjury.

Once the patient is permitted ambulation with crutches, usually partial weight bearing to tolerance, active range-of-motion exercises can begin. All exercises should be pain free and should not include motion beyond active abilities. The patient uses crutches for about 6 to 8 weeks postinjury, until he or she is able to ambulate normally and demonstrates good hip control. Closed kinetic chain exercises begin when the patient begins weight bearing, but hip flexion beyond 90° is avoided for up to 12 to 16 weeks postinjury. Machine squats and leg press and other resistive machines for the hip are appropriate after week 12. Pool exercises can be started around week 8; however, swimming should be avoided until week 12 when the hip strength is sufficient to provide hip stability against the water's resistance, and the breaststroke should be avoided until week 16. Stationary-bike exercise can begin at week 12 to 16; treadmill walking begins during week 10 and is performed without an incline until week 12. When the patient demonstrates good hip control, walking can progress to jogging after week 14 to 16. The patient transitions to running and to agility and sport-specific activities as he or she makes further gains in strength, control, and coordination, usually anywhere from week 20 to week 30.

Case Study

A 17-year-old, female, forward soccer player reports that she has had progressive anterior hip pain for the past four weeks. The pain has increased to the point that it bothers her on stairs and during walking and standing. She ambulates with an antalgic gait, using a shortened stride length and keeping the hip flexed and in a forward trunk lean. Your examination reveals tenderness to resisted hip flexion that increases with resisted knee extension applied simultaneously. Hip flexion is weak. Passive stretch of prone hip extension with knee flexion is more uncomfortable than hip extension with the knee extended. There is tenderness to palpation of the anterior inferior iliac spine, and pressure on this area reproduces the patient's pain.

Questions for Analysis

1. What do you suspect is the patient's problem?

2. What other differential diagnoses should you eliminate, and how would you accomplish this?

3. Explain what your treatment for her today will include.

4. What home instructions will you give the patient before she leaves today?

5. Outline the rehabilitation program you will place the patient on over the next two weeks. How will you decide when she is ready to resume full sport participation?

SUMMARY

1. *Discuss how anteversion and retroversion change lower-extremity mechanics.*

   Normal alignment places the neck in a line that is 15° anterior to the line of the femur in the adult. If the angle is greater than 15°, the hip is in anteversion. If it is less than 15°, the hip is in retroversion. Retroversion and anteversion alter knee alignment and change the forces acting throughout the entire lower extremity. Retroversion results in frog-eyed patellae, or calcaneal inversion, and causes the individual to ambulate with a toe-out gait. Anteversion causes squinting patellae, or foot pronation, and causes the individual to ambulate with a toe-in gait. Anteversion makes the hip susceptible to dislocation.

2. *Explain the mechanical factors involved in gait with hip abductor weakness and explain how a cane assists in normal gait.*

   When the person stands on the involved extremity, the abductors are not strong enough to counter the force of gravity pulling the non-weight-bearing hip downward and laterally rotating the pelvis, so a normal gait is not possible. The patient either drops the non-weight-bearing hip and downwardly rotates the pelvis to that side, or tilts the trunk to lurch over the weak hip during stance on the leg so that the center of gravity is closer to the fulcrum, the femoral head. If the center of gravity is moved far enough laterally to put it lateral to the fulcrum, the abductors do not have to work and the pelvis does not drop. If a cane is used on the side opposite the weakness, an upward force is transmitted through the cane to counterbalance the downward gravitational force on the same side. Because the lever-arm from the cane to the fulcrum is longer than the center of gravity's lever arm, the force that must be transmitted through the cane is relatively small.

3. *Identify a joint mobilization technique for the hip and explain its benefit.*

   Medial glide is used to increase hip extension and external rotation.

4. *Identify a flexibility and a strengthening exercise for the hip.*

Thomas stretch is used to gain hip extension. A rubber tubing exercise moving into extension is used to increase hip extensor strength.

5. *Identify a proprioceptive exercise for the hip and indicate its progression.*

In a proprioceptive exercise progression for the hip, the patient stork stands with eyes open, then with eyes closed, then on an unstable surface, then on an unstable surface while performing a distracting activity, and finally on the involved leg while performing a resisted exercise with the uninvolved extremity.

6. *List precautions for a hip-dislocation rehabilitation program.*

Activities that put the hip at risk for redislocation include hip adduction, hip flexion, and trunk forward bending. Therefore, the patient should not cross the legs, sit in a chair with the leg at 90° to the trunk, or bend over from the waist for 12 to 16 weeks postinjury.

CRITICAL THINKING QUESTIONS

1. If you were Dave in the opening scenario, how would you manage Jackson's injury? Would you insist that he take time off from his performances; would you rehabilitate the injury as if Jackson were not performing daily; would you treat the injury to keep it from getting worse until the season was over and fully rehabilitate it then; would you refuse to treat him unless he complied with your recommendations; or would you use some other approach? Give justifications for your decision and explain your treatment program.

2. If a patient complains of anterior hip pain, what possible diagnoses will you need to differentiate before beginning a rehabilitation program? (Hint: Do a mental review of all the structures from superficial to deep.) What differences would there be in the rehabilitation programs for those diagnoses?

3. If a gymnast sustained an anterior hip contusion on the bars, what possible secondary problems would cause her to require rehabilitation? What would be your rehabilitation approach to these problems?

REFERENCES

Cyriax, J.H. 1975. *Textbook of orthopaedic medicine. Vol. 1. Diagnosis of soft tissue lesions.* Baltimore: Williams & Wilkins.

Geraci, M.C. 1994. Rehabilitation of pelvis, hip, and thigh injuries in sports. *Physical Medicine and Rehabilitation Clinics of North America* 5:157–174.

Kapandji, 1978. *The physiology of the joints. Vol. 2. Lower limb.* New York: Churchill Livingstone.

Mellman, M.F., McPherson, E.J., Dorr, L.D., and P. Kwong. 1996. Differential diagnosis of back and lower extremity problems. In *The spine in sports,* ed. R.G. Watkins. St. Louis: Mosby.

Micheli, L.J., and C.M. Coady. 1997. Approaching hip, pelvis, and groin injuries in athletes. *Biomechanics* 4:22–26.

Travell, J.G., and D.G. Simons. 1992. *Myofascial pain and dysfunction. The trigger point manual.* Vol. 2. Baltimore: Williams & Wilkins.

GLOSSARY

A band—The portion of the sarcomere where the thick filaments interdigitate with the thin filaments.

ABCs of proprioception—Agility, balance and coordination.

abduction—Lateral movement of a limb or segment away from the midline of the body or part.

absolute refractory period—The time immediately following a stimulus when depolarization prevents another response of the muscle cell from occurring.

acceleration—Rate at which velocity increases.

acceleration phase—That portion of swing in which momentum is increased and the non-weight-bearing limb has propulsion forward.

accessory joint motion—Necessary mobility for normal joint motion that cannot be voluntarily performed or controlled.

accommodating resistance—An activity where the resistance provided a muscle changes as the muscle moves through its range of motion. Isokinetic activity.

acetylcholine—A neurotransmitter at the myoneural junction of striated muscles. Causes vasodilation.

actin—One of two primary proteins of the thin filament of the sarcomere.

action peak—The second ground reaction force peak. The peak occurs during the last half of support and is usually less than impact peak.

action potential—A brief nerve impulse created from a rapid change in the membrane potential to cause a muscle contraction.

active assistive range of motion (AAROM)—Range of motion that is performed with a combination of voluntary activity of the muscles and passive assistance from an outside source.

active range of motion (AROM)—The amount of movement produced at a joint by the patient without assistance.

active stretch—A stretch that uses the patient's active muscle force to control and provide the force for the stretch.

active trigger point—A trigger point that is always tender and that can produce referred pain whether the muscle is active or inactive.

adduction—Lateral movement of a limb or segment toward the midline of the body or part.

adenosine diphosphate (ADP)—A phosphate compound that, when combined with a phosphate, forms adenosine triphosphate (ATP) for energy production. It is also the product of the breakdown of ATP during energy production.

adenosine triphosphate (ATP)—A phosphate compound that provides energy for muscle activity.

adrenaline—See *epinephrine.*

afferent muscle nerve fiber—A sensory nerve fiber from the muscle spindle and Golgi tendon organ. There are two primary types, A and C fibers. C fibers are pain receptors; A fibers are tension and length receptors. Group III delta are A receptors that responds to pressure pain. Group I are A receptors: Group Ia form muscle spindle primary endings and Group Ib form Golgi tendon organs. Group II are A receptors and form muscle spindle secondary endings.

afferent receptors—Sensory receptors that transmit information from the periphery to the central nervous system.

agility—The ability to control the direction of a body or its parts during rapid movement.

agonist(ic)—A muscle acting as a prime mover to produce a motion.

all-or-none principle—A motor unit does not respond until the stimulus is sufficient to produce an action potential. The action potential produces a reaction from the entire motor unit.

alpha motor neuron—An efferent nerve from the ventral horn of the spinal cord to the muscle.

amortization phase—The second phase of a plyometric activity that is the rapid transition from eccentric to concentric motion.

angiogenesis—Formation of new blood vessels.

angle of pull of a muscle—Angle formed by the muscle's line of pull and the line of the bone. Maximal isometric force occurs at a 90° angle of pull.

angular motion—Rotational movement on an axis through an arc.

antagonist(ic)—A muscle that opposes the motion of another muscle.

anteversion—Excessive anterior angulation of the femoral head, resulting in a toe-in gait.

arachidonic acid—An unsaturated essential fatty acid. Works as a precursor in the production of substances, including leukotrienes, prostaglandins, and thromboxanes.

Archimedes' principle of buoyancy—Principle stating that a body partially or fully immersed in a fluid will experience an upward thrust of that fluid that is equal to the weight of the fluid the body displaces.

areolar connective tissue—Loose connective tissue with unorganized structure and relatively long distances between cross-links.

arthrokinematics—The motions between the bones that make up a joint, including roll, slide, spin, compression, and distraction.

arthroscopy—Use of an endoscope to examine or surgically treat the interior aspect of a joint.

assessment—A conclusion based on the gathering of information through an evaluation.

ATPase (adenosine triphosphatase)—Myosin enzyme that is a catalyst the body uses to break down ATP into ADP and phosphate for energy production.

atrophy—Wasting away of tissue with a decrease in size and strength, especially from lack of use.

autogenic inhibition—A protective mechanism provided by the Golgi tendon organ, in which a Golgi tendon organ stimulus facilitated by a sudden stretch causes a reflex activation of the antagonist and relaxation of the agonist.

balance—The body's ability to maintain an equilibrium by controlling the body's center of gravity over its base of support.

ballistic stretching—A rapid stretch or bouncing technique used primarily in sport activities but seldom used in rehabilitation because of the increased risk of injury.

Bankart lesion—Tear of the capsulolabral complex from the glenoid rim.

barrier—A resistance that is felt when a part is moved through its passive range of motion in muscle energy techniques.

Barton's fracture—A fracture of the wrist that occurs with a sudden, violent wrist extension and pronation.

base of support—Two-dimensional area that lies within the points of contact between an object and the supporting surface.

basophil—See *granular leukocyte*.

Bennett's fracture—A fracture of the first metacarpal.

boutonniere deformity—Deformity characterized by flexion of the PIP joint and hyperextension of the DIP joint.

boxer's fracture—Fracture of the metacarpals secondary to a compressive force.

bradykinin—A local tissue hormone that is activated by the interaction of proteases upon the Hageman factor. A very potent local vasodilator. It increases vascular permeability and stimulates local pain receptors.

brain stem—Includes the midbrain, pons, medula oblongata, and diencephalon to form the stem of the brain between the spinal cord and cerebrum.

Brannock measuring device—Used to determine shoe size (length and width).

bursa—Synovial-filled membrane that lies between adjacent structures to limit friction and ease movement.

bursitis—Inflammation or swelling of a bursa.

callus—Fibrous matrix formed at a bone's fractured sites. Immobilizes the bone fragments and serves as the foundation for eventual bone replacement.

capsular pattern—A characteristic pattern of motion unique to each joint when a loss of motion is caused by capsular tightness.

carpal tunnel syndrome—A condition of the wrist and hand characterized by compression of the median nerve as it passes through the carpal tunnel.

center of buoyancy—The center of gravity of the fluid displaced by a body in water and the point at which the buoyant force acts on the body.

center of gravity—The point on an object around which its weight is balanced.

central nervous system—The brain and spinal cord comprise the central nervous system.

cerebellum—That section of the brain that lies below the posterior cerebrum and behind the brain stem and is connected to the brain stem by paired peduncles.

cerebral cortex—The surface of the brain that contains primarily gray matter and nerve cell bodies.

cerebrum—The largest portion of the brain encompassing most of the skull.

chemoattractant—See *chemotactic factor*.

chemotactic factor—A chemical gradient. Also referred to as a *chemotactin* or *chemoattractant*. Occurs after an injury. Cells either become oriented along a chemical concentration gradient or move in the direction of that gradient. Example: Chemicals attract platelets, red blood cells, and polymorphonuclear leukocytes into an injured area.

chemotactin—See *chemotactic factor*.

chemotaxis—Movement of cells or chemicals in response to a chemical stimulus. Vital activities in wound healing that occur through complex and not totally understood processes.

claw toes—Toes that are extended at the metatarsophalangeal joints and flexed at the proximal and distal interphalangeal joints.

closed kinetic chain—Characterizing a motion in which the distal segment of an extremity is weight bearing and the body moves over the hand or foot.

close-packed position—The joint position in which the joint surfaces are most congruent with each other.

Codman's exercises—Low-level passive flexibility exercises for the shoulder that are performed by the patient. Also known as *pendulum exercises*.

cogwheel resistance—An abnormal response during muscle testing that is observed as a series of catch-and-release tensions rather than a smooth resistance, indicative of the individual's providing a less than maximal effort.

collagen—Major structure of the body's protein. There are five types in the body: type I, the most abundant type, is high in tensile strength and is found in dermis, fascia, and bone; type II is found in cartilage; type III is found in embryonic connective tissue; types IV and V are found in basement membranes. Forms inelastic bundles to provide structure, integrity, and tensile strength to tissues.

collagenase—An enzyme produced by newly formed epithelial cells and fibroblasts. Involved in the degradation of collagen during tissue repair. It is important in controlling the collagen content in a wound.

collar—The top rim of the shoe that is often padded to reduce friction on the Achilles.

Colles fracture—A fracture in which the distal radius proximal to the wrist is fractured and is displaced dorsally.

comparable sign—A sign produced by an active or passive movement or test that reproduces a patient's symptom, such as pain or protective muscle spasm.

compartment syndrome—A significant rise in intracompartmental pressure caused by severe bleeding within a muscular compartment that can compromise neurovascular structures.

complement system—Various proteins found in serum. Act as chemotactic factors for neutrophils and phagocytosis.

concave-convex rule—Roll and slide occur in the same direction when a concave surface moves on a convex surface.

concentric motion—Dynamic activity in which the muscle shortens.

concentric phase—The third phase of a plyometric activity, resulting from the combined eccentric and amortization phases. The concentric phase is the outcome phase. If the eccentric activity has been quickly performed and the amortization has occurred rapidly, the concentric phase will produce the desired powerful outcome.

contact pressure—Pressure that occurs between two objects in contact with each other.

contractility—The ability of a muscle fiber to contract.

contraction phase—That part of the mechanical response of a muscle twitch that follows the latency period during which the sarcomere's actin and myosin cross-bridge activity occurs.

contracture—Failure of a muscle to relax. Can occur after fatigue.

convex-concave rule—Roll and slide occur in opposite directions when a convex surface moves on a concave surface.

coordination—The ability of muscles and muscle groups to perform complicated movements.

coxa valga—Femoral neck angulation greater than 135°.

coxa vara—Femoral neck angulation less than 120°

creep—Permanent tissue elongation caused by low-level stress applied over an extended period.

crepitus—A cracking or grating sound or sensation caused by inflammation or degenerative changes.

cross-bridges—The "head" projections from the myosin filaments that link the thick filaments to the thin filaments through a complex process.

De Quervain's disease—Tenosynovitis of the abductor pollicis longus and extensor pollicis brevis tendons and their sheaths on the radial side of the thumb.

deceleration—Negative acceleration.

deceleration phase—That portion of swing in which the limb slows down in preparation for making initial contact with the ground. Also known as *terminal swing*.

dense connective tissue—Connective tissue with highly organized, parallel collagen fibers and more cross-links than loose connective tissue.

depression—A downward movement of the scapula.

dislocation—Complete disassociation or displacement of one joint surface on another.

dorsiflexion—The sagittal plane movement in which the ankle joint angle is decreased as the dorsal foot is moved upward toward the anterior surface of the lower leg.

double-crush syndrome—A condition in which an injury at one site produces signs and symptoms at another site.

double float—The nonsupport phase in a running stride.

double-limb support—The point of the gait cycle that occurs at the beginning of the stance phase during heel strike for one leg and the end of the stance phase just before toe-off for the other.

downward rotation—A movement of the scapula that causes the glenoid to face downward and backward. The inferior angle of the scapula moves medially, and the scapula slides backward.

drag—The water's resistance to a body moving through it. There are three types of drag: form drag, wave drag, and frictional drag.

drug interaction—A reaction in which one drug either enhances or reduces the effectiveness of other drugs that are also being taken.

duration of drug action—Amount of time the blood level of a drug is at or above the level needed to obtain a minimum therapeutic effect. Determined by the drug's half-life.

dynamic activity—Activity in which movement occurs.

dynamic restraint—One of two systems a joint has for its stability. Dynamic restraints are the neuromuscular components that provide movement.

dynamic splint—Splint used to increase motion or limit unwanted activity. It incorporates springs, rubber bands, or other elastic elements to provide a continual low-grade passive stretch, passive assistive motion, or active assistive motion to an area.

dynamometer—A device used to measure strength.

eccentric motion—A dynamic activity in which the muscle lengthens.

eccentric phase—The first phase of a plyometric activity during which the muscle is prestretched as it actively lengthens in preparation for performing the activity. The slack is taken out of the muscle, and its elastic components are put on stretch.

eddy—Circular motion of water layers pulling against a moving object.

elasticity—An object's ability to return to normal shape or size after a deforming force is applied.

elastin—An essential protein of connective-tissue elastic structures. Arranged in a wavy orientation. The wavy arrangement allows tissue to change with stress and to resume normal conditions after stress removal. It plays an as yet unknown role in the remodeling phase.

electrothermally assisted capsular shift—A relatively recently developed arthroscopic procedure used in the shoulder to reduce joint laxity.

elevation—An upward movement of the scapula.

end-feel—The nature of resistance that is felt at the end of joint movement.

endomysium—Connective-tissue layer covering a muscle fiber and continuous with the muscle fiber's membrane.

endothelial cells—Large flat cells that line blood and lymphatic vessels.

endothelial leukocyte—A large white blood cell that circulates in the bloodstream and tissues. Acts as a phagocyte to remove debris from an injured area.

endurance limit—See *fatigue failure*.

energy—The capacity to do work.

engram—A memory trace of an activity accomplished through repetitive application of stimuli.

eosinophil—See *granular leukocyte*.

epicondylitis—An overuse injury to the tendinous attachments of the flexor/pronator group at the medial epicondyle or the extensor/supinator group at the lateral epicondyle. Also referred to as *tennis elbow*.

epimysium—Connective-tissue layer covering an entire muscle.

epinephrine—A hormone. Also called *adrenaline*. A potent stimulator of the sympathetic nervous system. It is also a powerful vasopressor, increasing blood pressure, stimulating the heart muscle, accelerating the heart rate, and increasing cardiac output. It also increases such metabolic activities as glycogenolysis and glucose release.

erythrocyte—An element of blood. Also known as a *red blood cell* or *corpuscle*. Used by the body for oxygen transport.

evaluation—The means by which a sport rehabilitation specialist seeks information on the severity, irritability, nature, and stage of a patient's injury.

eversion—Outward-turning motion of the foot that causes the bottom of the foot to face laterally.

excursion—Amount of movement from one point to another.

extension—Straightening of a joint so that the two body segments move apart and increase the joint angle.

extensible—Able to lengthen. When muscle temperature increases, the muscle fibers and its connective tissue become more easily stretched.

extensor lag—Inability to fully extend the knee during active motion, but full passive motion is present.

external rotation (ER)—Rotation of a joint around its axis in a transverse plane away from the midline of the body. Also called *lateral rotation*.

extracellular matrix—The basic material from which tissue develops. Produced by fibroblasts in wounds. Composed of fibers and ground substance. Serves as a foundation on which anything is cast.

extrafusal fiber—A regular muscle fiber. Also known as a *myofibril*.

extrinsic foot muscles—Muscles that provide function of the toes, foot, and ankle but originate in the lower leg and terminate in the foot.

extrinsic muscles—Muscles that originate proximally from the hand or foot and terminate within the hand or foot.

exudate—Material that escapes from blood vessels following an injury. It contains high concentrations of protein, cells, and other materials from injured cells. As polymorphonuclear leukocytes die and decompose, the exudate may resemble pus although no infection is present.

factor XII—See *Hageman factor*.

fast-twitch fiber—A muscle fiber, also called a *type II fiber* or *fast oxidative fiber*, that is lighter in color than a slow-twitch fiber and that reaches its maximum tension approximately 50 ms after being stimulated.

fatigue—An inability to continue an activity.

fatigue failure—The point at which the cumulative stress of a repetitive submaximal load results in tissue failure. Also called *endurance limit*.

Feiss line—A line from the tip of the medial malleolus to the first metatarsal head. It is used as a point of reference to determine relative position of the navicular tubercle.

fibrin—Insoluble fibrous protein. Formed by fibrinogen. Important in clotting.

fibrinogen—A globulin present in plasma. Converts to fibrin to form a fibrin plug at the injury site.

fibrinolysin—An enzyme in plasma that is released in later healing. Converts fibrin into a soluble substance to unplug lymphatics.

fibroblast—A connective-tissue cell. Fibroblasts differentiate into chondroblasts, osteoblasts, and collagenoblasts. They form the fibrous tissues to support and bind a variety of the body's tissues.

fibrocyte—An inactive fibroblast. See *fibroblast*.

fibronectin—An adhesive glycoprotein found in most body tissues and serum. Fibronectin is plentiful in early granulation tissue formation but gradually disappears during the remodeling phase. Fibronectins cross-link to collagen in connective tissue, thereby playing a role in the adhesion of fibroblasts to fibrin. They are also involved in the collection of platelets in an injured area, and enhance myofibroblast activity.

first-class lever—A lever in which the fulcrum is between the resistance and the force.

first ray—The joint between the first metatarsal and the medial cuneiform. This is the primary weight-bearing ray of the foot and has triplanar motion.

flexibility—Mobility of a body segment, dependent on soft-tissue tolerance to movement and the ability of soft tissue to move with forces applied to it. Flexibility can involve soft-tissue mobility alone or in combination with joint motion. Used interchangeably with *range of motion*.

flexion—Bending of a joint so that the two body segments approach each other and decrease the joint angle.

fixation—A state of stabilization in which motion is restricted or prevented.

foam roller—Cylindrical therapeutic tool made of Ethafoam or polyurethane and used in rehabilitation in neurological, orthopedic, and sports medicine facilities.

foot abduction—The transverse plane movement of the foot in which the lateral foot is moved away from the midline.

foot adduction—The transverse plane movement of the foot in which the medial foot is moved toward the midline.

foot eversion—The frontal-plane movement in which the plantar foot rotates inward so that the medial border is lifted upward.

foot flat—That portion of the stance phase of the gait cycle in which the foot is flat on the floor. Also known as *loading response*.

foot inversion—The frontal-plane movement in which the plantar foot rotates outward so that the lateral border is lifted upward.

foot strike—Initial foot contact with the ground in running. The term replaces *initial contact* or *heel strike*.

force—A strength or energy that causes movement and has direction and magnitude.

force couple—Two equal forces acting in opposite but parallel directions to create a rotatory motion.

force deformation—The amount of force applied to maintain a change of length or deformation of tissue.

forefoot valgus—An eversion deformity of the midtarsal joint causing the medial forefoot to be lower than the lateral forefoot in non-weight bearing when viewed in the same plane as a perpendicular line bisecting the calcaneus.

forefoot varus—An inversion deformity of the midtarsal joint causing the medial forefoot to be higher than the lateral forefoot in non-weight bearing when viewed in the same plane as a perpendicular line bisecting the calcaneus.

form drag—The resistance an object encounters in a fluid, as determined by the object's size and shape.

foxing—An additional piece of the heel counter that is often seen in athletic shoes to further reinforce the rearfoot in order to help maintain the heel counter's shape.

free nerve endings—Small-diameter, unmyelinated afferent nerve endings located throughout soft-tissue and articular structures that perceive pain and temperature. They are nociceptors that are stimulated by pain and inflammation. Although they do not play a role in proprioception, they respond to any extreme joint position.

friction—Resistance to movement between two surfaces.

frictional drag—The result of water's surface tension. This is not a factor in therapeutic exercise.

frog's eye—Condition in which the patellae face outward in relation to each other rather than forward.

frontal (coronal) plane—Any vertical plane that divides the body into front and back parts.

functional evaluation—An assessment of the patient's ability to perform accurately and safely an exercise or skill drill before that patient is allowed to advance to the next level.

functional exercise—Activities that mimic the stresses, demands, and skills of the sport and advance a patient toward a safe and prompt return to sport participation.

gait cycle—The time from the point at which the heel of one foot touches the ground to the point at which it touches the ground again.

genu recurvatum—Excessive knee hyperextension.

genu valgus—Knee alignment in which the knees are angled toward each other. Also called *genu valgum*.

genu varum—Knee alignment in which the knees are bowed outward. Also called *genu varus*.

glycoprotein—One of a number of protein-carbohydrate compounds that are elements of ground substance. Includes fibronectin. Probably cross-links with collagen so that tissue is able to withstand pressure without harming tissue integrity.

glycosaminoglycan (GAG)—One of a number of compounds occur-ring mostly in proteoglycans. Glycosaminoglycans are nonfibrous elements of ground substance in the extracellular matrix. Examples: hyaluronic acid, proteoglycans. Different glycosamino-glycans have different functions—for example, stimulating fibroblast proliferation, promoting collagen synthesis and maturation, contributing to tissue resilience, and regulating cell function.

Golgi-Mazzoni corpuscles—These afferent receptors are located in joint capsules. They are stimulated by joint compression but not by joint motion. Any weight-bearing activity stimulates these slowly adapting receptors. They are not believed to play a role in proprioception except in identification of joint compression.

Golgi tendon organ (GTO)—A stretch receptor found in series within the musculotendinous structure. It responds to muscle contraction more than to muscle stretch to signal force.

goniometer—A tool used to measure joint range of motion. The device uses either a 180° or a 360° system.

goniometric terms—See *abduction, adduction, depression, dorsiflexion, downward rotation, elevation, eversion, extension, external rotation, flexion, frontal (coronal) plane, horizontal extension, horizontal flexion, internal rotation, inversion, opposition, plantar flexion, pronation, protraction, radial deviation, retraction, sagittal plane, supination, transverse (horizontal) plane, ulnar deviation, upward rotation*.

granular leukocyte—White blood cells, divided into three groups: neutrophils, eosinophils, and basophils. Among their functions are chemotaxis and phagocytosis, as well as release of histamine and serotonin to produce vasoactive reactions following injury.

granulation tissue—Newly formed vascular tissue that is produced during wound healing. Consists of fibroblasts, macrophages, and neovascular structure within a base of connective-tissue matrix of collagen, hyaluronic acid, and fibronectin. It has the velvety appearance of small, red, nodular masses seen in new tissue. It eventually forms the cicatrix of the wound.

granuloma—Hard mass of fibrous tissue. Occurs in chronic inflammatory conditions when the body produces collagen around a foreign substance to protect itself from that substance.

grasshopper eye—See *frog's eye.*

ground substance—Gel-like material in which connective-tissue cells and fibers are embedded. Part of the connective tissue or extracellular matrix. Reduces friction between the connective-tissue fibers when forces are applied to the structure. Adds to the area's density.

growth factor—A factor released by platelets and macrophages. Growth factors perform complex and numerous roles, including the stimulation of reepithelialization, and are chemotactic for macrophages, monocytes, and neutrophils. The role of growth factors is not thoroughly understood but is believed to be important throughout tissue repair. Also referred to as *growth hormone factor.*

H band—That portion of the sarcomere that contains only thick filaments.

Hageman factor—An enzyme present in the blood. It initiates the blood coagulation process by converting prothrombin to thrombin following trauma to an area.

half-life—Amount of time it takes for the level of a drug in the bloodstream to diminish by one half. Determines the frequency with which a medication is taken.

hallux valgus—A condition also known as a *bunion.* Present when the first metatarsophalangeal joint is greater than 10° in valgus, so that the first toe points laterally toward the other toes.

hammertoe—Condition in which the toe is extended at the metatarsophalangeal joint, flexed at the proximal interphalangeal joint, and extended at the distal interphalangeal joint.

heel counter—The portion of a shoe that circles the calcaneus and serves as an important rearfoot stabilizer.

heel-off—The portion of the stance phase of the gait cycle in which the weight begins to transfer to the front of the foot and the heel is lifted off the floor. Also known as *terminal stance.*

heel strike—The portion of the stance phase of the gait cycle in which the heel first comes in contact with the floor. Also known as *initial contact.*

hip pointer—a contusion along the iliac crest.

histamine—A local tissue hormone released by mast cells and granulocytes. Increases vascular permeability to proteins and fibronectin.

Hooke's law—Law stating that the stress applied to a body to deform it is proportional to the strain as long as the body's elasticity limit is not exceeded.

horizontal extension—A motion of the upper extremity in a transverse plane away from the midline of the body. Also called *horizontal abduction.*

horizontal flexion—A motion of the upper extremity in a transverse plane toward the midline of the body. Also called *horizontal adduction.*

hyaluronic acid—See *glycosaminoglycan.* A major component of early granulation tissue. Greatest amounts are seen in a wound during the first four to five days. Promotes cell movement and migration during repair. Stimulates fibroblast proliferation. Produces edema by absorbing large amounts of water to increase fibroblast migration.

hypertrophy—An increase in muscle bulk from an increase in size of the muscle fibers, not the number of muscle fibers. Hypertrophy occurs with strength gains.

hysteresis—The process of tissue lengthening that results when the tissue is unable to withstand forces that are progressively applied to it.

I band—The portion of the sarcomere that contains only thin filaments.

impact peak—The ground reaction force that is a rapid peak occurring very quickly with impact at the foot's initial contact with the ground.

inertia—The tendency of an object at rest or in uniform motion to remain in that state until an external force is applied. See also *Newton's first law of motion.*

inflare—A pelvic girdle dysfunction in which the iliosacral joint is medially rotated.

inhibition—Transmission of an impulse that results in the cessation or decrease of an activity.

initial contact—See *heel strike.*

initial swing—The portion of the swing phase that includes early swing and acceleration.

insole board—The part of a shoe that lies between the upper and lower segments and that serves as the attachment for the two segments. Also called *last.*

internal rotation (IR)—Rotation of a joint around its axis in a transverse plane toward the midline of the body. Also called *medial rotation.*

internuncial transmission—Transmission of a message by a neuron that is interposed between two other neurons. The transmission rate is slower than that for monosynaptic transmission.

intrafusal muscle fiber—Modified muscle fiber that lies within a muscle spindle. The two types of muscle fibers are nuclear bag fibers and nuclear chain fibers.

intrinsic foot muscles—Muscles that control the foot and toes and originate and terminate within the foot.

intrinsic muscles—Muscles that originate and terminate within the hand or foot.

inversion—An inward-turning motion of the foot that causes the bottom of the foot to face medially.

irritability—The amount of stimulation that is required to initiate a response, such as pain.

isokinetic—Characterizing a dynamic activity in which the velocity of movement remains the same and the resistance varies.

isometric—Characterizing an activity produced when muscle tension is created without a change in the muscle's length. An isometric activity is a static activity.

isotonic—Characterizing an activity during which a muscle's length changes.

joint reaction force—Forces that are transmitted from one segment to another through the connecting joint.

jump sign—A reflex response to a trigger point palpation that includes a wincing or withdrawal reaction by the patient.

juncturae tendinum—A fibrous band that limits independent motion of the extensor tendons of the hand.

kallikrein—A proteolytic enzyme found in blood plasma, lymph, and other exocrine secretions. Activated by the Hageman factor. Forms kinins and activates plasminogen, a precursor of plasmin. Increases vascular permeability and vasodilation.

kinetic energy—Energy that a body has because of its motion.

kinin—A generic term for polypeptides related to bradykinin. Kinins are potent local tissue hormones and are found in injured tissue, released from plasma proteins. Examples: bradykinin, kallidin. Kinins mediate the classic signs of inflammation. Their action in the microvascular system is similar to that of histamine and serotonin in the early inflammation phase to cause increased microvascular permeability.

lactic acid—A by-product of muscle activity that leads to fatigue by reducing the muscle's calcium-binding capacity and impairing glycogen breakdown.

last—An important component of a shoe that determines the shoe's shape, size, style, and fit. It can be straight or curved. A shoe is constructed around a last that can be formed as a board last, slip last, or combination last.

latent trigger point—A trigger point that is painful only when it is palpated.

leukocyte—White blood cell or corpuscle. Types include polymorphonuclear leukocytes and mononuclear cells. These cells have notable phagocytic properties for removal of debris from an injury site.

leukotriene—A compound formed from arachidonic acid. Leukotrienes regulate inflammatory reactions. Some stimulate the movement of leukocytes into the area.

lever—A simple machine with a rigid bar and a fulcrum.

linear motion—Movement in a straight line.

line of gravity—Imaginary line through an object's center of gravity to the center of the earth.

line of pull of a muscle—The long axis of the muscle along which it exerts force.

lipid—A heterogeneous group of fats and fatlike substances, including fatty acids and steroids. Lipids serve as a source of fuel and are important to the structure and makeup of cells.

Little League elbow—A valgus traction force injury of the medial elbow that may start out as an inflammatory response or apophysitis and progress to an avulsion of the apophysis if the repetitive stress continues.

loading response—See *foot flat*.

local twitch response—An involuntary contraction of the muscle fibers in response to the snapping palpation.

loose-packed position—A joint position in which there is not complete congruency of joint surfaces with each other. Also called *open-packed position*. A joint demonstrates its greatest laxity in a loose-packed position.

lordosis—Excessive anterior convexity of the cervical and lumbar spine.

lymphocyte—A nonphagocytic leukocyte found in blood and lymph. These cells serve as important structures in the body's immune system by producing antibodies.

M band—The center of the A band where the thick filaments are attached.

macrophages—Mononuclear phagocytes that arise from stem cells in bone marrow. Considered one of the regulators of the repair process. They serve to phagocytize injury areas of debris, kill microorganisms, and secrete substances into an injury site, including enzymes, fibronectin, and coagulation factors. They play a role in keeping the inflammatory process localized and enhance collagen deposition and fibroblast proliferation.

mallet deformity—Avulsion of the extensor digitorum longus from the distal phalanx. Also known as *baseball finger*.

manipulation—Passive joint movement used to increase joint mobility. It incorporates a sudden, forceful thrust that is beyond the patient's control.

manual muscle test—An evaluation technique that uses manual resistance against a muscle or muscle group to provide a grade for that muscle or muscle group. Muscle grades range from 0 (zero) to 5 (normal).

manual therapy—The use of hands-on techniques for evaluating, treating, and improving the status of neuromusculoskeletal conditions.

massage—Manual manipulation of soft tissue to effect changes in the neuromuscular, lymph, cardiovascular, and connective-tissue systems.

mast cells—Connective-tissue cells. Also referred to as *mastocytes* and *labrocytes*. Store and produce various mediators of inflammation. Through their release of histamine, enzymes, and other mediators, mast cells cause increased local blood flow, attract immune cells, stimulate cell production of fibroblasts and endothelial cells, and promote and control remodeling of extracellular matrix.

matrix—Substance of a tissue. Can refer to intracellular or extracellular structure. Forms the basis from which a structure develops.

Meissner's corpuscles—Sensory nerve endings that transmit light-touch sensation.

midsole—The middle portion of a shoe's outer sole that can be composed of a variety of substances. It can also include a wedge. The midsole provides shock attenuation, stability, and control.

midstance—The portion of the stance phase of the gait cycle in which the foot is directly under the body's weight and the entire foot is in contact with the floor. Also known as *single-leg support*.

midswing—Also known as *swing-through*.

mitochondria—Organelles of a cell that are the primary energy source for the cell and that contain the enzyme used to metabolize lactic acid for energy to form adenosine triphosphate.

mobilization—Passive joint movement for increasing joint mobility or reducing pain. The applied force is light enough that the patient can stop the movement at any time.

modality—A physical agent used to relieve pain, improve circulation, reduce spasm, and promote healing.

momentum—Amount of motion that a moving object has.

monocyte—Mononuclear phagocytic leukocyte. Monocytes are formed in the bone marrow and transported to tissues to become macrophages. They debride an injury site.

mononuclear phagocyte—Any cell capable of ingesting particulate matter. The term usually refers to macrophages (polymorphonuclear leukocytes) and monocytes (mononuclear phagocytes). These ingest microorganisms and debride an injury site.

monosynaptic response—A reflex response involving only one synapse that is between the afferent and efferent nerves.

monosynaptic transmission—The direct connection between a sensory nerve and a motor neuron. Also called a *monosynaptic reflex*.

motor unit—A neuromuscular unit composed of the nerve, or motor neuron, and the muscle fibers that it innervates.

mucopolysaccharide—Polysaccharide. Also called *GAG*. See *glycosaminoglycan*.

muscle endurance—Ability of a muscle or muscle group to perform repeated contractions against a less-than-maximal load.

muscle energy—A manual therapy technique using precisely applied active muscle contraction against a counterforce to correct alignment and improve function.

muscle energy technique—The use of muscle contraction to precipitate a correction of a joint's malalignment.

muscle spasm—Prolonged reflex muscle contraction.

muscle spindle—A neuromuscular spindle, composed of intrafusal muscle fibers, that lies between regular muscle fibers. With its complex afferent and efferent supply, it provides the body with sensory stimulation and motor responses. The muscle spindle is sensitive to stretch, and signals muscle length and rate of change in the muscle's length.

muscle stiffness—The change in a muscle's tension that occurs as the muscle's length changes; related to the strength of the muscle's cross-bridge connections and the amount of muscle hypertrophy. The more stiffness a muscle has, the more resistant it is to stretching. Muscle stiffness is related to muscle tone.

muscular endurance—A muscle or muscle group's ability to sustain a submaximal force during either static or dynamic activity over time.

muscular strength—The amount of force a muscle or muscle group exerts. The ability to resist or produce a force.

myoblast—A cell formed from myogenic cells in muscle. Myoblasts form myotubes that eventually evolve into muscle fiber.

myofibroblasts—Fibroblasts that have the ultrastructural features of a fibroblast as well as the qualities of a smooth muscle cell. They are responsible for wound contraction.

myogenic cells—Cells that arise from muscle and later become myoblasts. See *myoblast*.

myosin—The chief protein structure of the thick filament of the sarcomere.

myotatic reflex—See *stretch reflex*.

neural mobilization—A manual therapy technique that stretches neural and connective tissue structures to affect neural symptoms, restore tissue balance, and improve function.

neurotransmitters—Hormones such as norepinephrine, epinephrine, and acetylcholine that are found in capillary, arteriole, and artery walls. They are released at the injury site to enhance platelet and leukocyte adherence to the vessel surface.

neutral spine—See *pelvic neutral*.

neutrophil—See *polymorphonuclear leukocyte*.

Newton's first law of motion—Law stating that a body remains at rest or in uniform motion until an outside force acts on it.

Newton's second law of motion—Law stating that acceleration of an object is directly proportional to the force causing the motion and inversely proportional to the mass of the object being moved.

Newton's third law of motion—Law stating that for every action there is an equal and opposite reaction.

nociceptors—Afferent nerve endings that transmit pain stimuli.

norepinephrine—A hormone that acts as a powerful vasoconstrictor at the immediate onset of injury. It may last from a few seconds to a few minutes.

nuclear bag fiber—One of two intrafusal muscle fibers within a muscle spindle, named for its nuclei arrangement. The nuclei are bunched together in the middle of the fiber's central region.

nuclear chain fiber—One of two intrafusal muscle fibers within a muscle spindle. Its nuclei are arranged in a chain or row. It is the smaller of the intrafusal muscle fibers.

nystagmus—A reflexive attempt to keep the eyes steady during body motion.

objective evaluation—An examination to discover the observable signs and effects of an injury; it involves observation, testing for quality and quantity of movement, strength assessment, neurological and other special testing, and palpation.

oculomotor system—An afferent system for balance that uses the eyes to provide the central nervous system with information regarding the body's relative position in space.

open kinetic chain—Characterizing a motion in which the distal segment of an extremity moves freely in space.

open reduction internal fixation (ORIF)—Surgical reduction of a fracture with application of a fixation device, such as a pin or screw, to stabilize the fracture site.

opposition—A diagonal movement of the thumb across the palm of the hand to permit the thumb to make contact with one of the other fingers.

orthotic—In reference to the foot, an appliance designed to correct body-segment or foot alignment or function, absorb stress, or reduce pressure or symptoms. Orthotics can be custom made or preformed and can vary in composition, degree of control, and type of correction.

Osgood-Schlatter disease—An inflammation or avulsion of the tibial apophysis, occurring in active, prepubescent children.

osteitis pubis—An inflammatory condition of shear stresses caused by either repeated trauma or strain on the symphysis pubis joint.

osteoblasts—Osteogenic cells from periosteum. Lay down the callus of fractured bone. Convert later to chondrocytes.

osteochondritis dissecans—Avascular necrosis of a joint's articular surface.

osteoclasts—Large multinuclear cells. Resorb dead, necrotic bone tissue.

osteocyte—A cell characteristic of adult bone. Maintains new bone mineralization.

outsole—The portion of a shoe that includes the lower segment and is in contact with the ground.

overflow—Also known as *irradiation*. With increased voluntary effort or prolonged effort, motor activity spreads to additional motor units of the same muscle and to motor untis of other muscles.

overload principle—To gain strength, a muscle must be overloaded beyond its accustomed level.

overpressure—Movement of a joint beyond its normal mobility to assess and feel or produce a comparable sign.

pacinian corpuscles—Afferent nerve endings that lie throughout the joint capsule and periarticular structures. They are rapidly adapting receptors thought to be compression sensitive, especially during high-velocity changes when the joint accelerates or decelerates as it moves into its limits of motion.

paratendinitis—An inflammation and thickening of the paratenon sheath of tendons that do not have synovial sheaths.

Pascal's law—Law stating that pressure from a fluid is exerted equally on all surfaces of an immersed object at any given depth (i.e., the deeper the object is immersed, the greater the pressure it encounters).

passive physiological range of motion—The amount of range of motion achieved without the assistance of the patient.

passive range of motion (PROM)—See *passive physiological range of motion*.

passive stretch—A stretch for which application relies on an outside force. The patient remains relaxed throughout the stretch.

patella alta—Position of the patella higher than normal in the patellofemoral groove.

patella baja—Position of the patella lower than normal in the patellofemoral groove.

pathoneurodynamics—A term coined by David Butler to describe pathological conditions that produce referral patterns proximally and distally from the site of pathology.

pelvic neutral—The position in which the spine and sacrolumbar junction incur the least stress. This is usually a midposition between the extremes of anterior and posterior pelvic tilt. Because of its impact on spine position, the position is also referred to as *neutral spine* or *straight spine*.

periarticular connective tissue—Soft tissue surrounding a joint, such as ligaments, the joint capsule, fascia, tendons, and synovial membranes.

perimysium—Connective-tissue layer covering a group of muscle fibers (fascicle).

pes cavus—An abnormal condition in which the foot has an abnormally high longitudinal arch. Associated with a rigid foot.

pes planus—An abnormal condition in which the foot has a low longitudinal arch. Associated with a hypomobile foot. Also known as a *pancake arch, flatfoot,* or *excessive pronation.* Associated with a flexible foot.

phagocyte—Any cell that ingests particulate matter. Commonly referred to as *polymorphonuclear leukocyte* and *mononuclear phagocyte,* otherwise known as *macrophage* and *monocyte.* These cells ingest microorganisms and other particulate antigens to debride an area.

phospholipids—Lipids that contain phosphoric acid. Found in all cells and in layers of plasma membranes. Stimulate the clotting mechanism.

physically active—Characterizing an individual who engages in occupational, recreational, or athletic activities that require physical skills and utilize strength, power, endurance, speed, flexibility, range of motion, or agility. (Based on the National Athletic Trainers' Association definition.)

physiological advantage—A muscle's ability to shorten. A muscle has its greatest physiological advantage when at its resting length.

physiological joint motion—Joint motion that can be performed voluntarily, such as shoulder flexion and ankle inversion.

plan of treatment program—The components, frequency, and duration of a treatment program. Includes the establishment of short-term and long-term goals.

plantar flexion—An extension of the ankle that causes the dorsum (top) of the foot to move away from the lower leg so that the angle of the ankle increases.

plasmin—An enzyme that occurs in plasma as plasminogen. It is activated by kallikrein and other activators. It converts fibrin to soluble substances.

plasminogen activator—An enzyme. See *fibrinolysin.* Converts fibrin to a soluble substance.

plasticity—In muscle physiology, a permanent change in length that occurs after an elongation force is applied.

platelet-derived growth factor (PDGF)—Substance found in platelets. It is essential for the growth of connective-tissue cells and stimulates the migration of polymorphonuclear leukocytes.

platelets—Irregular cell fragments found in blood. The first cells seen at an injury site, platelets are classified as regulatory cells of healing. Release growth factors. Form a plug at the injury to stop bleeding.

plica—A redundant fold in the knee's synovial lining, palpated as a band extending medially from the patella.

plumb line—A string with a weight (formerly a lead weight, but any weight object will do) at the end. When suspended, the string forms a vertical line.

plyometric exercise—A lengthening of a muscle followed by a sudden shortening to produce increased power. Also called *stretch-shortening exercise.*

polymorphonuclear leukocytes—One of the granular leukocytes. Also referred to as *PMNs* or *neutrophils.* These cells are chemotactic and phagocytic in the healing process.

posture—The relative alignment of the various body segments with one another.

potential energy—Energy that is stored in a body.

power—Work produced over time.

preswing—See *toe-off.*

primary intention—Healing that occurs with minor or surgical wounds. Reepithelialization closes the wound within 48 h. Scarring is minimal when healing by primary intention occurs.

procedure (vs. modality)—A treatment technique that involves the sport rehabilitation specialist's active participation or supervision.

pronation—Movement of the palm backward or downward so that the palm faces in a posterior direction, opposite the anatomical position. Also, a multiplanar rotation of the subtalar and transverse tarsal joints that is the combination of dorsiflexion, abduction, and eversion.

proprioception—The body's ability to transmit afferent information regarding position sense, to interpret the information, and to respond consciously or unconsciously to stimulation through appropriate execution of posture and movement.

proprioceptive neuromuscular facilitation (PNF)—A combined movement pattern that uses neural stimulation to facilitate a proper muscle response.

prostaglandins (PGs)—Components stemming primarily from arachidonic acid. Release of these substances requires the presence of the complement system and follows kinin formation. Specific PG compound compositions are designated by adding a letter, "A" through "I," and a subscript number, 1 through 3, to designate the number of hydrocarbon bonds. Examples: PGE_1 and PGE_2. Prostaglandins mediate cell migration during inflammation and modulate serotonin and histamine. Some PGs increase pain sensitivity, induce fever, and suppress lymphocyte transformation, thereby inhibiting the inflammatory reaction. Mediate myofibroblasts. Prostaglandins initiate early phases of injury repair as well as playing a role in the later stages of inflammation.

protease—An enzyme that acts as a catalyst to split interior peptide bonds in protein. Activates kallikrein to release bradykinin, ultimately causing increased vascular permeability to result in an increase in concentration of proteins and cells in the wound spaces.

proteoglycan—Substances found in tissues, including synovial fluid and connective-tissue matrix. Proteoglycan solutions are very viscous lubricants and are sulfated glycosaminoglycans. See *glycosaminoglycan.* A proteoglycan provides a resilient matrix for inhibiting cell migration. Regulates cell function and proliferation and regulates collagen fibrillogenesis.

protraction—A forward movement of the scapula. Also called *scapular abduction.*

pump bump—Increased prominence of the posterior calcaneal tuberosity. Also know as a *calcaneal exostosis.*

Q-angle—The angle formed by a line from the anterior superior iliac spine to the middle patella and a line from the middle patella to the tibial tubercle.

radial deviation—A movement of the wrist toward the thumb side of the forearm. Also called *radial flexion.*

range of motion—Amount of movement within a joint. Range of motion is affected by soft-tissue mobility and can be influenced by strength when performed actively. Used interchangeably with *flexibility.*

rearfoot valgus—An abnormal condition in which the calcaneus is everted relative to the tibia.

rearfoot varus—An abnormal condition in which the calcaneus is inverted relative to the posterior bisection of the lower leg.

refraction—When a light ray moves from air through water, it bends as it moves from the air, which has a lower density than the water does, into the water with its higher density. This makes the pool bottom appear closer than it actually is and makes objects within the water appear distorted.

refractory period—The time immediately following a stimulation, when the muscle fiber is unable to respond to additional stimuli. It is divided into an absolute refractory period and a relative refractory period.

rehabilitation clinician—The medical professional responsible for the design, progression, supervision, and administration of a rehabilitation program for individuals involved in physical activity. Medical professionals who most often assume these responsibilities include certified athletic trainers and physical therapists.

relative density—See *specific gravity.*

relative refractory period—A period that follows depolarization after a membrane has become partially repolarized. During this period the membrane is able to respond again if the stimulus is stronger than the normal threshold level.

resisted range of motion (RROM)—Motion that occurs with resistance applied to the movement. Also referred to as *strengthening exercises* or *progressive resistive exercises.*

resting membrane potential—The electrical potential difference across an inactive cell's membrane.

reticulin—A collagen-like fiber. Some consider reticulin a type III collagen fiber. Forms the early framework for collagen deposition in a wound.

retraction—A backward movement of the scapula. Also called *scapular adduction.*

retroversion—Decreased anterior angulation of the femoral neck, resulting in a toe-out gait.

Romberg test—A test for balance in which a patient stands with feet together and eyes closed. Increased postural sway compared to when eyes are open is a positive sign.

Ruffini nerve endings—These afferent receptors are in the joint capsule on the flexion side of the joint. They are slowly adapting and respond more to loads on the connective tissue in which they are contained than to displacement of that connective tissue. These receptors are stimulated by extreme joint motion when the capsule is stressed in extension with rotation.

saddle—The portion of a shoe that includes the midsection along the longitudinal arch, usually reinforced to assist in supporting the midfoot.

sagittal plane—The anterior-posterior vertical plane through which the longitudinal axis passes and which divides the body into right and left halves.

SAID principle—specific adaptation to imposed demands. Tissue will adapt to the specific stresses applied to it. This is a principle upon which a therapeutic exercise program is designed.

sarcomere—The smallest contractile element of a muscle fiber.

sarcoplasmic reticulum—A highly specialized intracellular membrane system that stores and transports calcium.

satellite cells—Cells present in muscle. Regenerate new muscle tissue.

scaption—Elevation of the shoulder in the scapular plane 30° forward of the frontal plane. This alignment of the glenohumeral joint with the scapula on the rib cage places the rotator cuff in the least stressful position for exercise.

scoliosis—A lateral or S curvature of the spinal column.

secondary intention—Healing that occurs in large wounds associated with soft-tissue loss. The wound heals with granulation tissue from the bottom and sides of the wound. Epithelial tissue does not form until granulation tissue has filled the wound. Larger scar formation occurs with healing by secondary intention. Wound contraction is evident with this healing.

second-class lever—A lever in which the resistance is between the fulcrum and the force.

serotonin—A hormone released by mast cells and platelets. Produces vasoconstriction in small vessels after norepinephrine activity is completed; occurs only when blood vessel endothelial walls are damaged. In later phases, it is responsible for initiating reactions leading to collagen cross-linking. It also is involved in granuloma formation.

shinsplints—A general term used to describe pain and inflammation of the musculotendinous unit and/or periosteum along the anteromedial border of the tibia. Also know as *medial tibial stress syndrome.*

single-leg support—The portion of the gait cycle in which the body weight is transferred entirely to the one supporting leg and the other leg is in the middle of its swing phase. Also known as *midstance.*

slow-twitch fiber—A muscle fiber that is a type I fiber or slow oxidative fiber, is darker in color than the fast-twitch fiber, and takes about 110 ms to reach its peak tension when stimulated.

Smith's fracture—A type of fracture in which the distal radius is fractured and the fragment is displaced palmarly.

sock liner—The portion of a shoe that lies on top of the insole board, used for shock absorption and friction reduction for the foot.

somatosensory system—Another term for the body's proprioceptive system.

specific gravity—The ratio of an object's weight to the weight of an equal volume of water. The term refers to the density of an object relative to that of water. This ratio is also called *relative density.* The specific gravity of water is 1.

spinal cord—Part of the central nervous system that extends from the brain to the second lumbar vertebra and contains a cervical and a lumbar enlargement where the dorsal and ventral roots leading to the extremities are contained.

spinal reflex—When an impulse goes from a dorsal root afferent nerve either to an internuncial connecting nerve or directly to an efferent nerve in the spinal cord, and then immediately out the ventral root to the muscle.

sprain—Stretching or tearing of a ligament or capsular structure.

squinting patellae—Patellae that are angled toward each other rather than facing forward.

stance phase—The portion of the gait cycle during which the foot is in contact with the floor and the extremity is bearing partial or total body weight.

static activity—An isometric activity in which no movement occurs.

static progressive splint—Change of static splints as motion of a segment changes so the desired goals, usually including increased motion, are achieved.

static restraint—One of two systems a joint has for its stability. Static restraints include ligaments, capsule, and other inert structures such as the glenoid labrum in the shoulder and the meniscus in the knee.

static splint—Splint used to support, protect, or restrict motion. It does not have any moving parts.

steady state of a drug—The state in which the average level of a drug remains constant in the blood: The amount of drug leaving the body is equal to the amount being absorbed. On average, a steady state occurs after five doses equal to the drug's half-life are administered.

step length—The distance from heel strike of one foot to heel strike of the other foot in one gait cycle.

strain—Amount of change in size or shape of an object caused by stress.

strength—A muscle's relative ability to resist or produce a force.

stress—Force required to change the shape or form of a body.

stretch reflex—The most basic sensorimotor response. Does not involve an internuncial neuron, but instead goes directly from the afferent sensory nerve (muscle spindle) to the spinal cord, where it makes contact with the motor nerve to permit a rapid muscle response.

stride length—The distance from heel strike of one foot to heel strike of the same foot in one gait cycle.

stride width—The body's side-to-side movement as weight is shifted from one lower extremity to the other.

structural fatigue—The point at which stress exceeds the tissue's ability to resist it and breakdown occurs.

subjective evaluation—The history of an injury, including the mechanism of injury, the patient's experience of pain and other symptoms, prior injuries, medical conditions, medications, and other pertinent social and medical factors.

subtalar joint—The joint formed by the talus and calcaneus. This joint allows inversion and eversion motion of the rearfoot.

subtalar neutral—The position in which the talus is palpable from its medial or its lateral aspect within the subtalar joint. The point at which the talus and navicular are most congruent and the alignment of the subtalar bones is optimal.

summation of forces—Sequential movement of body segments to increase force production for a desired motion.

supination—Movement of the palm forward or upward into the anatomical position. Also, the multiplanar rotation of the subtalar and transverse tarsal joints that includes plantar flexion, adduction, and inversion.

swan-neck deformity—A deformity caused by hyperextension at the PIP joint and hyperflexion at the DIP joint due to disruption of the volar plate and tensioning of the flexor tendons.

swing phase—The time during which the foot is not in contact with the floor and no weight is borne on the extremity.

swing-through—The middle of the swing phase, also called *midswing*.

Swiss ball—A large, vinyl ball developed by an Italian toy manufacturer that is used in physical therapy and therapeutic exercise programs.

synergist(ic)—A muscle that assists an agonist muscle.

talocrural joint—The true ankle joint that is formed by the talus and tibia with the fibula. The joint allows dorsiflexion and plantar flexion motions.

tarsal tunnel—Formed by the medial malleolus, calcaneous, talus, and deltoid ligament's posterior aspect.

tendinitis—The global term used to identify an inflammation of a tendon. Also spelled **tendonitis.**

tendinosis—A condition that involves microscopic tears of the tendon caused by repeated trauma.

tenocyte—Tendon cell. Converts to fibroblasts during healing of tendons.

tenosynovitis—An inflammation of the synovial sheath that surrounds a tendon.

tensile strength—Maximal amount of stress or force that a structure is able to withstand before tissue failure occurs. Tensile strength varies as tissue healing proceeds. One must take tensile strength of an injured structure into account when determining appropriate stress application in rehabilitation.

terminal stance—See *heel-off.*

terminal swing—The portion of the swing phase that includes late swing, or deceleration.

tetanus—An intermittent contraction of a muscle that is demonstrated as a fibrillation of the muscle.

tetany—A sustained maximal contraction of a muscle.

third-class lever—A lever in which the force is between the fulcrum and the resistance.

thoracic kyphosis—Excess posterior convexity of the thoracic spine.

thoracic outlet syndrom (TOS)—A clinical term that describes compression of the neurovascular structures as they exit through the thoracic outlet at the base of the neck.

threshold stimulation—The minimal stimulation required to initiate a muscular response.

thrombin—An enzyme that converts fibrinogen to fibrin to form a fibrin plug early in the inflammation phase. In later inflammation, it stimulates fibronectin production and fibroblast proliferation.

thromboxane—A compound that is produced by platelets and is unstable. Its half-life is 30 s. Related to prostaglandins. Acts as a vasoconstrictor and is a potent inducer of platelet aggregation.

tibial torsion—An abnormal structural condition in which the tibia is rotated along its longitudinal axis so that the foot is rotated laterally beyond the normal 15° in relation to the patella's midline.

tibial varum—An abnormal condition in which the distal tibia is closer to the midline than the proximal tibia.

toe box—The upper portion of the shoe that covers the toes. It varies in width and height, and functions to retain the shape of the shoe's forefoot and provide room for the toes.

toe-off—The portion of the gait cycle during which the foot comes off the floor and the swing phase begins. Also called *push-off* or *preswing.*

torque—The ability of a force to produce rotational movement.

transverse (horizontal) plane—A plane that divides the body or a body part into upper and lower parts. It is parallel to the horizon.

Trendelenburg gait—An abnormal gait secondary to gluteus medius weakness. The gait is also known as a *gluteus medius gait* and is seen as a drop of the pelvis on the uninvolved side during weight bearing on the involved side.

trigger point—According to Travell and Simons (1983, p. 3), a "focus of hyperirritability in a tissue that, when compressed, is locally tender and, if sufficiently hypersensitive, gives rise to referred pain and tenderness, and sometimes to referred autonomic phenomena and distortion of proprioception." A myofascial trigger point includes a taut band of muscle with its surrounding fascia.

tropomyosin—One of two primary proteins of the thin filament of the sarcomere.

troponin—A protein on the actin filament to which calcium ions bind during a sarcomere's cross-bridging process.

ulnar deviation—A movement of the wrist toward the little-finger side of the forearm. Also called *ulnar flexion.*

ultimate strength—The greatest load a tissue can tolerate before it reaches failure.

upward rotation—A movement of the scapula that causes the glenoid to face forward and upward. The inferior angle of the scapula moves laterally away from the spine, and the scapula slides forward.

Valsalva maneuver—When the breath is held, intrathoracic pressure is increased. This can lead to impeded venous return to the right atrium, causing increased peripheral venous pressure, increasing blood pressure and reducing cardiac output because of diminished cardiac volume.

vamp—The upper portion of a shoe that covers the toes and forefoot and includes the toe box.

velocity—Rate of change of position.

vestibular system—An afferent system within the inner ear that is responsible for sending messages to the central nervous system regarding vertical and horizontal position and motion.

viscoelasticity—The property of being both viscous and elastic.

viscosity—The resistance to movement within a fluid or fluidlike substance that is caused by the friction of the fluid's molecules. Viscosity limits the rate of muscle contraction: The faster the contraction, the greater the internal resistance and the less the force that can be generated.

volitional—The conscious performance or an activity.

wave drag—The water's resistance as a result of turbulence.

work—Product of a force and the distance through which it is applied.

Z disk—The end of the sarcomere element where the thin filaments attach. Also known as the Z-line or Z-band.

BIBLIOGRAPHY

Ahmed, A.M., and D.L. Burke. 1983. In vitro measurement of static pressure distribution in synovial joints: I. Tibial surface of the knee. *Journal of Biomedical Engineering* 105:216–225.

Akeson, W.H., Woo, S.L.-Y., Amiel, D., Coutts, R.D., and D. Daniel. 1973. The connective tissue response to immobility: Biochemical changes in periarticular connective tissue of the immobilized rabbit knee. *Clinical Orthopaedics* 93:356–365.

Allerheiligen, B., and R. Rogers. 1995. Plyometrics program design. *Strength and Conditioning* 17:26–31.

Almekinders, L.C., and J.A. Gilbert. 1986. Healing of experimental muscle strains and the effects of non-steroidal antiinflammatory medication. *American Journal of Sports Medicine* 14:303–308.

Alon, R. 1990. *Mindful spontaneity: Moving in tune with nature: Lessons in the Feldenkrais method.* New York: Harper & Row.

American Academy of Orthopaedic Surgeons. 1965. *Joint motion: Method of measuring and recording.* New York: Churchill Livingstone.

Andriacchi, T.P., Sabiston, K., DeHaven, K., Dahners, L., Woo, S., Frank, C., Oakes, B., Brand, R., and J. Lewis. 1988. Ligament: Injury and repair. In *Injury and repair of the musculoskeletal soft tissues,* ed. S.L.-Y. Woo and J.A. Buckwalter. Park Ridge, IL: American Academy of Orthopaedic Surgeons.

Appell, H.-J. 1990. Muscular atrophy following immobilization: A review. *Sports Medicine* 10:42–58.

Archambault, J.M., Wiley, J.P., and R.C. Bray. 1995. Exercise loading of tendons and the development of overuse injuries. *Sports Medicine* 20:77–89.

Barber, F.A. 1994. Accelerated rehabilitation for meniscus repairs. *Arthroscopy: The Journal of Arthroscopic and Related Surgery* 10:206–210.

Barlow, W. 1977. *The Alexander Technique.* New York: Knopf.

Barrack, R.L., Lund, P.J., and H.B. Skinner. 1994. Knee joint proprioception revisited. *Journal of Sport Rehabilitation* 3:18–42.

Baumhauer, J., Shereff, M., and J. Gould. 1997. Ankle pain in runners. In *Running injuries,* ed. G.N. Guten. Philadelphia: Saunders.

Beard, G., and E.C. Wood. 1969. *Massage principles and techniques.* Philadelphia: Saunders.

Berger, R.A. 1962. Optimal repetitions for the development of strength. *Research Quarterly* 33:334–338.

Bernier, J.N., and D.H. Perrin. 1998. Effect of coordination training on proprioception of the functionally unstable ankle. *Journal of Orthopaedic and Sports Physical Therapy* 27:264–275.

Betz, P., Norlich, A., Wilske, J., Tubel, J., Penning, R., and W. Eisenmenger. 1992. Time-dependent appearance of myofibroblasts in granulation tissue of human skin wounds. *International Journal of Legal Medicine* 150:99–103.

Beynnon, B.D., Fleming, B.C., Johnson, R.J., Nichols, C.E., Renstrom, P.A., and M.H. Pope. 1995. Anterior cruciate ligament strain behavior during rehabilitation exercises in vivo. *American Journal of Sports Medicine* 23:24–34.

Billeter, H., and H. Hoppeler. 1992. Muscular basis of strength. In *Strength and power in sport,* ed. P.V. Komi. Boston: Blackwell Scientific.

Bockrath, K., Wooden, C., Worrell, T., Ingersoll, C.D., and T. Farr. 1993. Effects of patellar taping on patella position and perceived pain. *Medicine and Science in Sports and Exercise* 25:989–992.

Bogduk, N., and L.T. Twomey. 1987. *Clinical anatomy of the lumbar spine.* New York: Churchill Livingstone.

Bolgla, L.A., and D.R. Keskula. 1997. Reliability of lower extremity functional performance tests. *Journal of Orthopaedic and Sports Physical Therapy* 26:138–142.

Bowers, W.H., and S.M. Tribuzi. 1992. Functional anatomy. In *Concepts in hand rehabilitation,* ed. B.G. Stanley and S.M. Tribuzi. Philadelphia: Davis.

Boyes, J.H. 1970. *Bunnell's surgery of the hand.* Philadelphia: Lippincott.

Braatz, J.H., and P. P. Gogia. 1987. The mechanics of pitching. *Journal of Orthopaedic and Sports Physical Therapy* 9:56–69.

Bradley, J.P., and J.E. Tibone. 1991. Electromyographic analysis of muscle action about the shoulder. *Clinics in Sports Medicine* 10:789–805.

Brittberg, M., Lindahl, A., Nilsson, A., Ohlsson, C., Isaksson, O., and L. Peterson. 1994. Treatment of deep cartilage defects in the knee with autologous chondrocyte transplantation. *New England Journal of Medicine* 331:889–895.

Brown, C.H., Steiner, M.E., and E.W. Carson. 1993. The use of hamstring tendons for anterior cruciate ligament reconstruction. Technique and results. *Clinics in Sports Medicine* 12:723–756.

Brown, D.R. 1980. *Neurosciences for allied health therapies.* St. Louis: Mosby.

Brownstein, B., Mangiene, R.E., Noyes, F.R., and S. Kryer. 1988. Anatomy and biomechanics. In *Physical therapy of the knee,* ed. R.E. Mangiene. New York: Churchill Livingstone.

Buckwalter, J.A. 1996. Effects of early motion on healing of musculoskeletal tissues. *Hand Clinics* 12:13–24.

Buckwalter, J.A., Rosenberg, L., Coutts, R., Hunziker, E., Reddi, A.H., and V. Mow. 1988. Articular cartilage: Injury and repair. In *Injury and repair of the musculoskeletal soft tissues,* ed. S.L.-Y. Woo and J.A. Buckwalter. Park Ridge, IL: American Academy of Orthopaedic Surgeons.

Butler, D.L., Grood, E.S., Noyes, F.R., and R.F. Zernicke. 1978. Biomechanics of ligaments and tendons. *Exercise and Sport Sciences Reviews* 6:125–281.

Butler, D.L., Noyes, F.R., and E.S. Grood. 1980. Ligamentous restraints to anterior-posterior drawer in the human knee. *Journal of Bone and Joint Surgery* 62A:259–270.

Butler, D.S. 1991. *Mobilization of the nervous system.* New York: Churchill Livingstone.

Butler, D.S. 1994. *Mobilization of the nervous system. Level II. 1996/97 course handbook.* Marina Del Rey, CA: Neuro Orthopedic Insitute.

Caplan, A.B., Carlson, J., Faulkner, J., Fischman, D., and W. Garrett, Jr. 1988. Skeletal muscle. In *Injury and repair of the musculoskeletal soft tissues,* ed. S.L.-Y. Woo and J.A. Buckwalter. Park Ridge, IL: American Academy of Orthopaedic Surgeons.

Christie, A.L. 1991. The tissue injury cycle and new advances toward its management in open wounds. *Athletic Training* 26:274–277.

Chu, D. 1989. *Plyometric exercises with medicine balls.* Livermore, CA: Bittersweet.

Chu, D. 1992. *Jumping into plyometrics.* Champaign, IL: Leisure Press.

Cipriani, D.J., Armstrong, C.W., and S. Gaul. 1995. Backward walking at three levels of treadmill inclination: An electromyographic and kinematic analysis. *Journal of Orthopaedic and Sports Physical Therapy* 22:95–102.

Clarke, D.H. 1971. The influence on muscular fatigue patterns of the intercontraction rest interval. *Medicine and Science in Sports* 3:83–88.

Clarke, D.H. 1975. *Exercise physiology.* Englewood Cliffs, NJ: Prentice Hall.

Close, J.R. 1964. *Motor function in the lower extremity: Analysis by electronic instrumentation.* Springfield, IL: Charles C Thomas.

Connolly, J.F. 1988. *Fracture complications, recognition, prevention, and management.* Chicago: Year Book Medical.

Corrigan, B., and G.D. Maitland. 1989. *Practical orthopedic medicine.* London: Butterworth.

Curwin, S., and W.D. Stanish. 1984. *Tendinitis: Its etiology and treatment.* Lexington, MA: Heath.

Cyriax, J.H. 1975. *Textbook of orthopaedic medicine. Vol. 1. Diagnosis of soft tissue lesions.* 6th ed. Baltimore: Williams & Wilkins.

Cyriax, J.H. 1977. *Textbook of orthopaedic medicine. Vol. 2. Treatment by manipulation, massage and injection.* Baltimore: Williams & Wilkins.

Daniels, L., and C. Worthingham. 1972. *Muscle testing.* Philadelphia: Saunders.

Davis, B.C., and R.A. Harrison. 1988. *Hydrotherapy in practice.* New York: Churchill Livingstone.

deAndrade, J.R., Grant, C., and A.S.-J. Dixon. 1965. Joint distension and reflex muscle inhibition in the knee. *Journal of Bone and Joint Surgery* 47A:313–322.

DeLorme, T.L., and A.L. Watkins. 1948. Technics of progressive resistance exercise. *Archives of Physical Medicine* 29:263–273.

Denegar, C. 2000. *Therapeutic modalities for athletic injuries: Modalities.* Champaign, IL: Human Kinetics.

Dillman, C.J. 1975. Kinematic analyses of running. *Exercise and Sport Sciences Reviews.* 3:193–218.

DiPietro, L.A. 1995. Wound healing: The role of the macrophage and other immune cells. *Shock* 4:233–240.

Dommissee, G.F. 1975. Morphological aspects of the lumbar spine and lumbosacral region. *Orthopedic Clinics of North America* 6:163–175.

Donatelli, R., and A. Owens-Burkhart. 1981. Effects of immobilization on the extensibility of periarticular connective tissue. *Journal of Orthopaedic and Sports Physical Therapy* 9:67–72.

Donkers, M.J., An, K.N., Chao, E.Y., and B.F. Morrey. 1993. Hand position affects elbow joint load during push-up exercise. *Journal of Biomechanics* 26:625–632.

Doucette, S.A., and D.D. Child. 1996. The effect of open and closed chain exercise and knee joint position on patellar tracking in lateral patellar compression syndrome. *Journal of Orthopaedic and Sports Physical Therapy* 23:104–110.

Doucette, S.A., and E.M. Goble. 1992. The effect of exercise on patellar tracking in lateral patellar compression syndrome. *American Journal of Sports Medicine* 20:434–440.

Doyle, J.R., and W.F. Blythe. 1975. The finger flexor tendon sheaths and pulleys. Anatomy and reconstruction. In *A.A.O.S. Symposium on Tendon Surgery of the Hand.* St. Louis: Mosby.

Duran, R.J., and R.G. Houser. 1975. Controlled passive motion following flexor tendon repair in zones 2 and 3. In *A.A.O.S. Symposium on Tendon Surgery of the Hand.* St. Louis: Mosby.

Durselen, L., Claes, L., and H. Kiefer. 1995. The influence of muscle forces and external loads on cruciate ligament strain. *American Journal of Sports Medicine* 23:129–136.

Dye, S.F., and W.D. Cannon. 1988. Anatomy and biomechanics of the anterior cruciate ligament. *Clinics in Sports Medicine* 7:715–725.

Edlich, R.F., Towler, M.A., Goitz, R.J., Wilder, R.P., Buschbacher, L.P., Morgan, R.F., and J.G. Thacker. 1987. Bioengineering principles of hydrotherapy. *Journal of Burn Care and Rehabilitation* 8:580–584.

Eldred, E. 1967. Peripheral receptors: Their excitation and relation to reflex patterns. *American Journal of Physical Medicine* 46:69–87.

Ellenbecker, T.S., and A.J. Mattalino. 1997. *The elbow in sport.* Champaign, IL: Human Kinetics.

Ellenbecker, T.S., and A.J. Mattalino. 1999. Glenohumeral joint range of motion and rotator cuff strength following arthroscopic anterior stabilization with thermal capsulorraphy. *Journal of Orthopaedic and Sports Physical Therapy* 29:160–167.

Elliot, D.H. 1965. Structure and function of mammalian tendon. *Biology Review* 40:392–421.

Enwemeka, C.S. 1989. Inflammation, cellularity, and fibrillogenesis in regenerating tendon: Implications for tendon rehabilitation. *Physical Therapy* 69:816–825.

Esch, D., and M. Lepley. 1974. *Evaluation of joint motion: Methods of measurement and recording.* Minneapolis: University of Minnesota Press.

Evans, R.B. 1989. Clinical application of controlled stress to the healing extensor tendon: A review of 112 cases. *Physical Therapy* 69:1041–1049.

Evans, R.B., and W.E. Burkhalter. 1986. A study of the dynamic anatomy of extensor tendons and implications for treatment. *Journal of Hand Surgery (Am)* 11:774–779.

Evans, R.B., Eggers, G.W.N., Butler, J.K., and J. Blumel. 1960. Experimental immobilization and remobilization of rat knee joints. *Journal of Bone and Joint Surgery* 42A:737–758.

Feltner, M., and J. Dapena. 1986. Dynamics of the shoulder and elbow joints of the throwing arm during a baseball pitch. *International Journal of Sport Biomechanics* 2:235–259.

Finsterbush, A., and B. Friedman. 1975. Reversibility of joint changes produced by immobilization in rabbits. *Clinics in Orthopaedics and Related Research* 111:290–298.

Fisher, A.C., Mullins, S.A., and P.A. Frey. 1993. Athletic trainers' attitudes and judgments of injured athletes' rehabilitation adherence. *Journal of Athletic Training* 28:43–47.

Forkin, D.M., Koczur, C., Battle, R., and R.A. Newton. 1996. Evaluation of kinesthetic deficits indicative of balance control in gymnasts with unilateral chronic ankle sprains. *Journal of Orthopaedic and Sports Physical Therapy* 23:245–250.

Freeman, M.A., and B. Wyke. 1967. The innervation of the knee joint. An anatomical and histological study in the cat. *Journal of Anatomy* 101:505–532.

Fritz, J.M., Irrgang, J.J., and C.D. Harner. 1996. Rehabilitation following allograft meniscal transplantation: A review of the literature and case study. *Journal of Orthopaedic and Sports Physical Therapy* 24:98–106.

Galloway, M.T., and P. Jokl. 1990. Patella plica syndrome. *Annals of Sports Medicine* 5:34–41.

Gambetta, V. 1986. In roundtable discussion: Blelik, E., Chu, D.A., Costello, F., Gambetta, V., Lundin, P., Rogers, R., Santos, J., and F. Wilt. 1986. Practical considerations for utilizing plyometrics. Part 1. *National Strength Coaches Association Journal* 8:14–22.

Garn, S.N., and R.A. Newton. 1988. Kinesthetic awareness in subjects with multiple ankle sprains. *Physical Therapy* 68:1667–1671.

Garrett, W.E., Jr. 1990. Muscle strain injuries: Clinical and basic aspects. *Medicine and Science in Sport and Exercise* 22:436–443.

Gelberman, R., An, K.-A., Banes, A., and V. Goldberg. 1988. Tendon. In *Injury and repair of the musculoskeletal soft tissues*, ed. S.L.-Y. Woo and J.A. Buckwalter. Park Ridge, IL: American Academy of Orthopaedic Surgeons.

Gelberman, R.H., Woo, S.L.-Y., Lothringer, K., Akeson, W.H., and D. Amiel. 1982. Effects of early intermittent passive mobilization on healing canine flexor tendons. *Journal of Hand Surgery* 7:170–175.

Geraci, M.C. 1994. Rehabilitation of pelvis, hip, and thigh injuries in sports. *Physical Medicine and Rehabilitation Clinics of North America* 5:157–174.

Gerhardt, J.J., and O.A. Russe. 1975. *International SFTR method of measuring and recording joint motion*. Bern: Huber.

Gilleard, W., McConnell, J., and D. Parsons. 1998. The effect of patellar taping on the onset of vastus medialis obliquus and vastus lateralis muscle activity in persons with patellofemoral pain. *Physical Therapy* 78:25–32.

Glascoe, W.M., Allen, M.K., Awtry, B.F., and H.J. Yack. 1999. Weight-bearing immobilization and early exercise treatment following a grade II lateral ankle sprain. *Journal of Orthopaedic and Sports Physical Therapy* 29:394–399.

Gough, J.V., and G. Ladley. 1971. An investigation into the effectiveness of various forms of quadriceps exercises. *Physiotherapy* 57:356–361.

Greenman, P.E. 1996. *Principles of manual medicine*. Baltimore: Williams & Wilkins.

Grelsamer, R.P., and J.R. Klein. 1998. The biomechanics of the patellofemoral joint. *Journal of Orthopaedic and Sports Physical Therapy* 28:286–298.

Grigg, P. 1994. Peripheral neural mechanisms in proprioception. *Journal of Sport Rehabilitation* 3:2–17.

Grood, E.S., Suntay, W.J., Noyes, F.R., and D.L. Butler. 1984. Biomechanics of the knee-extension exercise. Effect of cutting the anterior cruciate ligament. *Journal of Bone and Joint Surgery* 66A:725–734.

Groppel, J.L., and R.P. Nirschl. 1986. A mechanical and electromyographical analysis of the effects of various joint counterforce braces on the tennis player. *American Journal of Sports Medicine* 14:195–200.

Gross, M.T. 1992. Chronic tendinitis: Pathomechanics of injury, factors affecting the healing response, and treatment. *Journal of Orthopaedic and Sports Physical Therapy* 16:248–261.

Gross, M.T., Bradshaw, M.K., Ventry, L.C., and K.H. Weller. 1987. Comparison of support provided by ankle taping and semirigid orthosis. *Journal of Orthopaedic and Sports Physical Therapy* 9:33–39.

Harrison, R.A., Hillman, M., and S. Bulstrode. 1992. Loading of the lower limb when walking partially immersed: Implications for clinical practice. *Physiotherapy* 78 (3):164–167.

Hay, J. 1978. *The biomechanics of sports techniques*. Englewood Cliffs, NJ: Prentice Hall.

Hayashi, K., Thabit, G., III, Bogdanske, J.J., Mascio, L.N., and M.D. Markel. 1996. The effect of nonablative laser energy on the ultrastructure of joint capsular collagen. *Arthroscopy: The Journal of Arthroscopic and Related Surgery* 12:474–481.

Hayashi, K., Thabit, G., III, Massa, K.L., Bogdanske, J.J., Cooley, A.J., Orwin, J.F., and M.D. Markel. 1997. The effect of thermal heating on the length and histologic properties of the glenohumeral joint capsule. *American Journal of Sports Medicine* 25:107–112.

Heppenstall, R.B. 1980. Fracture healing. In *Fracture treatment and healing*, ed. R.B. Heppenstall. Philadelphia: Saunders.

Hertling, D., and R.M. Kessler. 1990. *Management of common musculoskeletal disorders.* 2nd ed. Philadelphia: Lippincott.

Hettinger, T., and E. Müller. 1953. Muscle strength and muscle training. *Arbeitsphysiologie* 15:111–126.

Hillman, S. 2000. *Introduction to athletic training.* Champaign, IL: Human Kinetics.

Hom, D.B. 1995. Growth factors in wound healing. *Otolaryngologic Clinics of North America* 28:933–953.

Hoppenfeld, S. 1976. *Physical examination of the spine and extremities.* New York: Appleton-Century-Crofts.

Hortobagy, T., and F.I. Katch. 1990. Eccentric and concentric torque–velocity relationships during arm flexion and extension. *European Journal of Applied Physiology* 60:395–401.

Host, H.H. 1995. Scapular taping in the treatment of anterior shoulder impingement. *Journal of Orthopaedic and Sports Physical Therapy* 75:803–812.

Houglum, J.E. 1998. Pharmocologic considerations in the treatment of injured athletes with non-steroidal anti-inflammatory drugs. *Journal of Athletic Training* 33:259–263.

Houglum, P.A. 1992. Soft tissue healing and its impact on rehabilitation. *Journal of Sport Rehabilitation* 1:19–39.

Huberti, H.H., and W.C. Hayes. 1984. Patellofemoral contact pressures. The influence of Q-angle and tendofemoral contact. *Journal of Bone and Joint Surgery* 66A:715–724.

Hunter, G.R. 1994. Muscle physiology. In *Essentials of strength training and conditioning,* ed. T.R. Baechle. Champaign, IL: Human Kinetics.

Iqbal, S., Schwellnus, M.P., Noakes, T., and C. Lombard. 1994. A fivefold reduction in the incidence of recurrent ankle sprains in soccer players using the Sport-Stirrup orthosis. 1994. *American Journal of Sports Medicine* 22:601–606.

Irrgang, J.J., Harner, C.D., Fu, F.H., Silbey, M.B., and R. DiGiacomo. 1997. Loss of motion following ACL reconstruction: A second look. *Journal of Sport Rehabilitation* 6:213–225.

Isear, J.A., Jr., Erickson, J.C., and T.W. Worrell. 1997. EMG analysis of lower extremity muscle recruitment patterns during an unloaded squat. *Medicine and Science in Sports and Exercise* 29:532–539.

Jenkins, W.L., Munns, S.W., Jayaraman, G., Wertzberger, K.L., and K. Neely. 1997. A measurement of anterior tibial displacement in the closed and open kinetic chain. *Journal of Orthopaedic and Sports Physical Therapy* 25:49–56.

Jobe, F.W., Moynes, D.R., and D.J. Antonelli. 1985. Rotator cuff function during the golf swing. *American Journal of Sports Medicine* 14:388–392.

Kaltenborn, F.M. 1980. *Mobilization of the extremity joints.* Oslo: Olaf Norlis Bokhandel.

Kamkar, A., Irrgang, J.J., and S.L. Whitney. 1993. Nonoperative management of secondary impingement syndrome. *Journal of Orthopaedic and Sports Physical Therapy* 17:212–224.

Kapandji, I.A. 1978. *The physiology of the joints. Vol. 2. Lower limb.* New York: Churchill Livingstone.

Karlsson, J., Thomee, R., and L. Sward. 1996. Eleven year follow-up of patello-femoral pain syndrome. *Clinical Journal of Sport Medicine* 6:22–26.

Karpovich, P.V., Herden, E.L., Jr., Asa, M.M., and G.P. Karpovich. 1959. Electrogoniometer: A new device for study of joints in action. *Federation Proceedings* 18:79.

Kaufman, K.R., An, K.-N., Litchy, W.J., Morrey, B.F., and Chao, E.Y.S. 1991. Dynamic joint forces during knee isokinetic exercise. *American Journal of Sports Medicine* 19:305–316.

Keith, R.H., Granter, C.V., Hamilton, B.B., and F.S. Sherwin. 1987. The functional independence measure: A new tool for rehabilitation. In *Advances in clinical rehabilitation,* ed. M.G. Eisenberg and R.C. Grzesink. New York: Springer.

Kelley, M.J. 1995. Anatomic and biomechanical rationale for rehabilitation of the athlete's shoulder. *Journal of Sports Rehabilitation* 4:122–154.

Kendall, F.P., McCreary, E.K., and P.G. Provance. 1993. *Muscles: Testing and function.* 4th ed. Baltimore: Williams & Wilkins.

Kessler, R.M., and D. Hertling. 1983. *Management of common musculoskeletal disorders.* Philadelphia: Harper & Row.

Kettenbach, G. 1990. *Writing S.O.A.P. notes.* Philadelphia: Davis.

Kibler, W.B. 1990. Concepts in exercise rehabilitation of athletic injury. In *Sports-induced inflammation,* ed. W.B. Leadbetter, J.A. Buckwalter, and S.L. Gordon. Park Ridge, IL: American Academy of Orthopaedic Surgeons.

Kibler, W.B. 1995a. Biomechanical analysis of the shoulder during tennis activities. *Clinics in Sports Medicine* 14:79–85.

Kibler, W.B. 1995b. Pathophysiology of overload injuries around the elbow. *Clinics in Sports Medicine* 14:447–457.

Kimura, I.F., Nawoczenski, D.A., Epler, M., and M.G. Owen. 1987. Effect of the AirStirrup in controlling ankle inversion stress. *Journal of Orthopaedic and Sports Physical Therapy* 9:190–193.

Kirsner, R.S., and W.H. Eaglstein. 1993. The wound healing process. *Dermatological Clinics* 11:629–638.

Klein, L., Heiple, K.G., Torzilli, P.A., Goldberg, V.M., and A.H. Burstein. 1989. Prevention of ligament and meniscus atrophy by active joint motion in a non–weight bearing model. *Journal of Orthopaedic Research* 7:80–85.

Klingman, R.E., Liaos, S.M., and K.M. Hardin. 1997. The effect of subtalar joint posting on patellar glide position in subjects with excessive rearfoot pronation. *Journal of Orthopaedic and Sports Physical Therapy* 25:185–191.

Knight, K.L. 1985. Guidelines for rehabilitation of sports injuries. *Clinics in Sports Medicine* 4:405–416.

Knight, K.L., Martin, J.A., and B.R. Londeree. 1979. EMG comparison of quadriceps femoris activity during knee extension and straight leg raises. *American Journal of Physical Medicine and Rehabilitation* 58:57–67.

Knott, M., and D.E. Voss. 1968. *Proprioceptive neuromuscular facilitation.* New York: Harper & Row.

Knuttgen, H.G. 1976. Development of muscular strength and endurance. In *Neuromuscular mechanisms for therapeutic and conditioning exercises,* ed. H.G. Knuttgen. Baltimore: University Park Press.

Kohn, H.S. 1997. Shin pain and compartment syndromes in running. In *Running injuries,* ed. G.N. Guten. Philadelphia: Saunders.

Konradsen, L., Holmer, P., and Sondergaard, L. 1991. Early mobilizing treatment for grade III ankle ligament injuries. *Foot & Ankle* 12:69–73.

Koopman, C.F. 1995. Cutaneous wound healing: An overview. *Otolaryngologic Clinics of North America* 28:835–845.

Kottke, F.J. 1982. Therapeutic exercise to develop neuromuscular coordination. In *Krusen's handbook of physical medicine and rehabilitation,* ed. F.J. Kottke, G.K. Stillwell, and J.F. Lehmann. Philadelphia: Saunders.

Kottke, F.J., Pauley, D.L., and R.A. Ptak. 1966. The rationale for prolonged stretching for correction of shortening of connective tissue. *Archives of Physical Medicine and Rehabilitation* 47:345–352.

Koury, J.M. 1996. *Aquatic therapy programming.* Champaign, IL: Human Kinetics.

Koutedakis, Y. 1989. Muscle elasticity—plyometrics: Some physiological and practical considerations. *Journal of Applied Research in Coaching and Athletics* 4:35–49.

Kowall, M.G., Kolk, G., Nuber, G.W., Cassisi, J.E., and S.H. Stern. 1996. Patellar taping in the treatment of patellofemoral pain. A prospective randomized study. *American Journal of Sports Medicine* 24:61–66.

Kubler-Ross, E. 1969. *On death and dying.* New York: Macmillan.

Lane, J.M., and J.R. Werntz. 1987. Biology of fracture healing. In *Fracture healing,* ed. J.M. Lane. New York: Churchill Livingstone.

Lange, G.W., Hintermeister, R.A., Schlegel, T., Dillman, C.J., and J.R. Steadman. 1996. Electromyographic and kinematic analysis of graded treadmill walking and the implications for knee rehabilitation. *Journal of Orthopaedic and Sports Physical Therapy* 23:294–301.

Lattanza, L., Gray, G.W., and R.M. Kantner. 1988. Closed versus open kinetic chain measurements of subtalar joint eversion: Implications for clinical practice. *Journal of Orthopaedic and Sports Physical Therapy* 9:310–314.

Lattanzio, P.-J., Petrella, R.J., Sproule, J.R., and P.J. Fowler. 1997. Effects of fatigue on knee proprioception. *Clinical Journal of Sport Medicine* 7:22–27.

Leadbetter, W.B. 1994. Soft tissue athletic injury. In *Sports injuries: Mechanisms, prevention, treatment,* ed. F.H. Fu and D.A. Stone. Baltimore: Williams & Wilkins.

Leanderson, J., Eriksson, E., Nilsson, C., and A. Wykman. 1996. Proprioception in classical ballet dancers. *American Journal of Sports Medicine* 24:370–374.

Lear, L.J., and M.T. Gross. 1998. An electromyographical analysis of the scapular stabilizing synergists during a push-up progression. *Journal of Orthopaedic and Sports Physical Therapy* 28:146–157.

Lehmann, J.F. 1982. Gait analysis: Diagnosis and management. In *Krusen's handbook of physical medicine and rehabilitation,* ed. F.J. Kottke, G.K. Stillwell, and J.F. Lehmann. Philadelphia: Saunders.

Leib, F.J., and J. Perry. 1971. Quadriceps function. An electromyographic study under isometric conditions. *Journal of Bone and Joint Surgery* 53A:749–758.

Lephart, S.M., and T.J. Henry. 1996. The physiological basis for open and closed kinetic chain rehabilitation for the upper extremity. *Journal of Sport Rehabilitation* 5:71–87.

Lephart, S.M., Kocher, M.S., Fu, F.H., Borsa, P.A., and C.D. Harner. 1992. Proprioception following ACL reconstruction. *Journal of Sport Rehabilitation* 1:188–196.

Light, K.E., Nuzik, S., Personius, W., and A. Barstrom. 1984. Low-load prolonged stretch vs. high-load brief stretch in treating knee contractures. *Physical Therapy* 64:330–333.

Lind, A.R. 1959. Muscle fatigue and recovery from fatigue induced by sustained contractions. *Journal of Physiology (London)* 147:162–171.

Lofvenberg, R., Karrholm, J., Sundelin, G., and O. Ahlgren. 1995. Prolonged reaction time in patients with chronic lateral instability of the ankle. *American Journal of Sports Medicine* 23:414–417.

Lundin, P. 1985. A review of plyometric training. *National Strength Coaches Association Journal* 7:69–74.

MacDougall, J.D., Elder, G.C.B., Sale, D.G., Moroz, J.R., and J.R. Sutton. 1980. Effect of training and immobilization on human muscle fibers. *European Journal of Applied Physiology* 43:25–34.

Madding, S.W., Wong, J.G., Hallum, A., and Medeiros, J.M. 1987. The effect of duration of passive stretch on hip abduction range of motion. *Journal of Orthopaedic and Sports Physical Therapy.*

Maitland, G.D. 1990. *Vertebral manipulation.* Boston: Butterworth-Heinemann.

Maitland, G.D. 1991. *Peripheral manipulation.* London: Butterworth-Heinemann.

Manheim, C.J. 1994. *The myofascial release manual.* Thorofare, NJ: Slack.

Mann, R.A. 1980. Biomechanics of walking, running, and sprinting. *American Journal of Sports Medicine* 8:345–350.

Markolf, K.L., Gorek, J.F., Kabo, J.M., and M.S. Shapiro. 1990. Direct measurement of resultant forces in the anterior cruciate ligament. An in vitro study performed with a new experimental technique. *Journal of Bone and Joint Surgery* 72A:557–567.

Martinez-Hernandez, A., and P.S. Amenta. 1990. Basic concepts in wound healing. In *Sports-induced inflammation,* ed. W.B. Leadbetter, J.A. Buckwalter, and S.L. Gordon. Park Ridge, IL: American Academy of Orthopaedic Surgeons.

Massie, D.L., and J.C. Spiker. 1990. *Foot biomechanics and the relationship to rehabilitation of lower extremity injuries.* Berryville, VA: Forum Medicum.

McNair, P.J., and S.N. Stanley. 1996. Effect of passive stretching and jogging on the series elastic muscle stiffness and range of motion of the ankle joint. *British Journal of Sports Medicine* 30:313–317.

McQuade, K.J., Dawson, J., and G.L. Smidt. 1998. Scapulothoracic muscle fatigue associated with alterations in scapulohumeral rhythm kinematics during maximum resistive shoulder elevation. *Journal of Orthopaedics and Sports Medicine* 28:74–80.

McWaters, G. 1988. *Deep water exercise for health and fitness.* Laguna Beach, CA: Publitech Editions.

Mellman, M.F., McPherson, E.J., Dorr, L.D., and P. Kwong. 1996. Differential diagnosis of back and lower extremity problems. In *The spine in sports,* ed. R.G. Watkins. St. Louis: Mosby.

Melzak, R. 1973. *The puzzle of pain.* New York: Basic Books.

Mero, A., Komi, T.V., Korjus, T., Navarro, E., and R.J. Gregor. 1994. Body segment contributions to javelin throwing during final thrust phase. *Journal of Applied Biomechanics* 10:166–177.

Micheli, L.J., and C.M. Coady. 1997. Approaching hip, pelvis, and groin injuries in athletes. *Biomechanics* 4:22–26.

Moll, J., and V. Wright. 1971. Normal range of spinal mobility: A clinical study. *Annals of Rheumatic Diseases* 30:381–386.

Montgomery, J.B., and J.R. Steadman. 1985. Rehabilitation of the injured knee. *Clinics in Sports Medicine* 4:333–343.

Morin, G.E., Tiberio, D., and G. Austin. 1997. The effect of upper trapezius taping on electromyographic activity in the upper and middle trapezius region. *Journal of Sports Rehabilitation* 6:309–318.

Moritani, T., and H.A. deVries. 1979. Neural factors versus hypertrophy in the time course of muscle strength gain. *American Journal of Physical Medicine* 58:115–130.

Moynes, D.R., Perry, J., Antonelli, D.J., and F.W. Jobe. 1986. Electromyography and motion analysis of the upper extremity in sports. *Journal of the American Physical Therapy Association* 66:1905–1911.

Muller, E.A. 1970. Influence of training and of inactivity on muscle strength. *Archives in Physical Medicine and Rehabilitation* 51:449–462.

National Athletic Trainers' Association Board of Directors. 1999. From the field. *NATA News*, March, 7.

Nirschl, R.P. 1977. Tennis elbow. *Primary Care* 4:367–382.

Nuber, G.W., Jobe, F.W., Perry, J., Moynes, D.R., and D. Antonelli. 1985. Fine wire electromyography analysis of muscles of the shoulder during swimming. *American Journal of Sports Medicine* 14:7–11.

Orchard, J.W., Fricker, P.A., Abud, A.T., and B.R. Mason. 1996. Biomechanics of iliotibial band friction syndrome in runners. *American Journal of Sports Medicine* 24:375–379.

Ounpuu, S. 1994. The biomechanics of walking and running. *Clinics in Sports Medicine* 13:843–862.

Pappas, A.M., Zawacki, R.M., and T.J. Sullivan. 1985. Biomechanics of baseball pitching, a preliminary report. *American Journal of Sports Medicine* 13:216–222.

Paris, S.V., and C. Patla. 1988. *E1 course notes: Extremity dysfunction and manipulation.* St. Augustine, FL: Patris.

Peacock, E.E. 1965. Physiology of tendon repair. *American Journal of Surgery* 109:283.

Peacock, E.E. 1984. *Wound repair.* 3rd ed. Philadelphia: Saunders.

Perlan, R., Frank, C., and G. Fick. 1995. The effect of elastic bandages on human knee proprioception in the uninjured population. *American Journal of Sports Medicine* 23:251–255.

Perry, J. 1978. Normal upper extremity kinesiology. *Physical Therapy* 58:265–278.

Perry, J. 1983. Anatomy and biomechanics of the shoulder in throwing, swimming, gymnastics, and tennis. *Clinics in Sports Medicine* 2:247–270.

Perry, J. 1990. Gait analysis in sports medicine. *Instructional Course Lectures* 39:319–324.

Perry, J. 1992. Gait analysis—normal and pathological function. Thorofare, NJ: Slack.

Peterson, P. 1986. The grief response and injury. *Athletic Training* 21:312–314.

Pink, M., Perry, J., Browne, A., Scovazzo, M.L., and J. Kerrigan. 1991. The normal shoulder during freestyle swimming. *American Journal of Sports Medicine* 19:569–576.

Posner-Mayer, J. 1995. *Swiss ball applications for orthopedic and sports medicine.* Denver: Ball Dynamics International.

Powers, C.M., Maffucci, R., and S. Hampton. 1995. Rearfoot posture in subjects with patellofemoral pain. *Journal of Orthopaedic and Sports Physical Therapy* 22:155–160.

Ray, R. 2000. *Management strategies in athletic training.* 2nd ed. Champaign, IL: Human Kinetics.

Reider, B. 1996. Medial collateral ligament injuries in athletes. *Sports Medicine* 21:147–156.

Reilly, D.T., and M. Martens. 1972. Experimental analysis of the quadriceps muscle force and patellofemoral joint reaction force for various activities. *Acta Orthopaedica Scandinavica* 43:126–137.

Richardson, A.B., Jobe, F.W., and H.R. Collins. 1980. The shoulder in competitive swimming. *American Journal of Sports Medicine* 8:159–164.

Risberg, M.A., Holm, I., Tjomsland, O., Ljunggren, E., and A. Ekeland. 1999. Prospective study of changes in impairments and disabilities after anterior cruciate ligament reconstruction. *Journal of Orthopaedic and Sports Physical Therapy* 29:400–412.

Rodgers, M.M. 1988. Dynamic biomechanics of the normal foot and ankle during walking and running. *Physical Therapy* 68:1822–1830.

Rotella, R.J. 1985. The psychological care of the injured athlete. In *Sports psychology: Psychological consideration in maximizing sport performance.* Ann Arbor, MI: McNaughton & Gun.

Rovere, G.D., Clarke, T.J., Yates, C.S., and K. Burley. 1988. Retrospective comparison of taping and ankle stabilizers in preventing ankle injuries. *American Journal of Sports Medicine* 16:228–233.

Ryu, R.K.N., McCormick, J., Jobe, F.W., Moynes, D.R., and D.J. Antonelli. 1988. An electromyographic analysis of shoulder function in tennis players. *American Journal of Sports Medicine* 16:481–485.

Saal, J.S. 1987. Flexibility training. In *Rehabilitation of sport injuries,* ed. J.A. Saal. Philadelphia: Hanley & Belfus.

Salter, R.B., Simmons, D.F., Malcom, B.W., Rumble, E.J., Macmichael, D., and N.D. Clements. 1980. The biological effect of continuous passive motion on the healing of full-thickness defects in articular cartilage. *Journal of Bone and Joint Surgery* 62A:1232–1251.

Scott, G.A., Jolly, B.L., and C.E. Henning. 1986. Combined posterior incision and arthroscopic intra-articular repair of the meniscus. *Journal of Bone and Joint Surgery* 68A:847–861.

Seto, J.L., and C.E. Brewster. 1994. Treatment approaches following foot and ankle injury. *Clinics in Sports Medicine* 13:695–719.

Shelbourne, K.D., Patel, D.V., Adsit, W.S., and D.A. Porter. 1996. Rehabilitation after meniscal repair. *Clinics in Sports Medicine* 15:595–612.

Shellock, F.G., and Prentice, W.E. 1985. Warming-up and stretching for improved physical performance and prevention of sports-related injuries. *Sports Medicine* 2:267–278.

Shultz, S.J., Houglum, P.A., and D.H. Perrin. 2000. *Assessment of athletic injuries.* Champaign, IL: Human Kinetics.

Silver, F.H., and A.I. Glasgold. 1995. Cartilage wound healing. *Otolaryngologic Clinics of North America* 28:847–864.

Simons, D.G. 1981. Myofascial trigger points: A need for understanding. *Archives of Physical Medicine and Rehabilitation* 62:97–99.

Sinacore, D.R., Bander, B.L., and A. Delitto. 1994. Recovery from a 1-minute bout of fatiguing exercise: Characteristics, reliability, and responsiveness. *Physical Therapy* 74:234–244.

Sitler, M., Ryan, J., Wheeler, B., McBride, J., Arciero, R., Anderson, J., and M.B. Horodyski. 1994. The efficacy of a semirigid ankle stabilizer to reduce acute ankle injuries in basketball. *American Journal of Sports Medicine* 22:454–461.

Somes, S., Worrell, T.W., Corey, B., and C.D. Ingersoll. 1997. Effects of patellar taping on patellar position in the open and closed kinetic chain: A preliminary study. *Journal of Sport Rehabilitation* 6:299–308.

Spencer, J.D., Hayes, K.C., and I.J. Alexander. 1984. Knee joint effusion and quadriceps reflex inhibition in man. *Archives of Physical Medicine and Rehabilitation* 65:171–177.

Stamford, B. 1985. The difference between strength and power. *Physician and Sportsmedicine* 13:155.

Stanton, P., and C. Purdam. 1989. Hamstring injuries in sprinting—the role of eccentric exercise. *Journal of Orthopaedic and Sports Physical Therapy* 17:343–349.

Staron, R.S., Leonardi, M.J., Karapondo, D.L., Malicky, E.S., Falkel, J.E., Hagerman, F.C., and R.S. Kikada. 1991. Strength and skeletal muscle adaptations in heavy-resistance-trained women after detraining and retraining. *Journal of Applied Physiology* 70:631–640.

Steadman, J.R., Forster, R.S., and J.P. Silferskiold. 1989. Rehabilitation of the knee. *Clinics in Sports Medicine* 8:605–627.

Stewart, K.M. 1992. Tendon injuries. In *Concepts in hand rehabilitation,* ed. B.G. Stanley and S.M. Tribuzi. Philadelphia: Davis.

Stone, M.H., and M.S. Conley. 1994. Bioenergetics. In *Essentials of strength training and conditioning,* ed. T.R. Baechle. Champaign, IL: Human Kinetics.

Stone, R.G., Frewin, P.R., and S. Gonzales. 1990. Long-term assessment of arthroscopic meniscus repair: A two- to six-year follow-up study. *Arthroscopy: The Journal of Arthroscopic and Related Surgery* 6:73–78.

Strasmann, T., van der Wal, J.C., Halata, Z., and J. Drukker. 1990. Functional topography and ultrastructure of periarticular mechanoreceptors in the lateral elbow region of the rat. *Acta Anatomica* 138:1–14.

Sutherland, D.H., Kaufman, K.R., and J.R. Moitoza. 1994. Kinematics of normal human walking. In *Human walking,* 2nd ed., ed. J. Rose and J.G. Gamble. Baltimore: Williams & Wilkins.

Sutton, G.S., and M.R. Bartel. 1994. Soft-tissue mobilization techniques for the hand therapist. *Journal of Hand Therapy* 7:185–192.

Taylor, D.C., Dalton, J.D., Jr., Seaber, A.V., and W.E. Garrett, Jr. 1990. Viscoelastic properties of muscle–tendon units. The biomechanical effects of stretching. *American Journal of Sports Medicine* 18:300–309.

Tenuta, J.J., and R.A. Arciero. 1994. Arthroscopic evaluation of meniscal repairs. Factors that effect healing. *American Journal of Sports Medicine* 22:797–802.

Thein, J.M., and L.T. Brody. 1998. Aquatic-based rehabilitation and training for the elite athlete. *Journal of Orthopaedic and Sports Physical Therapy* 27:32–41.

Thigpen, C.M. 1983. Early management of fractures of the foot and ankle. *Current Concepts in Trauma Care* 6:4–8.

Tiberio, D. 1987. The effect of excessive subtalar joint pronation on patellofemoral mechanics: A theoretical model. *Journal of Orthopaedic and Sports Physical Therapy* 9:160–165.

Travell, J. 1976. Myofascial trigger points: Clinical view. In *Advances in pain research and therapy,* vol. 1, ed. J.J. Bonica and D. Albe-Fessard. New York: Raven Press.

Travell, J.G., and D.G. Simons. 1983. *Myofascial pain and dysfunction. The trigger point manual.* Vol. 1. Baltimore: Williams & Wilkins.

Travell, J.G., and D.G. Simons. 1992. *Myofascial pain and dysfunction. The trigger point manual.* Vol. 2. Baltimore: Williams & Wilkins.

Upton, A.R.M., and A.J. McComas. 1973. The double crush in nerve entrapment syndromes. *Lancet* 2:359–362.

Warren, C.G., Lehmann, J.K., and Koblanski, J.N. 1976. Heat and stretch procedures: An evaluation using rat tail tendon. *Archives of Physical Medicine and Rehabilitation* 57:122–126.

Wathen, D. 1994. Load assignment. In *Essentials of strength training and conditioning,* ed. T.R. Baechle. Champaign, IL: Human Kinetics.

Wegener, L., Kisner, C., and D. Nichols. 1997. Static and dynamic balance responses in persons with bilateral knee osteoarthritis. *Journal of Orthopaedic and Sports Physical Therapy* 25:13–18.

Wells, K.F., and K. Luttgens. 1976. *Kinesiology: Scientific basis of human motion.* 6th ed. Philadelphia: Saunders.

Wilk, K.E., Arrigo, C., Andrews, J.R., and W.G. Clancy, Jr. 1999. Rehabilitation after anterior cruciate ligament reconstruction in the female athlete. *Journal of Athletic Training* 34:177–193.

Wilk, K.E., Voight, M.L., Keirns, M.A., Gambetta, V., Andrews, J.R., and C.J. Dillman. 1993. Stretch-shortening drills for the upper extremities: Theory and clinical application. *Journal of Orthopaedic and Sports Physical Therapy* 17:225–239.

Williams, K.R. 1985. The biomechanics of running. *Exercise and Sport Sciences Reviews* 13:389–441.

Wilmore, J.H., and D.L. Costill. 1994. *Physiology of sport and exercise.* Champaign, IL: Human Kinetics.

Wilt, F. 1975. Plyometrics. What it is—how it works. *Athletic Journal* 55:76–90.

Winter, D.A. 1987. *The biomechanics and motor control of human gait.* Waterloo, ON: University of Waterloo Press.

Witvrouw, E., Sneyers, C., Roeland, L., Victor, J., and J. Bellemans. 1996. Reflex response times of vastus medialis oblique and vastus lateralis in normal subjects and in subjects with patellofemoral pain syndrome. *Journal of Orthopaedic and Sports Physical Therapy* 24:160–165.

Woodall, W., and J. Welsh. 1990. A biomechanical basis for rehabilitation programs involving the patellofemoral joint. *Journal of Orthopaedic and Sports Physical Therapy* 11:535–542.

Worrell, T.W., Crisp, E., and C. LaRosa. 1998. Electromyographic reliability and analysis of selected lower extremity muscles during lateral step-up conditions. *Journal of Athletic Training* 33:156–162.

Worrell, T.W., Ingersoll, C.D., Bockrath-Pugliese, K., and P. Minis. 1998. Effect of patellar taping and bracing on patellar position as determined by MRI in patients with patellofemoral pain. *Journal of Athletic Training* 33:16–20.

Young, A., Stokes, M., and J.F. Iles. 1987. Effects of joint pathology on muscle. *Clinical Orthopaedics* 219:21–27.

Zinovieff, A.N. 1951. Heavy-resistance exercises. The "Oxford Technique." *British Journal of Physical Medicine* 14:129–132.

SUGGESTED READING

Adriani, E., Luziatelli, S., and P.P. Mariani. 1993. Medial instability of the elbow: Surgical management and rehabilitation. *Journal of Sports Traumatology and Related Research* 15:45–52.

Allegrucci, M., Whitney, S.L., and J.J. Irrgang. 1994. Clinical implications of secondary impingement of the shoulder in freestyle swimmers. *Journal of Orthopaedic and Sports Physical Therapy* 20:312–318.

Andrews, J.R., and J.A. Whiteside. 1993. Common elbow problems in the athlete. *Journal of Orthopaedic and Sports Physical Therapy* 17:289–295.

Andrews, J.R., and K.E. Wilk. 1994. *The athlete's shoulder.* New York: Churchill Livingstone.

Åstrand, P.O., and K. Rodahl. 1977. *Textbook of work physiology.* New York: McGraw Hill.

Barker, C. 1988. Evaluation, treatment, and rehabilitation involving a submuscular transposition of the ulnar nerve at the elbow. *Athletic Training* 23:10–12.

Basmajian, J.V. 1973. Electromyographic analysis of basic movement patterns. In *Exercise and Sport Sciences Reviews,* vol. 1, ed. J.H. Wilmore. New York: Academic Press.

Batt, M.E. 1995. Shin splints—a review of terminology. *Clinical Journal of Sports Medicine* 5:53–57.

Berardi, G. 1995. Proprioceptive training following acute Achilles injury in dance. *Impulse* 3:200–213.

Bonci, C.M., Sloane, B., and K. Middleton. 1992. Nonsurgical/surgical rehabilitation of the unstable shoulder. *Journal of Sport Rehabilitation* 1:146–171.

Borsa, P.A., Lephart, S.M., Kocher, M.S., and S.P. Lephart. 1994. Functional assessment and rehabilitation of shoulder proprioception for glenohumeral instability. *Journal of Sport Rehabilitation* 3:84–104.

Braatz, J.H., and P.P. Gogia. 1987. The mechanics of pitching. *Journal of Orthopaedic and Sports Physical Therapy* 9:56–69.

Breig, A. 1978. *Adverse mechanical tension in the nervous system.* Stockholm: Almqvist & Wiksell.

Brewster, C., and D.R. Moynes Schwab. 1993. Rehabilitation of the shoulder following rotator cuff injury or surgery. *Journal of Orthopaedic and Sports Physical Therapy* 18:422–426.

Brunet, M.E., Haddad, R.J., Sanchez, J., and E. Leonard. 1984. How I manage sprained finger in athletes. *Physician and Sportmedicine* 12:99–108.

Brunnstrom, S., Lehmkuhl, L.D., and L.K. Smith. 1983. *Clinical kinesiology.* Philadelphia: Davis.

Burnett, W.R. 1992. Rehabilitation techniques for ligament injuries of the hand. *Hand Clinics* 8:803–815.

Cibulka, M.T. 1992. The treatment of the sacroiliac joint component to low back pain: A case report. *Physical Therapy* 72:917–922.

Clemens, S., and B. Foss-Campbell. 1993. Rehabilitation following traumatic hand injury: Hand therapists' perspective. Part 1: Acute phase of hand rehabilitation. *Plastic Surgical Nursing* 13:129–139.

Cordova, M.L., and C.W. Armstrong. 1996. Reliability of ground reaction forces during a vertical jump: Implications for functional strength assessment. *Journal of Athletic Training* 31:342–345.

Cornwall, M.W. 1984. Biomechanics of non contractile tissue. *Physical Therapy* 64:1869–1873.

Corrigan, B., and G.D. Maitland. 1989. *Practical orthopaedic medicine.* Boston: Butterworth.

Craeger, C.C. 1996. *Therapeutic exercises using foam rollers.* Berthoud, CO: Executive Physical Therapy.

Culham, E., and M. Peat. 1993. Functional anatomy of the shoulder complex. *Journal of Orthopaedic and Sports Physical Therapy* 18:342–350.

Daniels, L., and C. Worthingham. 1977. *Therapeutic exercise for body alignment and function.* Philadelphia: Saunders.

Davies, G.J., and S. Dickoff-Hoffman. 1993. Neuromuscular testing and rehabilitation of the shoulder complex. *Journal of Orthopaedic and Sports Physical Therapy* 18:449–458.

Dillman, C.J., Fleisig, G.S., and J.R. Andrews. 1993. Biomechanics of pitching with emphasis upon shoulder kinematics. *Journal of Orthopaedic and Sports Physical Therapy* 18:402–408.

Dovelle, S., and P.K. Heeter. 1985. Early controlled mobilization following extensor tendon repair in zone V–VI of the hand: Preliminary report. *Contemporary Orthopaedics* 11:41–44.

Dumbelton, J.H., and J. Black. 1975. *An introduction to orthopedic materials.* Springfield, IL: Charles C Thomas.

Ellenbecker, T.S. 1995. Rehabilitation of shoulder and elbow injuries in tennis players. *Clinics in Sports Medicine* 14:87–104.

Erhard, R.E., Delitto, A., and M.T. Cibulka. 1994. Relative effectiveness of an extension program and a combined program of manipulation and flexion and extension exercises in patients with acute low back syndrome. *Physical Therapy* 74:1093–1100.

Evans, R.B., and D.E. Thompson. 1992. An analysis of factors that support early active short arc motion of the repaired central slip. *Journal of Hand Therapy* 5:187–201.

Feldenkrais, M. 1973. *Body and mature behavior.* New York: International Universities Press.

Feldenkrais, M. 1990. *Awareness through movement.* San Francisco: Harper.

Foster, D.N., and M.N. Fulton. 1991. Back pain and the exercise prescription. *Clinics in Sports Medicine* 10:197–209.

Frankel, V.H., and M. Nordin. 1980. *Basic biomechanics of the skeletal system.* Philadelphia: Lea & Febiger.

Frost, H.M. 1973. *Orthopedic biomechanics.* Springfield, IL: Charles C Thomas.

Gardiner, M.D. 1981. *The principles of exercise therapy.* London: Bell.

Greenman, P.E. 1996. *Principles of manual medicine.* Baltimore: Williams & Wilkins.

Grieve, G.P. 1984. *Mobilisation of the spine.* New York: Churchill Livingstone.

Groves, R., and D.N. Camaione. 1983. *Concepts in kinesiology.* Philadelphia: Saunders.

Grubbs, N. 1993. Frozen shoulder syndrome: A review of literature. *Journal of Orthopaedic and Sports Physical Therapy* 18:479–487.

Grundnes, O., and O. Reikeras. 1992. Blood flow and mechanical properties of healing bone. *Acta Orthopaedica Scandinavica* 63:487–491.

Halikis, M.N., and J. Taleisnik. 1996. Soft-tissue injuries of the wrist. *Clinics in Sports Medicine* 15:235–259.

Hartley-O'Brien, S.J. 1980. Six mobilization exercises for active range of hip flexion. *Research Quarterly for Exercise and Sport* 51:625–635.

Hodges, P.W., and C.A. Richardson. 1997. Contraction of the abdominal muscles associated with movement of the lower limb. *Physical Therapy* 77:132–144.

Holt, L.E., Travis, T.M., and T. Okita. 1970. Comparative study of three stretching techniques. *Perceptual and Motor Skills* 31:661–616.

Hopkins, T.J., and A.A. White. 1993. Rehabilitation of athletes following spine injury. *Clinics in Sports Medicine* 12:603–618.

Hunter, J.M., Schneider, L.H., Mackin, E.J., and A.D. Callahan, eds. 1990. *Rehabilitation of the hand: Surgery and therapy.* St. Louis: Mosby.

Institute of Physical Art. 1991. *Integrating function: The foam roll approach.* Steamboat Springs, CO: Author.

Irrgang, J.J., Whitney, S.L., and E.D. Cox. 1994. Balance and proprioceptive training for rehabilitation of the lower extremity. *Journal of Sport Rehabilitation* 3:68–83.

Janisse, D.J. 1994. Indications and prescriptions for othoses in sports. *Orthopedic Clinics of North America* 25:95–107.

Jobe, F.W., and J.P. Bradley. 1989. The diagnosis and nonoperative treatment of shoulder injuries in athletes. *Clinics in Sports Medicine* 8:419–438.

Jobe, F.W., Moynes, D.R., and C.E. Brewster. 1987. Rehabilitation of shoulder joint instabilities. *Orthopedic Clinics of North America* 18:473–482.

Jobe, F.W., and G. Nuber. 1986. Throwing injuries of the elbow. *Clinics in Sports Medicine* 5:621–636.

Johannsen, F., Remvig, L., Kryger, P., Beck, P., Warming, S., Lybeck, K., Dreyer, V., and L.H. Larsen. 1995. Exercises for chronic low back pain: A clinical trial. *Journal of Orthopaedic and Sports Physical Therapy* 22:52–59.

Jones, F.P. 1978. *Body awareness in actions.* New York: Schocken Books.

Kapandji, I.A. 1980. *The physiology of the joints. Vol. 1. Upper limb.* New York: Churchill Livingstone.

Kegerreis, S. 1983. The construction and implementation of functional progressions as a component of athletic rehabilitation. *Journal of Orthopaedic and Sports Physical Therapy* 5:14–19.

Kegerreis, S., Malone, T., and J. McCarroll. 1984. Functional progressions: An aid to athletic rehabilitation. *Physician and Sportsmedicine* 12:67–71.

Kegerreis, S., and T. Wetherald. 1987. The utilization of functional progressions in the rehabilitation of injured wrestlers. *Athletic Training* 22:32–35.

Kendall, H.O., Kendall, F.P., and D.A. Boynton. 1970. *Posture and pain.* Huntington, NY: Robert E. Krieger.

Kenneally, M., Rubenach, H., and R. Elvey. 1988. The upper limb tension test: The SLR of the arm. In *Physical therapy of the cervical and thoracic spine,* ed. R. Grant. New York: Churchill Livingstone.

Keskula, D.R., Duncan, J.B., Davis, V.L., and P.W. Finley. 1996. Functional outcome measures for knee dysfunction assessment. *Journal of Athletic Training* 31:105–110.

Kleinert, H.E., and C. Verdan. 1983. Report of the committee on tendon injuries. *Journal of Hand Surgery (Am)* 7:794–798.

Kottke, F.J. 1982. Therapeutic exercise to maintain mobility. In *Krusen's handbook of physical medicine and rehabilitation,* ed. F.J. Kottke, G.K. Stillwell, and J.F. Lehmann. Philadelphia: Saunders.

Kuzmich, D. 1994. The levator scapulae: Making the con-NECK-tion. *Journal of Manual and Manipulative Therapy* 2:43–54.

Leanderson, J., Eriksson, E., Nilsson, C., and A. Wykman. 1996. Proprioception in classical ballet dancers. A prospective study of the influence of an ankle sprain on proprioception in the ankle joint. *American Journal of Sports Medicine* 24:370–373.

Lee, D. 1986. Principles and practice of muscle energy and functional techniques. In *Modern manual therapy of the vertebral column,* ed. G. Grieves. New York: Churchill Livingstone.

Lee, D.G. 1986. "Tennis elbow": A manual therapist's perspective. *Journal of Orthopaedic and Sports Physical Therapy* 8:134–142.

Lee, H.W.M. 1994. Progressive muscle synergy and synchronization in movement patterns: An approach to the treatment of dynamic lumbar instability. *Journal of Manual and Manipulative Therapy* 2:133–142.

Leibowitz, J. 1990. *The Alexander Technique.* New York: Harper & Row.

Lephart, S.M., and T.J. Henry. 1995. Functional rehabilitation for the upper and lower extremity. *Orthopedic Clinics of North America* 26:579–592.

Lephart, S.M., Perrin, D.H., Fu, F.H., and K. Minger. 1991. Functional performance tests for the anterior cruciate ligament insufficient athlete. *Athletic Training* 26:44–50.

Levine, W.R. 1992. Rehabilitation techniques for ligament injuries of the wrist. *Hand Clinics* 8:669–677.

Litchfield, R., Hawkins, R., Dillman, C.J., Atkins, J., and G. Hagerman. 1993. Rehabilitation for the overhead athlete. *Journal of Orthopaedic and Sports Physical Therapy* 18:433–442.

Loudin, J.K., and S.L. Bell. 1996. The foot and ankle: An overview of arthrokinematics and selected joint techniques. *Journal of Athletic Training* 31:173–178.

Mackinnon, S.E. 1992. Double and multiple crush syndromes. *Hand Clinics* 8:369.

Maitland, G.D. 1990. *Vertebral manipulation.* Boston: Butterworth-Heinemann.

Maitland, G.D. 1991. *Peripheral manipulation.* Boston: Butterworth-Heinemann.

Manheim, C.J. 1994. *The myofascial release manual.* 2nd ed. Thorofare, NJ: Slack.

Mascaro, T.B., and L.E. Swanson. 1994. Rehabilitation of the foot and ankle. *Orthopedic Clinics of North America* 25:147–160.

May, E.J., Silfverskiold, K.L., and C.J. Sollerman. 1992. Controlled mobilization after flexor tendon repair in zone II: A prospective comparison of three methods. *Journal of Hand Surgery* 5:942–952.

McPoil, T.G. 1988. Footwear. *Physical Therapy* 68:1857–1865.

McQuade, K.J., and G.L. Smidt. 1998. Dynamic scapulohumeral rhythm: The effects of external resistance during elevation of the arm in the scapular plane. *Journal of Orthopaedic and Sports Physical Therapy* 27:125–133.

Meister, K., and J.R. Andrews. 1993. Classification and treatment of rotator cuff injuries in the overhand athlete. *Journal of Orthopaedic and Sports Physical Therapy* 18:413–421.

Miller, A.S., and T.M. Narson. 1995. Protocols for proprioceptive active retraining boards. *Chiropractic Sports Medicine* 9:52–55.

Morris, M., Jobe, F.W., Perry, J., Pink, M., and B.S. Healy. 1989. Electromyographic analysis of elbow function in tennis players. *American Journal of Sports Medicine* 17:241–247.

Moynes, D.R. 1983. Prevention of injury to the shoulder through exercises and therapy. *Clinics in Sports Medicine* 2:413–422.

Murray, M.P., Drought, A.B., and R.C. Kory. 1964. Walking patterns of normal men. *Journal of Bone and Joint Surgery* 46A:335–360.

Nordin, M., and V.H. Frankel. 1980. Biomechanics of collagenous tissues. In *Basic biomechanics of the skeletal system*, ed. V.H. Frankel and N. Nordin. Philadelphia: Lea & Febiger.

Oliver, J. 1994. *Back care: An illustrated guide.* Boston: Butterworth-Heinemann.

Ollivierre, C.O., and R.P. Nirschl. 1996. Tennis elbow. Current concepts of treatment and rehabilitation. *Sports Medicine* 22:133–139.

Pappas, A.M., Zawacki, R.M., and C.F. McCarthy. 1985. Rehabilitation of the pitching shoulder. *American Journal of Sports Medicine* 13:223–235.

Payne, R.M., and M. Voight. 1993. The role of the scapula. *Journal of Orthopaedic and Sports Physical Therapy* 18:386–391.

Pezzullo, D.J., Karas, S., and J.J. Irrgang. 1995. Functional plyometric exercises for the throwing athlete. *Journal of Athletic Training* 30:22–26.

Plancher, K.D., Litchfield, R., and R.J. Hawkins. 1995. Rehabilitation of the shoulder in tennis players. *Clinics in Sports Medicine* 14:111–137.

Rasch, P.J., ed. 1989. *Kinesiology and applied anatomy.* Philadelphia: Lea & Febiger.

Reynolds, N.L., and T.W. Worrell. 1991. Chronic Achilles peritendinitis: Etiology, pathophysiology, and treatment. *Journal of Orthopaedic and Sports Physical Therapy* 13:171–176.

Rubin, D. 1981. Myofascial trigger point syndromes: An approach to management. *Archives of Physical Medicine and Rehabilitation* 62:107–110.

Safran, M.R., Caldwell, G.L., Jr., and F.H. Fu. 1994. Proprioception considerations in surgery. *Journal of Sport Rehabilitation* 3:105–115.

Saudek, C.E., and K.A. Palmer. 1987. Back pain revisited. *Journal of Orthopaedic and Sports Physical Therapy* 8:556–566.

Sisto, D.J., Jobe, F.W., Moynes, D.R., and D.J. Antonelli. 1987. An electromyographic analysis of the elbow in pitching. *American Journal of Sports Medicine* 15:260–263.

Smith, K.F. 1979. The thoracic outlet syndrome: A protocol of treatment. *Journal of Orthopaedic and Sports Physical Therapy* 1:89–99.

Snyder-Mackler, L., DeLuca, P.F., Williams, P.R., Eastlack, M.E., and A.R. Bartolozzi. 1994. Reflex inhibition of the quadriceps femoris muscle after injury or reconstruction of the anterior cruciate ligament. *Journal of Bone and Joint Surgery* 76A:555–560.

Stone, J.A., Lueken, J.S., Partin, N.B., Timm, K.E., and E.J. Ryan. 1993. Closed kinetic chain rehabilitation for the glenohumeral joint. *Journal of Athletic Training* 28:34–37.

Stone, J.A., Partin, N.B., Lueken, J.S., Timm, K.E., and E.J. Ryan, III. 1994. Upper extremity proprioceptive training. *Journal of Athletic Training* 29:15–18.

Strauss, R.H., ed. 1979. *Sports medicine and physiology.* Philadelphia: Saunders.

Stroyan, M., and K.E. Wilk. 1993. The functional anatomy of the elbow complex. *Journal of Orthopaedic and Sports Physical Therapy* 17:279–288.

Tan, J.C., and M. Nordin. 1992. Role of physical therapy in the treatment of cervical disk disease. *Orthopedic Clinics of North America* 23:435–449.

Tanigawa, M.C. 1972. Comparison of the hold-relax procedure and passive mobilization on increasing length. *Physical Therapy* 52:725–735.

Tippett, S.R., and M.L. Voight. 1995. *Functional progressions for sport rehabilitation.* Champaign, IL: Human Kinetics.

Walker, J.M. 1992. The sacroiliac joint: A critical review. *Physical Therapy* 72:903–916.

Wallin, D., Ekblom, B., Grahn, R., and T. Nordenborg. 1985. Improvement of muscle flexibility. A comparison between two techniques. *American Journal of Sports Medicine* 13:263–268.

Warren, C.G., Lehmann, J.K., and Koblanski, J.N. 1971. Elongation of rat tail tendon: Effect of load and temperature. *Archives of Physical Medicine and Rehabilitation* 52:465–474.

Wadsworth, C.T. 1983. Clinical anatomy and mechanics of the wrist and hand. *Journal of Orthopaedic and Sports Physical Therapy* 4:206–216.

Watkins, R.G. 1996. *The spine in sports.* St. Louis: Mosby.

Wehbe, M.A. 1996. Early motion after hand and wrist reconstruction. *Hand Clinics* 12:25–29.

Werner, S.L., Fleisig, G.S., Dillman, C.J., and J.R. Andrews. 1993. Biomechanics of the elbow during baseball pitching. *Journal of Orthopaedic and Sports Physical Therapy* 17:274–278.

Wilk, K.E., and C. Arrigo. 1993. Current concepts in the rehabilitation of the athletic shoulder. *Journal of Orthopaedic and Sports Physical Therapy* 18:365–378.

Wilk, K.E., C. Arrigo, and J.R. Andrews. 1993. Rehabilitation of the elbow in the throwing athlete. *Journal of Orthopaedic and Sports Physical Therapy* 17:305–317.

Wilk, K.E., Voight, M.L., Keirns, M.A., Gambetta, V., Andrews, J.R., and Dillman, C.J. 1993. Stretch shortening drills for the upper extremities: Theory and clinical application. *Journal of Orthopaedic and Sports Physical Therapy* 17:225–239.

Wilkerson, G.B., and A.J. Nitz. 1994. Dynamic ankle stability: Mechanical and neuromuscular interrelationships. *Journal of Sport Rehabilitation* 3:43–57.

Wilmore, J.H., and D.C. Costill. 1994. *Physiology of sport and exercise.* Champaign, IL: Human Kinetics.

Wood, E.C., and P.D. Becker. 1981. *Beard's massage.* Philadelphia: Saunders.

Zimmerman, G.R. 1994. Carpal tunnel syndrome. *Journal of Athletic Training* 29:22–30.

Zmierski, T., Kegerreis, S., and J. Scarpaci. 1995. Scapular muscle strengthening. *Journal of Sport Rehabilitation* 4:244–252.

INDEX

Note: Page numbers followed by *f* or *t* refer to figures or tables, respectively.

ABOUT THE AUTHOR

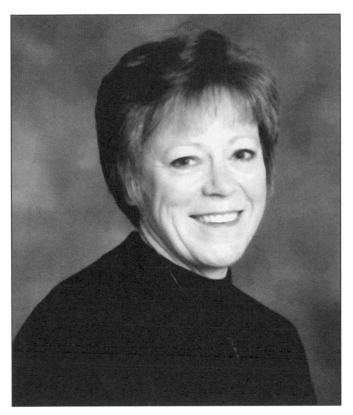

Peggy A. Houglum, MS, ATC, PT, has more than 28 years of experience in rehabilitation providing patient and athlete care since 1971. Her extensive background as a certified athletic trainer and physical therapist has provided her with a unique perspective regarding rehabilitation programs that make therapuetic exercise techniques meaningful and appropriate for athletic injury treatment.

Houglum has clinical experience with the United States Olympic Committee, the 1984 Olympics, the 1985 World University Games, and at universities and clinics.

A member of the National Athletic Trainers' Association and the Sports Section of the American Physical Therapy Association, Houglum received the NATA Most Distinguished Athletic Trainer Award in 1996. Presently chair of the NATA Continuing Education Committee, she also has served on the NATA Professional Education Committee, the NATA Education Council, and the NATA Clinical Education Committee.

Houglum attained her master's degree in athletic training from Indiana State University and is presently pursuing a PhD in Sports Medicine from the University of Virginia. She lives in Charlottesville, Virginia, and enjoys painting, cycling, and traveling in her spare time.

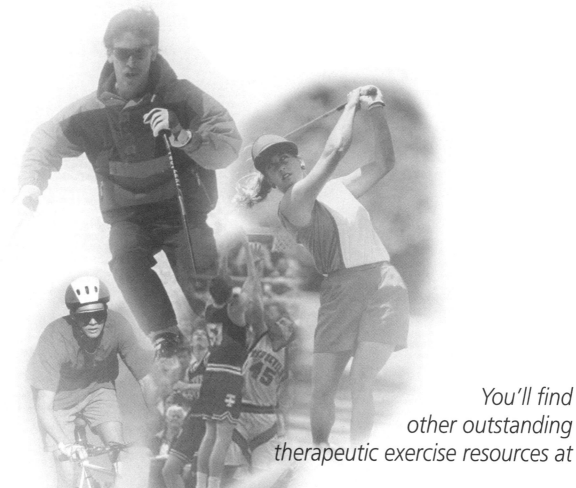